Dermatology Essentials

SECOND EDITION

Dermatology Essentials

Jean L. Bolognia MD
Professor of Dermatology
Yale Medical School
New Haven, CT, USA

Julie V. Schaffer MD
Professor of Pediatrics
Hackensack Meridian School of Medicine
Hackensack, NJ, USA

Karynne O. Duncan MD
Private Practice
St Helena, CA, USA

Christine J. Ko MD
Professor of Dermatology and Pathology
Yale Medical School
New Haven, CT, USA

For additional online content visit the expertconsult website:
www.expertconsult.com

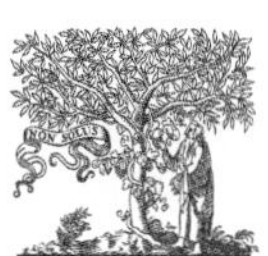

ELSEVIER London New York Oxford Philadelphia St Louis Sydney 2022

© 2022, Elsevier Inc. All rights reserved.
First edition 2014

No part of this publication may be reproduced or transmitted in any form or by any means, electronic or mechanical, including photocopying, recording, or any information storage and retrieval system, without permission in writing from the publisher. Details on how to seek permission, further information about the Publisher's permissions policies and our arrangements with organizations such as the Copyright Clearance Center and the Copyright Licensing Agency, can be found at our website: www.elsevier.com/permissions

This book and the individual contributions contained in it are protected under copyright by the Publisher (other than as may be noted herein).

Notices

Practitioners and researchers must always rely on their own experience and knowledge in evaluating and using any information, methods, compounds or experiments described herein. Because of rapid advances in the medical sciences, in particular, independent verification of diagnoses and drug dosages should be made. To the fullest extent of the law, no responsibility is assumed by Elsevier, authors, editors or contributors for any injury and/or damage to persons or property as a matter of products liability, negligence or otherwise, or from any use or operation of any methods, products, instructions, or ideas contained in the material herein.

ISBN: 978-0-323-62453-4

Cover Photograph Credits

Cover photographs from left to right are courtesy of: Julie V. Schaffer MD, Yale Dermatology Residents' Slide Collection, Yale Dermatology Residents' Slide Collection, and Mark D.P. Davis MD

Content Strategist: Charlotta Kryhl
Content Development Specialist: Joanne Scott
Project Manager: Joanna Souch
Design: Margaret Reid
Illustration Manager: Muthukumaran Thangaraj
Marketing Manager: Kate Bresnahan

Printed in India

Last digit is the print number: 9 8 7 6 5

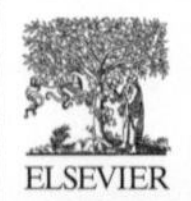

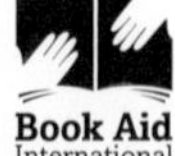

Working together to grow libraries in developing countries

www.elsevier.com • www.bookaid.org

Contents

Contents

SECTION 17

VASCULAR DISORDERS

SECTION 18

NEOPLASMS OF THE SKIN

For further reading and references, a cross-reference is made at the end of each chapter to the corresponding topic in *Dermatology, Fourth Edition,* Bolognia, Schaffer & Cerroni, editors. ISBN 9780702062759, published by Elsevier.

Preface

The goal of our *Dermatology Essentials* handbook is to present the broad spectrum of cutaneous diseases in a manner that is straightforward and logical while at the same time maintaining a necessary level of sophistication. The text portion of each section is relatively brief and easy to review, with schematics and tables providing additional and more detailed information. Throughout the handbook are algorithms that present a practical approach to evaluation, differential diagnosis, and treatment of skin disorders. The clinical photographs were chosen with two key objectives in mind – to provide characteristic examples of specific diseases and to offer key teaching points. It is our hope that this handbook will improve the dermatologic care of patients and provide clinicians with greater confidence as they approach patients with cutaneous diseases.

Acknowledgments

We wish to thank all the dermatologists whose clinical photographs are used in this handbook as well as the textbook *Dermatology*. In particular we thank Kalman Watsky, MD, whose photographs appear throughout the book. The team at Elsevier has provided enormous support, in particular Joanne Scott and Joanna Souch. Charlotta Kryhl also provided guidance for the project.

The following were sourced from the **Yale Dermatology Residents' Slide Collection (YDRSC)**:

1.3C, 1.3F, 1.4Aiii, 1.5B, 1.6Cii, 1.13A, 2.1B, 2.3, 4.8D, 5.7A, e5.12C, 6.4B, 6.9, 6.12A, 6.15, 6.16, 6.17A, 6.17C, e6.18, e6.20A, e6.21A, e6.22, e6.24, e6.25A, e6.35, 7.2A, 7.2B, 7.3C, 7.3D, 7.6A, 7.8, 7.9A, e7.14, e7.19, e7.20, 8.3B, 8.6, 8.8, e8.10, 9.5A, 9.5D, 9.5E, 9.5G, 9.6A, 9.6B, 9.6C, 9.7, 9.9A, 9.9B, 9.11A, e9.12, e9.13, e9.14, e9.17A, e9.17C, e9.18, 10.3A, 10.7, 10.8A (inset), 10.9A, 12.12B, 12.12E, 12.17, e12.26, 13.2B, 13.2I, 14.1B, 14.1C, 15.1A, 15.1B, 15.2A, 15.2B, 15.6, 16.1B, 16.1C, 16.1E, 16.2A, 16.4, 16.7A, 16.7B, 16.8, 16.9, 16.10A, 17.3, 17.7C, 17.8, 17.9B, 17.10A, 17.12, 17.13D, e17.18, e17.23A, e17.23B, e17.24A, e17.26, e17.27B, e17.28A, e17.35, 18.1D, 18.8, 18.9C, 18.11A, 18.12A, 18.18, 19.1C, 19.2B, 19.4A, 19.4B, 19.5B, 19.10A, 19.10B, 19.10D, e19.20, 20.2A, 21.5C, 21.6B, 21.7A, e21.12A, 22.1A, 22.1B, 22.1C, 22.1D, 22.7A, 22.7C, 23.6A, 24.2B, 24.5B, 24.10, e24.12, e24.16, e24.22, 25.2A, 25.2B, 26.3A, 26.5A, 26.6A, 26.6C, 26.8A, e26.10A, e26.11, 27.3, 27.4, 28.2A, 28.2B, 28.15, e28.17, e28.18, e28.19A, e28.19B, e28.21, e28.24, e28.25, 29.3C, 29.4B, e29.16, 30.6B, 30.12, e30.14, 31.2B, 31.3A, 31.4D, 31.5, 31.11C, 31.11D, e31.15A, e31.15B, 32.6, 32.7A, 33.3A, 33.3B, 33.3D, 33.3E, 33.3F, 33.3G, 33.4A, 33.5, 33.6, 33.7C, 33.10, 33.11, 34.2A, 34.11B, 35.4, e35.13, e35.15, e35.17C, 36.6B, e36.19, 37.1A, 38.6, 38.8B, e38.10A, e38.10B, 39.3A, 39.7A, 39.8B, e39.14A, 40.1, 41.2A, 41.5A, e41.10, 42.5C, 42.7B, 42.8B, 42.10, 43.7A, 43.8A, 43.9B, 43.9D, 43.9E, e43.15, e43.16A, e43.18A, 44.1A, e44.5B, e44.7C, 45.3B, 46.6A, 46.6B, 46.8C, 46.10C, 46.10D, e46.22, 47.3B, 47.4B, 47.9, 47.10A, e47.14B, e47.15C, e47.24A, 48.1B, 48.1D, 48.9, 48.10, 48.11A, 48.11B, e48.14, 49.4A, e50.19, e50.21, 51.2C, 51.2E, 51.3B, 51.3D, e51.11A, e51.18A, e51.18B, 52.2B, 52.8C, 53.2B, 53.15, e53.24, 54.14, 54.15A, 54.15E, 54.15F, 54.15G, 54.16, 54.17, 54.18A, 54.19, 54.23A, 54.23B, e54.28, e54.29A, e54.31, 55.3B, 55.8B, 55.17B, 56.4A, 56.4D, 56.11C, 56.11D, 56.11E, 56.11G, 56.11H, 56.11J, 56.11K, e56.17, e56.27, 57.6, e57.15B, e59.22 (inset 2), e59.31A, e59.32, Table 59.3 (insets), 60.9A, e60.21A, e60.22, 61.5, 61.9A, 61.9B, 61.12, 61.17, e61.22B, e61.30, e61.31, e61.37, e61.38, e61.40, e61.42, 62.9, 62.10, 62.11B, 62.13, 62.15, 62.16, 62.17A, 62.17B, 62.17C, e62.18, e62.19, 63.5, 63.6, 64.3D, 64.8A, 64.8C, 64.10, 64.13A, 64.13C, 64.13D, 64.13E, 64.13F, 64.15F, 64.19A, 64.25A, 64.25B, 64.25D, 64.25E, e64.26B, e64.27, e64.57, 65.7, 65.9A, 65.9B, 65.11A, 65.12, 65.14, 65.17, e65.30B, 67.4A, 67.6A, 67.6B, 67.6C, 67.9A, 67.9D, 67.9E, 67.9H, 67.11A, 67.11B, 67.13, 68.7A, 68.7C, 69.2B, 69.4A, 69.4B, 69.4C, 69.4D, 69.5A, 69.5B, 69.5C, 69.6A, 69.6B, 69.9, 69.13A, 69.13C, 70.1B, 71.1, 71.2D, 71.11, e71.18A, 72.7, e72.12, Table 72.1 (inset 1), 73.2C, 73.4C, 73.13, e73.24F, e73.27C, 74.7A, e74.26, 76.1A, 76.1C, 76.1E, 76.5, 76.8, 76.10, e76.12, e76.13, 77.2, 77.3A, 77.10, 78.1A, 78.1C, 78.1D, 78.1E, 78.2C, 78.2D, 78.3B, 78.4, 78.19, e78.22, e78.23, e78.25, e78.29, 79.2, 79.4A, 79.4B, 79.5, 80.2A, 80.2B,

81.4B, 81.7, e81.14, 82.2C, e82.11, 83.6A, e83.14, 84.6B, 85.3, 85.4C, 85.6A, 85.16A, 85.22, 85.26, e85.37B, e85.45, 86.2A, 86.2B, 86.3A, 86.4A, 86.5E, 86.10, 86.11B, 86.13B, 86.15A, 87.9, 87.12A, 87.14, 88.3A, 88.3C, 88.4, 88.6B, 88.6C, 88.7B, 88.9C, 89.2B, 89.6A, 89.8A, 90.1A, 90.2, 90.6B, 90.12, e90.15, 91.2, 91.3, 91.4A, 91.5, 91.6, 91.7A, 91.8A, 91.9A, 91.11, 91.13, 91.14, 91.15, e91.18, e91.20B, 92.1, 92.4, 92.6, 92.7, 92.10B, 93.6E, e93.21A, 94.3, 94.4, e94.17, 95.5, 95.11, 95.12, 95.17A, e95.23, e95.24, e95.25, 96.5, 96.6, e96.13C, e96.14B, 99.1, 99.3A, e99.14, 100.3B, 100.3C and e100.6.

The following were sourced from the **NYU Dermatology Slide Collection** (**NYUDSC**):

e7.13B, e7.23, e7.26, 8.3A, 8.4, 8.5, e8.14, 9.5C, 9.8B, e9.16, e9.17B, e9.24, 11.2C, 12.18, e14.14, e19.17, 20.3, 23.6B, 23.6C, 24.4, 36.5C, e36.13, e36.15, 40.4A, 46.7B, 53.11C, 55.3A, 55.4A, 55.4B, 56.6B, e56.14, 57.12, 59.6, 61.10C, 61.10D, 61.13, e61.35, 63.7A, 63.7B, 65.5, 65.11B, 68.6A, 68.6B, 69.8, e69.18, e71.19, 73.4B, 73.5B, e73.24C, 78.7A, 78.7B, e81.13, 95.6, 95.9, 95.10 and 95.20.

The following were sourced from the **USC Dermatology Residents' Slide Collection** (**USCDRSC**):

4.6, 36.10, 38.1, 51.7C, 54.13, e55.23B, e60.16C, e61.36, 64.16A, 64.16B, 64.18, 64.22A, 64.22B, 64.23, e64.33, e65.29, 71.2C, e71.18B, 82.2A, 85.28, 91.12, 94.11, and e99.16.

The following were sourced from the **SUNY Stony Brook Dermatology Residents' Slide Collection** (**SUNYSBDRSC**):

Figure 54.15C.

Chapter 58, Nail Disorders – Nail photos are courtesy of Antonella Tosti, YDRSC, Julie V. Schaffer, and Jean L. Bolognia.

Dedication

To our families, in particular our husbands – Dennis, Andy, David and Peter – who provided the indispensable support required to complete this book, from serving as sounding boards to creating quiet time in busy households.

List of Abbreviations

Ab	Antibody
ABI	Ankle–brachial index
ACE	Angiotensin-converting enzyme
AI-CTD	Autoimmune connective tissue disease
ALK	Anaplastic lymphoma kinase
AK	Actinic keratosis
ANA	Antinuclear antibody
ANCA	Antineutrophil cytoplasmic antibody
ART	Antiretroviral therapy
BB	Broadband
BCC	Basal cell carcinoma
BID	Two times daily
BSA	Body surface area
BUN	Blood urea nitrogen
CBC	Complete blood count
CDC	Centers for Disease Control and Prevention
CMV	Cytomegalovirus
CNS	Central nervous system
CO	Carbon monoxide
COPD	Chronic obstructive pulmonary disease
Cr	Creatinine
CRP	C-reactive protein
CS	Corticosteroids
CSF	Cerebrospinal fluid
CT	Computed tomography
CTCL	Cutaneous T-cell lymphoma
CXR	Chest X-ray
DDT	Dichlorodiphenyltrichloroethane (an insecticide)
Dx	Diagnosis
DDx	Differential diagnosis
DEET	N, N-diethyl-meta-toluamide
DFA	Direct fluorescence antibody
DHEAS	Dehydroepiandrosterone sulfate
DIHS	Drug-induced hypersensitivity syndrome (also known as DRESS)
DM	Diabetes mellitus
DRESS	Drug reaction with eosinophilia and systemic symptoms (also known as DIHS)
DVT	Deep vein thrombosis
EBV	Epstein–Barr virus
ECG	Electrocardiogram
EEG	Electroencephalogram
EGFR	Epidermal growth factor receptor
ELISA	Enzyme-linked immunosorbent assay
EMG	Electromyography
ESR	Erythrocyte sedimentation rate
FDA	US Food and Drug Administration
G6PD	Glucose-6-phosphate dehydrogenase
GI	Gastrointestinal
GM-CSF	Granulocyte–macrophage colony-stimulating factor
GVHD	Graft-versus-host disease
H&E	Hematoxylin and eosin
HBV	Hepatitis B virus

HCTZ	Hydrochlorothiazide
HCV	Hepatitis C virus
HIV	Human immunodeficiency virus
HPV	Human papillomavirus
HSCT	Hematopoietic stem cell transplant
HSV	Herpes simplex virus
ICU	Intensive care unit
IFE	Immunofixation electrophoresis
IL	Interleukin
IM	Intramuscularly
IV	Intravenous
IVIg	Intravenous immunoglobulin
KA	Keratoacanthoma
KOH	Potassium hydroxide
LDH	Lactate dehydrogenase
LE	Lupus erythematosus
LFTs	Liver function tests
LPLK	Lichen planus-like keratosis
MEN	Multiple endocrine neoplasia
MHC	Major histocompatibility complex
MRA	Magnetic resonance angiography
MRI	Magnetic resonance imaging
MRSA	Methicillin-resistant *Staphylococcus aureus*
NB-UVB	Narrowband UVB
NK	Natural killer
NMSC	Non-melanoma skin cancer
NSAIDs	Nonsteroidal anti-inflammatory drugs
OTC	Over-the-counter
PAS	Periodic acid Schiff
PCR	Polymerase chain reaction
PDGF	Platelet-derived growth factor
PDT	Photodynamic therapy
PET	Positron emission tomography
PO	Per os (oral administration)
PPD	Purified protein derivative
PUVA	Psoralen plus ultraviolet A light
RBC	Red blood cell
RPR	Rapid plasma reagin (test for syphilis)
Rx	Treatment
SC	Subcutaneous
SCC	Squamous cell carcinoma
SLE	Systemic lupus erythematosus
SPEP	Serum protein electrophoresis
SSRIs	Selective serotonin reuptake inhibitors
STIs	Sexually transmitted infections
TB	Tuberculosis
TCAs	Tricyclic antidepressants
TGF	Transforming growth factor
TID	Three times daily
TNF	Tumor necrosis factor
TPMT	Thiopurine methyltransferase
TSH	Thyroid stimulating hormone
TST	Tuberculin skin test
URI	Upper respiratory infection
UVA	Ultraviolet A
UVB	Ultraviolet B
UVA1	Ultraviolet A1 (340–400 nm)
UVR	Ultraviolet radiation
VDRL	Venereal Disease Research Laboratory (test for syphilis)
VEGFR	Vascular endothelial growth factor receptor
VZV	Varicella–zoster virus
WBC	White blood cell count
XRT	Radiation therapy

Basic Principles of Dermatology

1

• In the approach to the patient with a dermatologic disease, it is important to think initially of broad categories (Fig. 1.1); this allows for a more complete differential diagnosis and a logical approach.

• Key elements of any clinical description include distribution pattern (Table 1.1; Figs 1.2 and 1.3), type of primary lesion and its topography (Table 1.2; Fig. 1.4), secondary features (Table 1.3), and its consistency via palpation (Tables 1.4 and 1.5).

• If atrophy is present, it should be categorized as epidermal, dermal, and/or subcutaneous (Fig. 1.5).

• Color is also an important feature (Table 1.6), and this can be influenced by the skin phototype (Appendix) such that an inflammatory

MAJOR DISTRIBUTION PATTERNS
• Generalized versus localized (see Fig. 1.2) versus solitary
• Unilateral versus bilateral
• If bilateral, symmetric or asymmetric pattern
• Random versus linear (see Fig. 1.3) or grouped (e.g. herpetiform, clustered)
• Special patterns – acral sites (nose, ears, distal extremities); seborrheic region (scalp, face, upper trunk); sun-exposed versus sun-protected sites; along cleavage lines; areas of occlusion; areas of pressure; areas in contact with allergens or irritants

Table 1.1 Major distribution patterns. Occasionally, the pattern represents a locus minoris resistentiae.

CLASSIFICATION SCHEME FOR DERMATOLOGIC DISORDERS

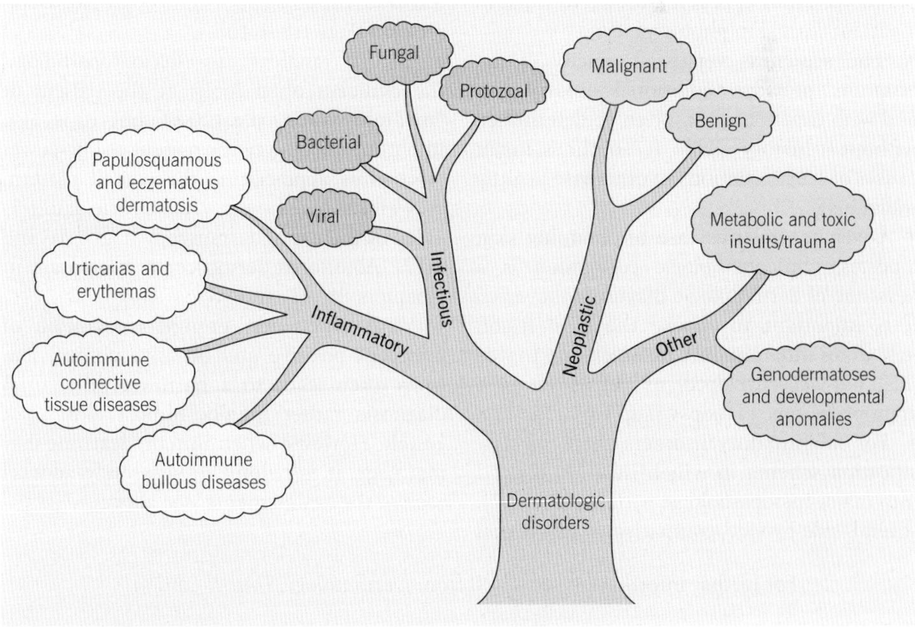

Fig. 1.1 Classification scheme for dermatologic disorders. This scheme is analogous to the structure of a tree with multiple branch points terminating in leaves.

EXAMPLES OF LOCALIZED DISTRIBUTION PATTERNS

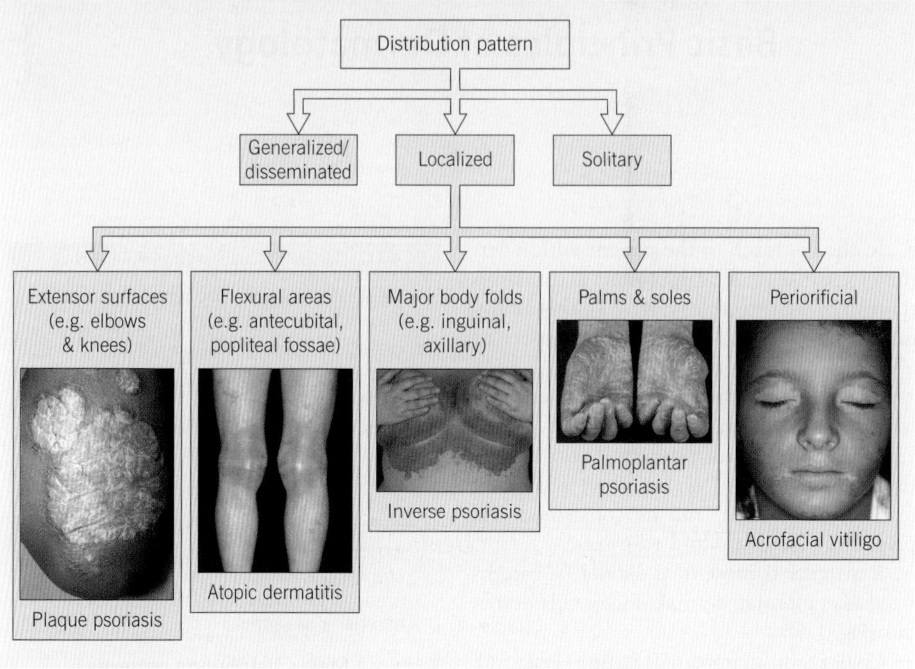

Fig. 1.2 Examples of localized distribution patterns. Additional patterns are outlined in Table 1.1. Generalized lesions are seen in morbilliform drug eruptions and viral exanthems. *Photographs, courtesy, Peter C. M. van de Kerkhof, MD, Thomas Bieber, MD, and Julie V. Schaffer, MD.*

lesion that appears pink in a patient with skin phototype I may appear red-brown to violet in a patient with skin phototype IV.

- The acuteness versus chronicity of the eruption provides additional information and with experience can often be determined without a history; Table 1.7 outlines major causes of acute eruptions in otherwise healthy individuals.
- Given the relative ease of obtaining skin biopsies, clinicopathologic correlation is a keystone of dermatologic diagnosis; however, it is important to choose the ideal lesion (e.g. in an inflammatory disorder, one that is fresh but well-developed), as well as the most appropriate type of biopsy (Fig. 1.6).
- For inflammatory disorders, there is a classification schema in which they are divided into major histopathologic patterns (Fig. 1.7); several side-by-side comparisons of clinical presentations with histopathologic findings illustrate the concept of clinicopathologic correlation (Figs 1.8–1.15).
- In an analogy to dermatopathology, the clinician often looks at the patient at "medium-power" (i.e. 20×), but it is also important to analyze the patient at low-power (4×), thus appreciating the overall pattern, as well as high-power (100×); the latter is aided by the use of dermoscopy (Figs 1.16 and 1.17). Additional dermoscopic images are in Chapters 88, 92, and 93.
- With experience, prompt recognition of pertinent positive and negative clinical features often leads to a narrower differential diagnosis rather rapidly, almost akin to a gestalt. However, when initially learning dermatology, it is helpful to separately address each of the key elements (see above).

For further information see Ch. 0 from *Dermatology, Fourth Edition*.

For additional online figures and tables visit www.expertconsult.com

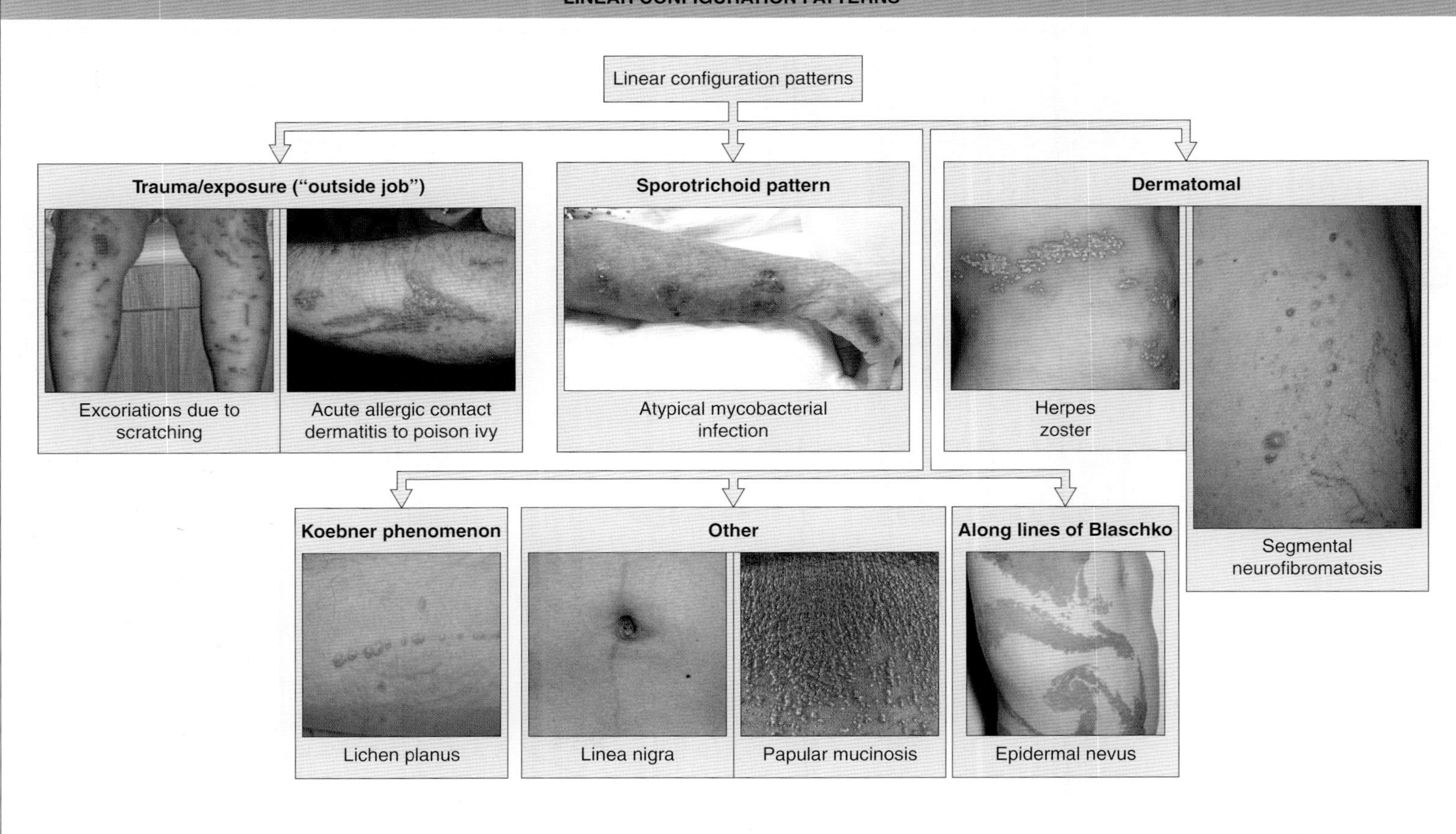

Fig. 1.3 Linear configuration patterns. *Photographs, courtesy, Kathryn Schwarzenberger, MD, Jean L. Bolognia, MD, Edward Cowen, MD, Whitney High, MD, Joyce Rico, MD, Louis A. Fragola, Jr., MD, and YDRSC.*

PRIMARY LESIONS – MORPHOLOGICAL TERMS					
	Term	**Clinical features**		**Clinical example**	**Clinical disorders**
Related by size	**Macule**	• Flat, circumscribed, non-palpable • <1 cm in diameter • Often hypo- or hyperpigmented • Also other colors (e.g. pink, red, violet) • It can be round, oval, or irregular in shape • May be sharply marginated or blend into the surrounding skin		Solar lentigines	• Ephelid (freckle) • Lentigo • Idiopathic guttate hypomelanosis • Petechiae • Flat component of viral exanthems • Junctional melanocytic nevus
	Patch	• Flat, circumscribed, non-palpable • >1 cm in diameter • Often hypo- or hyperpigmented • Also other colors (e.g. blue, violet)		Vitiligo	• Vitiligo • Melasma • Dermal melanocytosis (Mongolian spot) • Café-au-lait macule • Nevus depigmentosus • Solar purpura • Port-wine stain (early)
Related by size	**Papule**	• Elevated, circumscribed • <1 cm in diameter • Elevation due to increased thickness of the epidermis and/or cells or deposits within the dermis • May have secondary changes (e.g. scale, crust, erosion) • Need to distinguish from vesicle or pustule		Seborrheic keratosis	• Seborrheic keratosis • Cherry angioma • Compound or intradermal melanocytic nevus • Verruca or molluscum contagiosum • Acrochordon • Milium, fibrous papule (angiofibroma)

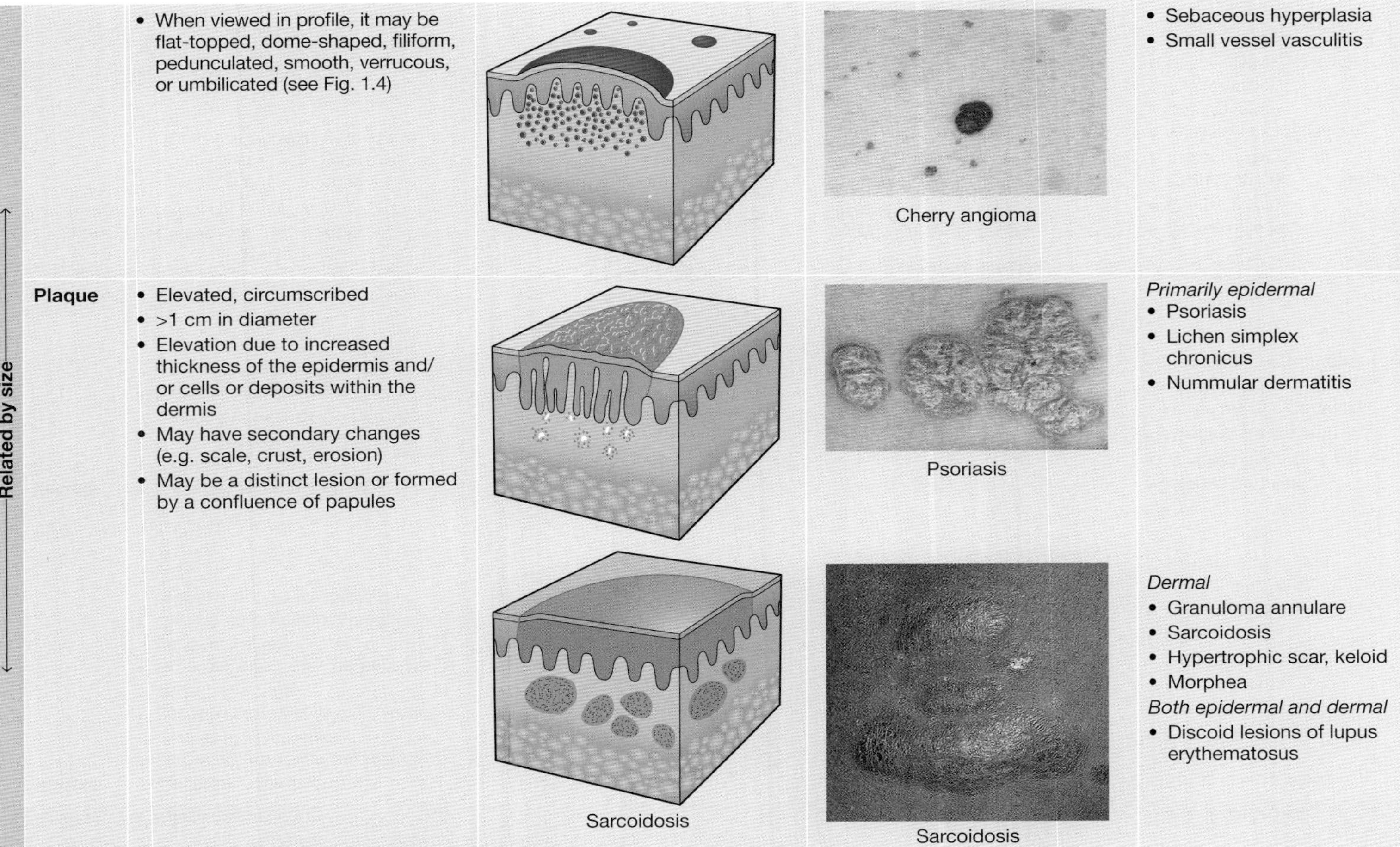

	• When viewed in profile, it may be flat-topped, dome-shaped, filiform, pedunculated, smooth, verrucous, or umbilicated (see Fig. 1.4)		Cherry angioma	• Sebaceous hyperplasia • Small vessel vasculitis
Plaque	• Elevated, circumscribed • >1 cm in diameter • Elevation due to increased thickness of the epidermis and/or cells or deposits within the dermis • May have secondary changes (e.g. scale, crust, erosion) • May be a distinct lesion or formed by a confluence of papules		Psoriasis	*Primarily epidermal* • Psoriasis • Lichen simplex chronicus • Nummular dermatitis
		Sarcoidosis	Sarcoidosis	*Dermal* • Granuloma annulare • Sarcoidosis • Hypertrophic scar, keloid • Morphea *Both epidermal and dermal* • Discoid lesions of lupus erythematosus

Table 1.2 Primary lesions – morphological terms. *Continued*

PRIMARY LESIONS – MORPHOLOGICAL TERMS

	Term	Clinical features	Clinical example	Clinical disorders
←Related by size→	**Nodule**	• Elevated, circumscribed • Larger volume than papule, often >1.5 cm in diameter • Located primarily in the dermis and/or subcutis • Greatest mass may be beneath the skin surface • Can be compressible, soft, rubbery, or firm to palpation	Epidermoid inclusion cysts	• Epidermoid inclusion cyst • Pilar cyst • Lipoma • Neurofibroma • Nodular melanoma • Metastases • Rheumatoid nodule • Panniculitis, e.g. erythema nodosum
	Vesicle	• Elevated, circumscribed • <1 cm in diameter • Fluid-containing, usually clear or serous but may be hemorrhagic • May become pustular, umbilicated, or an erosion	Herpes simplex	• Herpes simplex • Varicella or herpes zoster • Dyshidrotic eczema • Acute allergic contact dermatitis • Dermatitis herpetiformis

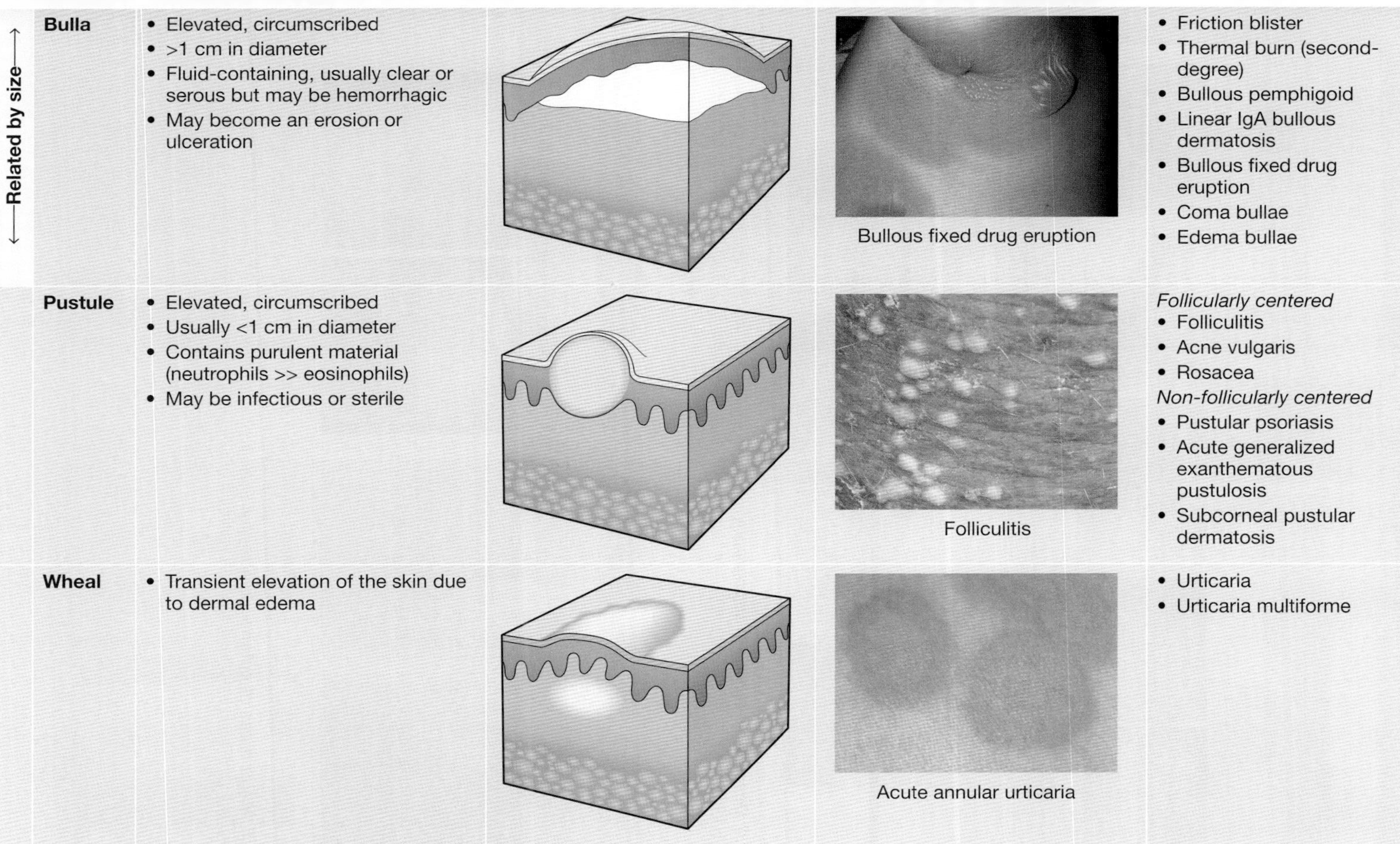

	Term	Description		Example	Related conditions
←Related by size→	**Bulla**	• Elevated, circumscribed • >1 cm in diameter • Fluid-containing, usually clear or serous but may be hemorrhagic • May become an erosion or ulceration		Bullous fixed drug eruption	• Friction blister • Thermal burn (second-degree) • Bullous pemphigoid • Linear IgA bullous dermatosis • Bullous fixed drug eruption • Coma bullae • Edema bullae
	Pustule	• Elevated, circumscribed • Usually <1 cm in diameter • Contains purulent material (neutrophils >> eosinophils) • May be infectious or sterile		Folliculitis	*Follicularly centered* • Folliculitis • Acne vulgaris • Rosacea *Non-follicularly centered* • Pustular psoriasis • Acute generalized exanthematous pustulosis • Subcorneal pustular dermatosis
	Wheal	• Transient elevation of the skin due to dermal edema		Acute annular urticaria	• Urticaria • Urticaria multiforme

Table 1.2 *Continued* **Primary lesions – morphological terms.** *Photographs, courtesy, Jean L. Bolognia, MD, Lorenzo Cerroni, MD, Edward Cowen, MD, Louis A. Fragola, Jr., MD, Whitney High, MD, Joyce Rico, MD, and Kalman Watsky, MD.*

DESCRIPTIVE TERMS FOR TOPOGRAPHY

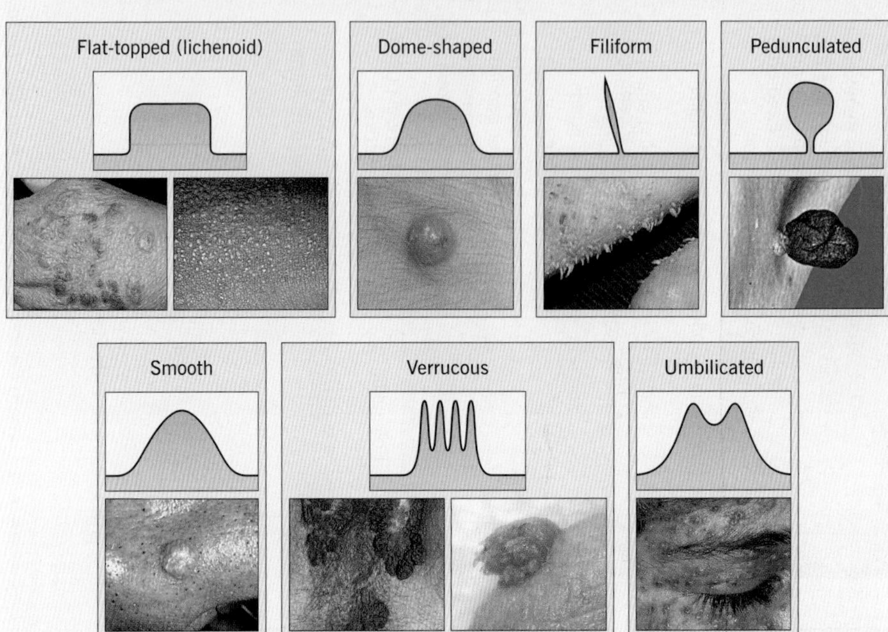

Fig. 1.4 Descriptive terms for topography. *Photographs, courtesy, Jennifer Choi, MD, Hideko Kamino, MD, Reinhard Kirnbauer, MD, Petra Lenz, MD, Frank Samarin, MD, Julie V. Schaffer, MD, Judit Stenn, MD, and YDRSC.*

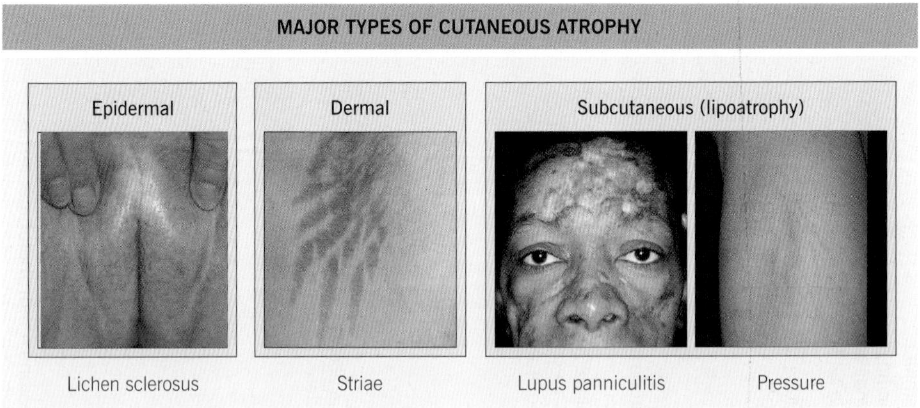

MAJOR TYPES OF CUTANEOUS ATROPHY

Epidermal | Dermal | Subcutaneous (lipoatrophy)

Lichen sclerosus | Striae | Lupus panniculitis | Pressure

Fig. 1.5 Major types of cutaneous atrophy. *Photographs, courtesy, Susan M. Cooper, MD, Fenella Wojnarowska, MD, Jean L. Bolognia, MD, and YDRSC.*

SECONDARY FEATURES – MORPHOLOGICAL TERMS			
Feature	**Description**		**Disorders**
Crust	• Dried serum (serous), blood (hemorrhagic), or pus on the surface • May include bacteria (usually *Staphylococcus*)	Secondarily infected hand dermatitis	• Eczema/dermatitis (multiple types) • Impetigo • Later phase of herpes simplex, varicella or zoster • Erythema multiforme
Scale	• Hyperkeratosis • Accumulation of stratum corneum due to increased proliferation and/or delayed desquamation • Represents a primary rather than a secondary feature in ichthyoses	Psoriasis	• Psoriasis (micaceous [silvery] scale) • Tinea (leading scale) • Erythema annulare centrifugum (trailing scale) • Actinic keratoses (gritty) • Pityriasis rosea (peripheral collarette and/or central scale) • Seborrheic (greasy) • Tinea versicolor (powdery [furfuraceous]) • Lamellar ichthyosis (plate-like)
Fissure	• Linear cleft in skin • Often painful • Results from marked drying, skin thickening, and loss of elasticity	Hand dermatitis	• Angular cheilitis • Hand dermatitis • Sebopsoriasis (intergluteal fold) • Irritant cheilitis
Excoriation	• Exogenous injury to all or part of the epidermis (epithelium) • Usually due to scratching	Neurotic excoriations	• A secondary feature of pruritic conditions, including arthropod bites and atopic dermatitis • Neurotic excoriations • Acne excoriée

Table 1.3 Secondary features – morphological terms. *Continued*

SECONDARY FEATURES – MORPHOLOGICAL TERMS			
Feature	**Description**		**Disorders**
Lichenification	• Thickening (acanthosis) of the epidermis, and accentuation of natural skin lines	Lichen simplex chronicus	• Lichen simplex chronicus, isolated or superimposed on a pruritic condition, e.g. atopic dermatitis
Erosion	• Partial, or sometimes complete, loss of the epidermis (epithelium) • A moist, oozing, and/or crusted lesion	Pemphigus foliaceus	• Impetigo • Friction • Trauma • Pemphigus, vulgaris and foliaceus • Staphylococcal scalded skin syndrome

Ulceration	• A deeper defect (compared to an erosion), with loss of at least the entire epidermis plus superficial dermis • May have loss of the entire dermis or even subcutis • Size, shape, and depth of the ulcer should be noted in addition to characteristics of the border, base, and surrounding skin 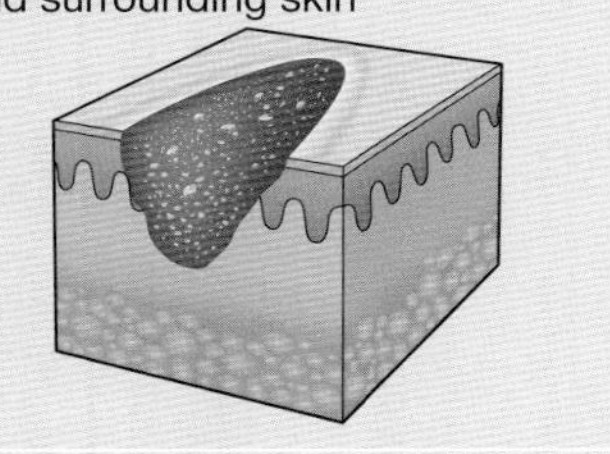	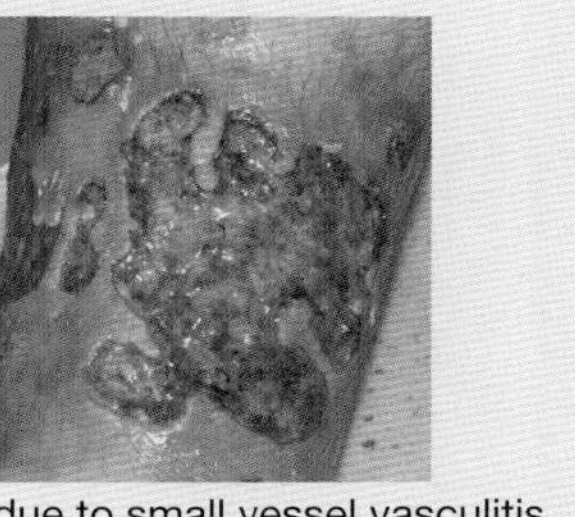 Ulcer due to small vessel vasculitis	• Venous (stasis) ulcer • Neuropathic ulcer • Arterial ulcer • Decubitus ulcer • Aphthous ulcer • Ecthyma gangrenosum • Ecthyma • Pyoderma gangrenosum
Atrophy	• Epidermal atrophy – thinning of the epidermis, leading to wrinkling and a shiny appearance • Dermal atrophy – loss of dermal collagen and/or elastin, leading to a depression (see Table 1.4)	 Striae secondary to potent corticosteroids	• Lichen sclerosus • Poikiloderma • Striae • Anetoderma • Focal dermal hyoplasia (Goltz syndrome)
Scar	• Increased thickness, usually of the dermis, due to enhanced production of collagen by fibroblasts 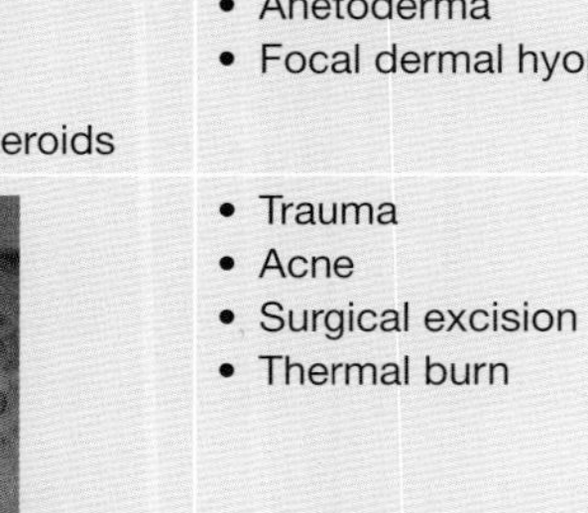	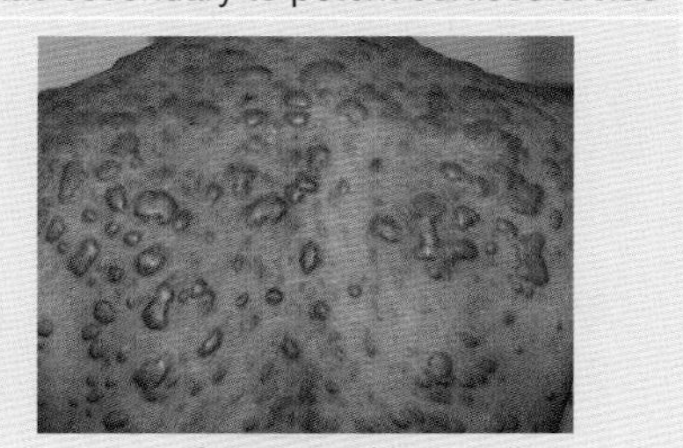 Acne scarring	• Trauma • Acne • Surgical excision • Thermal burn 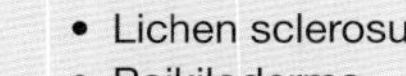

Table 1.3 *Continued* **Secondary features – morphological terms.** *Photographs, courtesy, Louis A. Fragola, Jr., MD, Jeffrey C. Callen, MD, Julie V. Schaffer, MD, and Whitney High, MD.*

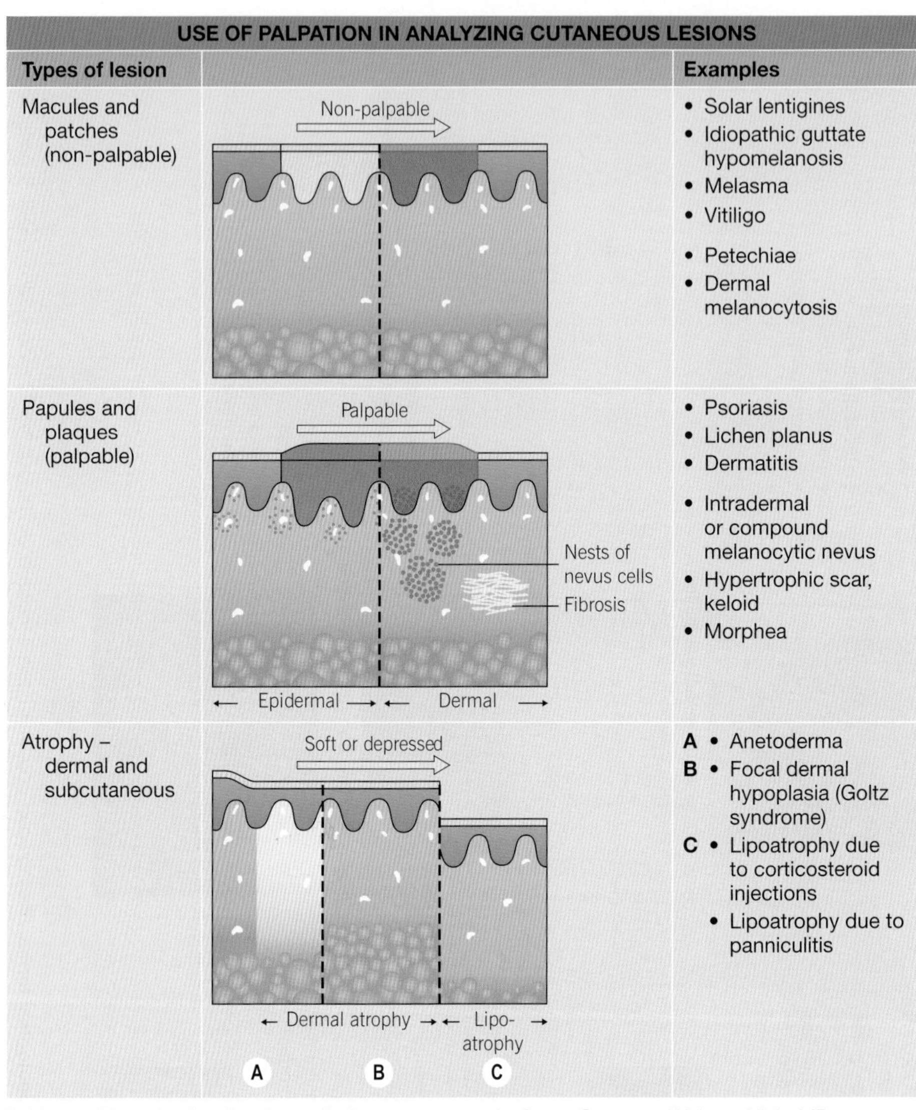

USE OF PALPATION IN ANALYZING CUTANEOUS LESIONS		
Types of lesion		**Examples**
Macules and patches (non-palpable)	Non-palpable	• Solar lentigines • Idiopathic guttate hypomelanosis • Melasma • Vitiligo • Petechiae • Dermal melanocytosis
Papules and plaques (palpable)	Palpable Nests of nevus cells Fibrosis ← Epidermal → ← Dermal →	• Psoriasis • Lichen planus • Dermatitis • Intradermal or compound melanocytic nevus • Hypertrophic scar, keloid • Morphea
Atrophy – dermal and subcutaneous	Soft or depressed ← Dermal atrophy → ← Lipo-atrophy → A B C	A • Anetoderma B • Focal dermal hypoplasia (Goltz syndrome) C • Lipoatrophy due to corticosteroid injections • Lipoatrophy due to panniculitis

Table 1.4 Use of palpation in analyzing cutaneous lesions. *Courtesy, Whitney High, MD.*

PALPATION OF CUTANEOUS LESIONS
• Soft (e.g. intradermal nevus) versus firm (e.g. dermatofibroma) versus hard (e.g. calcinosis cutis, osteoma cutis) • Compressible (e.g. venous lake) versus noncompressible (e.g. fibrous papule) • Tender (e.g. inflamed epidermoid inclusion cyst, angiolipoma, leiomyoma) versus nontender • Blanchable (e.g. erythema due to vasodilation) versus nonblanchable (e.g. purpura) – aided by diascopy • Rough versus smooth • Mobile versus fixed to underlying structures • Dermal versus subcutaneous • Temperature – normal versus elevated • Other, e.g. thrill, pulsatile

Table 1.5 Palpation of cutaneous lesions.

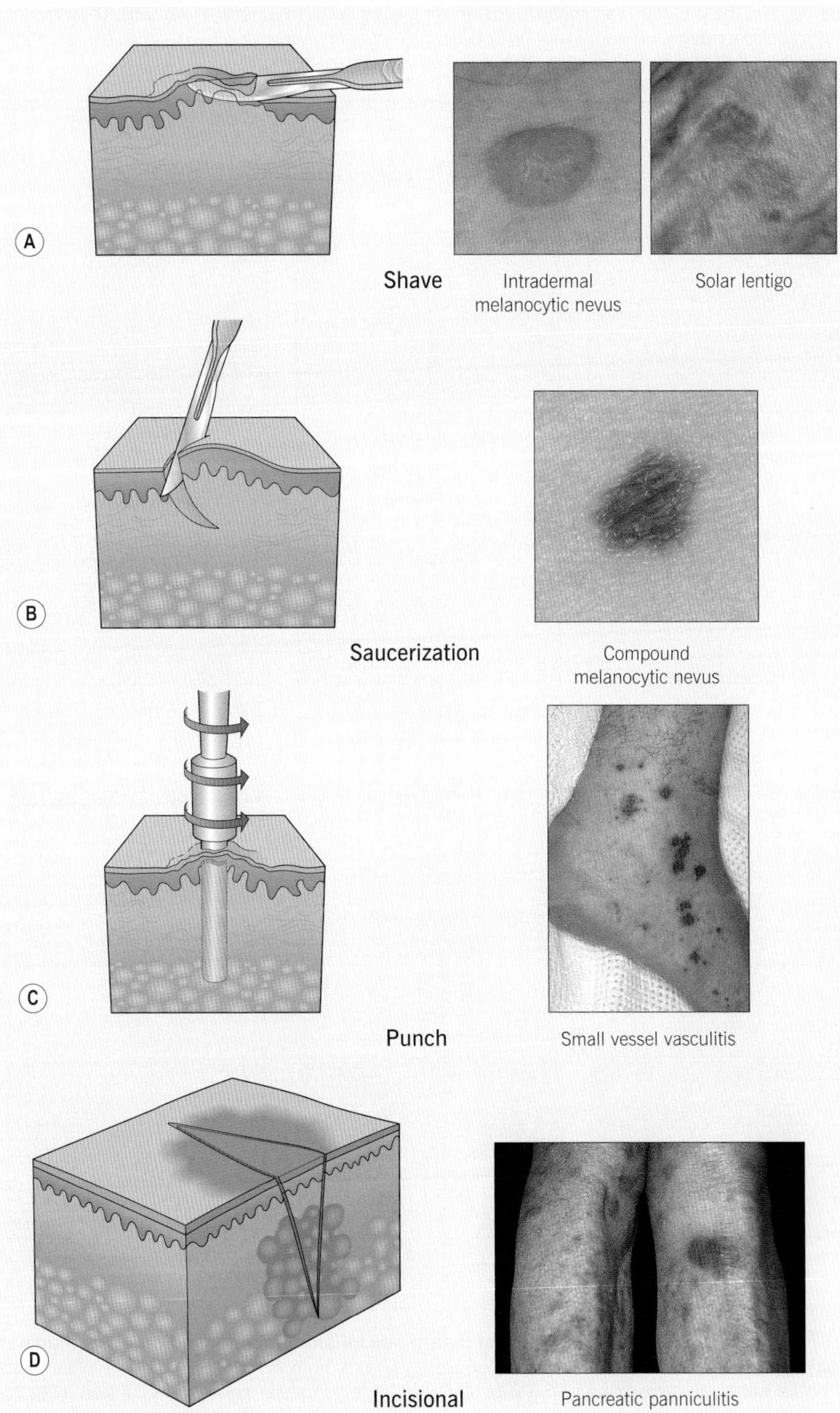

Fig. 1.6 Different cutaneous biopsy techniques. *See next page for figure legend.*

Fig. 1.6 Different cutaneous biopsy techniques. A Superficial shave biopsy can be performed to remove the elevated portion of an intradermal nevus or to distinguish a solar lentigo (pictured here) from lentigo maligna. **B** Deep shave biopsy (saucerization); performed to remove a compound melanocytic nevus or atypical melanocytic nevus. **C** Punch biopsy; performed to examine the dermis (as well as the epidermis) and the preferred technique for diagnosing cutaneous small vessel vasculitis. **D** Incisional biopsy; recommended for determining the specific type of panniculitis. *Courtesy, Suzanne Olbricht, MD, Raymond Barnhill, MD, Kenneth Greer, MD, Frank Samarin, MD, and YDRSC.*

MAJOR HISTOPATHOLOGIC PATTERNS OF CUTANEOUS INFLAMMATION

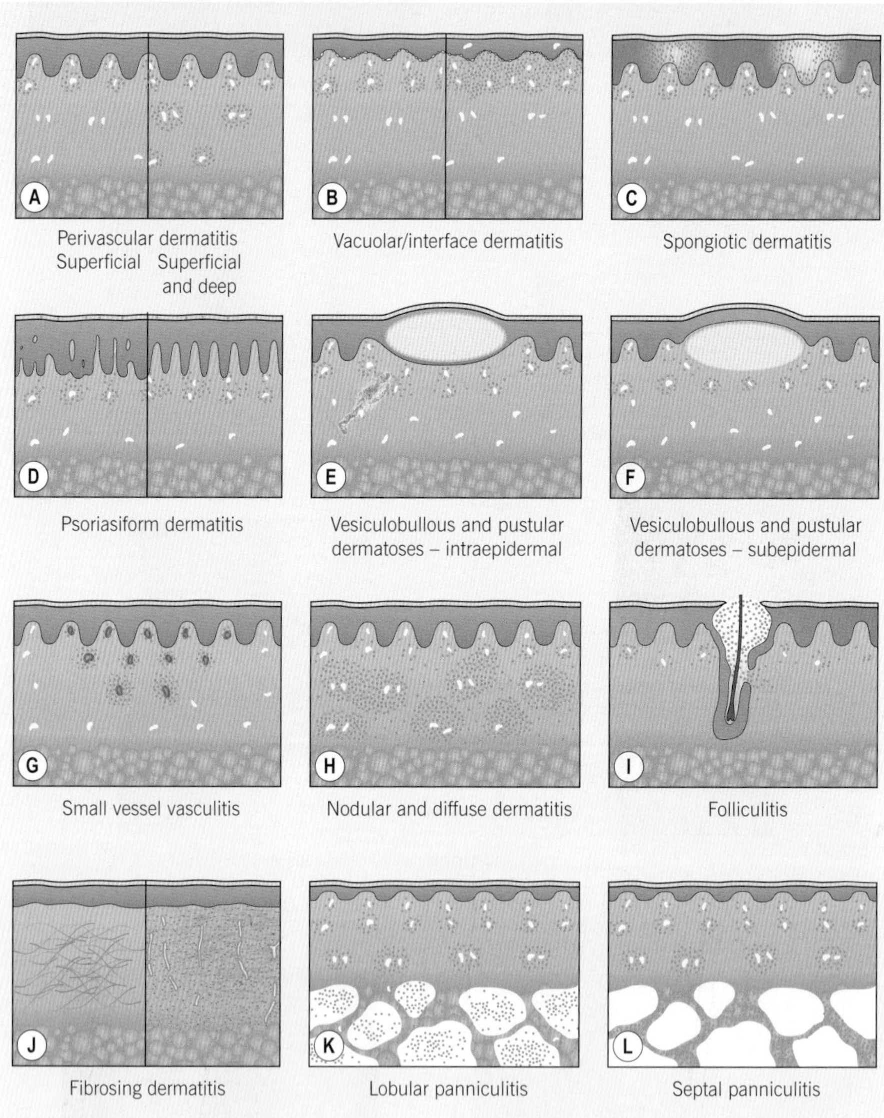

Fig. 1.7 Major histopathologic patterns of cutaneous inflammation (based on Ackerman's classification). Basic patterns of inflammation result primarily from the distribution of the inflammatory cell infiltrate within the dermis and/or the subcutaneous fat (e.g. nodular, perivascular). It also reflects the character of the inflammatory process itself (e.g. pustular), the presence of injury to blood vessels (e.g. vasculitis), involvement of hair follicles (e.g. folliculitis), abnormal fibrous dermal and/or subcutaneous tissue, and formation of vesicles and bullae. *Adapted from Ackerman AB. Histologic Diagnosis of Inflammatory Skin Diseases: A Method by Pattern Analysis. Philadelphia: Lea & Febiger, 1978.*

COLORS OF CUTANEOUS LESIONS	
Color	**Clinical examples**
White	Vitiligo, idiopathic guttate hypomelanosis, calcinosis cutis
Tan*	Postinflammatory hypopigmentation, nevus depigmentosus
Yellow	Sebaceous hyperplasia, carotenoderma, xanthoma
Pink to red-brown (range of erythema influenced by skin phototype)	Psoriasis, dermatitis, morbilliform drug eruption, viral exanthem
Orange-red (salmon)	Pityriasis rubra pilaris
Green	*Pseudomonas* infection or colonization (e.g. of onycholysis)
Blue	Ecchymosis, venous lake, dermal melanocytosis, blue nevus, cyanosis
Gray	Postinflammatory hyperpigmentation (dermal), erythema dyschromicum perstans, argyria
Purple/violaceous	Solar purpura, small vessel vasculitis, lichen planus, lymphoma cutis
Brown	Seborrheic keratosis, compound melanocytic nevus, melasma, postinflammatory hyperpigmentation (epidermal)
Black	Infarct with necrosis, melanoma

**Not to be confused with increase in pigmentation that follows exposure to ultraviolet irradiation.*

Table 1.6 Colors of cutaneous lesions.

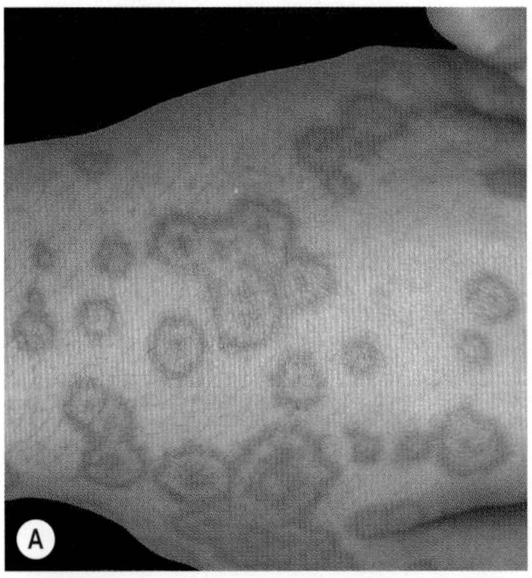

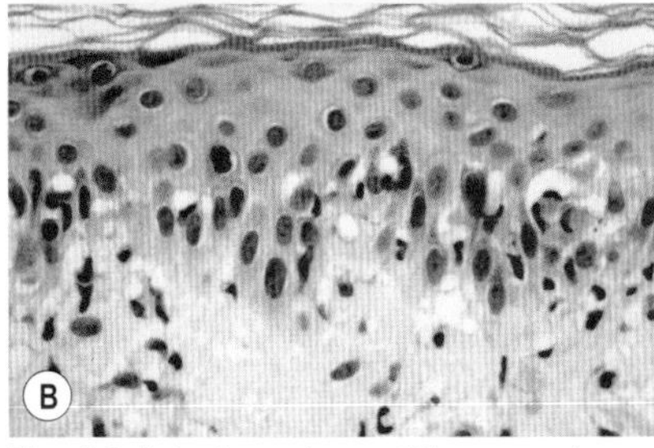

Fig. 1.8 Interface dermatitis, vacuolar type. A Erythema multiforme – edematous papules with central dusky erythema surrounded by an annulus of edema and then a peripheral rim of erythema, leading to a target-like appearance. **B** Vacuolar alteration along the dermal–epidermal junction in association with exocytosis of keratinocytes.
Courtesy, Carlo F. Tomasini, MD.

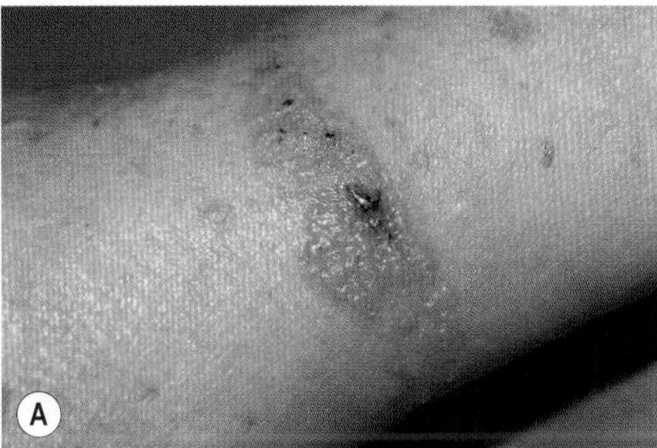

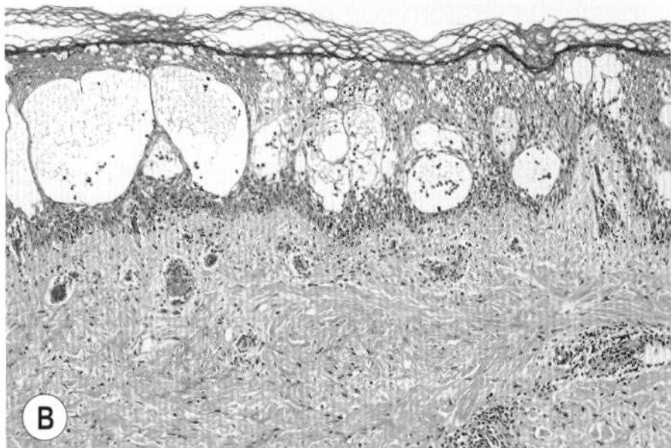

Fig. 1.9 Spongiotic dermatitis. A Acute allergic contact dermatitis to *Toxicodendron radicans* (poison ivy). The central black discoloration is due to the plant's resin. **B** Intercellular edema (spongiosis) and vesicle formation within the epidermis. Lymphocytes are also seen in both the epidermis and dermis.
A, Courtesy, Kalman Watsky, MD; B, Courtesy, James Patterson, MD.

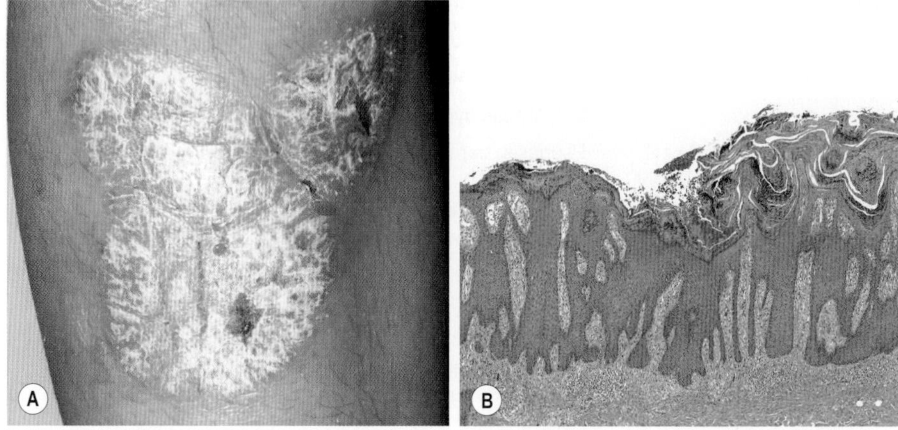

Fig. 1.10 Psoriasiform pattern. A Psoriasis vulgaris – pink plaques with silvery scale on the shin; this clinical description utilizes the key elements of color, primary lesion, secondary changes, and distribution pattern (extensor surfaces) in order to arrive at the diagnosis. **B** Regular epidermal hyperplasia and elongated dermal papillae with thin suprapapillary plates and confluent parakeratosis. The parakeratosis represents the histopathologic correlate of the visible scale. *A, Courtesy, Julie V. Schaffer, MD; B, Courtesy, Lorenzo Cerroni, MD.*

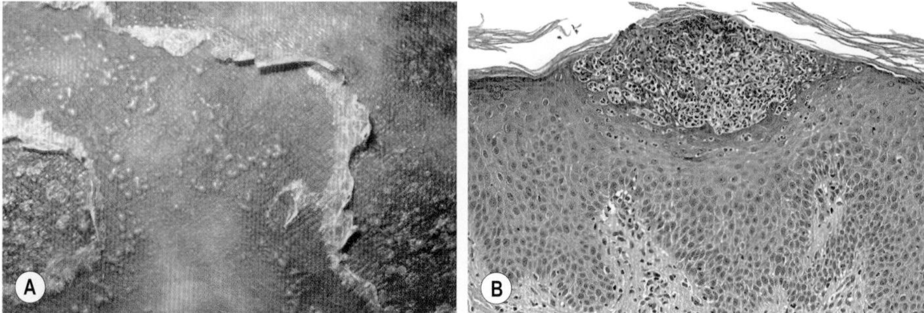

Fig. 1.11 Intraepidermal pustular dermatosis. A Pustular psoriasis. **B** Collection of neutrophils beneath the stratum corneum (subcorneal pustule). Scattered neutrophils are in the upper malpighian layer. *A, Courtesy, Kenneth Greer, MD; B, Courtesy, Lorenzo Cerroni, MD.*

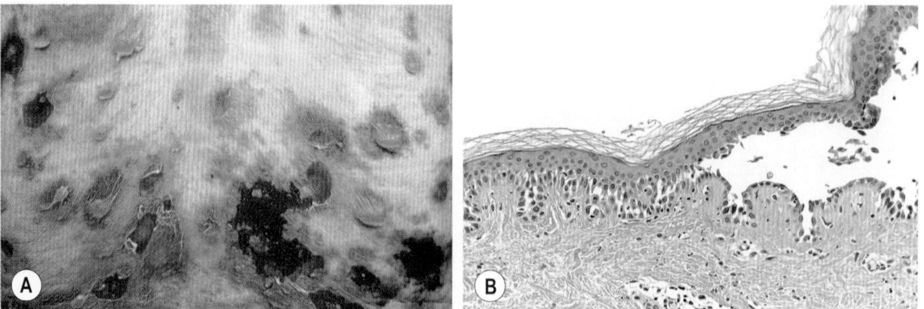

Fig. 1.12 Intraepidermal vesiculobullous dermatosis, acantholytic type. A Pemphigus vulgaris with flaccid bullae and erosions. Note the dependent location of the pustular contents of bullae. **B** The keratinocytes within the lower epidermis have lost their intercellular attachments and have separated from one another, resulting in an intraepidermal blister. *A, Courtesy, Carlo Francesco Tomasini, MD; B, Courtesy, Lorenzo Cerroni, MD.*

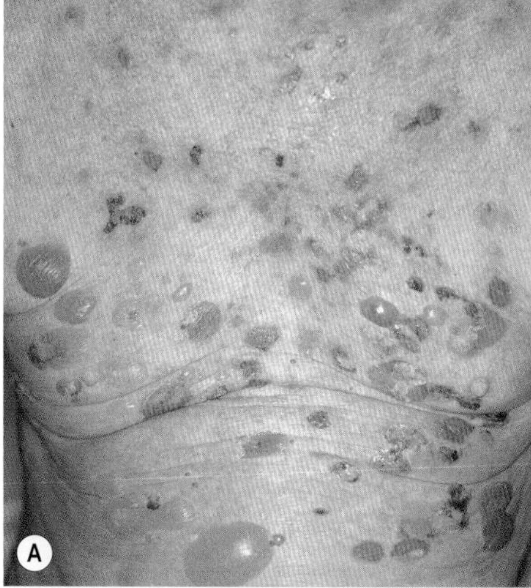

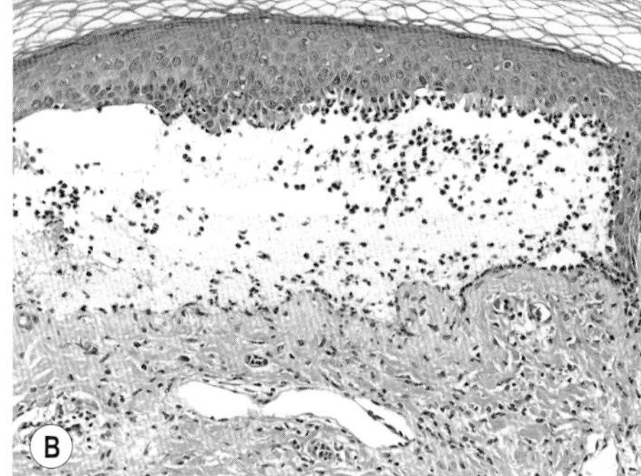

Fig. 1.13 Subepidermal vesiculobullous dermatosis. A Bullous pemphigoid with tense bullae. **B** Subepidermal blister with numerous eosinophils within the blister cavity. *A, Courtesy, YDRSC; B, Courtesy, Lorenzo Cerroni, MD.*

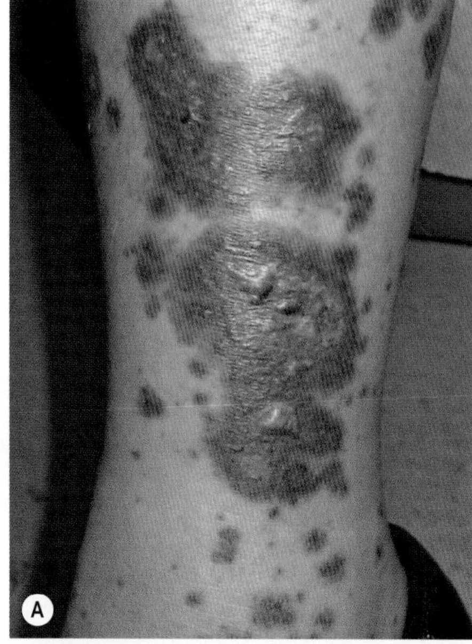

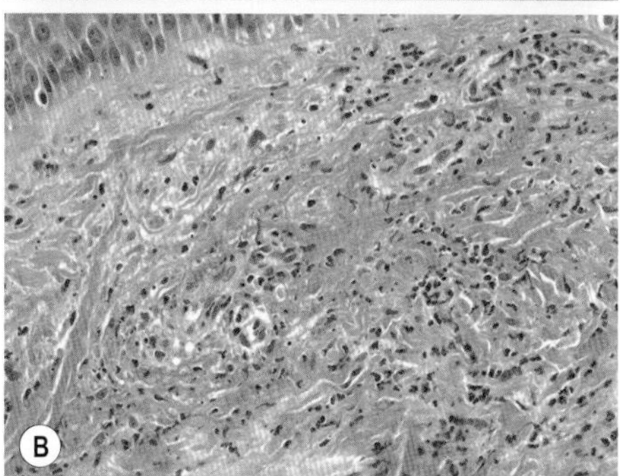

Fig. 1.14 Small vessel vasculitis. A Inflammatory palpable purpura of the leg. **B** Perivascular and interstitial infiltrate of neutrophils with nuclear dust (leukocytoclasia). Fibrin within the vessel wall and extravasation of erythrocytes is also seen. *A, Courtesy, Carlo F. Tomasini, MD; B, Courtesy, Christine Ko, MD.*

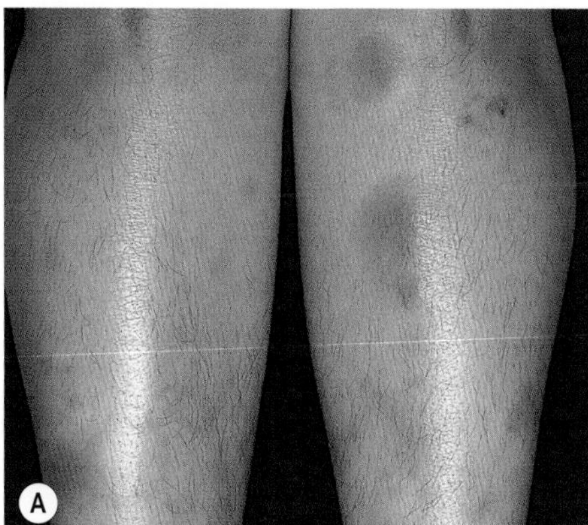

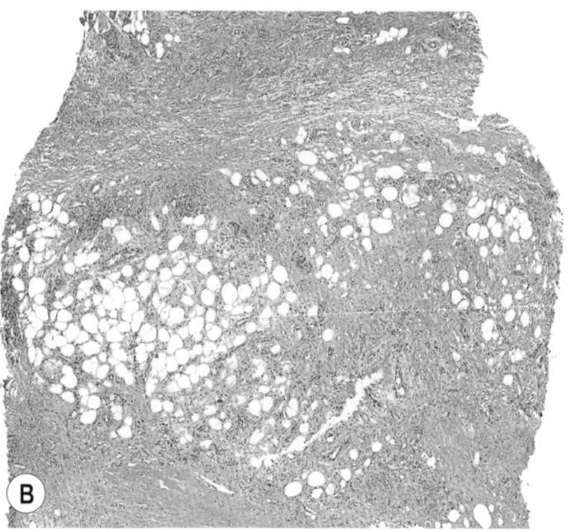

Fig. 1.15 Septal panniculitis. A Multiple red-brown nodules of erythema nodosum on the shins, admixed with healing bruise-like areas. **B** Predominantly septal granulomatous infiltrate with formation of characteristic Miescher's granulomas. *A, Courtesy, Kenneth Greer, MD; B, Courtesy, Christine Ko, MD.*

ACUTE CUTANEOUS ERUPTIONS IN OTHERWISE HEALTHY INDIVIDUALS	
Disorder	**Characteristic findings**
Urticaria (see Ch. 14)	• Pathogenesis involves degranulation of mast cells with release of histamine • Primary lesion: edematous wheal with erythematous flare • Widespread distribution • Very pruritic* • Individual lesions are transient (<24 hours in duration) • May become chronic (>6 weeks)
Acute allergic contact dermatitis (see Ch. 12)	• Immune-mediated and requires prior sensitization • Primary lesion: dermatitis, with vesicles, bullae, and weeping when severe • Primarily in sites of exposure; occasionally more widespread due to autosensitization • Pruritus, often marked • Spontaneously resolves over 2–3 weeks if no further exposure to allergen (e.g. poison ivy, nickel)
Acute irritant contact dermatitis (see Ch. 12)	• Direct toxic effect • Primary lesion: ranges from erythema to bullae (e.g. chemical burn) • At sites of exposure • Burning sensation • Spontaneously resolves over 2–3 weeks if no further exposure to irritant (e.g. strong acid, strong alkali)
Exanthematous (morbilliform) drug eruptions (see Ch. 17)	• Immune-mediated and requires prior sensitization • Pink to red-brown, blanching macules and papules; may become purpuric on distal lower extremities • Widespread distribution • May be pruritic • Spontaneously resolves over 7–10 days if no further exposure to inciting drug
Pityriasis rosea (see Ch. 7)	• May follow a viral illness • Primary lesion: oval-shaped, pink to salmon-colored papule or plaque with fine white scale centrally and peripheral collarette; occasionally vesicular • Initial lesion is often largest (herald patch) • Favors trunk and proximal extremities; may have inverse pattern (axillae and groin); long axis of lesions parallel to skin cleavage lines (see Fig. 7.7) • Spontaneously resolves over 6–10 weeks; exclude secondary syphilis
Viral exanthems (see Ch. 68)	• Due to a broad range of viruses, including rubeola, rubella, enteroviruses, parvovirus, adenovirus (see Fig. 68.1) • Often associated with fever, malaise, arthralgias, myalgias, nausea, upper respiratory symptoms • Primary lesions vary from blanching pink macules and papules to vesicles or petechiae • Distribution varies from acral to widespread; may have an enanthem • Spontaneously resolves over 3–10 days

**May have burning rather than pruritus with urticarial vasculitis, and individual lesions of urticarial vasculitis can last longer than 24 hours.*

Table 1.7 Acute cutaneous eruptions in otherwise healthy individuals.

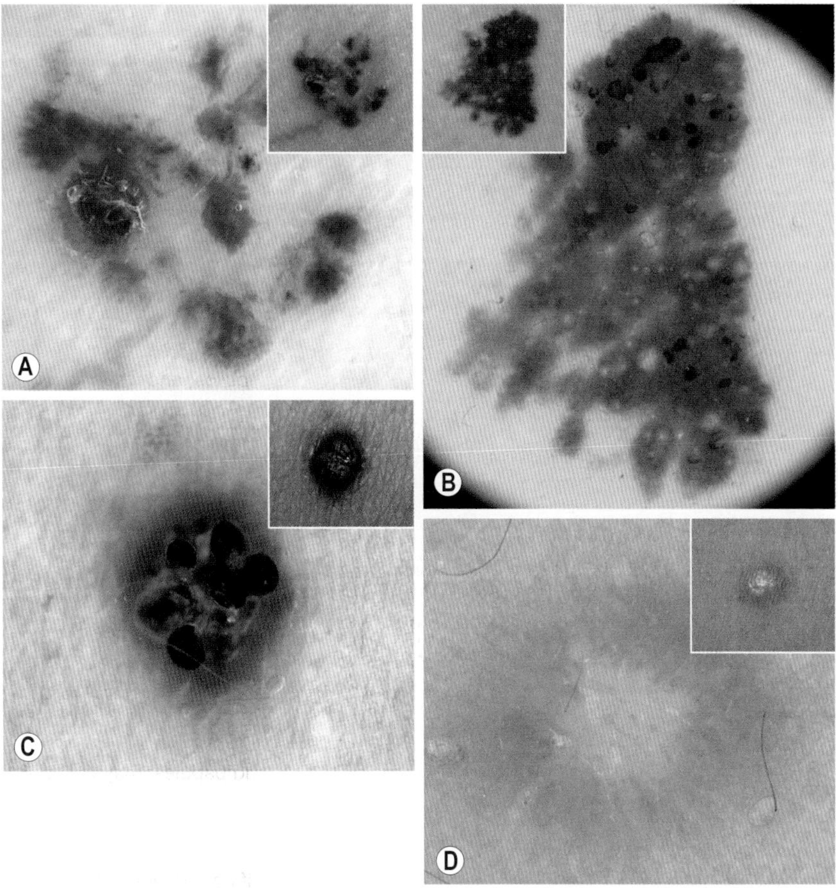

Fig. 1.16 Use of dermoscopy to aid in the diagnosis of four common pigmented (non-melanocytic) cutaneous lesions. A Pigmented basal cell carcinoma with leaf-like areas (islands of blue-gray color) at the periphery and a small erosion of reddish color at the left side of the lesion. **B** Seborrheic keratosis with typical milia-like cysts (white shining globules) and comedo-like openings (black targetoid globules). **C** Angiokeratoma with red-black lacunas clearly visible as well-demarcated roundish structures. **D** A dermatofibroma with characteristic central white patch and peripheral delicate pseudo-network. Dermoscopic features of melanocytic nevi and melanoma are reviewed in Chapters 92 and 93. *Courtesy, Giuseppe Argenziano, MD, and Iris Zalaudek, MD.*

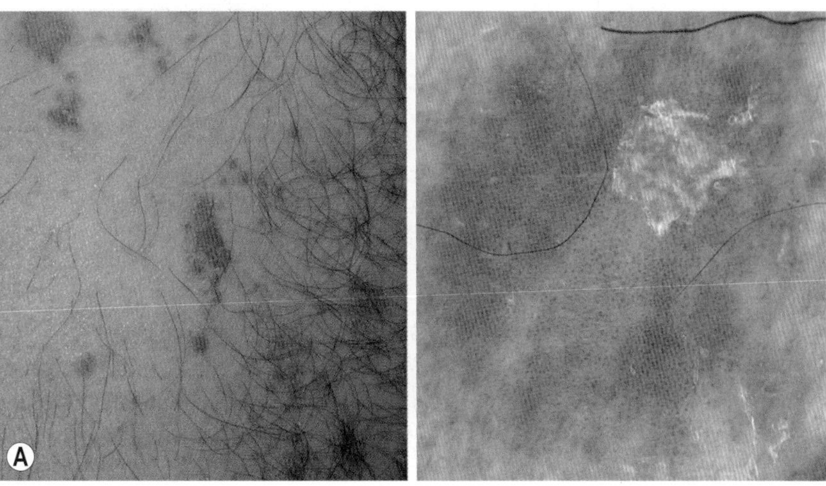

Fig. 1.17 Use of dermoscopy to aid in the diagnosis of inflammatory disorders. A By dermoscopy, classic psoriasis plaques exhibit regular dotted vessels. *Continued*

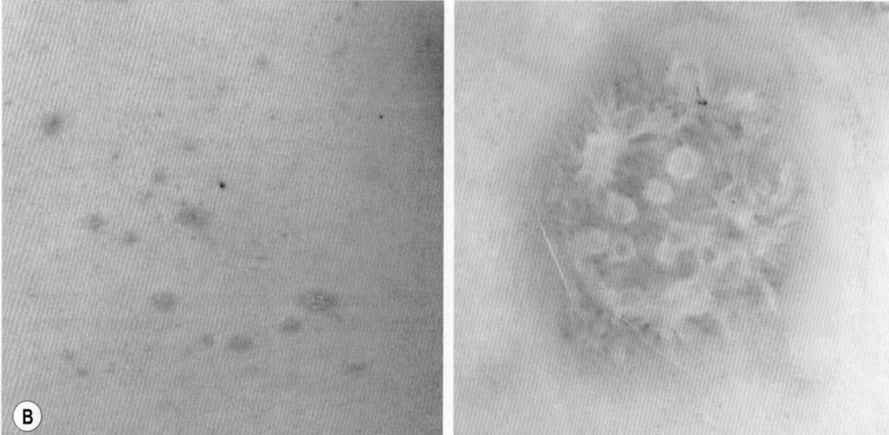

Fig. 1.17 *Continued* **B** The dermoscopic pattern of lichen planus is definitely different from the previous one. Here, dotted vessels are seen at the border of typical whitish lines and clods, which closely resemble the Wickham striae found in lichen planus of the oral mucosa. *Courtesy, Giuseppe Argenziano, MD, and Iris Zalaudek, MD.*

Bedside Diagnostics 2

• A range of bedside diagnostic procedures are performed to assist in the diagnosis of skin disorders.

• The most commonly performed procedures include microscopic examination of skin scrapings mounted in either potassium hydroxide (KOH) or mineral oil and microscopic examination of hair shafts.

Potassium Hydroxide (KOH) Preparation of Scale

• Microscopic examination of scale (stratum corneum), obtained via scraping with a metal blade or glass slide and mounted in KOH, is commonly performed to confirm superficial cutaneous fungal infections (Fig. 2.1).

• These fungal infections include tinea (pityriasis) versicolor, tinea corporis/faciei/manuum/cruris/pedis, and cutaneous candidiasis (see Ch. 64).

• Addition of chlorazol black to the KOH can improve detection (see Fig. 2.1B).

• Neither the genus nor the species of a dermatophyte can be determined by the KOH examination of scale.

• For onychomycosis, both nail plates and subungual debris are examined; in addition, nail plates can be fixed in formalin and stained with periodic acid Schiff (PAS) or Gomori methenamine silver stain (see Ch. 64).

Potassium Hydroxide (KOH) Preparation of Hair Shafts

• Tinea capitis is divided into two major forms: (1) endothrix – conidia occur within the hair shaft; and (2) ectothrix – while the fungus grows inside the hair shaft, conidia form on its surface (Figs 2.2 and 2.3; see Ch. 64).

• For KOH examination and fungal culture, fragile and broken hairs are preferred and can be obtained by scraping with a metal blade or glass slide or, in children, a sterile toothbrush or moistened cotton applicator (Q-tip®).

Mineral Oil Scraping for Suspected Scabies

• Place 2–3 drops of mineral oil on a glass slide. Dip the metal blade into the oil and then scrape suspicious lesions, e.g. burrows, inflammatory papules. Next place skin scrapings on a glass slide. Several skin lesions should be scraped. Dermoscopy can be performed to better identify burrows and an adult female mite at the end of the burrow prior to scraping (see Ch. 71). Sometimes, KOH is used rather than mineral oil. Firm application of transparent adhesive tape to suspicious lesions followed by rapid removal and transfer to a glass slide is an alternative technique, providing easier transport to a laboratory.

• In addition to adult mites, eggs and feces (scybala) can be seen when scrapings are examined microscopically (Figs 2.4 and 2.5).

Tzanck Smear

• The advent of direct fluorescent antibody (DFA) and polymerase chain reaction (PCR) assays to detect herpes simplex and varicella–zoster viral infections has led to a decline in the performance of Tzanck smears.

• Nonetheless, it can serve as an easy-to-perform bedside test with results available immediately, including during laboratory "off-hours". A Tzanck smear is most sensitive when an intact vesicle or bulla is present; in immunocompromised hosts, crusted lesions may also be positive.

• The roof is retracted and scraping of the base and angles of the vesicle should be performed in order to obtain virally infected keratinocytes, which are thinly spread onto a glass slide, allowed to dry, and then stained with Giemsa stain (Figs 2.6 and 2.7).

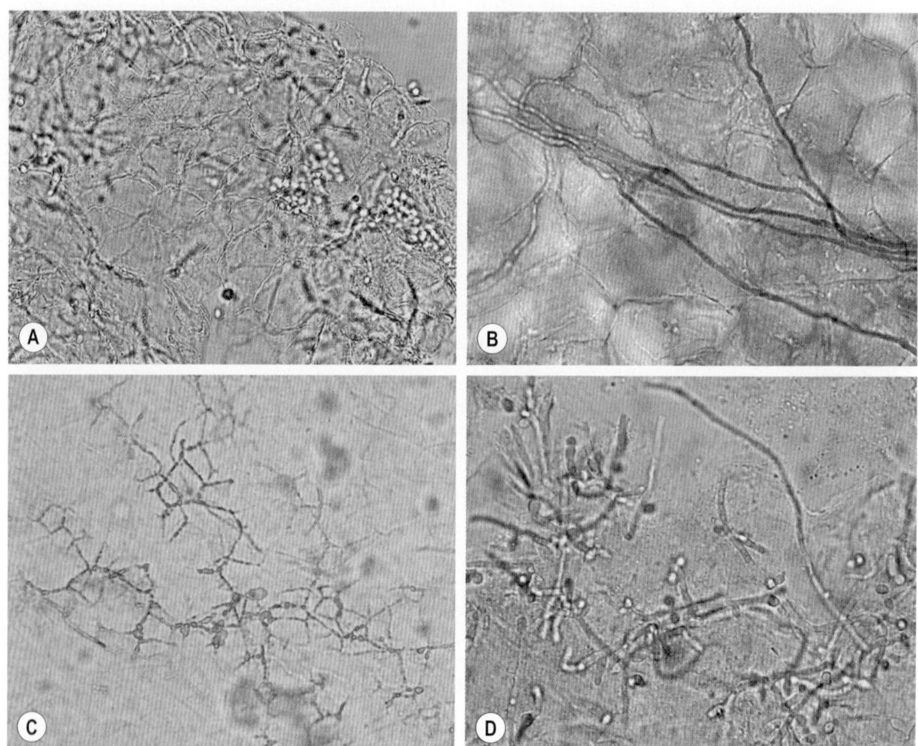

Fig. 2.1 Microscopic examination of potassium hydroxide (KOH) preparations of scale. **A** Tinea (pityriasis) versicolor due to *Malassezia* spp. with short mycelial forms and clusters of yeast forms. **B** Tinea corporis due to a dermatophyte with hyphae that cross over more than one cell (squame) and are branching. Chlorazol black has been added to the KOH and the stained hyphae are easier to detect. **C** Branching mosaic pattern that represents the junctures of normal epidermal cells; this is a cause of false-positive KOH exams. **D** Cutaneous candidiasis with yeast forms and pseudohyphae. Pseudohyphae can sometimes be difficult to distinguish from hyphae. *A, Courtesy, Ronald Rapini, MD; B, Courtesy, YDRSC; C, Courtesy, Louis A. Fragola, Jr., MD; D, Courtesy, Frank Samarin, MD.*

Microscopic Examination of Molluscum Bodies

- In some patients, lesions of molluscum contagiosum may not have a classic appearance – e.g. due to inflammation, previous treatments, large size – and confirmation of the diagnosis without performing a skin biopsy can be helpful.
- The center of the papulonodule, which is often paler in color, is gently curetted to remove a core composed of the viral particles, and the contents are then thinly spread onto a glass slide; saline or KOH can be added prior to placing the coverslip (Fig. 2.8).

Gram Stain

- Performed when pustular material is available and identifies both Gram-positive and Gram-negative bacteria (Fig. 2.9).
- In addition, fungal organisms (e.g. *Candida*) can be identified.

Dermal Scrapings and Touch Preps

- When there is suspicion of a septic embolus or a primary infection involving the dermis and/or subcutis (bacterial, fungal, parasitic), then in addition to a sterile skin biopsy (Fig. 2.10), a touch prep or a dermal scraping can be performed. Often, the patient is immunocompromised. If there is pustular drainage, then a Gram stain and KOH preparation are performed first.
- In a touch prep, the base of a skin biopsy which includes dermis ± subcutis is tapped multiple times against a glass slide. After drying for several minutes, the glass slide

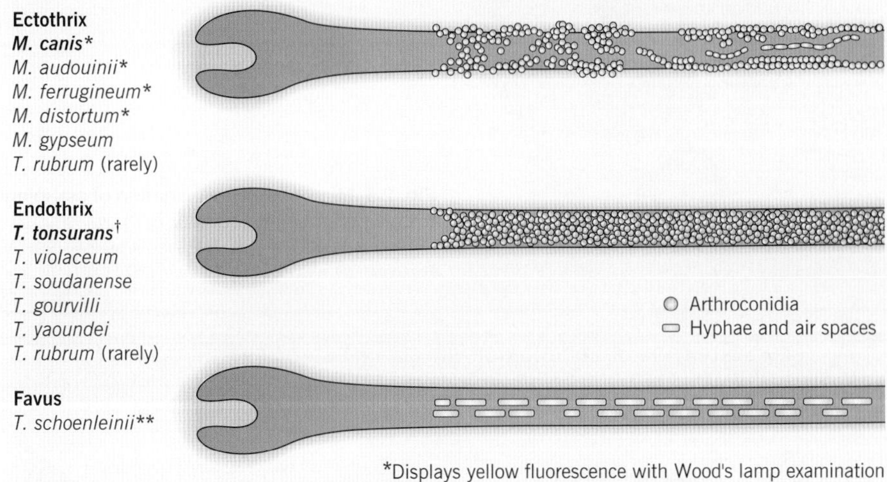

Fig. 2.2 The three patterns of hair invasion in tinea capitis and the causative dermatophytes. See Ch. 64 for additional details.

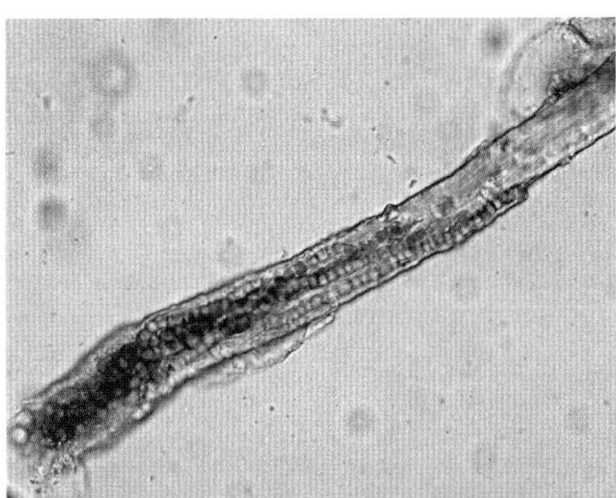

Fig. 2.3 Microscopic examination of a KOH preparation of a hair shaft with an endothrix dermatophyte infection (tinea capitis). The most common species for endothrix infections is *Trichophyton tonsurans*. Chlorazol black has been added to the KOH. *Courtesy, YDRSC.*

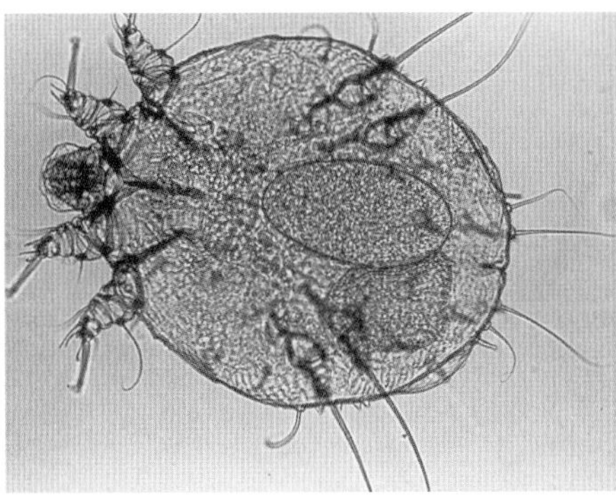

Fig. 2.4 Microscopic examination of scrapings from a patient with scabies. Female *Sarcoptes scabiei* var. *hominis* mite with eggs. There is a flattened, oval body with wrinkle-like corrugations and eight legs. *With permission from Taplin D, Meinking TL. Infestations. In: Schachner LA, Hansen RC (Eds.), Pediatric Dermatology, 4th edn. Edinburgh, UK: Mosby, 2011:1141–1180.*

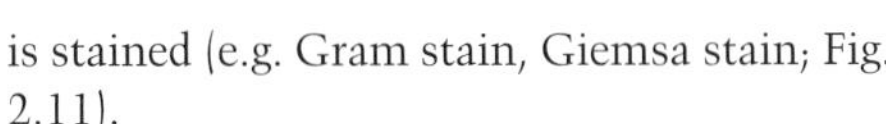

is stained (e.g. Gram stain, Giemsa stain; Fig. 2.11).

• In a dermal scraping, the epidermis (if present) is reflected back after injection of local anesthesia, and a curette is used to scrape dermal tissue onto a slide.

Giemsa Stain for Eosinophils or Amastigotes

• Identification of eosinophils can assist in distinguishing the pustulovesicular lesions of erythema toxicum neonatorum from neonatal pustular melanosis and congenital candidiasis.

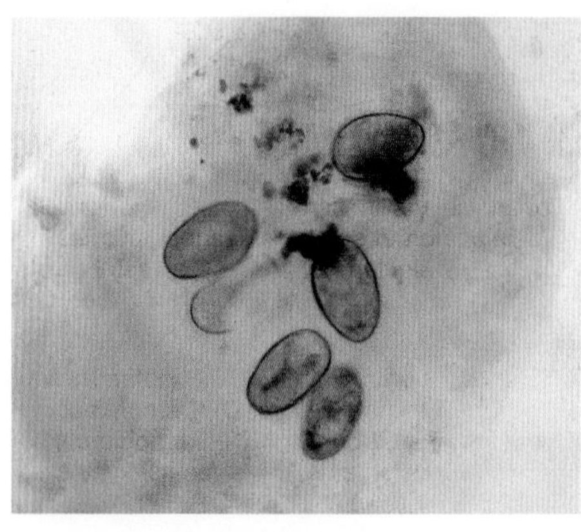

Fig. 2.5 Microscopic examination of scrapings from a patient with scabies. Both oval-shaped eggs and scybala (feces) are seen. *Courtesy, Craig N. Burkhart, MD, and Craig G. Burkhart, MD.*

DEMONSTRATION OF LOCATION OF VIRALLY INFECTED KERATINOCYTES IN VESICULOBULLOUS LESIONS OF HERPES SIMPLEX, VARICELLA AND HERPES ZOSTER

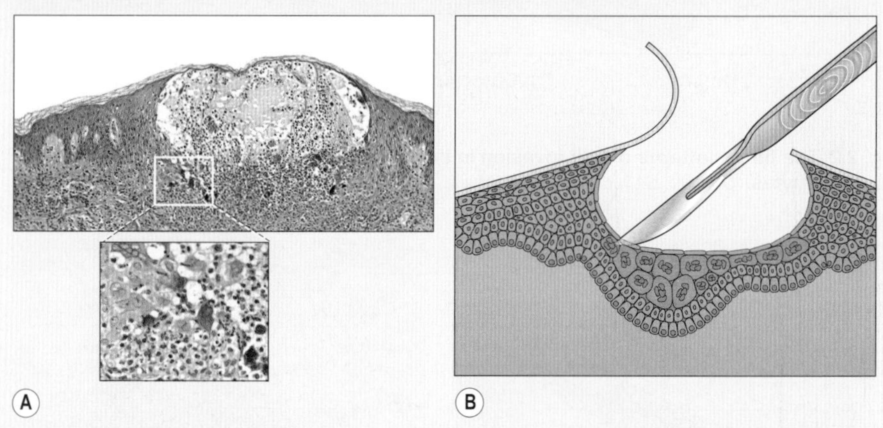

Fig. 2.6 Demonstration of location of virally infected keratinocytes in vesiculobullous lesions of herpes simplex, varicella, and herpes zoster. A Histologically, viral changes (e.g. multinucleated giant cells) are seen at the base of the vesicle; note their absence on the roof. **B** Scraping of the base of the vesicle is performed after the roof of the blister is reflected. *A, Courtesy, Lorenzo Cerroni, MD.*

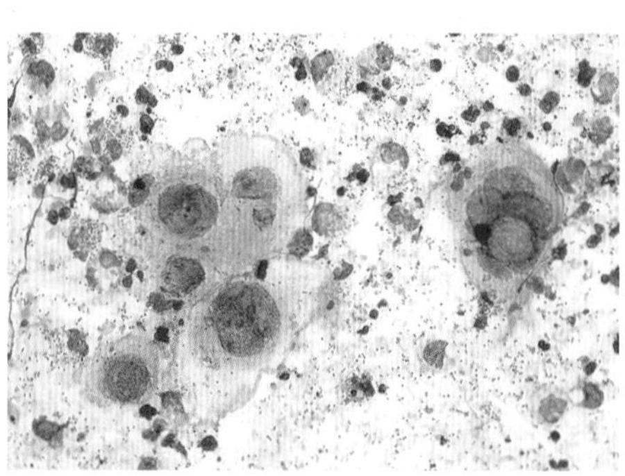

Fig. 2.7 Tzanck smear demonstrating multinucleated giant cells. Such cells are seen in herpes simplex, varicella, and herpes zoster viral infections (Giemsa stain). *Courtesy, Louis A. Fragola, Jr., MD.*

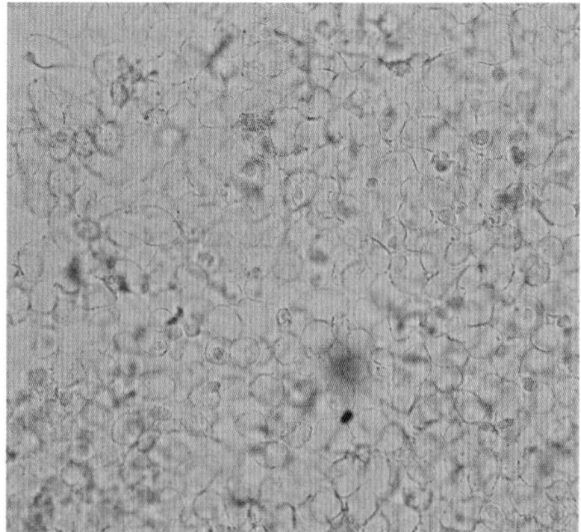

Fig. 2.8 Large, round molluscum bodies are present in a scraping of the center of a papulonodule. The scrapings can be mounted in saline or KOH solution. *Courtesy, Bradley Bloom, MD.*

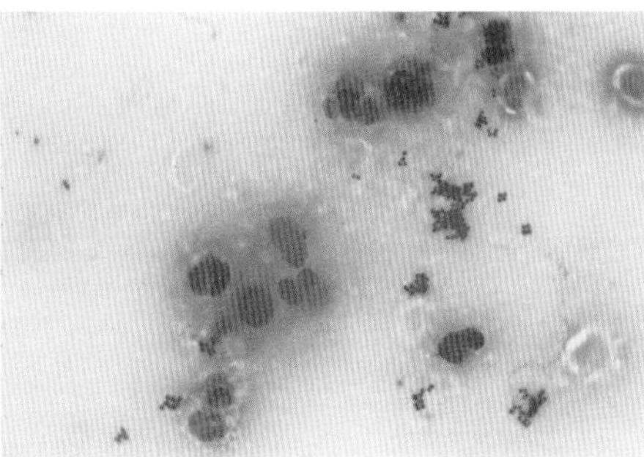

Fig. 2.9 Gram stain of pus demonstrating polymorphonuclear leukocytes (neutrophils) and Gram-positive cocci in clusters (*Staphylococcus aureus*). *From Ekkelenkamp, MB, Rooijakkers, SHM, Bonten, MJM. In: Cohen J, Powderly W, Opal S (Eds.), Infectious Diseases, 3rd edn. Edinburgh, UK: Mosby, 2010.*

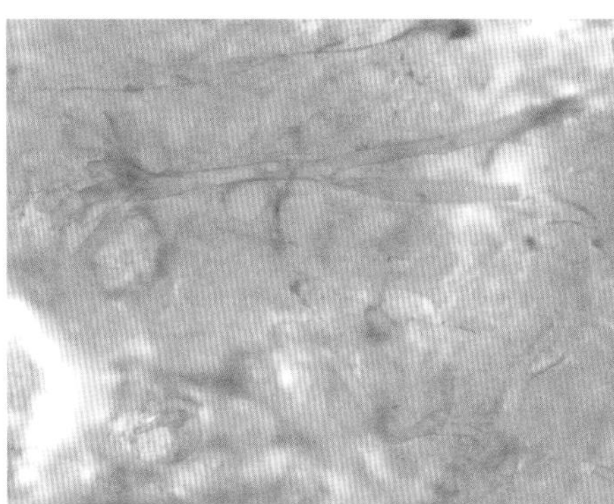

Fig. 2.11 Microscopic examination of a "touch prep" from an incisional biopsy performed of a necrotic lesion on the chest of an immunocompromised patient. Note the branching, ribbon-like, non-septate hyphae characteristic of *Rhizopus*. *Courtesy, Jean L. Bolognia, MD.*

PERFORMANCE OF A STERILE SKIN BIOPSY

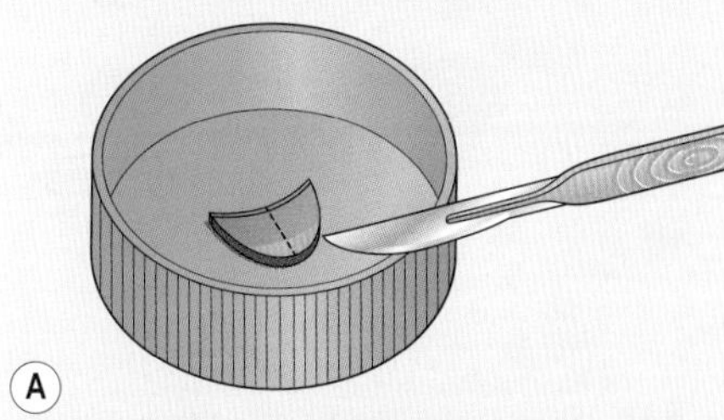

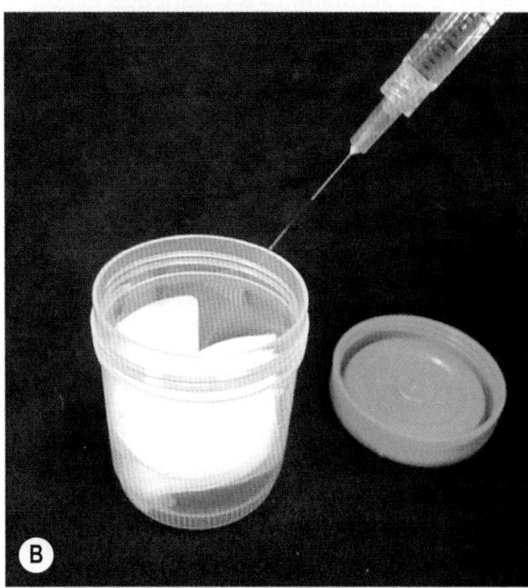

Fig. 2.10 Performance of a sterile skin biopsy. This is done when there is a suspicion of a septic embolus or primary skin infection of the dermis and/or subcutis. The equipment required includes a chemical antiseptic (e.g. chlorhexidine), alcohol pads, local anesthetic, punch biopsy instrument or scalpel, sterile scissors and forceps, sterile urine cup containing sterile gauze dampened with non-bacteriostatic saline, and glass slides. Following cleansing of the skin (antiseptic followed by alcohol), the skin is injected with local anesthesia, and a biopsy of dermis plus subcutaneous fat is performed (see Ch. 1). **A** The specimen is cut into two pieces on the sterile side of the urine container lid, while avoiding compression of the tissue. An alternative is to do two biopsies. **B** One piece or biopsy is placed in a sterile urine cup with moistened gauze, and the bottom of the second piece or second biopsy is tapped several times against a glass slide before being placed in formalin. The sealed sterile urine cup is hand-carried to the microbiology laboratory. Once the glass slide is dry, the touch prep can be stained to detect infectious organisms.

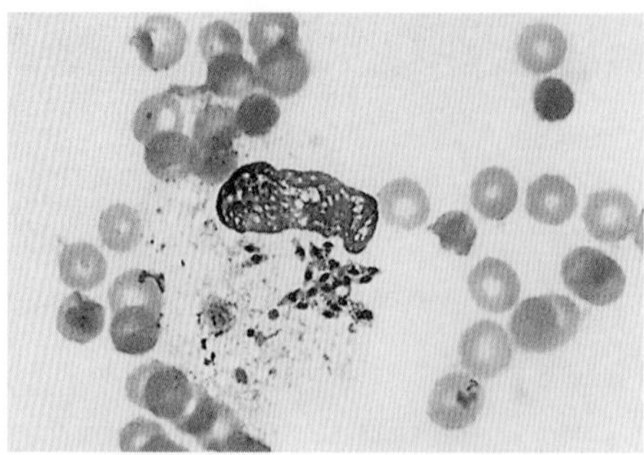

Fig. 2.12 Dermal tissue obtained from a skin slit and scraping of a cutaneous lesion of leishmaniasis shows amastigotes within macrophages. *From Peters W, Pasvol G. Tropical Medicine and Parasitology, 6th edn. London: Mosby, 2007.*

- A skin slit and scraping of cutaneous lesions of leishmaniasis demonstrate amastigotes in macrophages when stained with a Giemsa stain (Fig. 2.12).

Acid-Fast Stain for Leprosy

- When leprosy is suspected, a fold of skin is firmly squeezed and a small incision is made with a scalpel, with the liquid expressed smeared onto a slide, allowed to dry, and stained with a Fite or Ziehl–Neelsen stain (Fig. 2.13).
- For bacilloscopy, the skin sites that are examined include the earlobes, elbows, dorsal fingers, and lesions or infiltrated areas.
- While acid-fast *Mycobacterium leprae* organisms are found in ≤5% of patients with tuberculoid leprosy, they are seen in 100% of patients with lepromatous leprosy (see Ch. 62).

Dark Field Microscopy for Treponemal Infections

- Dark field microscopy is utilized for the examination of unstained live organisms and in dermatology, primarily for the diagnosis of primary syphilis and less often secondary cutaneous syphilis (see Ch. 69).
- Expressed serous exudate with a minimal number of red blood cells is placed onto a slide and then a coverslip applied.

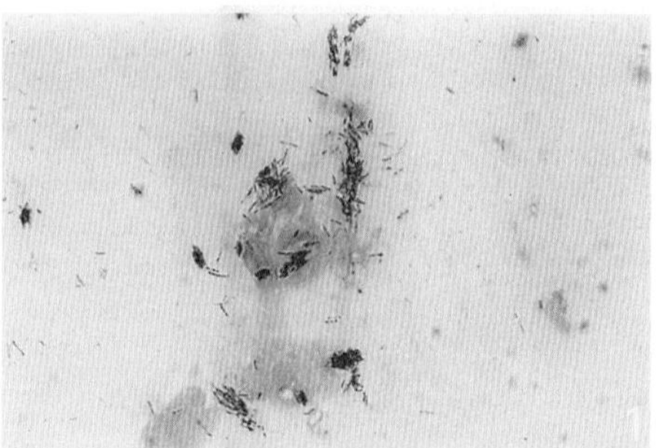

Fig. 2.13 Smear stained with a Ziehl–Neelsen stain demonstrating acid-fast bacilli in a patient with leprosy. *From Peters W, Pasvol G. Tropical Medicine and Parasitology, 6th edn. London: Mosby, 2007.*

- The *Treponema* spirochetes have a characteristic morphology and movement pattern (Fig. 2.14).

Evaluation of Folliculitis

- While the most common forms of folliculitis are associated with normal flora or *Staphylococcus aureus*, there are forms due to Gram-negative rods (e.g. *Pseudomonas*), *Malassezia* (*Pityrosporum*) spp., herpes simplex, and *Demodex* spp. (see Fig. 31.1).
- For bacteria, cultures are the primary means of diagnosis, but for *Pityrosporum* and *Demodex* folliculitis, bedside diagnosis is key (Fig. 2.15). In *Pityrosporum* folliculitis, only yeast forms are seen.

Hair Shaft Examination

- Assessment of hair thinning, which may be due to miniaturization, shedding, or breakage, most commonly includes a gentle hair pull and a hair shaft examination of cut, rather than pulled, hairs; some clinicians also do a vigorous hair pluck referred to as a trichogram (20–40 scalp hairs grasped by a hemostat with rubber-covered jaws).
- In general, telogen hairs are observed with a gentle hair pull, but in disorders such as loose anagen syndrome, anagen hairs may be seen (see Ch. 56).
- In a trichogram, the ratio of anagen : telogen hairs is determined by microscopic examination of the hair bulbs (Fig. 2.16). The

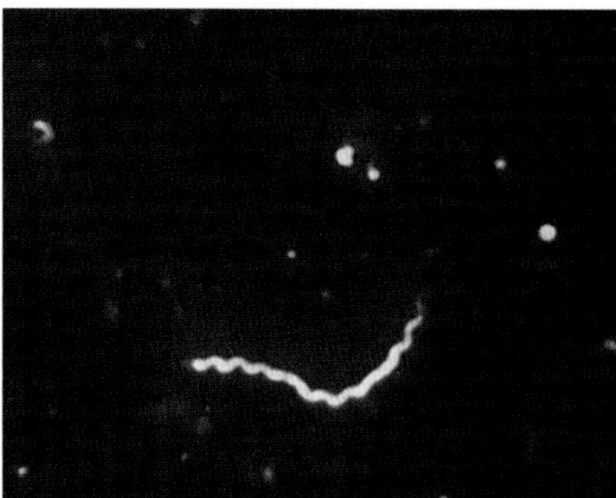

Fig. 2.14 Dark field microscopic examination of a spirochete. Treponemes are recognized by their characteristic corkscrew shape and deliberate forward and backward movement with rotation about the longitudinal axis. *From Morse et al. Atlas of Sexually Transmitted Diseases and AIDS, 3rd edn. London: Mosby; 2003.*

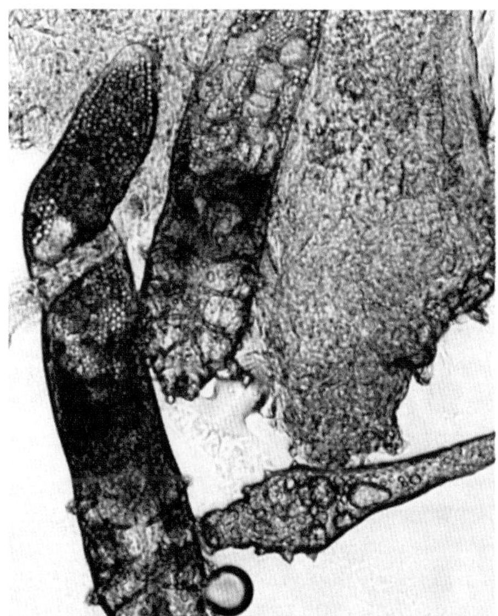

Fig. 2.15 Microscopic examination of follicular contents in a patient with *Demodex* folliculitis.

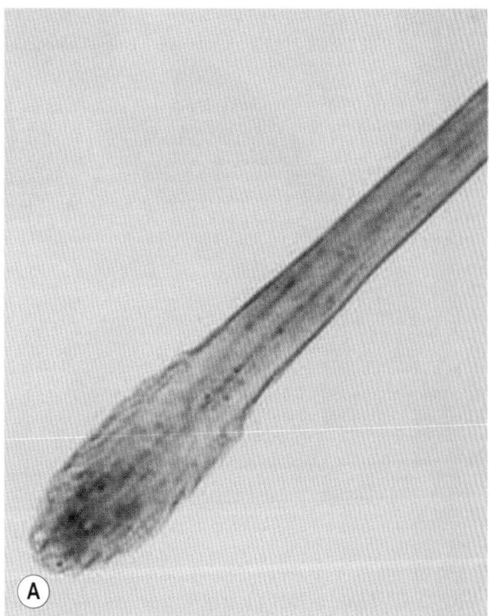

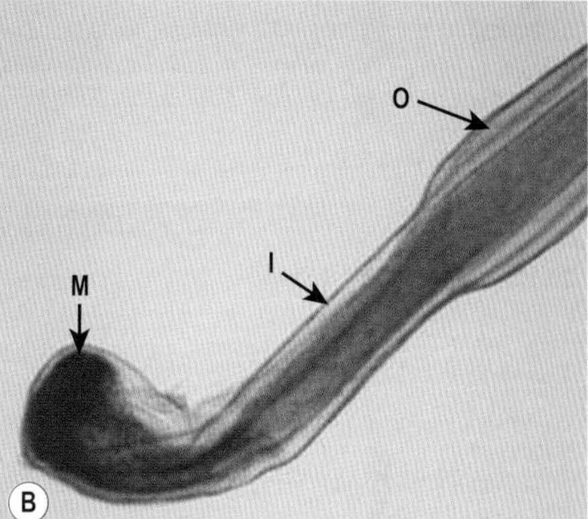

Fig. 2.16 Comparison of a telogen versus anagen hair shaft. A A telogen hair shaft has a club-shaped bulb. **B** An anagen hair has attached root sheaths as well as a pigmented and distorted bulb, sometimes resembling a hockey stick. M, matrix; I, inner root sheath; O, outer root sheath. *B, Courtesy, Leonard Sperling, MD.*

normal anagen-to-telogen ratio is 9:1, but in telogen effluvium, it can be 7:3 or less.

- Hair shaft examination can also detect bacterial and fungal infections (e.g. trichomycosis axillaris, white piedra, black piedra), hair casts, nits due to head lice infestation, and hair shaft abnormalities (e.g. trichorrhexis nodosa) (Fig. 2.17) (see Fig. 64.3 and Chs 56, 64, and 71).
- For optimal detection of hair shaft abnormalities, mounting in Permount™ (an adhesive composed of polymers dissolved in toluene) is performed.

Identification of Arthropods

- Another bedside diagnostic procedure is the identification of lice, insects (e.g. bedbugs), and arachnids (e.g. ticks). Chs 71 and 72 review their identification via macroscopic and microscopic findings.

Wood's Lamp Examination

- Table 2.1 outlines the fluorescent colors that are seen following absorption of UVA irradiation by different substances.

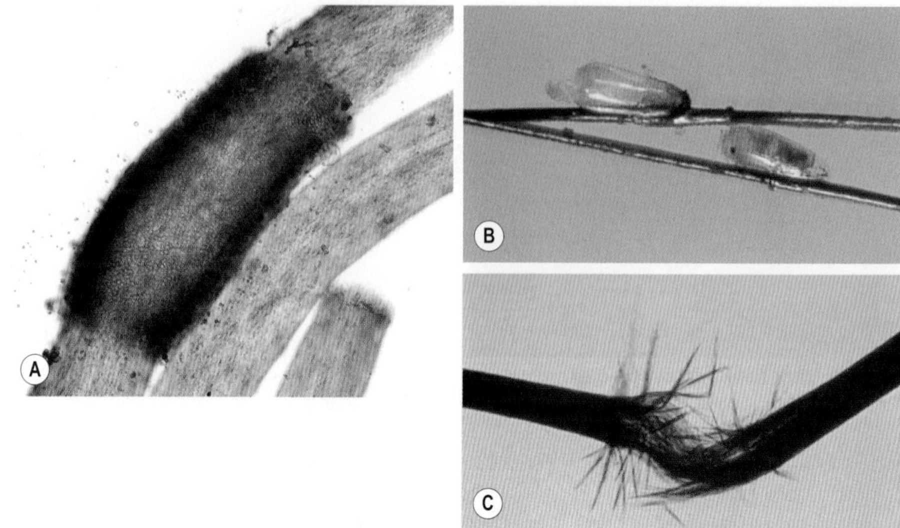

Fig. 2.17 Hair shaft examination as a diagnostic tool. A Nodule composed of numerous conidia of *Trichosporon inkin* in a patient with white piedra. **B** Two head louse egg casings (nits) are seen attached to hair shafts. **C** In trichorrhexis nodosa, the two ends of the hair shaft resemble opposing broomsticks. *B, With permission from Taplin D, Meinking TL. Infestations. In: Schachner LA, Hansen RC (Eds.), Pediatric Dermatology, 4th edn. Edinburgh, UK: Mosby, 2011:1141–1180; C, Courtesy, Christine Ko, MD.*

WOOD'S LAMP EXAMINATION	
Fluorescent color/change	**Clinical example(s)**
Chalk-white to blue-white	Vitiligo (well-developed lesion)
Coral pink	Erythrasma (see Fig. 61.10B)
Golden to yellow-green	Tinea (pityriasis) versicolor
Blue-green to yellow-green	Tinea capitis due to *Microsporum* spp.
Enhancement of hypopigmentation	Ash leaf spot
Enhancement of brown color	Lentigines, epidermal form of post-inflammatory hyperpigmentation
Brown to brown-gray color becomes less obvious	Dermal form of postinflammatory hyperpigmentation

Table 2.1 Wood's lamp examination. UVA irradiation (peak of ~365 nm) is emitted by a Wood's lamp. Colors within the visible spectrum have longer wavelengths and less energy than UVA.

Fever and Rash 3

• A variety of infectious and inflammatory conditions can present with fever and a rash (Fig. 3.1). The cutaneous findings range from a morbilliform eruption or urticaria (Figs 3.2 and 3.3) to petechial, vesiculobullous, and pustular lesions (Figs 3.4–3.7).

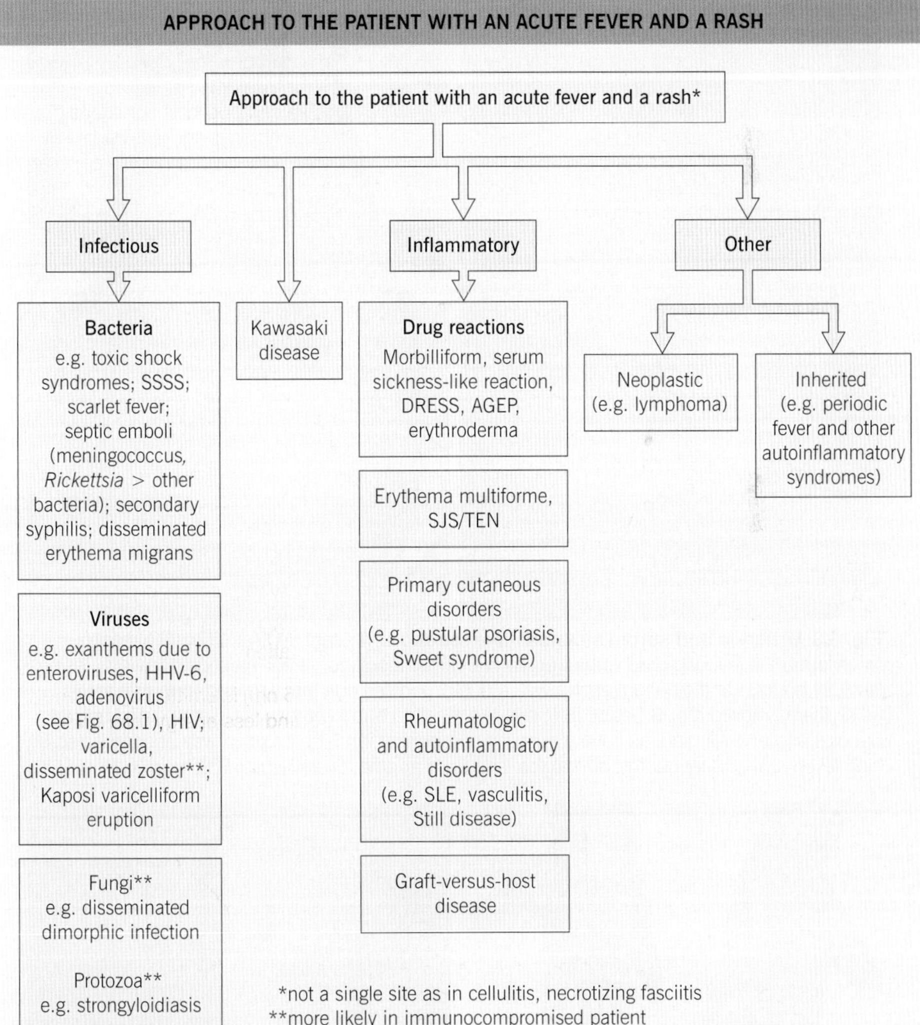

Fig. 3.1 Approach to the patient with an acute fever and a rash. AGEP, acute generalized exanthematous pustulosis; HHV, human herpes virus; SJS, Stevens–Johnson syndrome; SSSS, staphylococcal scalded skin syndrome; TEN, toxic epidermal necrolysis.

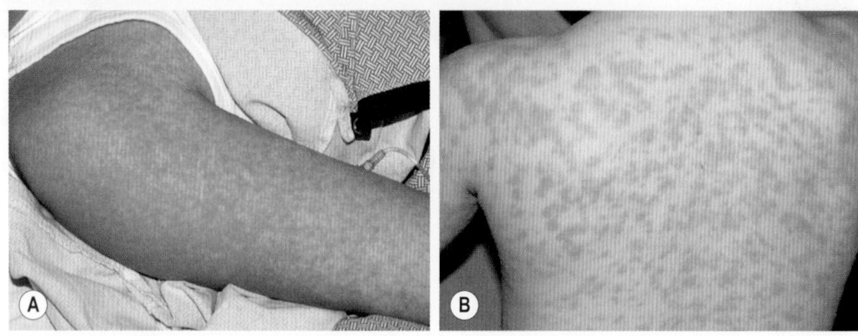

Fig. 3.2 Morbilliform drug eruptions. A Fine pink macules and thin papules, becoming confluent on the posterior upper arm, which is a dependent area in this hospitalized patient. **B** More edematous ("urticarial") pink papules; unlike true urticaria, these lesions are not transient. *Courtesy, Julie V. Schaffer, MD.*

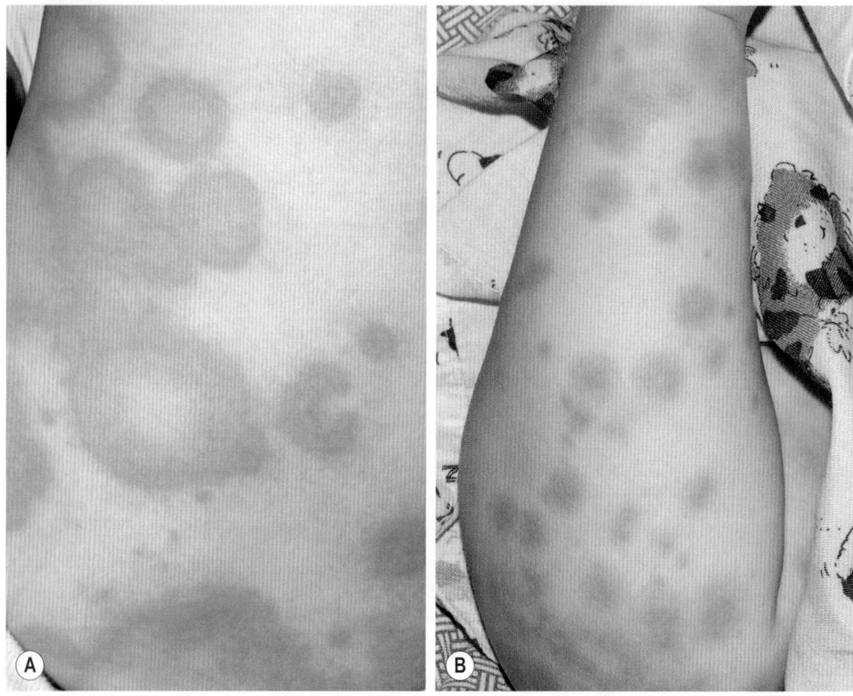

Fig. 3.3 Urticaria and serum sickness-like reaction. A Giant annular urticaria (urticaria "multiforme") in a young child with a recent viral upper respiratory tract infection. Individual lesions last <24 hours, but they often resolve with a dusky purplish hue that can lead to misdiagnosis as erythema multiforme. **B** Serum sickness-like reaction due to amoxicillin. Some of the urticarial papules and annular plaques have a purpuric component, and the eruption was accompanied by high fevers, lymphadenopathy, arthralgias, and acral edema. *Courtesy, Julie V. Schaffer, MD.*

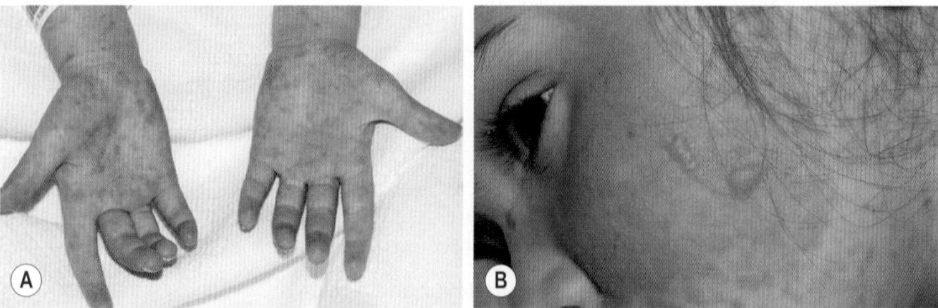

Fig. 3.4 Stevens–Johnson syndrome. The patient initially developed multiple small pink papules mimicking a morbilliform eruption, but with accentuation on the palms **(A).** A day later, confluent erythema and bullae had developed **(B),** and involvement of the vermilion lips and conjunctiva was evident. *Courtesy, Julie V. Schaffer, MD.*

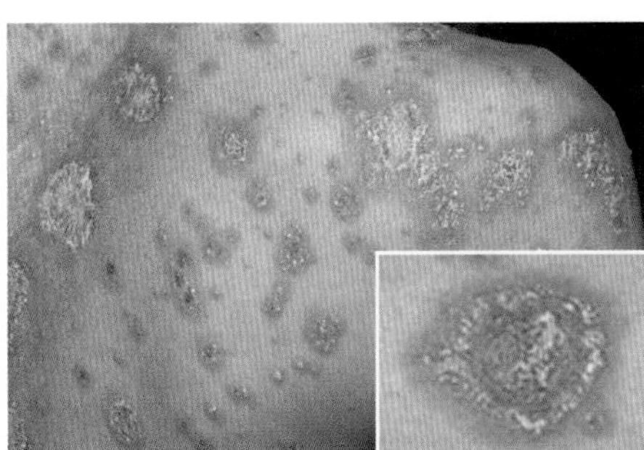

Fig. 3.5 Pustular psoriasis in a pediatric patient. Multiple sterile papulopustules and expanding annular red plaques with pustulation at the advancing edge. This eruption was widespread and associated with fever and malaise. *Courtesy, Julie V. Schaffer, MD.*

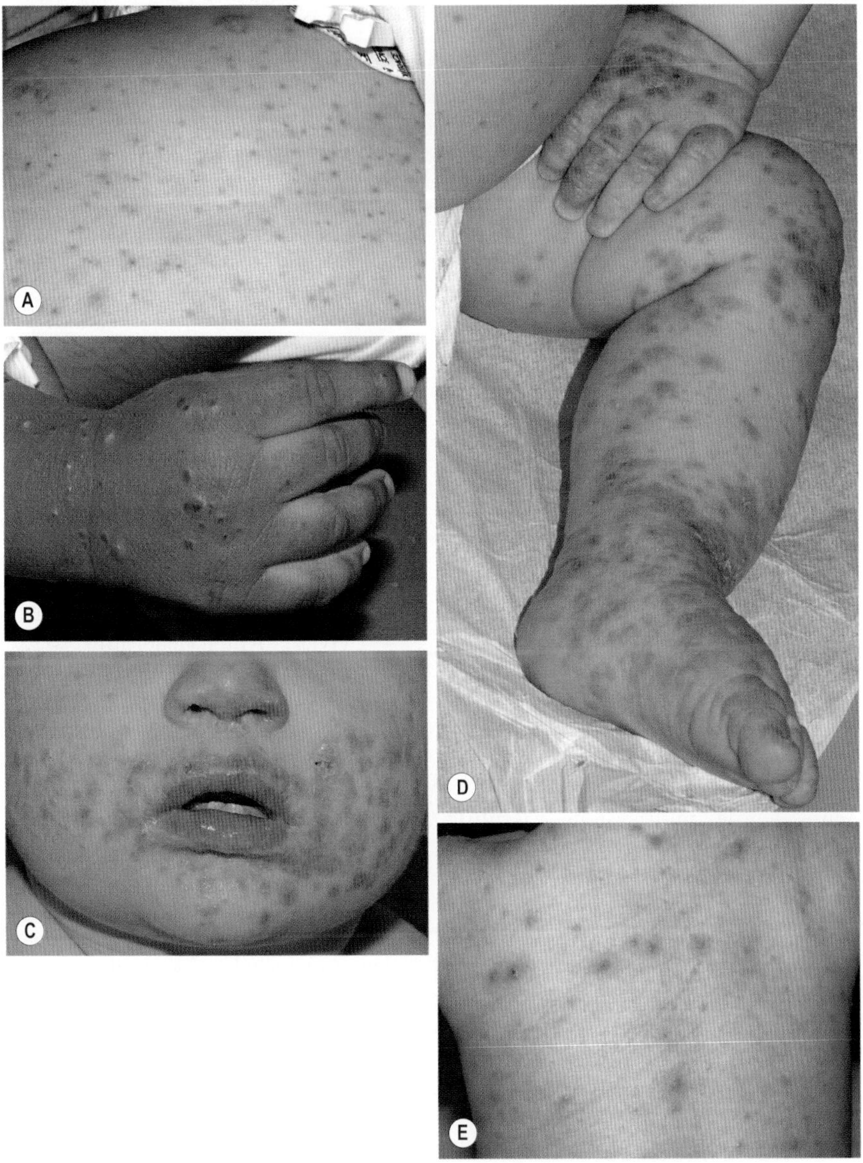

Fig. 3.6 Viral exanthems. A Enteroviral exanthem presenting as widespread small pink papules, many with petechiae centrally. **B–D** Vesicular eruptions with variable crusting due to coxsackievirus A6 infection, with characteristic perioral involvement (**C**) and widespread "eczema coxsackium" in an infant with atopic dermatitis (**D**). **E** Scattered vesicles on erythematous bases in varicella, with lesions in different stages of evolution. *Courtesy, Julie V. Schaffer, MD.*

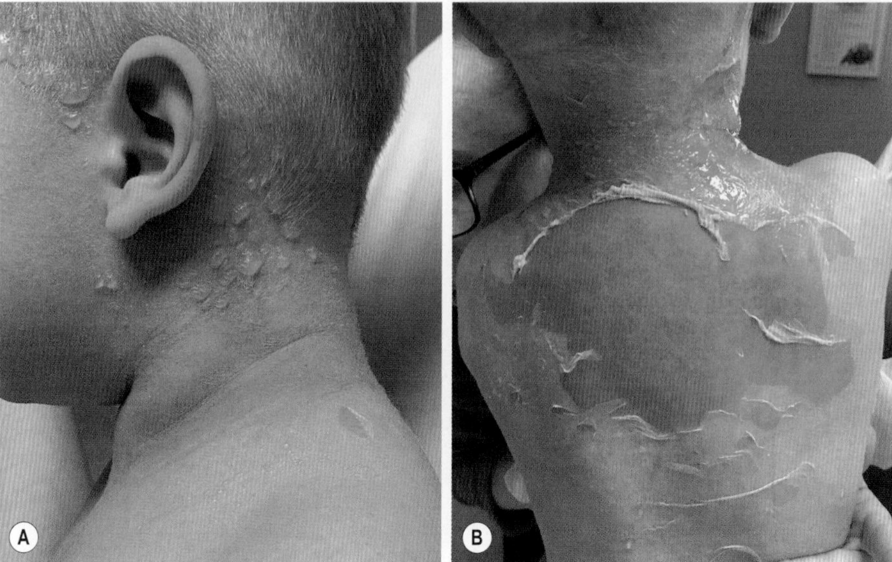

Fig. 3.7 Staphylococcal scalded skin syndrome in a 2-year-old child. A Diffuse, tender erythema with accentuation on the neck. Note the flaccid vesicles, skin wrinkling, and superficial erosion. **B** Later development of extensive superficial sloughing of the skin. *Courtesy, Julie V. Schaffer, MD.*

• Clinical features that distinguish entities within the differential diagnosis of an exanthematous drug eruption are summarized in Fig. 3.8.

• Although the initial skin findings of some potentially life-threatening disorders can mimic a more common benign disorder, the development of other cutaneous and extracutaneous features as the condition evolves points to the correct diagnosis (Table 3.1).

Kawasaki Disease

• Acute febrile multisystem vasculitic syndrome that primarily affects children <5 years of age (rarely adults), with ~3-fold higher incidence in Asians than Caucasians.

• Most common cause of pediatric acquired heart disease in the United States, with greatest morbidity from coronary artery aneurysms.

• Etiology remains unknown; factors include a genetic predisposition to immune activation and possibly an infectious trigger.

• Diagnostic criteria include fever (>39°C/102°F) for ≥5 days plus the presence of ≥4 of the following five criteria.
  - Bilateral non-purulent bulbar conjunctival injection
  - Oropharyngeal changes such as "chapped"/fissured lips (Fig. 3.9), a "strawberry" tongue, and diffuse hyperemia
  - Cervical lymphadenopathy (>1.5 cm; usually unilateral)
  - Erythema, edema, and (eventually) desquamation of the hands and feet (Fig. 3.10A)
  - Polymorphous exanthem – morbilliform or urticarial > erythema multiforme-like (Fig. 3.10B), scarlatiniform, or pustular

• Initial manifestation is often erythema in the perineal area, followed by desquamation (Fig. 3.10B–3.10D); subacute manifestations can include a psoriasiform eruption and transverse orange-brown (pseudo) chromonychia.

• "Incomplete" Kawasaki disease (more common in infants) is diagnosed if fever for ≥5 days and coronary artery abnormalities (via echocardiography or angiography) but <4 other criteria.

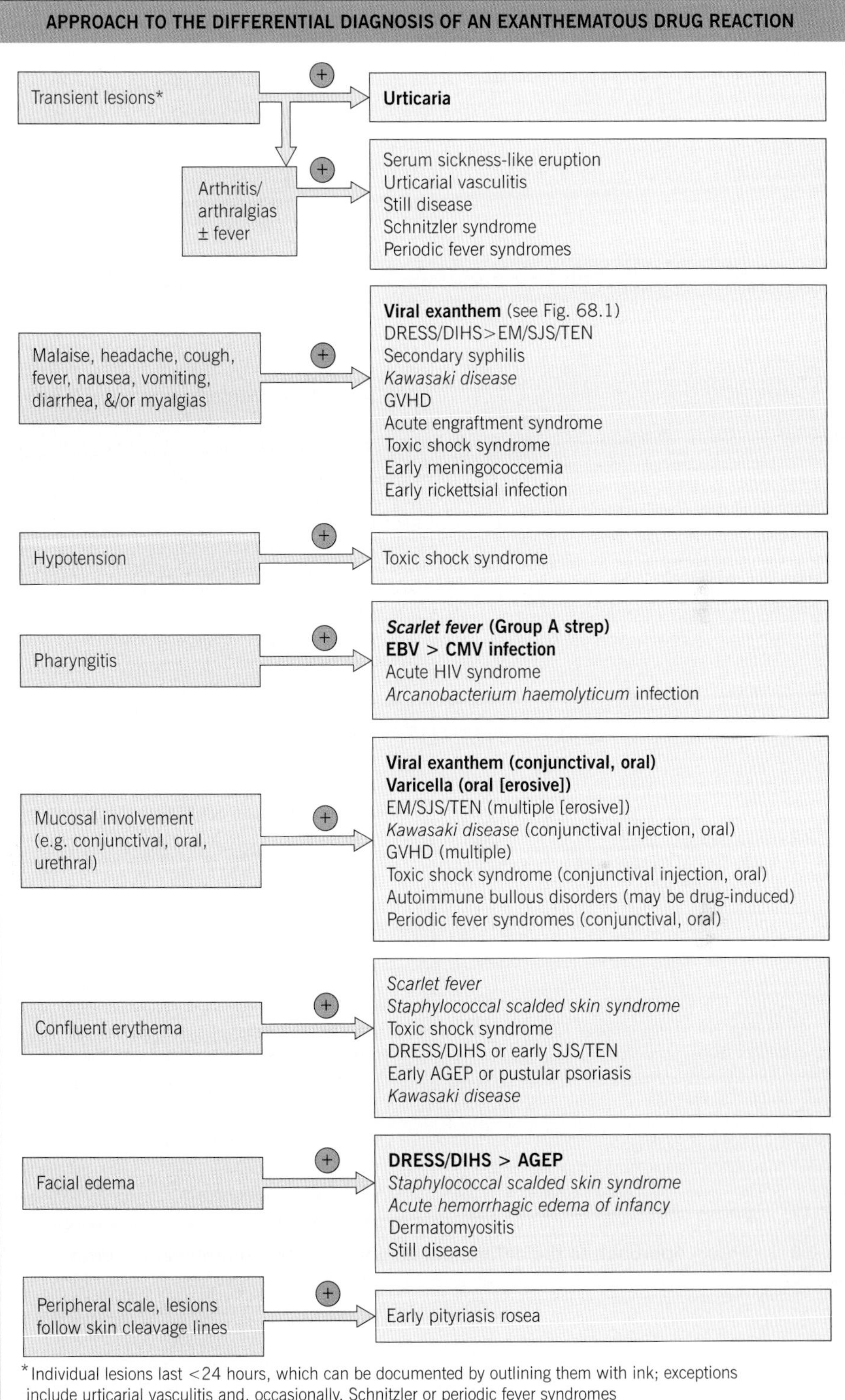

Fig. 3.8 Approach to the differential diagnosis of an exanthematous drug reaction. With a few exceptions (e.g., pityriasis rosea, autoimmune bullous disorders), patients with these entities may be febrile. *Entities in italics occur primarily in children*. Toxic shock syndrome can be staphylococcal or streptococcal (see Ch. 61). Acute generalized exanthematous pustulosis (AGEP) is also referred to as a pustular drug eruption. Autoimmune bullous disorders that may be drug-induced include bullous pemphigoid or linear IgA bullous dermatosis > pemphigus. *Continued*

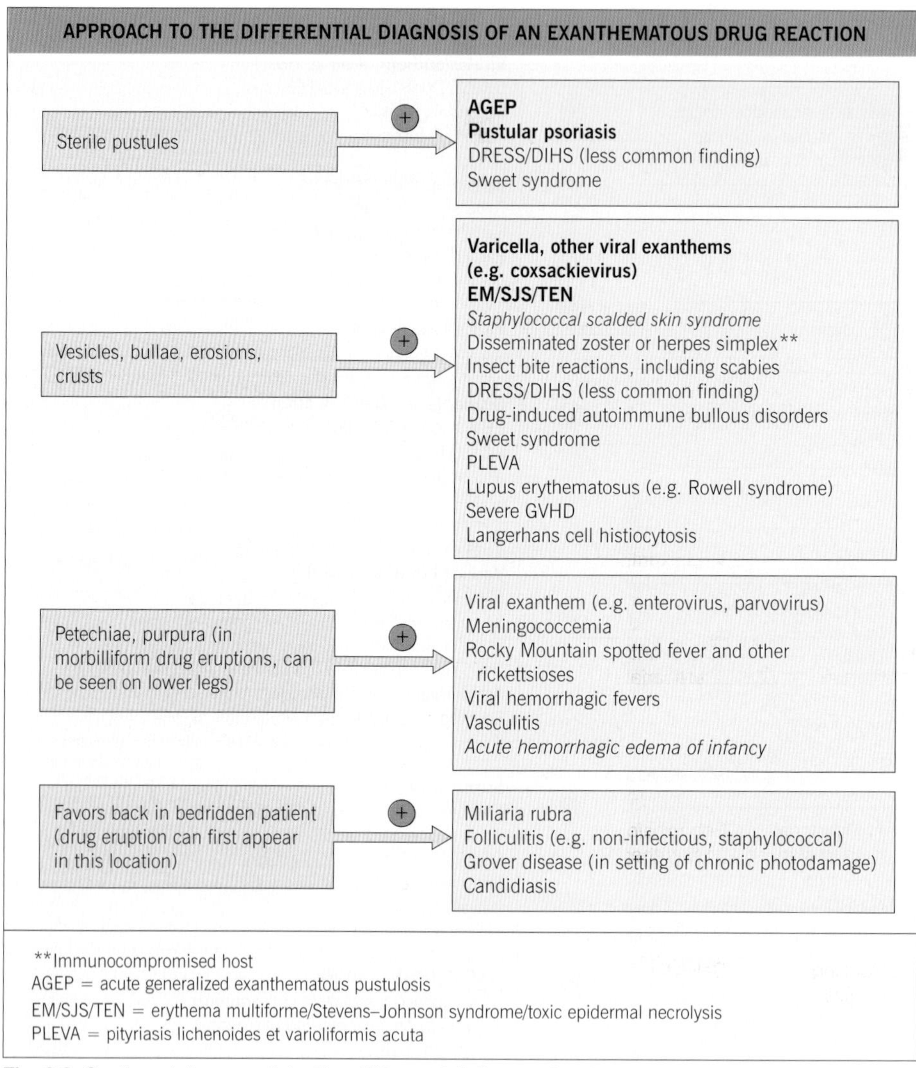

Fig. 3.8 *Continued* **Approach to the differential diagnosis of an exanthematous drug reaction.**

POTENTIALLY LIFE-THREATENING CONDITIONS WITH INITIAL SKIN FINDINGS THAT CAN MIMIC A MORE COMMON BENIGN DISORDER		
Potentially life-threatening condition	**Benign disorder that is mimicked early in the course**	**Clues to the diagnosis as the condition evolves**
DRESS/DIHS*	Morbilliform/urticarial drug eruption > viral exanthem	• Facial swelling • High fever • Prominent lymphadenopathy • Marked peripheral blood eosinophilia, atypical lymphocytes • Elevated transaminases, other signs of internal organ involvement
Stevens–Johnson syndrome/ toxic epidermal necrolysis	Morbilliform/urticarial drug eruption > viral exanthem	• Early involvement of palms & soles • Duskiness or blistering (often initially in the center of lesions) • Painful/tender skin • Mucosal erosions (oral, nasal, ocular, genital)
Rocky Mountain spotted fever (RMSF), other rickettsial spotted fevers	Viral exanthem (or severe viral syndromes)	• Potential exposure to ticks (e.g. season [spring–late summer for RMSF], geographic location) • High fever, myalgias, headache (often for 2–5 days prior to rash) • Rash begins on wrists/ankles → spreads centripetally (± palms/soles) • Petechiae within erythematous macules/ papules
Meningo-coccemia	Viral exanthem	• Petechiae → retiform purpura • Fever with chills, myalgias • Headache, stiff neck
Kawasaki disease	Viral exanthem, morbilliform/ urticarial drug eruption, erythema multiforme, "diaper dermatitis" (for early perineal eruption)	• Early perineal erythema → desquamation • Conjunctival injection • "Chapped" lips, "strawberry" tongue • Acral erythema and edema • Continued high-spiking fever • Prominent unilateral lymphadenopathy
Staphylococcal scalded skin syndrome (SSSS)	Seborrheic dermatitis, viral exanthem	• Painful/tender skin • Periorificial (around mouth & eyes) edema and (later) radial scale-crusts • Confluent erythema → superficial erosions/peeling, esp. in intertriginous sites
Necrotizing fasciitis	Cellulitis	• Tense, "woody" induration • Extreme pain *or* (later) anesthesia • Rapid evolution • Erythema → dusky gray color • Watery, malodorous discharge

**In general, begins ≥2 weeks after drug is initiated and has a relatively limited set of culprit medications (see Ch. 17).*

Table 3.1 Potentially life-threatening conditions with initial skin findings that can mimic a more common benign disorder. The cutaneous manifestations are most likely to resemble those of milder disorder during the first 24 hours. Diffuse erythema, often beginning on the trunk, or a scarlatiniform exanthem can also be early manifestations of toxic shock syndrome.

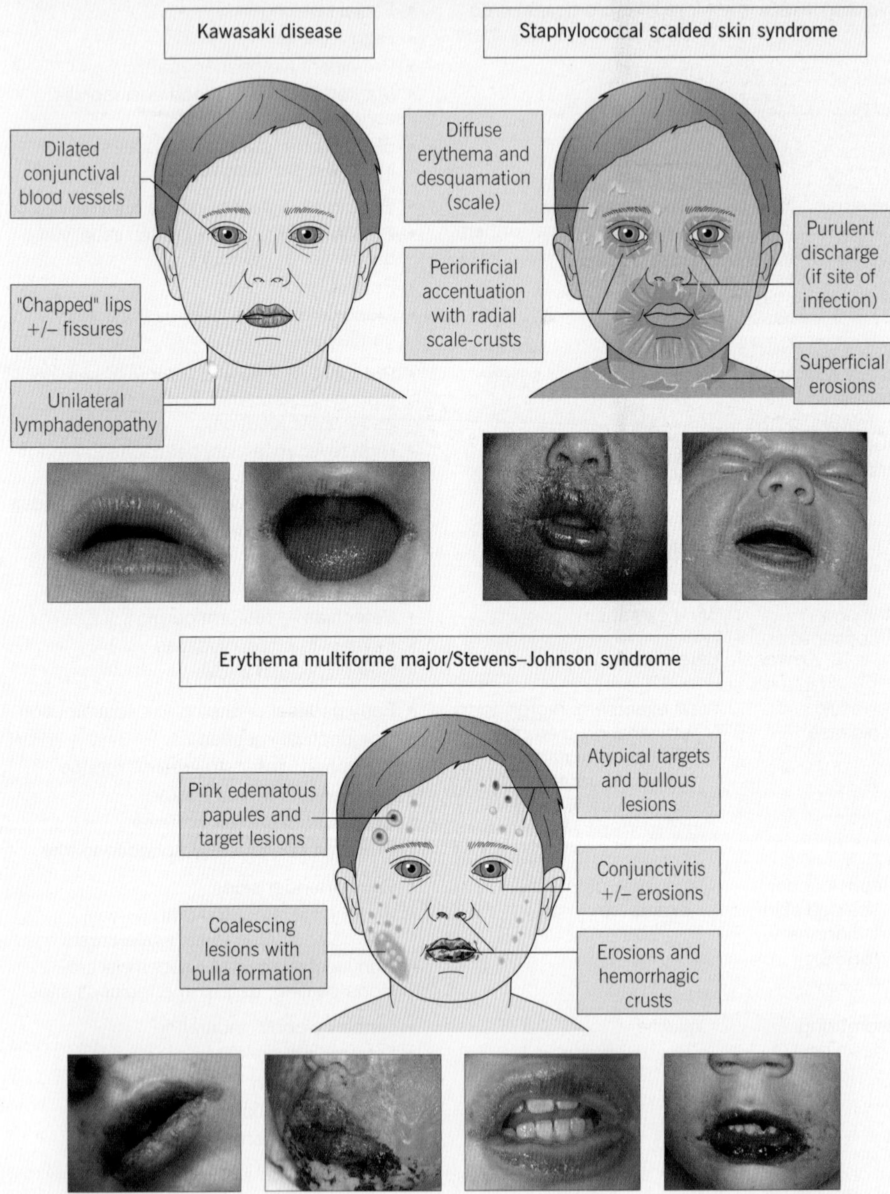

Fig. 3.9 Facial findings in Kawasaki disease, staphylococcal scalded skin syndrome, and erythema multiforme major/Stevens–Johnson syndrome. Hemorrhagic crusting and erosions of the vermilion portion of the lips can also be seen in primary gingivostomatitis due to herpes simplex virus, pemphigus vulgaris, and paraneoplastic pemphigus.

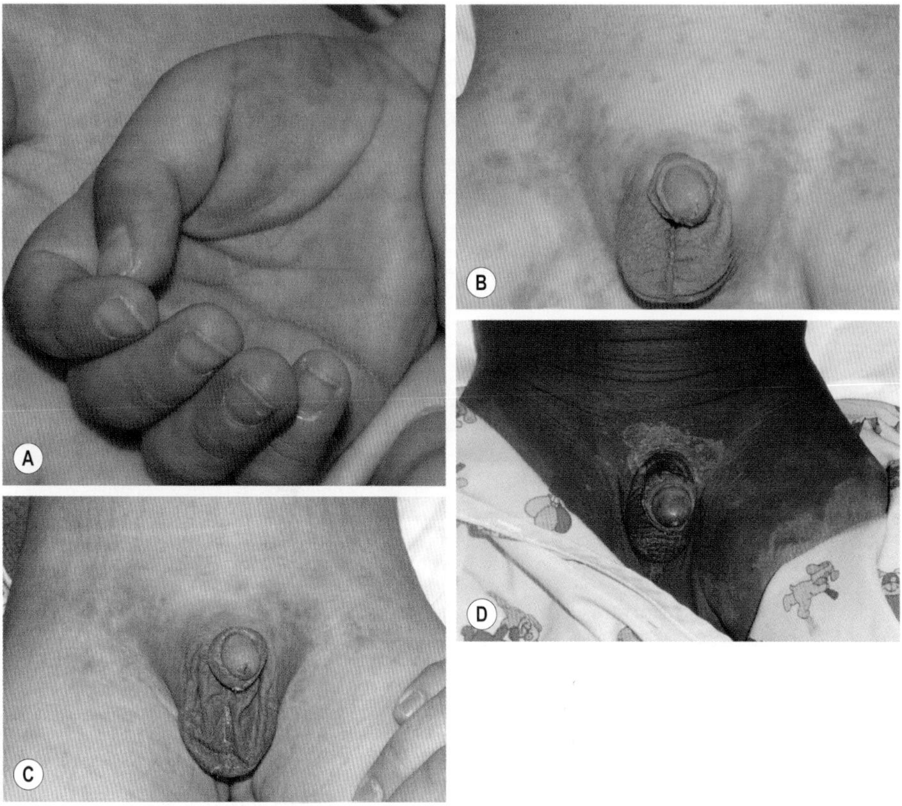

Fig. 3.10 Kawasaki disease. A Erythema and edema of the palm early in the disease course. **B, C** Erythema multiforme-like lesions becoming confluent in the perineal region on the second day of fever **(B)**, followed by desquamation 2 days later **(C)**. **D** Erythema (less evident due to the patient's darkly pigmented skin) and desquamation in the genital area. Involvement of the skin in this location is a characteristic early finding in Kawasaki disease. *A–C, Courtesy, Julie V. Schaffer, MD. D, Courtesy, Anthony Mancini, MD.*

- Other cardiac (e.g. myo-/pericarditis, valvular abnormalities), CNS (e.g. irritability, aseptic meningitis), musculoskeletal (e.g. arthritis), gastrointestinal, and genitourinary involvement can occur.
- Laboratory findings of acute disease include leukocytosis with neutrophilia, anemia, elevated ESR/CRP and hepatic transaminase levels, hypoalbuminemia and sterile pyuria; thrombocytosis typically develops by the 2nd or 3rd week (occasionally thrombocytopenia early).
- **DDx:** viral exanthem, multisystem inflammatory syndrome in children associated with COVID-19, scarlet fever, toxic shock syndrome, early staphylococcal scalded skin syndrome, drug reaction, erythema multiforme, Still disease, periodic fever syndrome.
- **Rx:** IVIg and aspirin are first-line; corticosteroids and infliximab are options for refractory disease.

Periodic Fever Syndromes

- Group of hereditary autoinflammatory disorders that feature recurrent episodes of fever and rash (Table 3.2).
- Cutaneous findings, which range from erysipeloid erythema to urticarial eruptions, represent clues to the underlying diagnosis.
- Acute inflammation in other organ systems can lead to manifestations such as arthritis, serositis, and conjunctivitis; over time, secondary systemic amyloidosis may develop.

For further information see Chs 20, 21, 45 and 81 from *Dermatology, Fourth edition*.

For additional online figures visit www.expertconsult.com 

HEREDITARY PERIODIC FEVER SYNDROMES THAT PRESENT WITH A RASH				
	Familial Mediterranean fever (FMF)	**Hyper-IgD with periodic fever syndrome (HIDS)**	**TNF receptor-associated periodic syndrome* (TRAPS)**	**Cryopyrin-associated periodic syndromes** (CAPS)**
Ethnic predilection	Armenians, Turks, Jews (especially Sephardic), Arabs, Italians	Dutch, northern Europeans	Variable	Variable
Inheritance	AR	AR	AD	AD
Gene	*MEFV*	*MVK*	*TNFRSF1A*	*NLRP3* > *NLRP12*
Protein	Pyrin	Mevalonate kinase	TNF receptor-1	Cryopyrin > monarch-1
Episode length	1–4 days	3–7 days	Often >7 days	<1–3 days
Mucocutaneous and ocular findings	Erysipeloid erythema and edema favoring leg/foot; ± palpable purpura (due to vasculitis)	Erythematous macules/papules; may become purpuric; ± oral or genital ulcers	Annular/serpiginous erythematous patches/plaques; distal migration on extremity; later ecchymotic; periorbital edema, conjunctivitis; ± oral ulcers	Urticarial papules and plaques; may be cold-induced; conjunctivitis > uveitis; ± oral ulcers
Musculoskeletal findings	Monoarthritis, myalgia	Arthralgia, oligoarthritis	Migratory myalgia > arthralgia > monoarthritis	Myalgia (limbs), arthralgia; arthritis and arthropathy in NOMID
Other clinical manifestations	Serositis (e.g., peritonitis mimicking acute abdomen, pleuritis), scrotal swelling, splenomegaly; amyloidosis	Abdominal pain, diarrhea, vomiting, cervical LAN, HSM	Serositis, scrotal pain, splenomegaly > LAN; amyloidosis	Hearing loss in MWS and NOMID; LAN, HSM, chronic aseptic meningitis & dysmorphic facies in NOMID; amyloidosis
Treatment	Colchicine prophylaxis; IL-1/IL-1R antag, TNF inhibitors, tocilizumab	CS for acute attacks; IL-1/IL-1R antag, TNF inhibitors, tocilizumab	CS for acute attacks; IL-1/IL-1R antag, etanercept, tocilizumab	CS for acute attacks; IL-1/IL-1R antag (rilonacept, canakinumab, anakinra)

**Includes familial Hibernian fever.*

***Cryopyrin-associated periodic syndromes (CAPS) include familial cold autoinflammatory syndrome, Muckle–Wells syndrome (MWS), and neonatal-onset multisystem inflammatory disease (NOMID; also known as chronic infantile neurologic, cutaneous and articular syndrome [CINCA]).*

Table 3.2 Hereditary periodic fever syndromes that present with a rash. In all of these disorders, episodic "attacks" are characterized by fever and may be associated with headache. Table 37.3 outlines the cutaneous findings in other inherited autoinflammatory diseases. AD, autosomal dominant; AR, autosomal recessive; HSM, hepatosplenomegaly; IL-1/IL-1R antag, IL-1/IL-1 receptor antagnoists; LAN, lymphadenopathy.

Pruritus and Dysesthesia 4

Definitions

• **Pruritus:** an unpleasant sensation of the skin that elicits a desire to scratch.
• **Dysesthesia:** an unpleasant, abnormal sensation that can be either spontaneous or evoked; abnormal, unpleasant sensations may include pain, pruritus ("neuropathic itch"), tingling, burning, "pins and needles".

Pruritus

• The most common skin-related symptom in dermatology; can have a profound negative impact on a patient's quality of life.
• Results from the activation of the sensory nervous system, involving four sequential levels: the peripheral nervous system → the dorsal root ganglia → the spinal cord → and the brain.
• There are multiple etiologies of pruritus, and it is often a major clinical challenge to diagnose the underlying etiology and to adequately treat.

Etiologies

• May arise ***secondary*** to a number of conditions:
  – Dermatologic disorders (Table 4.1, Fig. 4.1)
  – Allergic or hypersensitivity syndromes
  – Systemic diseases (10–25%) and malignancies (Figs 4.2 and 4.3)
  – Toxins associated with kidney or liver dysfunction
  – Medications (Table 4.2)
  – Neurologic disorders (see text below)
  – Psychiatric conditions (see Ch. 5)
• May also be ***primary*** or ***idiopathic*** – that is, no readily apparent skin disease, underlying etiology, or associated condition.
• Most patients with pruritus due to an underlying dermatologic disorder present with characteristic or diagnostic skin lesions (e.g. dermatitis of the flexures in atopic dermatitis; see Table 4.1).
• In ***primary*** pruritus and ***secondary*** pruritus NOT due to an underlying dermatologic disorder, the lesions are usually nonspecific (e.g. linear excoriations [see Fig. 4.1], prurigo simplex, prurigo nodularis [Figs 4.5 and 4.6]).

Diagnostic Pearls

• Patients with chronic, idiopathic pruritus need serial examinations because pruritus can antedate clinical manifestations of the underlying disorder (e.g. lymphoma) or with time, more specific lesions may appear (e.g. bullous pemphigoid).
• Sparing of the mid upper back, an area of patient-hand inaccessibility ('butterfly sign') (see Fig. 4.6), is suggestive of pruritus NOT associated with a dermatologic disorder; note, however, this sign is not seen in those who use back scratchers or similar devices.
• Aquagenic pruritus, provoked by cooling of the skin after emergence from a bath, is often idiopathic but may be a sign of polycythemia vera.
• Of note, some patients may have a combination of specific and nonspecific skin lesions and both may be due to an underlying systemic disorder (e.g. eosinophilic folliculitis associated with HIV infection/AIDS).

Approach to the Patient with Pruritus

• Identifying the underlying etiology of a patient's pruritus is important in determining the appropriate management.
• A simplified approach to the patient with pruritus is presented in Fig. 4.2 and Table 4.3.

Management of Pruritus

• General treatment measures for pruritus are outlined in Table 4.4.

COMMON DERMATOLOGIC DISEASES WITH PRURITUS AS A MAJOR SYMPTOM
Infestations/bites and stings
• Scabies, pediculosis, arthropod bites
Inflammation
• Dermatitis: atopic, stasis, allergic > irritant, seborrheic (especially of the scalp) • Psoriasis, parapsoriasis • Lichen planus • Urticaria, dermographism (Fig. 4.4), papular urticaria, urticarial dermatitis • Drug eruptions (e.g. morbilliform) • Bullous diseases (e.g. BP, DH) • Mastocytosis • Eosinophilic folliculitis • Pruritic papular eruption of HIV • LS (especially of the vulva), dermatomyositis, LE (systemic and cutaneous) • GVHD
Infection
• Bacterial (e.g. folliculitis) • Viral (e.g. varicella) • Fungal (e.g. inflammatory tinea) • Parasitic (e.g. schistosomal cercarial dermatitis)
Neoplastic
• Cutaneous T-cell lymphoma (e.g. mycosis fungoides, Sézary syndrome)
Other
• Xerosis/eczema craquelé • Scar-associated pruritus, post-burn pruritus • Fiberglass dermatitis • Lichen simplex chronicus, prurigo nodularis • Primary cutaneous amyloidosis (macular, lichenoid) • Pregnancy dermatoses • Neuropathic itch (e.g. notalgia paresthetica) • PMLE, actinic prurigo, chronic actinic dermatitis • Darier and Hailey–Hailey disease • Porphyrias • Ichthyoses

Table 4.1 Common dermatologic diseases with pruritus as a major symptom. BP, bullous pemphigoid; DH, dermatitis herpetiformis; LS, lichen sclerosus; PMLE polymorphous light eruption.

Classic Clinical Findings from Chronic Pruritus

LICHEN SIMPLEX CHRONICUS (LSC)

• Skin-colored to pink or hyperpigmented plaques with exaggerated skin lines and a leathery appearance due to repeated, often habitual, scratching or rubbing (Fig. 4.7).

• Favors the posterior neck and occipital scalp (see Fig. 4.7B), anogenital region (see Table 1.3), and ankles (see Fig. 4.7A) as well as the extensor surface of the forearms and shins.

• LSC may be superimposed upon a specific cutaneous disorder, most commonly atopic dermatitis.

• In addition to symptomatic relief (e.g. topical anesthetics such as pramoxine), disruption of the itch–scratch cycle requires discussion of possible psychosocial issues (e.g. stress, depression, anxiety).

• **Rx:** potent topical CS, often under occlusion (e.g. hydrocolloid dressings), can be helpful.

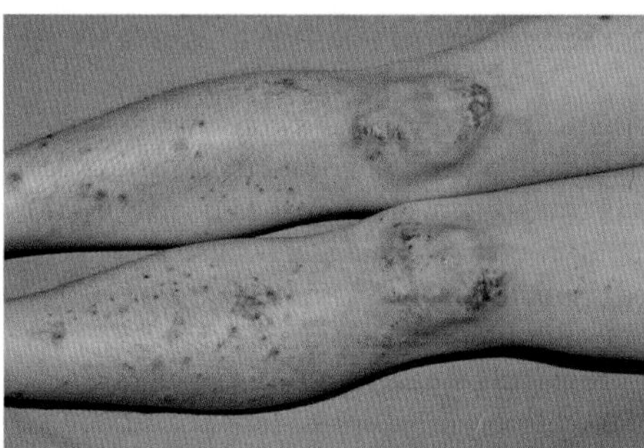

Fig. 4.1 Nonspecific lesions in atopic dermatitis. Prurigo simplex, prurigo nodularis-like lesions and angulated ulcerations; the latter two are primarily on the knees. Although this patient had atopic dermatitis, similar lesions can be seen in patients with "primary" or "idiopathic" pruritus. *Courtesy, Antonio Torrelo, MD.*

- **Other Rx:** intralesional CS or use of an office-applied dressing (e.g. Unna boot) may be required.

PRURIGO NODULARIS

- Multiple, discrete, firm papulonodules with central scale-crust due to chronic and repetitive scratching and picking.
- Degree of pruritus can vary from moderate to intense.
- Lesions usually favor the extensor surfaces of the extremities (see Fig. 4.5), upper back, and buttocks, but they can be widespread in easily reachable areas (see Fig. 4.6).
- Disruption of the itch–scratch cycle requires symptomatic relief and discussion of psychosocial issues as in LSC (see above).
- **Rx:** depending on the number of lesions, varies from superpotent topical or intralesional CS to phototherapy (UVB [broadband or narrowband] or PUVA) and thalidomide.
- Novel agents, especially monoclonal antibodies (e.g. nemolizumab, dupilumab), may be beneficial for recalcitrant disease.
- If no underlying reversible disorder is detected (see Table 4.3), prurigo nodularis can be difficult to treat.

Neurologic Etiologies of Pruritus and Dysesthesia

- The same neurological diseases that can cause neuropathic pain and dysesthesia can also cause neuropathic itch, with some differences (e.g. opioid pain relievers that help treat neuropathic pain may cause or worsen neuropathic itch).
- Neuropathic itch syndromes are typically due to either peripheral (PNS) or central nervous system (CNS) disorders and can be further categorized into focal or regional presentations.
- CNS-related neuropathic itch syndromes involve abnormalities of the brain.
- PNS-related neuropathic itch syndromes involve abnormalities of the spinal cord, cranial or spinal nerve roots, or peripheral nerves.
- Neuropathic itch is more likely to develop in the head and neck region than on the lower body (e.g. facial zoster is more likely to cause post-herpetic itch [PHI] than zoster on the torso).
- Neuropathic itch differs in quality from other forms of pruritus and often makes afflicted individuals want to "dig at" or "gouge out" their skin; it is not responsive to antihistamines, but patients may find relief with application of ice packs.
- Patients with neuropathic itch often present first to a dermatologist.

TRIGEMINAL TROPHIC SYNDROME (TTS)

- A type of intractable facial neuropathic itch characterized by "painless scratching" to the point of self-harm and cutaneous ulceration.
- Classically involves the nasal ala and typically results from impingement or damage to the sensory portion of the trigeminal nerve (Figs 4.8 and 4.9).
- Common inciting factors include iatrogenesis (ablation of the Gasserian ganglion to treat intractable trigeminal neuralgia), infection (varicella zoster virus [VZV], herpes simplex virus), stroke (infarction of the posterior cerebellar artery), CNS tumors or their resultant treatment.
- Clinically may present as a small crust that develops into a crescentic ulcer that may gradually extend to involve the cheek and upper lip.
- The nasal tip is usually spared because its nerve supply is derived from the external branch of the anterior ethmoidal nerve.
- Treatment is difficult and should involve protective barriers, patient education, and surgical consultation; gabapentin, amitriptyline, and carbamazepine have been anecdotally reported as helpful.

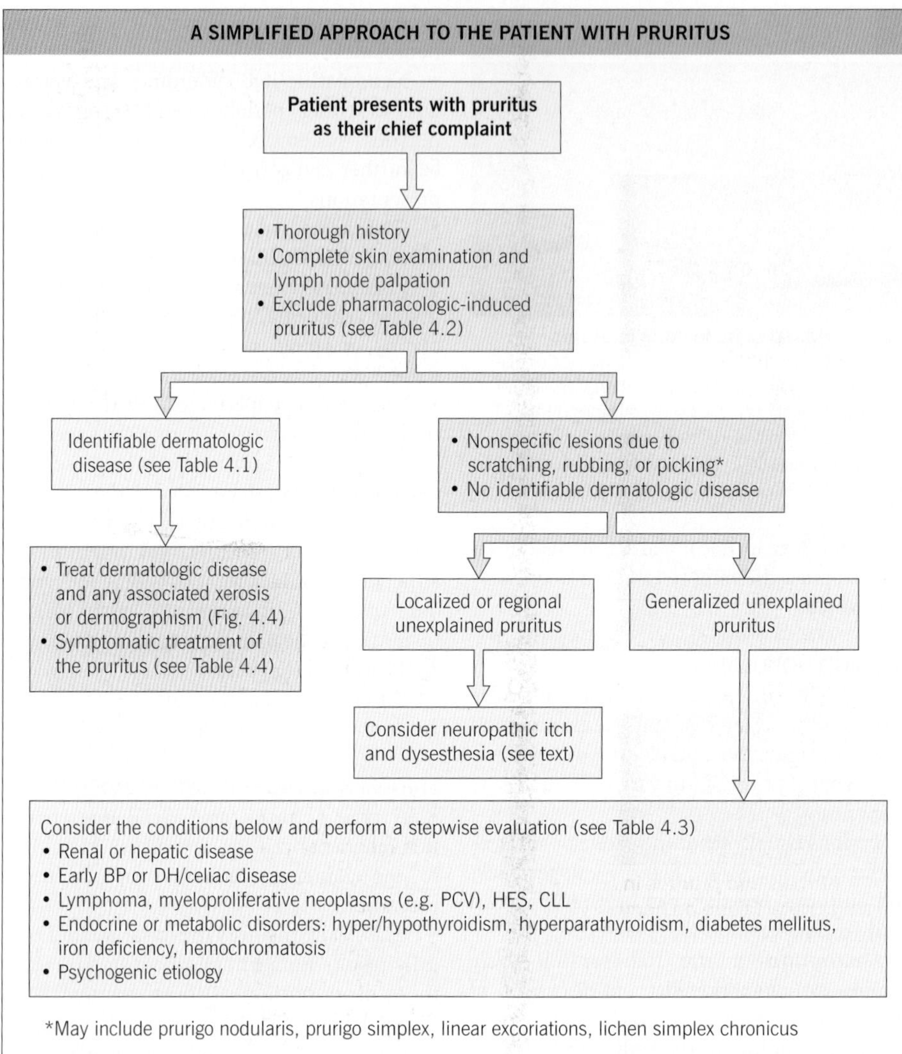

Fig. 4.2 A simplified approach to the patient with pruritus. BP, bullous pemphigoid; CLL, chronic lymphocytic leukemia; DH, dermatitis herpetiformis; HES, hypereosinophilic syndromes; PCV, polycythemia vera.

SENSORY (MONO)NEUROPATHIES WITH PRURITUS AND DYSESTHESIA (RADICULOPATHIES)

- Characterized by a pattern of focal or regional neurological dysfunction that is caused by "injury" to a single sensory nerve root (SNR) or less often to a few adjacent nerve roots, resulting in pruritus or dysesthesia.
- "Injuries" that can cause damage to these SNRs may include (1) impingement from spinal osteoarthritis; (2) distal impingement or irritation by inflamed muscles or connective tissues; (3) infections (e.g. VZV, Lyme disease, leprosy); and (4) other rare causes, such as tumors (schwannomas, metastases), vascular malformations, and cysts.
- The abnormal sensation (e.g. pruritus or other dysesthesia) is perceived in the skin area that is innervated by the damaged SNR(s), and these areas are known as dermatomes (see Fig. 67.10).
- Clinical presentations are usually unilateral and on the side of the damaged SNR, but occasionally may be bilateral.
- The evaluation of an unexplained radiculopathy should include a neurologic examination.

• If the symptoms are severe, sudden in onset, or worsen significantly, then radiologic imaging (MRI is most sensitive) of the appropriate area of the spine can be performed.

• If radiologic imaging is negative, electromyogram and nerve conduction studies can be considered.

• In general, symptomatic treatment may include (1) topical agents (e.g. anesthetics, capsaicin); (2) various oral neuromodulators (e.g. gabapentin, pregabalin, other anticonvulsants); (3) physical therapy and acupuncture (if underlying muscle or connective tissue inflammation); and (4) botulinum toxin injections to weaken impinging muscles, if deemed safe.

• Several classic radiculopathies encountered in dermatology are (1) "shingles" or post-herpetic neuralgia (PHN) or post-herpetic itch (PHI); (2) notalgia paresthetica; (3) brachioradial pruritus, and (4) meralgia paresthetica (see Fig. 4.8).

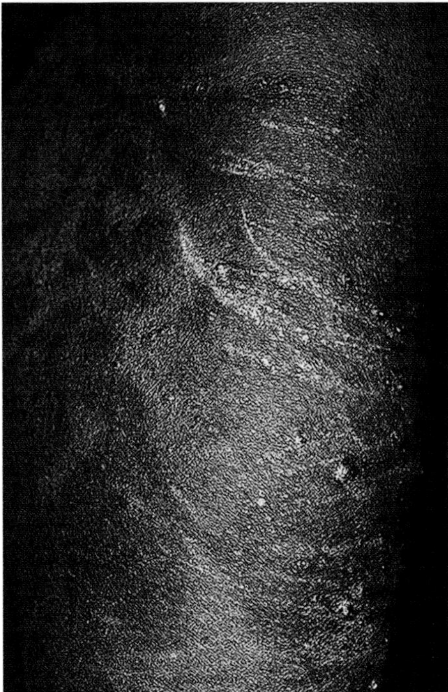

Fig. 4.3 Xerosis and pruritus in a patient with end-stage renal failure on hemodialysis. There are a few papules of acquired perforating dermatosis admixed with the scratch marks. *Courtesy, Jean L. Bolognia, MD.*

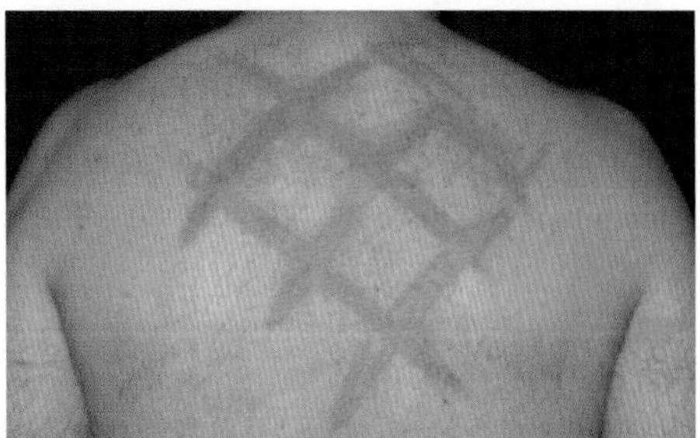

Fig. 4.4 Dermographism. Linear streaks of urticaria induced by scratching the skin. Assessment for dermographism should be performed in all patients with pruritus. *Courtesy, Franz J. Legat, MD.*

COMMON PHARMACOLOGIC ETIOLOGIES OF PRURITUS WITHOUT A RASH
Most common
• *Opioids:* tramadol, codeine, morphine*,**, butorphanol*, fentanyl*
• *Illicit drugs:* methamphetamine, cocaine
Less common
• *Antihypertensives:* calcium channel blockers
• *Antimalarials:* chloroquine (most common in individuals of African heritage)
• *Psychotropic drugs:* selective serotonin reuptake inhibitors
• *Anti-neoplastic agents*: CTLA-4 inhibitors, PD-1 inhibitors, EGFR inhibitors, selective BRAF or MEK inhibitors, tyrosine kinase inhibitors (e.g. sorafenib [especially scalp pruritus])
• *Other:* statins, hydroxyethyl starch, omeprazole, paclitaxel, tamoxifen, granulocyte–macrophage colony-stimulating factor, interferon

**Pruritus is more likely with intrathecal/epidural than systemic administration.*
***Also causes nonimmunologic release of histamine from mast cells.*

Table 4.2 Common pharmacologic etiologies of pruritus without a rash. Itch may also occur as a direct effect of interleukin 2 therapy. Additional drugs may cause pruritus secondary to cholestatic injury (e.g. sulfonamides, penicillins, erythromycin estolate). CTLA-4, cytotoxic T lymphocyte-associated antigen 4; PD-1, programmed cell death protein 1.

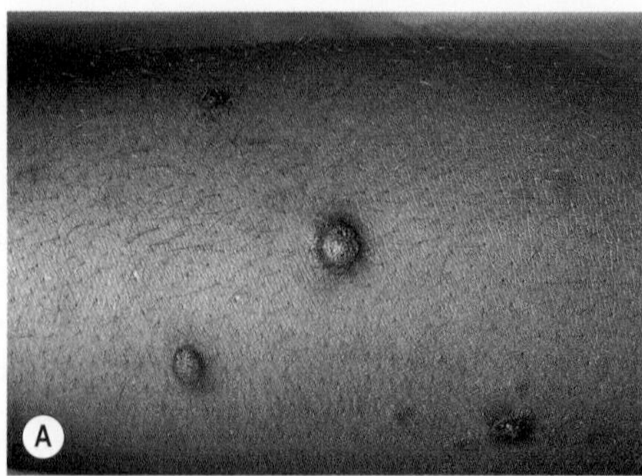

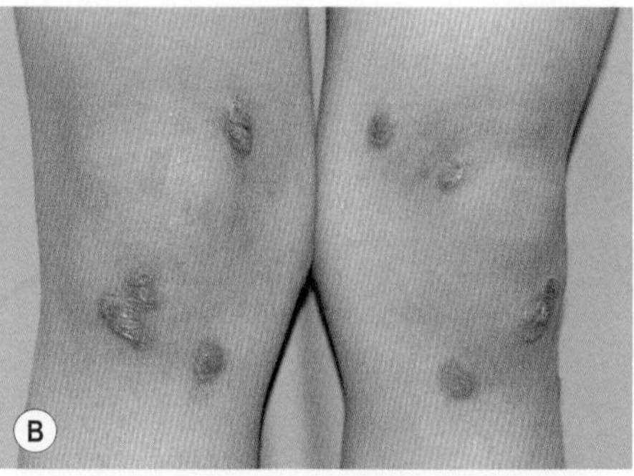

Fig. 4.5 Prurigo nodularis. A Firm hyperpigmented papulonodules on the extensor forearm due to repeated scratching and picking. **B** Papulonodules and plaques in various stages on the knees of a patient with atopic dermatitis. *A, Courtesy, Ronald P. Rapini, MD; B, Courtesy, Antonio Torrelo, MD.*

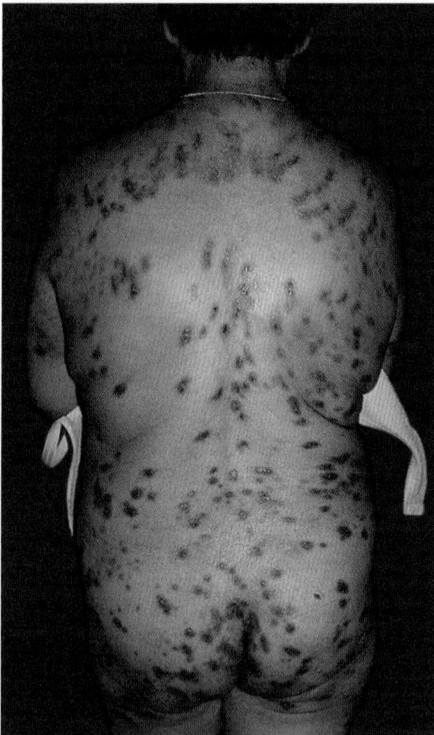

Fig. 4.6 Multiple lesions of prurigo nodularis. Note the sparing of the mid upper back ("butterfly sign"). *Courtesy, USCDRSC.*

NOTALGIA PARESTHETICA

- Affects roughly 10% of the adult population and thought to be related to SNR impingement at the level of the spinal cord due to osteoarthritis or more distally, due to impingement or irritation from inflamed muscles or other connective tissue.
- Presents with focal, intense pruritus of the upper back, most commonly along the medial scapular borders (see Fig. 4.8A and C); sometimes the pruritus is accompanied by other dysesthesias (e.g. pain, burning).
- Often, a hyperpigmented patch that is a result of chronic rubbing is seen in the area of pruritus (Fig. 4.8A and C).
- **DDx:** macular amyloidosis, which is also due to chronic rubbing and is probably a related entity; both disorders can be a cutaneous marker of Sipple syndrome, especially if the onset is during childhood or adolescence.
- **Rx:** topical capsaicin, a natural plant product that depletes substance P from cutaneous nerve endings, 5 times daily for 1 week followed by 3 times daily for 3–6 weeks may be effective.
- **Other Rx:** topical anesthetics, gabapentin, and acupuncture.

BRACHIORADIAL PRURITUS

- Chronic, intermittent pruritus or burning pain of the dorsolateral aspects of the forearms and elbows; sometimes more extensive area of involvement (e.g. shoulder region) (see Fig. 4.8A and B).
- Most patients have photodamaged skin and degenerative cervical spine disease, with UV light exposure and heat serving as triggers.
- The patient can often precisely delineate the affected area with a marking pen, and within this area are excoriations, prurigo simplex lesions, and sometimes even scarring (see Fig. 4.8B).

LABORATORY AND RADIOGRAPHIC EVALUATION OF THE PATIENT WITH GENERALIZED PRURITUS OF UNKNOWN ETIOLOGY
Basic initial evaluation
CBC with differential and platelet count ESR and CRP Creatinine, blood urea nitrogen, electrolytes Liver transaminases, alkaline phosphatase, bilirubin LDH Fasting glucose TSH ± free thyroxine
Possible additional evaluation
Skin biopsy
Routine histology (if skin lesions are present) Direct immunofluorescence studies*
Other laboratory tests
Serum total and/or allergen-specific IgE Serum ferritin, iron, total iron binding capacity Hemoglobin A1c Parathyroid function (calcium, phosphate and parathyroid hormone levels) Stool for ova/parasites and/or occult blood Viral hepatitis panel (including hepatitis B and C viruses) HIV testing Anti-tissue transglutaminase ± epidermal transglutaminase IgA antibodies** Anti-BP180 and anti-BP230 bullous pemphigoid IgG antibodies Anti-mitochondrial and anti-smooth muscle antibodies Serum tryptase, histamine, and/or chromogranin-A levels Urinalysis with sediment evaluation 24-hour urine collection for 5-hydroxyindoleacetic acid (5-HIAA; a serotonin metabolite) and porphyrins Serum protein electrophoresis, serum immunofixation electrophoresis
Radiographic studies
Chest X-ray or CT scan Abdominal and pelvic ultrasonography or CT scan Lymph node ultrasonography
Other investigations
Patch testing Prick testing for major atopy and relevant occupational allergens Age-appropriate cancer screening (in conjunction with primary care physician) If hydroxyethyl starch (HES)-induced pruritus is suspected, electron microscopy of a biopsy sample from normal-appearing skin

**Biopsy perilesional skin or normal-appearing skin (in vicinity of lesions if present) to assess for bullous pemphigoid and dermatitis herpetiformis, respectively.*
***Often performed in conjunction with serum total IgA; in patients with IgA deficiency, anti-tissue transglutaminase IgG antibodies should be assessed.*

Table 4.3 Laboratory and radiographic evaluation of the patient with generalized pruritus of unknown etiology. A general physical examination should also be performed by the patient's primary care physician. Selection of particular tests beyond the basic initial evaluation is based upon the patient's history, physical examination findings, and pruritus severity. The results of initial testing can also help to direct further evaluation.

- The "ice-pack sign" is another diagnostic clue, because application of ice is often reported as the only modality that provides relief.
- **Rx:** sun protection, cold packs, topical medications (pramoxine, capsaicin), oral neuromodulating drugs (gabapentin, amitriptyline).

MERALGIA PARESTHETICA

- Due to impingement of the lateral femoral cutaneous nerve as it passes through the

GENERAL MEASURES FOR THE TREATMENT OF PRURITUS AND DYSESTHESIA
Skin care
• Lukewarm baths or showers with minimal use of soap (use mild soaps or non-soap cleansers) • Moisturization twice a day, especially while skin still damp (ointment > cream) • Avoid woolens, harsh fabrics, fabric softeners • Keep nails cut short • Address any superimposed dermographism
Topicals
• *Cooling agents/counterirritants*: e.g. menthol, camphor, capsaicin (best for localized itch, especially of neuropathic origin) • *Anesthetics*: e.g. pramoxine, lidocaine, prilocaine, polidocanol, palmitoylethanolamine • *Anti-inflammatory agents*: corticosteroids, calcineurin inhibitors
Systemic medications
• *Antihistamines*: especially if there is a component of dermographism or urticaria; otherwise limited efficacy beyond sedative effects; consider doxepin (beginning with 10–25 mg at bedtime) • *Neuromodulators*: gabapentin, pregabalin (best for neuropathic pruritus, post-herpetic neuralgia, post-burn pruritus) • *Antidepressants:* SSRIs (e.g. fluoxetine, paroxetine, sertraline, venlafaxine), tricyclics (e.g. amitriptyline, doxepin), mirtazapine (sedative effects) • *Opioid antagonists/agonists:* e.g. naltrexone, naloxone, nalfurafine*, butorphanol nasal spray • *Other:* thalidomide, monoclonal antibodies (e.g. nemolizumab, dupilumab; especially for prurigo nodularis); aprepitant (reports of benefit in atopic dermatitis, CTCL, and itch induced by EGFR- and tyrosine kinase-inhibitors)
Physical modalities
• *Phototherapy*: UVB (broadband or narrowband), PUVA, UVA, UVA-1 • Acupuncture
Psychological approaches
• Behavior modification therapy, biofeedback • Support groups
Treatment for renal pruritus
• *Topical measures:* capsaicin, pramoxine, γ-linolenic acid, cromolyn sodium • *Systemic measures (first-line):* gabapentin, pregabalin, UVB (broadband or narrowband) • *Systemic measures (second-line):* naltrexone, nalfurafine*
Treatment for hepatic pruritus
• *Systemic measures (first-line):* cholestyramine, ursodeoxycholic acid • *Systemic measures (second-line):* rifampin • *Systemic measures (third-line):* naloxone, naltrexone, nalfurafine*

**Kappa-opioid receptor agonist; available in Japan.*

Table 4.4 General measures for the treatment of pruritus and dysesthesia. CTCL, cutaneous T-cell lymphoma.

inguinal ligament; rarely due to trauma or ischemia.

• Presents with pruritus or dysesthesia of the anterolateral thigh, most often numbness or burning pain (see Fig. 4.8D).

• Predisposing factors include obesity, pregnancy, tight clothing, and, rarely, mass effect from tumor or hemorrhage.

• **Rx:** removal of the cause of compression, focal nerve block at the inguinal ligament, and lastly surgical decompression.

• Neuromodulating medications are not typically helpful.

SMALL FIBER POLYNEUROPATHIES (SFPN)

• Perhaps the most common cause of chronic pruritus in the following areas: bilateral feet; feet and legs; hands and legs; or other widespread bilateral areas of the body.

• Typically presents with pruritus, dysesthesias, paresthesias, and/or neuropathic pain in a "stocking-glove" distribution; muscle function is usually intact.

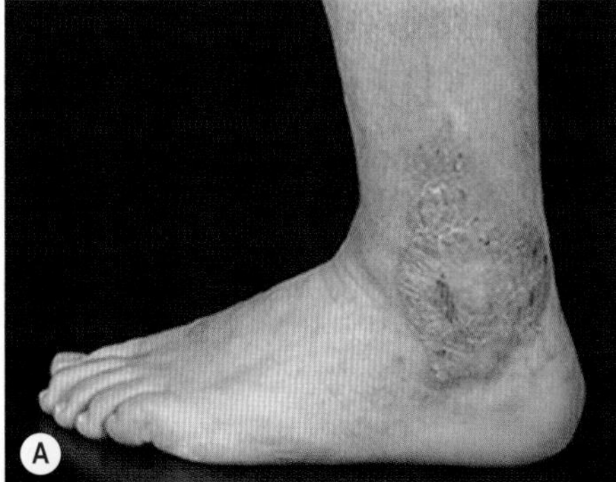

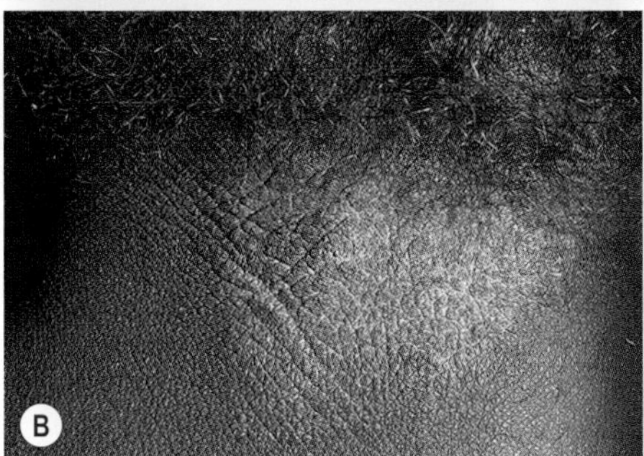

Fig. 4.7 Lichen simplex chronicus. A Lichenified plaque on the ankle of a young man. **B** Note the increased skin markings in this hyperpigmented plaque on the posterior neck.
A, Courtesy, Franz Legat, MD; B, Courtesy, Ronald P. Rapini, MD.

- If the diagnosis of SFPN is suspected based on history and neurologic examination, then potentially treatable causes should be identified, including:
  - Fasting blood glucose, HbA1c (diabetes mellitus)
  - Serum B_{12}, RBC folate, methylmalonic acid, homocysteine, and copper levels (B_{12}, folate, or copper deficiencies)
  - Serum (SPEP) and urine (UPEP) protein electrophoreses, immunofixation and serum-free light-chain analysis (monoclonal gammopathy)
  - CBC with differential and platelets (hematologic malignancies)
- For SFPN, there are two diagnostic tests:
  - Immunohistochemical staining (e.g. anti-PGP9.5) of a (non-traumatized) distal leg skin punch biopsy specimen to evaluate the small nerve fibers (requires a special fixative)
  - Autoimmune function testing (e.g. sweat functioning)

Regional Dysesthesia Syndromes

- Typically caused by an underlying neurological disorder (either peripheral or central), but it is not always identifiable.
- Several locoregional dysesthesia syndromes are encountered in dermatology: burning mouth syndrome (orodynia), burning scalp syndrome (scalp dysesthesia), and several dysesthetic anogenital syndromes.
- **DDx:** includes psychogenic pruritus/dysesthesia (see Ch. 5).

Burning Mouth Syndrome (Orodynia)

- Burning mucosal pain without clinically detectable oral lesions; most commonly affects middle-aged to elderly women.
- Typically bilateral, involving the anterior two-thirds of the tongue, palate, and lower lip.
- Diagnosis requires exclusion of secondary causes such as malignancy (e.g. oral SCC), vitamin deficiencies (e.g. folate, B_{12}), candidiasis, xerostomia (e.g. previous radiation therapy, Sjögren syndrome), contact stomatitis, and ill-fitting dentures.
- Depression and anxiety are more common in patients with burning mouth syndrome.
- **Rx:** oral tricyclic antidepressants and gabapentin in addition to topical anesthetics (e.g. lidocaine, dyclonine) and mouthwashes (various combinations of tetracycline, hydrocortisone, diphenhydramine, nystatin, and Maalox®).

Burning Scalp Syndrome (Scalp Dysesthesia)

- Diffuse scalp burning, pain, pruritus, numbness or tingling without any specific cutaneous lesions.
- Strongly correlated with underlying depression and anxiety.
- Occasionally associated with primary neurologic disorders (e.g. multiple sclerosis).
- Diagnosis requires exclusion and treatment of secondary causes, such as seborrheic dermatitis, folliculitis, lichen planopilaris, allergic or irritant contact dermatitis, dermatomyositis, and discoid lupus erythematosus.
- **Rx:** oral tricyclic antidepressants.

Dysesthetic Anogenital Syndromes

- Various names: pruritus ani, anodynia, pruritus vulvae, vulvodynia, pruritus scroti, scrotodynia, penile pain syndrome.

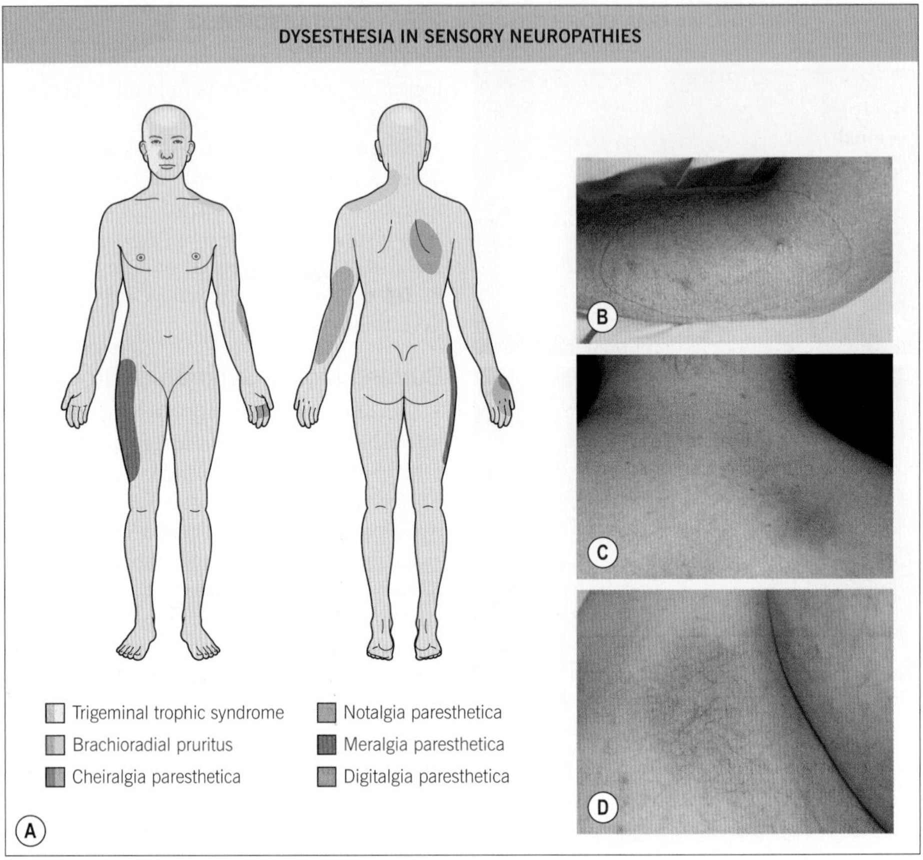

DYSESTHESIA IN SENSORY NEUROPATHIES

- Trigeminal trophic syndrome
- Brachioradial pruritus
- Cheiralgia paresthetica
- Notalgia paresthetica
- Meralgia paresthetica
- Digitalgia paresthetica

A B C D

Fig. 4.8 Dysesthesia in sensory neuropathies. A Distribution of dysesthesia in selected neuropathic conditions. Darker shades indicate more common areas of involvement. **B** Brachioradial pruritus with the affected area outlined by ink. **C** Classic notalgia paresthetica with hyperpigmentation on the right upper back at the medial scapular border. **D** Meralgia paresthetica presenting as hyperpigmentation and lichenification in a discrete area of dysesthesia on the anterior thigh. *A, Courtesy, Karynne O. Duncan, MD; B, Courtesy, Elke Weisshaar, MD and Jeffrey D. Bernhard, MD; C, Courtesy Lorenzo Cerroni, MD; D, Courtesy, YDRSC.*

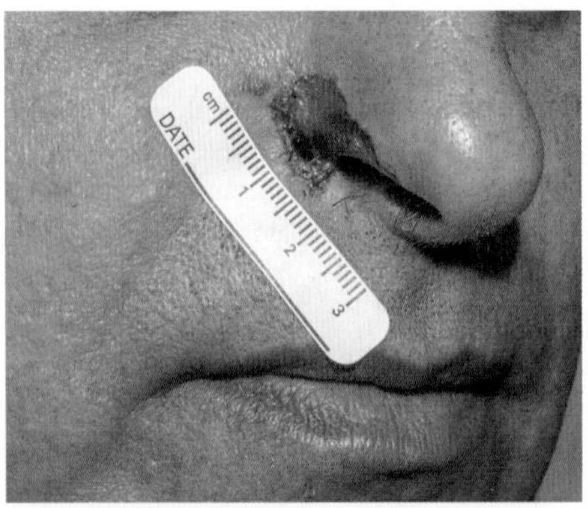

Fig. 4.9 Trigeminal trophic syndrome. Ulceration localized to the nasal ala and adjacent cheek. *Courtesy, Edward Cowen, MD.*

- Severe, intractable pruritus or dysesthesia despite either a normal clinical examination or the presence of nonspecific cutaneous findings.
- When all typical secondary causes of anogenital pruritus and dysesthesia have been investigated and treated (e.g. candidiasis, fecal incontinence; see Ch. 60), and the patient still has symptoms, consider lumbosacral radiculopathy (imaging studies), dermographism (trial of oral antihistamines), and contact dermatitis (patch testing).
- If no etiology detected, consider both psychiatric counseling and treatment with a neuromodulator medication (e.g. tricyclic antidepressant or gabapentin).

Complex Regional Pain Syndrome (CRPS)

- Previously known as reflex sympathetic dystrophy; characterized by continuing regional pain that is out of proportion to the usual course following trauma or other insults.
- The upper extremities, particularly the hands (Fig. 4.10) are most commonly affected but lower extremities may also be involved.
- Due to regional insult to nociceptive terminals that results in a signal cascade which ultimately amplifies the pain response in the CNS.
- Characteristic findings include burning pain, hyperalgesia, allodynia, vasomotor dysfunction (e.g. erythema, edema, livedo reticularis, cyanosis), hypertrichosis, hyperhidrosis, nail dystrophy, motor dysfunction and eventually atrophy.

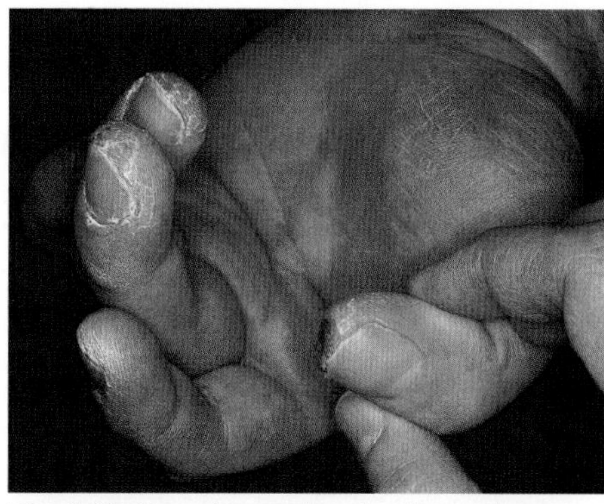

Fig. 4.10 Complex regional pain syndrome with scaling and erosions of the fingertips. *Courtesy, Kalman Watsky, MD.*

- Patients with suspected CRPS should be referred to a neurologist for further evaluation.

For further information see Ch. 6 from *Dermatology, Fourth Edition*.

For additional online figures and tables visit www.expertconsult.com 

5 Psychocutaneous Disorders

Introduction

• Psychodermatology refers to any aspect of dermatology in which psychological factors play a significant role.
• Psychodermatologic disorders can be classified in two ways: (1) by the specific psychodermatologic condition or (2) by the underlying psychopathology (Fig. 5.1).
• Treatment is simplified by basing the choice of psychotropic medication or therapy on the underlying psychopathology (Table 5.1).
• The more commonly encountered primary psychiatric disorders in dermatology include body dysmorphic disorder, excoriation (skin-picking) disorder, acne excoriée, trichotillomania, other body-focused repetitive behavior disorders (BFRBD), delusions of parasitosis, dermatitis artefacta, and nonsuicidal self-injury.
• Because many of these patients with primary psychiatric disorders present to the dermatologist and not the psychiatrist, it is important to establish the correct diagnosis and to offer appropriate treatment options.

The More Common Primary Psychiatric Disorders Seen in Dermatology

Obsessive–Compulsive and Related Disorders: General Features

• *Obsessions* are recurrent and persistent thoughts, images, or urges that are intrusive and unwanted.
• *Compulsions* are repetitive behaviors or mental acts that are performed in order to reduce anxiety or distress, especially that arising from obsessions.
• In all of these disorders, the preoccupations and/or behaviors lead to significant distress or impairment in social, occupational, or other areas of functioning.
• Some of these conditions feature *body-focused repetitive behaviors (BFRB;* e.g. hair-pulling, skin-picking; Table 5.2, Fig. 5.2).
• BFRB become *disorders* (BFRBD) when the following criteria are met: (1) the repetitive behavior causes skin lesions; (2) there are repeated attempts to decrease or stop the behavior; (3) the behavior causes significant distress or impaired functioning; (4) there is no other underlying medical condition or mental disorder to explain the behavior.

BODY DYSMORPHIC DISORDER

• Characterized by a distressing or impairing preoccupation with a nonexistent or slight defect in appearance.
• On a psychiatric spectrum from obsessional to delusional.
• Mean age of onset is 30–35 years; females = males; present in up to 10–15% of dermatologic patients.
• Patients usually concerned with nose, mouth, hair, breasts, or genitalia.
• Often adopt compulsive (e.g. numerous visits to physician for reassurance), ritualistic (e.g. excessive grooming routines), or delusional (e.g. multiple unnecessary surgeries) behaviors.
• Consider and assess for this diagnosis in patients seeking multiple cosmetic procedures.
• **Rx:** selective serotonin reuptake inhibitors (SSRIs) for obsessive–compulsive disorder (OCD) variant or antipsychotics for delusional variant.

EXCORIATION (SKIN-PICKING) DISORDER

• Previously known as *"neurotic excoriations;"* categorized in DSM-5™ as a BFRBD characterized by a conscious, repetitive, and uncontrollable desire to pick, scratch or rub the skin, resulting in skin lesions.

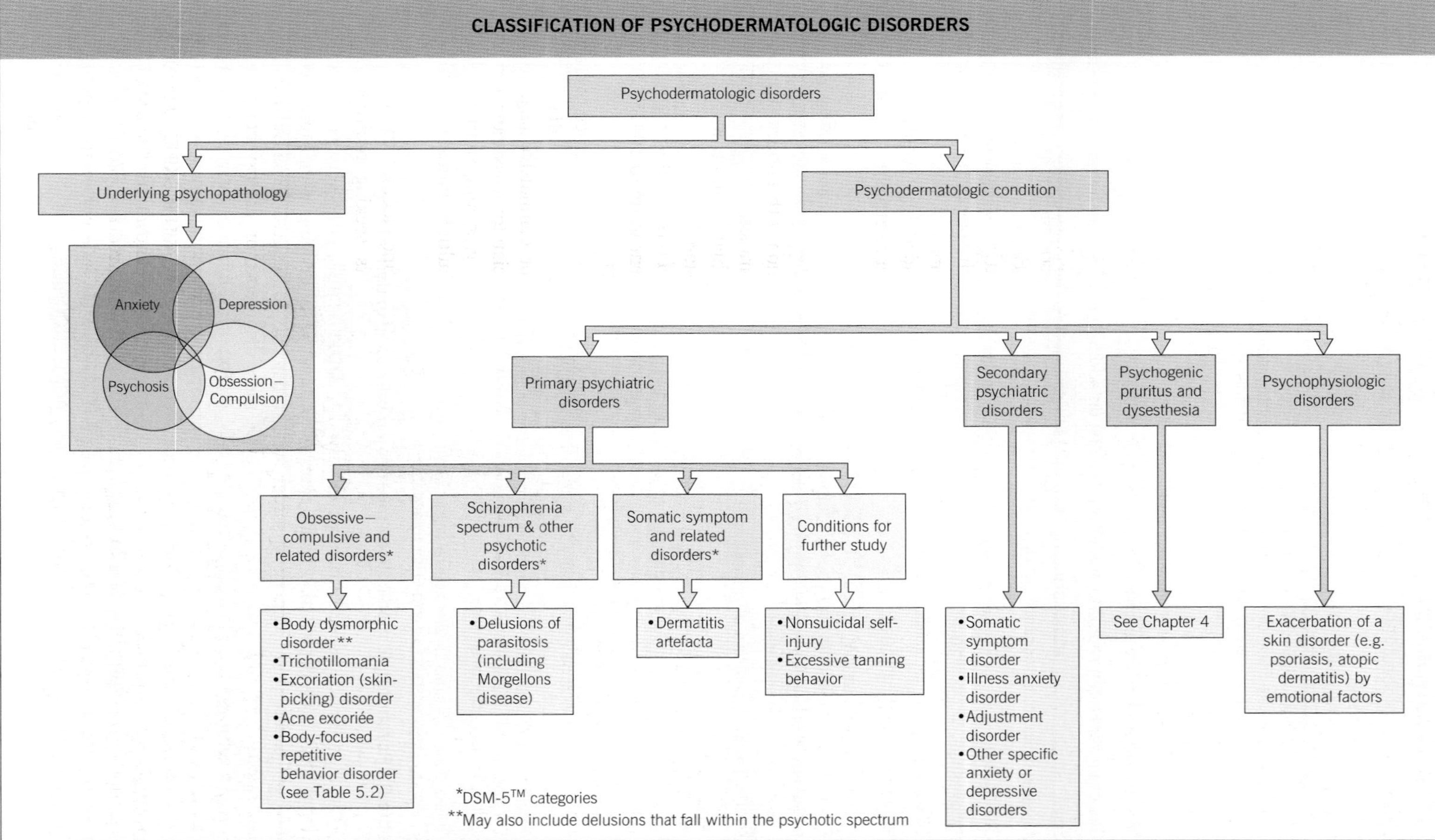

Fig. 5.1 Classification of psychodermatologic disorders.

PSYCHOTROPIC MEDICATIONS MOST COMMONLY USED IN DERMATOLOGY		
Treatment of procedural anxiety in adults (prior to procedure)		
Benzodiazepines Diazepam: 10 mg orally 30 minutes prior Alprazolam: 0.5 mg orally 30–60 minutes prior Lorazepam: 2 mg orally 30–60 minutes prior • An approximate 50% dose reduction necessary for older (age >60) or debilitated adults, patients with low cardiac output or hepatic insufficiency • Repeated dose, 50–100% of initial dose, may be repeated in 30–60 minutes if initial dose has no effect • Patients must have a driver to take them home		
Treatment of obsessive compulsive disorder (OCD)		
Selective serotonin reuptake inhibitors (SSRIs) (in addition to cognitive behavioral therapy)		
SSRI	**Initial dose**	**Maximum dose (via weekly dose escalation**)**
Fluoxetine	10–20 mg/day	60 mg/day*
Citalopram	10–20 mg/day	40 mg/day**
Paroxetine	10–20 mg/day	50 mg/day
Sertraline	25–50 mg/day	200 mg/day
Escitalopram	10 mg/day	20 mg/day**
• Clinical response may take 6–10 weeks to become apparent • Children, adolescents and young adults should be closely monitored for any suicidal ideation • N-acetylcysteine (up to 2400 mg/day) alone, or in combination with SSRIs has shown promise in treating OCD		
Treatment of delusions of parasitosis		
Antipsychotics Pimozide: initiate at 0.5–1 mg/day and gradually (every 2–4 weeks) titrate up to 2–6 mg/day, if needed Risperidone: initiate at 0.5 mg/day and titrate up to 1–4 mg/day, if needed Olanzapine: initiate at 2.5 mg/day and gradually titrate up to 5–15 mg/day, if needed • Response is often seen after ~2 weeks and treatment should be continued for several months, followed by gradual tapering • Side effects include extrapyramidal symptoms, QTc prolongation (significant risk, pimozide; moderate risk, risperidone); tardive dyskinesia (pimozide, if prolonged use); metabolic syndrome (risperidone, olanzapine), weight gain (olanzapine), and hyperprolactinemia (risperidone). Baseline ECG recommended (pimozide) if history of arrythmia or cardiac conduction abnormalities.		

**Make dose adjustments after several weeks of therapy*
***Higher doses associated with QTc prolongation*

Table 5.1 Psychotropic medications most commonly used in dermatology.

• On a psychiatric spectrum most closely related to OCD but may also be an expression of generalized anxiety disorder or depression.

• Most common in middle-age; females > males.

• Favors scalp, face, upper back, extensor forearms, shins, buttocks.

• Lesions usually in all stages of evolution: erosions (prurigo simplex) (Fig. 5.3A), deep circular or linear ulcerations with hypertrophic borders, hypo- or hyperpigmented scars (Fig. 5.3B); admixed well-healed scars point to chronicity.

• **DDx:** (1) underlying causes of pruritus (see Ch. 4); (2) underlying primary cutaneous disorder (e.g. folliculitis); (3) stereotypic movement disorders.

• **Rx:** symptomatic treatment of pruritus (topicals, oral antihistamines); tricyclic antidepressants (TCAs) or SSRIs (if underlying depression); SSRIs (if underlying OCD); consultation with a psychiatrist.

ACNE EXCORIÉE

• Considered a subset of excoriation (skin-picking) disorder, characterized by ritualistic picking of acne lesions (Fig. 5.4).

BODY-FOCUSED REPETITIVE BEHAVIORS (BFRBs) AND ASSOCIATED MUCOCUTANEOUS FINDINGS	
Body-focused repetitive behavior	**Associated mucocutaneous findings**
Lip licking	Irritant contact dermatitis, secondary bacterial or yeast infections
Lip picking or biting	Multiple erosions or ulcerations, recurrent HSV
Cheek chewing or biting	Bite fibroma, morsicatio buccarum
Cuticle pulling, picking, or biting (see Fig. 5.2)	Paronychia, nail surface irregularities
Nail biting (onychophagia) (see Fig. 5.2)	Paronychia, nail dystrophy, subungual hemorrhages
Nail picking or pulling (onychotillomania)	
Habit-tic deformity of the thumbnail	Multiple midline Beau's lines with prominent longitudinal central depression
Thumb or finger sucking	Skin maceration, dermatitis, secondary bacterial or yeast infections
Nose picking (rhinotillexomania)	Erosions, secondary bacterial infections
Trichotillomania	See text
Excoriation (skin-picking) disorder	See text

Table 5.2 Body-focused repetitive behaviors (BFRBs) and associated mucocutaneous findings. BFRBs occur on a chronic basis and present with characteristic mucocutaneous findings, depending on the body site and behavior type. These behaviors exist along a spectrum, with habits at one end and body-focused repetitive behavioral disorders (BFRBD) at the other end. The latter disorders continue despite repeated attempts to stop, and lead to impaired functioning (e.g. social, occupational) or to distress manifesting as feelings of loss of control, embarrassment, or shame.

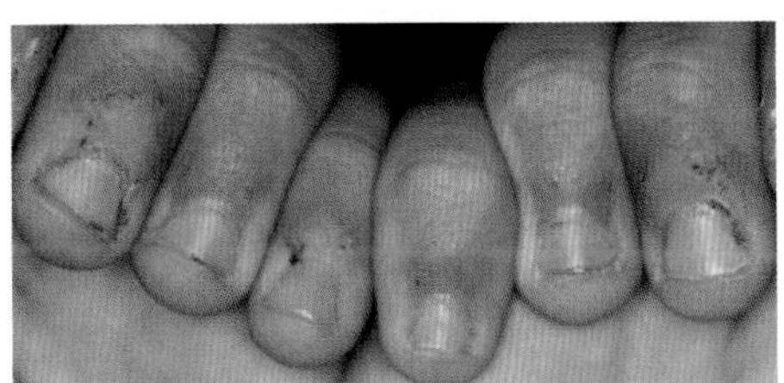

Fig. 5.2 Body-focused repetitive behaviors. Sequelae of nail biting (onychophagia) and cuticle picking. *Courtesy, Karynne O. Duncan, MD.*

- Often associated with OCD; most common in young females.
- **Rx:** aggressively treat underlying acne; TCAs or SSRIs (if underlying depression); SSRIs (if underlying OCD); consultation with a psychiatrist.

TRICHOTILLOMANIA

- Categorized in DSM-5™ as a BFRBD characterized by the recurrent pulling out of one's hair, resulting in hair loss.
- In dermatologic practice, often see cases of hair pulling that are on a spectrum from inattentive habitual hair pulling to obvious OCD psychopathology (BFRBD).
- Most helpful to approach the patient by age of onset, in terms of discussing prognosis and treatment.
  - ***Preschool onset:*** typically benign course; most children outgrow the habit; **Rx** involves bringing awareness to parents and patient
  - ***Pre-adolescent to young adult onset:*** more chronic, relapsing course; on a spectrum from habit/unawareness to underlying psychopathology; **Rx** includes bringing awareness, behavioral modification therapy, psychotropic medications as necessary
  - ***Adult onset:*** more protracted course; often due to underlying psychopathology; **Rx** most often entails referral to psychiatrist/psychologist and treatment of underlying psychiatric disorder
- Peak onset ages 8–12 years; females > males.
- Most commonly scalp hair, but also eyebrows, eyelashes, or pubic hair.

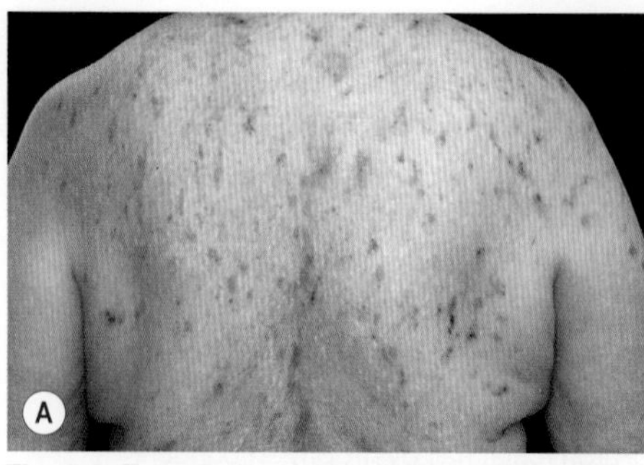
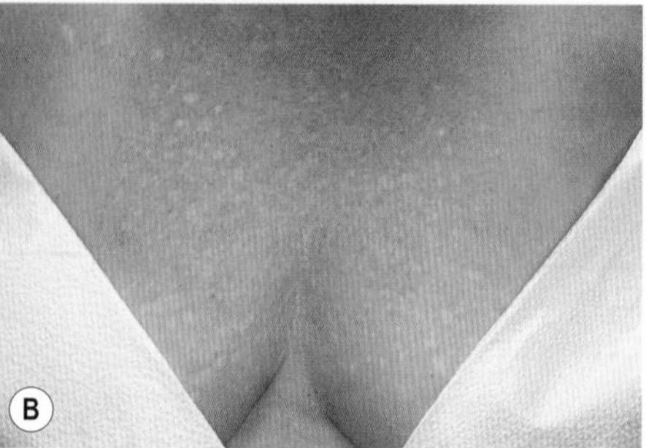

Fig. 5.3 Excoriation (skin-picking) disorder. A Multiple linear excoriations and prurigo simplex lesions on the back of this woman who picked at her skin for several hours each day, often using a kitchen table knife on her back. **B** Numerous hypopigmented scars on the chest of this woman from years of extensive skin picking. *Courtesy, Karynne O. Duncan, MD.*

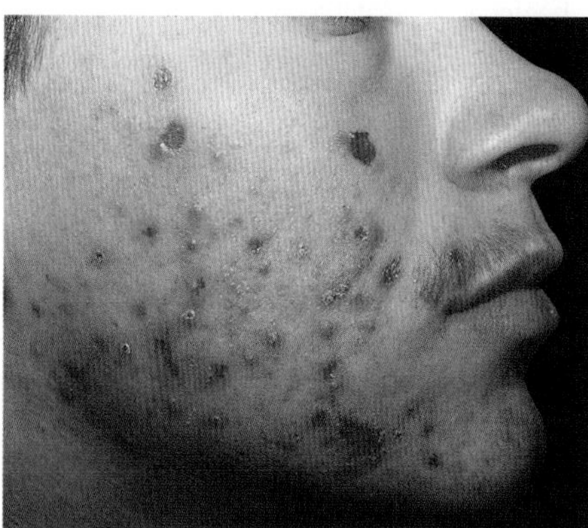

Fig. 5.4 Acne excoriée. This patient compulsively picked at his acne lesions. *Courtesy, Richard Odom, MD.*

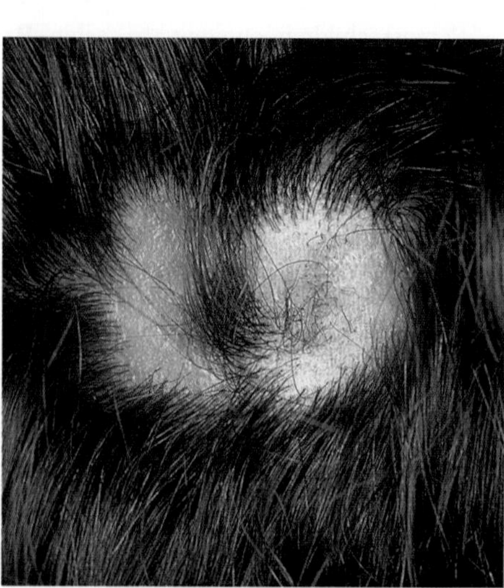

Fig. 5.5 Trichotillomania. Classic findings with small areas of sparing. *Courtesy, John Koo, MD.*

- Classically see hairs of varying lengths distributed within the area of alopecia; uninvolved areas are normal (Fig. 5.5).
- Sometimes associated ritualistic behavior or trichophagy.
- **DDx:** other causes of non-scarring alopecia (e.g. alopecia areata, tinea capitis).
- A helpful diagnostic test is the "clipped hair square," in which a small section of hair is clipped close to the scalp with scissors; in trichotillomania the hairs (being too short to pull out) display uniform hair regrowth.
- **Rx:** behavioral modification is primary treatment; psychosocial support; SSRIs; case reports of olanzapine, N-acetylcysteine (1200–2400 mg/day for adults) or inositol being helpful.

Schizophrenia Spectrum and Other Psychotic Disorders

DELUSIONS OF PARASITOSIS

- A *somatic type of delusional disorder* (within the broad group of *schizophrenia spectrum and other psychotic disorders*) in which patients have the isolated, fixed, false belief (delusion) that their skin is infested with parasites, despite any objective evidence of an infestation.
- DSM-5™ criteria for diagnosis include the following: (1) delusion has been present for ≥1 month; (2) patient has no other impaired functioning or bizarre behavior apart from the impact of the delusion; (3) the delusion cannot be attributed to the effects of a substance, medication, medical condition or other psychiatric disorder.

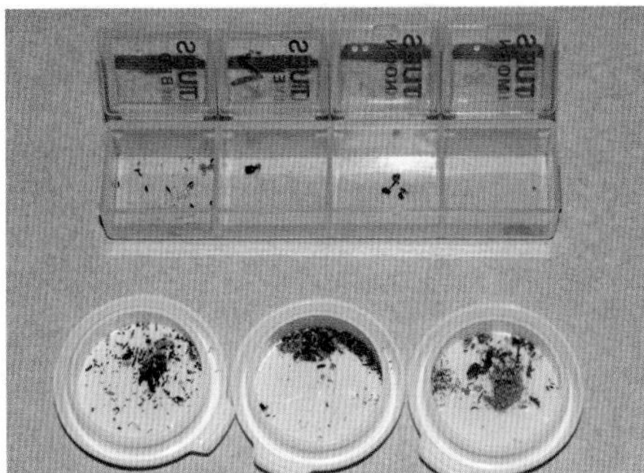

Fig. 5.6 Delusions of parasitosis. Samples of alleged "parasites" brought in by a patient ("matchbox sign"). *Courtesy, Kalman Watsky, MD.*

- Typical onset is in the mid 50s–60s.
- Patients often bring in bits of skin, lint, and other specimens to prove the existence of the supposed parasites (Fig. 5.6).
- Often experience cutaneous sensations of crawling, biting, and/or stinging.
- Skin findings, which are self-induced, range from none to excoriations, lichenification, prurigo nodularis, and ulcerations.
- **DDx:** true formication (tactile hallucination involving the sensation of bugs crawling or biting the skin) related to alcohol withdrawal or other drugs (e.g. amphetamines, cocaine), a medical condition (e.g. neurologic disorder), or other psychiatric disorder (e.g. schizophrenia).
- A recent investigation by the Centers for Disease Control and Prevention supported the categorization of Morgellons disease as a form of delusions of parasitosis; hallmark of Morgellons is that patients claim to observe "fibers" exuding from their skin.
- **Rx:** establish rapport with patient first; do not challenge their delusional belief; antipsychotics (see Table 5.1).

Somatic Symptom and Related Disorders

DERMATITIS ARTEFACTA

- A type of factitious disorder within the broad DSM-5™ category of somatic symptom and related disorders.
- Characterized by self-inflicted lesions as a means to satisfy a psychological need that is not consciously understood; self-denial.
- Rare disorder; many patients suffer from borderline personality disorder; may have underlying depression and/or anxiety.
- Onset typically in adolescence or young adulthood; females >> males.
- Lesions often appear in easy-to-reach areas and appear in bizarre shapes and configurations; may employ outside instruments (Fig. 5.7).
- **DDx:** (1) primary dermatologic disorder; (2) delusions of parasitosis; (3) malingering (conscious gain); (4) nonsuicidal self-injury (patients acknowledge they injured themselves); (5) factitious disorder imposed on another (previously called Munchausen syndrome by proxy).
- **Rx:** symptomatic treatment of wounds; psychosocial support; psychotropic medications tailored to underlying psychopathology.

Other/Conditions for Further Study

NONSUICIDAL SELF-INJURY (CUTTING)

- Repeated infliction of shallow injuries to the surface of the body, typically via cutting, stabbing or burning; often a sharp object (e.g. knife or razor), cigarette, or eraser is employed.
- No suicidal intent; purpose is usually to reduce negative emotions or to resolve an interpersonal difficulty; patients will admit to this behavior but often will not seek help.
- Often associated with depression, anxiety and sometimes with borderline personality disorder.
- Onset is typically in early adolescence; female : male ratio is about 1.5 : 1.
- Most common sites of involvement are the dorsal hands/arms and anterior thighs; lesions present as an admixture of linear erosions or well-healed scars (Fig. 5.8), often in an array of parallel lines (likened to "railroad ties"); some individuals will cut words into their skin; with time, the cutting will typically escalate to more frequent and numerous lesions.
- Unexplained, recurrent "cuts and scratches" on the forearms and legs of adolescents should arouse suspicion for this behavior.
- **DDx**: in contrast to dermatitis artefacta, patients acknowledge that they inflicted the lesions upon themselves.
- **Rx:** familial and psychological support; treatment of underlying psychopathology.

For further information see Ch. 7 from *Dermatology, Fourth Edition*.

For additional online figures visit www.expertconsult.com 

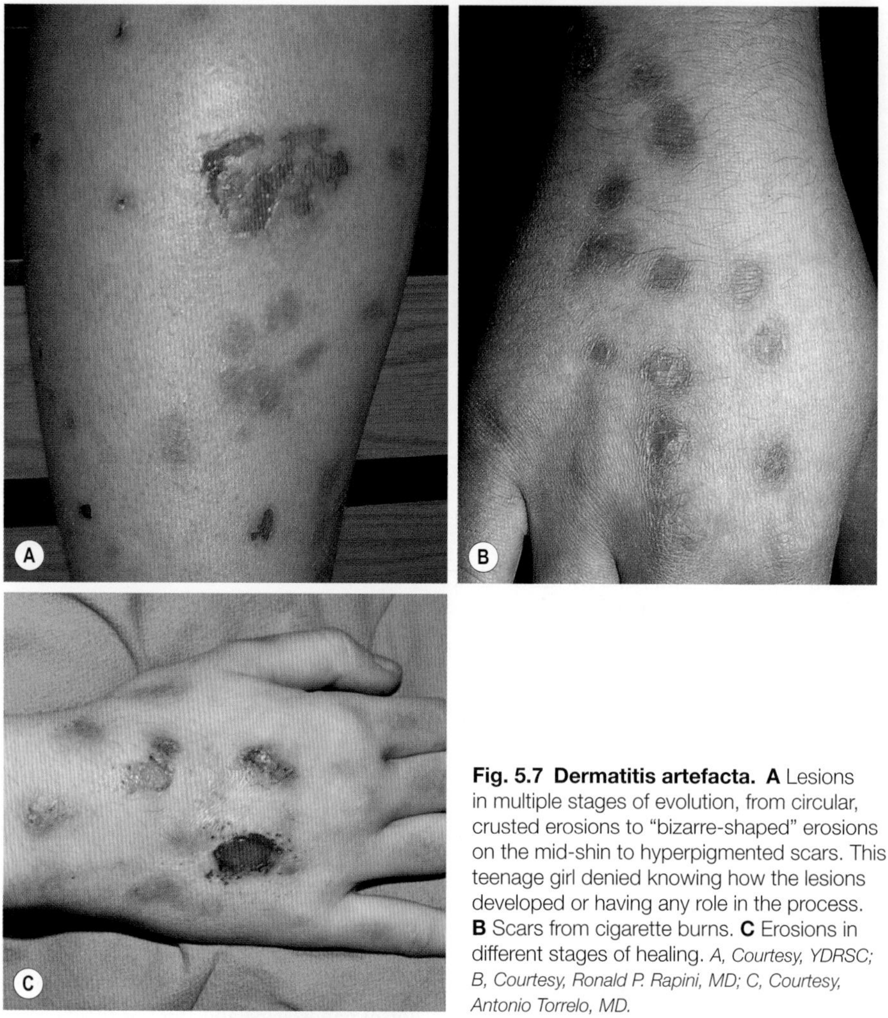

Fig. 5.7 Dermatitis artefacta. A Lesions in multiple stages of evolution, from circular, crusted erosions to "bizarre-shaped" erosions on the mid-shin to hyperpigmented scars. This teenage girl denied knowing how the lesions developed or having any role in the process. **B** Scars from cigarette burns. **C** Erosions in different stages of healing. *A, Courtesy, YDRSC; B, Courtesy, Ronald P. Rapini, MD; C, Courtesy, Antonio Torrelo, MD.*

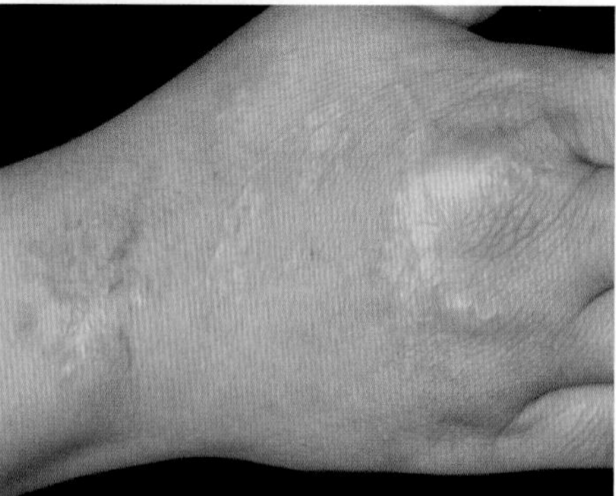

Fig. 5.8 Nonsuicidal self-injury. Repeated episodes of self-cutting with a razor blade caused these hypopigmented scars on the dorsal hand and forearm of this young woman. *Courtesy, Karynne O. Duncan MD.*

Psoriasis 6

Key Points

- Affects up to 2% of the population.
- Chronic disorder in those with a polygenic predisposition combined with triggering factors such as infections (especially streptococcal infection, but also HIV infection) or medications (e.g. interferon, β-blockers, lithium, or oral CS taper).
- Koebner phenomenon – elicitation of psoriatic lesions by traumatizing the skin.
- Common sites (Fig. 6.1)
  - Scalp
  - Elbows and knees
  - Nails, hands, feet, trunk (intergluteal fold)
- Skin lesions
  - Most commonly – well-demarcated, erythematous plaques with silvery scale (Fig. 6.2)
  - Other lesions include sterile pustules, glistening plaques in intertriginous zones
- Histopathologic findings
  - Regular acanthosis, confluent parakeratosis with neutrophils, hypogranulosis, dilated blood vessels (see Ch. 1)
- Major systemic association is psoriatic arthritis (Table 6.1), most commonly presenting as asymmetric oligoarthritis of hands/feet; the metabolic syndrome is also common.
- Pathogenesis
  - Regarded as a T-cell-driven disease involving cytokines, including TNF-α and IL-23 (stimulates Th17 cells)
  - Genes that have been associated with psoriasis include those encoding IL-12, IL-23, caspase recruitment domain family member 14 (CARD14, a regulator of NF-κB signaling) and, for generalized pustular psoriasis, the IL-36 receptor antagonist (a regulator of IL-8 production and IL-1β responses)

Variants

Chronic Plaque Psoriasis

- Typical lesion – well-demarcated, erythematous plaque with silvery scale.
- Often symmetrical lesions on the elbows and knees; additional sites include the scalp, presacrum, hands, feet, intergluteal fold, and umbilicus (Fig. 6.3, Fig. 6.4, Fig. 6.5).
- May be generalized (Fig. 6.6).
- Lesions may be surrounded by a peripheral, blanching ring (Woronoff's ring), especially when patient is receiving phototherapy.
- **DDx:** *for lesions on the elbows/knees* – dermatomyositis, pityriasis rubra pilaris (in children); *for truncal lesions* – various forms of dermatitis including nummular, parapsoriasis, mycosis fungoides, subacute cutaneous lupus erythematosus, drug-induced psoriasiform eruptions; *for palmoplantar lesions* (see Fig. 13.1 and Table 13.1) – tinea, keratotic eczema.

Guttate Psoriasis

- Typical lesion – small papule or plaque (3 mm to 1.5 cm) with adherent scale (Fig. 6.7).
- Generalized distribution.
- Affects children > adults.
- Often preceded by an upper respiratory tract infection.
- In children, may have spontaneous remission but often responds well to UVB phototherapy.
- **DDx:** pityriasis rosea, syphilis, id reaction to tinea pedis, and small plaque parapsoriasis.

Linear Psoriasis

- Linear, erythematous, scaly lesions that often follow the lines of Blaschko.
- **DDx:** inflammatory linear verrucous epidermal nevus (ILVEN; follows the lines of Blaschko; resistant to therapy), epidermal nevus with superimposed psoriasis.

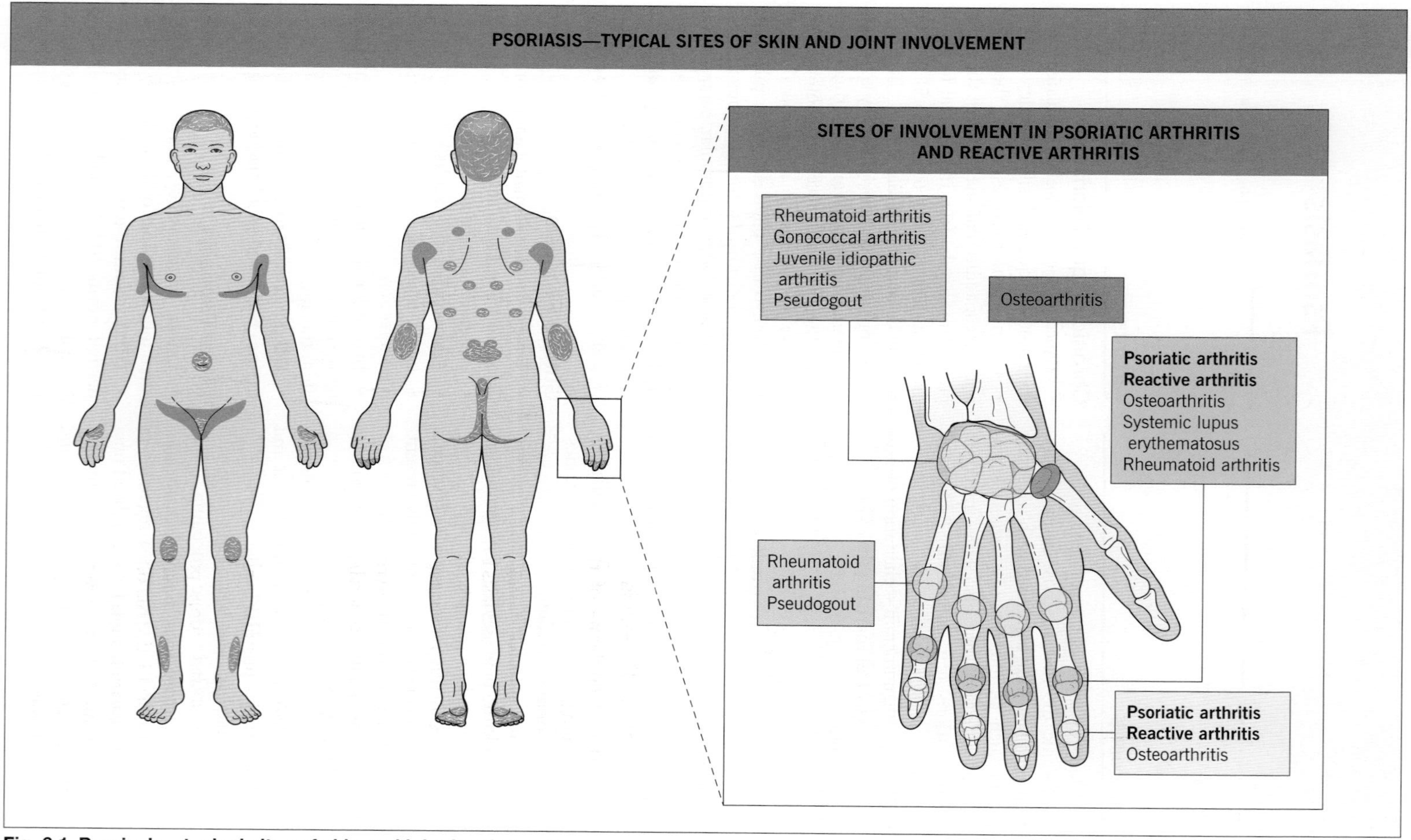

Fig. 6.1 Psoriasis – typical sites of skin and joint involvement.

FIVE TYPES OF PSORIATIC ARTHRITIS
• Mono- and asymmetric oligoarthritis
• Arthritis of distal interphalangeal joints
• Rheumatoid arthritis-like presentation
• Arthritis mutilans
• Spondylitis and sacroiliitis

Table 6.1 Five types of psoriatic arthritis.

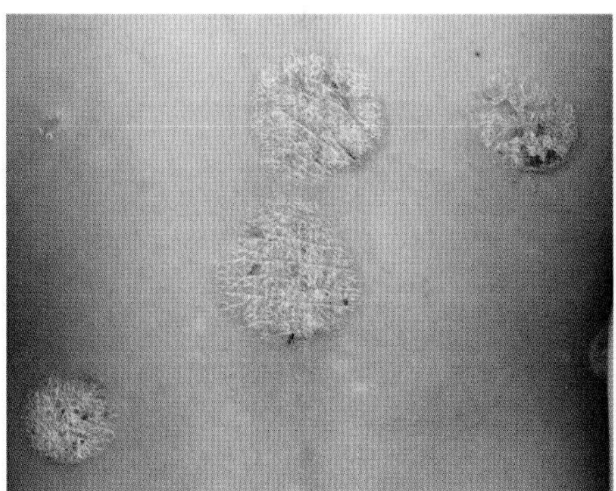

Fig. 6.2 Psoriatic plaques. Note the sharp demarcation and silvery scale. *Courtesy, Julie V. Schaffer, MD.*

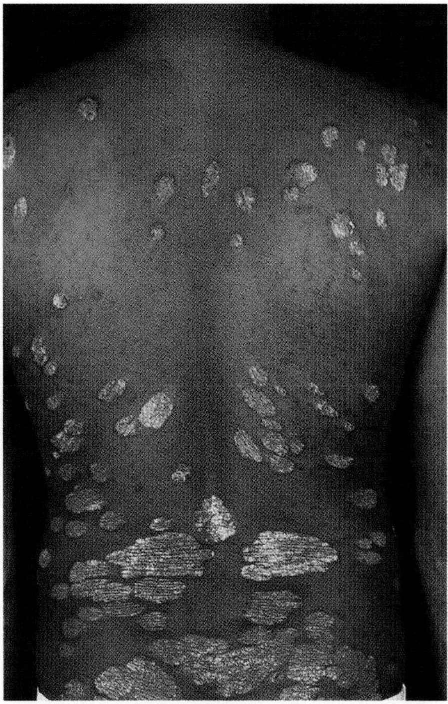

Fig. 6.3 Symmetric distribution of psoriatic plaques. *Courtesy, Peter C. M. van de Kerkhof, MD.*

Erythrodermic Psoriasis

- Generalized erythema of the skin, with areas of scaling.
- Gradual or acute onset.
- Nail changes, facial sparing, and a history of typical plaque-type psoriasis may be helpful clues.
- May be seen after abrupt tapering of medications, especially CS.
- **DDx:** other causes of erythroderma, e.g. pityriasis rubra pilaris, generalized atopic dermatitis, Sézary syndrome (see Table 8.2).

Pustular Psoriasis

- Generalized pustular psoriasis (von Zumbusch pattern)
  - Erythema and sterile pustules arising within erythematous, painful skin; lakes of pus characteristic (Fig. 6.8)
  - Often associated fever
  - Triggering factors – pregnancy (termed impetigo herpetiformis), rapid tapering of CS, hypocalcemia, infections
  - **DDx:** acute generalized exanthematous pustulosis (AGEP; pustular drug reaction) (see Ch. 17)
- Palmoplantar (pustulosis)
  - Sterile pustules on palms/soles (Fig. 6.9)
  - May have no evidence of psoriasis elsewhere
  - Triggering factors – infections, stress
  - May be aggravated by smoking
  - Associated with inflammatory bone lesions (see Ch. 21)
- Annular pattern (Fig. 6.10)
  - **DDx:** includes Sneddon–Wilkinson disease (see below)
- Exanthematic type
  - Significant overlap with AGEP
- Localized pattern – within plaques, often due to irritants (Fig. 6.11).
- Acrodermatitis continua (of Hallopeau)
  - Erythema and scale of distal digit with pustules (Fig. 6.12)
  - Often associated fever

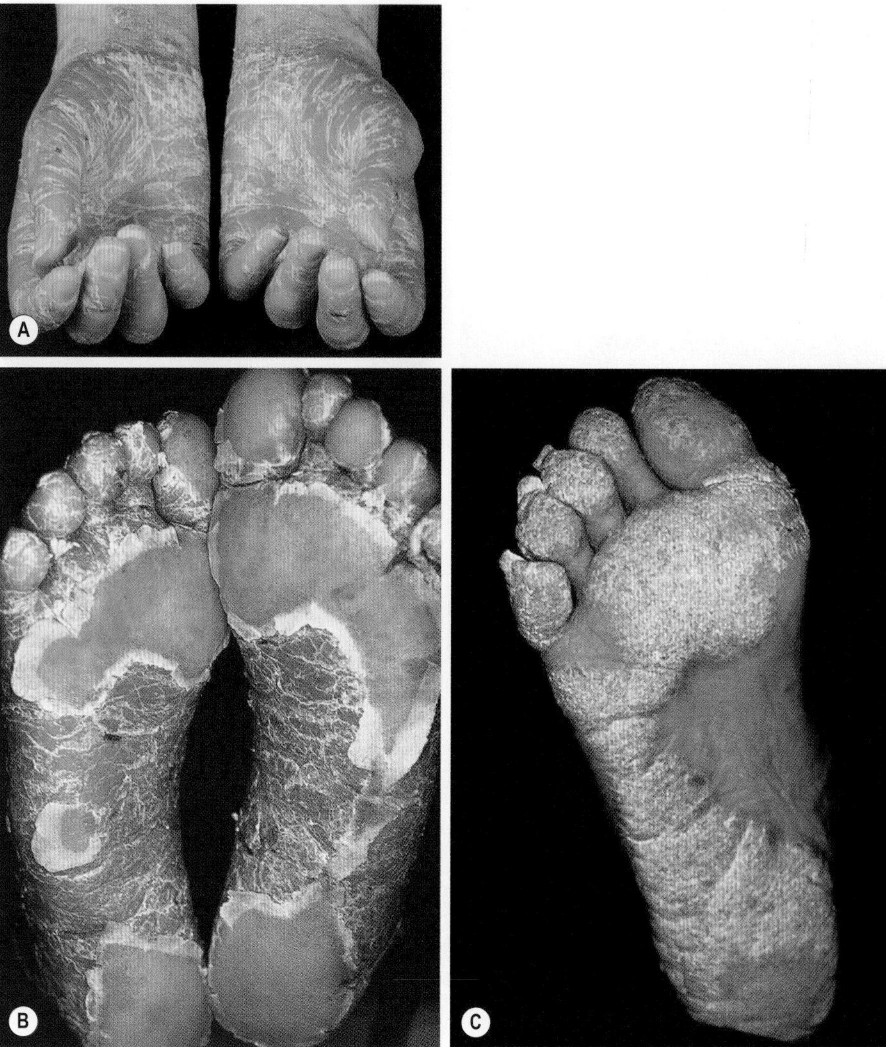

Fig. 6.4 Palmoplantar psoriasis. Erythematous scaling plaques of the palmar **(A)** and plantar surfaces **(B)**. Occasionally, there is well-demarcated hyperkeratosis with minimal erythema **(C)**. *A, Courtesy, Peter C. M. van de Kerkhof, MD; B, Courtesy, YDRSC.*

Special Sites

Scalp

- Well-demarcated, erythematous plaques with silvery scale.
- Scale may be attached for some distance onto scalp hairs, giving an asbestos-like appearance (pityriasis amiantacea).
- Occasionally alopecia may be seen within lesions.
- **DDx:** seborrheic dermatitis (more diffuse pattern), tinea capitis, dermatomyositis.

Flexural (Inverse Psoriasis)

- Shiny, pink, well-demarcated thin plaques with minimal scale (Fig. 6.13).
- Common sites include the axilla, inguinal crease, intergluteal cleft, inframammary area, and retroauricular fold.
- Sebopsoriasis – seborrheic dermatitis and psoriasis are at either ends of a spectrum, with intermediate forms termed sebopsoriasis.
- Additional **DDx:** seborrheic dermatitis, candidiasis, tinea cruris, erythrasma, granular parakeratosis (see Fig. 13.4).

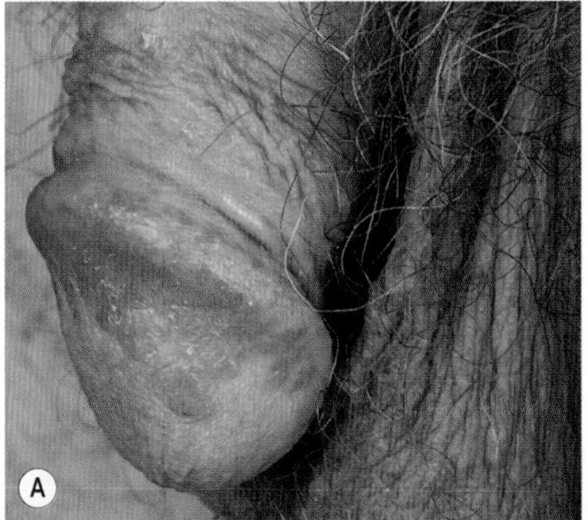

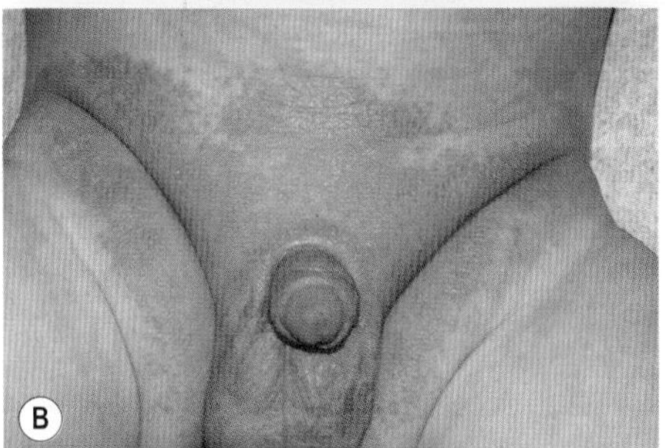

Fig. 6.5 Psoriasis of the genitalia. A Well-demarcated erythematous plaques with scale on the glans and shaft of the penis in an adult. **B** Infantile psoriasis with a well-demarcated erythematous plaque of the diaper area, along with involvement of the penis and scrotum. This is in contrast to atopic dermatitis where there is often sparing of the diaper area. *A, Courtesy, Lorenzo Cerroni, MD; B, Courtesy, Julie V. Schaffer, MD.*

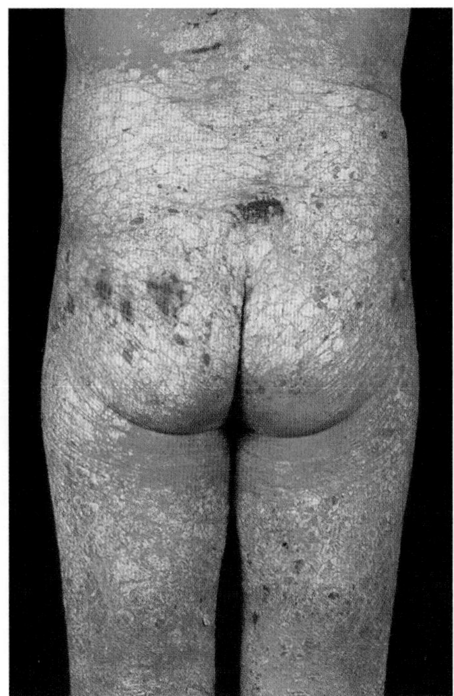

Fig. 6.6 Widespread chronic plaque psoriasis. *Courtesy, Peter C. M. van de Kerkhof, MD.*

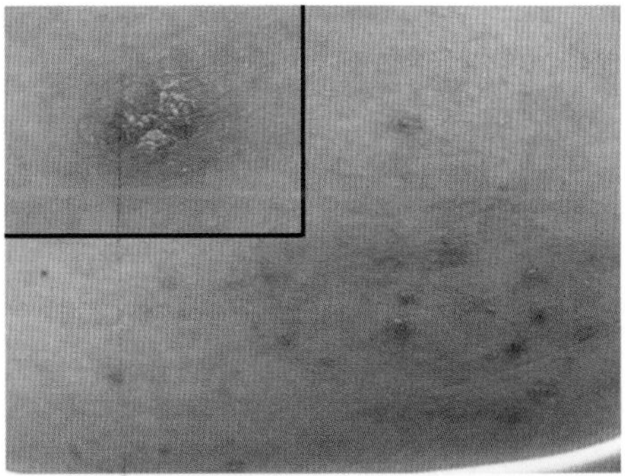

Fig. 6.7 Guttate psoriasis. Small discrete papules and plaques of guttate psoriasis. *Courtesy, Christine J. Ko, MD.*

Oral

- Migratory, annular lesions with central denuded areas and white borders.
- Similar to geographic tongue clinically and histopathologically.

Nail (see Ch. 58)

- Fingernails > toenails (Fig. 6.14).
- Associated with psoriatic arthritis.
- Findings include nail pitting, oil spots (salmon patch), onycholysis with proximal red rim, splinter hemorrhages, subungual debris.

Sneddon–Wilkinson Disease (Subcorneal Pustular Dermatosis)

- Often begins in body folds or major intertriginous zones.
- Lesions are annular with superficial pustules on the border.
- Classic sign is a half and half pustule with clear fluid superiorly and pus inferiorly (dependent portion).
- Two schools of thought – this disease is (1) a variant of psoriasis vs (2) a separate entity (Fig. 6.15).

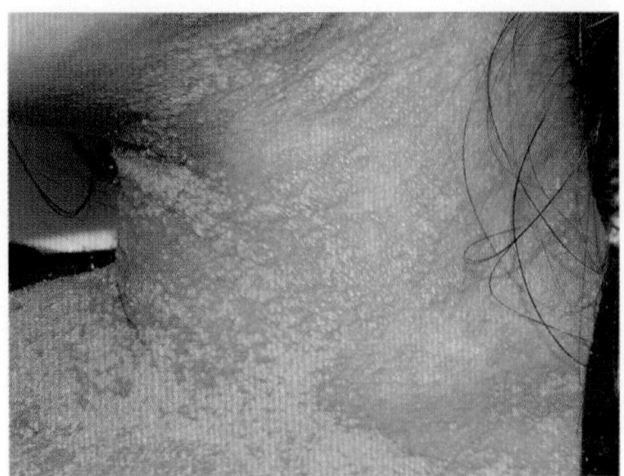

Fig. 6.8 Pustular psoriasis. Large areas of erythema with numerous pustules. Confluence of pustules creates lakes of pus. *Courtesy, Julie V. Schaffer, MD.*

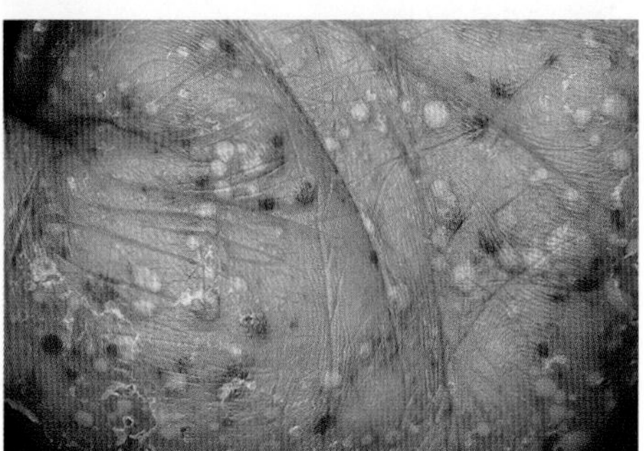

Fig. 6.9 Pustulosis of the palms and soles. Multiple sterile pustules are admixed with yellow-brown macules on the palm. *Courtesy, YDRSC.*

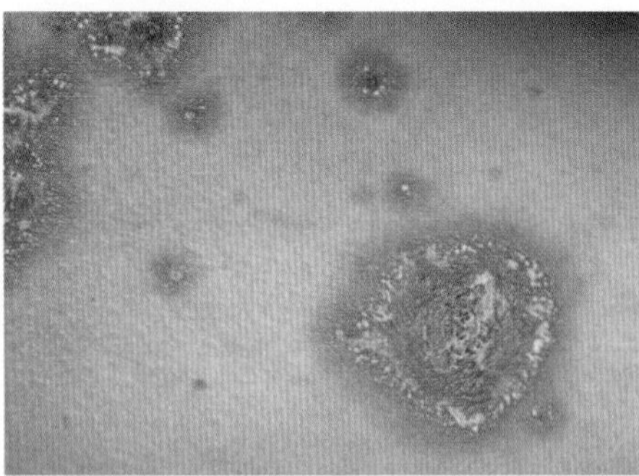

Fig. 6.10 Annular pustular psoriasis. Multiple annular inflammatory plaques studded with pustules. *Courtesy, Julie V. Schaffer, MD.*

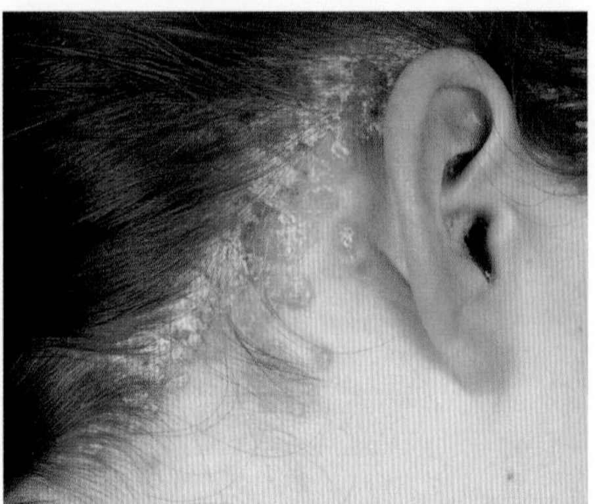

Fig. 6.11 Scalp psoriasis with extension onto the neck. Note the involvement of the external auditory canal. *Courtesy, Peter C. M. van de Kerkhof, MD.*

Psoriatic Arthritis

- Seen in 5–30% of patients with cutaneous psoriasis.
- Most commonly is an asymmetric oligoarthritis affecting the distal, or both proximal and distal ("sausage"), interphalangeal joints (Fig. 6.16).
- More rarely, but classically, is arthritis of all the distal interphalangeal joints of the fingers.
- Occasionally, presentation is rheumatoid arthritis-like, affecting small- and medium-sized joints symmetrically.
- Arthritis mutilans – rare form with acute, rapidly progressive joint inflammation and destruction; softening and telescoping of the digits.
- Spondylitis and sacroiliitis – axial arthritis as well as arthritis of the knees and sacroiliac joints; may be HLA-B27-positive and may have associated inflammatory bowel disease or uveitis.
- **DDx:** reactive arthritis (previously referred to as Reiter disease)
    - Urethritis, arthritis, ocular findings (e.g., conjunctivitis), and oral ulcers in addition to psoriasiform lesions, especially on the soles (keratoderma blennorrhagicum) or genitalia (balanitis circinata) (Fig. 6.17)
    - More common in men
    - Strongly associated with HLA-B27
    - Course is often self-limited
    - May be severe in HIV-positive individuals (see Table 6.1)

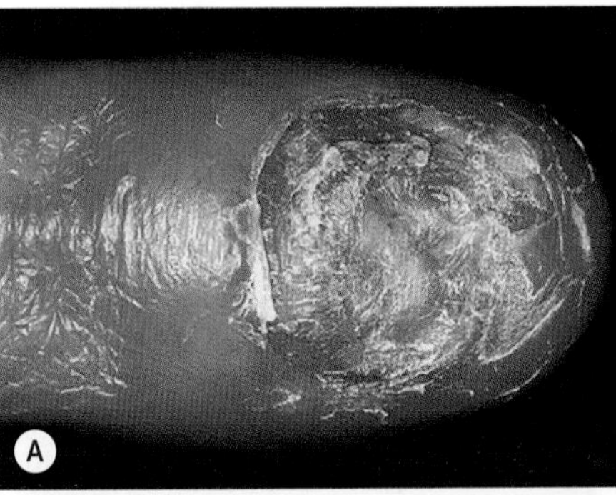

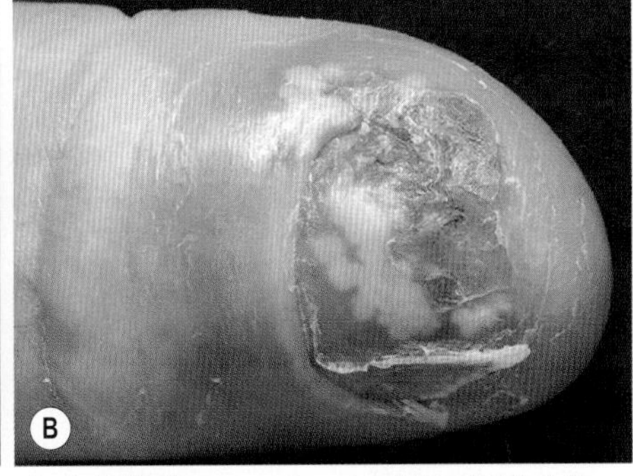

Fig. 6.12 Acrodermatitis continua (of Hallopeau). A, B Erythema and scale of the distal digit, pustules within the nail bed, and partial shedding of the nail plate. *A, Courtesy, YDRSC; B, Courtesy, Peter C. M. van de Kerkhof, MD.*

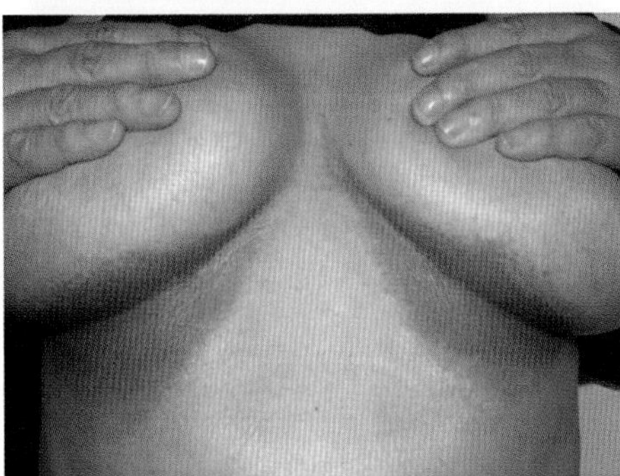

Fig. 6.13 Inverse psoriasis. Shiny erythematous plaques of the inframammary folds that lack scale. *Courtesy, Luis Requena, MD.*

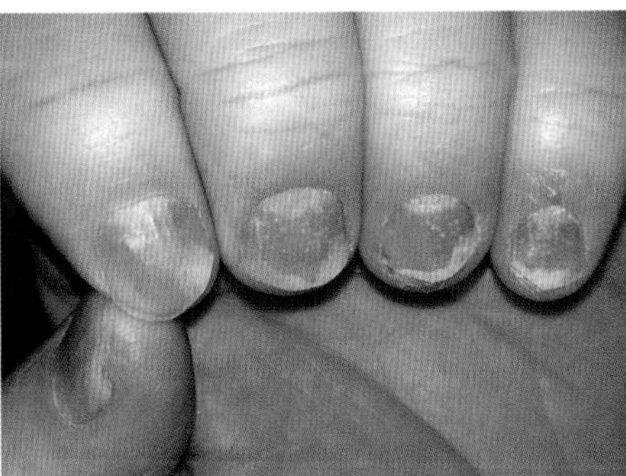

Fig. 6.14 Nail psoriasis. Changes include distal onycholysis, pitting, and "oil spot" (salmon patch) phenomenon.

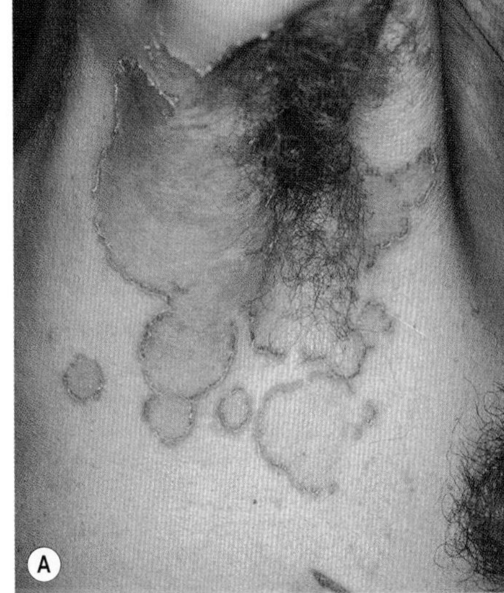

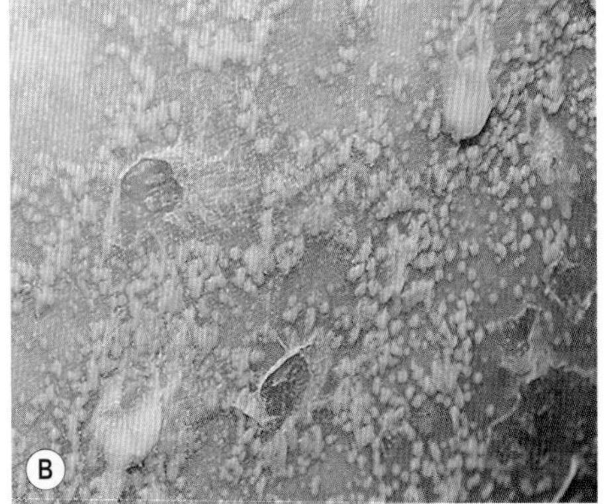

Fig. 6.15 Sneddon–Wilkinson disease.
A Annular and polycyclic plaques in the axilla.
B Numerous, fragile, subcorneal pustules arising within a background of erythema. There is dependent pooling of the pustular contents in some of the larger lesions. There is significant overlap with pustular psoriasis. *A, Courtesy, YDRSC; B, Courtesy, Department of Dermatology, Medical University of Graz.*

Treatment

- Topical agents
  - First-line
    - CS (Table 6.2)
    - Vitamin D_3 analogues (calcipotriene [calcipotriol], calcitriol) (Table 6.3)
  - Second-line
    - Calcineurin inhibitors (may be first-line for sensitive areas such as the face or flexures)
    - Tars (e.g. liquor carbonis detergens [LCD] 5%)
    - Anthralin
    - Tazarotene
- Phototherapy and systemic agents
  - First-line
    - Phototherapy – UVB (narrowband or broadband > PUVA) (Table 6.4); if thick keratotic plaques, can combine with oral retinoids. Oral PUVA – 0.6–0.8 mg/kg of 8-methoxypsoralen (MOP) orally 1–3 hours before light exposure; bath PUVA – 0.5–5 mg of 8-MOP/liter of bath water with immediate irradiation after soaking for 15–20 minutes; topical PUVA (e.g. for palms/soles) – 8-MOP 0.1–0.01% cream/ointment/lotion followed by UVA irradiation
    - Methotrexate (oral or intramuscular, occasionally subcutaneous) (Table 6.5)

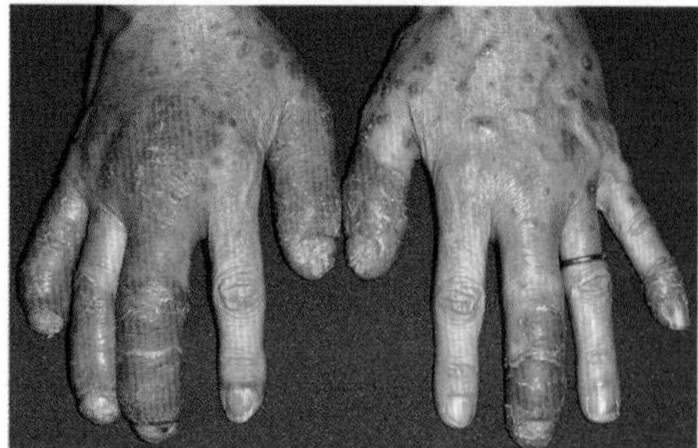

Fig. 6.16 Psoriatic arthritis. Asymmetric involvement of the distal interphalangeal (DIP) and proximal interphalangeal (PIP) joints. A "sausage" digit (third digit bilaterally) results from involvement of both the DIP and PIP joints. *Courtesy, YDRSC.*

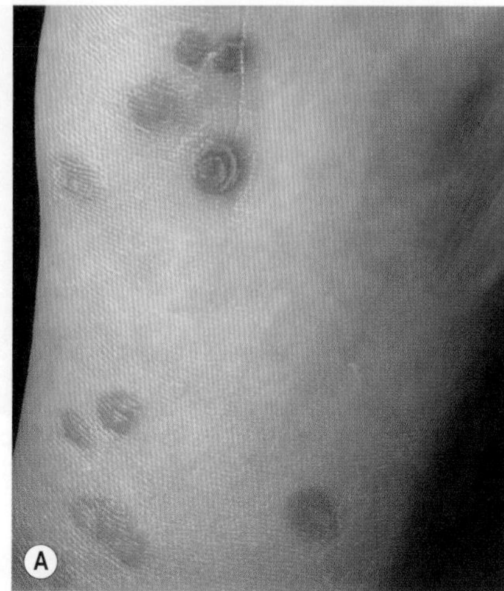

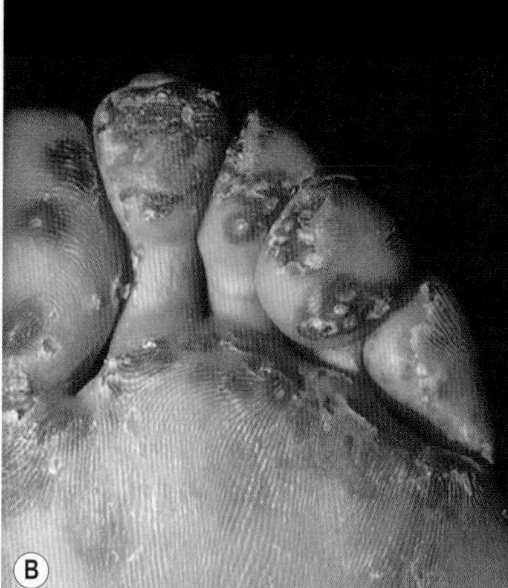

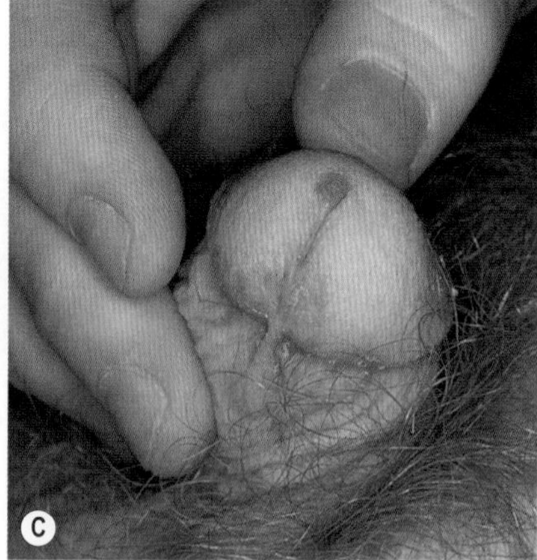

Fig. 6.17 Reactive arthritis (formerly Reiter disease). A, B Plantar lesions of keratoderma blennorrhagicum. **C** Papulosquamous lesions of balanitis circinata on the penis. *A, C, Courtesy, YDRSC; B, Courtesy, Eugene Mirrer, MD.*

INDICATIONS AND CONTRAINDICATIONS FOR TOPICAL CORTICOSTEROIDS
Indications
• Mild to moderate psoriasis: first-line treatment as monotherapy or in combination • Severe psoriasis: often in combination with a vitamin D_3 analogue, a topical retinoid, anthralin, or tar • Monotherapy for flexural and facial psoriasis (usually mild strength) • Recalcitrant plaques often require occlusion (plastic, hydrocolloid)
Contraindications
• Bacterial, viral, and mycotic infections • Atrophy of the skin • Allergic contact dermatitis due to corticosteroids or constituents of the formulation • Pregnancy or lactation*
**Relative; can consider limited use of mild- to moderate-strength corticosteroids.*

Table 6.2 Indications and contraindications for topical corticosteroids. Maximal quantities: 50 gm/week of a superpotent corticosteroid; 100 gm/week of a potent corticosteroid. *Courtesy, Peter C. M. van de Kerkhof, MD.*

INDICATIONS AND CONTRAINDICATIONS FOR VITAMIN D_3 ANALOGUES
Indications
• Mild to moderate psoriasis: first-line treatment as monotherapy or in combination • Severe psoriasis: combination treatment
Contraindications
• Involvement requiring more than the maximally recommended quantity, e.g. 100 gm/week of calcipotriene • Abnormality in bone or calcium metabolism* • Renal insufficiency • Allergy to the vitamin D_3 analogue or constituents of the preparation • Pregnancy or lactation
**For example, sarcoidosis and bone metastases.*

Table 6.3 Indications and contraindications for vitamin D_3 analogues. If used in conjunction with phototherapy, vitamin D_3 preparations need to be applied after UV irradiation or at least several hours prior, because they may reduce UV penetration into the skin. *Courtesy, Peter C. M. van de Kerkhof, MD.*

    - Oral retinoids (e.g. acitretin, isotretinoin)
  - Second-line systemic
    - Targeted immunomodulators ("biologic" agents) (Tables 6.6 and 6.7)
    - Cyclosporine

- See Table 6.8 for treatment options for special sites.
- See Table 6.9 for treatment options in patients with comorbidities or special situations.
- See Appendix for the recommended laboratory evaluation for patients receiving targeted immunomodulators.

For further information see Ch. 8 from *Dermatology, Fourth Edition*.

For additional online figures visit www.expertconsult.com 

INDICATIONS AND CONTRAINDICATIONS FOR PHOTOTHERAPY
Indications
• Moderate to severe psoriasis: first-line treatment as monotherapy or in combination
Contraindications (absolute or relative)
• Genetic disorders characterized by increased photosensitivity or an increased risk of skin cancer (UVB and PUVA)* • Skin type I (UVB and PUVA)† • Photosensitive dermatoses (UVB and PUVA)† • Unavoidable phototoxic systemic or topical medications (UVB and PUVA)† • Vitiligo (UVB and PUVA)† • Previous history of arsenic exposure, ionizing irradiation, or excessive phototherapy (UVB and PUVA) • High cumulative number of PUVA treatments, i.e. >150–200 individual treatments (PUVA)* • Treatment with cyclosporine (UVB and PUVA)* • Immunosuppressive medication (UVB and PUVA) • Previous history of skin cancers (PUVA > UVB) • Atypical melanocytic nevi (UVB and PUVA) • Seizure disorder (risk of fall/injury; UVB and PUVA) • Poor compliance (UVB and PUVA) • Men and women in reproductive years without contraception (PUVA) • Pregnancy or lactation (PUVA)* • Impaired liver function or hepatotoxic medication (PUVA) • Cataracts (PUVA)
**Absolute contraindication.* *†Need to adjust the dose and monitor closely.*

Table 6.4 Indications and contraindications for phototherapy. *Courtesy, Peter C. M. van de Kerkhof, MD.*

Supplementary Figures

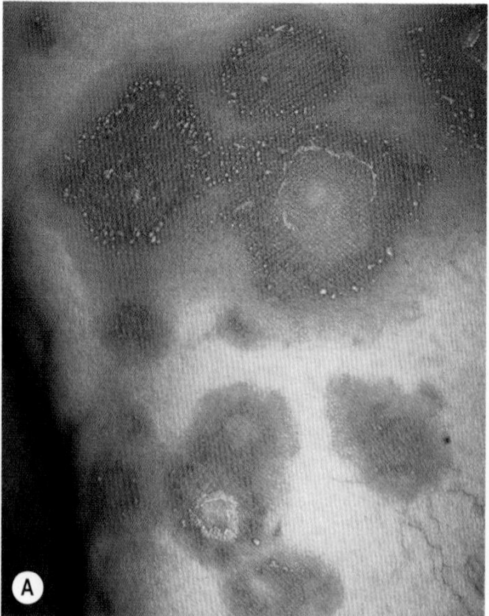

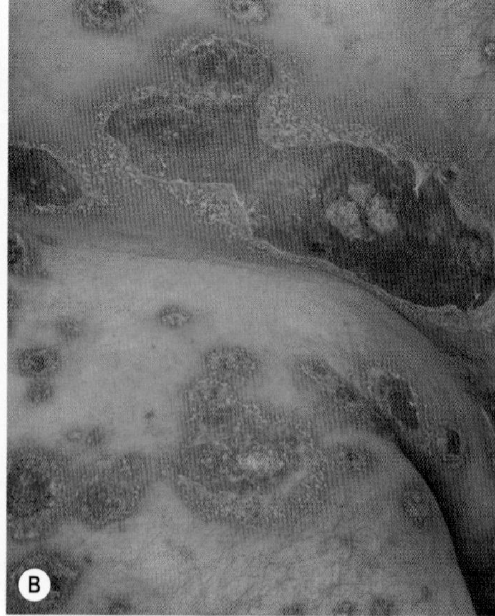

sFig. 6.1 Annular pustular psoriasis. Multiple annular inflammatory plaques studded with pustules. As the lesions enlarge, there can be central clearing, dry desquamation **(A)**, and/or moist desquamation that resembles wet cigarette paper **(B)**. *A, Courtesy, YDRSC; B, Courtesy, Peter C. M. van de Kerkhof, MD.*

INDICATIONS AND CONTRAINDICATIONS FOR METHOTREXATE (MTX)
Indications
• Severe psoriasis • Chronic plaque psoriasis (>10–15% BSA or interference with employment or social functioning) • Pustular psoriasis (generalized or localized) • Erythrodermic psoriasis • Psoriatic arthritis (moderate to severe) • Severe nail psoriasis • Psoriasis not responding to topical treatments, phototherapy, and/or systemic retinoids
Contraindications (absolute or relative)
• Impaired kidney function (creatinine clearance <60 ml/min)‡ • Severe anemia, leukopenia, and/or thrombocytopenia* • Significant liver function abnormalities, hepatitis (active and/or recent), severe fibrosis, cirrhosis, excessive alcohol intake* • Concomitant hepatotoxic medications • Concomitant medications that increase MTX levels, e.g. trimethoprim–sulfamethoxazole* • Significantly reduced pulmonary function* • Pregnancy or lactation* • Currently planning to have children (male and female patients)‡ • Immunodeficiency syndromes • Severe infections* • Active infections • Peptic ulcer (active)* • Gastritis • Concomitant radiation therapy • Pleural effusion or ascites‡ • Hypersensitivity to MTX* • Unreliable patient*
**Absolute contraindication.* *†Requires significant reduction in dosage.* *‡Because of possible mutagenic risk and teratogenicity, discontinue MTX 3 months prior to attempts to conceive; continue contraception during these 3 months.*

Table 6.5 Indications and contraindications for methotrexate (MTX). *Courtesy, Peter C. M. van de Kerkhof, MD.*

COMMERCIALLY AVAILABLE BIOLOGIC AGENTS FOR THE TREATMENT OF PSORIASIS		
Target		**Biologic agents (estimated % of patients who achieve PASI75)**
TNF		Etanercept (30–60), adalimumab (50–80), infliximab (75–85)
IL-12/IL-23	p40 subunit of IL-12/IL-23	Ustekinumab (65–80)
	IL-23	Guselkumab (80–90)
IL-17		Secukinumab (65–85), ixekizumab (85–90), risankizumab (63–98), tildrakizumab (61–66), brodalumab (60–85)

Table 6.6 Commercially available biologic agents for the treatment of psoriasis. Biosimilar products, e.g. adalimumab-atto, etanercept-szzs, infliximab-dyyb, are also commercially available. PASI, psoriasis area severity index.

FDA WARNINGS AND PRECAUTIONS FOR TARGETED IMMUNE MODULATORS USED FOR PSORIASIS
TNF inhibitors
• Increased risk of serious infections, including tuberculosis, bacterial sepsis, systemic fungal infections (e.g. histoplasmosis), and infections due to opportunistic pathogens
• Risk of hepatitis B virus reactivation
• Malignancies (especially lymphomas) have been reported in patients receiving these agents, including children and adolescents – For infliximab, lymphomas are seen more often than in the general population and fatal hepatosplenic T-cell lymphomas have developed in patients with inflammatory bowel disease who were also receiving azathioprine or 6-mercaptopurine – An increased risk of non-melanoma skin cancer and melanoma has been observed in patients with rheumatoid arthritis treated with TNF inhibitors
• Congestive heart failure (exacerbation or new onset) has been observed
• Demyelinating disease (exacerbation or new onset) has been observed
• Anaphylaxis or severe allergic reactions can occur, including serum sickness-like reactions to infliximab
• Other potential adverse events include autoimmune hepatitis, cytopenias, and a lupus-like syndrome
IL-12/IL-23 inhibitors
• Serious infections have been observed; may increase the risk of infection and reactivation of latent infections
• Patients genetically deficient in IL-12/IL-23 have an increased risk of severe infections with mycobacteria and *Salmonella*
• BCG vaccination should not be given in the year prior to initiation or the year following completion of ustekinumab therapy
• Could potentially increase the risk of malignancies
• Hypersensitivity reactions (e.g. angioedema, anaphylaxis) can occur
• Reversible posterior leukoencephalopathy syndrome has been reported
IL-17 inhibitors
• Serious infections have been observed; may increase the risk of infection and reactivation of latent infections – Patients genetically deficient in IL-17 are prone to chronic mucocutaneous candidiasis
• New onset and exacerbation of inflammatory bowel disease have occurred
• Hypersensitivity reactions (e.g. angioedema, anaphylaxis) can develop
• For brodalumab: suicidal ideation and behavior, including complete suicides, have occurred

Table 6.7 US Food and Drug Administration (FDA) warnings and precautions for targeted immune modulators used for psoriasis. Live vaccines should not be given to patients receiving these medications. BCG, bacillus Calmette-Guérin.

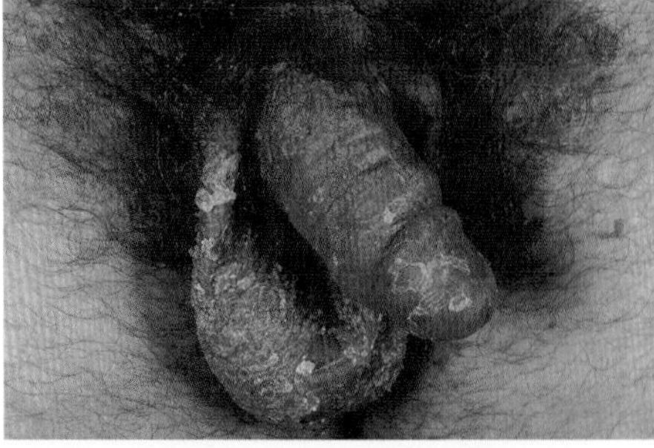

sFig. 6.2 Psoriasis of the genitalia. Erythematous plaques with scale on the penis and scrotum. *Courtesy, Peter C. M. van de Kerkhof, MD.*

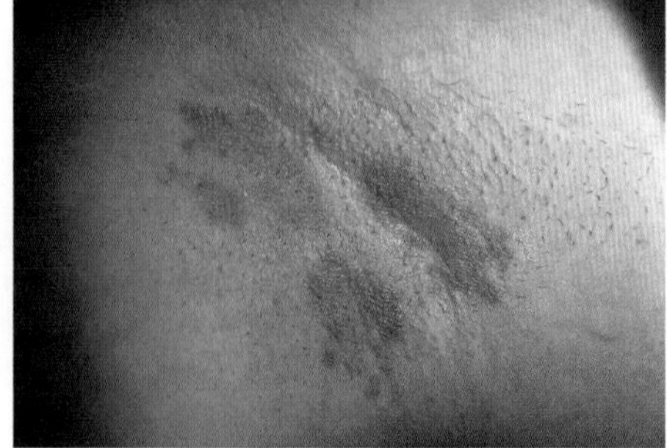

sFig. 6.3 Inverse psoriasis. Shiny erythematous plaques in the axilla that lack scale. *Courtesy, Ronald P. Rapini, MD.*

MANAGEMENT OF PSORIASIS AT SPECIFIC SITES	
Specific sites	**Special considerations and practical treatments**
Scalp	• Remove scale with topical 5–10% salicylic acid
	• Apply potent or ultrapotent corticosteroids in a lotion, gel foam or shampoo formulation, either alone or in combination with calcipotriene
Face; groin, axilla, and other body folds	• First-line: mild topical corticosteroids
	• Second-line: topical calcineurin inhibitors or tacalcitol/calcitriol in combination with a mild topical corticosteroid
Nail	• Differentiate proximal versus distal nail unit pathology due to nail matrix versus nail bed pathology, respectively; consider coexisting onychomycosis
	• For distal nail unit pathology: vitamin D_3 analogues topically (limited evidence)
	• For proximal pathology: intralesional corticosteroids and/or systemic antipsoriatic therapies

Table 6.8 Management of psoriasis at specific sites. These sites do improve with systemic therapies, but involvement of these sites alone is usually not a sufficient indication for a systemic therapy. *Courtesy, Peter C. M. van de Kerkhof.*

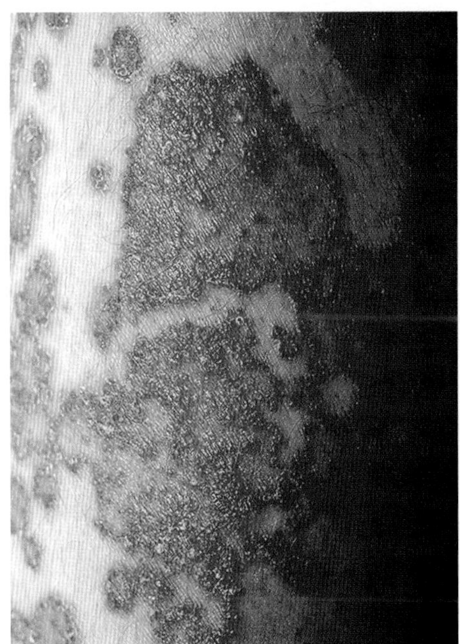

sFig. 6.4 "Localized" pattern of pustular psoriasis. The pustules are limited to pre-existing plaques of psoriasis. *Courtesy, YDRSC.*

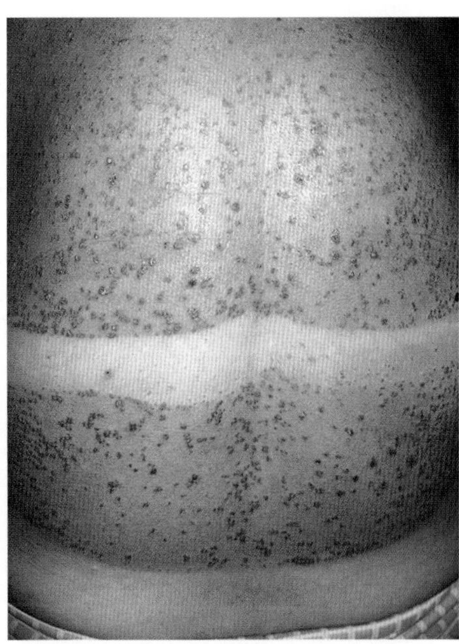

sFig. 6.5 Guttate psoriasis. Numerous papules due to the Koebner phenomenon after a sunburn. *Courtesy Ronald P. Rapini, MD.*

PREFERRED TREATMENTS FOR PSORIASIS IN THE SETTING OF COMORBIDITIES

Comorbidity or special situation	Topical therapies		Phototherapy	Systemic therapies				
	Corticosteroids	Other topical agents		Apremilast†	Retinoids	MTX†,^	CSA*	Immunomodulators ("biologics")**
Liver disease	✓	✓	✓ (UVB)	✓				✓
Hepatitis B viral infection	✓	✓	✓ (UVB)	✓				✓ (IL-17 inhibitors considered safer) Test for anti-HBc Ab, HBsAg; if latter +, measure HBV DNA Consult gastroenterologist re HBV pretreatment
Hepatitis C viral infection	✓	✓	✓ (UVB)	✓				✓ (TNF inhibitors > IL-17 or IL-23 inhibitors) Test for anti-HCV Ab, HCV RNA to assess need for HCV treatment
Metabolic syndrome	✓	✓	✓	✓	✓^	✓^	✓	✓ (infliximab and ustekinumab are dosed by weight)
Latent tuberculosis infection	✓	✓	✓	✓	✓			✓ (IL-17 inhibitors considered safer) Consult for pretreatment with INH
HIV/AIDS, well-controlled	✓	✓	✓ (UVB)	✓	✓			✓Co-management with infectious disease specialist
Pregnancy	✓ (mild to moderate strength)	✓ can use certain topicals with caution (e.g. anthralin, calcipotriene)	✓ (UVB)				✓ (pregnancy category C)	✓ (consider TNF inhibitors*** [especially certolizumab given minimal placental transfer], ustekinumab***, IL-17 inhibitors [e.g. secukinumab***], IL-23 inhibitors) Co-management with gynecologist

History of internal malignancy (e.g. lymphoma, lung cancer)	✓	✓	✓ (UVB)	✓	✓			Consult with oncologist
History of frequent skin cancers	✓	✓ (vitamin D_3 analogues, retinoids)		✓	✓			

†Renal dysfunction requires a dose adjustment.
**Contraindicated for patients with renal dysfunction.*
***TNF inhibitors are relatively contraindicated in lupus erythematosus patients; IL-17 inhibitors should be avoided in patients with inflammatory bowel disease (Crohn disease and ulcerative colitis).*
^Used with caution in patients with non-alcoholic steatohepatitis.
****Pregnancy category B.*

Table 6.9 Preferred treatments for psoriasis in the setting of comorbidities. INH, isoniazid.

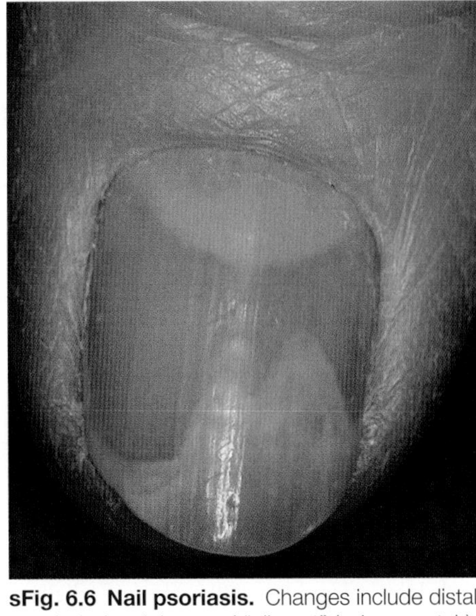

sFig. 6.6 Nail psoriasis. Changes include distal onycholysis, pitting, and "oil spot" (salmon patch) phenomenon. *Courtesy, YDRSC.*

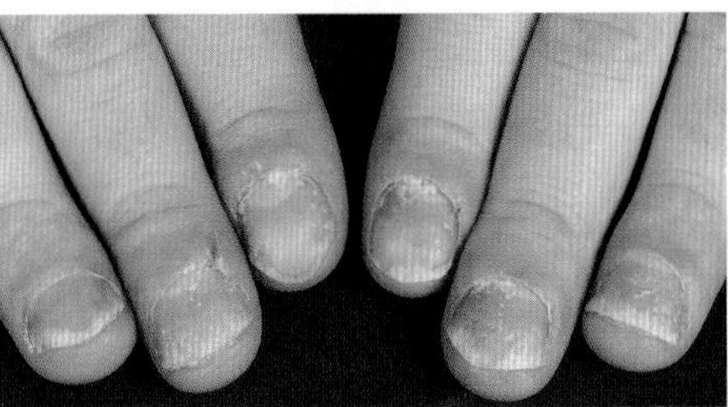

sFig. 6.7 Nail psoriasis. Nail plate pitting, distal onycholysis, oil drop changes, and subungual and proximal hyperkeratosis are seen. There is also proximal nail-fold inflammation with loss of the cuticle, especially of the forefingers. *Courtesy, Marcel C. Pasch, MD.*

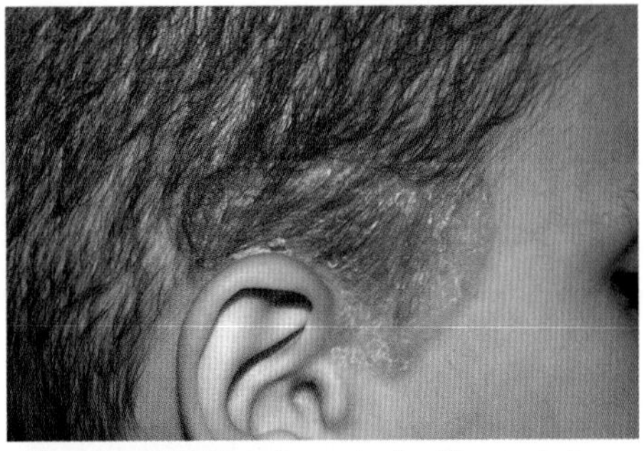

sFig. 6.8 Childhood psoriasis. The scalp is a common site of involvement and psoriasis is distinguished by its sharp demarcation. *Courtesy, Julie V. Schaffer, MD.*

7 Other Papulosquamous Disorders

Parapsoriasis

- Chronic, usually asymptomatic patches or thin plaques with fine scale whose color varies from pink to red-brown; may have associated epidermal atrophy and occasionally poikiloderma (large plaque parapsoriasis).
- Two major forms of parapsoriasis are small plaque (lesions usually <5 cm in diameter) and large plaque (usually >5 cm); digitate dermatosis is a form of the former, whereas retiform parapsoriasis is a variant of the latter (Figs 7.1 and 7.2).
- While the distribution may be limited or more generalized, there is a tendency for an increase in extent over time; large plaque parapsoriasis can favor the sun-protected "girdle" area; both forms usually occur in adults.
- Controversy exists regarding the percentage of cases of large plaque parapsoriasis that eventually evolve into mycosis fungoides.
- Histologically, parakeratosis and nonspecific spongiotic dermatitis is seen in small and large plaque; large plaque may have a more lichenoid infiltrate.
- An infiltrate of $CD4^+$ T lymphocytes, often clonal, in large plaque > small plaque parapsoriasis, leading to the term "clonal dermatitis".
- **DDx:** small plaque – pityriasis rosea (PR), PR-like drug eruption, pityriasis lichenoides chronica, guttate psoriasis, secondary syphilis; large plaque parapsoriasis – patch stage mycosis fungoides (MF), MF-like drug eruption; if a few lesions, consider tinea corporis.
- **Rx:** topical CS, sunlight, phototherapy (e.g. NB-UVB).

Pityriasis Lichenoides et Varioliformis Acuta (PLEVA) and Pityriasis Lichenoides Chronica (PLC)

- PLEVA, also known as Mucha–Habermann disease, and PLC exist along a clinicopathologic spectrum such that patients can have characteristic lesions of both disorders, either concurrently or in tandem.
- In both forms, there are recurrent crops of papules with individual lesions spontaneously resolving over weeks (PLEVA) to months (PLC); only occasionally is there an obvious trigger (e.g. viral infection, medication); the entire course of the disorder can last for years.
- PLEVA occurs more commonly in younger age groups; it is characterized by widespread erythematous papules that are often crusted but may be vesicular or pustular (Fig. 7.3A–C).
- The onset of PLEVA can be abrupt, and recurrences typically occur for months to years; there is an unusual ulcerative form that is accompanied by fever, lymphadenopathy, arthritis, and mucosal involvement.
- PLC is characterized by pink to red-brown papules with scale and can resolve with postinflammatory guttate hypopigmentation (Fig. 7.3D, E).
- Histologically, parakeratosis, an interface dermatitis with necrotic keratinocytes, and extravasation of red blood cells are seen; the infiltrate is composed of T cells that are often monoclonal; in PLEVA, the infiltrate may be wedge-shaped and neutrophils may be seen.
- **DDx:** PLEVA – varicella or other viral exanthem, e.g. coxsackievirus, disseminated zoster without a dermatome (more limited duration), lymphomatoid papulosis (often fewer larger lesions), arthropod reactions, small vessel vasculitis; PLC – small plaque parapsoriasis, pityriasis rosea, secondary syphilis, guttate psoriasis, lichen planus.
- **Rx:** topical CS, prolonged courses of antibiotics (e.g. erythromycin, tetracyclines), phototherapy (e.g. NB-UVB); severe cases may require methotrexate in consultation with a dermatologist.

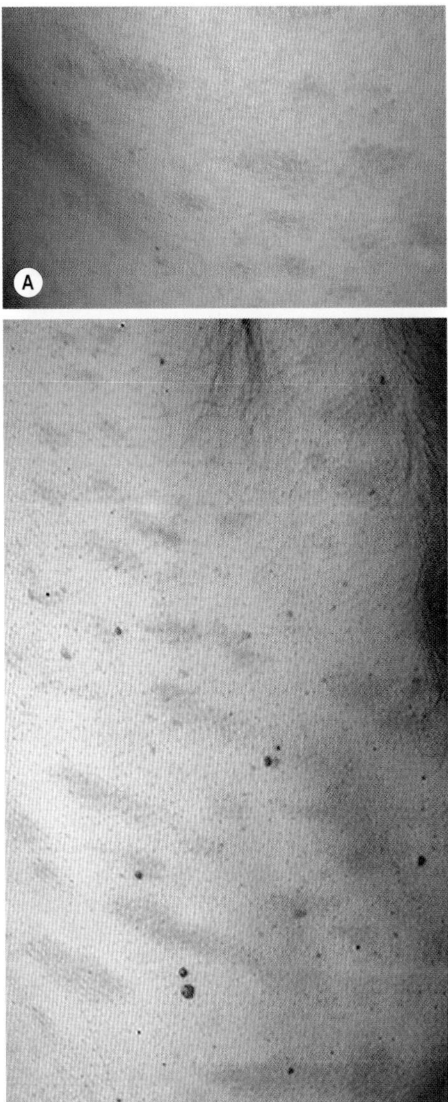

Fig. 7.1 Small plaque parapsoriasis.
A Small (<5 cm), dull pink, slight scaly patches on the trunk. **B** Digitate dermatosis with elongated finger-like lesions on the flank that are pink-brown to yellow-brown in color. Digitate dermatosis is the exception to the 5-cm rule as the lesions may measure 10 cm or more along their long axes. *A, Courtesy, Lorenzo Cerroni, MD; B, Courtesy, Gary Wood, MD, and George Reizner, MD.*

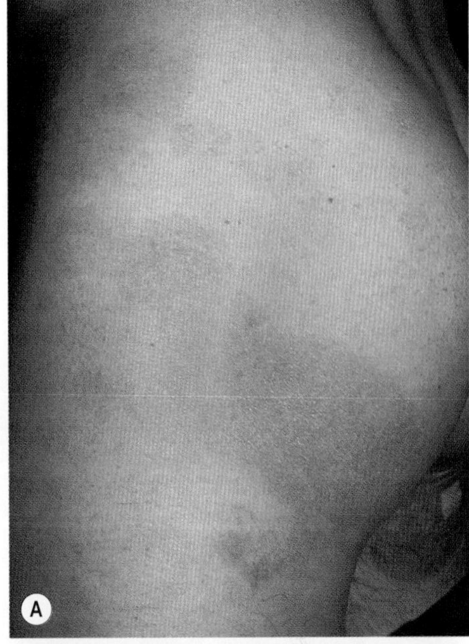

Fig. 7.2 Large plaque parapsoriasis. **A** Large, variably erythematous patches in the bathing trunk region – a classic clinical presentation. **B** Retiform parapsoriasis with pink-brown lesions forming a net-like pattern, hence the term retiform; note the associated wrinkling due to epidermal atrophy. *A, B, Courtesy, YDRSC.*

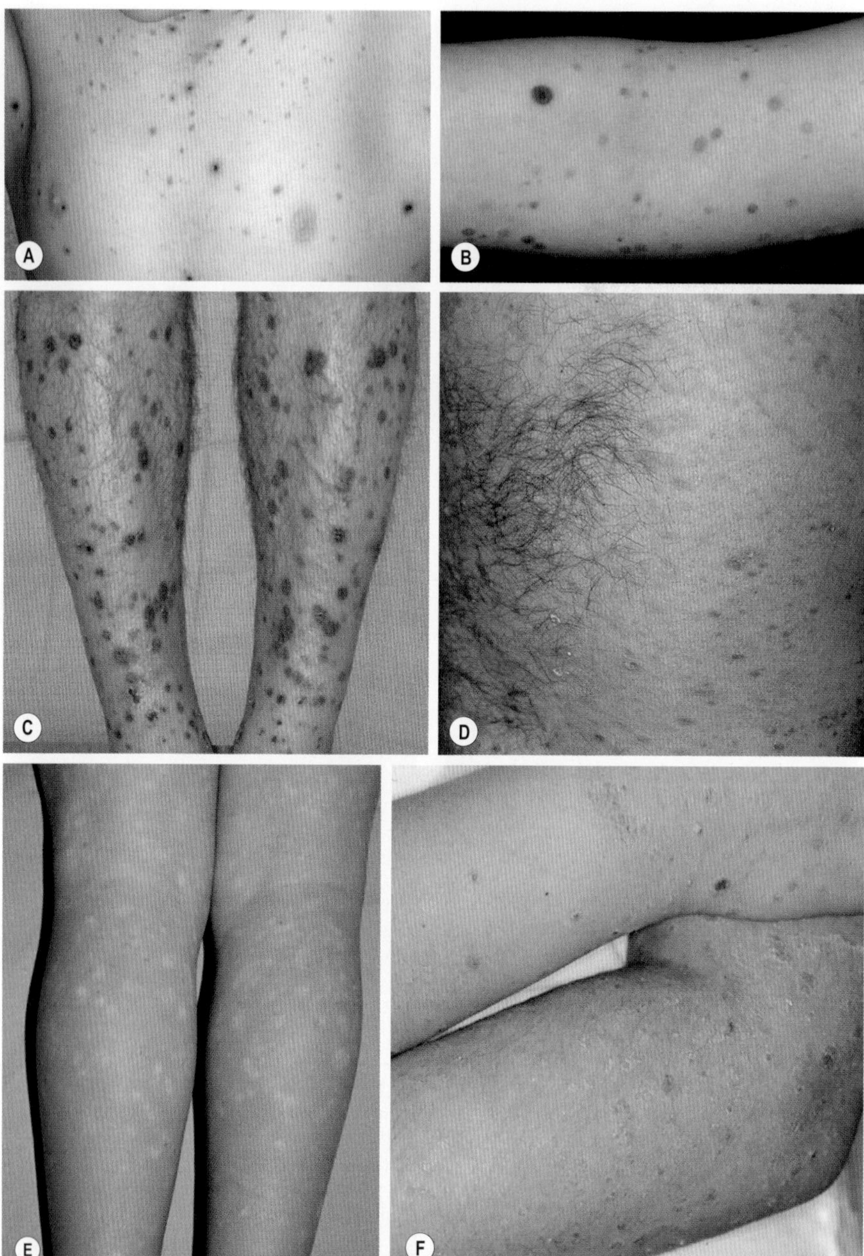

Fig. 7.3 Clinical spectrum of pityriasis lichenoides. In the acute form (PLEVA), widespread erythematous papules and papulovesicles are admixed with crusted lesions **(A, B)**; sometimes there can be an ulcerative component **(C)**. Lesions can heal with varioliform scars. Individuals with the chronic form (PLC) develop multiple red-brown papules, some of which have scale **(D)**; these lesions often heal with hypopigmentation, especially in patients with darkly pigmented skin **(E)**. **F** A number of patients will have lesions characteristic of both PLEVA and PLC. *A, Courtesy, Julie V. Schaffer, MD; B, Courtesy, Thomas Schwarz, MD; C, D, Courtesy, YDRSC; E, Courtesy, Antonio Torrelo, MD; F, Courtesy, Kalman Watsky, MD.*

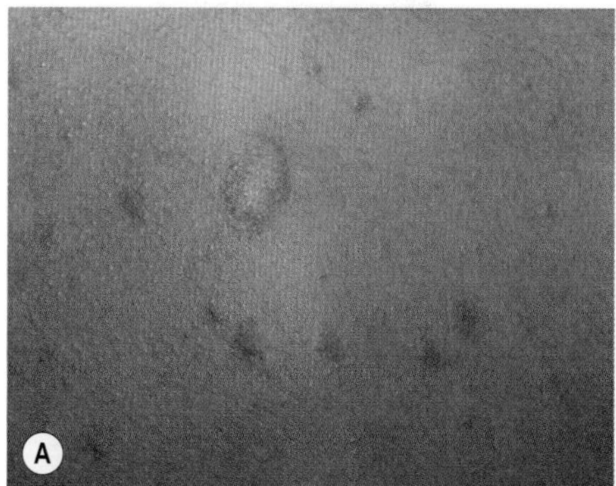

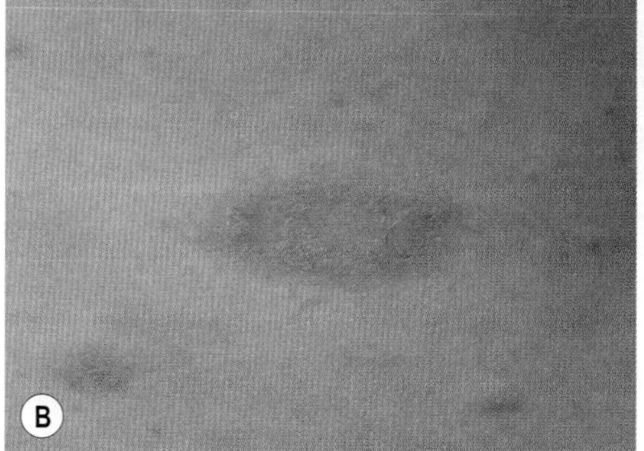

Fig. 7.4 Pityriasis rosea – herald patches in two patients with different skin phototypes. A, B A herald patch typically precedes the development of a more widespread eruption. Either central or peripheral white scale can be seen. *A, Courtesy, Kalman Watsky, MD; B, Used with permission of the Mayo Foundation for Medical Education and Research.*

Pityriasis Rosea

- Occurs more commonly in adolescents and young adults; in general, individuals are healthy and have no systemic complaints/ symptoms (see Table 1.7).
- The etiology is unknown, but viral infections may serve as a trigger.
- Lesions increase in number and extent over a few weeks but then spontaneously resolve; classically, the initial lesion, known as the "herald patch," is often the largest (Fig. 7.4).
- The distribution is that of a 1920s bathing suit – proximal extremities and trunk; occasionally, an inverse pattern is seen in which the majority of lesions are in the axillae and/ or groin (Fig. 7.5).
- Pink to salmon-colored papules or plaques are round or oval in shape (Fig. 7.6), with their long axes following Langer's lines of cleavage (Fig. 7.7), creating a "Christmas tree" pattern on the trunk; scale, both fine white centrally and as a collarette at the edge of the lesion, is the most common secondary change, but occasionally crusting, vesicles, purpura, or even pustules may be seen.

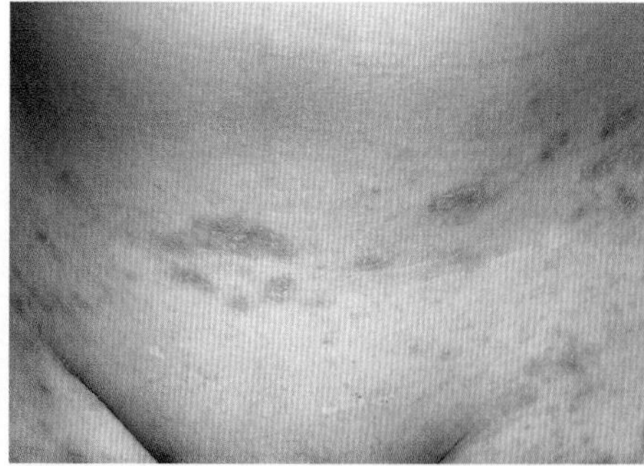

Fig. 7.5 Inverse pityriasis rosea. In this variant, the lesions are limited to the pelvic region and/or axillae. The long axes of the lesions follow the lines of cleavage. *Courtesy, Julie V. Schaffer, MD.*

- The average duration is 6–8 weeks, with some cases lasting for months.
- Histologically, mounds of parakeratosis are seen, accompanied by spongiosis and a mild perivascular and interstitial lymphocytic infiltrate; extravasation of red blood cells may occur.
- **DDx:** guttate psoriasis, secondary syphilis (preceding chancre, usually genital; accompanied by malaise, lymphadenopathy, other mucocutaneous signs such as condylomata lata, palmoplantar lesions; and positive Venereal Disease Research Laboratory [VDRL] or rapid plasma reagin [RPR] test), pityriasis lichenoides chronica (especially if persistent), nummular dermatitis (if vesicular), pityriasis rosea-like drug eruptions (e.g. ACE inhibitors, metronidazole).
- **Rx:** topical anti-pruritic lotions or CS (for the minority of patients with associated pruritus), natural sunlight, 14-day course of erythromycin, 10-day course of azithromycin, NB-UVB.

Pityriasis Rubra Pilaris (PRP)

- One of the dermatologic disorders that can lead to an erythroderma (Fig. 7.8), often with an onset in the head and neck region; peaks of incidence – first to second decade of life and sixth decade of life.

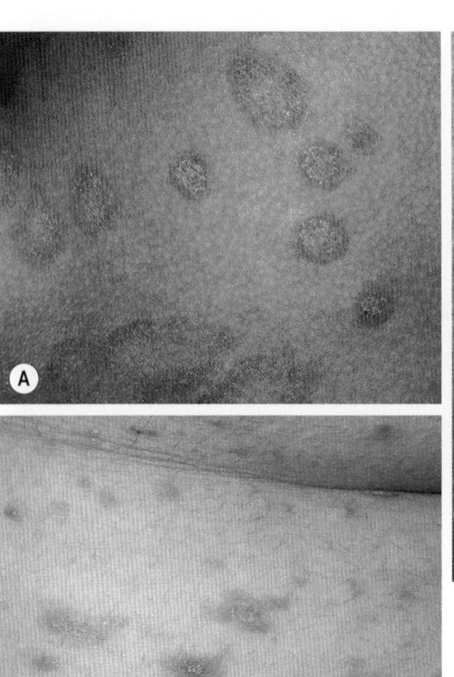

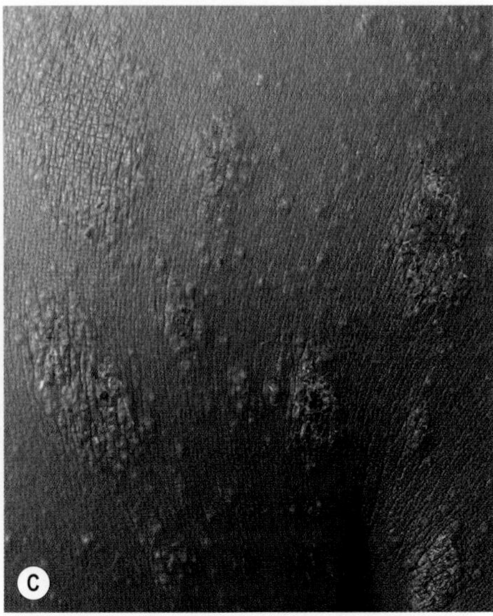

Fig. 7.6 Pityriasis rosea. A, B Both round and oval-shaped plaques can be seen as well as fine white scale and collarettes of scale. **C** In patients with more darkly pigmented skin, central hyperpigmentation can develop and there may be a more follicular pattern. *A, Courtesy, YDRSC; B, Courtesy, Julie V. Schaffer, MD; C, Courtesy, Aisha Sethi, MD.*

LESIONS OF PITYRIASIS ROSEA FOLLOWING THE SKIN TENSION LINES

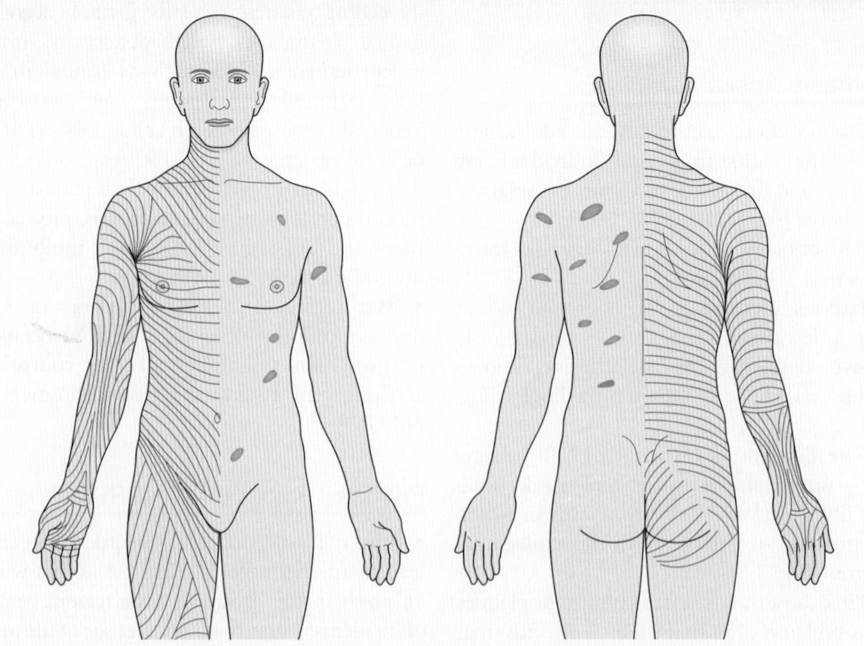

Fig. 7.7 Lesions of pityriasis rosea following the skin tension lines. These lines are often referred to Langer's lines of cleavage. The long axis of the individual lesions aligns with these lines.

- It is characterized by a salmon or orange-red color, islands of sparing, follicular papules (including within the relatively spared areas and on the dorsal fingers), and a waxy keratoderma (Fig. 7.9).
- May be exacerbated by exposure to UV irradiation and rarely triggered by medications (e.g. tyrosine kinase inhibitors); classic forms spontaneously resolve within 3–5 years.
- Five major forms plus an HIV-associated type have been described, with distinctions based on age of onset and distribution, with the adult classic form being the most common (Figs 7.10 and 7.11); occasionally PRP is familial and can be due to *CARD14* mutations.
- Histologically, there is alternating ortho- and parakeratosis, both vertically and horizontally, within the stratum corneum (checkerboard pattern); additional findings are follicular plugging with a shoulder of parakeratosis, acantholysis within the epidermis, and variable inflammation.
- **DDx:** other causes of erythroderma, in particular psoriasis and Sézary syndrome (see Table 8.2), and an unusual form of dermatomyositis seen more often in Asians (Wong type); in children, also progressive symmetric erythrokeratoderma; early on, seborrheic dermatitis.
- **Rx:** oral isotretinion, acetretin, methotrexate, TNF inhibitors (mixed results); response should be seen within 6 months.

Pityriasis Rotunda

- Seen primarily in the Far East, Mediterranean basin, and Africa; favors individuals with darker skin phototypes.
- Large, asymptomatic, circular and polycyclic patches with scale that are often hyperpigmented; the lesions are also well demarcated and lack inflammation clinically, occurring on the trunk and extremities.
- Associated with malnutrition and secondarily with internal malignancies or systemic infections; occasionally, familial, especially in Caucasians.
- Histologically, resembles ichthyosis vulgaris with hyperkeratosis and a reduced granular layer.
- **DDx:** leprosy, large plaque parapsoriasis, tinea corporis, tinea versicolor.

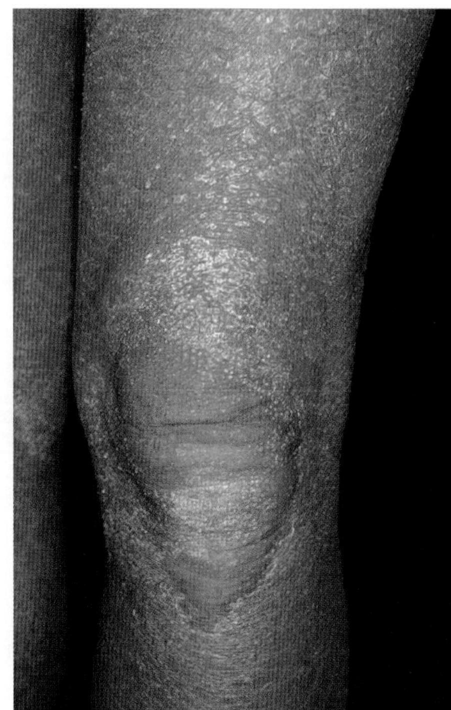

Fig. 7.8 Erythroderma due to pityriasis rubra pilaris. Within areas of erythema, follicular hyperkeratosis (knee) may be more difficult to appreciate than in areas of relative sparing (compare to Fig. 7.9A). *Courtesy, YDRSC.*

Granular Parakeratosis

- Originally described in the axillae of adults (primarily women), but can involve other intertriginous zones and in infants, the diaper area.
- Red-brown plaques with scale, often thick, that may be related to chronic irritation (Fig. 7.12); there may be secondary maceration and pruritus.
- Diagnostic histopathologic findings of marked compact parakeratosis with retained keratohyaline granules within the stratum corneum.
- **DDx:** other causes of intertrigo (e.g. seborrheic dermatitis, inverse psoriasis, candidiasis), irritant or allergic contact dermatitis, erythrasma, Hailey–Hailey disease.
- **Rx:** discontinuation of topical irritants (e.g. mineral salt-containing crystals used as "natural" deodorants, biodegradable diapers), mild topical CS.

For further information see Ch. 9 from *Dermatology, Fourth Edition*.

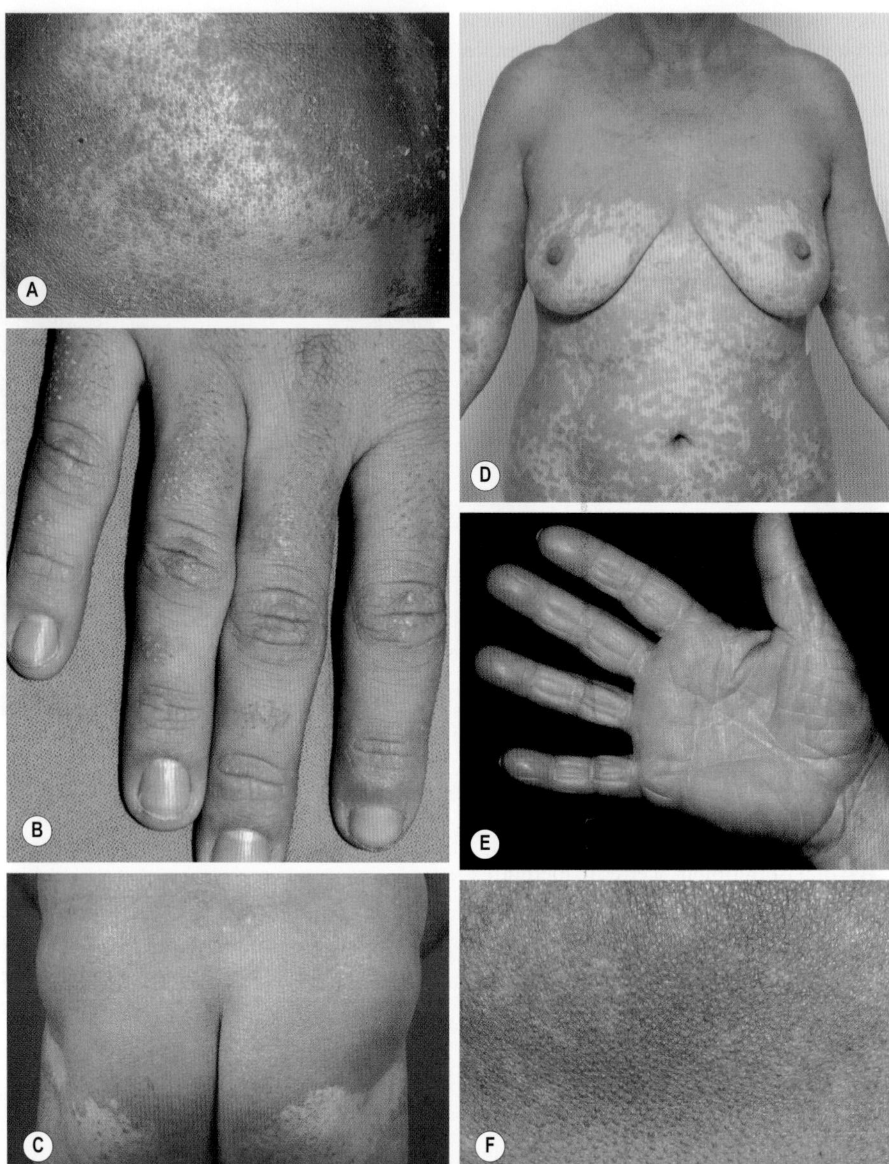

Fig. 7.9 Pityriasis rubra pilaris. A Orange-red follicular papules with coalescence into large scaly plaques, in addition to islands of sparing; follicular hyperkeratosis is often easier to appreciate within the relatively spared islands. **B** On the dorsal aspects of the digits, clustered keratotic follicular papules can resemble a "nutmeg grater". **C, D** The islands of sparing may be rather sharply demarcated; note the salmon color of the plaques. **E** Waxy keratoderma, again with an orange hue. **F** Orange-red keratotic follicular papules. *A, Courtesy, YDRSC; B, Courtesy, Antonio Torrelo, MD; C, Courtesy, NYUDSC; D, Used with permission of the Mayo Foundation for Medical Education and Research; E, F, Courtesy, Luis Requena, MD.*

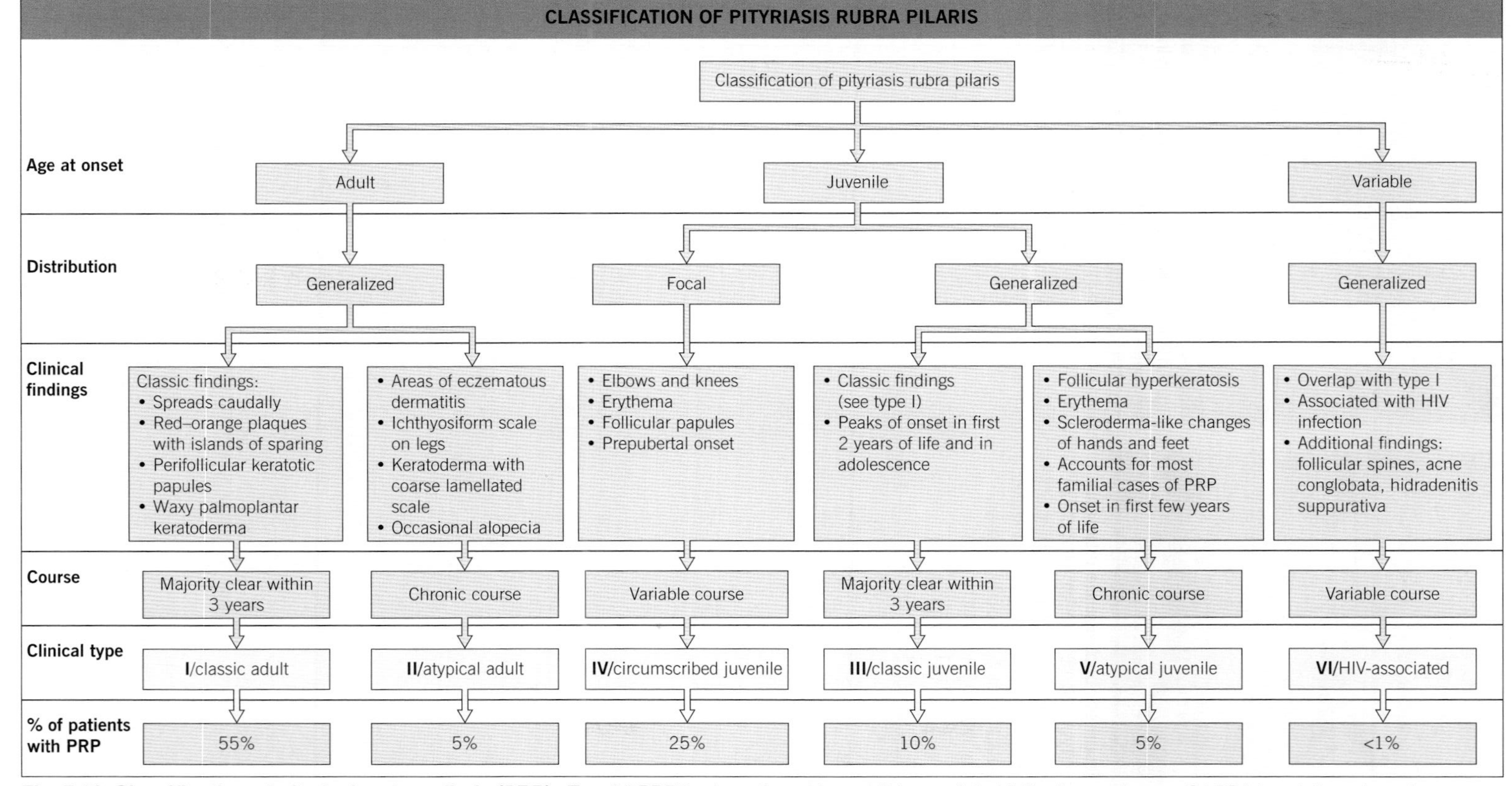

Fig. 7.10 Classification of pityriasis rubra pilaris (PRP). Type VI PRP is also referred to as HIV-associated follicular syndrome. *CARD14* mutations have been detected in patients with familial PRP.

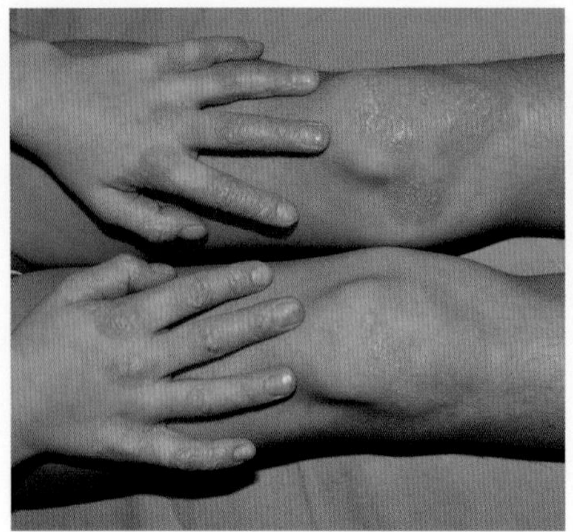

Fig. 7.11 Circumscribed juvenile pityriasis rubra pilaris (type IV). Symmetric pink plaques with scale are present on the dorsal aspect of the fingers, metacarpophalangeal joints, and knees. There are follicular keratotic papules on the knees. *Courtesy, Antonio Torrelo, MD.*

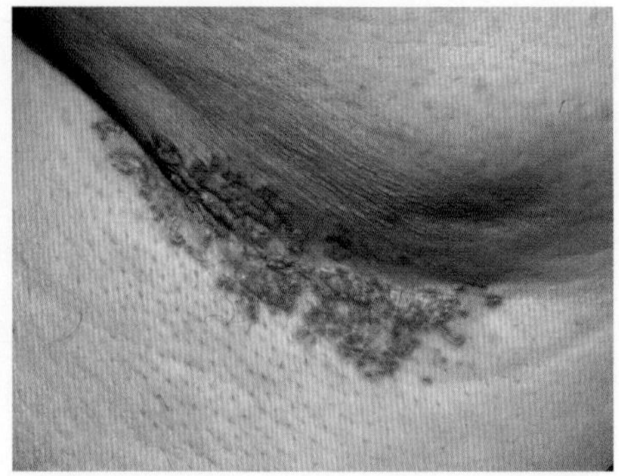

Fig. 7.12 Granular parakeratosis involving the axilla. Coalescing brown papules with hyperkeratosis and slight maceration. *Courtesy, Kalman Watsky, MD.*

Erythroderma 8

• Defined as generalized redness and scaling involving >80–90% of the body surface area (BSA).

• A clinical presentation that can arise from a variety of diseases, often divided into three major categories: (1) primary skin disorders; (2) drug-related (Table 8.1); and (3) malignancies, particularly Sézary syndrome and erythrodermic mycosis fungoides.

• In adults (Table 8.2), the most common primary skin disorders are psoriasis (Fig. 8.1) and atopic dermatitis (Fig. 8.2), with allergic contact dermatitis or pityriasis rubra pilaris (Fig. 8.3) less common.

• In addition to atopic dermatitis, causes in infants and neonates (Table 8.3) include inherited ichthyoses, immunodeficiencies, staphylococcal scalded skin syndrome (SSSS), and seborrheic dermatitis.

• Despite varied etiologies, patients have a number of clinical features in common: generalized erythema and desquamation (scaling) (Fig. 8.6), pruritus with secondary changes (e.g. lichenification), dyspigmentation, eruptive seborrheic keratoses (Fig. 8.7), secondary cutaneous infections, ectropion (Fig. 8.8) and purulent conjunctivitis; additional findings include palmoplantar keratoderma, nail dystrophy and alopecia.

DRUGS ASSOCIATED WITH ERYTHRODERMA	
Common	**Less common***
• Allopurinol • Beta-lactam antibiotics • Carbamazepine/oxcarbazepine • Gold • Phenobarbital • Phenytoins • Sulfasalazine • Sulfonamides** • Zalcitabine	• Captopril/lisinopril • Carboplatin/cisplatin • Checkpoint inhibitors*** • Cytarabine • Cytokines (IL-2/GM-CSF) • Dapsone • Diflunisal • Fluindione • Hydroxychloroquine/chloroquine • Isoniazid • Isotretinoin/acitretin • Lithium • Mercury compounds • Minocycline • Omeprazole/lansoprazole • Ribavirin • Telaprevir • Thalidomide • Tocilizumab • Vancomycin†

**Reference for additional drugs: Litt JZ, Shear NH. Drug Eruption & Reaction Manual, 23rd ed. Boca Raton: CRC Press; 2017.*
***Includes furosemide.*
****Ipilimumab, nivolumab, pembrolizumab.*
†Not to be confused with the infusion reaction due to rapid infusion of vancomycin.

Table 8.1 Drugs associated with erythroderma.

CAUSES OF ERYTHRODERMA IN ADULTS	
Underlying disease	**Major features**
Common	
Psoriasis (Ch. 6) (see Fig. 8.1)	• Pre-existing psoriatic plaques • Often spares face • Nail changes (pits, oil drop, onycholysis) • Subcorneal pustules (pustular psoriasis) • Inflammatory arthritis • Personal or family history of psoriasis • Onset after withdrawal of CS or methotrexate • On a medication that can exacerbate psoriasis (e.g. lithium)
Atopic dermatitis (Ch. 10) (see Fig. 8.2)	• Pre-existing lesions (e.g. in flexures) • Severe pruritus • Lichenification, including eyelids • Prurigo nodularis • Elevated serum IgE, eosinophilia • Personal or family history of atopy • Cataracts, keratoconus
Drug reactions (Ch. 17) (see Table 8.1)	• Often preceded by morbilliform or scarlatiniform exanthem • Typically more abrupt onset • Facial edema • In dependent areas, may become purpuric • No history of skin diseases • Usually resolves within 2–6 weeks after withdrawal of culprit drug; with the possible exception of DRESS/DIHS (see Ch. 17)
Idiopathic erythroderma (see Fig. 8.4)	• Elderly men • Chronic, relapsing • Severe pruritus • Palmoplantar keratoderma • Dermatopathic lymphadenopathy • Consider less commonly associated drugs (Table 8.1) • Continue to re-evaluate for cutaneous T-cell lymphoma
Less common	
Cutaneous T-cell lymphoma (CTCL) (Ch. 98)	• Sézary syndrome more common than erythrodermic mycosis fungoides or other forms of CTCL • Intense pruritus • Deep purple-red hue • Painful fissured keratoderma • Alopecia • Leonine facies • Lymphadenopathy • Elevated $CD4^{+}$:$CD8^{+}$ ratio (blood) • Detection of clonal T-cell population in skin and blood (flow cytometry)
Pityriasis rubra pilaris (Ch. 7) (see Fig. 8.3)	• Cephalocaudal progression • Salmon-colored erythema • Islands of sparing (*nappes claires*) • Waxy keratoderma • Perifollicular keratotic papules • Flare after sun exposure

Table 8.2 Causes of erythroderma in adults. *Continued*

CAUSES OF ERYTHRODERMA IN ADULTS	
Underlying disease	**Major features**
Dermatitis (non-atopic) • Contact (Ch. 12) • Seborrheic (Ch. 11) • Stasis with autosensitization (Ch. 11)	• Pre-existing localized disease • Distribution of initial lesions • Occupation and hobbies • Patch testing • Review oral medications (systemic contact dermatitis)
Rare	
Crusted (Norwegian) scabies (Ch. 71)	• Elderly, infants, immunocompromised • Crusted keratoderma
Chronic actinic dermatitis (Ch. 73)	• Initial lesions in photodistribution • Drug history • UVA, UVB, and visible light phototesting • Photopatch testing
Papuloerythroderma of Ofuji	• Widespread, pruritic, red-brown, flat-topped papules; may become confluent • Sparing of skin folds ("deck chair" sign) • Favors elderly men • May be associated with lymphoma or HIV infection
Paraneoplastic erythroderma	• Fine scaling, melanoerythroderma • Cachexia • Lymphoproliferative disorders (other than Sézary syndrome), including lymphomas and rarely thymomas • In the case of solid-organ malignancies, usually late-stage
Other	
• Hypereosinophilic syndrome (Ch. 20) • Lichen planus • Autoimmune connective tissue disease (dermatomyositis, lupus) • Autoimmune bullous dermatoses (e.g. pemphigus foliaceus [Fig. 8.5]) • Dermatophyte infection • Mastocytosis • GVHD	

Table 8.2 *Continued* **Causes of erythroderma in adults.**

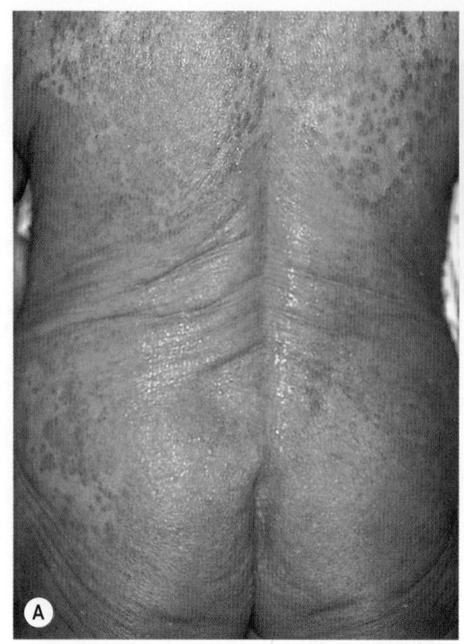

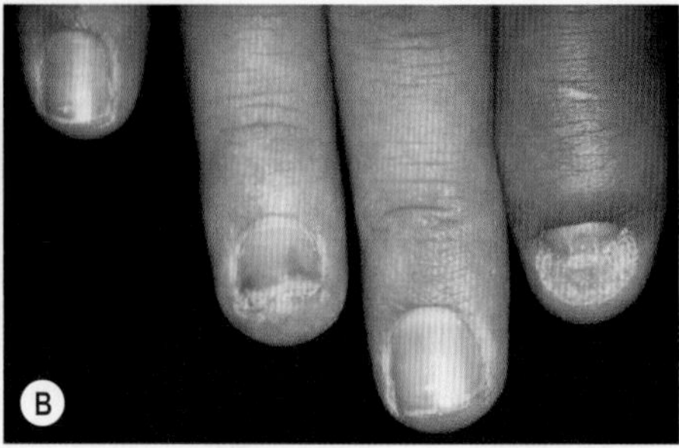

Fig. 8.1 Psoriatic erythroderma. A The disease flare correlated with the administration of lithium. **B** Nail findings (subungual hyperkeratosis, nail plate thickening, and oil-drop changes) point to the diagnosis of psoriasis. There is also soft tissue swelling of the forefinger due to psoriatic arthritis. *A, Courtesy, Jean L. Bolognia, MD; B, Courtesy, Wolfram Sterry, MD.*

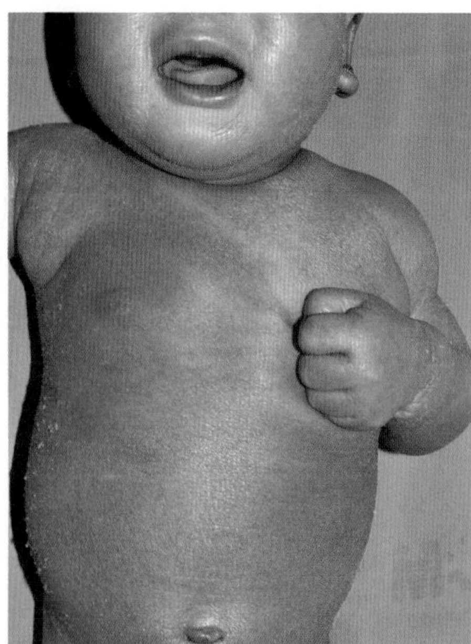

Fig. 8.2 Erythroderma due to atopic dermatitis. Widespread erythema, fine white scaling and obvious pruritus in addition to circumoral pallor in this infant. *Courtesy, Antonio Torrelo, MD.*

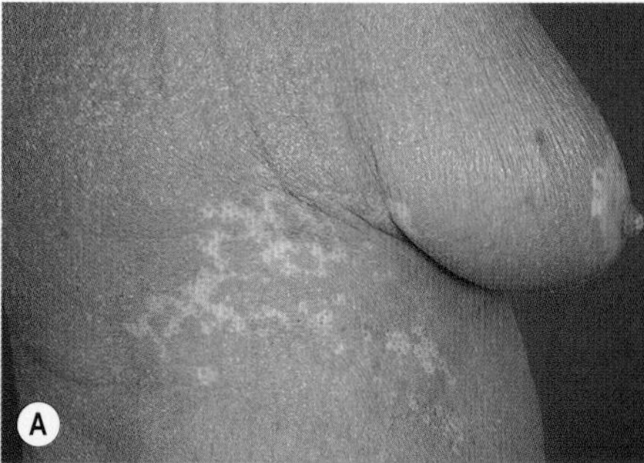

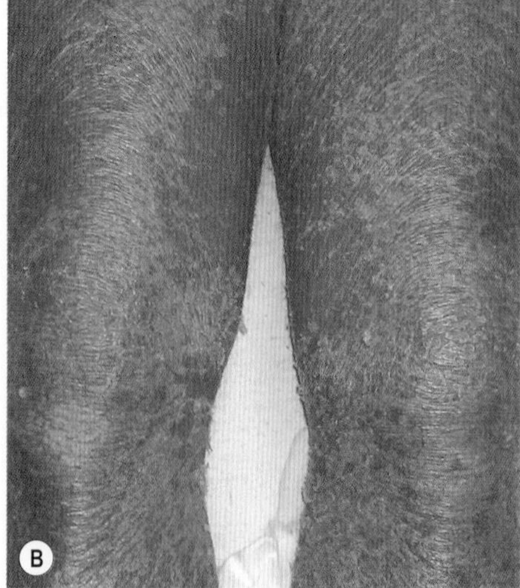

Fig. 8.3 Erythroderma secondary to pityriasis rubra pilaris. A few islands of sparing are noted on the flank and breast **(A)**. **B** Large thin scales are seen as well as the distinctive salmon to orange-red color. *A, Courtesy, NYUDSC; B, Courtesy, YDRSC.*

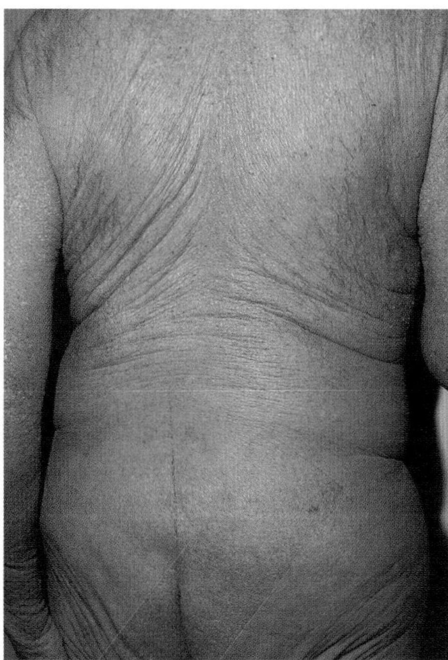

Fig. 8.4 Idiopathic erythroderma. This is the type of patient who requires longitudinal evaluation to exclude the development of cutaneous T-cell lymphoma. *Courtesy, NYUDSC.*

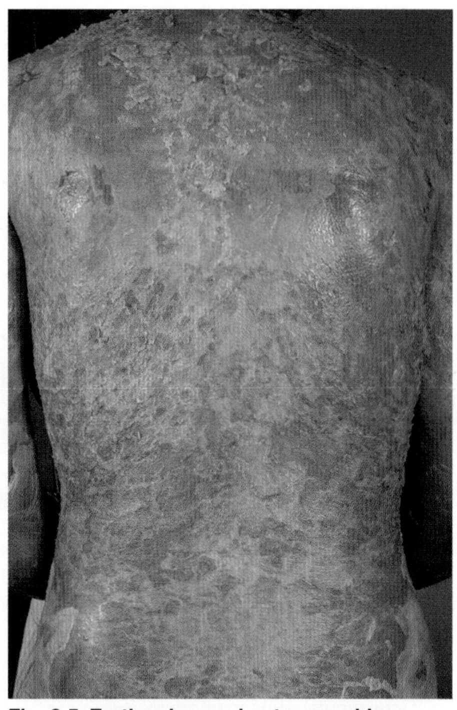

Fig. 8.5 Erythroderma due to pemphigus foliaceus. Generalized erythema with widespread scale-crusts and large areas of erosion. *Courtesy, NYUDSC.*

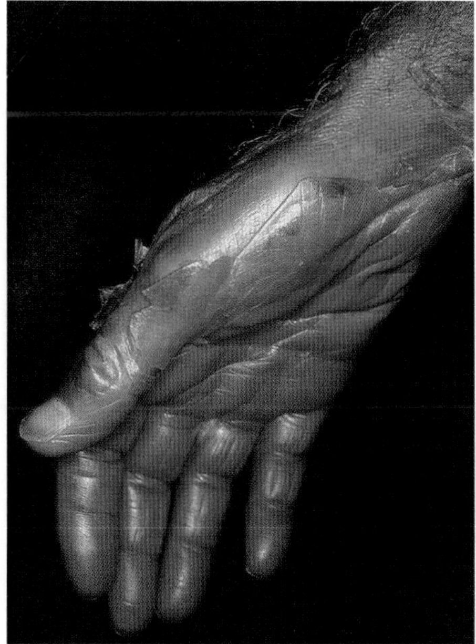

Fig. 8.6 Erythroderma with desquamation. Obvious exfoliation of scale with underlying erythema. *Courtesy, YDRSC.*

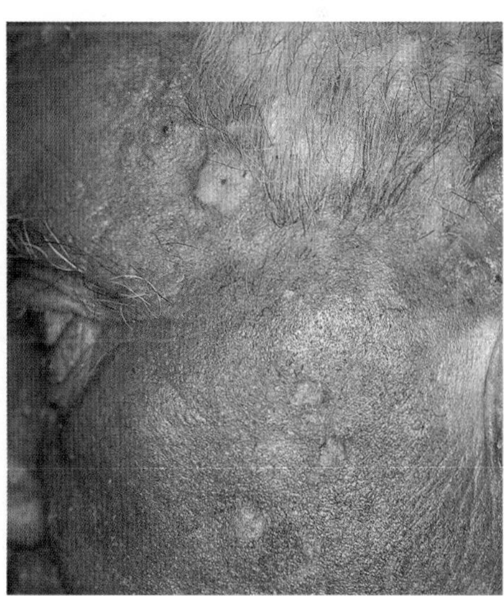

Fig. 8.7 Eruptive seborrheic keratoses in a patient with idiopathic erythroderma. *Courtesy, Jean L. Bolognia, MD.*

CAUSES OF ERYTHRODERMA IN NEONATES AND INFANTS
Inherited ichthyoses (Ch. 46)
• Epidermolytic ichthyosis (bullous congenital ichthyosiform erythroderma) • Congenital ichthyosiform erythroderma (CIE) (non-bullous form) • Netherton syndrome • Conradi–Hünermann–Happle syndrome (X-linked dominant chondrodysplasia punctata)
Immunodeficiencies (Ch. 49)
• Omenn syndrome • Other forms of SCID, agammaglobulinemia, complement deficiencies (e.g. C3, C5), IPEX syndrome • Wiskott–Aldrich syndrome, hyper-IgE syndrome
Primary dermatoses
• Atopic dermatitis • Seborrheic dermatitis • Psoriasis
Drug reactions (see Table 8.1)
Infections
• Staphylococcal scalded skin syndrome (Ch. 61) • Neonatal toxic shock-like exanthematous disease • Congenital cutaneous candidiasis
Other
• Diffuse cutaneous mastocytosis • Pityriasis rubra pilaris (Ch. 7) • GVHD • Rare ichthyoses • Ankyloblepharon, ectodermal dysplasia, and cleft lip/palate (AEC) syndrome (Ch. 52) • Nutritional dermatitis, including kwashiorkor

Table 8.3 Causes of erythroderma in neonates and infants. SCID, severe combined immunodeficiency; IPEX, immune dysregulation, polyendocrinopathy, enteropathy, X-linked.

• In addition to these shared features, more specific clinical findings and initial sites of involvement may suggest the underlying etiology (see Table 8.2).

• Potential systemic complications: generalized lymphadenopathy, edema, tachycardia, high-output cardiac failure, hepatomegaly, thermoregulatory disturbances, compensatory hypermetabolism, cachexia, hypoalbuminemia, and anemia.

• Dx is often challenging because both clinical and histologic features may be nonspecific; repeat clinical examinations, laboratory evaluations, and skin biopsies are often necessary (Fig. 8.9).

• Despite a thorough evaluation, the cause can remain unknown (idiopathic) in up to a third of patients (see Fig. 8.4).

• Some patients with idiopathic erythroderma eventually develop a cutaneous T-cell lymphoma (CTCL).

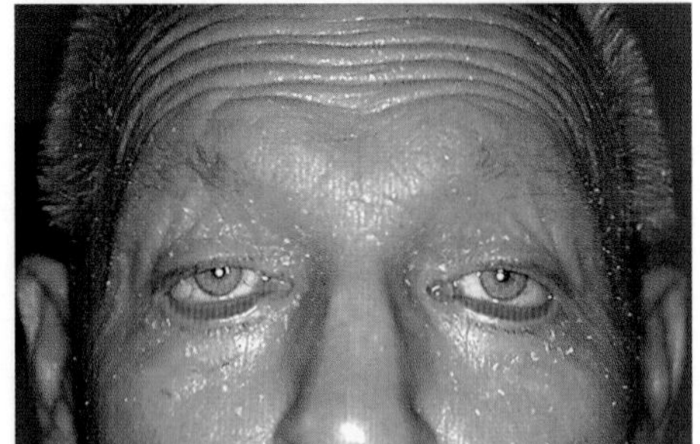

Fig. 8.8 Ectropion in the setting of erythroderma. *Courtesy, YDRSC.*

• Treatment strategies should address the dermatological symptoms, the underlying etiology, and the associated systemic complications (Table 8.4).

• May represent a serious medical threat to the patient and require hospitalization.

GENERAL TREATMENT STRATEGIES FOR ADULT ERYTHRODERMA
General measures
• Consider hospitalization • Nutritional assessment • Correct fluid/electrolyte imbalances • Prevent hypothermia • Treat secondary infections (e.g. *Staphylococcus aureus*) • Oral antihistamines to suppress pruritus (via sedation)
Topical measures
• Open wet dressings (see Appendix) • Bland emollients • Low- to mid-potency topical CS (ointments > creams) • Reserve high-potency topical CS for lichenified areas • Avoid coal tar ointments and anthralin, may aggravate condition
Additional measures
• Treat specific underlying disease, if known • Idiopathic and/or refractory to topical medications and general measures, consider: – Systemic CS (start dose of prednisone: 1 mg/kg/day with maintenance dose of ≤0.5 mg/kg/day with slow taper) – Methotrexate (7.5–10 mg/week) – Cyclosporine (initial dose of 4–5 mg/kg/day with reduction to 1–3 mg/kg/day) – Azathioprine (as dosed for atopic dermatitis; see Ch. 10) – Mycophenolate mofetil • Psoriasis – Avoid systemic CS – Consider methotrexate*, acitretin, cyclosporine, targeted immune modulators ("biologics") • Drug eruptions – Stop offending drug – In severe cases (e.g. DRESS/DIHS), may need to use systemic CS
**May take 4–6 weeks to see any significant improvement.*

Table 8.4 General treatment strategies for adult erythroderma.

For further information see Ch. 10 from *Dermatology, Fourth Edition*.

For additional online figures visit www.expertconsult.com 

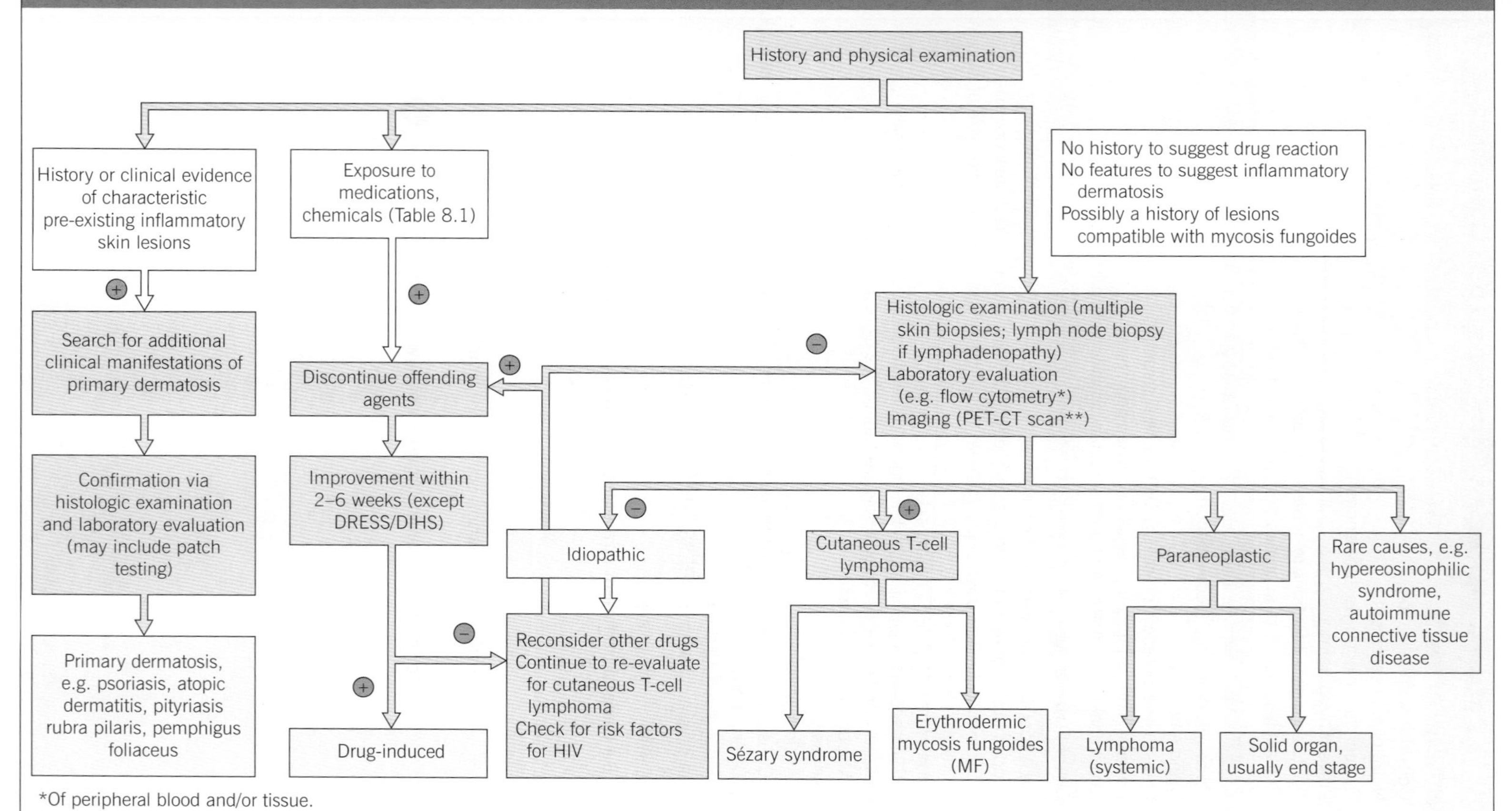

Fig. 8.9 Approach to the differential diagnosis of adult erythroderma. PET, positron emission tomography.

Lichen Planus and Lichenoid Dermatoses

9

Lichen Planus

- Idiopathic disorder that can affect the skin, hair, nails, and/or mucosae (oral, vulvovaginal) and most commonly affects adults.
- May represent a T-cell-mediated autoreactive disorder against keratinocytes whose self-antigens have been altered by trauma or infection (e.g. HCV).
- Flat-topped (lichenoid) papules that are often polygonal in shape and purple in color may coalesce into plaques (Fig. 9.1); lesions usually resolve with hyperpigmentation (Fig. 9.2).
- A characteristic finding is Wickham striae, a network of fine white lines on the surface of papules and plaques (Fig. 9.3).
- The most common cutaneous sites of involvement are the scalp, flexor wrists (Fig. 9.4), forearms, genitalia, distal lower extremities, in particular the shins, and presacral areas.
- There are multiple variants of lichen planus, from exanthematous to hypertrophic (Table 9.1; Figs 9.5 and 9.6).
- Histologically, a band-like infiltrate of lymphocytes is seen in the upper dermis abutting the epidermis, with apoptosis of keratinocytes (Civatte or colloid bodies) and hypergranulosis; the outline of the lower aspect of the epidermis may be sawtooth-like and melanophages are present in the upper dermis.
- **DDx:** lichenoid drug eruption, lupus erythematosus, pityriasis lichenoides chronica, lichen nitidus, GVHD, and a lichenoid "id" reaction due to acute contact dermatitis to nickel (children), as well as the entities in the comments section of Table 9.1.
- **Rx:** topical or intralesional CS, topical calcineurin inhibitors, phototherapy (NB-UVB), and if severe, consider systemic therapy, e.g. oral CS, hydroxychloroquine [scalp disease], acitretin, JAK inhibitors, apremilast. Topical options for oral lichen planus are outlined in Table 59.2.

Lichenoid Drug Eruption

- A drug-induced eruption that has an appearance similar to lichen planus; frequently more generalized or in a photodistribution (e.g. HCTZ-induced [Fig. 9.7]).
- Often a latent period of months after instituting drug.
- Lesions tend to be more eczematous, psoriasiform, or pityriasis rosea-like.

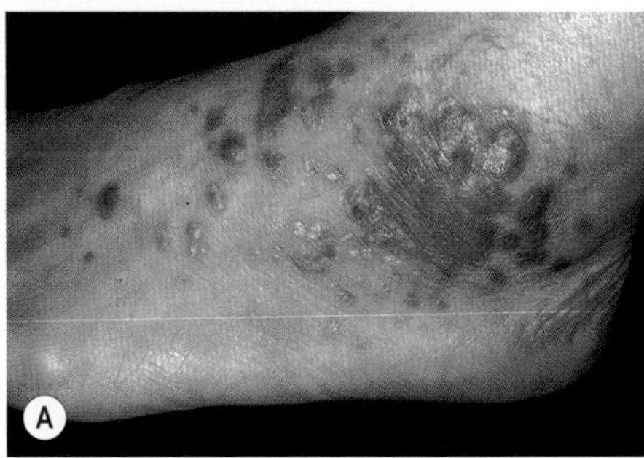

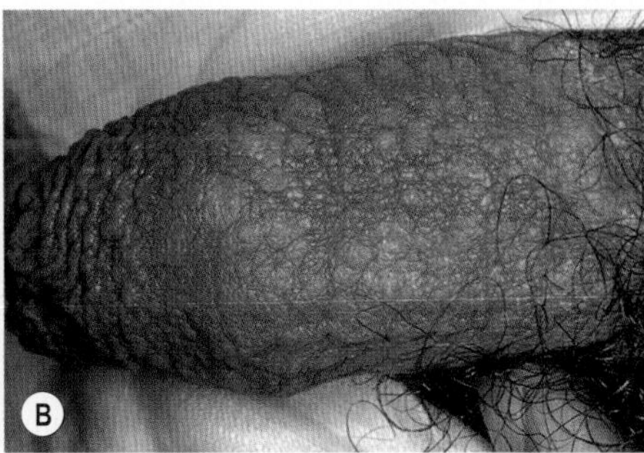

Fig. 9.1 Lichen planus. A Violaceous papules and plaques with white scale and Wickham striae on the dorsal foot. **B** Note the flat-topped (lichenoid) nature of the violaceous papules on the penis.
A, Courtesy, Tetsuo Shiohara, MD. B, Courtesy, Louis A. Fragola, Jr, MD.

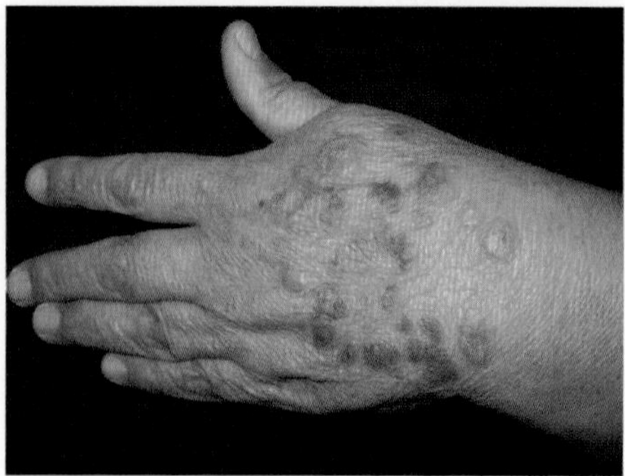

Fig. 9.2 Lichen planus of the dorsal hand. Note the flat-topped nature of the lesions and the postinflammatory hyperpigmentation. *Courtesy, Frank Samarin, MD.*

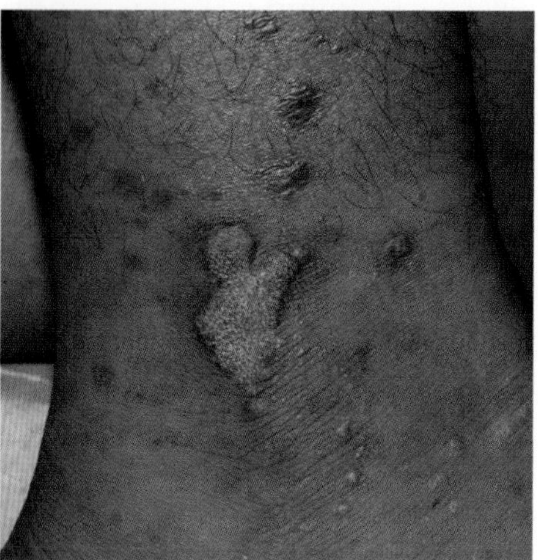

Fig. 9.3 Wickham striae in lichen planus. This patient has a hypertrophic lesion in addition to classic lesions. *Courtesy, Julie V. Schaffer, MD.*

- Most commonly incriminated drugs are angiotensin-converting enzyme (ACE) inhibitors, thiazide diuretics, antimalarials, β-blockers, TNF inhibitors, quinidine and immune checkpoint inhibitors (e.g. nivolumab).
- Despite discontinuation of the offending drug, the eruption may be persistent, requiring treatments employed for lichen planus (e.g. topical corticosteroids).

Lichen Striatus

- Linear array of small, 2–4 mm, flat-topped (lichenoid) papules whose color ranges from skin-colored to pink to tan (i.e. hypopigmented, especially in darkly pigmented patients) (Fig. 9.8).

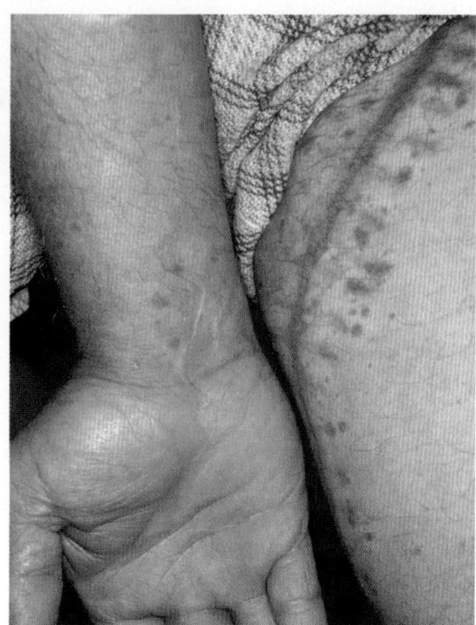

Fig. 9.4 Koebnerization of lichen planus into the site of the excision of the saphenous vein. Lesions also appeared where Steri-Strips™ had been applied. Note the pink to light violet color of the flexor wrist lesions in this lightly pigmented patient. *Courtesy, Robert M. Hartman, MD.*

- Lesions appear over several days to weeks along the lines of Blaschko (see Ch. 51) and are usually asymptomatic.
- Favors children (median age = 2–3 years), with a single streak along one extremity; spontaneously resolves over months to a few years.
- Acral streaks can be associated with nail dystrophy (e.g. onycholysis, splitting).
- No consistently identified trigger and mosaicism for a particular gene not detected to date.
- **DDx:** linear lichen planus, Blaschkitis (multiple streaks; adults; relapsing course; trunk > extremities), subtle or inflamed epidermal nevus > linear GVHD (specific setting), linear porokeratosis, linear psoriasis.
- **Rx:** no specific effective therapy; observation given spontaneous resolution; can try topical corticosteroids or topical calcineurin inhibitors.

Lichen Nitidus

- Multiple, tiny, discrete, flat-topped papules that are uniform in size and usually

VARIANTS OF LICHEN PLANUS		
Type	**Clinical aspects**	**Comments**
Actinic LP	Sun-exposed sites, especially face, neck, dorsal aspect of arms Red-brown annular plaques or melasma-like appearance	Middle East Young adults, children
Acute (exanthematous; eruptive) LP (Fig. 9.5A)	Abrupt onset Widespread distribution	Usually self-limited (3–9 months) Exclude lichenoid drug eruption, pityriasis rosea, secondary syphilis
Annular LP (Fig. 9.5B)	Thin raised border, with hyperpigmented or skin-colored center	Favors axillae, groin/penis, extremities
Atrophic LP (Fig. 9.5C)	Large plaques with epidermal atrophy Later stage of disease	**DDx:** lichen sclerosus Annular variant with loss of elastic fibers centrally
Bullous LP (Fig. 9.5D)	Bullae within pre-existing lesions	Separation of epidermis from dermis with underlying lichenoid lymphocytic infiltrate
Hypertrophic LP (Figs 9.3 & 9.5E)	Favors shins and dorsal feet Thick pruritic plaques with scale Can develop SCC	Average duration – 6 years **DDx:** lichen amyloidosis, LSC, rupioid psoriasis
Inverse LP (Fig. 9.5F)	Violaceous plaques Axillae > inguinal or other major body folds	Overlap with LP pigmentosus as lesions resolve with hyperpigmentation
LP pemphigoides	Variable distribution of vesicobullae, including previously uninvolved skin	Routine histopathology and DIF of bullous lesions – similar to BP; IIF: autoAb to BPAG2
LP pigmentosus (Fig. 9.5G)	Brown to gray-brown macules and patches in sun-exposed areas of the face and neck *or* intertriginous zones Inflammatory phase usually absent	Skin phototypes III and IV Coexisting LP lesions in 20% of patients **DDx:** erythema dyschromicum perstans, resolved inverse LP
Lichen planopilaris (see Ch. 56)	Keratotic plugs within hair follicles with narrow surrounding red to violet-colored rim Hair-bearing sites, especially the scalp	A form of scarring alopecia Variant – frontal fibrosing alopecia (see Ch. 56) **DDx** for scalp: discoid LE
Linear LP (Fig. 9.5H)	Need to distinguish Koebner phenomenon from lesions following lines of Blaschko	See Chs 1 and 51 **DDx:** lichen striatus if along lines of Blaschko
LP/LE overlap	Lesions favor acral sites Overlapping features	Spectrum – from only cutaneous LE to systemic LE
Nail LP (Fig. 9.6A,B); (see Ch. 58)	Lateral thinning, longitudinal ridging, fissuring Dorsal pterygium	Variant – twenty-nail dystrophy (more common in children)
Oral LP (Fig. 9.6C,D)	Reticular form – white lacy lines or circle with short radiating spikes (buccal mucosa) Erosive form* – includes chronic desquamative gingivitis	Patients can have both gingival and vulvovaginal involvement May be associated with HCV infection
Ulcerative LP	Plantar surface > palms	
Vulvovaginal LP (see Ch. 60)	Inner aspects of labia minora Glazed erythema that easily bleeds	**DDx:** lichen sclerosus

**If erosive variant plus lichenoid cutaneous lesions, DDx includes paraneoplastic pemphigus.*

Table 9.1 Variants of lichen planus (LP). AutoAb, autoantibody; BP, bullous pemphigoid; BPAG2, bullous pemphigoid antigen 2 (type XVII collagen); DIF, direct immunofluorescence; HCV, hepatitis C virus; IIF, indirect immunofluorescence; LSC, lichen simplex chronicus.

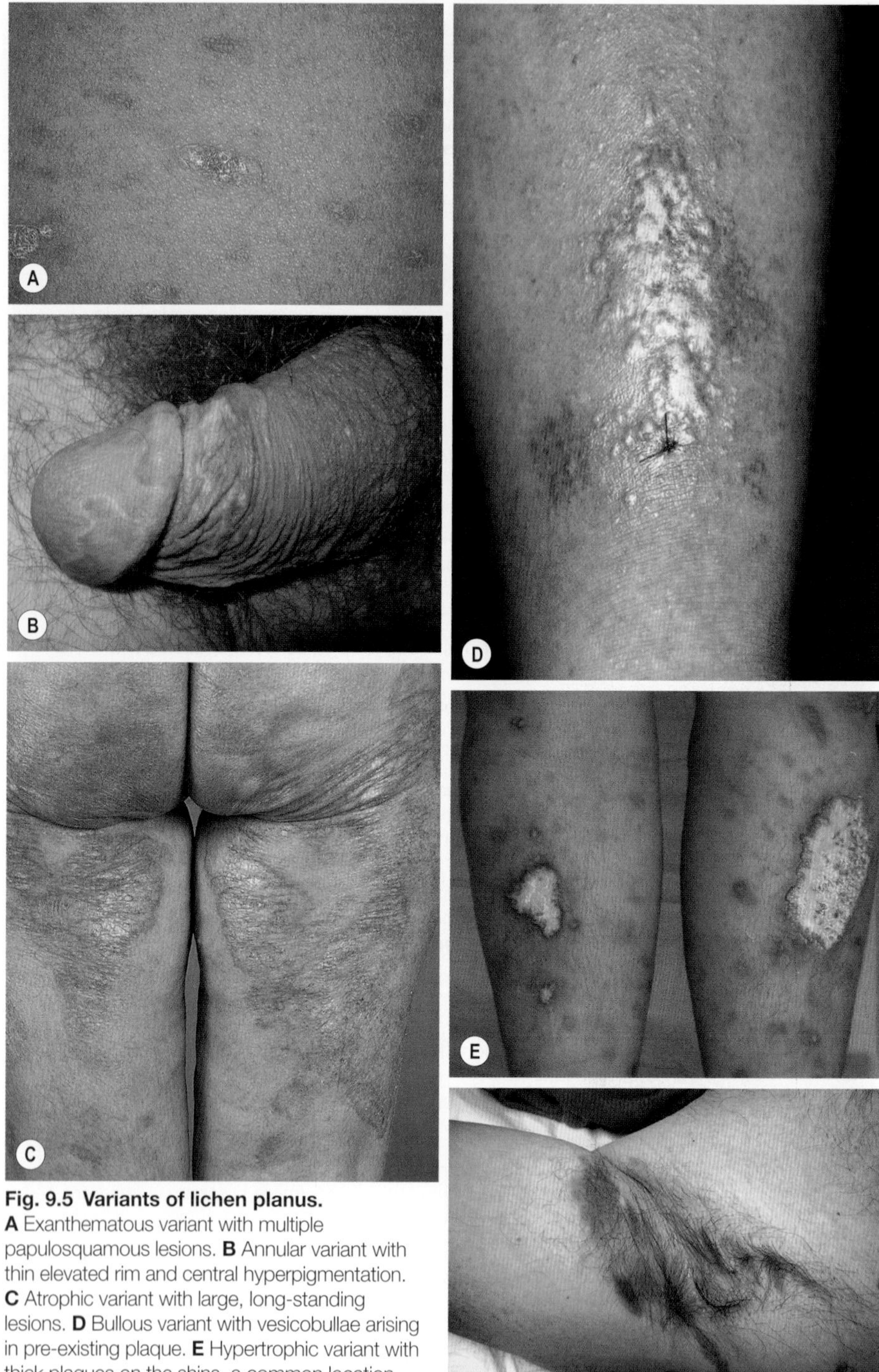

Fig. 9.5 Variants of lichen planus.
A Exanthematous variant with multiple papulosquamous lesions. **B** Annular variant with thin elevated rim and central hyperpigmentation. **C** Atrophic variant with large, long-standing lesions. **D** Bullous variant with vesicobullae arising in pre-existing plaque. **E** Hypertrophic variant with thick plaques on the shins, a common location for this variant. **F** Inverse variant of the axillae; note the purple color. *Continued*

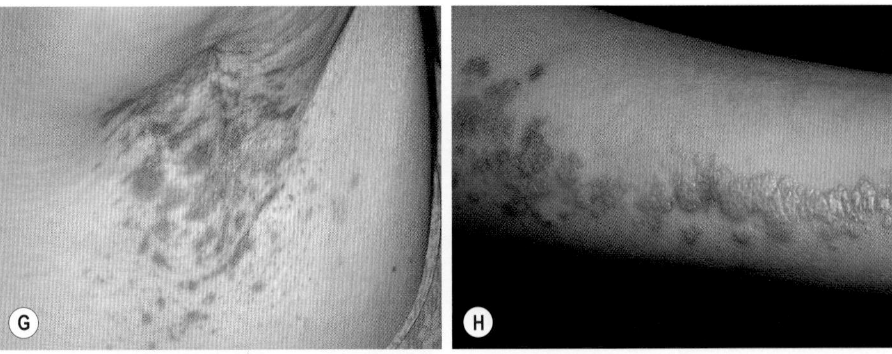

Fig. 9.5, cont'd G Pigmentosus variant with only hyperpigmented lesions in an intertriginous zone. **H** Linear variant with coalescence of violaceous lesions with Wickham striae along the lines of Blaschko on an extremity. Note the postinflammatory hyperpigmentation proximally. *A, D, E, G, Courtesy, YDRSC; B, Courtesy, Frank Samarin, MD; C. Courtesy, NYUDSC; F, Courtesy, Jeffrey Callen, MD; H, Courtesy, Joyce Rico, MD.*

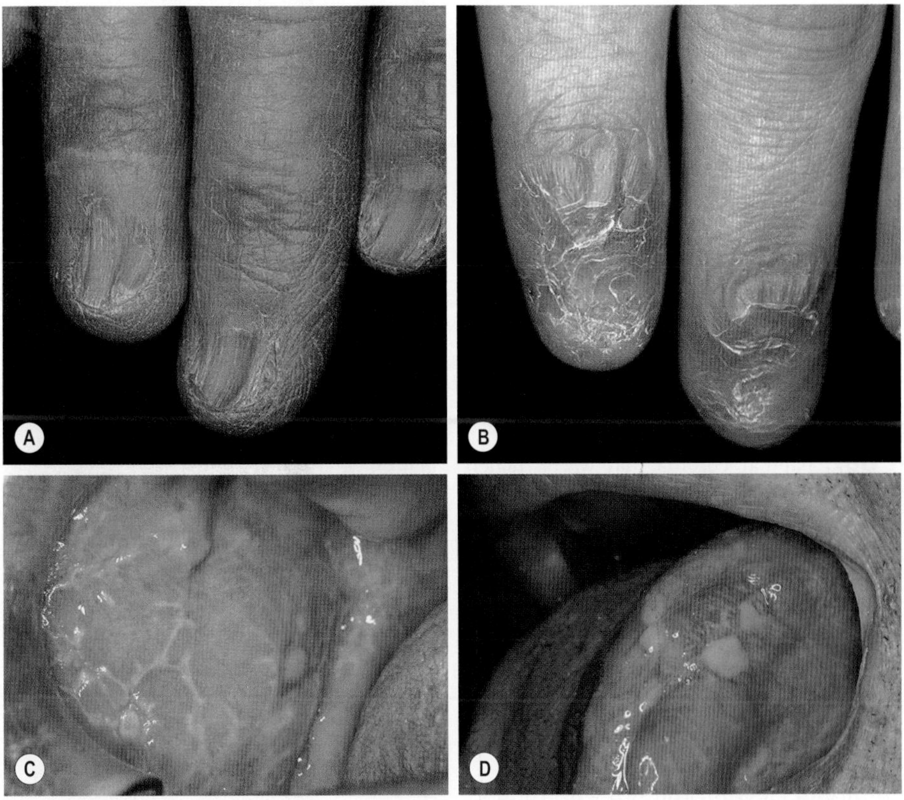

Fig. 9.6 Lichen planus of the nails and oral mucosa. A Thinning of the nail plate with lateral loss. **B** Violaceous discoloration of the periungual area with pterygium formation. **C** Reticular oral form characterized by a white lacy pattern composed of rings with short radiating spikes; there is also an erosion of the buccal mucosa. **D** Erosions, lacy pattern, and scarring of the tongue. *A–C, Courtesy, YDRSC; D, Courtesy, Louis A. Fragola, Jr., MD.*

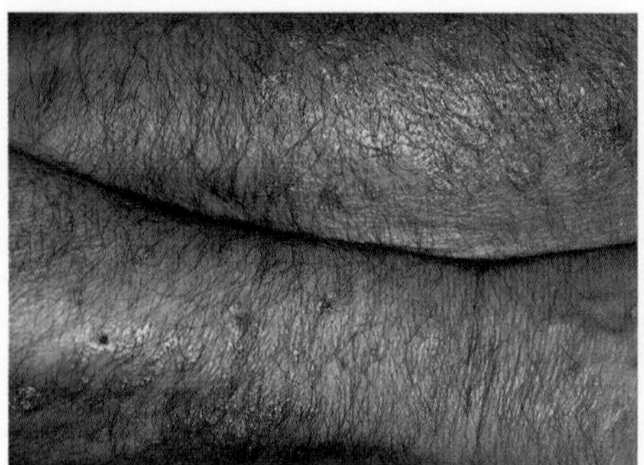

Fig. 9.7 Lichenoid drug eruption in a photodistribution. The patient was taking HCTZ. Note the sparing under the watchband. *Courtesy, YDRSC.*

skin-colored (Fig. 9.9); may occasionally be pink to brown in color or hypopigmented (darkly pigmented individuals).

- Lesions favor the anterior trunk, genitalia, and upper extremities and tend to cluster; variants include vesicular, hemorrhagic, linear, and spiny.
- A linear arrangement of papules may be seen, due to the Koebner phenomenon (Table 9.2).
- No consistently identified trigger and persists for months to years.
- Histologically, characteristic finding of a "ball" consisting of a superficial circumscribed infiltrate of lymphocytes and epithelioid cells (2–3 dermal papillae in width) surrounded by a "claw" of epidermis.
- **DDx:** papular eczema, flat warts, lichen planus, frictional lichenoid dermatitis of the elbows and knees, lichen striatus (when linear), secondary syphilis, lichen spinulosus, lichen scrofulosorum, actinic lichen nitidus (see below).
- **Rx:** no specific effective therapy; can try topical CS or topical calcineurin inhibitors and for extensive disease, phototherapy (e.g. NB-UVB).

Erythema Dyschromicum Perstans (EDP; Ashy Dermatosis)

- Symmetric distribution of multiple oval-shaped gray to gray-brown macules and patches (0.5–2.5 cm; Fig. 9.10); occasionally, a transient thin peripheral rim of erythema is present.

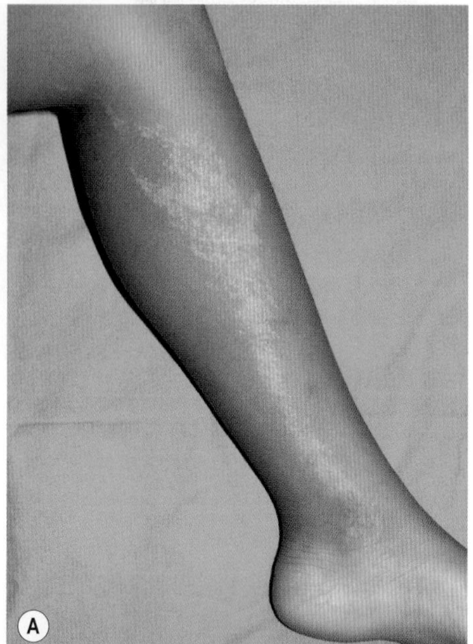

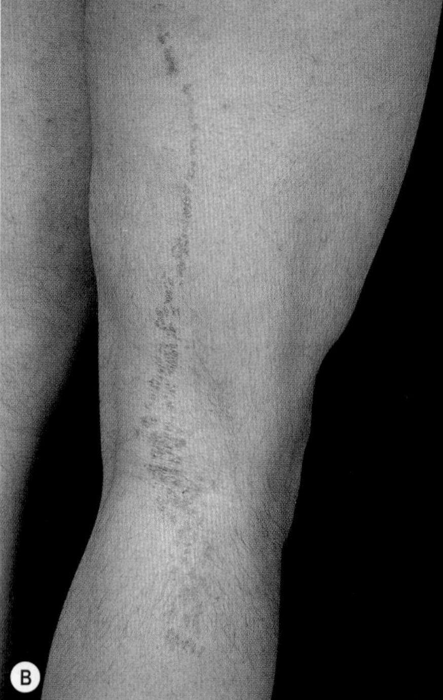

Fig. 9.8 Lichen striatus. A Linear streak on the leg that follows the lines of Blaschko. It is composed of numerous small, tan (hypopigmented), flat-topped papules. **B** Single streak on the posterior lower extremity composed of multiple pink flat-topped papules. The differential diagnosis would include Blaschkitis and linear lichen planus. *A, Courtesy, Antonio Torrelo, MD; B, Courtesy, NYUDSC.*

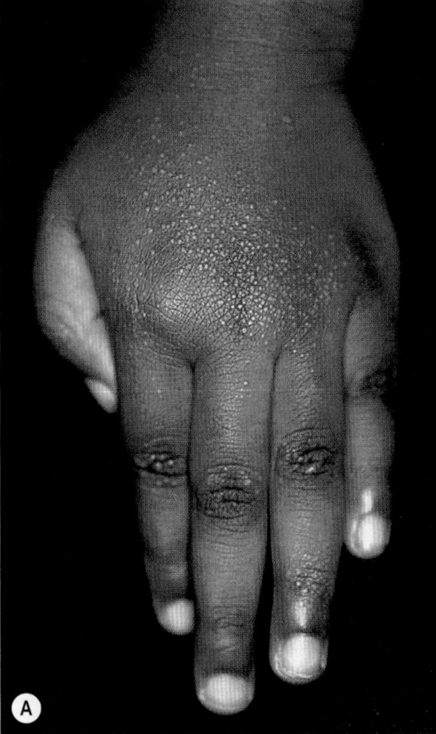

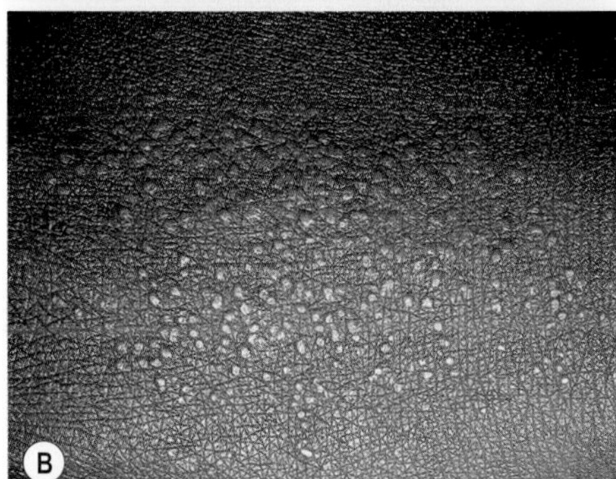

Fig. 9.9 Lichen nitidus. A Numerous tiny flat-topped papules on the hand. **B** A close-up view shows the shiny surface. *Courtesy, YDRSC.*

• Favors neck, trunk, and proximal upper extremities; as in pityriasis rosea, the long axis of lesions often follows skin cleavage lines, i.e. Langer's lines (see Fig. 7.7).

• Slowly progressive, asymptomatic disorder that favors children and young adults, in particular individuals from Latin America with skin phototypes III and IV.

• No consistently identified trigger.

• In children, may resolve after a few years (~70% of patients by 2 or 3 years), but often more chronic in adults.

CLINICAL ENTITIES THAT COMMONLY DISPLAY KOEBNER (ISOMORPHIC) PHENOMENON
• Psoriasis • Vitiligo • Lichen planus • Lichen niditus • Cutaneous small vessel vasculitis • Still disease • Inoculation* – verrucae, mollusca contagiosa
**Sometimes referred to as pseudo-Koebner phenomenon.*

Table 9.2 Clinical entities that commonly display Koebner (isomorphic) phenomenon. This is to be distinguished from Wolf isotopic response in which a second skin disease appears at the site of an initial unrelated and often healed skin disease (e.g. granuloma annulare at site of healed herpes zoster).

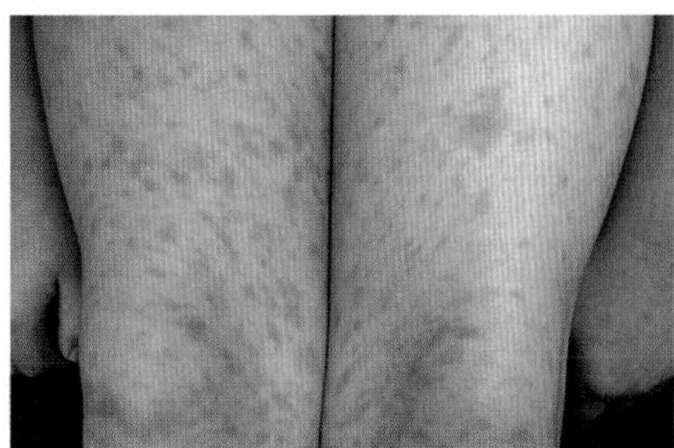

Fig. 9.10 Erythema dyschromicum perstans. Numerous oval to polygonal, gray-brown (ashy-colored) macules on the lower extremities. *Courtesy, Graham Dermatopathology Library Collection, Wake Forest University.*

• Histologically, melanin-containing dermal macrophages (melanophages; incontinent pigment) is predominant finding.

• **DDx:** multiple fixed drug eruption (lesions more circular and browner color), postinflammatory hyperpigmentation (e.g. previous lichenoid drug eruption, pityriasis rosea), lichen planus pigmentosus.

• Idiopathic eruptive macular pigmentation is often considered to be a variant of EDP.

• **Rx:** no specific effective therapy; can try sunscreens and mild topical CS.

Lichen Spinulosus

• Clusters of multiple follicular papules, each containing a keratotic spine.

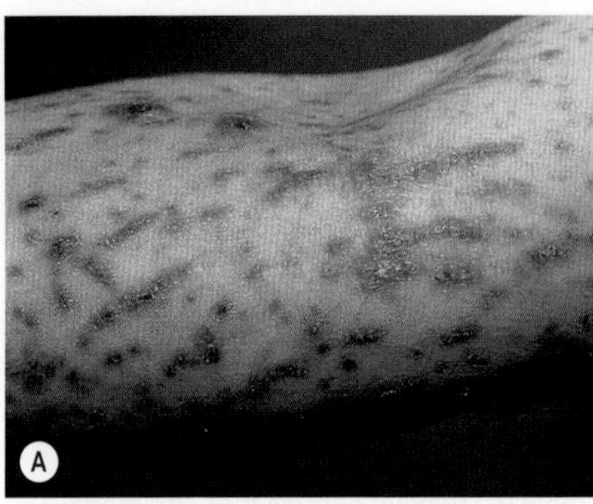

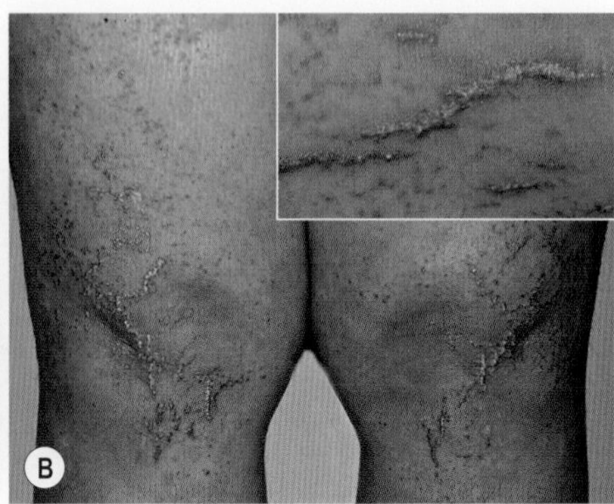

Fig. 9.11 Keratosis lichenoides chronica. A Linear and stellate keratotic plaques. **B** Symmetrical distribution of linear and reticulated keratotic plaques admixed with small violaceous lichenoid papules. *A, Courtesy, YDRSC; B, Courtesy, Kathy Schwarzenberger, MD.*

- Appears abruptly and usually no associated symptoms.
- Favors the neck, extensor arms, abdomen and buttocks of children and adolescents.

Keratosis Lichenoides Chronica

- Violaceous keratotic lichenoid papules are arranged in a linear or reticulated pattern (Fig. 9.11); can resemble Chinese characters.
- Involvement of the limbs and trunk in a symmetric fashion, in addition to facial plaques that may be psoriasiform.
- Tends to be chronic, progressive, and difficult to treat; occasionally responds to phototherapy (NB-UVB or PUVA) ± systemic retinoids.

Actinic Lichen Nitidus (Summertime Actinic Lichenoid Eruption)

- Pinhead-sized papules in sun-exposed sites in young adults with darker skin phototypes (IV, V); histopathologic features similar to lichen nitidus.
- Some clinicians have expanded the clinical spectrum such that it overlaps with actinic lichen planus.

Annular Lichenoid Dermatitis (of Youth)

- Limited number of annular red-brown lesions with central hypopigmentation; they are often 5–15 cm in diameter and favor the groin and flanks.
- More commonly seen in children and young adults.
- **DDx:** inflammatory morphea, mycosis fungoides, inflammatory vitiligo, figurate erythemas.

For further information see Ch. 11 from *Dermatology, Fourth Edition*.

For additional online figures visit www.expertconsult.com 

Atopic Dermatitis 10

Introduction

- Common inflammatory skin disease that affects 10–25% of children and 2–10% of adults in most high-income and some low-income countries.
- Eczematous dermatitis characterized by intense pruritus and a chronic or chronically relapsing course.
- Sequelae often include sleep disturbances, psychological distress, disrupted family dynamics, and impaired functioning at school or work.
- Onset usually in infancy or early childhood, with development in the first year of life in >50% and before 5 years of age in >85% of affected individuals.
- Often accompanied by other atopic disorders such as asthma and allergic rhinoconjunctivitis (hay fever), which develop in an age-dependent sequence referred to as the atopic march (Fig. 10.1).
- Atopy is linked to the presence of allergen-specific serum IgE antibodies, which exist in ~70% of individuals who meet diagnostic criteria for atopic dermatitis (AD) (Table 10.1).
- The "hygiene hypothesis" postulates that decreased exposure to infectious agents in early childhood increases susceptibility to atopic diseases.
- Both a genetic predisposition and environmental triggers (e.g. irritation, epicutaneous sensitization, microbial colonization) have pathogenic roles in AD.
- Loss-of-function variants in the filaggrin gene (*FLG*), which encodes a protein important to epidermal barrier function, represent a major predisposing factor for AD that is present in 20–50% of AD patients of European or Asian descent; these *FLG* variants are also implicated in ichthyosis vulgaris.

Clinical Features and Disease Stages of AD

- Pruritic eczematous lesions are often excoriated and exist on a spectrum of acuity:
  - *Acute lesions*: edematous, erythematous papules and plaques that may have vesiculation, oozing, and crusting (Figs 10.2B and 10.3B, C)
  - *Subacute lesions:* erythematous patches or plaques with scaling and variable crusting (Fig. 10.4A)
  - *Chronic lesions:* thickened plaques with lichenification (increased skin markings) as well as scaling (Figs 10.3A and 10.4B–E)
- Regional variants of AD are depicted in Fig. 10.5.
- Small perifollicular papules (papular eczema) are especially common in patients with darkly pigmented skin (Fig. 10.6).
- Postinflammatory hyper-, hypo-, or (in severe cases) depigmentation may be seen upon resolution of AD lesions (see Fig. 10.8).
- **DDx:** outlined in Table 10.2.
- AD is divided into infantile, childhood, and adolescent/adult stages with characteristic morphologies and distributions (see Figs 10.2 and 10.5).

Infantile AD (Age <2 Years)

- Usually develops after 6 weeks of age and often features acute lesions.
- Frequently begins on the cheeks, forehead, and scalp (see Fig. 10.2); also favors the extensor aspects of the extremities and trunk (see Fig. 10.3A, B).
- The diaper area and central face tend to be spared.

Childhood AD (Age 2–12 Years)

- Lesions are less acute and typically become lichenified.

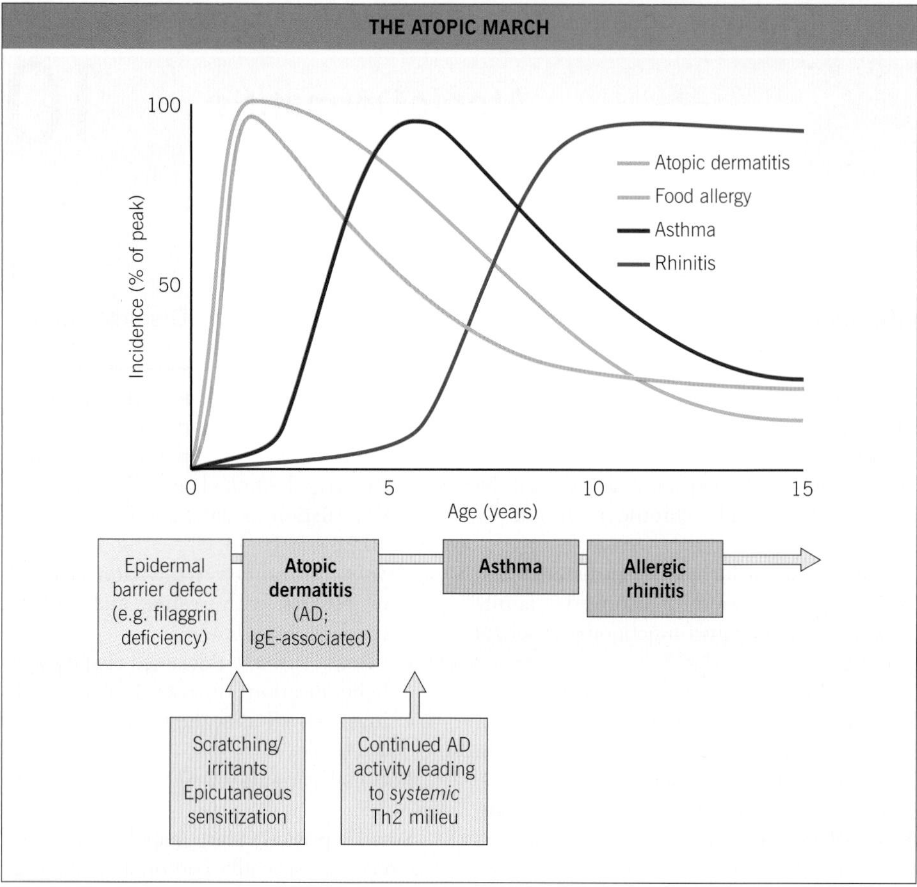

Fig. 10.1 The atopic march.

DIAGNOSTIC FEATURES AND TRIGGERS OF ATOPIC DERMATITIS
Essential features *(must be present and are sufficient for diagnosis)*
• Pruritus – Rubbing or scratching can initiate or exacerbate flares ("the itch that rashes") – Often worse in evening and triggered by exogenous factors (e.g. sweating, rough clothing) • Typical eczematous morphology and age-specific distribution patterns (see text and Figs 10.2 and 10.5) • Chronic or relapsing course
Important features *(seen in most cases, support the diagnosis)*
• Onset during infancy or early childhood • Personal and/or family history of atopy (IgE reactivity) • Xerosis – Dry skin with fine scale in areas *without* clinically apparent inflammation – Often leads to pruritus

Table 10.1 Diagnostic features and triggers of atopic dermatitis (AD). *Continued*

DIAGNOSTIC FEATURES AND TRIGGERS OF ATOPIC DERMATITIS
Associated features *(suggest the diagnosis, but less specific)* (see Figs 10.5 and 10.8)
• Other filaggrin deficiency-associated conditions: keratosis pilaris, hyperlinear palms, and ichthyosis vulgaris (IV; see Ch. 46; ~15% of patients with AD have moderate–severe IV, and >50% of patients with IV have AD) • Follicular prominence, lichenification, and prurigo lesions • Ocular conditions: recurrent conjunctivitis, anterior subcapsular cataract; periorbital changes: pleats, darkening • Other regional findings, e.g. perioral or periauricular dermatitis, pityriasis alba • Atypical vascular responses, e.g. mid facial pallor, white dermographism*, delayed blanch
Triggers
• *Climate:* extremes of temperature (winter or summer), low humidity • *Irritants:* wool/rough fabrics, perspiration, detergents, solvents • *Infections:* cutaneous (e.g. *Staphylococcus aureus*, molluscum contagiosum) or systemic (e.g. URI) • *Environmental allergies:* e.g. to dust mites, pollen, contact allergens; consider patch testing if recalcitrant AD, especially if in an atypical distribution • *Food allergies:* – Trigger in small minority of AD patients, e.g. 10–30% of those with moderate to severe, refractory AD – Common allergens: egg (most often linked to AD exacerbation), milk, peanuts/tree nuts, (shell)fish, soy, wheat – Limited food allergy testing is recommended in children <5 years of age who have moderate to severe AD with: (1) persistent activity despite optimized management; or (2) a history of an immediate allergic reaction after ingesting a particular food – Introduction of peanut-containing foods as early as 4–6 months of age is recommended to reduce risk of peanut allergy in infants with AD; prior peanut-specific IgE and/or skin prick testing should be performed in those with severe AD or egg allergy – Detection of allergen-specific IgE (via blood and skin-prick tests) does *not* necessarily mean that allergy is triggering the patient's AD; when relevant food allergens are identified and avoided, skin-directed AD therapy is still important

**Stroking the skin leads to a white streak that reflects excessive vasoconstriction.*

Table 10.1 *Continued* **Diagnostic features and triggers of atopic dermatitis (AD).**

DIFFERENTIAL DIAGNOSIS OF ATOPIC DERMATITIS		
Chronic dermatoses		
C	Seborrheic dermatitis	Common (especially in infants)
B	Contact dermatitis (allergic* or irritant)	Common
B	Psoriasis (especially palmoplantar)	Common
A>C	Nummular eczema	Uncommon (although nummular lesions can be seen in AD, true nummular eczema is uncommon)
A	Asteatotic eczema	Common
B	Lichen simplex chronicus	Common
Infections and infestations		
B	Scabies	Common
B	Dermatophytosis*	Common
B	Impetigo	Especially for nummular lesions
Primary immunodeficiencies e.g. hyper-IgE and Wiskott–Aldrich syndromes (C)		
Malignancies e.g. mycosis fungoides, Sézary syndrome (A > C)		
Genetic/metabolic disorders e.g. Netherton syndrome, ectodermal dysplasias		
Autoimmune disorders e.g. dermatitis herpetiformis, pemphigus foliaceus, dermatomyositis		
Other e.g. keratosis pilaris, photoallergic drug eruptions, eczematous drug eruptions**		

**Common causes of autosensitization dermatitis (id reaction).*
***Although drug eruptions are common, those resembling AD are uncommon.*

Table 10.2 Differential diagnosis of atopic dermatitis (AD). A, adults; B, both; C, children/infants.

INFANTILE ATOPIC DERMATITIS

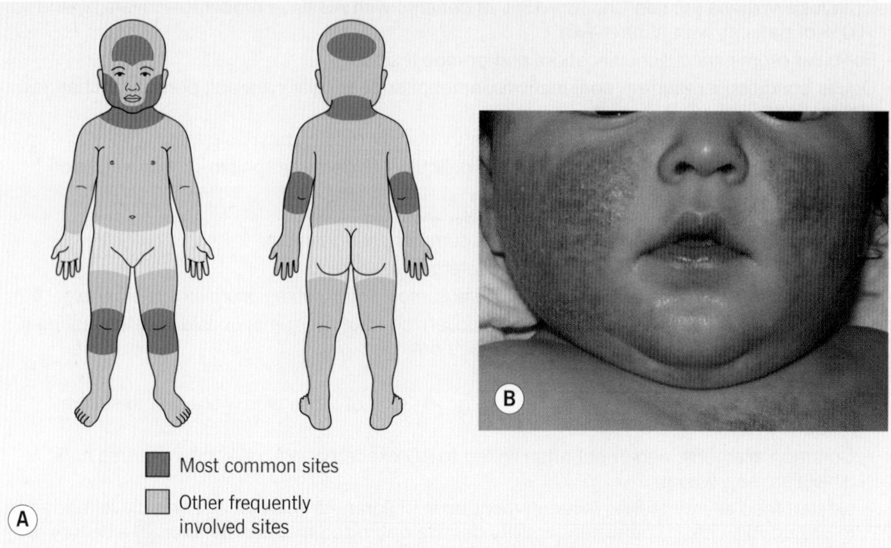

Fig. 10.2 Infantile atopic dermatitis. A Distribution pattern of infantile atopic dermatitis. **B** Erythema and scale-crust on the cheeks, with sparing of the central face.

• Favors the antecubital and popliteal fossae (flexural eczema), wrists/ankles, hands/feet, neck, and periorificial regions of the face (see Figs 10.4 and 10.5).
• Often associated with widespread xerosis.
• ≥50% of children with AD go into remission by 12 years of age.

Adolescent/Adult AD (Age >12 Years)

• Subacute to chronic, lichenified lesions with distribution similar to childhood AD.
• Some patients have chronic involvement limited to a particular site, e.g. the hands or face (especially the eyelids) (Fig. 10.7; see Fig. 10.5).
• Chronic papular lesions may develop due to habitual scratching or rubbing (see Fig. 10.6).
• More often extensive or even erythrodermic if continuous since childhood.

Associated Features of AD

• Figs 10.8 and 10.9 present findings that are frequently associated with AD.

Keratosis Pilaris

• Affects >40% of patients with AD and ~15% of the general population.
• Onset typically in childhood; may improve after puberty (especially facial involvement).
• Affects the lateral aspect of the upper arms, thighs, and lateral cheeks (especially in children); the trunk and distal extremities are much less common sites.
• Keratotic follicular papules, often with a rim of erythema (see Fig. 10.9A) or (especially on the cheeks) a background of patchy erythema.
• *Keratosis pilaris rubra* (KPR) has prominent, confluent background erythema (see Fig. 10.9B).
• *Keratosis pilaris atrophicans* is a rare atrophic variant that favors the lateral eyebrows.
• Keratolytic agents (e.g. lactic, glycolic, or salicylic acid) and topical retinoids are sometimes used to decrease the hyperkeratotic component, but the benefit is limited and irritation can occur, especially in AD patients.

Pityriasis Alba

• Common in children/adolescents, especially those with AD and tan or darkly pigmented skin.
• Ill-defined hypopigmented macules and patches (usually 0.5–3 cm) with subtle fine scaling.
• Located on face (especially cheeks) (see Fig. 10.9C) > shoulders and arms.

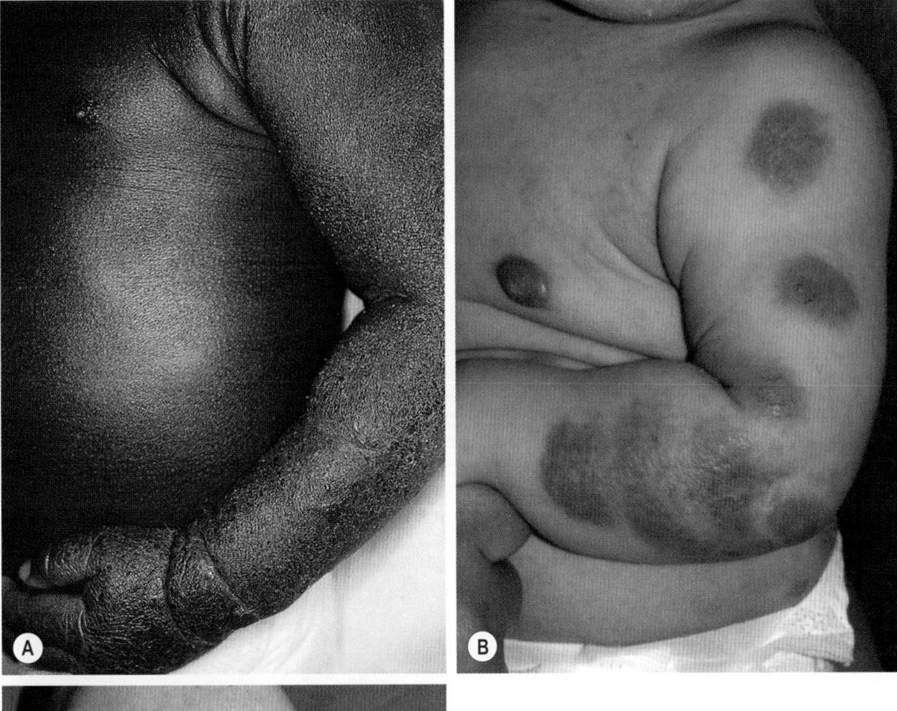

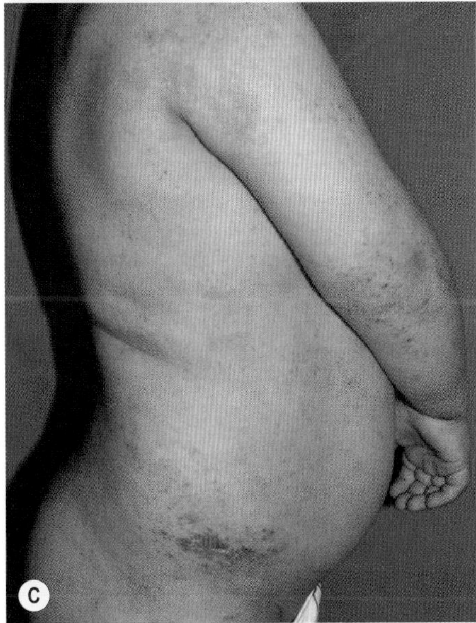

Fig. 10.3 Extensive atopic dermatitis (AD). **A** AD on the extensor surface of an infant's arm, which is a common site in this age group. Note the follicular prominence on the trunk. **B** Nummular lesions on the extensor aspect of the arm in an infant with widespread AD. Note the nipple eczema. **C** Widespread AD in a young child with excoriations, crusting, and lichenification. *A, Courtesy, YDRSC; B, Courtesy, Julie V. Schaffer, MD; C, Courtesy, Maeve McAleer, MD, Grainne O'Regan, MD, and Alan Irvine, MD.*

• Represents a low-grade eczematous dermatitis with postinflammatory hypopigmentation as the primary clinical manifestation.

• **DDx:** postinflammatory hypopigmentation (e.g. from AD, psoriasis, or pityriasis lichenoides chronica; usually also extrafacial lesions), tinea versicolor (individual lesions more sharply demarcated and smaller), vitiligo (depigmented).

• **Rx:** regular use of sunscreens may make pityriasis alba less noticeable.

Complications of AD

• An impaired skin barrier and modified immune milieu predispose AD patients to cutaneous infections.

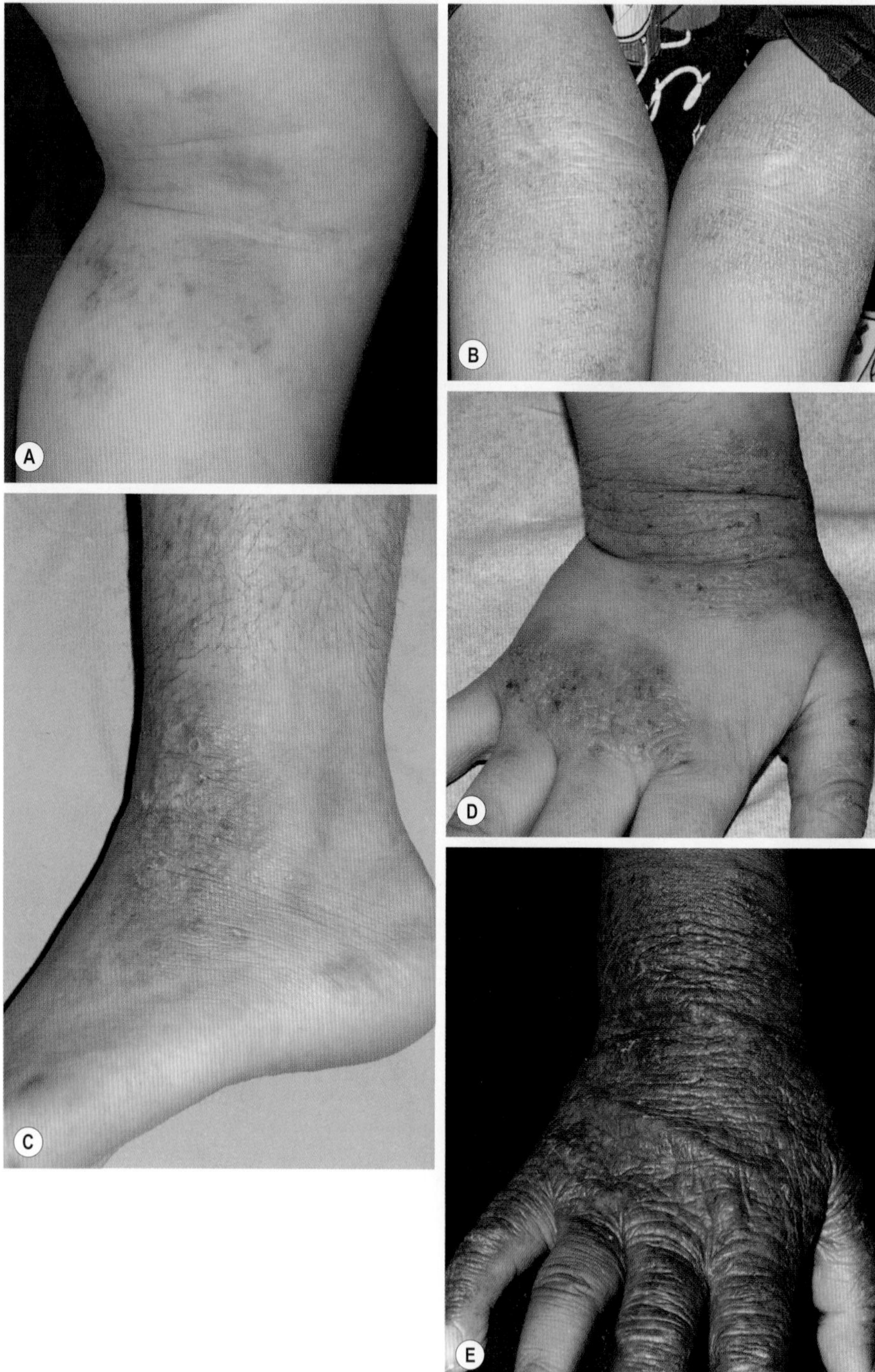

Fig. 10.4 Childhood atopic dermatitis. **A** Flexural eczema in the popliteal fossa with excoriations and hemorrhagic crusting. **B** Lichenification, scale, and punctate excoriations in the antecubital fossae. **C** Coalescing papules and lichenification on the ankle due to chronic scratching and rubbing. **D, E** Thick eczematous plaques with excoriations (**D**) and marked lichenification (**E**) on the dorsal hand and wrist. *A, B, D, E, Courtesy, Julie V Schaffer, MD; C, Courtesy, Antonio Torrelo, MD.*

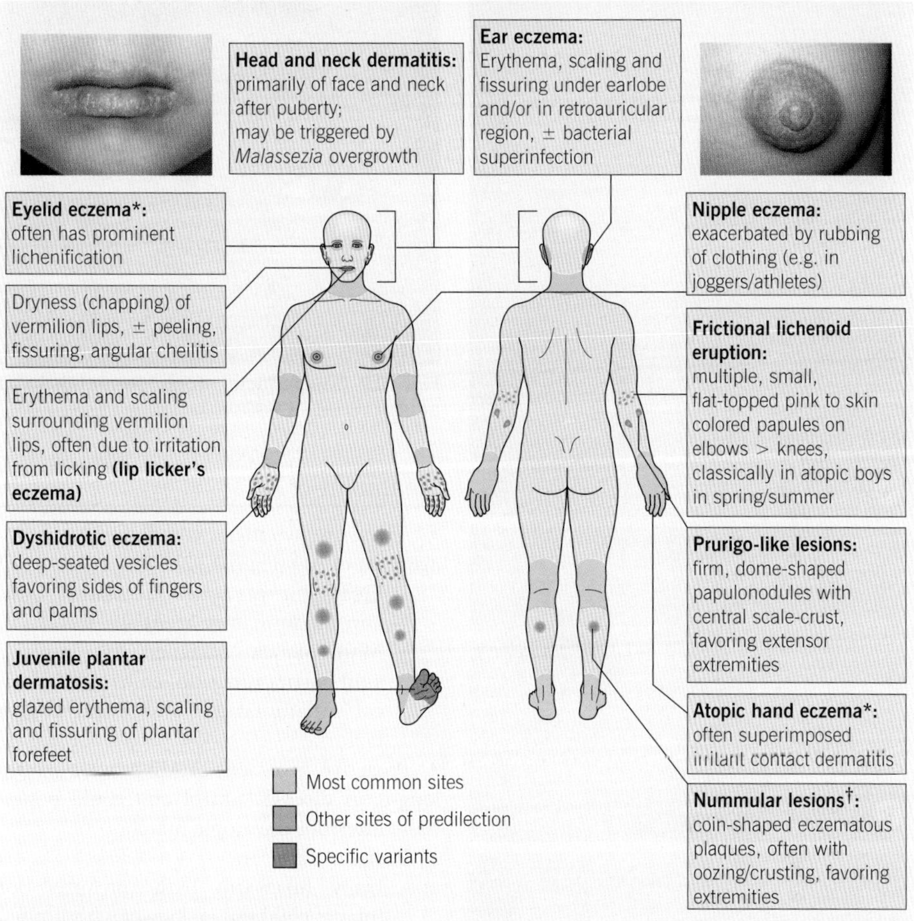

Fig. 10.5 Childhood and adolescent atopic dermatitis (AD): distribution patterns and regional variants.

- Affected skin is usually colonized by *Staphylococcus aureus*, and impetiginization (which can also result from *Streptococcus pyogenes*) (Fig. 10.10), folliculitis, and furunculosis frequently occur.
- Eczema herpeticum typically presents with rapid development of numerous monomorphic, punched-out erosions with hemorrhagic crusting (Fig. 10.11); vesicles may or may not be evident.
- Molluscum contagiosum infections result in an increased number of lesions, usually with associated dermatitis (see Ch. 68).
- Potential ocular complications of AD are listed in Table 10.1.

Triggers and Prevention of AD

- Multiple environmental and psychological factors can trigger or exacerbate AD (see Table 10.1).
- Avoidance of relevant triggers represents an important consideration in AD management.
- Administration of probiotics/prebiotics to pregnant mothers and infants may potentially help to prevent AD onset in high-risk individuals.

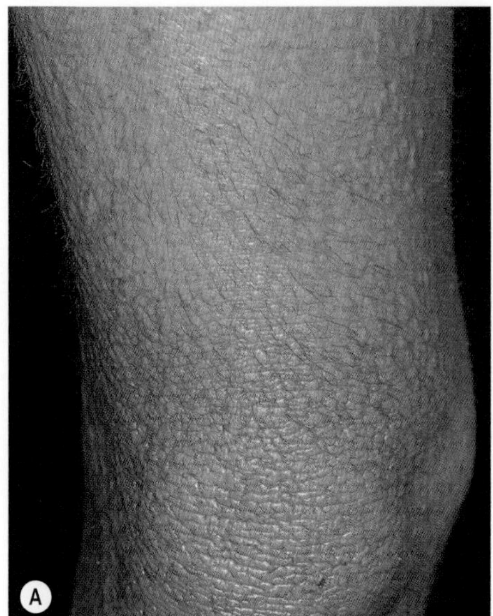

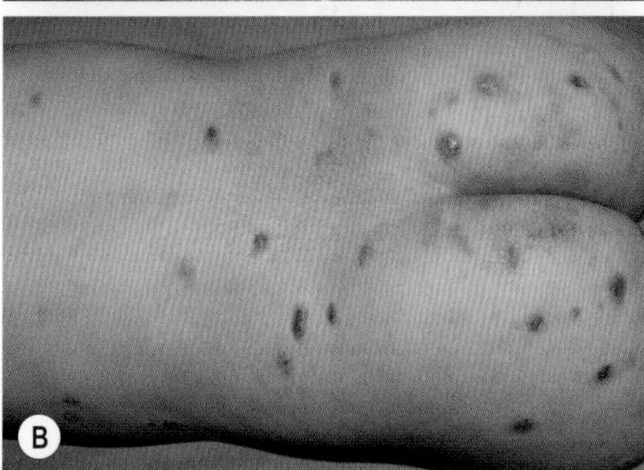

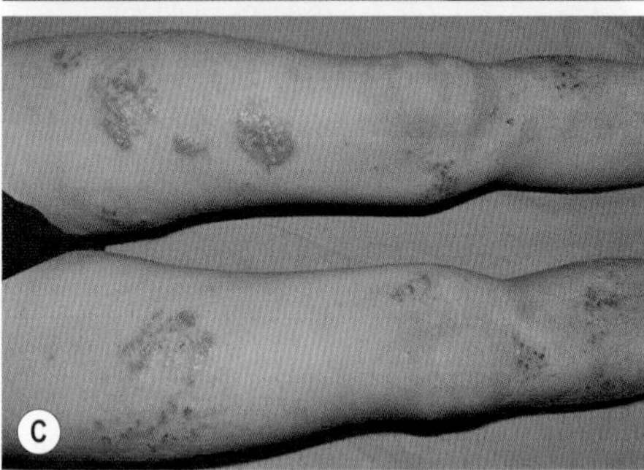

Fig. 10.6 Atopic dermatitis variants. **A** Chronic papular lesions resulting from habitual rubbing and scratching in the setting of longstanding disease. **B** Prurigo lesions presenting as firm, dome-shaped papules and nodules with central hemorrhagic crust. **C** Nummular plaques with oozing and crusting on the legs. *A, Courtesy, Thomas Bieber, MD, and Caroline Bussman, MD; B, C, Courtesy, Antonio Torrelo, MD.*

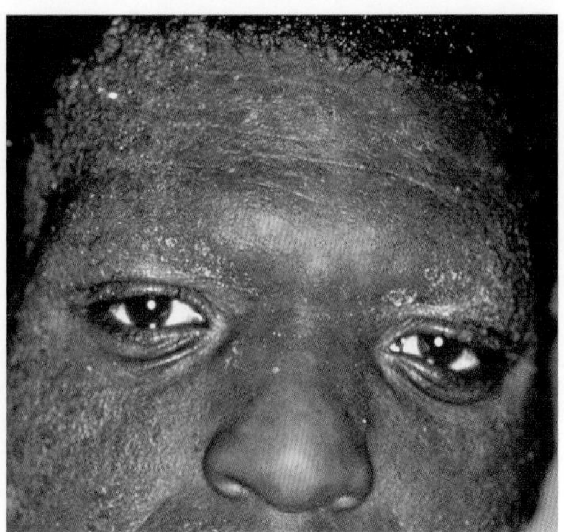

Fig. 10.7 Severe facial atopic dermatitis in an adult. *Courtesy, YDRSC.*

Treatment of AD

- There are two major components to management of AD (Fig. 10.12).
  - Treatment of active dermatitis with anti-inflammatory agent(s)
  - Maintenance designed to improve skin barrier function, control subclinical inflammation, and avoid trigger factors
- Proactive treatment of AD provides better long-term disease control and could potentially interrupt the atopic march.
- Basics of skin care.
  - Daily lukewarm bath (preferred for infants/children) or shower with limited use of a mild cleanser
  - Within 3 minutes of exit from bath/shower, application of (1) a topical CS (or calcineurin inhibitor/other anti-inflammatory agent) when/where indicated; and then (2) liberal use of an emollient to the entire skin surface
  - Ointments (minimize stinging) and creams (less greasy) are preferred to lotions as emollients and should be applied twice daily; products containing lactic or glycolic acid can lead to stinging and should be avoided
- Topical anti-inflammatory agents.
  - First-line: topical CS of appropriate strength used once or twice daily until eczema is clear (see Fig. 10.12)

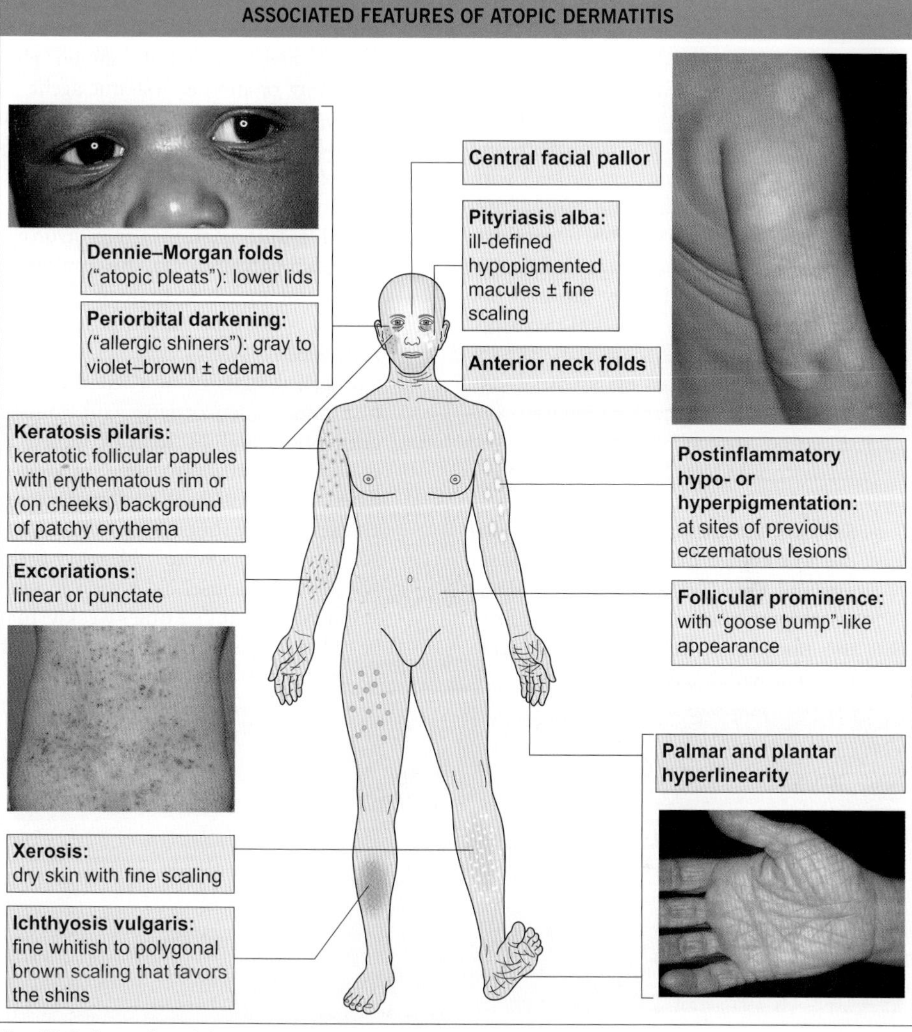

Fig. 10.8 Associated features of atopic dermatitis. *Inset of eyes: Courtesy, YDRSC. Inset of hand: Courtesy, Jean L. Bolognia, MD. Insets of excoriations and hypopigmentation: Courtesy, Antonio Torrelo, MD.*

  - CS ointments (minimize stinging) and creams are generally preferred, but CS solutions, foams, and oils are useful for AD on the scalp
  - Addressing patients'/parents' specific concerns about CS use helps to maximize adherence to the treatment plan
  - Tap water compresses followed by CS application or wet wraps after CS application can speed improvement of acute flares
- Second-line: topical calcineurin inhibitors (TCIs; e.g. tacrolimus, pimecrolimus) or crisaborole are helpful primarily for thinner lesions, especially on the face and in intertriginous areas
- High-level maintenance with intermittent use of a topical CS and/or TCI to usual sites of eczema once clear can help to control subclinical inflammation and prevent flares (see Fig. 10.12)

• Phototherapy and systemic anti-inflammatory agents.
- Narrowband UVB (often induces remission) > UVA1 (for acute flares) > UVA-broadband UVB combination
- Dupilumab, a monoclonal antibody that targets IL-4 and IL-13 signaling

involved in Th2 inflammation, is FDA-approved for the treatment of recalcitrant moderate-to-severe AD in patients ≥6 years of age (with studies in younger children in progress); it can be used with concurrent topical CS treatment and has a favorable side-effect profile, with injection site reactions and conjunctivitis each occurring in 5–10% of patients
  - Among other systemic anti-inflammatory agents traditionally utilized for severe, recalcitrant AD, oral cyclosporine has the most evidence for efficacy, but its use is limited by potential side effects such as nephrotoxicity; azathioprine, mycophenolate mofetil, and methotrexate have less dramatic benefit but better long-term safety profiles
  - Systemic CS therapy should be avoided due to the high likelihood of significant rebound flares (see Fig. 10.12) and the unacceptable side effects of long-term use; uncommon exception: severe acute flare (e.g. with a specific trigger) resistant to aggressive topical management – this short course of systemic CS must be transitioned to a topical regimen, phototherapy, or another systemic agent
- Emerging AD treatments include topical and oral JAK inhibitors and biologic agents targeting IL-13 or IL-31.
- Adjunctive pharmacologic therapy.
  - Sedating antihistamines (e.g. hydroxyzine, diphenhydramine, doxepin) given at bedtime may help to break the itch–scratch cycle, especially if pruritus disrupts sleep
  - Controlled trials of non-sedating antihistamines, leukotriene antagonists, antibiotics (oral or topical) aimed at reducing colonization, and probiotics have not consistently demonstrated efficacy as treatments of AD; dilute sodium hypochlorite (bleach) baths (¼–½ cup of household bleach in ~full standard bathtub 1–2 times weekly) may be of benefit, especially in patients with recent staphylococcal superinfections

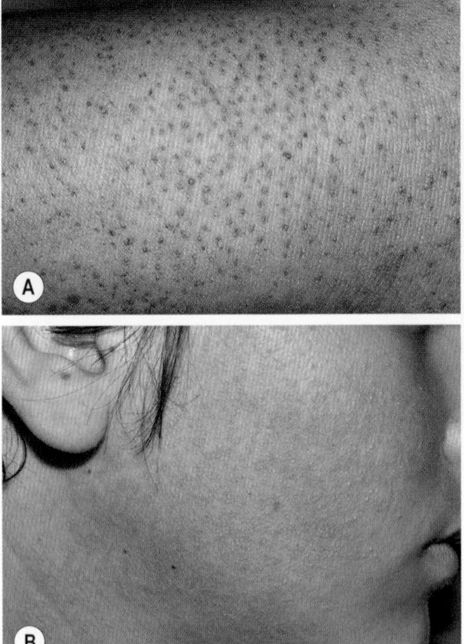

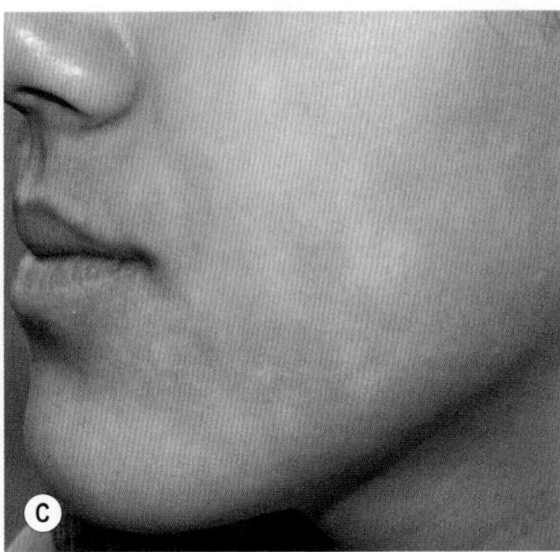

Fig. 10.9 Associated findings in patients with atopic dermatitis. A Keratosis pilaris. Note the discrete perifollicular papules with central keratotic cores on the extensor surface of the upper arm. Each papule has a rim of erythema. **B** Keratosis pilaris rubra on the lateral face. This variant is characterized by tiny, grain-like follicular papules superimposed on confluent erythema. **C** Pityriasis alba. Note the slight scale associated with the hypopigmented macules and patches on the cheek. *A, Courtesy, YDRSC. B, Courtesy, Angela Hernández-Martín, MD; C, Courtesy, Julie V. Schaffer, MD.*

For further information see Ch. 12 from *Dermatology, Fourth Edition*.

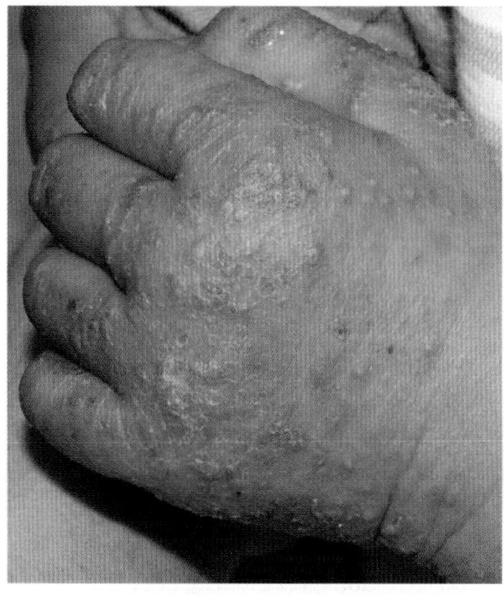

Fig. 10.10 Infected hand dermatitis in a patient with atopic dermatitis. There is impetigo-like crusting as well as pustules. *Courtesy, Julie V. Schaffer, MD.*

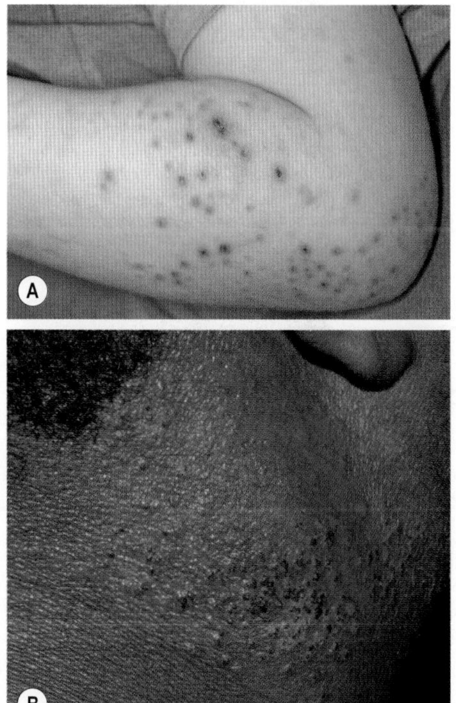

Fig. 10.11 Eczema herpeticum. Note the monomorphic erosions and hemorrhagic crusts on the arm (**A**) and posterior neck (**B**). Vesicles are rarely evident. *A, Courtesy, Maeve McAleer, MD, Grainne O'Regan, MD, and Alan Irvine, MD; B, Courtesy, Julie V. Schaffer, MD.*

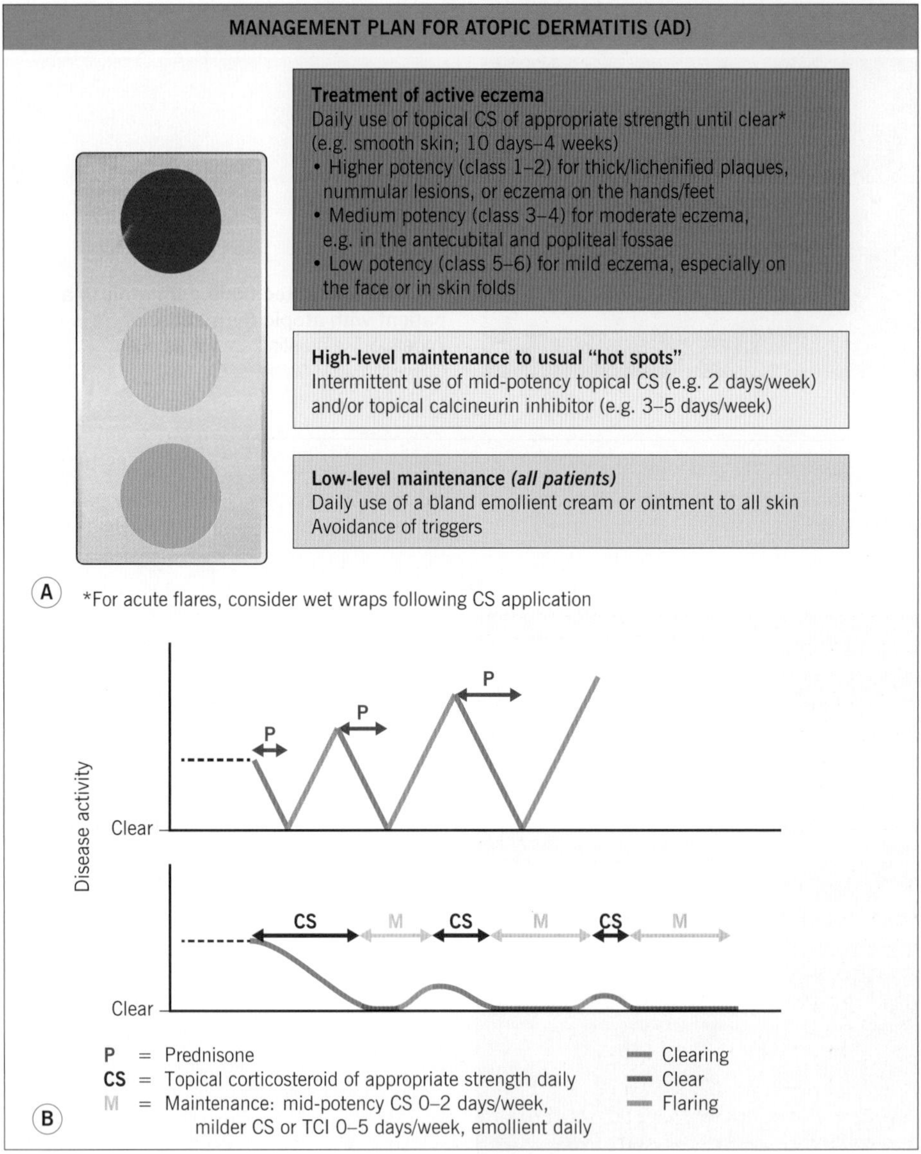

MANAGEMENT PLAN FOR ATOPIC DERMATITIS (AD)

Treatment of active eczema
Daily use of topical CS of appropriate strength until clear*
(e.g. smooth skin; 10 days–4 weeks)
- Higher potency (class 1–2) for thick/lichenified plaques, nummular lesions, or eczema on the hands/feet
- Medium potency (class 3–4) for moderate eczema, e.g. in the antecubital and popliteal fossae
- Low potency (class 5–6) for mild eczema, especially on the face or in skin folds

High-level maintenance to usual "hot spots"
Intermittent use of mid-potency topical CS (e.g. 2 days/week) and/or topical calcineurin inhibitor (e.g. 3–5 days/week)

Low-level maintenance *(all patients)*
Daily use of a bland emollient cream or ointment to all skin
Avoidance of triggers

A

*For acute flares, consider wet wraps following CS application

Disease activity
Clear
P
P
P
Clear
CS
M
CS
M
CS
M

P = Prednisone
CS = Topical corticosteroid of appropriate strength daily
M = Maintenance: mid-potency CS 0–2 days/week, milder CS or TCI 0–5 days/week, emollient daily

Clearing
Clear
Flaring

B

Fig. 10.12 Management plan for atopic dermatitis. **A** The therapeutic regimen should include both treatment of active eczema and maintenance (low-level in all and high-level in some patients). **B** Intermittent courses of a systemic CS result in rebound flares and worsening of disease over time. In contrast, a proactive regimen utilizing topical CS leads to longer clear periods and milder disease over time.

Other Eczematous Eruptions 11

The major forms of dermatitis include atopic (see Ch. 10), contact (see Ch. 12), seborrheic, asteatotic (xerotic), stasis, and nummular. Dermatitis of special sites – i.e. hands, feet, lips, eyelids, diaper area, and major body folds – is reviewed in Chapter 13, and pityriasis alba is reviewed in Chapters 10 and 54.

Seborrheic Dermatitis

- Common disorder with both an infantile and an adult form (Figs 11.1 and 11.2); unusual in children.
- Possibly related to components of sebum and *Malassezia* spp.
- Severe or recalcitrant seborrheic dermatitis can be a sign of underlying HIV infection or neurologic disorder.
- In adults, tends to be a chronic relapsing disorder; stress or tapering of systemic CS can lead to a flare.
- Symmetric distribution pattern that includes regions with greater sebum production – scalp, ears (external canal, retroauricular fold), medial eyebrows, upper eyelids, nasolabial folds, central chest – and major body folds.
- Lesions are pink-yellow to red-brown in color, depending on the underlying skin phototype, and they often have greasy scale, especially in the head and neck region; occasionally annular in configuration.
- On the scalp, involvement tends to be more diffuse, compared to the well-circumscribed plaques with thicker silvery scale that are more characteristic of scalp psoriasis.
- In some patients, the lesions of the scalp, ears, and major body folds have features of both seborrheic dermatitis and psoriasis, leading to the term "sebopsoriasis".
- **DDx:** psoriasis, contact dermatitis, other causes of diaper dermatitis (see Fig. 13.4), intertrigo (see Fig. 13.2) or blepharitis (see Fig. 13.6), tinea (pityriasis) versicolor (when presternal), tinea capitis (especially in children), atopic dermatitis, pityriasis amiantacea, and dermatomyositis (scalp); may coexist with rosacea.
- **Rx:** topical antifungal creams and daily shampooing (e.g. ketoconazole, ciclopirox, selenium sulfide or zinc-containing shampoo alternating with a gentle shampoo), mild topical CS on the face and in body folds and moderate-strength topical CS for the scalp and ears; topical calcineurin inhibitors (e.g. tacrolimus ointment).

Asteatotic Eczema (Xerotic Eczema, Eczema Craquelé)

- Arises in areas of dry skin, especially during winter months, in dry climates, and in older adults.
- The areas of dermatitis resemble a "dried riverbed" or "crazy-paving" with superficial cracking of the skin (Fig. 11.3).
- May be associated with pruritus; stinging can occur with application of water-based topical agents, including those that contain lactic or glycolic acid.
- Favors the shins, thighs, lower flanks, and posterior axillary line; may become more widespread but with sparing of the face, palms, and soles.
- Involvement of the posterior axillary line seen in chronic GVHD; when widespread, consider the possibility of an underlying systemic lymphoma.
- **DDx:** stasis dermatitis ± autosensitization, ichthyosis vulgaris, adult atopic dermatitis, allergic or irritant contact dermatitis.
- **Rx:** decrease frequency of bathing and use of soaps, liberal use of water-in-oil emollients, mild topical CS ointments.

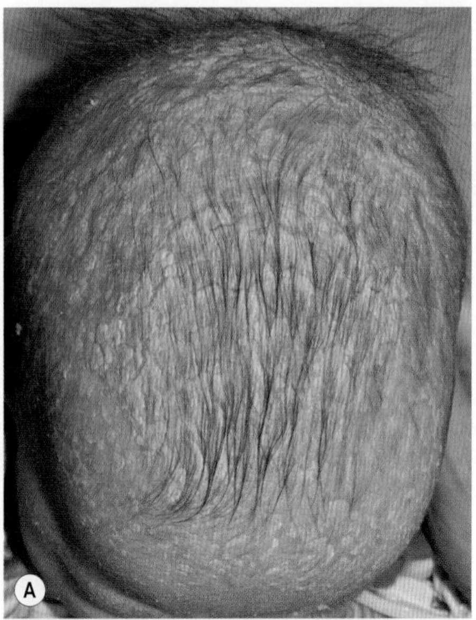

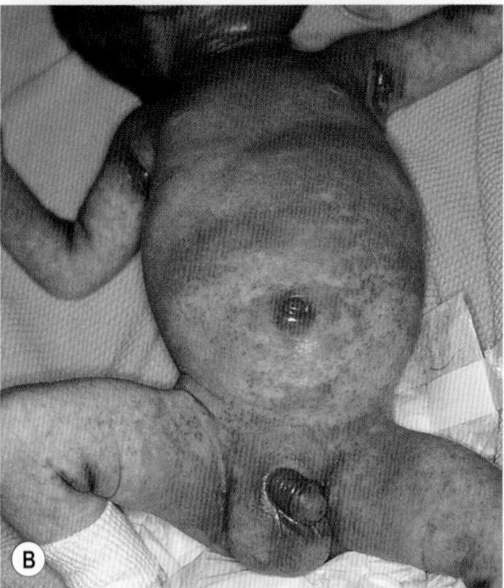

Fig. 11.1 Infantile seborrheic dermatitis. **A** Involvement of the scalp with thick adherent yellow scale overlying mild inflammation is often referred to as "cradle cap". **B** Glistening red plaques of the neck, axillary and inguinal folds as well as the penis and umbilicus. Note disseminated lesions on the trunk and extremities. *A, Courtesy, Antonio Torrelo, MD; B, Courtesy, Robert Hartman, MD.*

Stasis Dermatitis

- Pruritic dermatitis with scale-crust and sometimes oozing that favors the shins and calves (see Fig. 86.5D); historically often begins near the medial malleolus.
- Patients often have a history of chronic lower extremity edema and may have a history of deep vein thromboses and/or recurrent cellulitis.
- Often accompanied by other signs of chronic venous hypertension (Table 11.1).
- One of the more common causes of autosensitization (Fig. 11.4).
- **DDx:** allergic contact dermatitis, irritant contact dermatitis, asteatotic eczema, nummular dermatitis; may accompany other causes of the red leg, especially cellulitis and acute or chronic lipodermatosclerosis (Fig. 11.5), but the latter lack the clinical and histopathologic findings of dermatitis.
- **Rx:** exclude superimposed allergic contact dermatitis (e.g. neomycin, preservatives in topical creams) or component of infectious eczematous dermatitis if draining ulcer; open wet dressings for a few days, mild topical CS ointments, leg elevation, pressure stockings (after excluding arterial insufficiency via ankle–brachial index), endovascular ablation of large varicosities, water-in-oil emollients for maintenance therapy.

Autosensitization Dermatitis (Id Reaction)

- More widespread distribution of dermatitis that follows by days to weeks the development of localized areas of dermatitis, e.g. allergic contact dermatitis, stasis dermatitis, inflammatory tinea infections.
- Can also represent a rebound phenomenon when there has been too rapid a taper of systemic CS, as in 6-day taper of prednisone or methylprednisolone (Medrol® dose pack) for poison ivy dermatitis.
- Favored sites of involvement (in addition to primary site): extensor aspects of extremities (see Fig. 11.4), palms and soles, usually in a symmetric pattern.
- In children with tinea capitis, the id reaction often involves the head and neck region.
- Areas of dermatitis, often ill-defined, can be accompanied by excoriated papules (Fig. 11.6).
- **DDx:** atopic dermatitis, widespread contact dermatitis (e.g. textiles), Gianotti–Crosti syndrome (children), drug eruption to systemic antifungal medication (tinea capitis id),

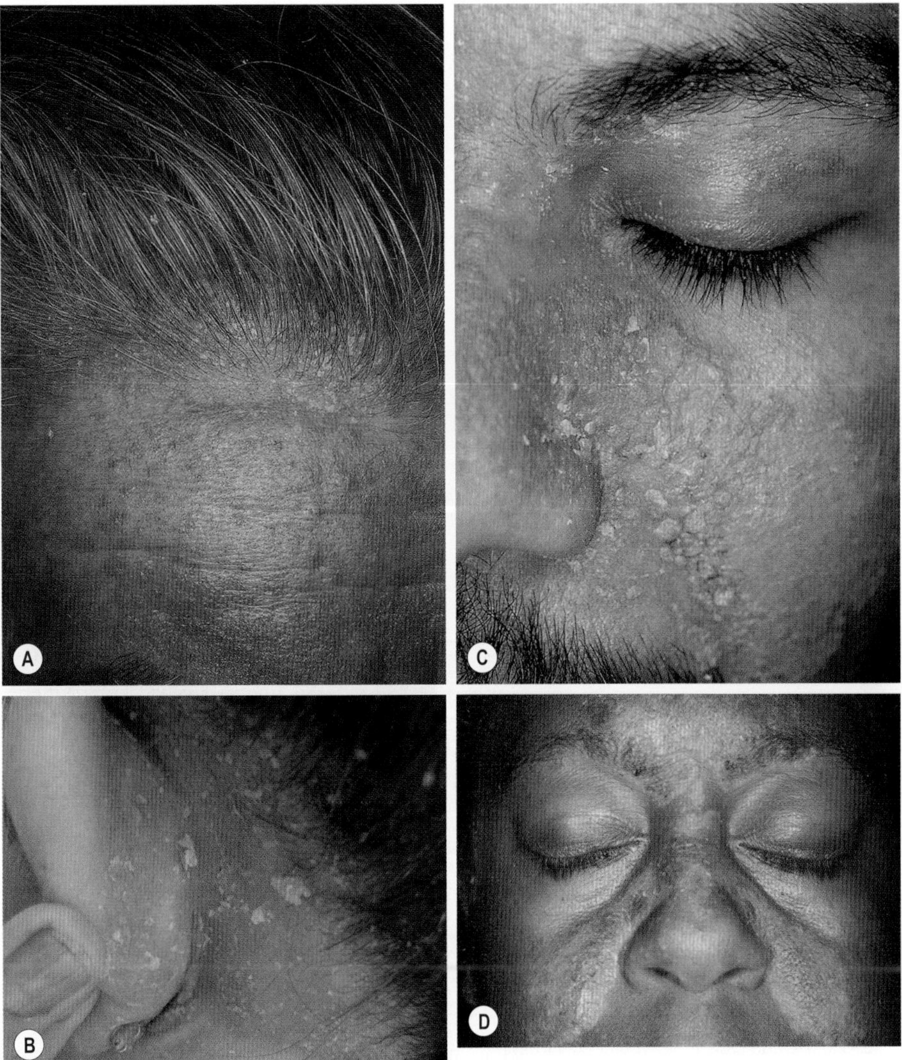

Fig. 11.2 Adult seborrheic dermatitis of the scalp, ear, and face. **A** Diffuse scaling of the scalp in addition to erythema of the forehead. **B** Fairly sharply demarcated pink plaque with white and greasy scale. Note the fissure in the retroauricular fold. **C** Thin pink-orange plaques with yellow, greasy scale, especially of the melolabial fold and eyebrows. When this degree of severity is seen, the possibility of underlying HIV infection needs to be considered. **D** Symmetric red-brown to violet plaques of the central forehead, nasal bridge, and medial cheeks with an associated hypopigmented figurate rim. *A, Courtesy, Jean L. Bolognia, MD; B, Courtesy, Norbert Reider, MD, and Peter O. Fritsch, MD; C, Courtesy, NYUDSC; D, Courtesy, Jeffrey Callen, MD.*

eczematous drug eruptions (e.g. calcium channel blockers [unusual]). When palmoplantar, dyshidrotic eczema, inflammatory tinea.

- **Rx:** in addition to aggressively treating the primary dermatitis, topical CS and oral antihistamines usually suffice; occasionally, when severe, systemic CS.

Infectious Eczematous (Eczematoid) Dermatitis

- Dermatitis that initially involves the skin surrounding a site of infection, usually bacterial, which is weeping or has drainage (e.g. otitis externa, infected leg ulcer, toe web infection) (Fig. 11.7).

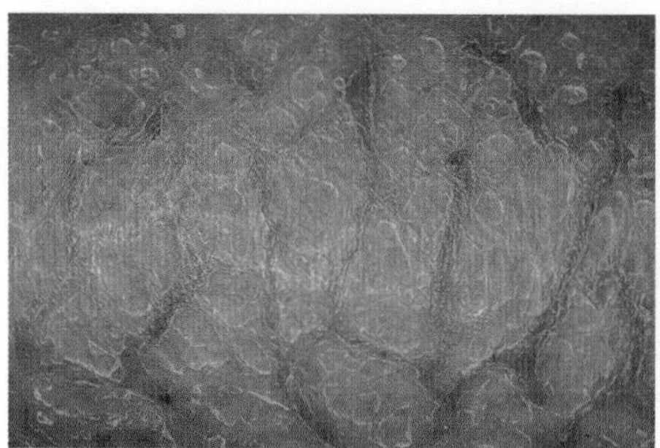

Fig. 11.3 Asteatotic eczema (eczema craquelé). The distal lower extremity has obvious inflammation and xerosis with adherent white scale (pseudo-ichthyosis) as well as a criss-cross pattern of superficial cracks and fissures said to resemble a dried riverbed. *Courtesy, Louis A. Fragola, Jr., MD.*

CUTANEOUS SIGNS OF CHRONIC VENOUS HYPERTENSION
• Edema, often tender • Varicosities • Stasis dermatitis • Petechiae superimposed on a yellow-brown discoloration due to hemosiderin deposits (stasis purpura) • Lipodermatosclerosis, acute and chronic • Stasis ulcerations, in particular above the medial malleolus • Acroangiodermatitis (pseudo-Kaposi sarcoma) • Livedoid vasculopathy (porcelain-white scars surrounded by punctate telangiectasias, small irregularly shaped purpuric macules due to infarcts, and painful ulcerations)*
**Need to exclude causes of hypercoagulability/thrombophilia.*

Table 11.1 Cutaneous signs of chronic venous hypertension.

• An id reaction can develop and treatment of both the infection and the dermatitis is recommended.

Nummular Dermatitis (Nummular Eczema)

• Markedly pruritic, coin-shaped lesions of dermatitis, usually measuring 2 or 3 cm in diameter (Fig. 11.8).

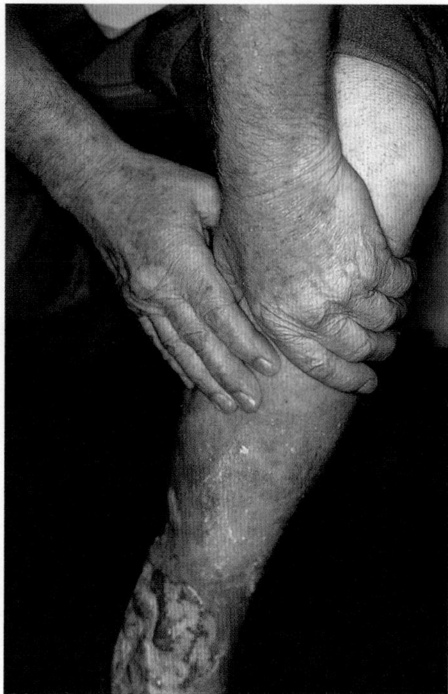

Fig. 11.4 Autosensitization dermatitis. There is dermatitis of the extensor surfaces of the upper extremities in this patient with allergic contact dermatitis to neomycin as well as stasis dermatitis and venous ulceration. *Courtesy, Jean L. Bolognia, MD.*

• Occurs primarily on the extremities, classically the legs in men and the arms in women.

• Favors adults and can develop in the absence of an atopic diathesis; a chronic relapsing course is common.

• **DDx:** coin-shaped lesions of atopic dermatitis, autosensitization dermatitis, impetigo, stasis dermatitis, allergic contact dermatitis, tinea corporis, vesicular pityriasis rosea, mycosis fungoides.

• **Rx:** in addition to topical CS and calcineurin inhibitors, often requires phototherapy to clear.

Dyshidrotic Eczema (Acute and Recurrent Vesicular Hand Dermatitis)

• Firm, pruritic vesicles of the palms > soles as well as the lateral and medial aspects of the digits (Fig. 11.9); tends to be recurrent.

APPROACH TO THE "RED LEG"

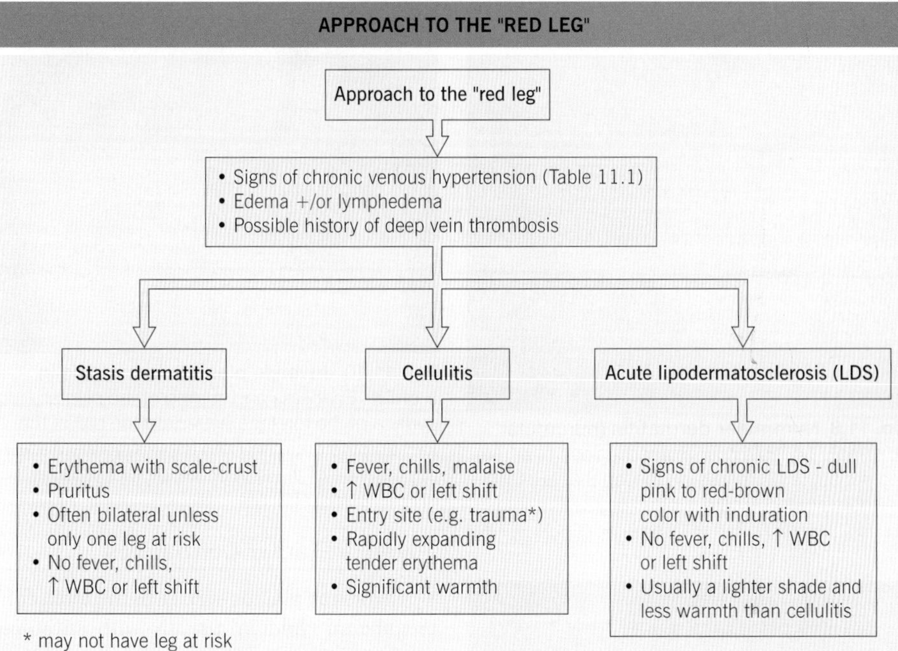

Fig. 11.5 Approach to the "red leg." Patients with lower extremity edema can have baseline tenderness with palpation.

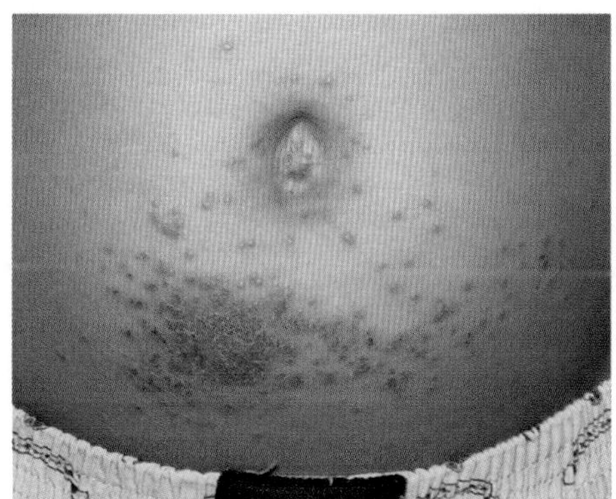

Fig. 11.6 Id reaction in a child due to allergic contact dermatitis (ACD) to nickel. Square-shaped area of ACD due to nickel in a buckle surrounded by multiple crusted edematous papules. *Courtesy, Julie V. Schaffer, MD.*

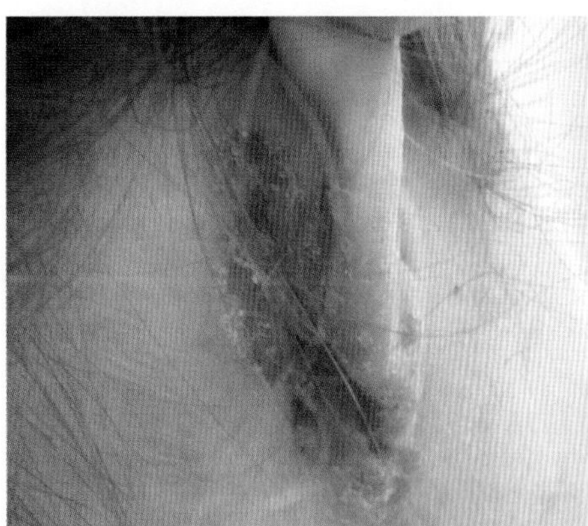

Fig. 11.7 Infectious eczematous dermatitis. Crusting and scaling at the periphery of otitis externa due to *Staphylococcus aureus*. *Courtesy, Norbert Reider, MD, and Peter O. Fritsch, MD.*

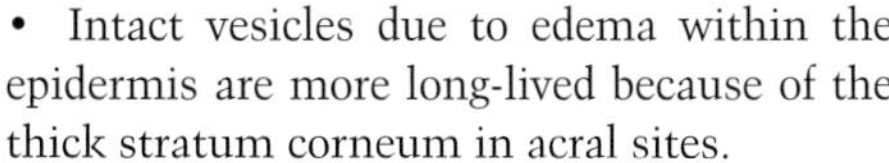

• Intact vesicles due to edema within the epidermis are more long-lived because of the thick stratum corneum in acral sites.
• When the vesicles are small and grouped, they are said to have an appearance similar to tapioca pudding.
• When larger vesicles develop, the term pompholyx is sometimes used.

• Can flare with stress, allergic or irritant contact dermatitis, and administration of IVIg; seen in patients with atopic dermatitis and hyperhidrosis.
• **DDx:** id reaction (can have overlap), inflammatory tinea pedis or manuum, allergic contact dermatitis, scabies,

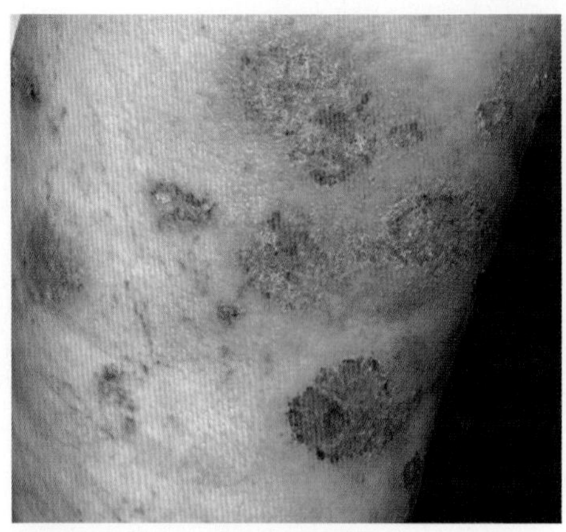

Fig. 11.8 Nummular dermatitis (nummular eczema). Multiple coin-shaped lesions of acute and subacute dermatitis on the leg that are fairly well demarcated. There is often marked pruritus. *Courtesy, Norbert Reider, MD, and Peter O. Fritsch, MD.*

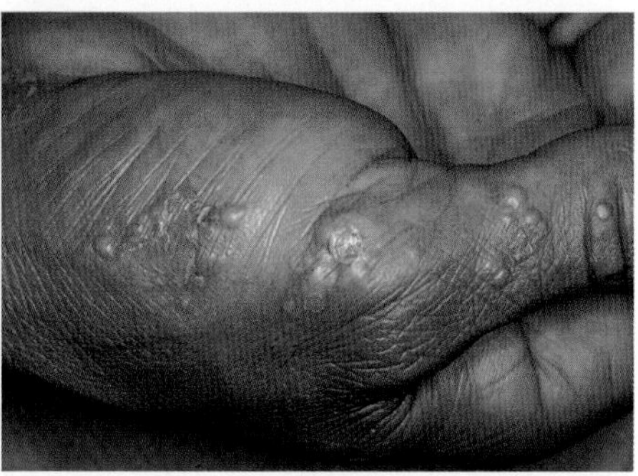

Fig. 11.9 Dyshidrotic eczema (pompholyx). Clusters of firm vesicles along the lateral aspect of the thumb and hypothenar eminence. *Courtesy Louis A. Fragola, Jr., MD.*

dyshidrosiform bullous pemphigoid; if secondarily infected, palmoplantar pustulosis; when localized to a single digit, whitlow (herpes simplex infection) or blistering digital dactylitis (staphylococcal or group A streptococcal infection).

• **Rx:** exclude allergic or irritant contact dermatitis; topical CS, topical calcineurin inhibitors, bath PUVA; occasionally, when severe, systemic CS.

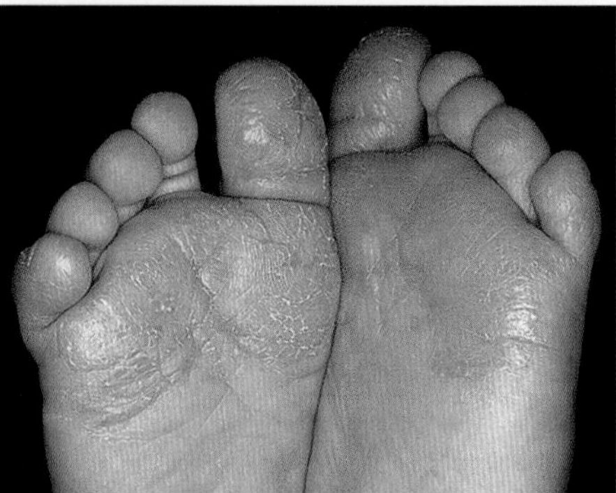

Fig. 11.10 Juvenile plantar dermatosis in a child. Erythema and scaling of the plantar surface of the forefoot, especially the ball of the foot and the great and fifth toes. Note the glazed appearance of the skin of the left foot. *Courtesy, Kalman Watsky, MD.*

Juvenile Plantar Dermatosis

• Favors the plantar surface of the forefeet in prepubertal children, usually with an atopic diathesis.

• The skin is dry and scaly with mild inflammation and a characteristic glazed appearance (Fig. 11.10).

• Thought to be related to hydration of the stratum corneum from wearing shoes made of impermeable materials and subsequent shearing of skin due to friction.

• **DDx:** other causes of foot dermatitis (see Table 13.1), especially psoriasis, allergic contact dermatitis (e.g. rubber, chromates in leather), tinea pedis (interdigital toe webs involved), atopic dermatitis.

• **Rx:** permeable socks and shoes, emollients, CS ointments, keep feet dry including removal of wet socks and wet shoes.

Infective Dermatitis

• Rare disorder of childhood or adolescence associated with human T-cell lymphotropic virus type 1 (HTLV-1) infection.

• Dermatitis of the scalp, ears, eyelid margins, paranasal skin, axillae, and groin that clears with oral antibiotics.

For further information see Ch. 13 from *Dermatology, Fourth Edition*.

For additional online figures visit www.expertconsult.com 

Irritant and Allergic Contact Dermatitis, Occupational Dermatoses, and Dermatoses Due to Plants

12

Key Points

- Irritant contact dermatitis (ICD)
  - Accounts for 80% of all causes of contact dermatitis
  - Secondary to a local toxic effect caused by a topical substance or physical insult
- Allergic contact dermatitis (ACD)
  - Accounts for 20% of all causes of contact dermatitis
  - A delayed-type hypersensitivity reaction to a substance to which the individual has been previously sensitized
  - Compared to ICD, more commonly presents with pruritus during the acute phase
- One of the most common occupational dermatoses is ICD.
- Plants can cause a variety of skin reactions, the most common in North America being ACD to poison ivy.

Irritant Contact Dermatitis

- Localized, non-immunologically mediated cutaneous inflammatory reaction (Figs 12.1–12.5).
- Secondary to a direct toxic effect
  - Chronic – erythema, fissures, and scale which is oftentimes thick
  - Acute – erythema, edema, and vesiculation followed by erosions and scaling; in severe cases may lead to epidermal necrosis (a "chemical burn")
- Commonly affects the hands (see Fig. 13.1); Table 12.1 reviews pertinent questions for when environmental exposures are suspected.
- A common cause of cheilitis (lip-licking; see Fig. 13.5).
- May be secondary to an occupational exposure (Table 12.2)

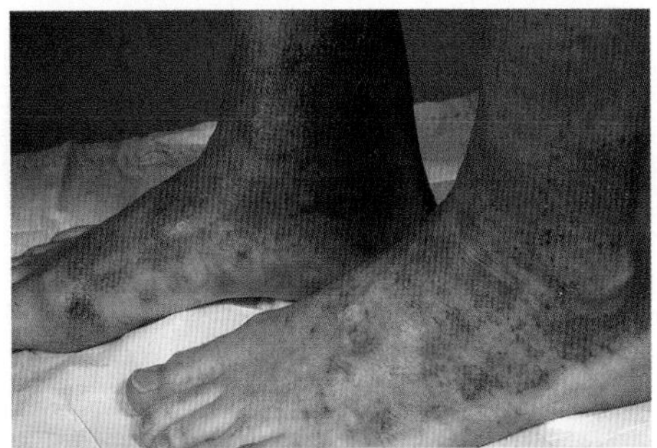

Fig. 12.1 Bilateral irritant contact dermatitis of the feet and ankles due to chronic occlusive footwear. *Courtesy, David Cohen, MD.*

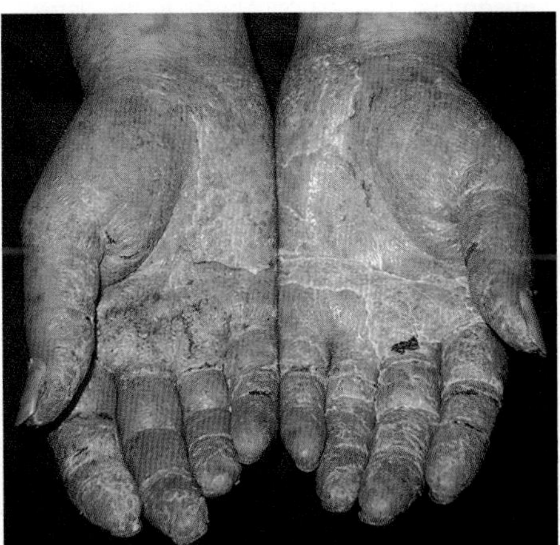

Fig. 12.2 Bilateral irritant contact dermatitis of the palms secondary to repeated contact with paint solvents. Extensive patch testing excluded allergic contact dermatitis in this professional paint and crayon illustrator. *Courtesy, Kalman Watsky, MD.*

  - Common causes are soaps and wet work, and less often petroleum products, cutting oils, and coolants

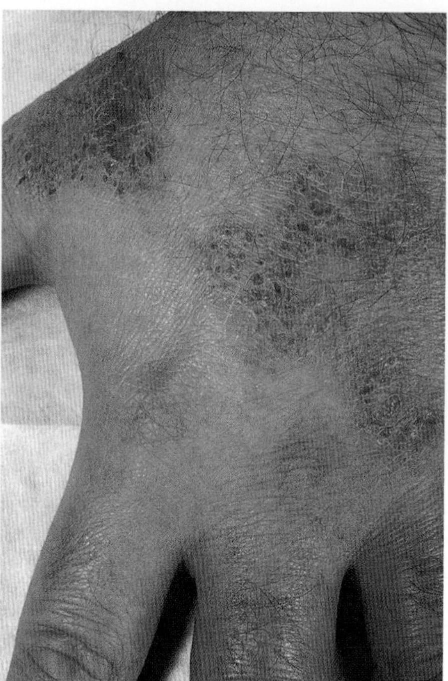

Fig. 12.3 Moderately severe irritant contact dermatitis of the hands due to chronic exposure to disinfecting solutions and antiseptics. The results of patch testing, latex challenge testing, and RAST testing were negative in this practicing dentist. *Courtesy, David Cohen, MD.*

- **DDx:** when severe, thermal burn; ACD and other dermatitides; there may be a combination of causes, e.g. ICD and ACD, ICD and atopic dermatitis.
- **Rx:** primarily avoidance of the irritant.

Allergic Contact Dermatitis

- In contrast to ICD, more commonly presents with pruritus during the acute phase; the chronic phase has significant overlap with ICD (Fig. 12.6).
- Initially, well demarcated and localized to site of contact with the allergen (Figs 12.7–12.12).
  - Acute – in addition to erythema and edema, vesicobullae and weeping may develop (Fig. 12.7)
  - Chronic – often lichenified with scale (Figs 12.6B and 12.9)
- Can have autosensitization with extension beyond original site (see Ch. 11); airborne allergens primarily contact exposed skin and can mimic (or overlap) photoallergic or phototoxic reactions (Fig. 12.11).

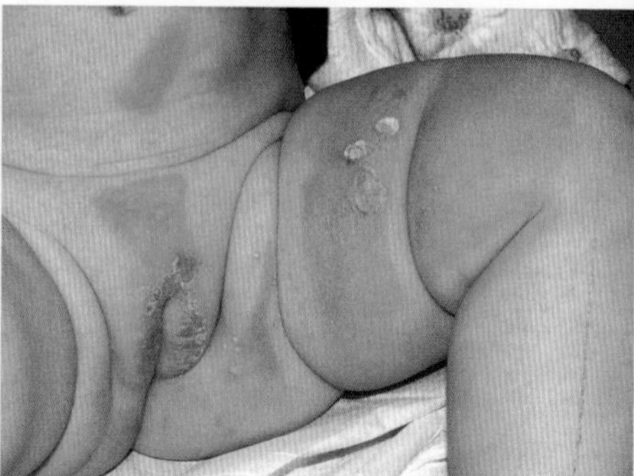

Fig. 12.4 Chemical burn from topical application of apple cider vinegar mimicking child abuse in an infant. Note the sharply demarcated erythema with angular borders and sparing of the skin folds, as well as the superficial blistering and desquamation. *Courtesy, Julie V. Schaffer, MD.*

- Occasionally, there is a diffuse, patchy distribution, depending on the allergen (e.g. body wash or shampoo) and/or concomitant atopic dermatitis.
- Common allergens are metals, fragrances, preservatives, and topical antibiotics, as well as plants, in particular poison ivy/oak (see below) (Fig. 12.12).
- Common causes of occupational ACD are rubber, nickel, epoxy resin, and aromatic amines.
- Suspected allergens should be avoided; a repeat open application test can be tried first but patch testing is required for accurate diagnosis; detailed lists of allergen-containing products are available.
- In patch testing, specific concentrations of allergens are dissolved in petrolatum or water and placed in wells that are then applied to the patient's back for 48 hours (Figs 12.13 and 12.14); grading of reactions is performed at two time points (Table 12.3).
- **DDx:** other forms of dermatitis (ICD, atopic dermatitis, stasis dermatitis, seborrheic dermatitis), erythematotelangiectatic rosacea, dermatophyte infection.
- **Rx:** short term: topical and systemic CS depending on severity; long term: avoidance of allergen(s).

Common Allergens

Metals

- Cross-reactivity not uncommon within each broad category.
- Nickel – found in costume jewelry, snaps on jeans, backs of watches, belt buckles

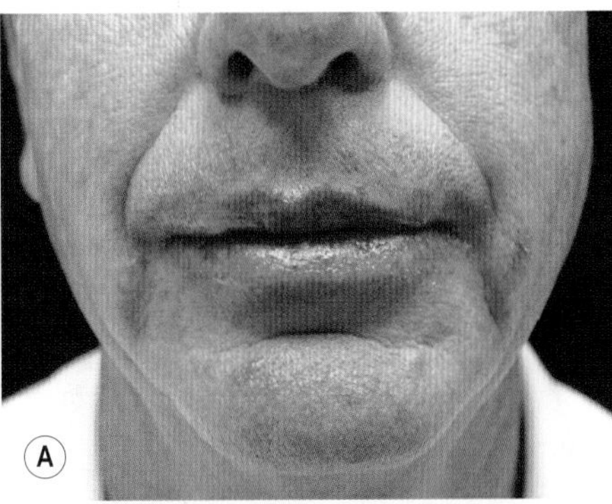

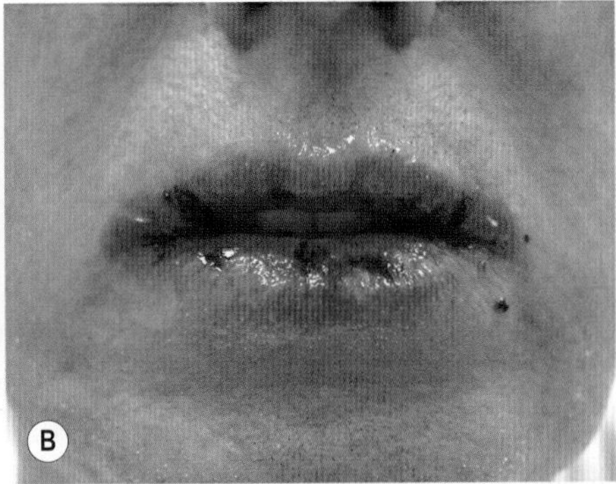

Fig. 12.5 Cheilitis due to irritant versus allergic contact dermatitis. A Irritant contact dermatitis – this patient had the habit of licking his lips and there is involvement of the vermilion and cutaneous lips as well as the perioral region. **B** Allergic contact dermatitis to oxybenzone with involvement of the upper and lower lips. *A, Courtesy, Jeffrey P. Callen; B, Courtesy, Kalman Watsky, MD.*

POINTS TO CONSIDER WHEN EVALUATING HAND DERMATITIS AND ENVIRONMENTAL EXPOSURES ARE SUSPECTED	
Occupation	Are findings consistent with work exposure as a cause?
	Does time off result in improvement?
Materials handled	Do labels and material safety data sheets (MSDS) list potential irritants or allergens?
	Is there a relationship to handling food?
	Other persons in workplace affected?
	Protective equipment (e.g. gloves) used?
Previous skin disease or history of atopy	Is there a history of eczema as a child?
Known allergies	Is there unrecognized exposure?
Treatment	May cause allergic contact dermatitis
Hobbies	Including exposure to plants

Table 12.1 Points to consider when evaluating hand dermatitis and environmental exposures are suspected. *Courtesy, Peter S. Friedmann, MD.*

(Figs 12.15 and 12.16); dimethylglyoxime test (Fig. 12.15 inset) identifies objects that release nickel (can purchase dimethylglyoxime at nonickel.com).

- Chromate – found in metals, leather, cement.
- Cobalt – used to harden metals; cosmetics, enamel, ceramics, hair dyes, and joint replacements; the cobalt spot test can be used.
- Gold – found in jewelry, dental fillings, and some electronics.

Topical Antibiotics

- Neomycin sulfate – found in many over-the-counter preparations (e.g. hemorrhoid creams).
- Bacitracin – in many products.

Fragrances

- Balsam of Peru (*Myroxylon pereirae*) – one of the naturally occurring fragrances; also found in spices (cloves, Jamaican pepper, cinnamon); fragrance can be used to mask odors in products, including some that are labeled "unscented". Allergic individuals should look for "fragrance-free" products, being aware that unfortunately even those products may be labeled as such despite containing some fragrance that is being used as a preservative.

Preservatives

- Formaldehyde – cosmetics and textiles (permanent press), medications, paints.

COMMON IRRITANTS AND EXAMPLES OF MAJOR EXPOSURE(S)	
Irritant	**Examples of major exposure(s)**
Inorganic acids	
Hydrofluoric acid	Etching of glass/metal/stone; rust/stain/limescale removers
Sulfuric acid	Manufacturing of fertilizers, textile fibers, explosives, paper
Hydrochloric acid	Production of fertilizers, dyes, paints; used in food processing
Chromic acid	Used in metal treatments
Nitric acid	Production of fertilizers and explosives; in cleaning products
Phosphoric acid	Used in fertilizer, pharmaceuticals, water treatment
Organic acids	
Formic acid	Used as a neutralizer in leather manufacturing
Alkalis	
Sodium hydroxide	Used in the manufacture of bleaches, dyes, vitamins, pulp, paper, plastics, soaps and detergents
Calcium oxide	
Metal salts	
Arsenic trioxide	Aerosolized in the smelting of metals
Beryllium compounds	Used in the production of hard, corrosion-resistant alloys
Solvents	
Stoddard solvent	Used in dry cleaning
Water	Ubiquitous
Alcohols	
Glycols	Commonly used in cosmetic products
Detergents and cleansers	
Sodium lauryl sulfate	Detergents and cleansers
Cocamidopropyl betaine	Detergents, therapeutic formulations, personal care products
Disinfectants	
Ethylene oxide	Medical sterilization
Chloroxylenol	Baby powders and shampoos
Iodines	Surgical scrub, shampoo, skin cleansers
Benzalkonium chloride	Used for instrument cleansing; in ophthalmic solutions
Food	Pineapples, garlic, mustard
Plants	Thistles, prickly pears, grasses
Plastics	
Bodily fluids	
Fabric/man-made vitreous fibers (e.g. fiberglass)	

Table 12.2 Common irritants and examples of major exposure(s). *Courtesy, David Cohen, MD.*

- Thimerosal – found as a preservative in vaccines, contact lens solution, antiseptics, and cosmetics.
- Quaternium-15 – formaldehyde-releasing preservative; found in shampoos, moisturizers, cosmetics, and soaps.
- Methylisothiazolinone (MI)/methylchloroisothiazolinone (MCI) – MI is sometimes present in combination with MCI or alone in sanitary wet wipes, make-up removal wipes (see Fig. 12.8), liquid soaps, as well as paints.

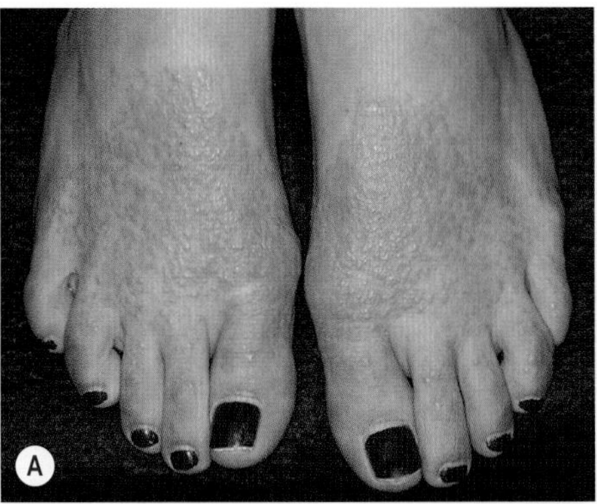

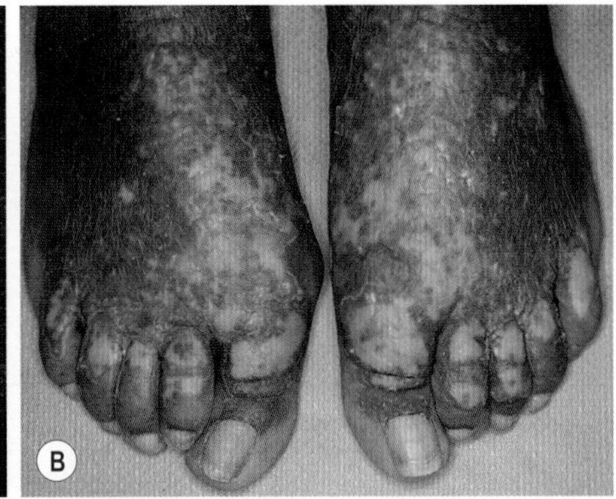

Fig. 12.6 Allergic contact dermatitis to shoes – acute versus chronic. A Extremely pruritic erythematous papules and papulovesicles appeared within days of wearing new sneakers; note the distribution pattern. **B** Pebbled and lichenified plaques with both hypo- and hyperpigmentation. The patient had a positive patch test to potassium dichromate. *Courtesy, Louis A. Fragola, Jr., MD.*

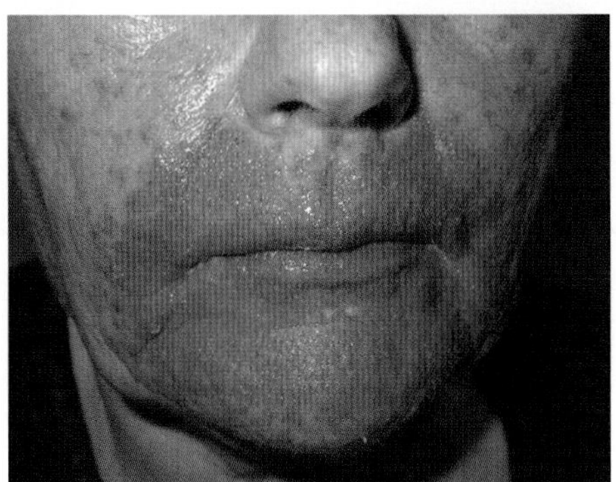

Fig. 12.7 Acute vesiculobullous allergic contact dermatitis. The allergen was neomycin from a topical antibiotic ointment. *Courtesy, Jonathan Chan, MD.*

Other Important Allergens

Topical Corticosteroids

- Can cause ACD in up to 6% of patients.
- Consider CS allergy if an existing dermatitis worsens with CS use or fails to clear; testing with topical tixocortol pivalate (group 1) and budesonide (group 1) will detect ~75% of CS allergy.
- If CS allergy is suspected/confirmed, use of a CS from a different class can be considered (see Appendix).

Other

Additional allergens include paraphenylenediamine in temporary tattoos (see Fig. 12.10) and hair dyes, propolis in lip balms, acrylates in artificial nails, thiuram in rubber and makeup applicators, formaldehyde resin in nail polish, components of adhesives, and blue dyes in textiles.

Systemic Contact Dermatitis

- Systemic exposure to a chemical/allergen to which the patient has had prior sensitization (Table 12.4; Fig. 12.17); e.g. administration of oral diphenhydramine to a patient previously sensitized to the topical formulation.

Occupational Dermatoses

- Most commonly an irritant (e.g. to soaps) > allergic contact dermatitis (e.g. to rubber).
- Other occupational dermatoses include contact urticaria (see Ch. 14), skin cancer, folliculitis (see Ch. 31), contact leukoderma (see Ch. 54), foreign body reactions, and infections (Table 12.5).

Plant Dermatoses

- Plants can cause a variety of skin reactions, including ACD (Fig. 12.12), ICD, urticaria, and phytophotodermatitis (Table 12.6).
- ACD to plants that contain urushiol.
  - Commonly secondary to poison ivy, genus *Toxicodendron* (Fig. 12.20) – compound leaves with three leaflets and flowers/fruits arising from the

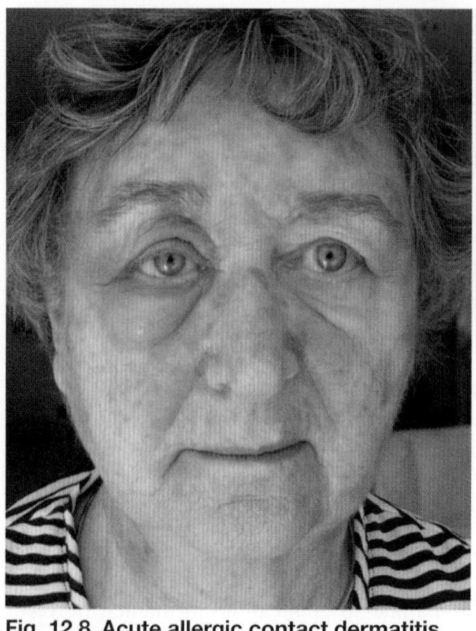

Fig. 12.8 Acute allergic contact dermatitis with a prominent component of edema. The allergen was methylisothiazolinone in a wet wipe used to remove make-up. *Courtesy, Rosemary L. Nixon, MD.*

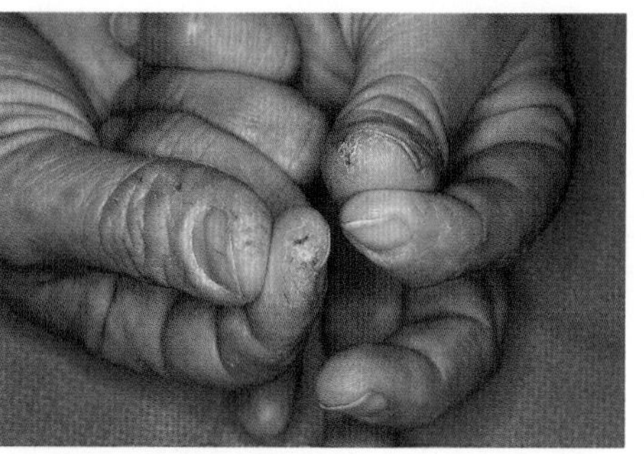

Fig. 12.9 Chronic allergic contact dermatitis due to glutaraldehyde. The patient was an optometrist. This presentation can also be seen in irritant contact dermatitis and distinction can be difficult without patch testing. *Courtesy, Kalman Watsky, MD.*

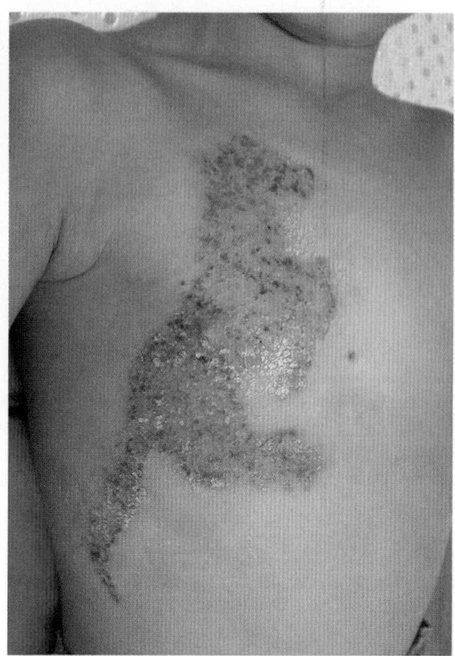

Fig. 12.10 Allergic contact dermatitis to *p*-phenylenediamine in a temporary tattoo. *Courtesy, Rosemary L. Nixon, MD.*

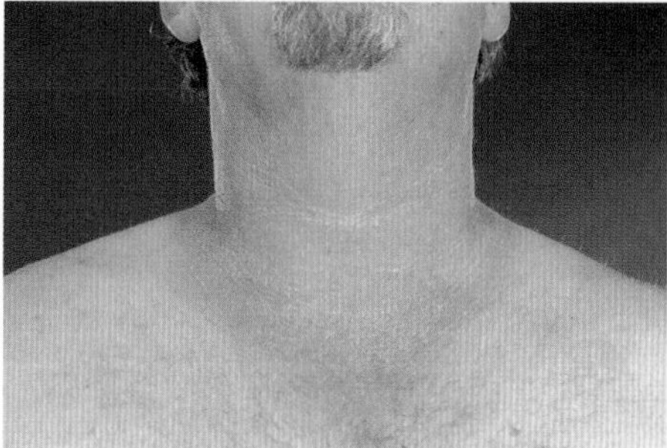

Fig. 12.11 Airborne contact dermatitis. The allergen was an epoxy resin. *Courtesy, Rosemary L. Nixon, MD.*

axillary position; black dots of urushiol often present on leaves

- Chemicals that cross-react with urushiol are found in the cashew nut tree (nutshell oil and bark), mango tree (leaves, bark, stems, fruit skin), Brazilian pepper tree (sap and crushed berries), Japanese lacquer tree (bark sap), Indian marking tree nut (black juice), and Ginkgo tree (seed coat)
- Allergen-containing smoke can cause respiratory tract inflammation, systemic contact dermatitis, and temporary blindness
- After contact with urushiol, a sensitized person develops erythema, vesicles/bullae, and edema within 2 days; the reaction can last 2 or 3 weeks (see Fig. 12.12)
- **Rx:** topical, or if severe, systemic CS; treatment should be for at least 2 weeks, otherwise rebound phenomenon common (i.e. avoid the use of a 6-day Medrol® dose pack)

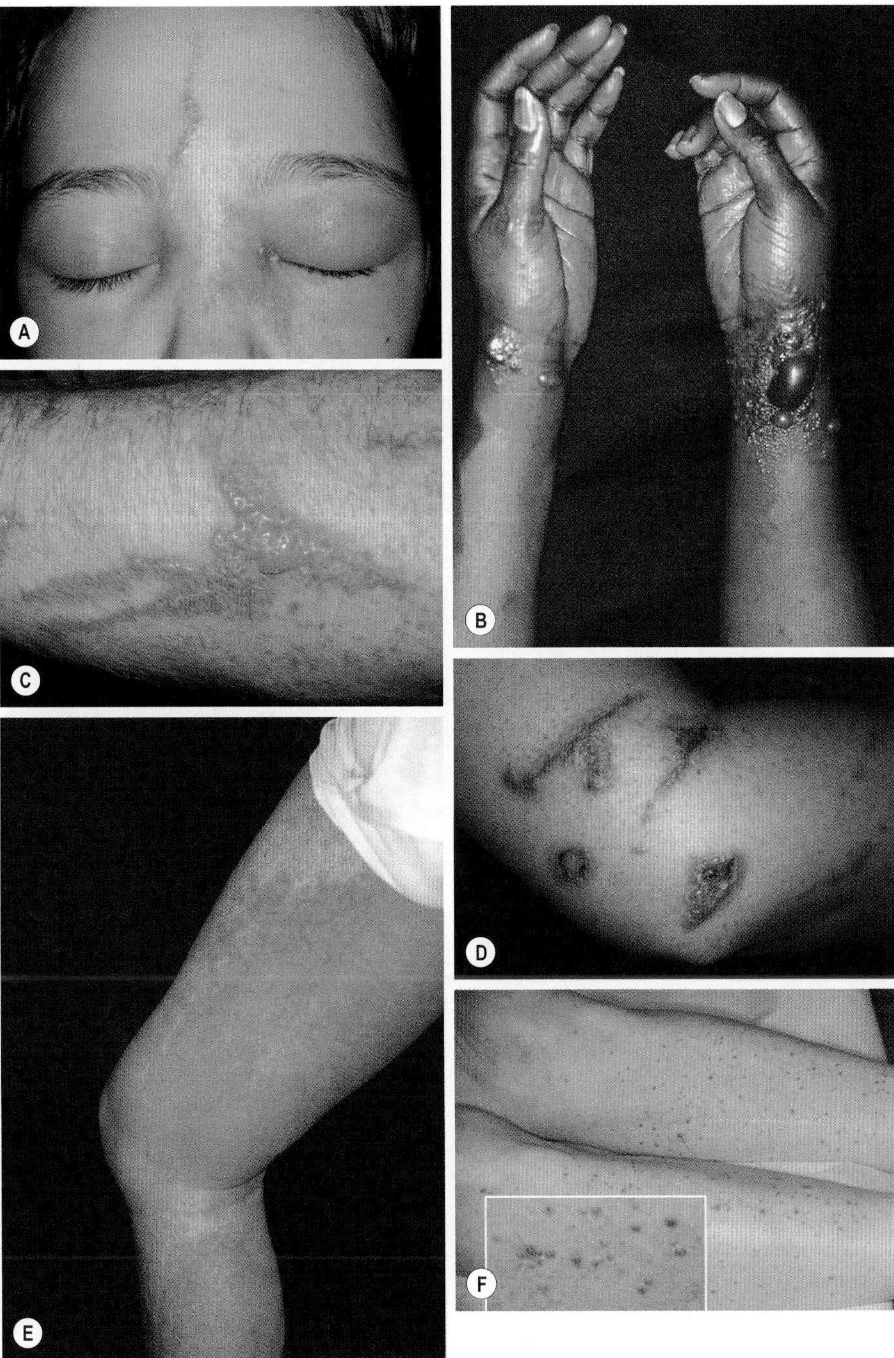

Fig. 12.12 Clinical manifestations of Anacardiaceae dermatitis. *Acute poison ivy dermatitis:* **A** Periorbital edema, in addition to crusted and weeping linear streaks and plaques. **B** This distribution pattern is seen in patients who wear gloves. **C** Erythematous streaks with linear vesicles. **D** "Black-spot" dermatitis: Note the black discoloration in the central portion of the edematous plaques due to plant resin. *Other:* **E** Allergic contact dermatitis due to cashew nut shell oil. This represented an occupational exposure. **F** Weed-whacker dermatitis with widespread spotted pattern. *A, F, Courtesy Louis A. Fragola, Jr., MD; B, E, Courtesy, YDRSC; C, Courtesy, Joyce Rico, MD; D, Courtesy, Kalman Watsky, MD.*

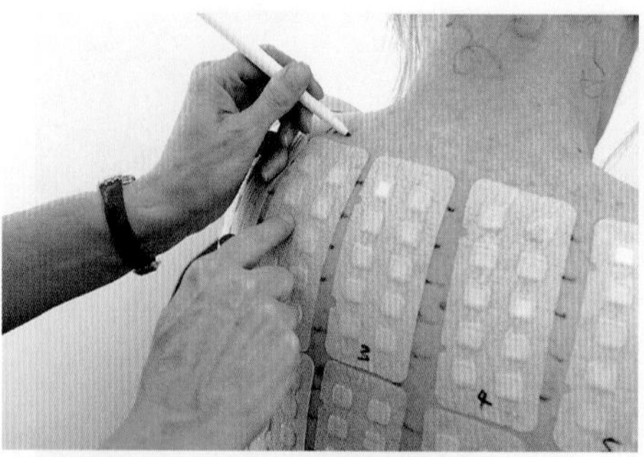

Fig. 12.13 Placement of allergens to the patient's back utilizing AllergEAZE™ chambers. *Courtesy, Rosemary L. Nixon, MD.*

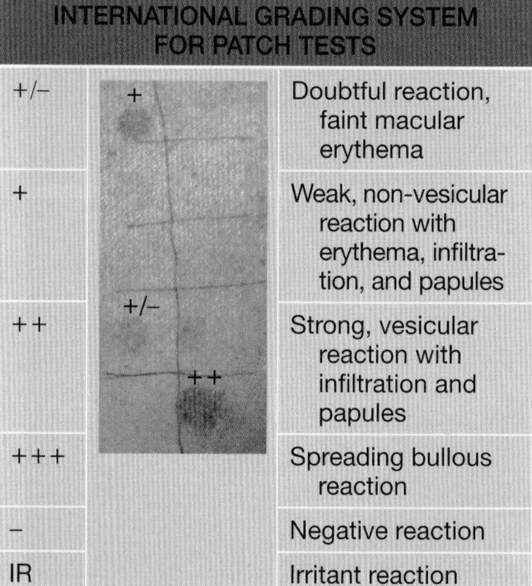

INTERNATIONAL GRADING SYSTEM FOR PATCH TESTS		
+/–		Doubtful reaction, faint macular erythema
+		Weak, non-vesicular reaction with erythema, infiltration, and papules
++		Strong, vesicular reaction with infiltration and papules
+++		Spreading bullous reaction
–		Negative reaction
IR		Irritant reaction

Grading is performed at two time points after the patch tests have been in place for 48 hours (then removed; see Fig. 12.14): initially after removal and then 1–7 days later.

Table 12.3 International grading system for patch tests.

- Phytophotodermatitis
  - Non-immunologic reaction to topical contact with a photosensitizer and subsequent exposure to ultraviolet A light

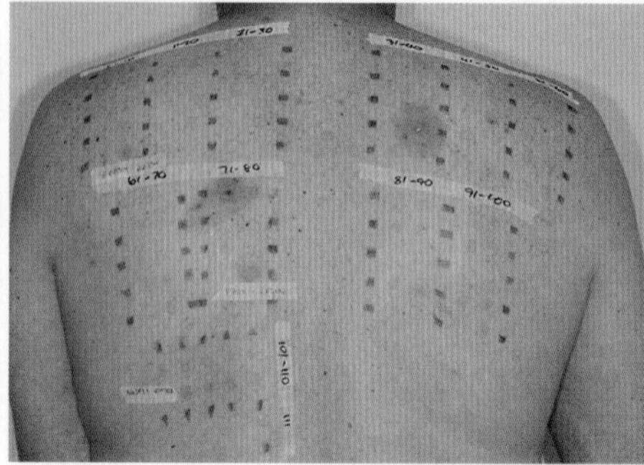

Fig. 12.14 Sites of specific patch tests labelled for future reference following removal of the chambers. *Courtesy, Rosemary L. Nixon, MD.*

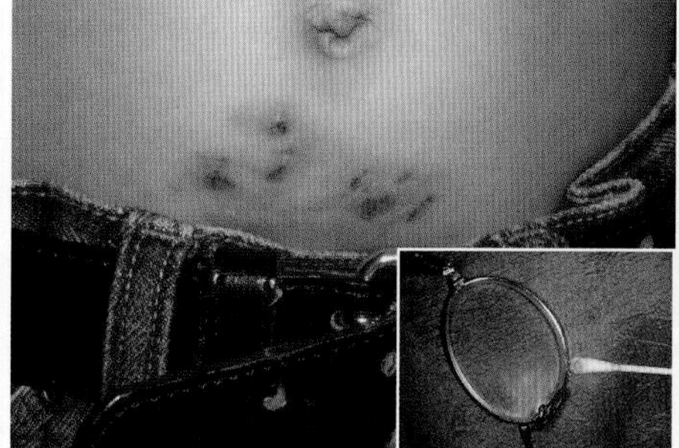

Fig. 12.15 Allergic contact dermatitis to nickel. Excoriated pink plaques due to nickel within the belt buckle. Inset: A positive dimethylglyoxime test in which the pink color indicates the presence of nickel. *Courtesy, Julie V. Schaffer, MD; Inset: Courtesy, Rosemary L. Nixon, MD.*

  - Erythema, vesicles/bullae, and subsequent hyperpigmentation; often in linear streaks or bizarre configurations; however, hyperpigmentation may be the only clinical finding (Figs 12.21 and 12.22)
  - Commonly secondary to furocoumarins (psoralens and angelicins) in plants, e.g. limes, celery, false Bishop's weed, and rue

For further information see Chs 14–17 from *Dermatology, Fourth Edition*.

For additional online figures and tables visit www.expertconsult.com 

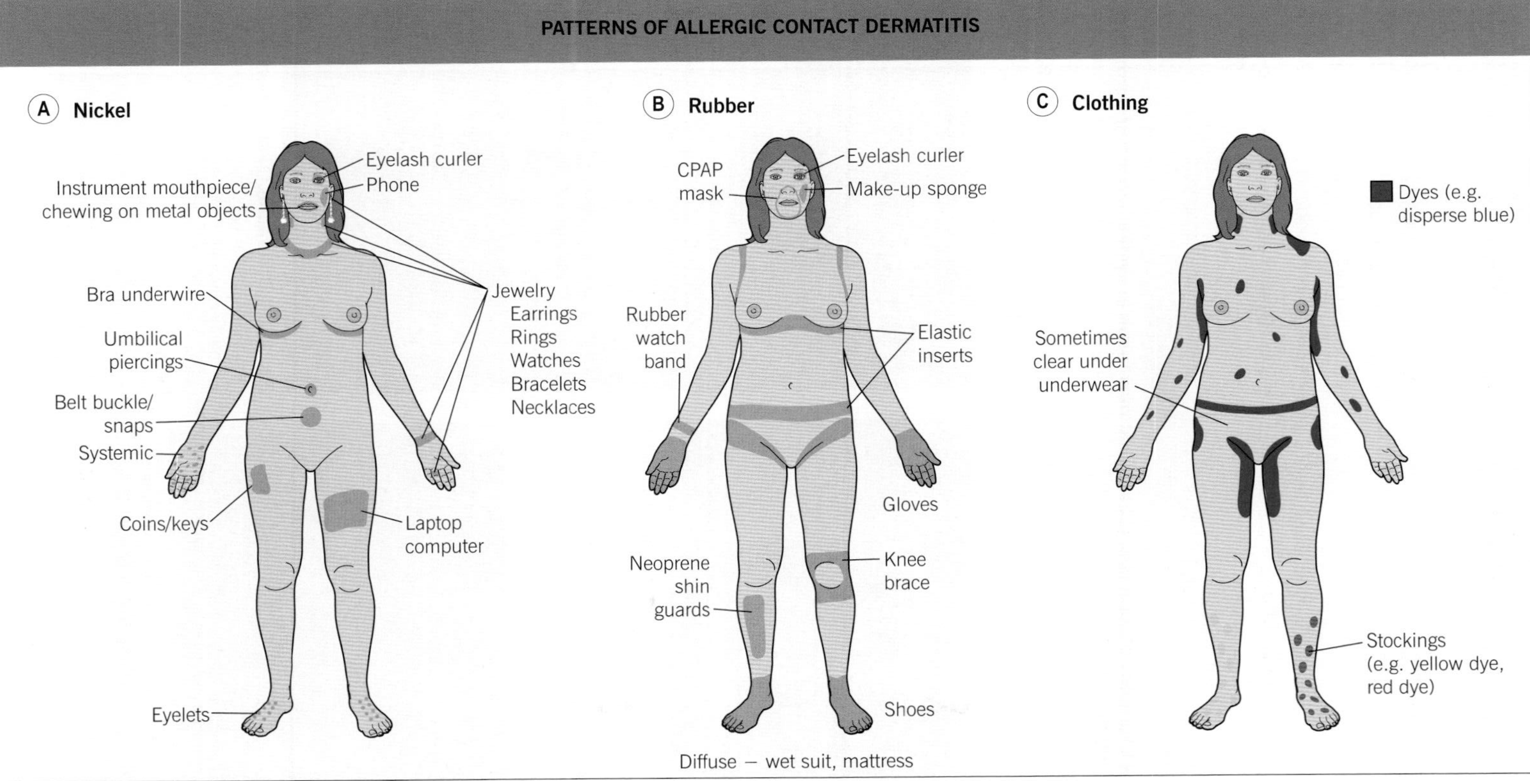

Fig. 12.16 Patterns of allergic contact dermatitis. A Due to nickel; lesions can also arise from metal braces and on the back at the site of bra clasps. **B** Due to rubber. **C** Due to dyes and resins in clothing. CPAP, continuous positive airway pressure. *Courtesy, Jean L. Bolognia, MD.*

EXAMPLES OF TOPICAL ALLERGENS THAT MAY RESULT IN SYSTEMIC CONTACT DERMATITIS AFTER SYSTEMIC EXPOSURE	
Cutaneous allergen	**Systemic exposure**
Ethylenediamine hydrochloride	Aminophylline, hydroxyzine/cetirizine
Poison ivy	Cashews, mango peel
Fragrance (balsam of Peru)	Foods, sodas, mouthwashes, spices
Sorbic acid	Preservative in food
Nickel and other metal salts	Nickel (and other metal salts) in food
Quinolones	Oral antibiotics
Neomycin	Streptomycin, kanamycin
Thiuram	Disulfiram

Table 12.4 Examples of topical allergens that may result in systemic contact dermatitis after systemic exposure.

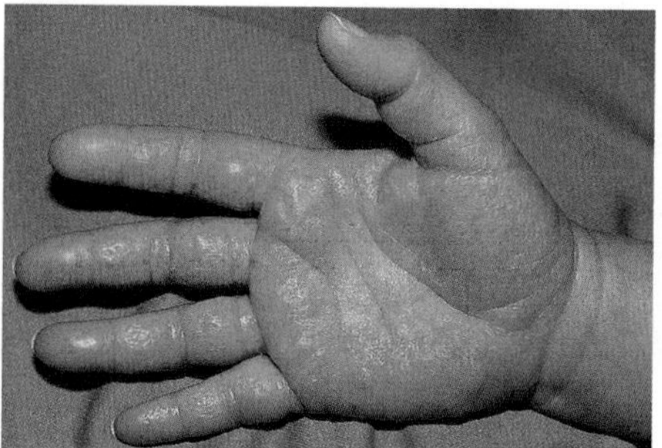

Fig. 12.17 Systemic contact dermatitis. This patient, who was previously sensitized to ethylenediamine, received intravenous aminophylline. *Courtesy, YDRSC.*

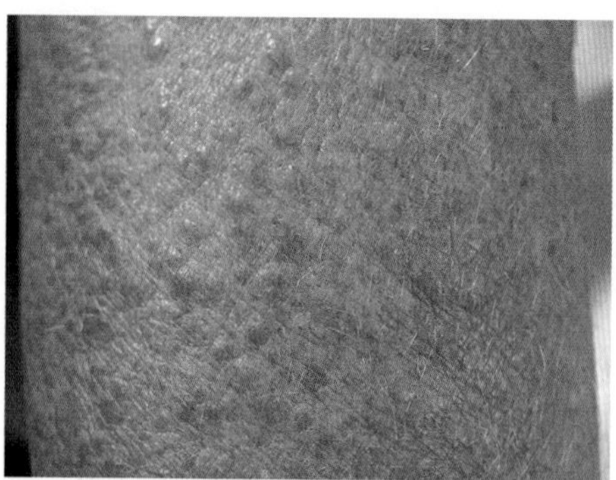

Fig. 12.18 Fiberglass dermatitis. Multiple pruritic pink papules at the site of exposure. *Courtesy, NYUDSC.*

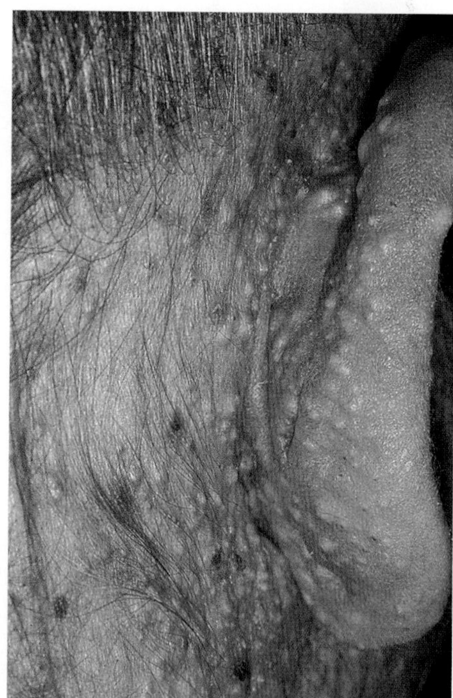

Fig. 12.19 Chloracne. Note involvement of retroauricular skin with numerous comedones (primarily closed) and cysts. The clinical differential diagnosis includes folliculotropic mycosis fungoides.

SELECTED OCCUPATIONAL DERMATOSES	
Dermatosis	**Key features**
Fiberglass dermatitis (Fig. 12.18)	Pruritus, tingling
	Erythematous papules (sometimes with follicular accentuation)
	Paronychia
Skin cancer	Major hazards are ultraviolet radiation, ionizing radiation, and carcinogenic chemicals
	Most common tumor is squamous cell carcinoma
Acne	Clinical features similar to non-occupationally related acne
	In addition, unusual sites may be affected (arms, abdomen)
	Inciting factors – exposures to oils, halogenated polycyclic hydrocarbons (chloracne), and repeated frictional trauma
	Chloracne – open comedones predominate; concentration of lesions on malar cheeks and behind ears (Fig. 12.19)
White finger(s)	Workers at risk include operators of chainsaws and pneumatic tools with exposures to vibrations from 30 to 300 Hz and cold
	Transient loss of sensation with possible permanent neuropathy
Orf	Seen in farmers, slaughterhouse workers, veterinarians
	Secondary to a parapoxvirus from exposure to sheep, goats, or reindeer
Herpetic whitlow	Exposure to herpes simplex virus, e.g. health care workers
Erysipeloid	Seen in farmers, fishermen, butchers
	Exposure to *Erysipelothrix rhusiopathiae* in shellfish, fish, birds, and mammals, especially pigs

Table 12.5 Selected occupational dermatoses.

MOST COMMON SKIN REACTIONS TO PLANTS		
Reaction type	**Plants/fruit**	**Inciting agent**
Allergic contact dermatitis	Poison ivy	Alkyl-catechols and resorcinols in urushiol
	Peruvian lily	Tulipalin A > B
	Chrysanthemum	Sesquiterpene lactones*
Irritant contact dermatitis	Dumb cane	Calcium oxalate
	Daffodils	Calcium oxalate
	Prickly pear	Glochids
Urticaria	Stinging nettle	Histamine
Phytophotodermatitis	Persian lime	Furocoumarins (psoralens and angelicins)
	Celery	Same
	Rue	Same
Other – burning/edema	Hot peppers	Capsaicin

**Can cause airborne contact dermatitis and positive in chronic actinic dermatitis.*

Table 12.6 Most common skin reactions to plants. Some plants can cause more than one reaction; e.g. garlic can cause ACD (diallyldisulfide), ICD, and urticaria.

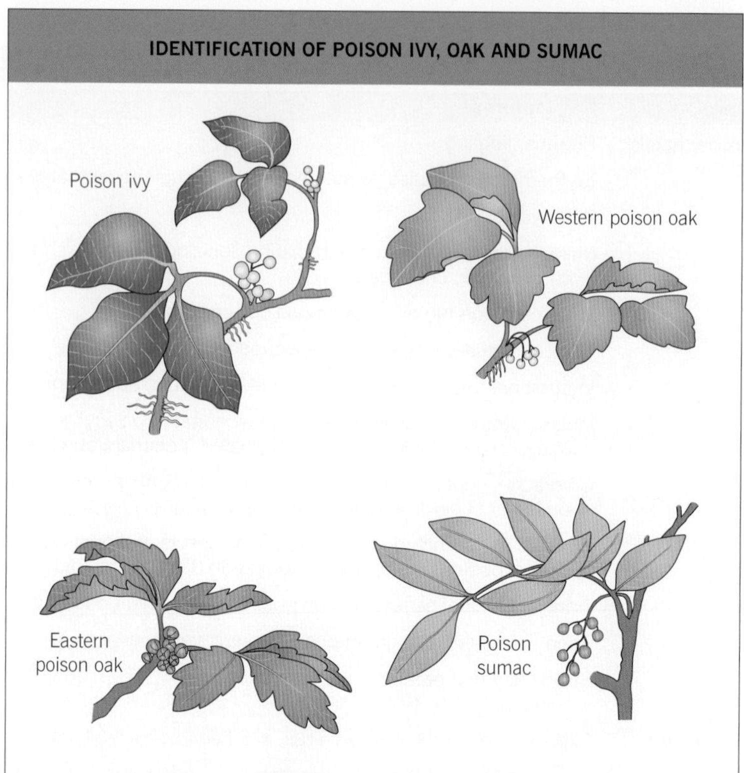

Fig. 12.20 Characteristic features useful for identifying poison ivy, poison oak, and poison sumac. *With permission from the American Journal of Contact Dermatitis.*

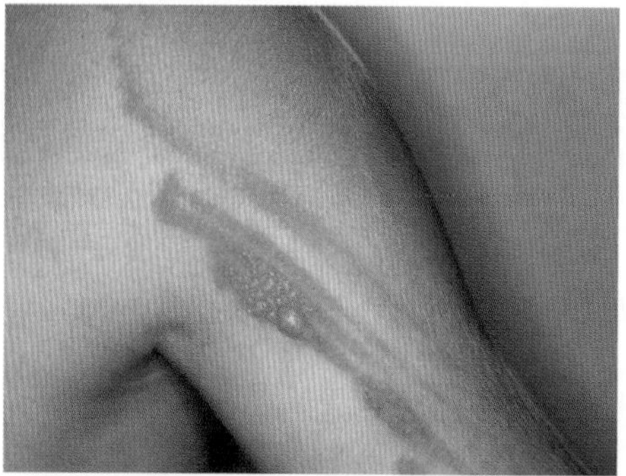

Fig. 12.21 Bullous phase of phytophotodermatitis. There was associated burning but no pruritus, and the linear bullae were replaced by hyperpigmentation. *Courtesy, Jean L. Bolognia, MD.*

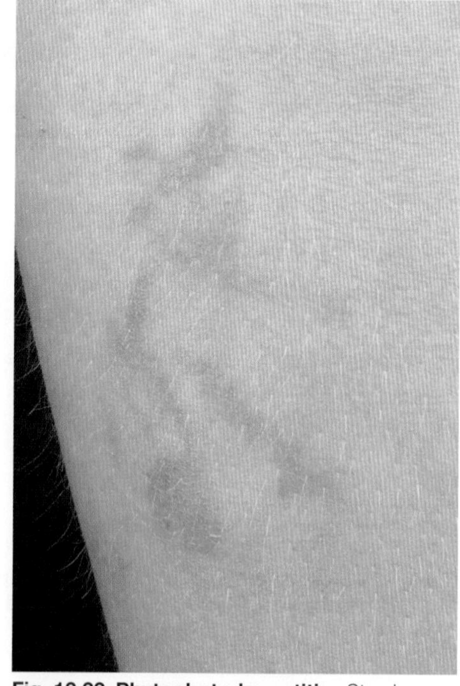

Fig. 12.22 Phytophotodermatitis. Streaky hyperpigmentation due to contact with a psoralen-containing plant followed by exposure to sunlight. *Courtesy, Lorenzo Cerroni, MD.*

Clinical Approach to Regional Dermatoses

13

• Some inflammatory, infectious, metabolic, neoplastic, and genetic skin conditions have a predilection for particular areas of the body.
• This chapter addresses the diagnosis and treatment of regional dermatoses affecting the hands, feet, intertriginous regions, diaper area, lips, and eyelids.

Dermatitis of the Hands and Feet

• An approach to the classification of hand dermatitis is presented in Fig. 13.1, and the differential diagnosis of foot dermatitis is summarized in Table 13.1.
• Because the hands and feet have a thicker stratum corneum than other areas of the body, percutaneous absorption of topical medications is decreased.
• High-potency topical CS or the use of occlusion may be needed to effectively treat inflammatory dermatoses in these sites.

Intertriginous Dermatitis

• Intertriginous areas include the inguinal creases, gluteal cleft, axillae, inframammary folds, and beneath pannus in obese patients.
• The differential diagnosis of dermatitis in the major skin folds is presented in Fig. 13.2.
• Other conditions with a predilection for intertriginous regions include skin tags, acanthosis nigricans, hidradenitis suppurativa, Fox–Fordyce disease, scabies, erythema migrans, variants of lichen planus (e.g. inverse, pigmentosus), inverse pityriasis rosea, vitiligo, lentigines in the setting of neurofibromatosis type 1, Dowling–Degos disease, and pseudoxanthoma elasticum.
• Occlusion and a high level of cutaneous hydration in intertriginous sites increase the absorption of topical medications.
• Low-potency topical CS are often effective for dermatoses in these areas, and prolonged use of more potent agents (including antifungal combination products; see below) has increased potential to result in side effects such as cutaneous atrophy (Fig. 13.3).

Diaper Dermatitis

• Develops in >50% of infants and has a variety of causes (Fig. 13.4).
• Dampness and exposure to urine and feces represent factors in the etiology of irritant and infectious forms of diaper dermatitis.
• Frequent changing of highly absorbent disposable diapers decreases the incidence and severity of diaper dermatitis.
• Seborrheic dermatitis and psoriasis in the diaper area predispose infants and toddlers to other forms of diaper dermatitis.
• An exuberant, multifactorial diaper dermatitis (e.g. sebopsoriasis with *Candida* or bacterial superinfection) can trigger the rapid development of numerous small, scaly erythematous papules in a widespread distribution on the trunk and extremities (psoriasiform "id" reaction).
• Mild topical CS are helpful for the inflammatory component of irritant dermatitis and primary dermatoses in the diaper area, while topical imidazole creams treat candidiasis and have additional anti-inflammatory effects; these agents can be used together for seborrheic dermatitis or psoriasis.
• Combination products containing a potent CS (e.g. Lotrisone® [clotrimazole + betamethasone dipropionate], Mycolog® [nystatin + triamcinolone]) and long-term daily use of any CS in the diaper area should be avoided (see above).
• Barrier ointments containing zinc oxide provide protective and soothing effects; a thick layer should be used (following application of anti-inflammatory/antimicrobial agents if needed) with each diaper change in patients with diaper dermatitis.

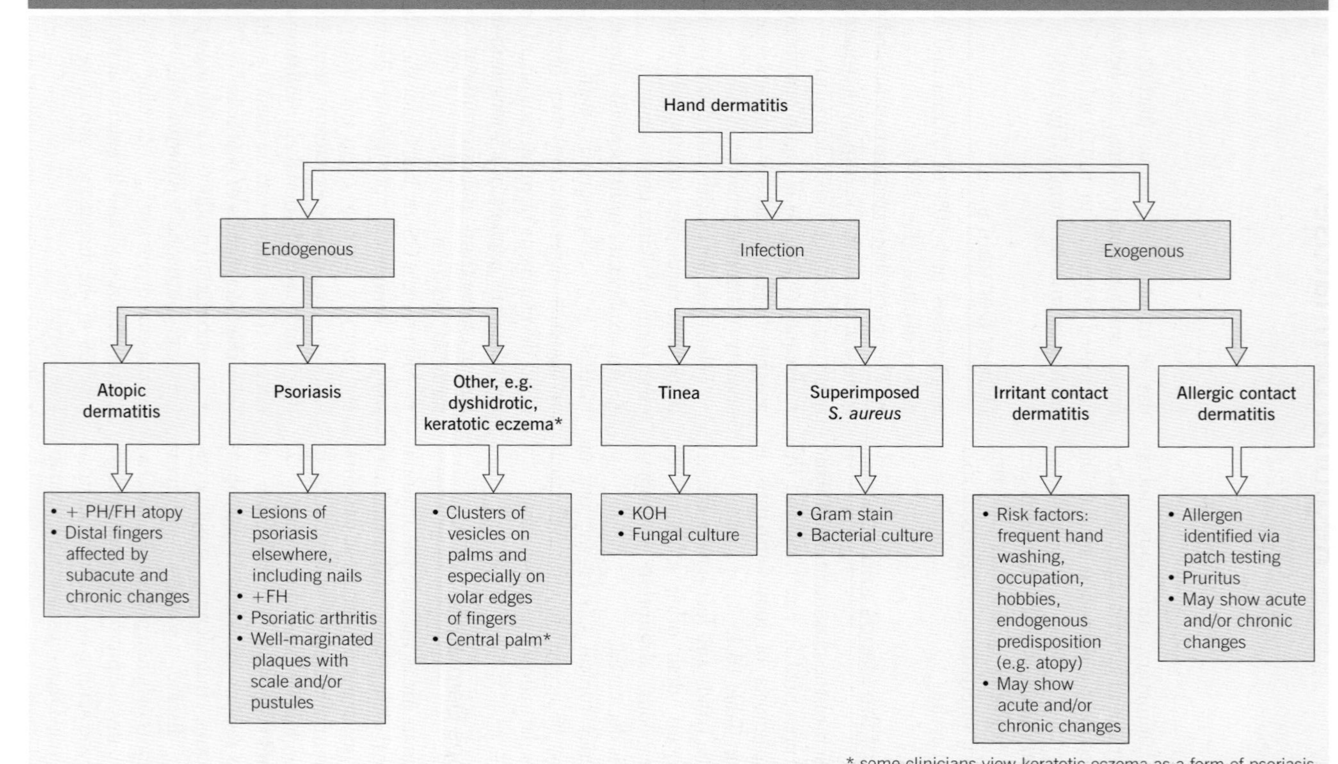

Fig. 13.1 Classification of hand dermatitis. More than one etiology may be present, e.g. atopic dermatitis plus irritant contact dermatitis. FH, family history; PH, personal history. *Courtesy, David E. Cohen, MD.*

DIFFERENTIAL DIAGNOSIS OF FOOT DERMATITIS
Allergic contact dermatitis
• Location of the dermatitis on the dorsal surface versus plantar surface (especially weight-bearing areas) of the feet can reflect an allergen in the top portion or sole of the shoe, respectively • Common shoe allergens include dichromate (used to tan leather), adhesive components (e.g. formaldehyde resins, colophony), rubber accelerators, and dyes; allergens implicated in foot dermatitis also include topical antibiotics (e.g. bacitracin) • Often associated with atopy and/or hyperhidrosis • Lesions extend more proximally in sock/stocking dermatitis, where the most common allergen is azo dyes
Dyshidrotic eczema
• Pruritic, deep-seated vesicles (often pinhead-sized) on the palms/soles and sides of the fingers/toes • Referred to as "pompholyx" when larger vesicles/bullae are present • Frequently associated with atopy or contact dermatitis (allergic and irritant)
Juvenile plantar dermatosis
• "Glazed" erythema, scale and fissuring on the balls of the feet and plantar aspect of the toes • Usually occurs in prepubertal children • Associated with atopic dermatitis, sweaty feet, and occlusive footwear
Tinea pedis (athlete's foot)
• Dermatophyte infections of the plantar skin are usually accompanied by involvement of the interdigital spaces (e.g. maceration) • A "moccasin" distribution of diffuse scaling/erythema and a vesicular inflammatory variant favoring the medial foot can also occur • Lesions on the lateral and dorsal aspects of the feet tend to have an annular configuration • Often associated with tinea unguium
Psoriasis
• Usually well-demarcated areas of erythema, adherent scale, and often fissuring • Psoriasiform plaques elsewhere (e.g. dorsal hands/feet, elbows/knees, scalp) and nail involvement (e.g. pitting, oil spots)
Pustulosis of the palms and soles
• "Sterile" pustules admixed with yellow-brown macules favoring the instep • Often *not* associated with plaque psoriasis elsewhere • Keratoderma blennorrhagicum occurs in the setting or reactive arthritis
Keratolysis exfoliativa (recurrent focal palmar and plantar peeling)
• Circinate pattern of superficial desquamation (collarettes) on the palms and/or soles • Worsens in warm weather and is associated with low-grade irritation/friction
Keratoderma climactericum
• Mechanically induced hyperkeratosis and fissuring on the heels and weight-bearing areas of the soles • Typically occurs in women >45 years of age • Predisposing factors include obesity and a cold, dry climate
Other
• Atopic dermatitis • Irritant contact dermatitis (e.g. related to occlusive footwear) • Crusted scabies • Pityriasis rubra pilaris • Inherited palmoplantar keratoderma (diffuse or focal) • Acquired keratoderma, e.g. associated with hypothyroidism

Table 13.1 Differential diagnosis of foot dermatitis.

DIFFERENTIAL DIAGNOSIS OF INTERTRIGINOUS DERMATOSES IN ADULTS

Common → Less common → Uncommon

Common

Irritant/frictional intertrigo*
- Ill-defined erythema/maceration
- Predisposing factors: obesity, heat & humidity, hyperhidrosis, diabetes mellitus, poor hygiene
- Secondary infections common

Seborrheic dermatitis**
- Well-demarcated, pink to red, moist patches/plaques
- Centered along inguinal creases
- Involvement of scalp, face, ears

Inverse psoriasis**
- Well-demarcated, pink to red plaques
- Shiny with little scale in folds
- Centered along inguinal creases
- Psoriasiform plaques elsewhere (e.g. genitals, intergluteal cleft, scalp, elbows/knees, hands/feet)
- Nail psoriasis (pitting, oil spots)

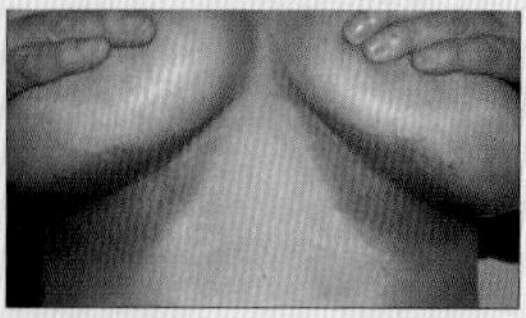

Dermatophytosis (tinea cruris)
- Less often centered along inguinal creases
- Expanding annular lesions with scaly erythematous border that may contain pustules or vesicles
- Extension to inner thigh, buttock; usually spares scrotum
- Coexisting tinea pedis/unguium very common

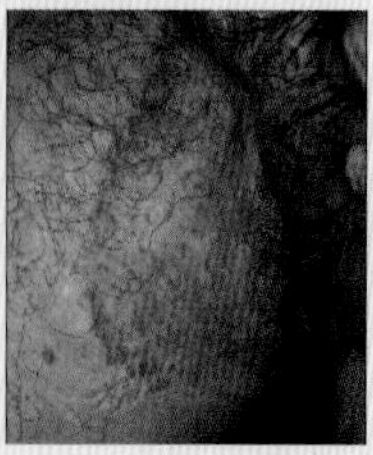

Less common

Candidiasis
- Intense erythema with desquamation and satellite papules/pustules
- Often involves scrotum as well as skin folds
- Predisposing factors: occlusion, hyperhidrosis, diabetes mellitus, antibiotic or corticosteroid use, immunosuppression

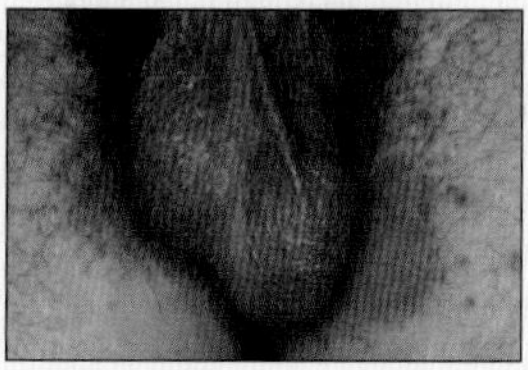

Erythrasma
- Pink–red to brown patches with fine scale
- Coral-red fluorescence with Wood's lamp illumination

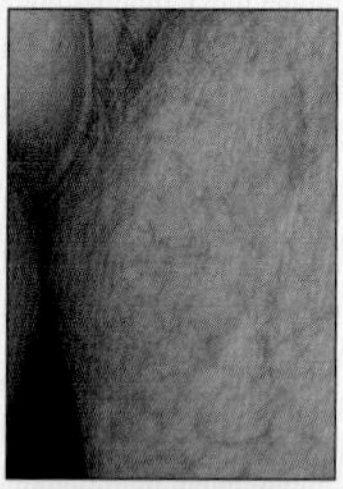

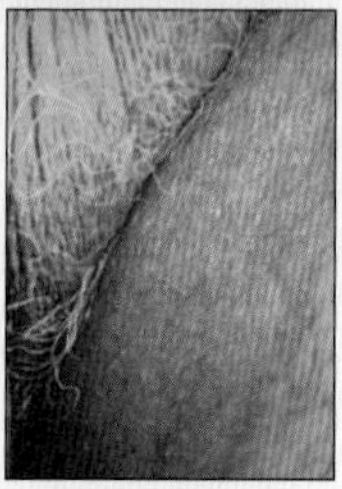

Allergic contact dermatitis
- Consider if fails to respond to usual therapy

Uncommon

Granular parakeratosis

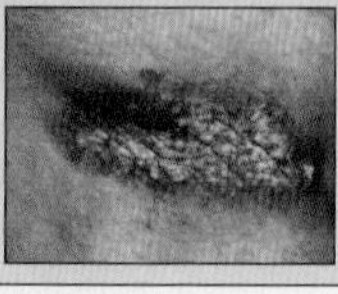

Systemic contact dermatitis, symmetrical drug-related intertriginous and flexural exanthema (Table 13.2), toxic erythema of chemotherapy

Hailey–Hailey disease, Darier disease (depicted), **pemphigus vegetans**

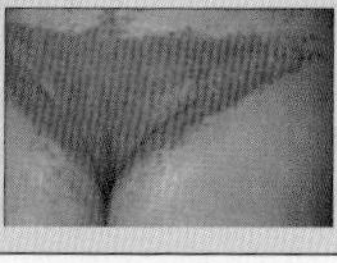

Zinc deficiency, necrolytic migratory erythema, other "nutritional dermatitis"

Cutaneous Crohn disease

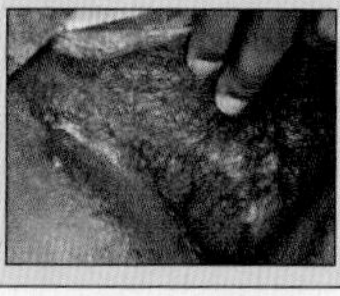

Langerhans cell histiocytosis

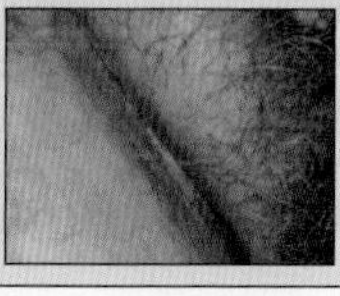

Extramammary Paget disease

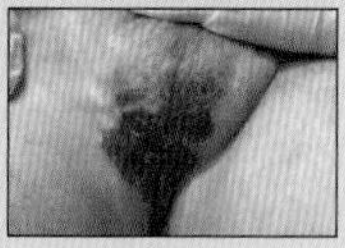

*Also referred to more nonspecifically as intertriginous dermatitis or intertrigo.
**The term "sebopsoriasis" may be used when features of both seborrheic dermatitis and psoriasis are present.

Fig. 13.2 Differential diagnosis of intertriginous dermatitis in adults. Individual patients often have multiple disorders superimposed upon one another. Bullous impetigo and streptococcal intertrigo are considerably more common in children than adults (see Fig. 13.4). *Insets: Courtesy, Luis Requena, MD; YDRSC; Eugene Mirrer, MD; Louis A. Fragola, Jr., MD; David Mehregan, MD and Robert Hartman, MD.*

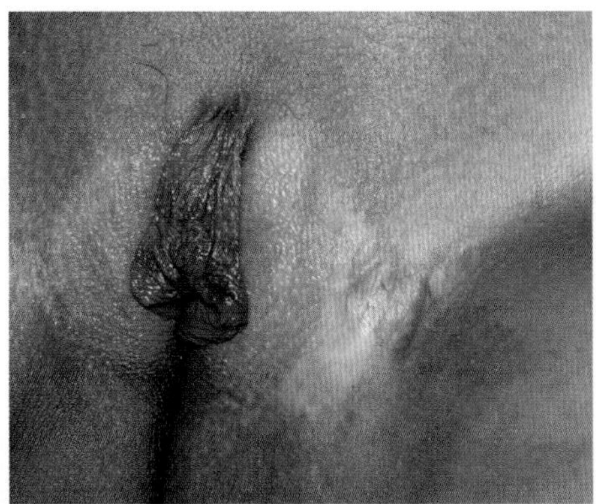

Fig. 13.3 Cutaneous atrophy in the inguinal fold from chronic use of a topical CS. This 10-year-old girl's seborrheic dermatitis had been treated with a mid-potency topical CS on a daily basis for several years, resulting in the development of striae. *Courtesy, Julie V. Schaffer, MD.*

Cheilitis

• The differential diagnosis of cheilitis and clues to determining the etiology are outlined in Fig. 13.5.

Eyelid Dermatitis

• An approach to the classification of eyelid dermatitis is presented in Fig. 13.6.

SYMMETRICAL DRUG-RELATED INTERTRIGINOUS AND FLEXURAL EXANTHEMA (SDRIFE): CLINICAL CRITERIA
• Exposure to a systemically administered drug*, occurring with either the initial or a repeated dose (excluding contact allergens)
• Sharply demarcated erythema of the gluteal/perianal area and/or V-shaped erythema of the inguinal/genital area
• Involvement of at least one other intertriginous site/flexural fold
• Symmetric involvement in affected areas
• Absence of systemic symptoms and signs
**Not a chemotherapeutic agent, so distinct from toxic erythema of chemotherapy.*

Table 13.2 Symmetrical drug-related intertriginous and flexural exanthema (SDRIFE): clinical criteria. This entity is also referred to as drug-induced intertrigo, flexural drug eruption, and baboon syndrome. The latter term is also used for a form of systemic contact dermatitis. *Adapted from Häusermann P, Harr TH, Bircher AJ. Baboon syndrome resulting from systemic drugs: Is there strife between SDRIFE and allergic contact dermatitis syndrome? Contact Dermatitis 2004;51:297–310.*

• Low-potency topical CS are often effective for dermatitis on the eyelids because of the delicate skin in this site, and prolonged CS use (especially of more potent agents) may potentially lead to ocular side effects.

For further information see Chs 13 and 15 from *Dermatology, Fourth Edition*.

For additional online figures and tables visit www.expertconsult.com 

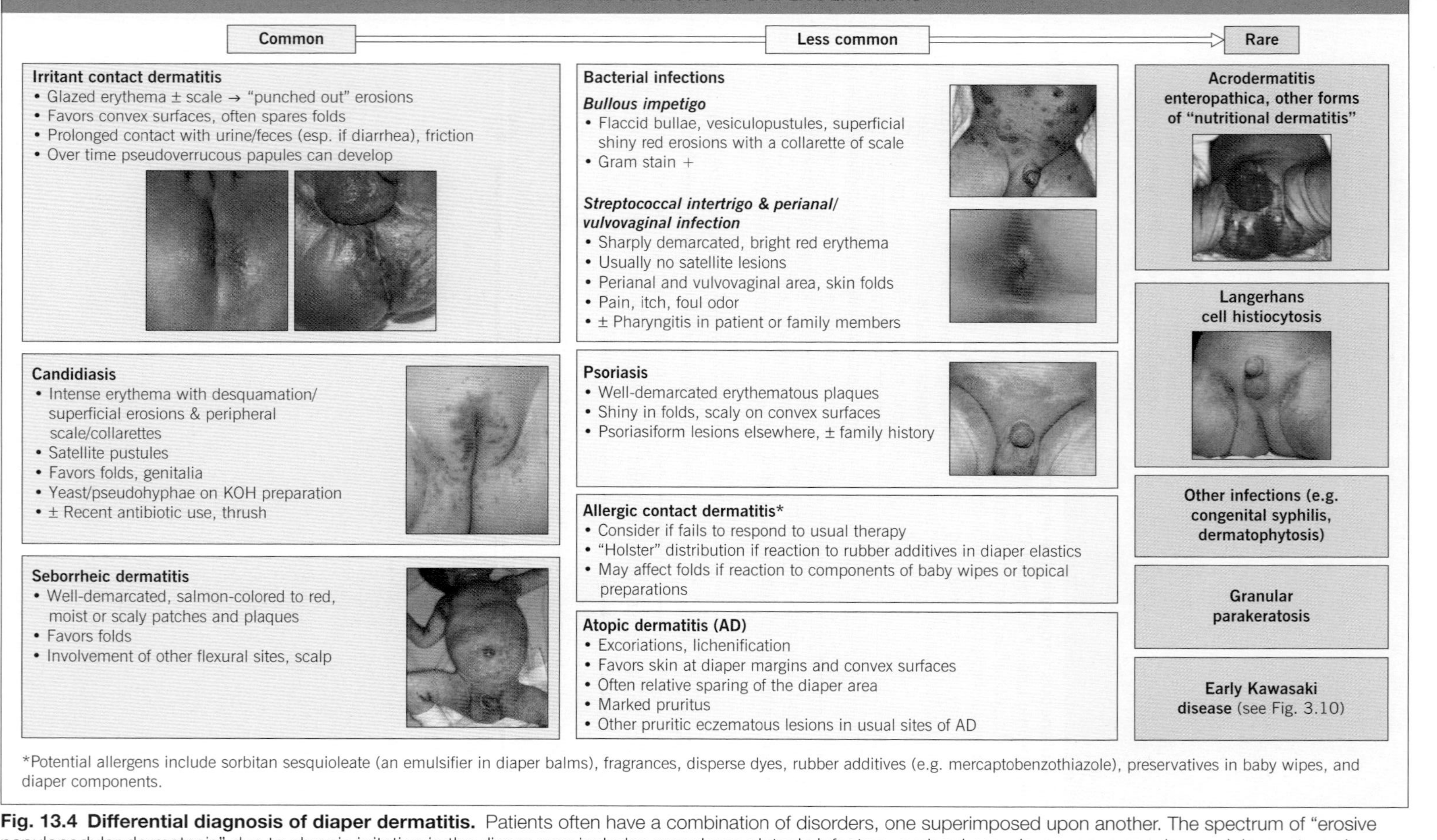

Fig. 13.4 Differential diagnosis of diaper dermatitis. Patients often have a combination of disorders, one superimposed upon another. The spectrum of "erosive papulonodular dermatosis" due to chronic irritation in the diaper area includes granuloma gluteale infantum, perianal pseudoverrucous papules, and Jacquet erosive dermatitis. Discrete papules or nodules can also be seen in scabies. Coxsackievirus infection and congenital syphilis may present with erosions in this location. *Insets:*

(A)

Common → Less common

Actinic cheilitis

- Lower >> upper vermilion lip (see Fig. 88.2F)
- Background of photodamage
- History of AKs, BCC, SCC
- May have diffuse hyperkeratosis and/or discrete AKs

Irritant contact dermatitis

- Both lower & upper lip involved
- Often extends onto cutaneous lip **(B)**
- Lip-licking most common cause

Atopic dermatitis

- Atopic diathesis, xerosis
- Lesions of atopic dermatitis elsewhere
- Angular fissures

Allergic contact dermatitis

- Both upper and lower lip involved
- Allergens include: fragrances/flavorings (e.g. in oral hygiene products and cosmetics), preservatives, sunscreens **(C)** > metals (e.g. nickel; perioral area > vermilion lips), topical antibiotics, propolis, topical corticosteroids

Candidal cheilitis

- Predisposing factors: dentures/orthodontic appliances, inhaled/oral corticosteroids, diabetes mellitus, HIV infection, deep oral commissure grooves, drooling
- May have erosions
- Angular fissures
- More likely to have oral thrush **(D)**

Lichen planus (LP) & GVHD

- Lacy pattern on lips and oral mucosa (LP, **E**; see Fig. 44.4C)
- Oral ulcerations
- Lesions of LP or GVHD elsewhere

Granulomatous cheilitis

- Diffuse enlargement of lips (see Fig. 59.12)
- Superimposed processes may lead to secondary changes
- May be associated with scrotal tongue, 7th nerve palsy
- Subset of patients have underlying Crohn disease, which can also present with angular fissures, linear ulcers of the buccal vestibule, and oral aphthae

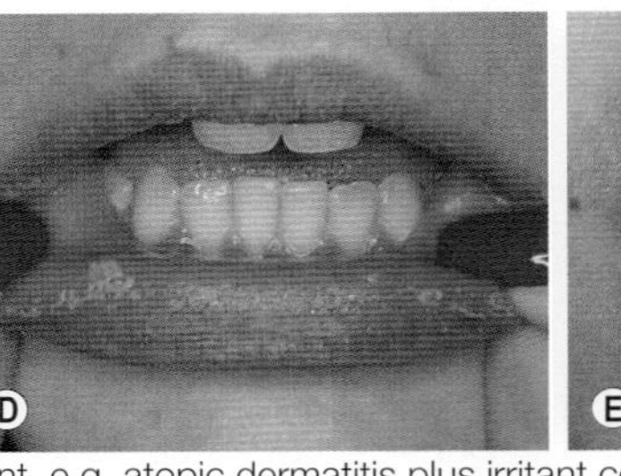
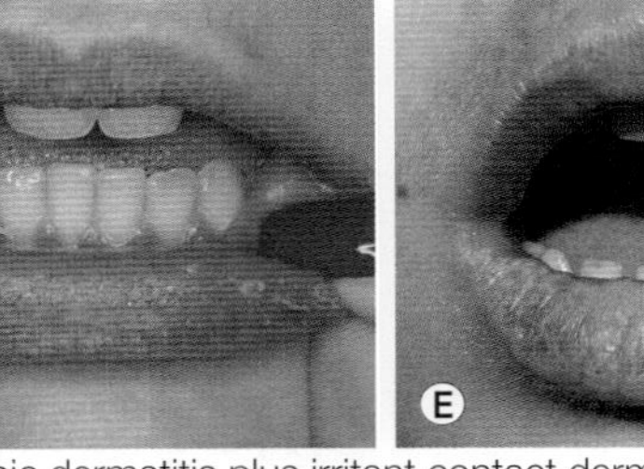
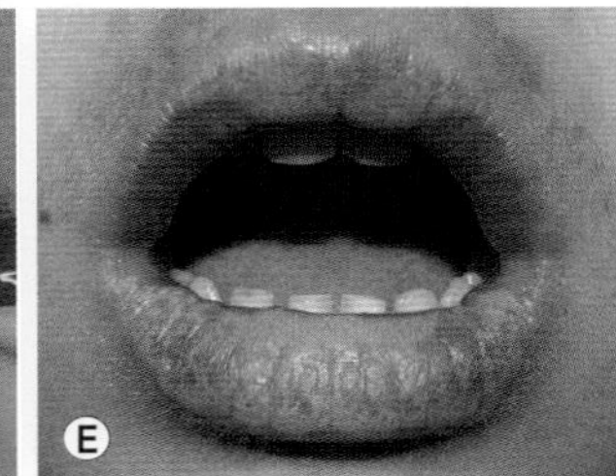

Fig. 13.5 Differential diagnosis of cheilitis. **A** Multiple etiologies are often present, e.g. atopic dermatitis plus irritant contact dermatitis. Other uncommon causes include cheilitis glandularis, actinic prurigo, lichen sclerosus, and nutritional deficiencies. **B** Irritant contact dermatitis – this patient had the habit of licking his lips and there is involvement of the vermilion and cutaneous lips as well as the perioral region. **C** Allergic contact dermatitis to oxybenzone with involvement of the upper and lower lips. **D** Thrush and candidal cheilitis. **E** Lichen planus presenting with a lacy pattern on the lips in a young boy. *A, Courtesy, Jean L. Bolognia, MD; B, Courtesy Jeffrey Callen, MD; C, Courtesy, Kalman Watsky, MD; D, Courtesy, Louis A. Fragola, Jr., MD; E, Courtesy, Julie V. Schaffer, MD.*

CLASSIFICATION OF EYELID DERMATITIS

Eyelid dermatitis

- **Endogenous***
  - **Seborrheic dermatitis > psoriasis**
    - Greasy scale
    - Affects eyelid margins & creases
  - **Atopic dermatitis**
    - Marked lichenification
    - Dennie–Morgan folds, periorbital darkening
  - **Ocular rosacea**
    - Eyelid margins only
    - Conjunctival injection, recurrent "styes"
  - **Dermatomyositis**
    - Purple-violet color (heliotrope)
    - Periorbital edema
- **Exogenous**
  - **Allergic contact dermatitis**
    - + Patch testing
    - Most often to preservatives, fragrances; consider nail products
    - Consider airborne contact dermatitis (e.g. to Compositae plants) if involves other exposed sites
  - **Irritant contact dermatitis**
    - Topical medications (e.g. for acne), anti-aging creams, cosmetics, occupational exposures

(A) *Diagnostic clues include a history of the condition and characteristic lesions elsewhere

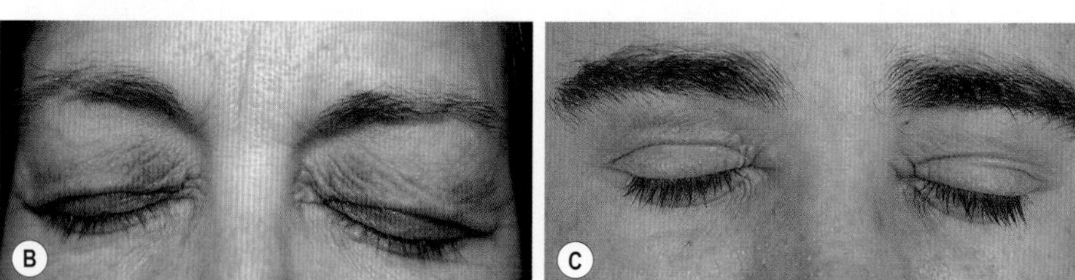

Fig. 13.6 Classification of eyelid dermatitis. A More than one etiology may be present, e.g. atopic dermatitis plus irritant contact dermatitis. **B** Allergic contact dermatitis to neomycin. **C** Airborne contact dermatitis to an epoxy resin.

Urticaria and Angioedema 14

- Urticaria and angioedema can occur at any age and are estimated to have an overall lifetime prevalence of 10–25%.
- Urticaria (hives) is characterized by *wheals*: evanescent, pale to pink-red, edematous papules or plaques (Fig. 14.1); lesions often have central clearing, a peripheral erythematous flare, and associated pruritus.
- Individual wheals last <24 hours, which can be documented by outlining them with ink.
- Angioedema represents deeper dermal and subcutaneous or submucosal swelling (Fig. 14.2); affected areas are ill-defined, have minimal or no overlying erythema, and may be painful as well as pruritic.
- In addition to the skin/subcutis, angioedema can affect the mouth and respiratory or gastrointestinal tract; an area of swelling may persist for several days.
- A classification scheme and **DDx** for urticaria and angioedema are presented in Table 14.1; patients with angioedema may have associated urticaria, including physical urticaria.
- Urticaria and urticaria-associated angioedema result from the release of histamine and other proinflammatory and vasoactive

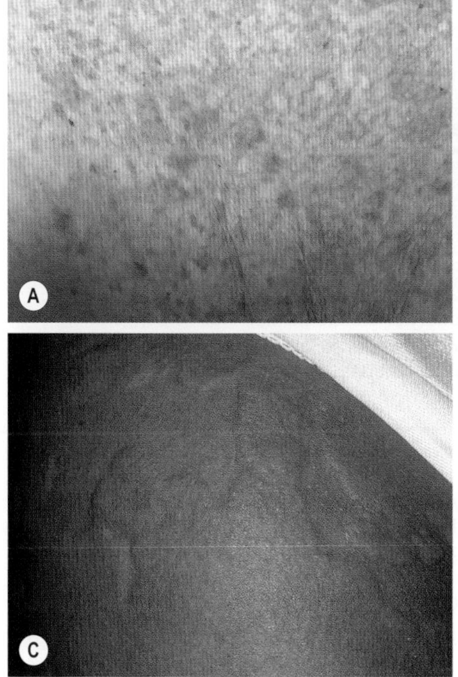

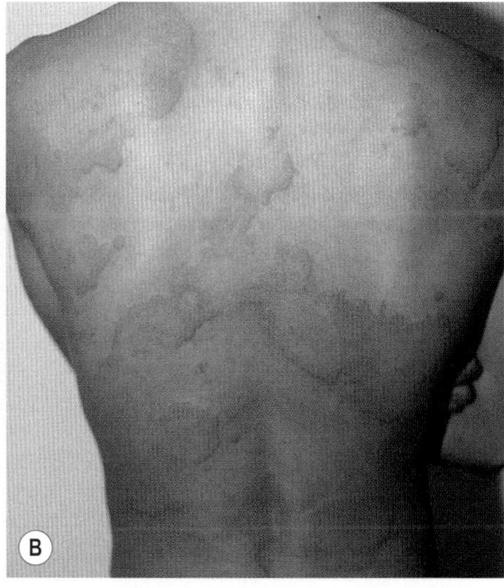

Fig. 14.1 Wheals. Wheals can be small **(A)** or large and annular **(B),** but they still retain the classic central pallor and erythematous flare. **C** Occasionally, more uniform edematous plaques are seen. *A, Courtesy, Jean L. Bolognia, MD; B, C, Courtesy, YDRSC.*

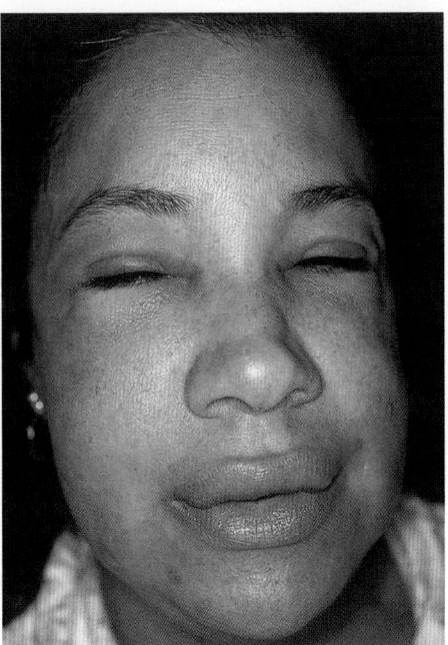

Fig. 14.2 **Angioedema.** The swelling is deeper than in wheals and may affect mucosal surfaces. Note the swelling of the lips and periorbital region and the lack of erythema. *Courtesy, Clive E. H. Grattan, MD.*

substances from mast cells; this leads to extravasation of plasma, vasodilatation, and pruritus.

- Stimuli for mast cell degranulation are shown in Fig. 14.3.

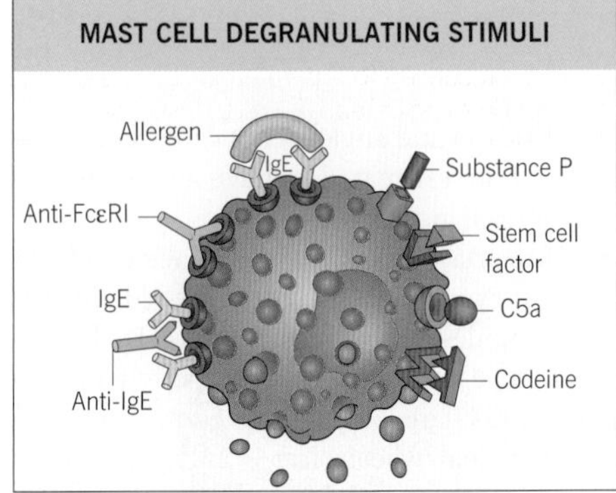

Fig. 14.3 Mast cell degranulating stimuli. Both immunologic and non-immunologic stimuli can lead to release of mediators. Stem cell factor is also known as KIT ligand. Autoantibodies against the high-affinity IgE receptor (FcεRI) and the Fc portion of IgE are implicated in chronic autoimmune urticaria.

CLASSIFICATION AND DIFFERENTIAL DIAGNOSIS OF URTICARIA AND ANGIOEDEMA

- **Spontaneous ("ordinary") urticaria**
  - Acute (duration <6 weeks)
  - Chronic (occurring at least twice weekly for ≥6 weeks*): median duration of ~2–5 years; includes an autoimmune form
- **Inducible urticaria (including physical urticaria)**
  - *Due to mechanical stimuli*: dermographism, delayed pressure urticaria†
  - *Due to temperature changes*: cold > heat-induced urticaria
  - *Due to sweating/physical exertion:* cholinergic > adrenergic urticaria, exercise-induced anaphylaxis
  - *Due to sun or water exposure:* solar and aquagenic urticaria
  - Contact urticaria (immunologic or non-immunologic)
- **Angioedema without wheals** (including hereditary angioedema; see Fig. 14.10)
- Related conditions in **DDx****: Schnitzler syndrome, serum sickness-like reaction (see Ch. 17), urticarial vasculitis† (see Ch. 19), hereditary autoinflammatory (e.g. periodic fever) syndromes (see Table 3.2)
- Additional **DDx:**
  - *For transient urticarial lesions*: Still disease, scombroid poisoning, erythema marginatum, cutaneous mastocytosis (also persistent red-brown papules/plaques)
  - *For urticarial lesions lasting >24 hours*: urticarial drug eruption, viral exanthem, erythema multiforme (central duskiness/vesiculation rather than clearing), insect bite reactions, Sweet syndrome, urticarial bullous pemphigoid, acute hemorrhagic edema of infancy, Kawasaki disease
  - *For angioedema*: early airborne or allergic contact dermatitis, insect bite reaction

**Urticaria occurring less frequently than this over a long period is referred to as episodic or recurrent.*
†Individual lesions tend to last >24 hours; urticarial vasculitis features burning/pain, purpura upon resolution, and a subgroup associated with hypocomplementemia and autoimmune connective tissue disease (e.g. SLE).
***Consider for chronic urticaria with associated symptoms such as fevers, pain, and arthralgias.*

Table 14.1 Classification and differential diagnosis of urticaria and angioedema.

CAUSES OF ACUTE AND CHRONIC SPONTANEOUS URTICARIA	
Acute urticaria	**Chronic urticaria**
• Infection (e.g. URI) (~40%) • Drug (~10%) • Food (≤1%) • Idiopathic (~50%)	• Autoimmune (histamine-releasing autoantibodies against FcεRI or the Fc portion of IgE; see Fig. 14.3) (40–50%) • Chronic infection (e.g. parasitic) (≤5%) • Pseudoallergic (≤5%) • Idiopathic (~50%)

Table 14.2 Causes of acute and chronic spontaneous urticaria. Acute urticaria data is for patients presenting to a dermatologist or emergency department. FcεRI, high-affinity IgE receptor (present on mast cells); IgE, immunoglobulin E.

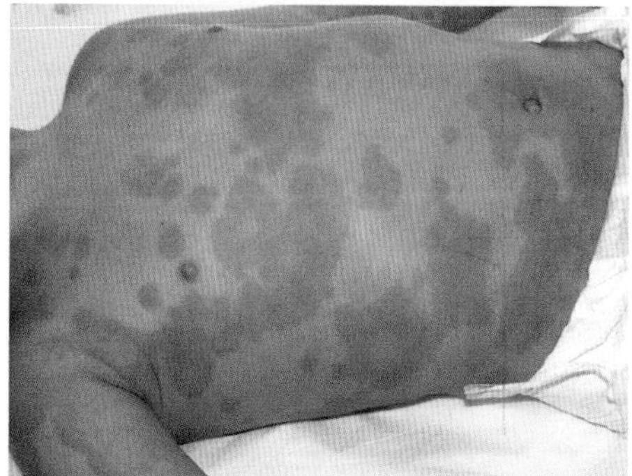

Fig. 14.4 Urticaria in a young child. This clinical presentation of urticaria, which is referred to as "urticaria multiforme", is sometimes misdiagnosed as erythema multiforme because of the dusky centers. As lesions expand, central clearing can occur, which is not seen in erythema multiforme. *Courtesy, Luis Requena, MD.*

Spontaneous ("Ordinary") Urticaria: Acute and Chronic

- Although both can occur at any age, acute urticaria is most common in children, whereas chronic urticaria has a peak in the fourth decade of life and a female:male ratio of ~2:1.
- The most frequent causes of acute and chronic urticaria are listed in Table 14.2.
- Acute urticaria in young children often presents with large annular or polycyclic lesions (urticaria "multiforme"; Fig. 14.4; see Fig. 3.3A) that tend to resolve with a transient dusky purplish hue, which can lead to misdiagnosis as erythema multiforme.
- Urticaria can result in sleep disturbances and anxiety.
- Chronic autoimmune urticaria is associated with an increased risk of other autoimmune conditions, such as thyroid disorders and celiac disease.
- An approach to the diagnosis of chronic urticaria is outlined in Fig. 14.5; extensive laboratory evaluations (e.g. for food allergies) are extremely low-yield and are not recommended.
- **Rx:** a stepwise therapeutic approach is presented in Fig. 14.6; long-acting antihistamines are the mainstay of treatment, and systemic corticosteroids should be avoided.

Inducible Urticaria

- Different forms of physical urticaria and other inducible urticaria variants may coexist with one another and/or chronic spontaneous urticaria.
- **Rx:** see Fig. 14.6.

Dermographism ("Skin Writing")

- Affects at least 10% of the general population; may lead to symptoms such as pruritus.
- Linear or irregularly shaped wheals develop at sites of scratching or friction (Fig. 14.7); lesions typically resolve within an hour.
- Can elicit via stroking the skin, e.g. with a thin wooden stick or tongue depressor.

Delayed Pressure Urticaria

- Pruritic and/or painful erythema and swelling (Fig. 14.8) develop 0.5–12 hours after sustained pressure to the skin (e.g. due to tight clothing or shoes); may last several days, sometimes with associated arthralgias and malaise.

Cold Urticaria

- Wheals ± angioedema develop within minutes of cold exposure, with maximal hiving upon rewarming; systemic reactions (e.g. anaphylaxis) may occur with aquatic activities.

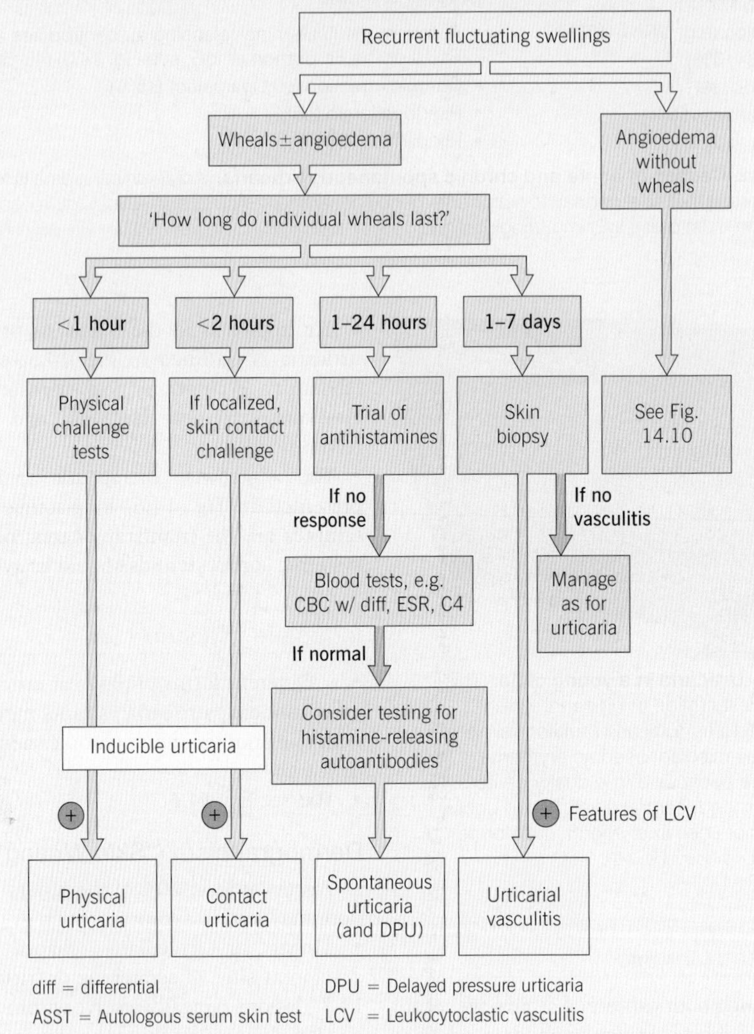

Fig. 14.5 Approach to the diagnosis of chronic urticaria. In a positive ASST, a localized wheal and flare response occurs upon intradermal injection of autologous serum, providing evidence of functional histamine-releasing factors in the blood. Regulations regarding blood products limit the availability of this test. *Courtesy, Clive E. H. Grattan, MD.*

- Can elicit via ice cube test (Fig. 14.9; 1- to 10-minute application within glove, then rewarming).
- Usually primary; <5% of cases are associated with cryoglobulins or cryofibrinogen.
- Rare early-onset variants with autosomal dominant inheritance and a negative ice cube test: cryopyrin-associated periodic syndrome (see Table 3.2), familial atypical cold urticaria (wheals upon evaporative cooling; *PLCG2* mutations).

Cholinergic Urticaria

- Multiple small (2–3 mm), monomorphic, pruritic wheals with an erythematous flare develop within 15 minutes of sweat-inducing stimulus (e.g. physical exertion, emotional stress, hot bath); favors the upper body but may be widespread.
- **DDx:** adrenergic urticaria (blanched halo rather than flare), heat urticaria (can occur without sweating), exercise-induced urticaria/anaphylaxis (only with exercise, not a hot

MANAGEMENT OF SPONTANEOUS AND PHYSICAL URTICARIAS

- Eliminate any modifiable cause
- Avoid physical triggers and drugs that stimulate mast cell degranulation (e.g. aspirin, NSAIDs, codeine, morphine)

↓

Scheduled administration of long-acting, low-sedating H1 antihistamine(s)
- Increasing to 2- to 4-times the standard dose, especially of (levo)cetirizine, can maximize benefit

↓ If response is not adequate

Combination therapies
- Consider adding another H1 antihistamine; low-dose doxepin* (10–50 mg in adults) at bedtime is particularly helpful
- Consider adding an H2 antihistamine (e.g. famotidine)
- If aspirin/NSAID sensitive, consider adding a leukotriene inhibitor

↓ If response is not adequate

Additional considerations for refractory disease
- Omalizumab (anti-IgE monoclonal antibody)
- Dapsone or colchicine (especially if neutrophilic component)
- Mycophenolate mofetil, methotrexate, cyclosporine

Treatments in specific acute circumstances
- Diphenhydramine for immediate initial treatment of acute urticaria
- Epinephrine (SC or IM) for anaphylaxis or severe pharyngeal angioedema
- In general, prednisone is not recommended, with the exception of a 2–3 week course for severe acute urticaria with systemic manifestations (e.g. serum sickness-like reactions), with co-administration of antihistamines

*A tricyclic antidepressant with potent H1 and H2 antihistamine effects; contraindications include narrow-angle glaucoma, urinary retention and recent MAOI administration

Fig. 14.6 Management of spontaneous and physical urticarias. MAOI, monoamine oxidase inhibitor.

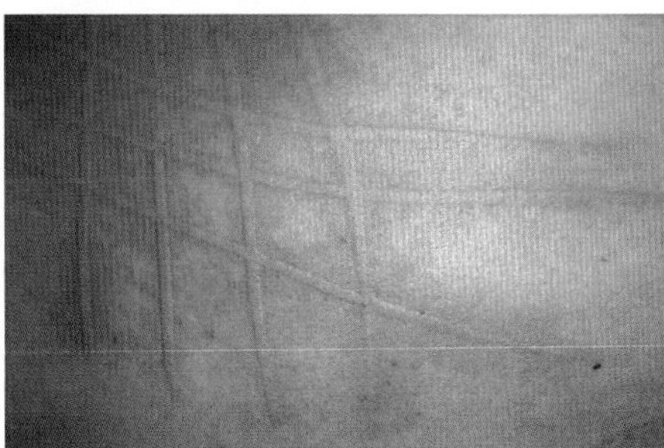

Fig. 14.7 Symptomatic dermographism within minutes of scratching. Dermographism can be a contributing factor in a number of dermatoses. *Courtesy, Jean L. Bolognia, MD.*

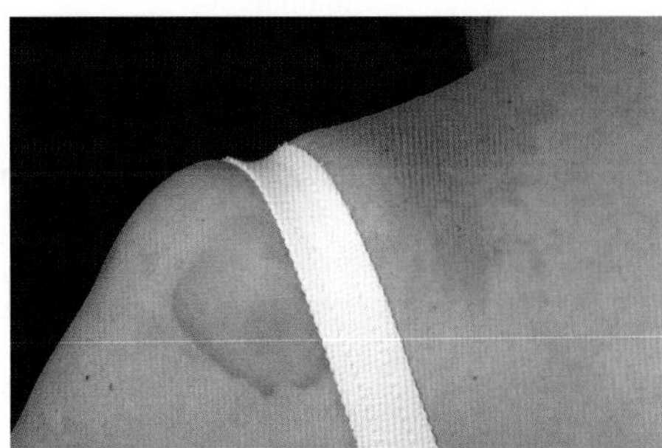

Fig. 14.8 Delayed pressure urticaria. *Courtesy, Clive E. H. Grattan, MD.*

bath), aquagenic urticaria (upon contact with water of any temperature).

Solar Urticaria

• Pruritus and wheals within 5–10 minutes of exposure to UVA and/or visible light > UVB (see Ch. 73).

Contact Urticaria

• *Immunologic contact urticaria* presents with localized pruritus and hives within 30 minutes of handling fresh vegetables/fruits or contact with latex in sensitized individuals; occasionally generalizes, and "protein contact dermatitis" may occur with repeated exposure (especially in atopic patients).
• Evaluation of suspected type 1 latex allergy initially involves a blood test for specific IgE; if negative, a prick test with latex extract can be performed in a controlled setting and, if there is no reaction, confirmed with a usage test (e.g. wearing the suspect glove).
• *"Oral allergy syndrome"* presents with intraoral itching and swelling in individuals with a pollen allergy upon ingestion of cross-reacting fresh fruits or vegetables.
• *Non-immunologic contact urticaria* results from exposure to plants containing toxins (e.g. histamine) within sharp "hairs" on their leaves (e.g. stinging nettles).

Schnitzler Syndrome

• Chronic urticaria ± pruritus associated with a monoclonal gammopathy (IgM >> IgG).
• Other features include fevers, arthralgias, bone pain, lymphadenopathy, leukocytosis, and an increased ESR; patients may develop a lymphoproliferative malignancy.
• **Rx:** prednisone, anakinra, and rituximab, as well as treatment of the underlying disorder.

Hereditary Angioedema (HAE)

• HAE due to deficiency (type I) or dysfunction (type II) of the complement C1 esterase inhibitor (C1 inh) is an uncommon autosomal dominant disorder that presents with episodic nonpruritic angioedema lasting 2–3 days, often beginning in early childhood and triggered by trauma; although not associated with true urticaria, attacks are occasionally preceded or accompanied by transient, nonpruritic, serpiginous erythematous patches.
• Type I/II HAE favors the extremities and gastrointestinal tract (may mimic an acute abdomen), and airway compromise due to laryngeal edema can occur.
• HAE with normal C1 inh (previously known as type III HAE) is a later-onset form with more frequent facial involvement that develops primarily in teenage girls and young women.
• Pathogenesis of HAE is related to excessive generation of bradykinin, which leads to increased vascular permeability.
• Evaluation and **DDx:** outlined in Fig. 14.10.
• **Rx:** *acute attacks* – IV C1 inhibitor concentrate, SC ecallantide (kallikrein inhibitor) or SC icatibant (bradykinin B_2 receptor antagonist); *short-term* (e.g. for surgical or dental procedures) or *long-term prophylaxis* – IV or SC C1 inhibitor concentrate, SQ lanadelumab (kallikrein inhibitor; long-term) > androgens (e.g. oral danazol), antifibrinolytic agents (long-term); antihistamines, epinephrine, and corticosteroids are *not* effective.

For further information see Ch. 18 from *Dermatology, Fourth Edition*.

For additional online figures and a table on antihistamines visit www.expertconsult.com 

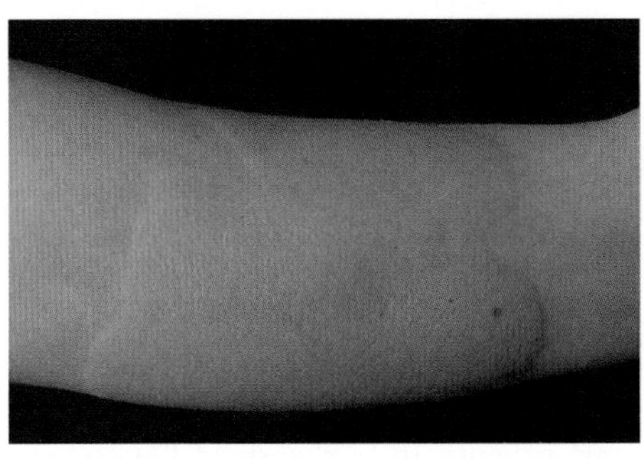

Fig. 14.9 Cold urticaria. Wheals developed on the forearm after placement of an ice cube for 10 minutes, followed by rewarming. *Courtesy, Thomas Schwarz, MD.*

ALGORITHM FOR THE DIAGNOSIS OF ANGIOEDEMA

- Angioedema
  - Without wheals
    - Low C4
      - Hereditary, type I → ↓ C1 inh protein levels; ↓ C1 inh function
      - Hereditary, type II → Normal C1 inh protein levels; ↓ C1 inh function
      - Acquired* → Normal or ↓ C1 inh protein levels; ↓ C1 inh function; ↓ C1q levels
        - Acquired, type I → Immune complex-mediated C1 and C1 inh consumption
        - Acquired, type II → Anti-C1 inh antibodies
    - Normal C4
      - Idiopathic
      - Drug-induced, e.g. ACE inhibitor
      - Episodic angioedema with eosinophilia
      - Hereditary, with normal C1 inh
      - Capillary leak syndrome (Clarkson syndrome)
  - With wheals
    - Diagnose and manage as for urticaria (see Fig. 14.5)

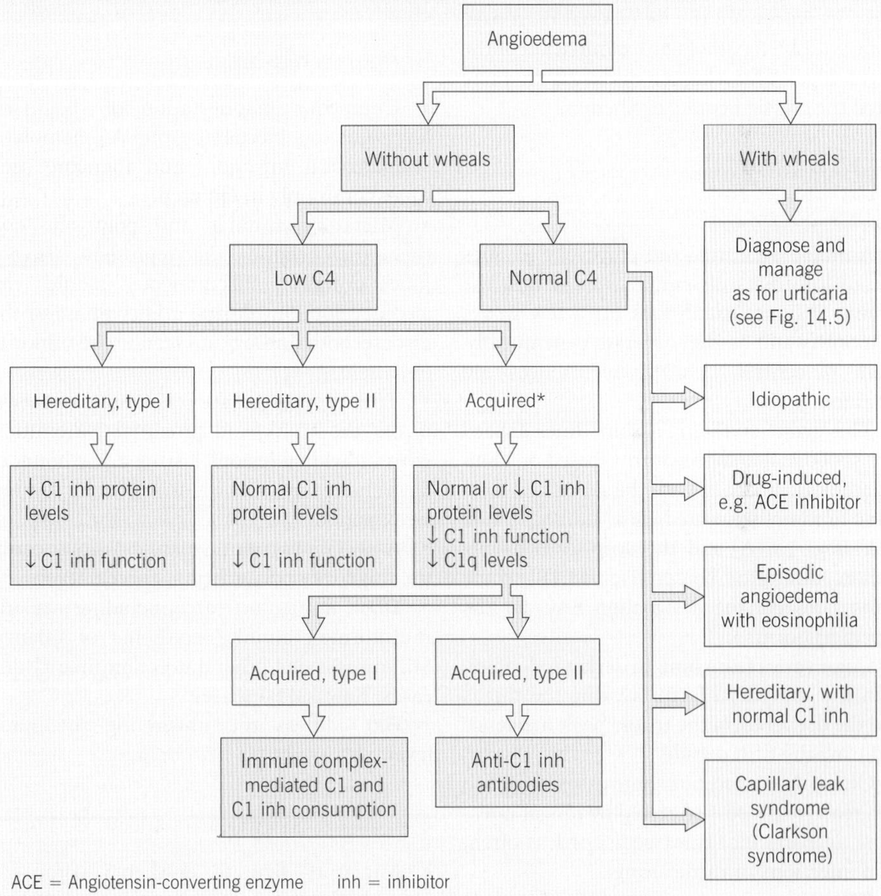

ACE = Angiotensin-converting enzyme   inh = inhibitor

* Associated with B-cell lymphoproliferative disorders (e.g. lymphomas, monoclonal gammopathy of undetermined significance)

Fig. 14.10 Algorithm for the diagnosis of angioedema. Genetic testing may help to confirm the diagnosis of hereditary angioedema with normal C1 inhibitor, with implicated genes including *F12* (factor XII) > *PLG* (plasminogen), *KNG1* (kininogen 1), and *ANGPT1* (angiopoietin-1). Episodic angioedema with eosinophilia as well as weight gain and fever is known as Gleich syndrome. Systemic capillary leak syndrome can lead to life-threatening hypotension and is associated with an IgG monoclonal gammopathy.

15 Figurate Erythemas

A number of cutaneous diseases can have an annular, arciform, or polycyclic configuration, from urticaria to granuloma annulare and tinea corporis (Table 15.1). Sites of involvement, rate of expansion, and characteristics of the border assist in narrowing the differential diagnosis, along with histopathologic examination of the active edge. This chapter discusses in more detail the classic figurate erythemas.

Erythema Annulare Centrifugum (EAC)

- Annular, arciform, and polycyclic plaques due to infiltrates of lymphocytes within the dermis; lesions usually last for a few weeks to months and as they migrate centrifugally, there is central clearing; recurrences are common.
- This gyrate erythema is sometimes divided into superficial and deep forms, based on clinicopathologic findings, with the superficial form being minimally elevated with "trailing" white scale (Fig. 15.1A) and the deep form having a more infiltrated border (Fig. 15.1B); some authors reserve the designation EAC for the superficial form.
- Color varies from pink to darker red-violet, with the superficial form favoring the thighs and the deeper form the trunk; peak incidence is during the fifth decade.
- Often idiopathic, but some cases appear to be a reactive process triggered by fungal infections, in particular tinea pedis, or less often, viral infections or medications.
- **DDx:** Tinea corporis (especially if scale is present); if no surface changes, annular urticaria (Fig. 15.2), benign lymphocytic infiltrate (of Jessner), cutaneous lymphoid hyperplasia, cutaneous lupus erythematosus (tumidus), and lymphoma cutis as well as the other entities covered in this chapter and Table 15.1; in some patients, the diagnosis of EAC is rendered after exclusion of other disorders.
- **Rx:** if trigger identified, it should be treated; if no trigger is identified, topical CS may be of some benefit.

Erythema Marginatum

- Cutaneous manifestation of rheumatic fever (due to a preceding group A β-hemolytic streptococcal infection) and therefore seen more commonly in children.
- Migratory annular and polycyclic erythematous eruption that represents a major Jones criterion; subcutaneous nodules can also develop, but during a later phase of the disease; both findings are seen in the minority of patients.
- This asymptomatic figurate erythema favors the trunk and proximal extremities, with individual lesions lasting a few hours to days and recurrences occurring over a several-week period.
- Associated systemic manifestations: carditis, migratory polyarthritis, chorea, fever.
- **DDx:** annular urticaria (including urticaria multiforme), annular erythema of infancy, Still disease and other autoinflammatory diseases, Kawasaki disease.
- **Rx:** address the underlying rheumatic fever.

Erythema Gyratum Repens

- Migratory figurate erythema composed of multiple concentric rings that is said to resemble the grain of wood (Fig. 15.3); the lesions can migrate up to 1 cm per day and may have associated scale or pruritus.
- Paraneoplastic dermatosis in the vast majority of patients, with lung cancer and breast cancer representing the most common

ADDITIONAL ENTITIES THAT CAN HAVE AN ANNULAR, ARCIFORM, OR POLYCYCLIC CONFIGURATION	
No epidermal (surface) changes	
Annular urticaria	Individual lesions are transient, lasting <24 hrs
Urticaria multiforme	Migratory edematous plaques that may have dusky centers; edema of the face, hands and feet can develop; primarily in infants and young children, often following a viral or bacterial infection
Serum sickness-like eruption	Urticarial (or morbilliform) eruption due to a systemic medication; may be accompanied by arthralgias, arthritis, and fever
Urticarial vasculitis	Individual lesions usually last >24 hrs and may resolve with petechiae
Granuloma annulare	Skin-colored to dull pink elevated border, often composed of coalescing papules; favors acral sites, elbows
Annular elastolytic giant cell granuloma	Chronically sun-exposed sites with significant photodamage; hypopigmented centrally as expands
Interstitial granulomatous dermatitis	Associated with autoimmune connective tissues diseases, e.g. rheumatoid arthritis, and systemic medications, e.g. TNF inhibitors
Sarcoidosis	Skin-colored to red-brown; with pressure (diascopy), has a yellow-brown color; face > trunk, extremities; sometimes has scale
Leprosy	Primarily tuberculoid and borderline forms, with the former often having central hypopigmentation
Syphilis	Secondary stage, in particular on the face, and tertiary stage (gummas); facial lesions may have central hyperpigmentation
Annular erythema of infancy	Slowly expanding with an urticarial border; individual lesions spontaneously resolve over a few days
Benign lymphocytic infiltrate (of Jessner)	Favors the head, neck, and upper trunk; erythematous papules and plaques last weeks to months
LE tumidus	Firm erythematous plaques that favor the face and upper trunk
Lymphoma cutis, both B- and T-cell	Pink to violet papules and plaques; may be primary cutaneous or related to a systemic lymphoma; some subtypes of CTCL, e.g. mycosis fungoides, can have scale
Scale and/or crust	
Tinea corporis	Scale and pustules in the advancing border; KOH examination is positive for hyphae
Seborrheic dermatitis	Lesions on the face and central chest; associated scale
Annular psoriasis	Scale is silvery; associated scalp, intergluteal, and nail involvement
Subacute cutaneous LE	Primarily sun-exposed sites, especially upper trunk and upper outer arms; hypopigmented centrally
Elastosis perforans serpiginosa	Border contains keratotic papules and lesions favor flexural sites

Table 15.1 Additional entities that can have an annular, arciform, or polycyclic configuration. *Continued*

ADDITIONAL ENTITIES THAT CAN HAVE AN ANNULAR, ARCIFORM, OR POLYCYCLIC CONFIGURATION	
Wickham striae within border	
Annular lichen planus	The elevated border is string-like
Petechiae within border	
Annular capillaritis	Both petechiae and yellow-brown hue due to hemosiderin
Vesicobullae within border	
Linear IgA bullous dermatosis	Border may resemble "string of pearls"; DIF required
More serpiginous border	
Cutaneous larva migrans	Favors feet, buttocks, and areas in contact with sandy ground

Table 15.1 *Continued* **Additional entities that can have an annular, arciform, or polycyclic configuration.** These disorders are covered in other chapters. See text for discussion of the classic figurate erythemas. Both erythema multiforme and erythema migrans can have a bull's-eye appearance. CTCL, cutaneous T-cell lymphoma; DIF, direct immunofluorescence.

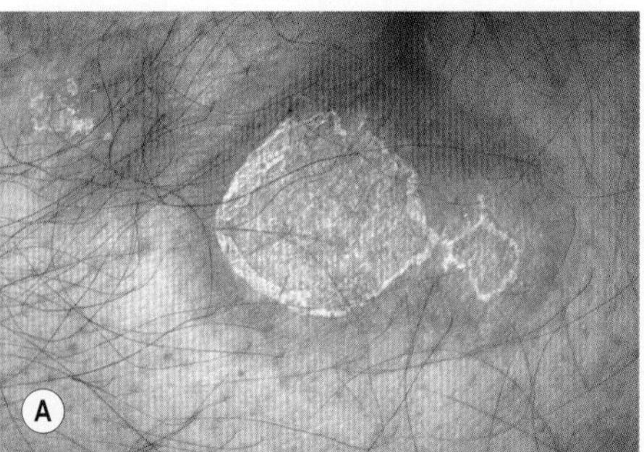

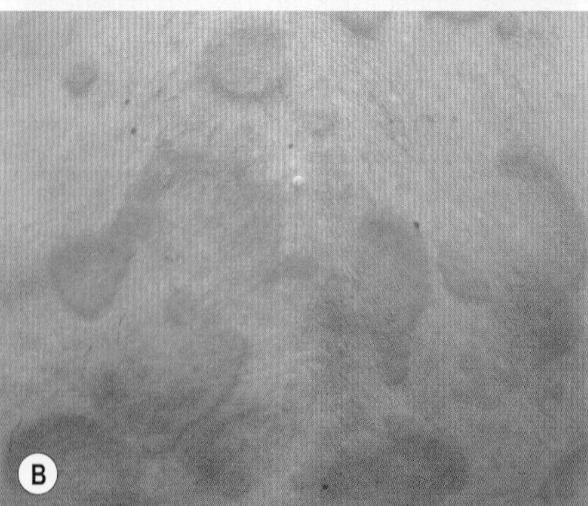

Fig. 15.1 Erythema annulare centrifugum. **A** Superficial form, with polycyclic plaques and delicate scale on the inner margin of the advancing edge (trailing scale). The scale is detached centrally. **B** Deep form, with obvious elevation of advancing edges and without trailing scale. *Courtesy, YDRSC.*

underlying malignancies; patients may have other paraneoplastic phenomena, e.g. acquired ichthyosis, palmoplantar keratoderma.

- Occasionally, patients have no underlying disease or an underlying infection, e.g. pulmonary tuberculosis.
- **DDx:** EAC (slower migration and usually not concentric), tinea imbricata, the resolving phase of pityriasis rubra pilaris, erythrokeratodermia variabilis, mycosis fungoides.
- **Rx:** address the underlying malignancy; if antineoplastic treatment is successful, the eruption will resolve.

Erythema Migrans (EM; Erythema Chronicum Migrans [ECM])

- Cutaneous manifestation of the earlier stages of infection with *Borrelia burgdorferi* spirochetes; seen in 60–80% of patients diagnosed with Lyme borreliosis.
- Occurs most commonly in the United States (northeast, upper Midwest, west coast), Scandinavia, and central Europe; natural hosts are white-footed mice and white-tailed deer.
- Can be localized to the site of the bite of an infected *Ixodes* tick (Figs 15.4 & 15.5) or as the disease progresses, becomes disseminated with multiple secondary lesions (Fig. 15.6); several species of *Ixodes* can transmit disease, including *I. scapularis*, *I. pacificus*, *I. ricinus*.
- At the site of the tick bite, usually after a period of 1 or 2 weeks (range 2–28 days),

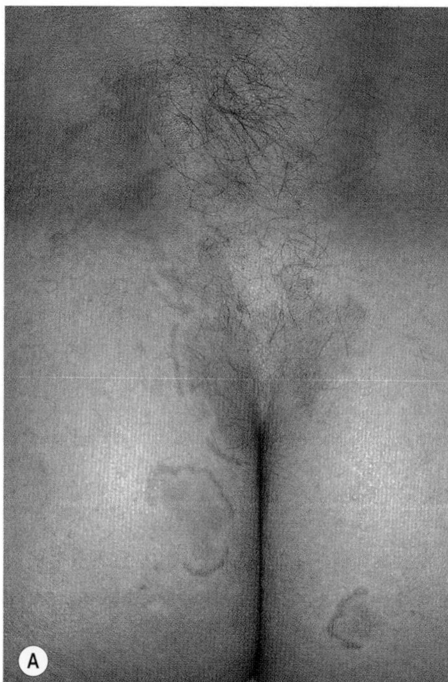

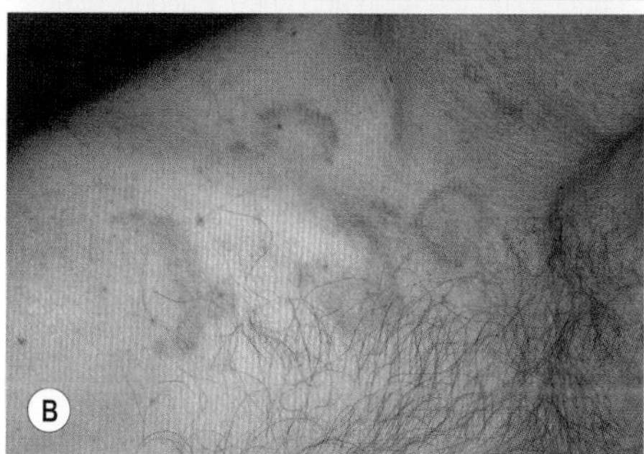

Fig. 15.2 A comparison of erythema annulare centrifugum and urticaria. The lesions in **A** have no scaling and may be confused with annular urticaria **(B)**. However, *individual* lesions of urticaria are evanescent, lasting <24 hours. Placement of an ink circle around a lesion, followed by longitudinal observation, allows this distinction. *Courtesy, YDRSC.*

an erythematous patch or plaque appears that expands over days to weeks to reach a diameter of at least 5 cm; central clearing can result in an annular lesion and sometimes the lesion has a bull's-eye appearance; occasionally, vesicles are seen.

• Primary lesions often favor body folds, are frequently asymptomatic and spontaneously resolve (without treatment) within 6 weeks; primary, and especially disseminated, lesions can be accompanied by flu-like symptoms – headache, malaise, arthralgia, myalgia, and fever.

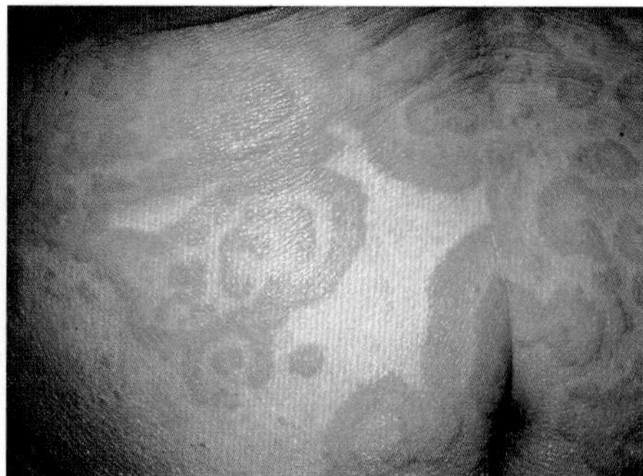

Fig. 15.3 Erythema gyratum repens. Multiple concentric annular plaques, with a wood-grain appearance. *Courtesy, Agustin Alomar, MD.*

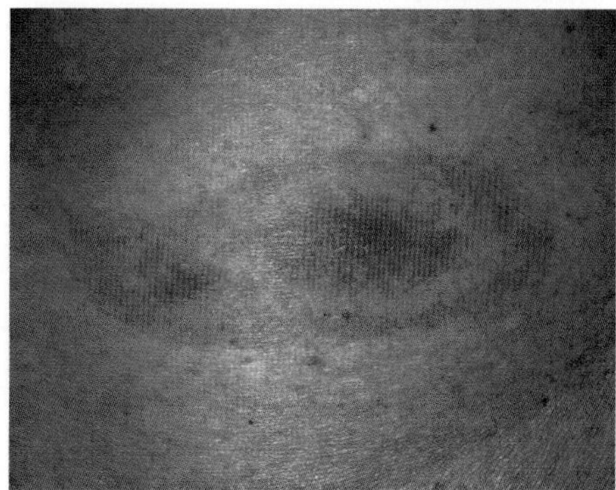

Fig. 15.4 Erythema migrans. Expanding annular plaque that has a bull's-eye appearance. *Courtesy, YDRSC.*

• Transmission usually requires attachment of the infected *Ixodes* tick for over 24 hours; if untreated, sequelae include arthritis, Bell palsy, and atrioventricular heart block (Table 15.2); *Ixodes* ticks may also transmit babesiosis, anaplasmosis, *Borrelia miyamotoi*, or Powassan virus.

• Development of additional cutaneous findings (e.g. pseudolymphoma, acrodermatitis chronica atrophicans; Fig. 15.7) is seen in individuals infected outside the United States and reflects the geographic distribution of different genospecies of *Borrelia*, e.g. *B. afzelii* is found in Europe but not the United States.

• **DDx:** exaggerated local reaction to an arthropod bite, cellulitis, allergic contact dermatitis, southern tick-associated rash illness (STARI or Masters disease), nonpigmented fixed drug eruption, and other causes of pseudocellulitis (see Table 61.2); of note,

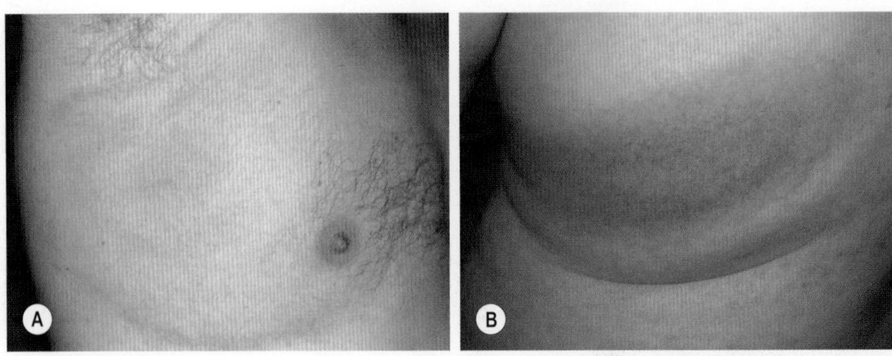

Fig. 15.5 **Erythema migrans.** **A**,**B** The lesions spread centrifugally, sometimes becoming >10 cm in diameter and may develop a violaceous color centrally. *A, Courtesy, Lorenzo Cerroni, MD; B, Courtesy, Dennis Cooper, MD.*

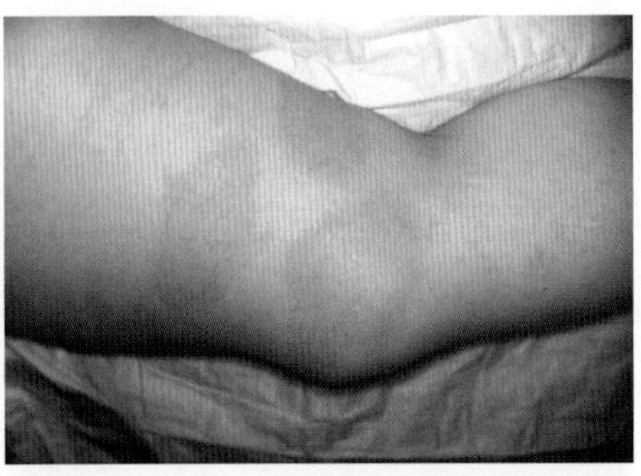

Fig. 15.6 Disseminated erythema migrans. Multiple circular pink plaques are scattered on the thigh and knee. Patients often have flu-like constitutional symptoms. *Courtesy, YDRSC.*

STAGES AND MAJOR ORGAN MANIFESTATIONS OF LYME BORRELIOSIS			
Organ	**Early localized disease**	**Early disseminated disease**	**Chronic disease**
Skin	Erythema migrans		Acrodermatitis chronica atrophicans (Europe)
	Disseminated erythema migrans		
	Borrelial lymphocytoma (Europe)		
Nervous system		Meningo-polyradiculoneuritis Cranial neuritis Bell palsy	Encephalopathy Encephalomyelitis Neuropathy
Musculoskeletal system		Arthralgias, arthritis Myositis	Chronic arthritis
Heart		Atrioventricular block Myopericarditis, pancarditis Tachycardia	
Lymphatic	Regional lymphadenopathy	Regional or generalized lymphadenopathy	
Other		Conjunctivitis, iritis Hepatitis Nonproductive cough Microscopic hematuria or proteinuria	

Table 15.2 Stages and major organ manifestations of Lyme borreliosis. *Adapted from Müllegger RR. Dermatological manifestations of Lyme borreliosis. Eur J Dermatol. 2004;14:296–309.*

peak specific IgM antibodies usually appear at 3–6 weeks into infection so they may not be detected in patients with early EM (false-negative rate as high as 60%).

- **Rx** is outlined in Table 15.3; for patients who: (1) live in an endemic area; (2) had a tick attached for >36 hours; (3) removed the tick within the past 72 hours; and (4) if possible, had the tick identified as *I. scapularis*, a single dose of oral doxycycline (200 mg) may reduce the risk of developing Lyme borreliosis from 3.2% to 0.4%.

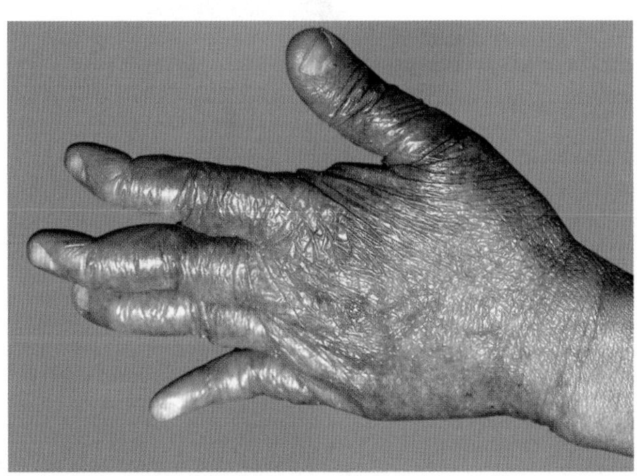

Fig. 15.7 Acrodermatitis chronica atrophicans is another manifestation of Lyme borreliosis. Note the shiny and wrinkled skin plus more visible superficial veins – signs of atrophy. *Courtesy, YDRSC.*

TREATMENT OPTIONS FOR BORRELIOSIS				
Manifestation	**Drug**	**Dose (pediatric dose*)**	**Duration (days)**	**Comments**
Erythema migrans	Doxycycline	100 mg (2 mg/kg) po BID	14 (range, 10–21)	• Not preferred in children <8 yrs of age**, or pregnant or lactating women • Good CNS penetration • Also treats human granulocytic anaplasmosis
	Amoxicillin	500 mg (16 mg/kg) po TID	14 (range, 14–21)§	
	Cefuroxime axetil	500 mg (15 mg/kg) po BID	14 (range, 14–21)	

**The maximum pediatric dose is the adult dose.*
***The American Academy of Pediatrics considers use of doxycycline for ≤21 days to be acceptable in children <8 years of age.*
§Recommended for 21 days for pregnant women.

Table 15.3 Treatment options for borreliosis. *Continued*

For further information see Ch. 19 from *Dermatology, Fourth Edition*.

For additional online figures and CDC Lyme disease surveillance case definition table visit www.expertconsult.com 

TREATMENT OPTIONS FOR BORRELIOSIS			
Manifestation	**Drugs**	**Duration (days)**	**Comments**
Meningitis	Ceftriaxone (iv), cefotaxime (iv)	14 (range, 10–28)	
Cranial nerve palsy (without meningitis)	Same drugs and dosages as for erythema migrans	14 (range, 14–21)	• May not affect outcome of facial palsy
Carditis	If symptomatic, initiate treatment with parenteral antibiotic (e.g. ceftriaxone) then based upon clinical response, finish course with oral agents	14 (range, 14–21)	• Advanced heart block may require a pacemaker
Arthritis	Same parenteral agents as for meningitis and same oral agents as for erythema migrans	28	• If persists or recurs, a second course of antibiotics

Table 15.3 *Continued* **Treatment options for borreliosis.** A Jarisch–Herxheimer-like reaction with an increase in systemic symptoms and in the size or intensity of the inflammation of the erythema migrans lesion occurs in ~15% of patients within 24 hours after the initiation of antimicrobial therapy. If all three antibiotics for erythema migrans are contraindicated, then macrolides (e.g. clarithromycin, azithromycin, erythromycin) can be prescribed but the cure rates are ~80% yrs, years.

Erythema Multiforme, Stevens–Johnson Syndrome, and Toxic Epidermal Necrolysis

16

Erythema Multiforme

- Self-limited, but potentially recurrent, disease.
- Two forms: erythema multiforme (EM) major and EM minor (Table 16.1).
- Both forms have an abrupt onset of papular 'target' lesions that favor acrofacial sites.
- Two types of target lesions: (1) typical targets, with at least three different zones; (2) atypical papular targets, with only two different zones and/or a poorly defined border (Fig. 16.1).
- EM minor: typical > atypical *papular* target lesions, little or no mucosal involvement, and no systemic symptoms.
- EM major: typical > atypical *papular* target lesions, moderate to severe mucosal involvement (Fig. 16.2), and some systemic symptoms (fever, asthenia, arthralgia).
- Preceding HSV infection is the most common precipitating factor; less often other infections, in particular *Mycoplasma pneumoniae* (Table 16.2 and see Fig. 16.2B); rarely drug exposure.
- The term *Mycoplasma*-induced rash and mucositis (MIRM) has been proposed to describe a clinical presentation with significant mucositis (oral, ocular and anogenital) ± more limited cutaneous involvement; some authors consider this entity to simply be a variant of EM.
- Diagnosis is based on clinicopathologic correlation and not solely histopathologic findings.
- EM is a distinct disorder from Stevens–Johnson syndrome (SJS) and toxic epidermal necrolysis (TEN) (see Table 16.1).
- EM does not progress to TEN.
- **DDx:** annular urticaria/urticaria multiforme (Fig. 16.3; Table 16.3), morbilliform drug reaction (Fig. 16.4), multiple fixed drug eruption (FDE), acute hemorrhagic edema of infancy, Kawasaki disease, small vessel vasculitis (classic and urticarial), Rowell syndrome, acute GVHD, drug reaction with eosinophilia and systemic symptoms (DRESS) (for EM major).
- **Rx** *mild* disease: symptomatic and supportive care, treat underlying infection if detected, ophthalmology consultation if ocular involvement.
- **Rx** *recurrent* disease: oral antiviral drug as prophylaxis for HSV infections, administered for at least 6 months (acyclovir 10 mg/kg/day, valacyclovir 500–1000 mg/day, or famciclovir 250 mg BID).
- **Rx** *severe recurrent* disease or *failure to respond* to prophylactic (anti-HSV) treatment: double the antiviral dose and if this fails, then consider referral to a dermatologist for possible immunosuppressive treatment.

Stevens–Johnson Syndrome (SJS) and Toxic Epidermal Necrolysis (TEN)

- SJS and TEN are considered the same disease, but along a clinical spectrum of severity and distinct from EM (see Table 16.1).
- Most likely etiology for both is an adverse reaction to a medication.
- Most common culprit drugs (Table 16.4): NSAIDs, antibiotics (in particular, sulfonamides and penicillins), aromatic anticonvulsants, and allopurinol.
- Increased risk in certain patient groups: immunocompromised (e.g. HIV infection), patients undergoing radiotherapy while concomitantly receiving anticonvulsants, patients with slow acetylator genotypes, and in patients who have specific HLA alleles (see Table 17.1); HLA genotyping is now recommended for all Asians prior to administering carbamazepine (*HLA-B*15:02*) and for Asians and African Americans prior to receiving allopurinol (*HLA-B*58:01*).
- Mucocutaneous tenderness, erythema, and varying degrees of epidermal detachment are characteristic features.

COMPARISON OF ERYTHEMA MULTIFORME (EM) MINOR, EM MAJOR, STEVENS–JOHNSON SYNDROME (SJS), SJS/TOXIC EPIDERMAL NECROLYSIS (TEN) OVERLAP, AND TEN						
Clinical entity	**Type of skin lesions**	**Distribution**	**Mucosal involvement**	**Systemic symptoms**	**Progression to TEN**	**Precipitating factors**
EM minor (Figs 16.1 & 16.4)	• Typical targets • ± *Papular* atypical targets	Extremities (especially elbows, knees, wrists, hands), face	Absent or mild	Absent	No	• Herpes simplex virus • Other infectious agents
EM major (Fig. 16.2)	• Typical targets • ± *Papular* atypical targets • Occasionally bullous lesions	Extremities, face	Severe	Usually present • Fever • Arthralgias	No	• Herpes simplex virus • *Mycoplasma pneumoniae* • Other infectious agents • Rarely, drugs
SJS (Figs 16.6 & 16.7)	• Dusky and/or dusky-red *macules* with epidermal detachment and erosions • *Macular* atypical targets • Bullous lesions • <10% BSA detachment	Isolated lesions Confluence (+) Trunk, face	Severe	Usually present • Fever • Lymphadenopathy • Hepatitis • Cytopenias	Possible	• Drugs • Occasionally, *Mycoplasma pneumoniae** • Rarely, immunizations
SJS/TEN overlap (Fig. 16.9)	• Similar to SJS • 10–30% BSA detachment	Isolated lesions Confluence (++) Trunk, face, neck	Severe	• Same as SJS	Likely	• Drugs
TEN (Figs 16.8, 16.10 & 16.11)	• Similar to SJS • >30% BSA detachment	Confluence (+++) Isolated lesions rare Trunk, face, neck, elsewhere	Severe, with involvement of respiratory and gastrointestinal mucosa	• Same as SJS plus nephritis		• Drugs

**Occasionally, also subcorneal pustules.*

Table 16.1 Comparison of erythema multiforme (EM) minor, EM major, Stevens–Johnson syndrome (SJS), SJS/toxic epidermal necrolysis (TEN) overlap, and TEN.

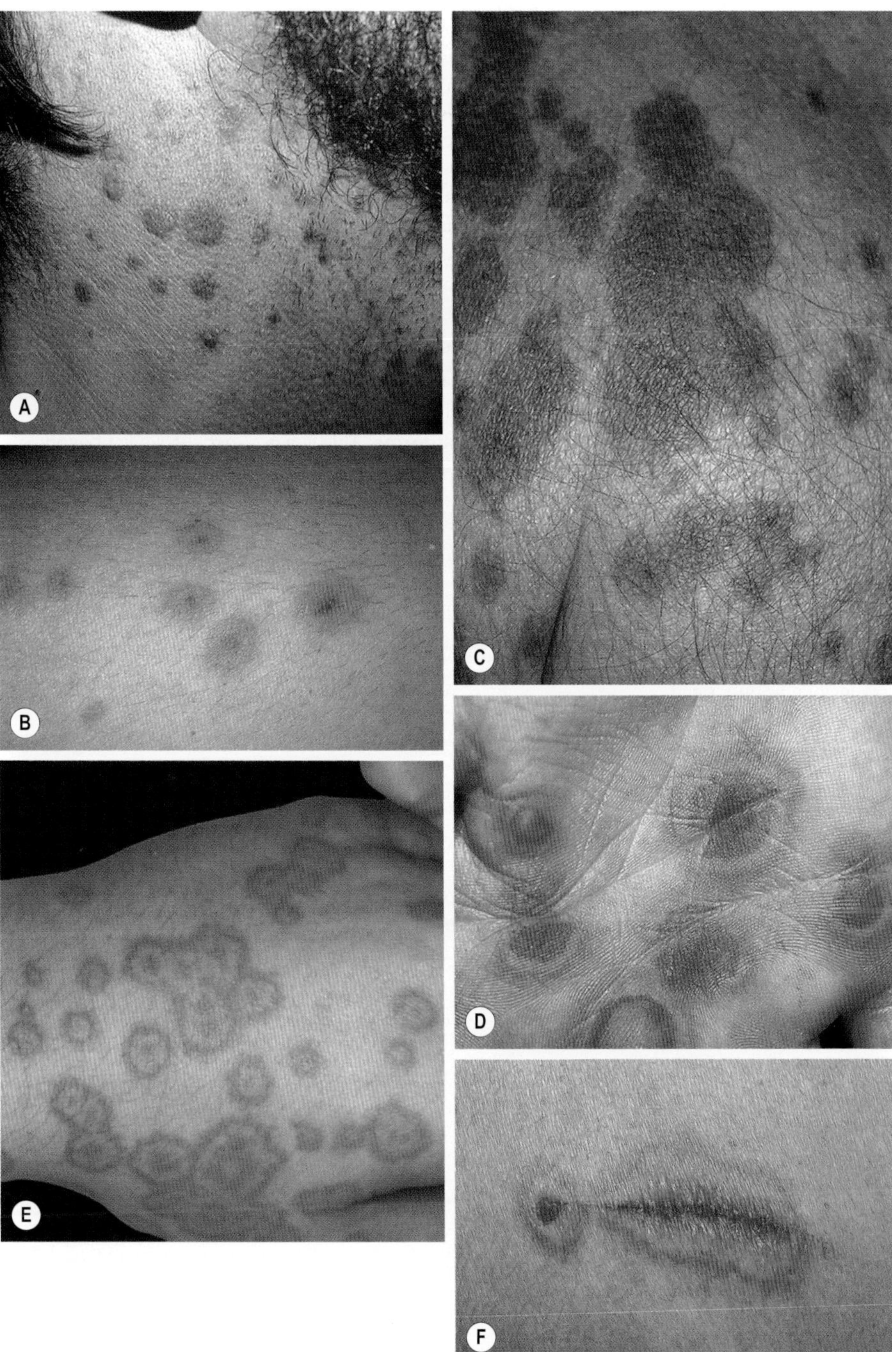

Fig. 16.1 Phenotypic variety in lesions of erythema multiforme (EM). A Edematous/urticarial. **B** Urticarial with central crusting. **C** Erythematous plaques with dusky centers; coalescence of the lesions leads to a well-defined polycyclic outline. **D, E** Typical (classic) target lesions on the palms and dorsal hand, with three zones of color change ("bull's eye"); note the central vesicles in **(D)**. **F** Isomorphic response with crust formation. *A, D, F Courtesy, William Weston, MD; B, C, E, Courtesy, YDRSC.*

PRECIPITATING FACTORS IN ERYTHEMA MULTIFORME		
Infections (~90% of cases)	Viral	• Herpes simplex virus (HSV-1, HSV-2) • Parapoxvirus (orf) • Vaccinia (smallpox vaccine) • Varicella zoster virus (chickenpox) • Adenovirus • Cytomegalovirus • Epstein–Barr virus • Hepatitis virus • Coxsackievirus • Parvovirus B19 • Human immunodeficiency virus
	Bacterial	• ***Mycoplasma pneumoniae*** (see Fig. 16.2B) • *Chlamydophila* (formerly *Chlamydia*) *psittaci* (ornithosis) • *Salmonella* • *Mycobacterium tuberculosis*
	Fungal	• *Histoplasma capsulatum* • Dermatophytes

Table 16.2 Precipitating factors in erythema multiforme. This is a *non-exhaustive* list based primarily on case reports and small series of cases. The most common causes are in bold.

COMPARISON OF URTICARIA AND ERYTHEMA MULTIFORME	
Urticaria	**Erythema multiforme**
Central zone is normal skin or transient duskiness	Central zone is damaged skin (dusky, bullous, or crusted)
Lesions are transient, lasting less than 24 hours*	Individual lesions "fixed" for at least 7 days
New lesions appear daily	All lesions appear within first 72 hours
May be associated with swelling of face, hands, or feet (angioedema)	No edema

**Confirmed with "circle test" – circle a given urticarial lesion with pen/marker and re-check to see if still there in 24 hours.*

Table 16.3 Comparison of urticaria and erythema multiforme.

MEDICATIONS MOST FREQUENTLY ASSOCIATED WITH STEVENS–JOHNSON SYNDROME (SJS) AND TOXIC EPIDERMAL NECROLYSIS (TEN)	
Allopurinol	Chlormezanone*,‡
Aminopenicillins	Lamotrigine (risk may be increased when co-administered with valproic acid)
Amithiozone (thioacetazone)*,†	Phenylbutazone*,§
Antiretroviral drugs, especially NNRTIs (e.g. nevirapine, efavirenz, etravirine)	Piroxicam
Aromatic anticonvulsants (e.g. phenobarbital, phenytoin, carbamazepine)	Quinolones
Cephalosporins	Sulfasalazine
Checkpoint inhibitors (e.g. ipilimumab, nivolumab)	Sulfonamide antibiotics (e.g. sulfamethoxazole**, sulfadiazine*,†, sulfadoxine†)

**Not available in the United States.*
†Antibacterial.
‡Sedative/hypnotic.
§Nonsteroidal anti-inflammatory drug.
***Usually in combination with trimethoprim.*

Table 16.4 Medications most frequently associated with Stevens–Johnson syndrome (SJS) and toxic epidermal necrolysis (TEN). For a complete updated list of drugs associated with SJS and TEN, refer to Litt JZ, Shear N. Litt's Drug Eruption and Reaction Manual, 26th ed. London: CRC Press, 2019. NRTIs, non-nucleoside reverse transcriptase inhibitors.

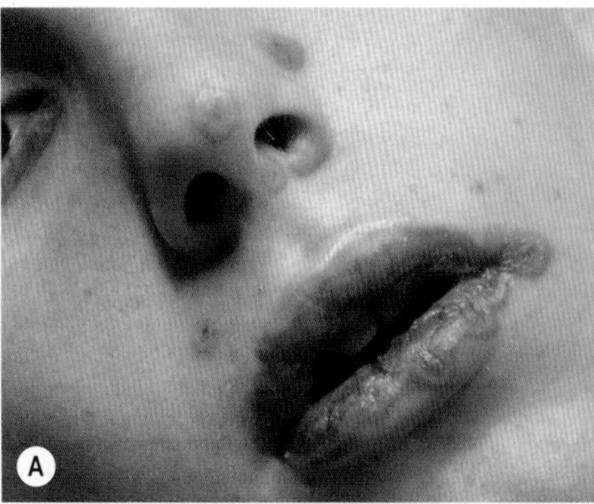

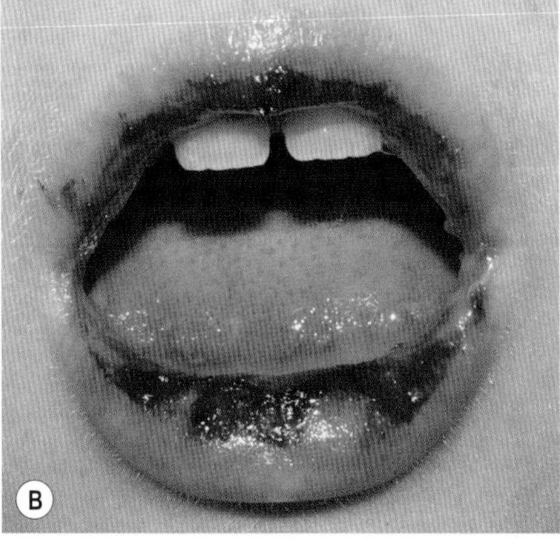

Fig. 16.2 Mucosal involvement in erythema multiforme (EM) major. A Typical target lesions are seen as well as serous crusting of the vermilion lips and eyelid margin. At the margin of the serous crusting of the lip, there are two zones of color with a polycyclic outline. **B** Erosions and hemorrhagic crusting of the lips in a child with the acro-mucosal variant associated with *Mycoplasma pneumoniae* infection. *A, Courtesy, YDRSC; B, Courtesy, Julie V. Schaffer, MD.*

- SJS is characterized by <10% body surface area (BSA) epidermal detachment, SJS–TEN overlap by 10–30% BSA epidermal detachment, and TEN by >30% BSA epidermal detachment (Fig. 16.5).
- Onset is usually 7–21 days after starting culprit medication.
- Symptoms that typically precede skin findings by 1–3 days: prodromal flu-like syndrome, sore throat, fever, painful skin.
- Tender cutaneous lesions are most prominent on the trunk (see Fig. 17.3), followed by extension to the face (Fig. 16.6A), neck and proximal extremities.

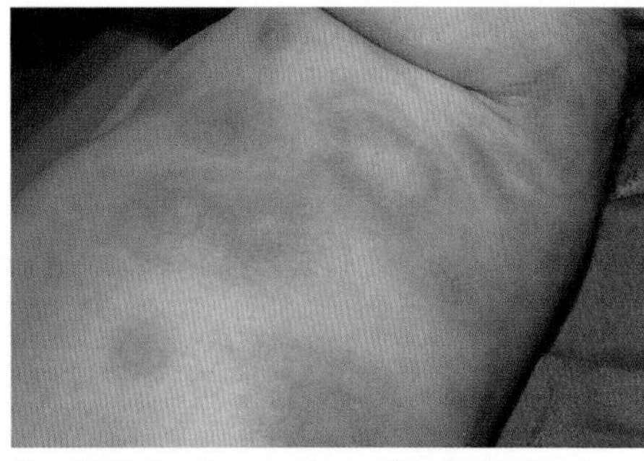

Fig. 16.3 Acute annular urticaria (urticaria multiforme) in an infant misdiagnosed as erythema multiforme. These migratory, annular plaques are markedly edematous. Some of the lesions have an erythematous or dusky center while others have central clearing with two shades of peripheral rings. There are no crusts or blisters. The term "urticaria multiforme" has been used to describe these skin findings, which are often preceded by a viral or bacterial infection and accompanied by angioedema of the face, hands, and/or feet. *Courtesy, Julie V. Schaffer, MD.*

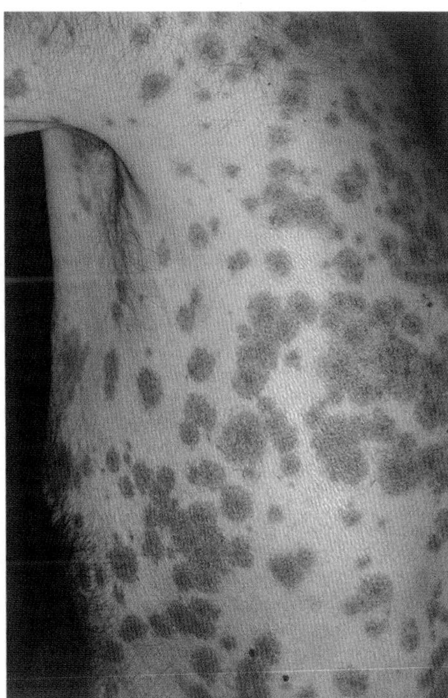

Fig. 16.4 Multiple lesions of erythema multiforme (EM) on the trunk. The dusky or crusted centers within the papules help to differentiate EM from a morbilliform drug eruption. *Courtesy, YDRSC.*

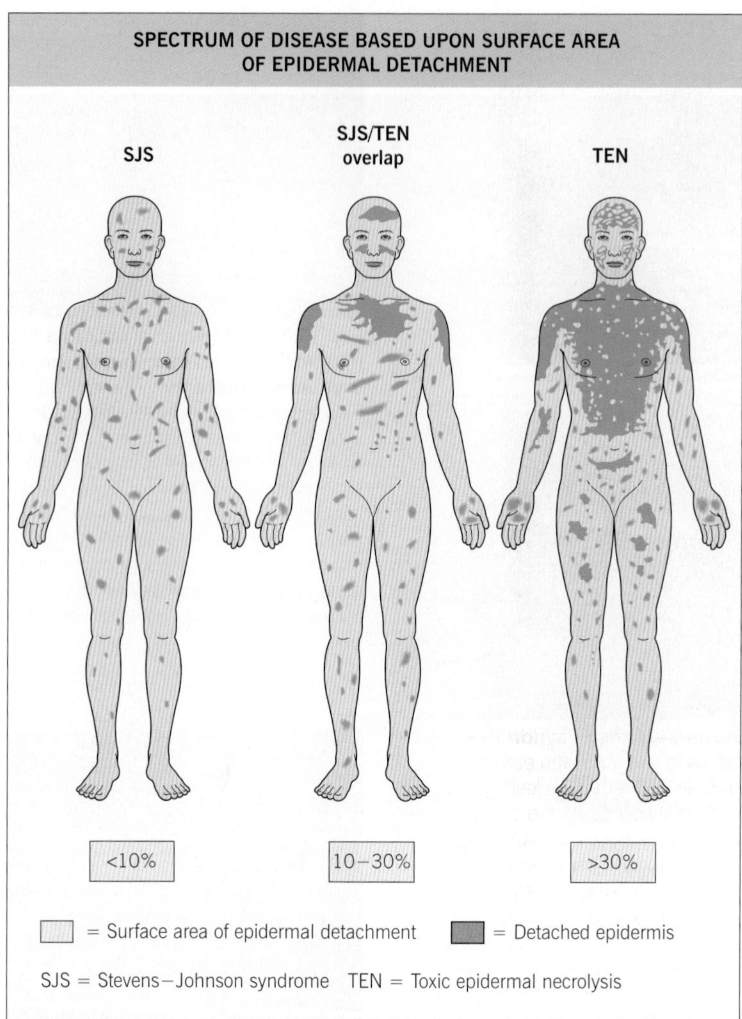

Fig. 16.5 Spectrum of disease based upon surface area of epidermal detachment.

- Painful erythema and erosions of buccal, ocular, and genital mucosa are seen in >90% of patients (Fig. 16.7 and see Fig. 16.6B).
- Morphologic progression of skin lesions: dusky red or purpuric *macules* (macular atypical targets) of various sizes and shapes that begin to coalesce (Fig. 16.8); the gray-colored centers become wrinkled and begin to slough due to the development of flaccid bullae and poor attachment of the necrotic epidermis (likened to wet cigarette paper) (Fig. 16.9); the result is raw, denuded, bright red dermis (scalding) (Fig. 16.10).
- Additional systemic findings: fever, lymphadenopathy, hepatitis, cytopenias, erosions of epithelium in the gastrointestinal and respiratory tracts.
- Unpredictable course; worse prognosis in the elderly and with increasing BSA involvement (Table 16.5).
- Mortality rate in SJS is 1–5% and in TEN, 25–35%; survivors may have both ocular (e.g. symblepharon, conjunctival synechiae, entropion, ingrowth of eyelashes) and cutaneous (e.g. scarring, dyspigmentation, eruptive melanocytic nevi) sequelae, as well as persistent erosions of the mucous membranes, urethral stenosis, phimosis, nail dystrophy, and diffuse hair loss (Fig. 16.11).
- Most important factor in improving outcome is withdrawal of the culprit medication.
- Epidermal detachment is due to extensive keratinocyte death via apoptosis, which is

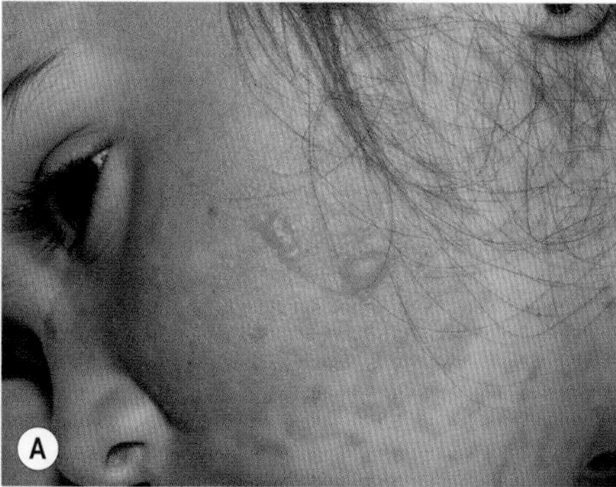

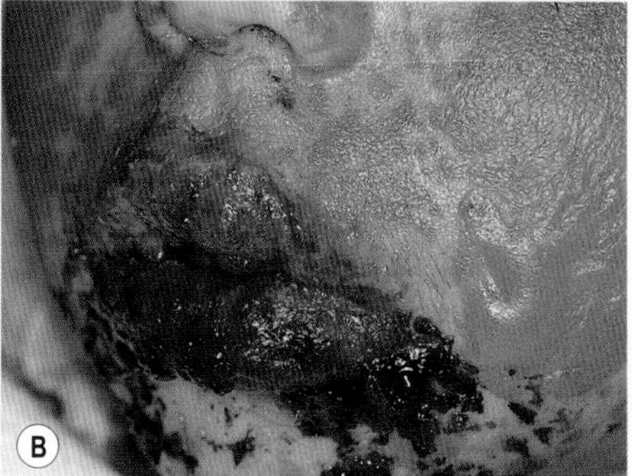

Fig. 16.6 Stevens–Johnson syndrome (SJS) in childhood. A In this child with early SJS, there are individual erythematous lesions on the lower face, but coalescence on the cheeks. The two fresh bullae on the cheek are still intact. **B** Hemorrhagic crusts and denudation of the lips in a child with SJS secondary to trimethoprim-sulfamethoxazole therapy; note the bullous cutaneous lesions. *A, Courtesy, Julie V. Schaffer, MD; B, Courtesy, William Weston, MD.*

mediated by interaction of the death receptor-ligand pair Fas–Fas ligand; perforin, granzyme B, and granulysin also play a role.

- **DDx:** EM major, drug-induced linear IgA bullous dermatosis (LABD), acute generalized exanthematous pustulosis (AGEP), generalized fixed drug eruption (FDE), severe acute GVHD, Rowell syndrome, paraneoplastic pemphigus, toxic erythema of chemotherapy (TEC), disseminated intravascular coagulation/purpura fulminans; in children can consider staphylococcal scalded skin syndrome (SSSS) and Kawasaki disease.
- **Rx:** stop the culprit medication, rapid initiation of supportive care, consider specific therapy (no evidence-based treatment) (Fig. 16.12).

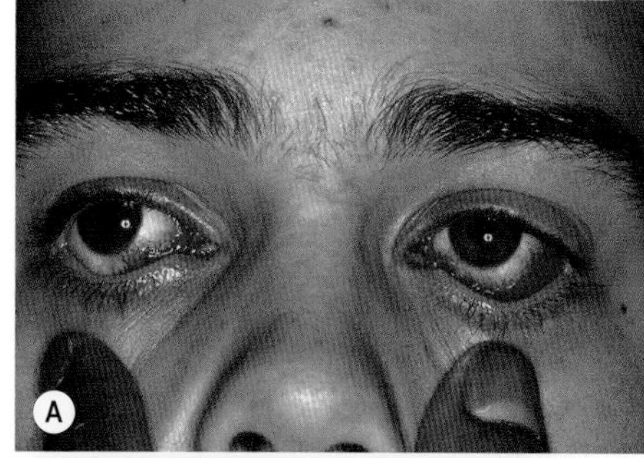

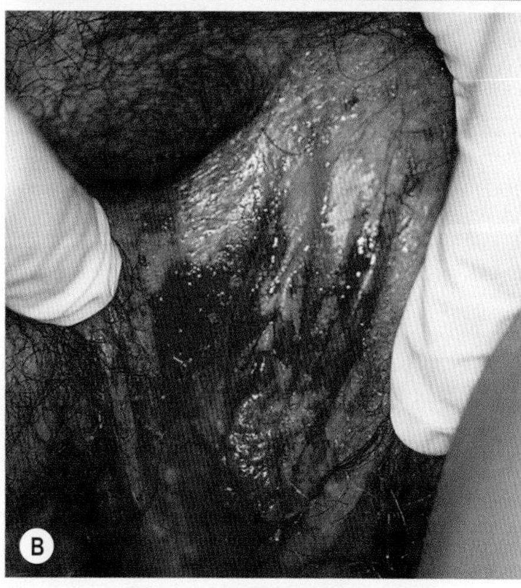

Fig. 16.7 Mucosal involvement in Stevens–Johnson syndrome (SJS). A Erythema and conjunctival erosions. **B** Erosions of the genital mucosa. *A, B, Courtesy, YDRSC.*

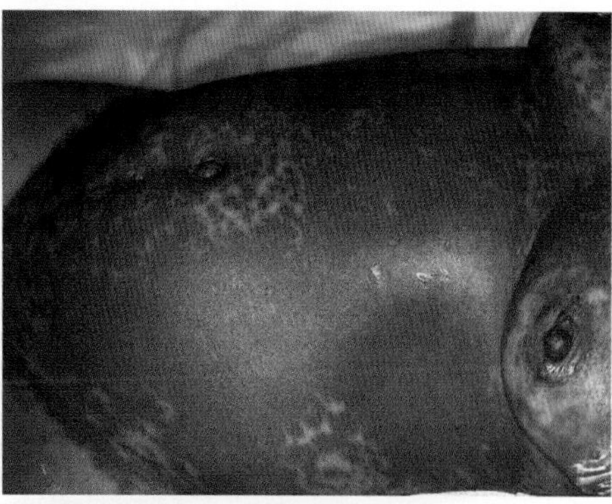

Fig. 16.8 Cutaneous features of toxic epidermal necrolysis (TEN). Characteristic dusky red color of the early macular eruption in TEN. Lesions with this color often progress to full-blown necrolytic lesions with dermal–epidermal detachment. *Courtesy, YDRSC.*

For further information see Ch. 20 from *Dermatology, Fourth Edition*.

For additional online figures visit www.expertconsult.com 

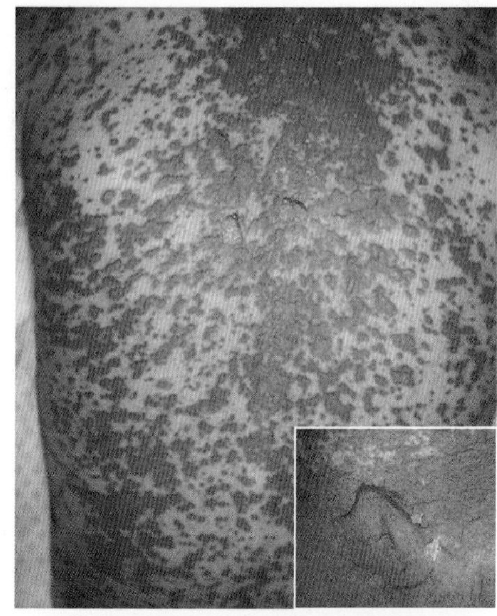

Fig. 16.9 Stevens–Johnson syndrome (SJS) versus SJS–TEN overlap. In addition to mucosal involvement and numerous dusky lesions with flaccid bullae, there are areas of coalescence and multiple sites of epidermal detachment. Because the latter involved >10% body surface area, the patient was classified as having SJS–TEN overlap. Note the epidermal detachment (inset), whose appearance has been likened to wet cigarette paper. *Courtesy, YDRSC.*

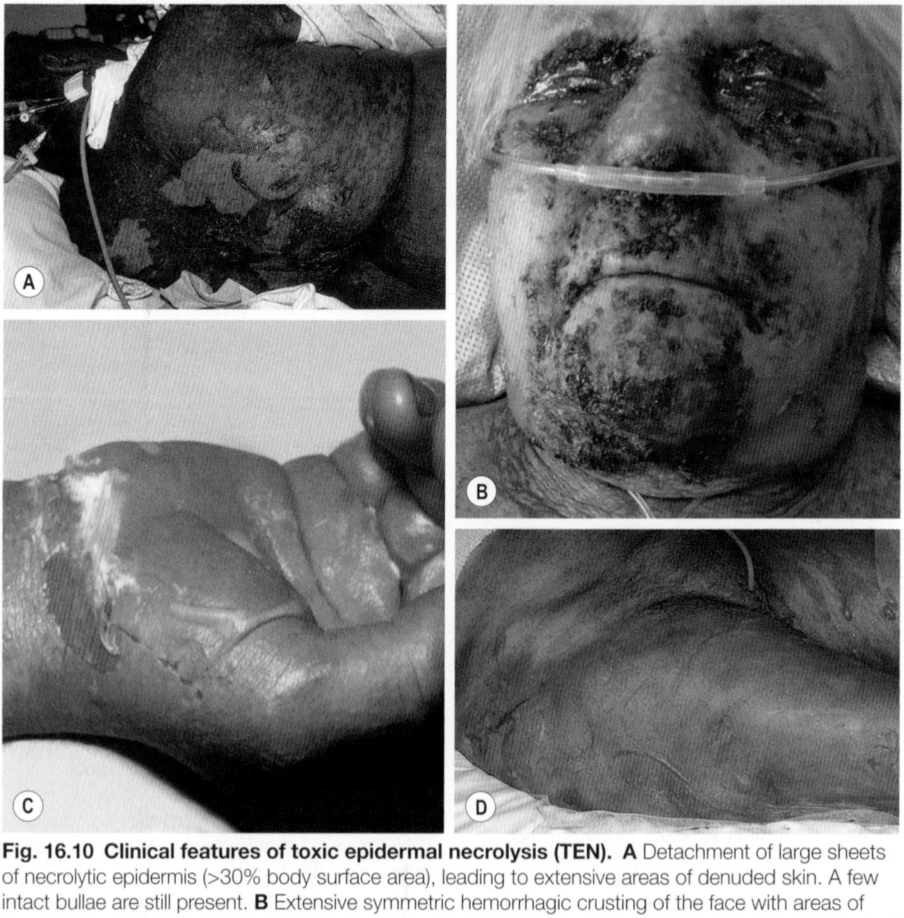

Fig. 16.10 Clinical features of toxic epidermal necrolysis (TEN). A Detachment of large sheets of necrolytic epidermis (>30% body surface area), leading to extensive areas of denuded skin. A few intact bullae are still present. **B** Extensive symmetric hemorrhagic crusting of the face with areas of denudation. **C** Epidermal detachment of palmar skin. **D** Note the rolled and folded sheets of detached epidermis at the edge of denuded skin in addition to widespread erythema and intact bullae. *A, Courtesy, YDRSC; B, Courtesy, Wolfram Hötzenecker, MD, Christina Prins, MD, Lars E. French, MD; C, Courtesy, Lars E. French, MD; D, Courtesy, Luis Requena, MD.*

SCORTEN SCALE	
Prognostic factors	**Points**
Age >40 years	1
Heart rate >120 bpm	1
Cancer or hematologic malignancy	1
BSA involved on day 1 above 10%	1
Serum urea level (>10 mmol/l)	1
Serum bicarbonate level (<20 mmol/l)	1
Serum glucose level (>14 mmol/l)	1
SCORTEN	**Mortality rate (%)**
0–1	3.2
2	12.1
3	35.8
4	58.3
≥5	90

Table 16.5 SCORTEN scale.

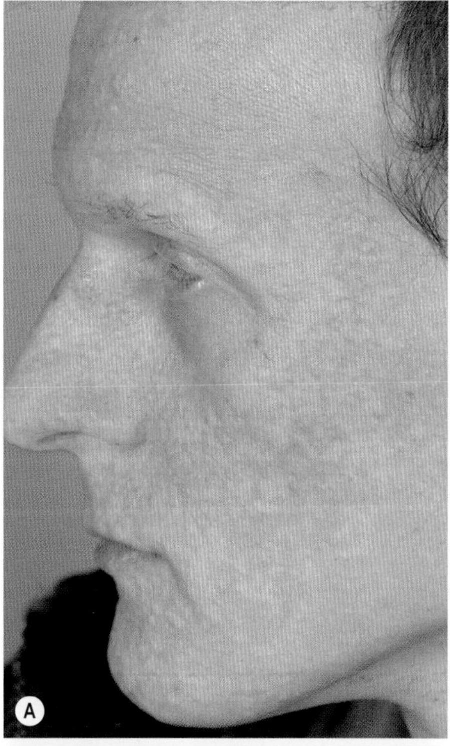

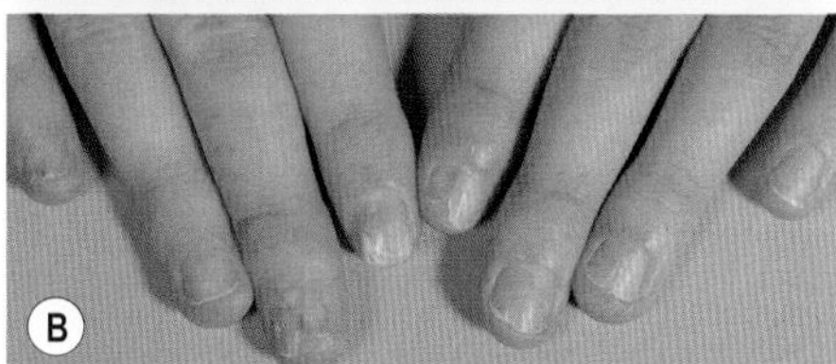

Fig. 16.11 Sequelae of toxic epidermal necrolysis. A Symblepharon, erosion of lower lateral eyelid margin and sparse eyelashes; the patient also had entropion with an ingrowth of eyelashes and pebble-like scarring of facial skin. **B** Nail dystrophy consisting of longitudinal ridging and fissuring, fragility and distal notching.
A,B, Courtesy, Wolfram Hötzenecker, MD, Christina Prins, MD, Lars E. French, MD.

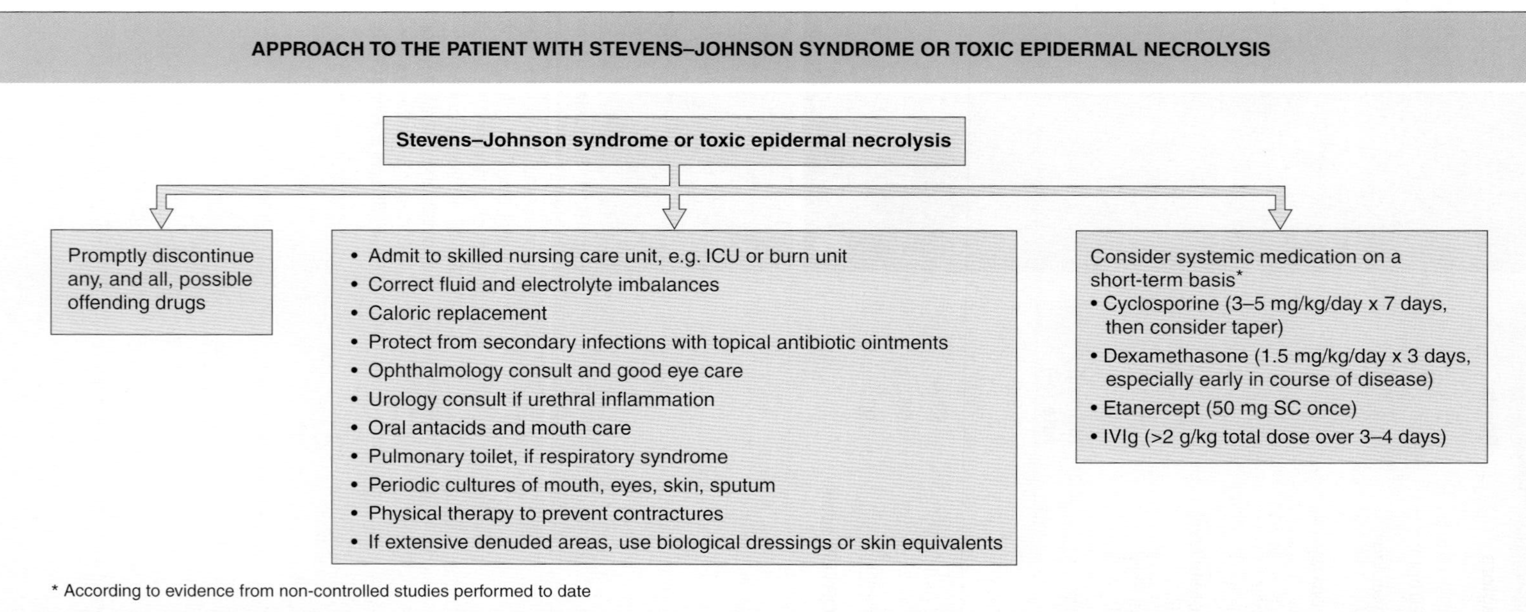

Fig. 16.12 Management of the patient with Stevens–Johnson syndrome or toxic epidermal necrolysis. ICU, intensive care unit.

Drug Reactions 17

AGEP, acute generalized exanthematous pustulosis;
DRESS, drug reaction with eosinophilia and systemic symptoms;
SJS, Stevens–Johnson syndrome;
TEN, toxic epidermal necrolysis

- The skin is one of the most common targets for adverse drug reactions.
- Risk factors for developing an adverse cutaneous drug reaction (ACDR) include: female gender, immunosuppression (e.g. HIV infection), specific HLA alleles (Table 17.1); the risk increases as the number of drugs taken increases.
- Pathogenesis of ACDRs is not totally understood but can involve immunologic, nonimmunologic, and idiosyncratic mechanisms (Table 17.2).

SPECIFIC HLA ALLELES THAT INCREASE THE RISK OF SEVERE CUTANEOUS DRUG REACTIONS			
Drug	**Higher risk population(s)**	**HLA allele**	**Type of drug reaction**
Abacavir**	All patients	**B*5701**	DRESS
Allopurinol**	Asians, US Blacks > Europeans	**B*5801**	SJS/TEN, DRESS
Carbamazepine**, lamotrigine, phenytoin	Han Chinese and other Asians	**B*1502**	SJS/TEN
Carbamazepine	Europeans, Japanese, Han Chinese	**A*3101**	DRESS
Dapsone	Chinese	B*1301	DRESS
Nevirapine	French	DRB1*01:01	DRESS

***It is recommended that patients in at-risk populations be screened for the presence of these HLA alleles prior to initiating treatment with these medications.*

Table 17.1 Specific HLA alleles that increase the risk of severe cutaneous drug reactions. Highest relative risks are in bold.

MECHANISMS OF CUTANEOUS DRUG-INDUCED REACTIONS	
Immunologic mechanism (unpredictable)	• IgE-dependent drug reactions • Cytotoxic drug-induced reactions • Immune complex-dependent drug reactions • Cell-mediated reactions
Nonimmunologic mechanism (sometimes predictable)	• Overdose • Pharmacologic side effects • Cumulative toxicity • Delayed toxicity • Drug–drug interactions • Alterations in metabolism • Exacerbation of disease
Idiosyncratic with a possible immunologic mechanism (unpredictable)	• DRESS • SJS/TEN • Drug reactions in the setting of HIV infection • Drug-induced lupus erythematosus

Table 17.2 Mechanisms of cutaneous drug-induced reactions.

SELECTED MOST AND LEAST LIKELY DRUGS TO CAUSE ADVERSE CUTANEOUS REACTIONS	
Most likely culprit drugs	**Least likely culprit drugs***
Antibiotics (e.g. penicillins, aminopenicillins, sulfonamides, cephalosporins, tetracyclines, fluoroquinolones)	Acetaminophen Aspirin* Diphenhydramine Opioids* (e.g. meperidine, codeine, morphine) Vitamins (e.g. multivitamins, thiamine, folic acid, ferrous sulfate) Potassium Magnesium Digoxin Aminophylline Spironolactone Nitroglycerin Lidocaine Insulin, regular Prednisone
Aromatic anticonvulsants (e.g. carbamazepine, phenytoin, phenobarbital, lamotrigine)	
Targeted therapies (e.g. EGFR inhibitors, BRAF inhibitors [when used alone])	
Checkpoint inhibitors (e.g. anti-CTLA-4 antibodies, anti-PD-1 antibodies, anti-PD-L1 antibodies)	
Other Packed red blood cells NSAIDs Allopurinol	

With the exception of urticaria with opioids and aspirin.

Table 17.3 Selected most and least likely drugs to cause adverse cutaneous reactions.

- Some of the most and least likely culprit drugs are listed in Table 17.3.
- Most common types of ACDRs: morbilliform > urticaria > vasculitis or fixed drug eruption (FDE) (Table 17.4).
- Severe cutaneous adverse drug reactions (SCARs) cause significant morbidity and potential mortality, but fortunately only constitute ~2% of ACDRs.
- SCARs that require immediate attention: SJS/TEN, DRESS (also referred to as drug-induced hypersensitivity syndrome [DIHS]), vasculitis, serum sickness, serum sickness-like reaction, angioedema/anaphylaxis, warfarin-induced skin necrosis, and heparin-induced thrombocytopenia and thrombosis syndrome (HIT) (see Table 17.4 and Fig. 17.1).
- Features that should alert one to the presence of a SCAR are outlined in Table 17.5.
- A practical approach in determining the cause of an ACDR is outlined in Table 17.6.
- Organizing pertinent information into a drug chart (see Fig. 17.2 and Appendix) can be helpful in synthesizing the available information.
- The most important step in the treatment of SCARs is early identification and withdrawal of the culprit drug.
- In non-life-threatening morbilliform drug eruptions, the culprit drug is ideally stopped, but if vitally important to the patient's health and no alternative drug is available, one can consider "treating through" the eruption with supportive care (e.g. topical CS and oral antihistamines).
- An approach to the management of a suspected ACDR is presented in Fig. 17.1.
- Additional reviews of specific types of drug reactions can be found in other chapters (Table 17.7).
- The use of both targeted therapies and immune checkpoint inhibitors to treat various malignancies has expanded rapidly. The more common mucocutaneous side effects of these agents are listed in Tables 17.8 and 17.9, respectively.
- Selected drug-induced eruptions due to chemotherapeutic agents are listed in Table 17.10.
- Localized injection site reactions to selected medications are outlined in Table 17.11.

For further information see Ch. 21 from *Dermatology, Fourth Edition*.

For additional online figures and tables visit www.expertconsult.com

CHARACTERISTICS OF SELECTED ADVERSE CUTANEOUS DRUG REACTIONS (ACDR)							
Diagnosis/ ***% drug-induced***	**Selected responsible drugs**	**Time interval to onset**	**Mucocutaneous features**	**Systemic features**	**Other helpful hints**	**Differential diagnosis**	**Treatment (in addition to withdrawal of culprit drug)**
Severe cutaneous adverse reactions to drugs (SCARs) (Fig. 17.1)							
SJS *80–90+%* **TEN** *80–90+%* (Fig. 17.3) (see Ch. 16)	• Antibiotics (e.g. sulfonamides, aminopenicillins, cephalosporins, quinolones) • Aromatic anticonvulsants* • NSAIDs • Allopurinol • Antiretroviral drugs (especially NNRTIs [nevirapine]) • Checkpoint inhibitors (e.g. ipilimumab, nivolumab)	• 7–21 days	• Mucosal erosions • Dusky macular atypical targets • Necrosis and epidermal detachment • SJS <10% BSA • SJS/TEN overlap 10–30% BSA • TEN >30% BSA	• Prodromal URI symptoms • Fever • Skin pain	• Leukopenia • Skin biopsy • Frozen section to differentiate from SSSS	• EM major • LABD • SSSS • AGEP • Severe acute GVHD • Rowell syndrome • Kawasaki disease • Generalized FDE • Paraneoplastic pemphigus	Mild disease • Hospitalization • Wound care • Ophthalmology consult Severe disease • ICU/burn care • Consider other systemic therapy (see Fig. 16.12)

Table 17.4A Characteristics of selected adverse cutaneous drug reactions (ACDR). *Continued*

CHARACTERISTICS OF SELECTED ADVERSE CUTANEOUS DRUG REACTIONS (ACDR)							
Diagnosis/ ***% drug-induced***	**Selected responsible drugs**	**Time interval to onset**	**Mucocutaneous features**	**Systemic features**	**Other helpful hints**	**Differential diagnosis**	**Treatment (in addition to withdrawal of culprit drug)**
DRESS *80–90+%* (Fig. 17.4)	• Aromatic anticonvulsants* • Antimicrobials (e.g. dapsone, sulfonamides) • Allopurinol • Antiretrovirals (e.g. abacavir, nevirapine)	• 15–40 days	• Facial edema • Edematous morbilliform eruption with follicular accentuation • Face, upper trunk, and extremities favored initially • Occasionally other skin findings: vesicles, bullae, pustules, erythroderma, purpura	(Always present to some degree) • Fever • Lymphadenopathy • Arthralgias/arthritis • Hepatitis • Myocarditis • Pneumonitis • Nephritis • Thyroiditis • Gastrointestinal bleeding (allopurinol)	• Marked eosinophilia • Lymphocytosis with increased atypical lymphocytes • Increased liver enzymes • Consider skin biopsy • Consider laboratory testing for reactivation of HHV6 in immunocompromised host • Cutaneous and visceral involvement may persist for weeks to months after withdrawal of culprit drug • With rapid taper of CS may see rebound	• Viral exanthem • Other ACDR • Cutaneous lymphoma • Pseudolymphoma • Idiopathic hypereosinophilic syndrome	• Oral CS with a long course (often several months for more severe disease) and slow taper • Topical CS may relieve symptoms • Longitudinal evaluation for up to a year, given delayed manifestations, e.g. thyroiditis, myocarditis

Table 17.4A *Continued* **Characteristics of selected adverse cutaneous drug reactions (ACDR).** *Continued*

CHARACTERISTICS OF SELECTED ADVERSE CUTANEOUS DRUG REACTIONS (ACDR)							
Diagnosis/ *% drug-induced*	**Selected responsible drugs**	**Time interval to onset**	**Mucocutaneous features**	**Systemic features**	**Other helpful hints**	**Differential diagnosis**	**Treatment (in addition to withdrawal of culprit drug)**
Cutaneous small vessel vasculitis (CSVV) *~10%*	• Penicillins • NSAIDs • Antibiotics (e.g. sulfonamides, cephalosporins, quinolones) • Diuretics (e.g. furosemide, hydrochlorothiazide) • Allopurinol • Phenytoin • Levamisole • Bortezomib • Systemic immunomodulators (e.g. G-CSF, GM-CSF, interferons, TNF inhibitors)	• 7–21 days (initial) • <3 days (rechallenge)	• Purpuric papules, most often on lower extremities • Hemorrhagic blisters • Urticaria-like lesions • Pustules	(Not always present) • Fever • Myalgias • Arthralgias/arthritis • Headache • Peripheral edema • Peripheral neuropathy • Glomerulonephritis	• Urinalysis and BUN/Cr to exclude active urine sediment/kidney involvement • Check stools for evidence of GI bleeding • Skin biopsy of early lesion for H&E and DIF	• CSVV that is idiopathic or due to infection, autoimmune connective tissue or disease, malignancy	Mild disease • Observation • High-potency topical CS Severe or systemic disease • Oral CS • Steroid-sparing immunosuppressive agents

Table 17.4A *Continued* **Characteristics of selected adverse cutaneous drug reactions (ACDR).** *Continued*

CHARACTERISTICS OF SELECTED ADVERSE CUTANEOUS DRUG REACTIONS (ACDR)							
Diagnosis/ ***% drug-induced***	**Selected responsible drugs**	**Time interval to onset**	**Mucocutaneous features**	**Systemic features**	**Other helpful hints**	**Differential diagnosis**	**Treatment (in addition to withdrawal of culprit drug)**
Cutaneous medium vessel vasculitis (CMVV)	• Hydralazine • Propylthiouracil • Methimazole • Minocycline • Penicillamine • Allopurinol • Sulfasalazine • Levamisole	• Hours to years	• Purpuric plaques and nodules (favors face, ears, breasts, and extremities) • Ulcers • Livedo reticularis • Digital necrosis • Occasionally palpable purpura, mimicking a CSSV	(Often present) • Fever • Arthralgias/arthritis • Necrotizing glomerulonephritis • Pulmonary hemorrhage • Peripheral neuropathy	• Skin biopsy may reveal leukocytoclastic vasculitis of superficial and deep vessels • ANCA (+) with propylthiouracil, hydralazine, minocycline, levamisole	• Polyarteritis nodosa (classic or cutaneous) • Granulomatosis with polyangiitis • Microscopic polyangiitis • Eosinophilic granulomatosis with polyangiitis	Mild, early disease • Drug withdrawal is often adequate Severe disease with systemic involvement or late withdrawal of culprit drug • May require immunosuppressive therapy
"True" serum sickness (due to nonhuman proteins) *>90%*	• Anti-thymocyte globulin • Tositumomab • Infliximab	• 7–21 days	• Morbilliform eruption • Urticaria • Purpuric papules/ plaques	• Fever • Arthralgias/ arthritis • Lymphadenopathy • Renal disease	• Hypocomplementemia • Circulating immune complexes • Vasculitis seen in skin biopsy	• Viral exanthem • Other ACDR	Mild disease • Supportive care Severe disease • Oral CS • Steroid-sparing immunosuppressive agents
Serum sickness-like reaction *>90%* (see Fig. 3.3B)	• Cefaclor • Minocycline • Penicillins • Sulfonamides • Bupropion • Propranolol • Phenytoin • NSAIDs	• 7–21 days	• Morbilliform eruption • Urticaria, acral edema • Urticarial papules and plaques with a purpuric component	• Fever • Arthralgia/arthritis • Lymphadenopathy	• *No* hypocomplementemia, circulating immune complexes, vasculitis or renal disease	• Urticaria multiforme • Viral exanthem • DRESS • Acute hemorrhagic edema of infancy • EM or early SJS • Kawasaki disease	• Long-acting oral antihistamines, especially if urticaria • Oral CS if significant symptoms

Table 17.4A *Continued* **Characteristics of selected adverse cutaneous drug reactions (ACDR).** *Continued*

CHARACTERISTICS OF SELECTED ADVERSE CUTANEOUS DRUG REACTIONS (ACDR)							
Diagnosis/ ***% drug-induced***	**Selected responsible drugs**	**Time interval to onset**	**Mucocutaneous features**	**Systemic features**	**Other helpful hints**	**Differential diagnosis**	**Treatment (in addition to withdrawal of culprit drug)**
Angioedema/ anaphylaxis *30%*	• Penicillins • Radiocontrast media • Monoclonal antibodies	• Minutes to hours	• Acute pale or pink subcutaneous swelling • Favors face (eyelids, ears, lips, nose) • Less often extremities and genitalia • Associated with urticaria 50% of the time	• Involvement of oropharynx, larynx, epiglottis, and surrounding tissues may impair breathing and swallowing • Intestinal wall edema can cause nausea, vomiting, diarrhea, pain • Hypotension and circulatory collapse with anaphylaxis		• Severe insect bite reaction • Food allergies • Hereditary angioedema • Acquired angioedema • Estrogen-dependent angioedema	Mild disease • Oral antihistamine Severe disease • Hospitalization • SC epinephrine (adrenaline) • IV/oral antihistamines • IV/oral CS
	• NSAIDs	• 1–7 days					
	• ACE inhibitors • Angiotensin II receptor blockers	• 1 day to several years					
Warfarin (Coumadin®)-induced skin necrosis *100%* (Fig. 17.5)	• Warfarin	• 2–5 days	• Red to violaceous painful plaques evolving into hemorrhagic blisters and necrotic ulcers • Favors areas of greatest subcutaneous fat, e.g. breasts, thighs, buttocks	• Extreme pain at affected site	• Protein C deficiency	• DIC • Septicemia	• Vitamin K • IV heparin • IV protein C concentrate

Table 17.4A *Continued* **Characteristics of selected adverse cutaneous drug reactions (ACDR).** *Continued*

CHARACTERISTICS OF SELECTED ADVERSE CUTANEOUS DRUG REACTIONS (ACDR)							
Diagnosis/ ***% drug-induced***	**Selected responsible drugs**	**Time interval to onset**	**Mucocutaneous features**	**Systemic features**	**Other helpful hints**	**Differential diagnosis**	**Treatment (in addition to withdrawal of culprit drug)**
Heparin-induced thrombocytopenia with thrombosis (HIT) *100%* (Fig. 17.6) (see Fig. 18.2)	• Heparin – all forms (IV, SC, LMWH; and in heparin flushes used for dialysis and IV catheters)	• 5–10 days (initial) • Early-onset, occurs within 24 hours (rechallenge within ~100 days of last exposure) • Delayed-onset, occurs ~9 days after stopping heparin • Anaphylactoid reaction, occurs within 30 minutes of IV bolus	• Skin necrosis at sites of injection and at distant sites (e.g. distal extremities, nose) • Digital ischemia • Petechiae	• Venous and arterial systemic thrombosis • In anaphylactoid reaction, see acute inflammatory (fever, chills) and cardiorespiratory (hypertension, shortness of breath) symptoms	• Thrombocytopenia or decrease in platelets by >50% • Positive functional assay (serotonin release assay or heparin-induced platelet aggregation assay) • Positive ELISA immunoassay for antiplatelet factor 4/heparin antibodies	• DIC • Septicemia • Antiphospholipid antibody syndrome	• Change to another, non-heparin anticoagulant, e.g. • Argatroban • Danaparoid • Fondaparinux • Bivalirudin • Direct acting oral anticoagulants • Once the thrombocytopenia is resolved, most patients are then transitioned to warfarin or other outpatient anticoagulant

Aromatic anticonvulsants (e.g. carbamazepine, phenytoin, phenobarbital, lamotrigine [especially in combination with valproic acid] are most often implicated).

Table 17.4A *Continued* **Characteristics of selected adverse cutaneous drug reactions (ACDR).** 5-FU, 5-fluorouracil; ACE, angiotensin-converting enzyme; DIC, disseminated intravascular coagulation; DIF, direct immunofluorescence; G-CSF and GM-CSF, granulocyte and granulocyte–macrophage colony-stimulating factors; LABD, linear IgA bullous dermatosis; LMWH, low-molecular-weight heparin; NNRTIs, non-nucleoside reverse transcriptase inhibitors; SSSS, staphylococcal scalded skin syndrome.

CHARACTERISTICS OF SELECTED ADVERSE CUTANEOUS DRUG REACTIONS (ACDR)							
Diagnosis/ ***% drug-induced***	**Selected responsible drugs**	**Time interval to onset**	**Mucocutaneous features**	**Systemic features**	**Other helpful hints**	**Differential diagnosis**	**Treatment (in addition to withdrawal of culprit drug)**
Less severe cutaneous adverse reactions to drugs							
Morbilliform/ exanthematous/ maculopapular drug eruption *Child: 10–20%* *Adult: 50–70%* (Fig. 17.7) (see Fig. 3.2)	• Aminopenicillins • Sulfonamides • Cephalosporins • Aromatic anticonvulsants* • Allopurinol • Abacavir • Nevirapine	• 4–14 days (occasionally sooner with rechallenge)	• Erythematous macules and subtle papules that often become confluent • Symmetric distribution favoring trunk, upper extremities • Dependent areas in bed-ridden patients • Purpuric lesions on lower legs and feet • Sometimes annular or targetoid plaques • Typically no mucosal involvement	• Pruritus • Low-grade fever	• Mild eosinophilia • May get a bit worse before getting better upon withdrawal of culprit drug • Eruption resolves in 1–2 weeks after withdrawal of culprit drug	• Viral exanthem	• Supportive care with oral antihistamines and mild topical CS • Can treat through eruption if culprit drug is crucially important to patient and no adequate alternative

Table 17.4B Characteristics of selected adverse cutaneous drug reactions (ACDR). Less severe adverse cutaneous reactions to drugs. *Continued*

CHARACTERISTICS OF SELECTED ADVERSE CUTANEOUS DRUG REACTIONS (ACDR)							
Diagnosis/ ***% drug-induced***	**Selected responsible drugs**	**Time interval to onset**	**Mucocutaneous features**	**Systemic features**	**Other helpful hints**	**Differential diagnosis**	**Treatment (in addition to withdrawal of culprit drug)**
Urticaria *<10%* (Fig. 17.8) (see Fig. 3.3A)	• Penicillins • Cephalosporins • NSAIDs • Monoclonal antibodies • Radiocontrast media**	• Minutes to hours	• Transient erythematous, edematous papules and plaques with central pallor • Varied sizes and configurations, including annular; sometimes transient central duskiness in children (urticaria "multiforme")	• Pruritus	• Individual lesions last <24 hours • Normal skin left behind when lesions resolve	• Other causes of urticaria (e.g. virus, food allergy, idiopathic) • Urticarial vasculitis • Serum sickness-like reaction • EM	• Oral antihistamines with a longer half-life, e.g. cetirizine
AGEP *70–90%* (Fig. 17.9)	• Antibiotics (e.g. aminopenicillins, penicillins, cephalosporins, clindamycin, macrolides, sulfonamides) • Calcium channel blockers (especially diltiazem)	• <4 days	• Numerous, small, mostly non-follicular, sterile pustules that arise within large areas of edematous erythema • Often begins on face and in intertriginous areas, and then becomes widespread • In 50% of patients, additional skin lesions: petechiae, purpura, atypical target-like lesions, vesicles	• Fever • Pruritus or burning	• Leukocytosis with neutrophilia • Transient renal dysfunction • Hypocalcemia • Skin biopsy helpful • Resolves with superficial desquamation	• Acute pustular psoriasis • DRESS • Morbilliform drug eruption • TEN	• Supportive care • Mild topical CS • Antipyretics

Table 17.4B *Continued* **Characteristics of selected adverse cutaneous drug reactions (ACDR).** Less severe adverse cutaneous reactions to drugs. *Continued*

CHARACTERISTICS OF SELECTED ADVERSE CUTANEOUS DRUG REACTIONS (ACDR)							
Diagnosis/ ***% drug-induced***	**Selected responsible drugs**	**Time interval to onset**	**Mucocutaneous features**	**Systemic features**	**Other helpful hints**	**Differential diagnosis**	**Treatment (in addition to withdrawal of culprit drug)**
Fixed drug eruption (FDE) *99%* (Fig. 17.10)	• Sulfonamides • NSAIDs • Tetracyclines • Pseudoephedrine (non-pigmenting FDE)	• 7–14 days (first exposure) • Within 24–48 hours (rechallenge)	• One or a few round, sharply demarcated erythematous and edematous plaques • Sometimes with a dusky violaceous hue, central blister, or detached epidermis • Favors lips, face, hands, feet, genitalia • Fades over several days; residual postinflammatory brown pigmentation Variants • Generalized FDE (numerous lesions) • Non-pigmenting FDE • Linear FDE		• Upon rechallenge lesions recur at exact same sites ± new lesions • Skin biopsy helpful	• Arthropod or spider bite (single lesion) • EM (generalized FDE) • SJS (generalized FDE plus mucosal involvement) • TEN (generalized FDE with blisters/ epidermal detachment) • Cellulitis (non-pigmenting FDE) • Lichen planus (linear FDE)	• Supportive care

Aromatic anticonvulsants (e.g. carbamazepine, phenytoin, phenobarbital, lamotrigine).
**Often anaphylactoid reaction.*

Table 17.4B *Continued* **Characteristics of selected adverse cutaneous drug reactions (ACDR).** Less severe adverse cutaneous reactions to drugs. 5-FU, 5-fluorouracil, EM, erythema multiforme.

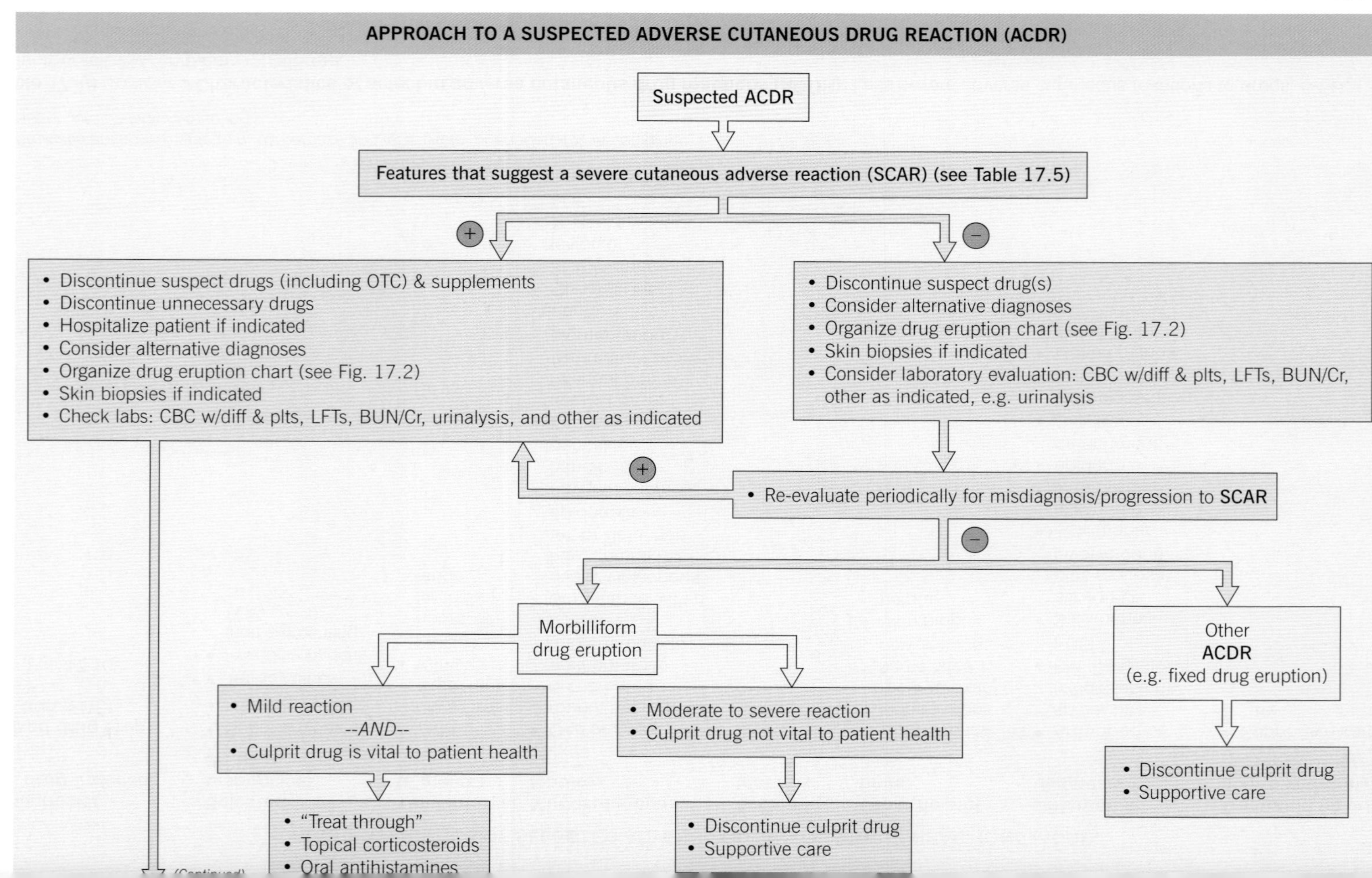
APPROACH TO A SUSPECTED ADVERSE CUTANEOUS DRUG REACTION (ACDR)
Suspected ACDR
Features that suggest a severe cutaneous adverse reaction (SCAR) (see Table 17.5)
+
• Discontinue suspect drugs (including OTC) & supplements
• Discontinue unnecessary drugs
• Hospitalize patient if indicated
• Consider alternative diagnoses
• Organize drug eruption chart (see Fig. 17.2)
• Skin biopsies if indicated
• Check labs: CBC w/diff & plts, LFTs, BUN/Cr, urinalysis, and other as indicated
−
• Discontinue suspect drug(s)
• Consider alternative diagnoses
• Organize drug eruption chart (see Fig. 17.2)
• Skin biopsies if indicated
• Consider laboratory evaluation: CBC w/diff & plts, LFTs, BUN/Cr, other as indicated, e.g. urinalysis
• Re-evaluate periodically for misdiagnosis/progression to SCAR
+
−
Morbilliform drug eruption
• Mild reaction
--AND--
• Culprit drug is vital to patient health
• "Treat through"
• Topical corticosteroids
• Oral antihistamines
• Moderate to severe reaction
• Culprit drug not vital to patient health
• Discontinue culprit drug
• Supportive care
Other ACDR (e.g. fixed drug eruption)
• Discontinue culprit drug
• Supportive care

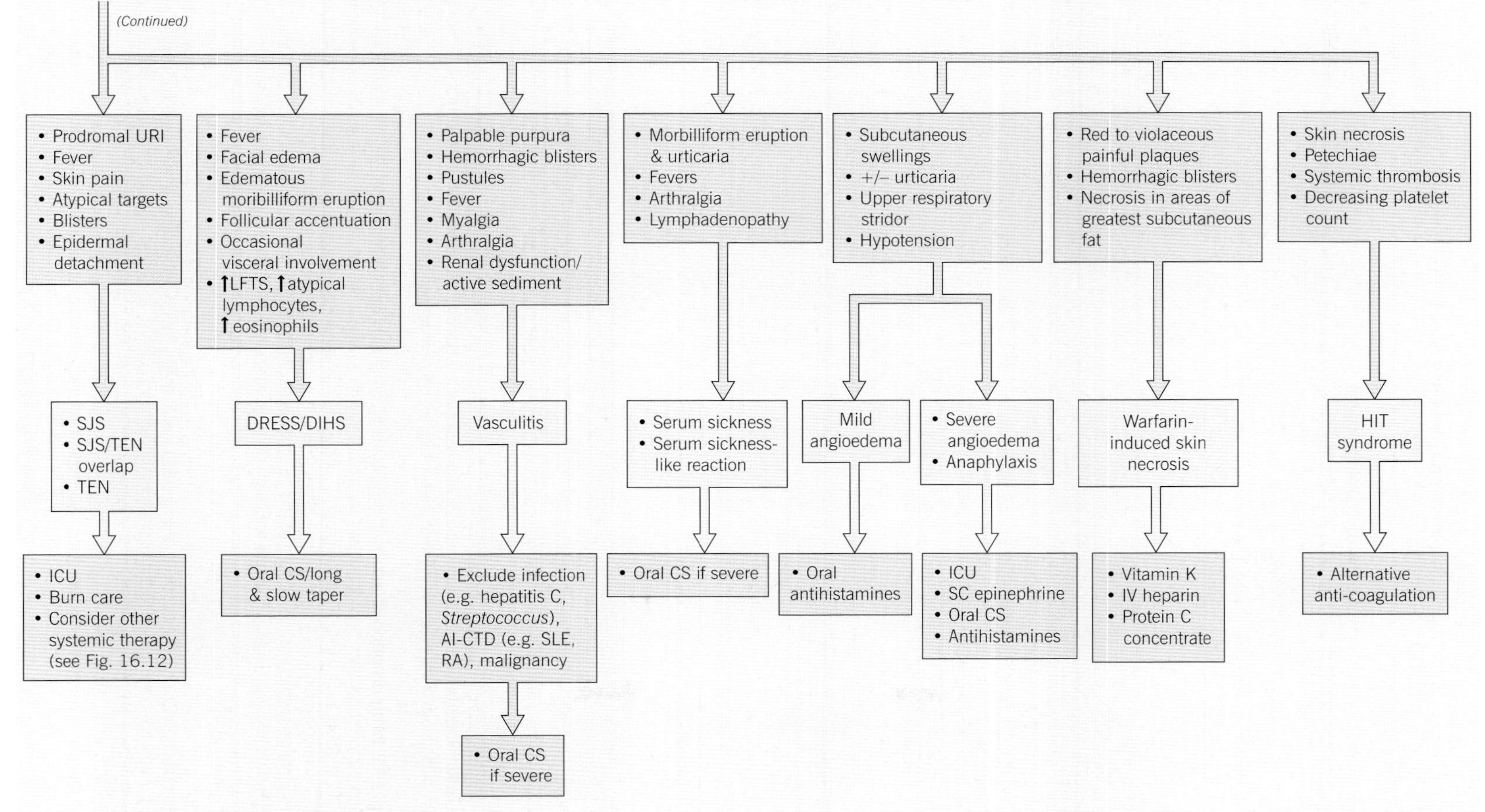

Fig. 17.1 Approach to a suspected adverse cutaneous drug reaction (ACDR). diff, differential; HIT, heparin-induced thrombocytopenia and thrombosis syndrome; plts, platelets; RA, rheumatoid arthritis; SCAR, severe cutaneous adverse reaction to a drug.

DRUG ERUPTION CHART - SAMPLE

	Dates drug(s) administered							Rash onset ↓	Derm consult ↓		Rash worse ↓			Rash better ↓		
Drugs	Pre-hospital Duration (years)	6/15	6/16	6/17	6/18	6/19	6/20	6/21	6/22	6/23	6/24	6/25	6/26	6/27	6/28	6/29
Aspirin	x 10	X	X	X	X	X	X	X	X	X	X	X	X	X	X	X
Heparin SC			X	X	X	X	X	X	X	X	X	X	X	X	X	X
Famotidine		X	X	X	X	X	X	X	X							
Insulin	x 5	X	X	X	X	X	X	X	X	X	X	X	X	X	X	X
Digoxin	x 8	X	X	X	X	X	X	X	X	X	X	X	X	X	X	X
Diltiazem	x 6	X	X	X	X	X	X	X	X	X	X	X	X	X	X	X
Multivitamin	x 5	X	X	X	X	X	X	X	X							
Thiamine		X	X	X												
Folate		X	X	X	X	X	X	X	X							
Lorazepam		X	X	X	X	X	X	X	X	X	X	X				
Zolpidem		X	X		X	X		X								
Acetaminophen		X	X													
Ibuprofen				X	X											
Tramadol HC						X	X	X								
Maalox®			X	X	X											
Lactulose						X	X	X								
Diphenhydramine								X	X	X	X	X	X			
Ampicillin/sulbactam		X	X													
Vancomycin				X	X	X	X	X	X							
Ceftazidime				X	X	X	X	X	X							
Levofloxacin										X	X					
Linezolid												X	X	X	X	X
Laboratory																
WBC		20.2	16.5	7.0	7.6	8.1	10.2	11.3	11.5	11.2	11.5	10.5	9.2	7.0	7.0	6.5
% Eosinophils		0%	0%	<1%	<1%	3%	5%	7%	9%	9%	8%	7%	5%	3%	1%	1%
% Atypical lymphocytes		0%	→													
Platelets		nl	→													
AST		nl	→													
ALT		nl	→													
BUN/Cr		nl	→													
Temperature (°C)		40			38			38.3		38.5			37.5			
Physical exam*		nl	→													
Type of rash								Morbilliform → Confluence								

*Checking for the presence of lymphadenopathy, arthritis, wheezing, hypotension

Fig. 17.2 Drug eruption chart. This is a helpful working template for organizing all of the available patient information into one document for a patient with a suspected adverse cutaneous drug reaction (ACDR). **Step 1:** Compile all of the recently consumed or administered drugs (including prescription, OTC, and supplements) into the chart. **Step 2:** Review and list the pertinent laboratory information and physical findings at the bottom of the chart. **Step 3:** Referring to Fig. 17.1, exclude a SCAR and categorize the type of ACDR. **Step 4:** Based on time intervals (see Table 17.4) and the most and least likely drugs to cause ACDR (see Table 17.3), begin to formulate the most likely culprit drugs and recommend their discontinuation. In addition, discontinue unnecessary drugs. **Step 5:** Longitudinal evaluation of the patient is necessary to (1) exclude progression to a SCAR, (2) determine the response upon discontinuation of the culprit drug (noting that it might "get worse before it gets better"), and (3) provide supportive care to the patient. In this sample patient, the most likely culprit drugs are ceftazidime > ampicillin/sulbactam > vancomycin; however, the multivitamin, folate, famotidine, zolpidem, acetaminophen, ibuprofen, tramadol, Maalox®, and lorazepam (must taper off and not abruptly stop) were also discontinued. Note that the discontinuation of levofloxacin by the primary physicians was not necessary. Refer to www.expertconsult.com for a blank template of the drug eruption chart. ALT, alanine aminotransferase; AST, aspartate aminotransferase.

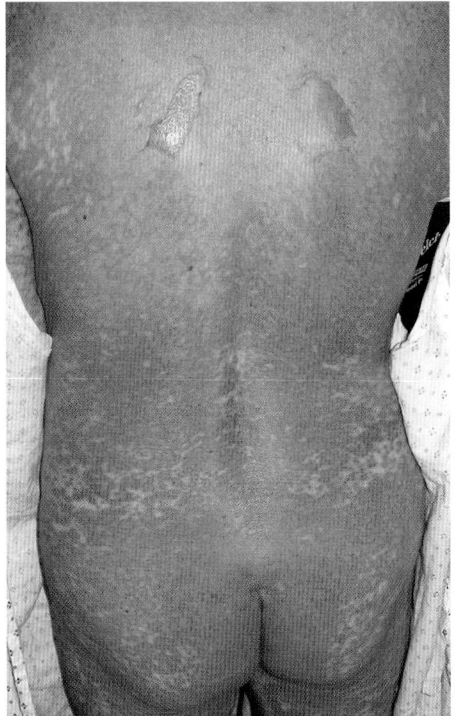

Fig. 17.3 Early Stevens–Johnson syndrome. This patient was originally diagnosed with a severe morbilliform drug eruption from penicillin, but then areas of epidermal detachment due to friction developed. *Courtesy, YDRSC.*

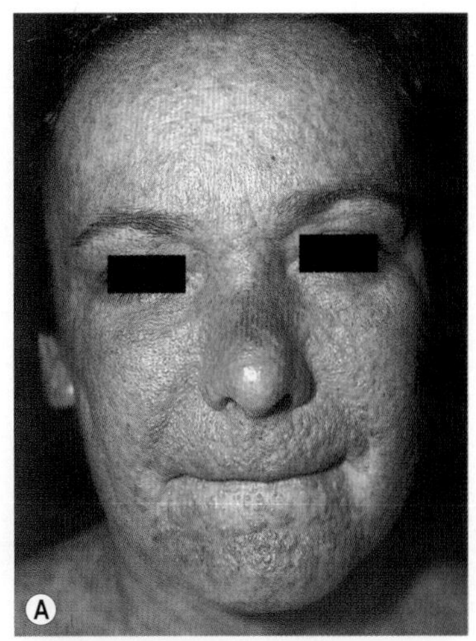

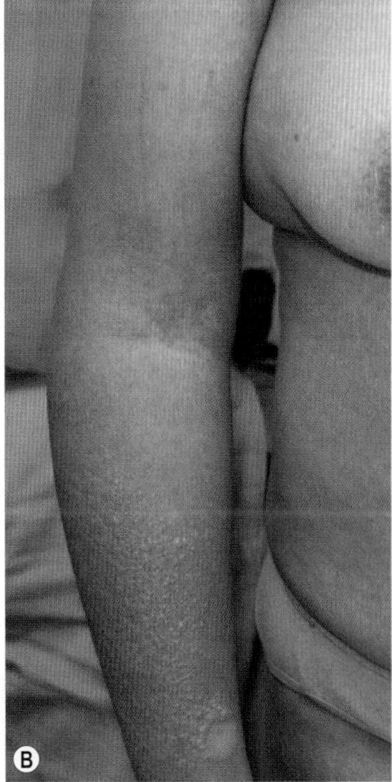

Fig. 17.4 Drug reaction with eosinophilia and systemic symptoms (DRESS). Also known as drug-induced hypersensitivity syndrome (DIHS). **A** Facial edema and multiple edematous papules are present. **B** Exanthematous eruption with confluence, edema and vesiculation on the forearm. *A, Courtesy, Kenneth Greer, MD; B, Courtesy Alicia Little, MD.*

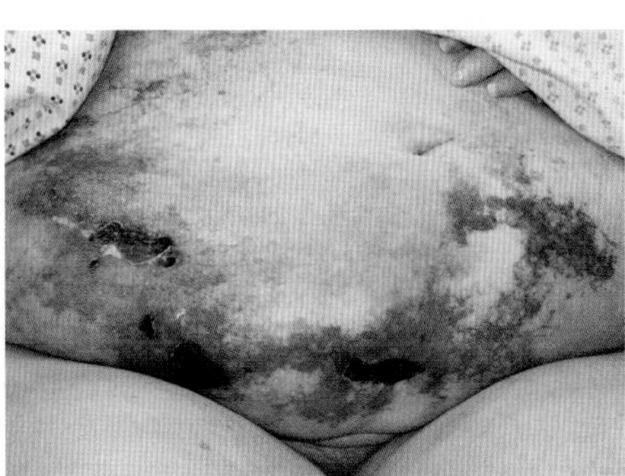

Fig. 17.5 Warfarin (Coumadin®)-induced skin necrosis. Retiform purpuric plaques with large hemorrhagic crusts and underlying ulcers on the abdominal pannus of a woman who recently initiated warfarin treatment. *Courtesy, Jean L. Bolognia, MD.*

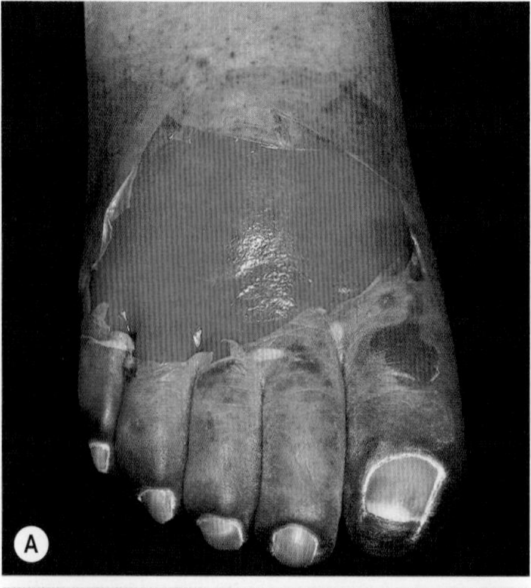

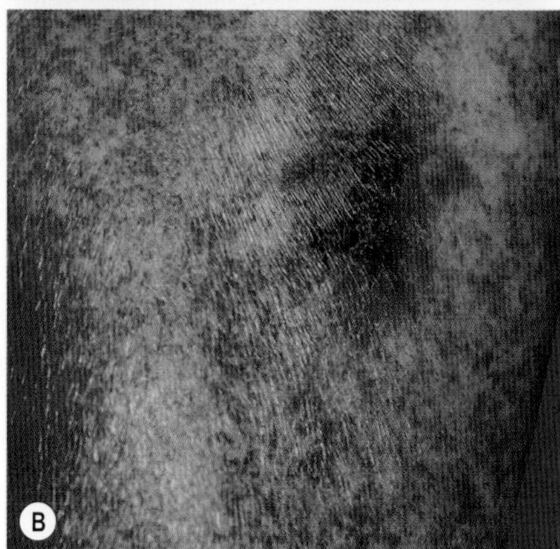

Fig. 17.6 Heparin-induced thrombocytopenia with thrombosis syndrome (HIT). A Ischemia and necrosis of the foot. **B** Petechiae due to thrombocytopenia and an irregular area of cutaneous necrosis. *A, Courtesy, Kalman Watsky, MD; B, Courtesy, Jean L. Bolognia, MD.*

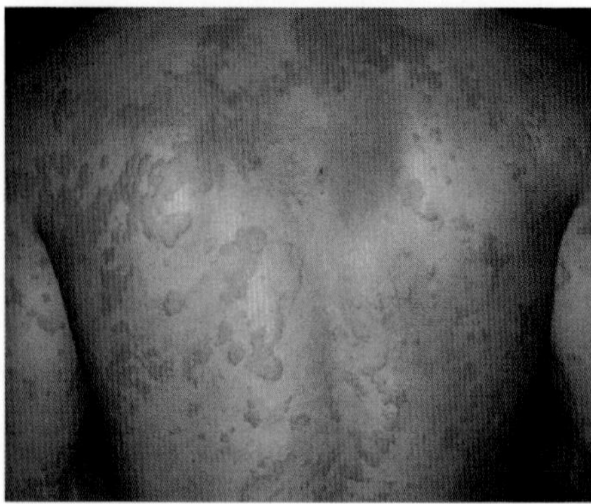

Fig. 17.8 Urticaria secondary to penicillin. Several of the lesions have a figurate appearance. *Courtesy, YDRSC.*

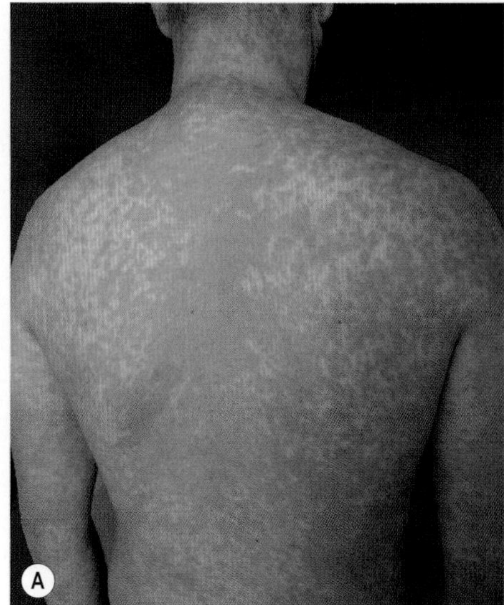

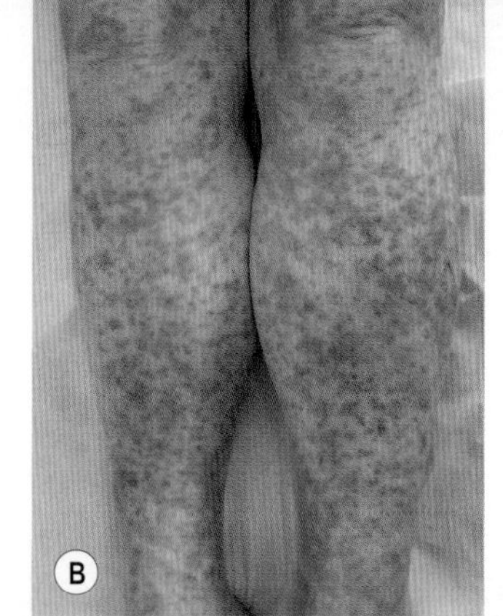

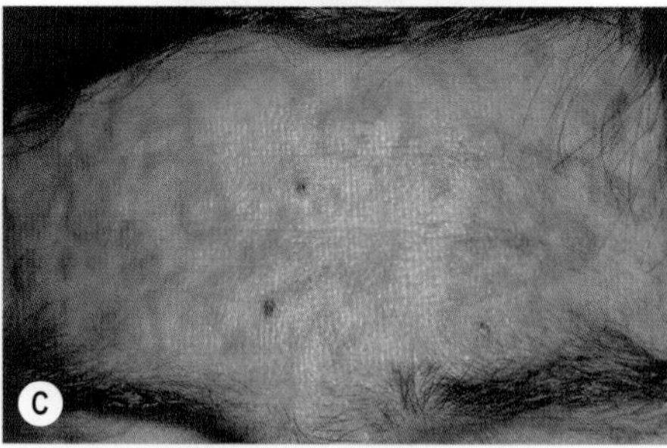

Fig. 17.7 Morbilliform (exanthematous) drug eruptions. A Erythematous papules and urticarial lesions with confluence on the mid back induced by amoxicillin. **B** Due to dependency, lesions on the distal lower extremities can become petechial or purpuric. **C** Pink papules and annular lesions on the forehead due to phenobarbital. *A, B, Courtesy, Laurence Valeyrie-Allanore, MD; C, Courtesy, YDRSC.*

FEATURES THAT SUGGEST A SEVERE CUTANEOUS ADVERSE REACTION TO A DRUG		
Cutaneous features	**Systemic features**	**Laboratory findings**
• Skin pain • Confluent erythema • Facial edema • Blisters or epidermal detachment • Mucosal erosions • Necrosis • Palpable purpura • Urticaria • Swelling of lips/tongue	• High fever • Lymphadenopathy • Arthralgia/arthritis • Shortness of breath, wheezing, stridor, hypotension • Other visceral involvement	• Marked eosinophilia • Lymphocytosis with atypical lymphocytes • Leukopenia • Abnormal liver or renal function tests • Thrombocytopenia

Table 17.5 Features that suggest a severe cutaneous adverse reaction (SCAR) to a drug.

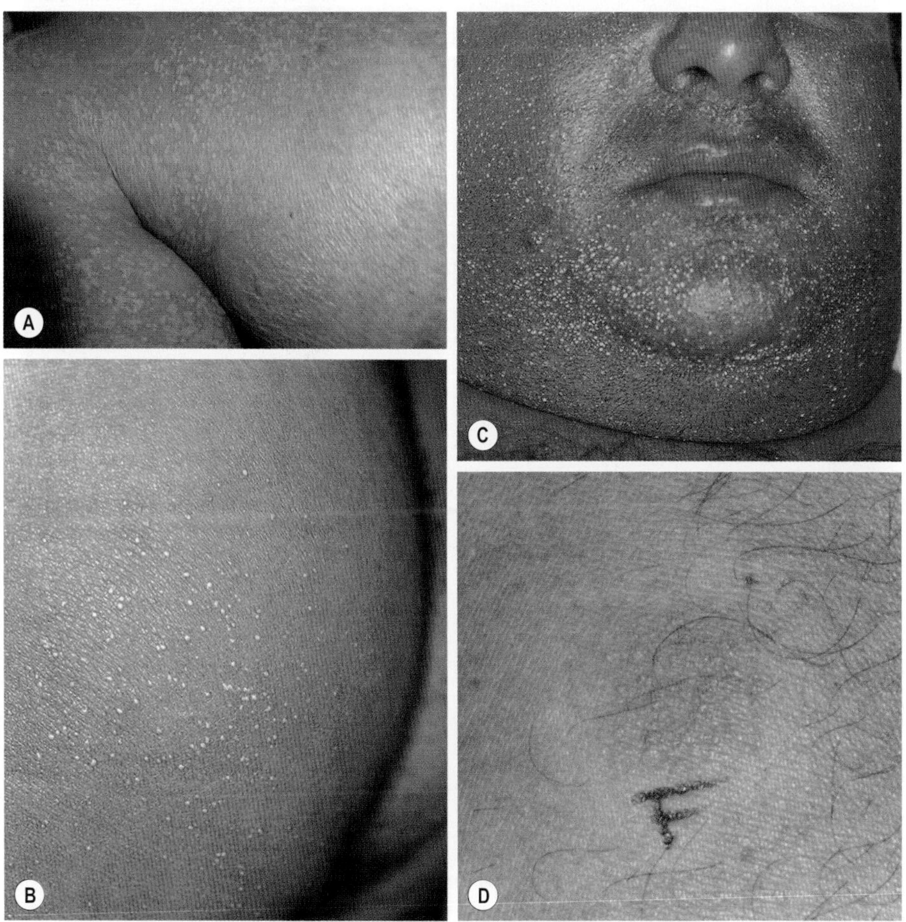

Fig. 17.9 Acute generalized exanthematous pustulosis (AGEP). A Numerous sterile pustules with superficial epidermal detachment in areas where the pustules have become confluent in a patient receiving amoxicillin. **B** Diffuse erythema of the buttock with multiple small sterile pustules due to a cephalosporin, and face (**C**) due to metronidazole. **D** Positive patch test result 4 days following the application of 0.75% metronidazole in a patient with a previous pustular drug eruption to that medication. *A, Courtesy, Laurence Valeyrie-Allanore, MD; B, Courtesy, YDRSC; C, D, Courtesy, Kalman Watsky, MD.*

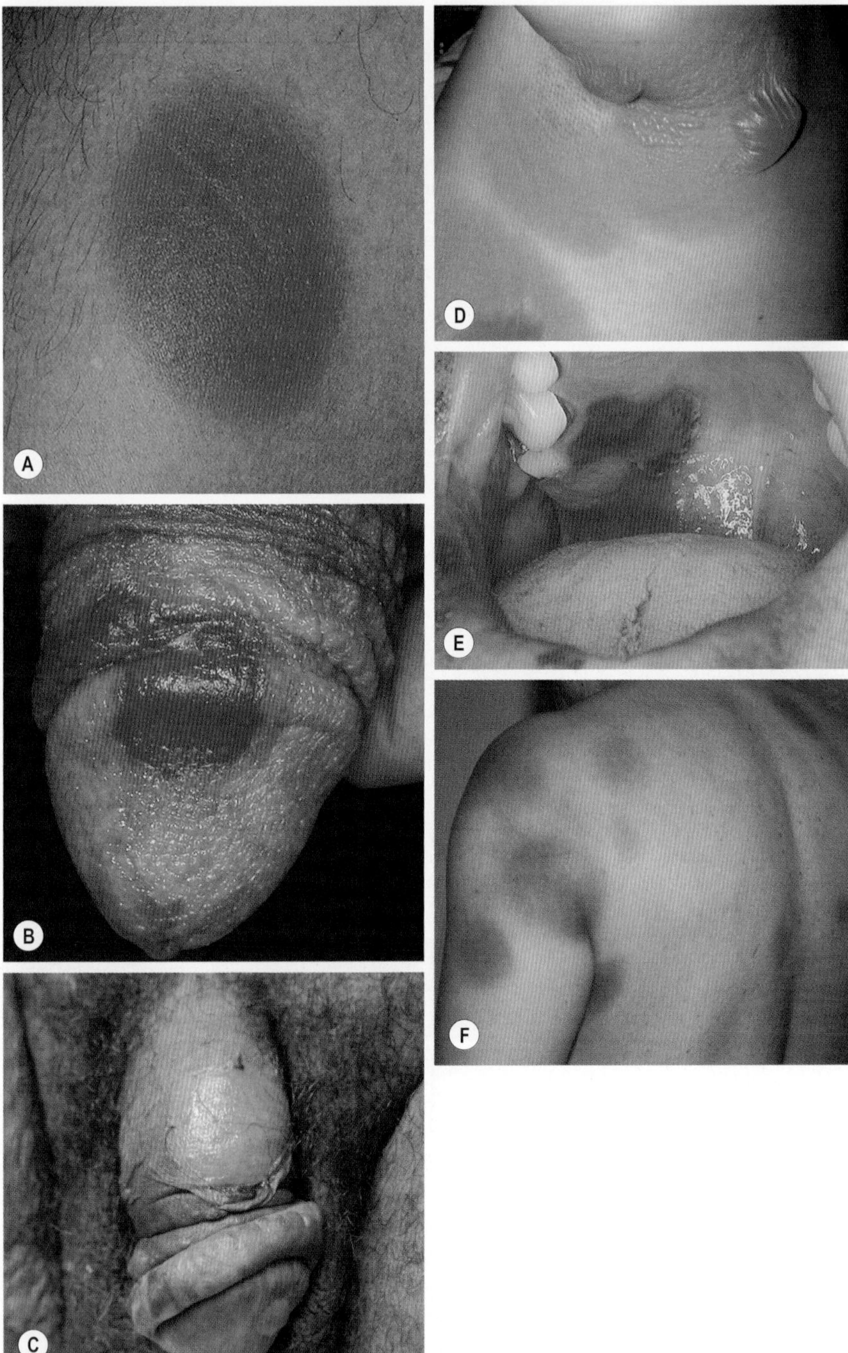

Fig. 17.10 Fixed drug eruptions (FDE). A An oval, well-demarcated red-brown plaque with a more erythematous border. **B** Erosive lesion of the penis due to epidermal detachment; this clinical presentation is sometimes misdiagnosed as recurrent HSV infection. **C, D** Generalized bullous FDE with involvement of the genitalia and intertriginous zones; erosions are seen following rupture of the bullae. Because of its more widespread distribution, this variant can be confused with SJS/TEN. **E** In the mouth, mucosal detachment leads to erosions. **F** Once inflammation is completely resolved, circular or oval areas of hyperpigmentation are commonly seen. Responsible drugs were phenolphthalein (**A**), ciprofloxacin (**B**), naproxen (**C**), pseudoephedrine (**D**), allopurinol (**E**), trimethoprim-sulfamethoxazole (**F**). *A, Courtesy, YDRSC; B, E, Courtesy, Kalman Watsky, MD; C, Courtesy, Sara Perkins, MD; D, Courtesy, Edward W Cowen, MD; F, Courtesy, Mary Stone, MD.*

DRUG RESPONSIBILITY ASSESSMENT	
Clinical characteristics	• Type of primary lesion (e.g. urticaria, erythematous papule, pustule, purpuric papule, vesicle or bulla) • Distribution and number of lesions • Mucous membrane involvement, facial edema • Associated signs and symptoms: fever, pruritus, lymph node enlargement, visceral involvement
Chronological factors	• Document all drugs to which the patient has been exposed (including OTC and complementary) and the dates of administration • Date of eruption • Time interval between drug introduction (or reintroduction) and skin eruption • Response to removal of the suspected agent • Consider excipients (e.g. soybean oil) • Response to rechallenge*
Literature search	• Bibliographic research (e.g. PubMed, Micromedex, Litt's Drug Eruption and Reaction Database) • Drug Alert Registry or MedWatch • Data collected by pharmaceutical companies • In the case of more recently released medications, extrapolation based on the class of drug and in particular the first drug released in the class

**Often inadvertent.*

Table 17.6 Logical approach to determine the cause of a drug eruption.

ADDITIONAL REVIEWS OF SPECIFIC TYPES OF DRUG REACTIONS	
Psoriasiform (Fig. 17.11)	Ch. 6
Erythroderma	Ch. 8, Table 8.1
Lichenoid (Fig. 17.12)	Ch. 9
Urticaria	Ch. 14
Stevens–Johnson syndrome and toxic epidermal necrolysis	Ch. 16
Warfarin- and heparin-induced necrosis	Ch. 18
Vasculitis	Ch. 19
Sweet syndrome	Ch. 21
Pemphigus and bullous pemphigoid	Chs 23 and 24
Linear IgA bullous dermatosis (LABD)	Ch. 25, Table 25.1
Acneiform/folliculitis	Chs 29 and 31
Hyper- and hypohidrosis	Ch. 32
Lupus erythematosus (systemic and cutaneous)	Ch. 33, Tables 33.4 and 33.5
Granulomatous (interstitial)	Ch. 37
Pseudoporphyria	Ch. 41, Table 41.2
Hypopigmentation (skin and hair)	Ch. 54
Hyperpigmentation and dyschromatosis	Ch. 55
Hypertrichosis and hirsutism	Ch. 57
Nail abnormalities	Ch. 58, Table 58.4
Gingival enlargement	Ch. 59, Table 59.3
Phototoxic and photoallergic	Ch. 73, Table 73.4
Cutaneous lymphoid hyperplasia (pseudolymphoma)	Ch. 99

Table 17.7 Additional reviews of specific types of drug reactions.

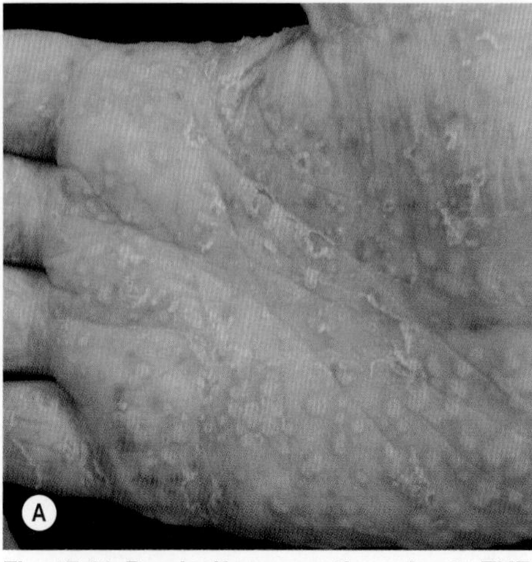

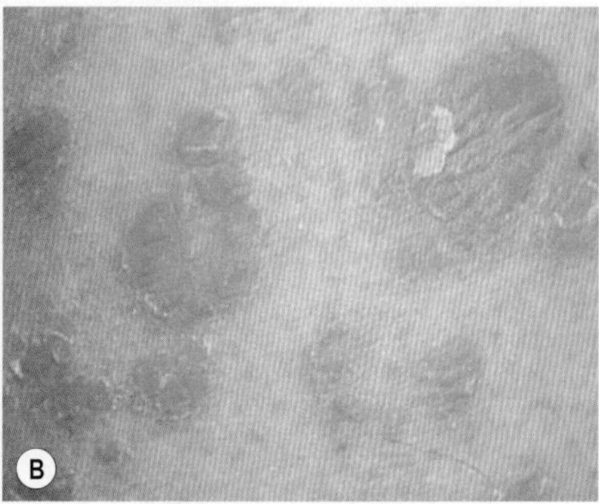

Fig. 17.11 Psoriasiform eruptions due to TNF inhibitors. A Palmoplantar pustulosis that developed as a complication of infliximab. **B** Eruption of plaque-type psoriasis in a patient receiving infliximab for GVHD of the gastrointestinal tract. *A, Courtesy, J. Mark Jackson, MD and Jeffrey P. Callen, MD; B, Courtesy, Dennis Cooper, MD.*

THE MORE COMMON MUCOCUTANEOUS SIDE EFFECTS OF TARGETED THERAPIES	
Mucocutaneous side effect	**General management recommendations**
Xerosis Pruritus Papulopustular eruption (Fig. 17.12) Morbilliform eruption Photosensitivity Palmoplantar hyperkeratosis Acral erythema (may be bullous) Paronychia Stomatitis Alopecia Curly, brittle hair Eyelash trichomegaly &/or facial hair growth Skin growths: squamous papillomas, KAs, SCCs*	• *EGFR inhibitor-induced papulopustular reaction prophylaxis (P) and treatment (T):* – Gentle cleansers, moisturization, sun avoidance/protection (P) – Topical antibiotics (e.g. clindamycin, erythromycin) twice daily (P, T) – Oral antibiotics (e.g. doxycycline [100 mg twice daily] or minocycline [50–100 mg twice daily]) (P, typically for 6–8 weeks; T) – Topical low to mid-potency CS twice daily (T) – Oral CS (e.g. prednisone 0.5 mg/kg/day × 7 days) if more severe or unresponsive to above measures (T) • *Management of hand-foot eruptions:* – Limit exposure to heat, hot water, tight clothing/shoes, chemical irritants – Topical high-potency CS ointments to inflamed areas twice daily – Topical keratolytic agents or humectants (e.g. 10–20% urea cream, ammonium lactate) to hyperkeratotic areas twice daily • *Management of stomatitis:* – See Table 59.2 – Morbilliform eruptions, such as those from selected BRAF inhibitors, may require a drug holiday or reduced dose

Most often seen when BRAF inhibitors are given alone; incidence can be significantly reduced when BRAF inhibitors are combined with MEK inhibitors.

Table 17.8 The more common mucocutaneous side effects of targeted therapies. Targeted therapies include: (1) various inhibitors of VEGFR (e.g. sorafenib, sunitinib, vandetanib, pazopanib, bevacizumab, ranibizumab) and EGFR (e.g. erlotinib, gefitinib, cetuximab, panitumumab, canertinib, lapatinib); (2) multi-kinase inhibitors that target the KIT receptor (e.g. imatinib, dasatinib, nilotinib) and MAP kinase pathway (vemurafenib, dabrafenib, cobimetinib); and (3) mTOR (e.g. sirolimus, everolimus, temsirolimus) and proteasome inhibitors (e.g. bortezomib, carfilzomib).

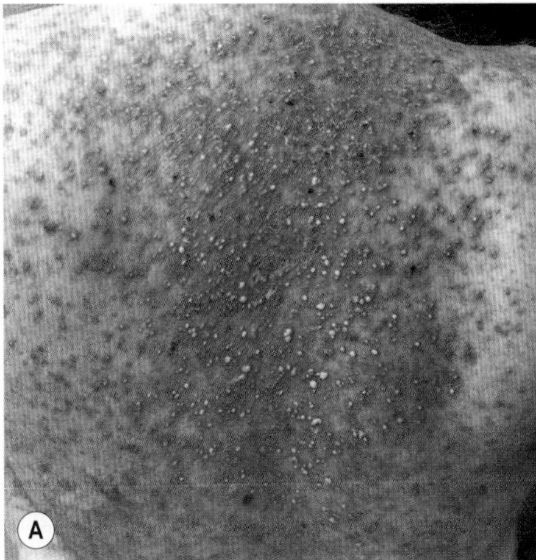
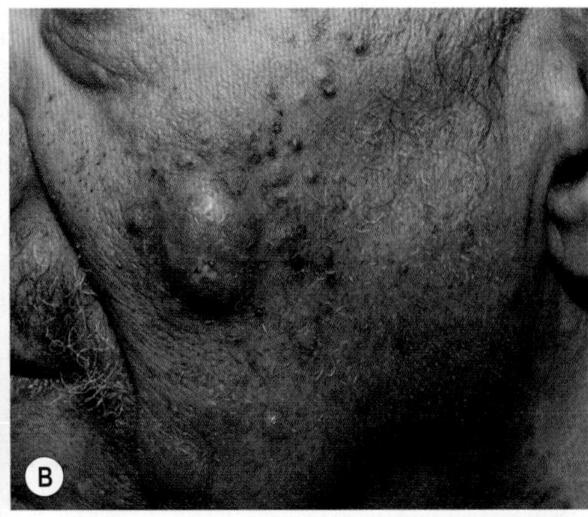

Fig. 17.12 Papulopustular (acneiform) reactions to epidermal growth factor receptor (EGFR) inhibitors. A Numerous pustules on an erythematous base with coalescence on the central upper back. **B** Multiple follicular papulopustules, hyperpigmented scars, and a large multiloculated inflamed cyst on the cheek. *A, Courtesy, Lauren Levy, MD and Jonathan Leventhal, MD; B, Courtesy, Kalman Watsky, MD.*

THE MORE COMMON MUCOCUTANEOUS SIDE EFFECTS OF IMMUNE CHECKPOINT INHIBITORS*	
Mucocutaneous side effect	**General management recommendations**
Xerosis	• General measures: gentle cleansers and daily moisturization; sun avoidance/protection • For pruritus, try long-acting, non-sedating antihistamines in the daytime (e.g. cetirizine) and more sedating antihistamines at bedtime (e.g. hydroxyzine, doxepin) • Morbilliform, eczematous, lichenoid and psoriasiform eruptions (grade 1 or grade 2***) can be treated with mid- to high-potency topical CS creams and ointments, respectively • More severe (grade 3 or 4***) or recalcitrant to topical treatment eruptions may require oral CS • Suspicion of SCAR requires biopsy, discontinuation of checkpoint inhibitor and possible hospitalization
Pruritus	
Morbilliform eruption**	
Dermatitis, eczematous or psoriasiform**	
Lichenoid eruption**	
Bullous pemphigoid, lichen planus pemphigoides	
Photosensitivity	
Vitiligo-like leukoderma, poliosis	
Alopecia areata, alopecia universalis	
Dermatomyositis, SCLE	
SCARs (e.g. SJS–TEN, DRESS, vasculitis, AGEP)	
Psoriasis flare	
Eruptive KAs	
Uveitis, episcleritis	
Sarcoid-like reaction	

**In addition to these mucocutaneous side effects, autoimmune-like inflammation of internal organs may often occur (e.g. enteritis/colitis, hepatitis, thyroiditis, myocarditis, pneumonitis, etc).*
***May be accentuated in sun-exposed sites; for lichenoid, may be intraoral.*
****Refer to https://www.asco.org/management-immune-related-adverse-events-patients-treated-immune-checkpoint-inhibitor-therapy.*

Table 17.9 The more common mucocutaneous side effects of immune checkpoint inhibitors. Dermatologic toxicity is the most common immune-related adverse event with checkpoint inhibitors, including anti-CTLA-4 (e.g. ipilimumab, tremelimumab), anti-PD-1 (e.g. nivolumab, pembrolizumab), and anti-PD-L-1 (e.g. atezolizumab, avelumab, durvalumab) antibodies. SCARs, severe cutaneous adverse reactions to medications; SCLE, subacute cutaneous lupus erythematosus.

MUCOCUTANEOUS SIDE EFFECTS OF CHEMOTHERAPEUTIC AGENTS	
Reactions	**Responsible drugs**
Alopecia, reversible	Alkylating agents: cyclophosphamide, ifosfamide, mechlorethamine (nitrogen mustard) Anthracyclines: daunorubicin, doxorubicin, idarubicin, mitoxantrone Taxanes: paclitaxel, docetaxel Topoisomerase 1 inhibitors: topotecan, irinotecan Etoposide, vincristine, vinblastine, actinomycin D, busulfan, MTX, gemcitabine
Alopecia, irreversible	Busulfan, thiotepa, cyclophosphamide (conditioning regimens); docetaxel, paclitaxel
Mucositis	Daunorubicin, doxorubicin, high-dose MTX, high-dose melphalan, topotecan, cyclophosphamide, taxanes, hydroxyurea, continuous infusions of 5-FU and prodrugs of 5-FU
Extravasation reactions (e.g. chemical cellulitis, ulceration)	Anthracyclines, carmustine, 5-FU, vinblastine, vincristine, mitomycin C
Chemotherapy recall (tender sterile inflammatory nodules at sites of previous chemotherapy extravasation or administration)	5-FU, mitomycin C, paclitaxel, doxorubicin, epirubicin
Hyperpigmentation (see Ch. 55) (Fig. 17.13E)	Alkylating agents: busulfan, cyclophosphamide, cisplatin, mechlorethamine, melphalan, bendamustine Antimetabolites: 5-FU, 5-FU prodrugs (e.g. capecitabine, tegafur), MTX, hydroxyurea Antibiotics: bleomycin, doxorubicin
Mucosal hyperpigmentation	Busulfan, 5-FU, hydroxyurea, cyclophosphamide
Nail hyperpigmentation (Fig. 17.13A)	5-FU, cyclophosphamide, daunorubicin, doxorubicin, hydroxyurea, MTX, bleomycin
Onycholysis	Paclitaxel, docetaxel (along with photosensitivity)
Radiation recall	MTX, doxorubicin, daunorubicin, taxanes, etoposide, dacarbazine, melphalan, capecitabine, gemcitabine, 5-FU, pemetrexed, actinomycin D, hydroxyurea
Radiation enhancement	Doxorubicin, hydroxyurea, taxanes, 5-FU, etoposide, gemcitabine, MTX
Photosensitivity	5-FU and 5-FU prodrugs, MTX, hydroxyurea, dacarbazine, mitomycin C, docetaxel
Inflammation of "keratoses" (Fig. 17.13B)	Actinic keratoses: 5-FU and 5-FU prodrugs, pentostatin, interleukin-2 Seborrheic keratoses: cytarabine, taxanes Disseminated superficial actinic porokeratosis: 5-FU and 5-FU prodrugs, taxanes
Toxic erythema of chemotherapy (Figs 17.14 and 17.15) • Acral erythema (erythrodysesthesia)	Cytarabine, anthracyclines, 5-FU and 5-FU prodrugs, taxanes, MTX, busulfan, cysplatin
• Eccrine squamous syringometaplasia	Cytarabine, busulfan, cyclophosphamide, carmustine, taxanes
Neutrophilic eccrine hidradenitis (Fig. 17.13C)	Cytarabine, bleomycin, anthracyclines, cyclophosphamide, cisplatin, topotecan
Ulcerations	Hydroxyurea (lower extremities)
Squamous cell carcinoma	Fludarabine, hydroxyurea, topical BCNU

Table 17.10 Mucocutaneous side effects of chemotherapeutic agents. 5-FU, 5-fluorouracil; BCNU, carmustine; MTX, methotrexate.

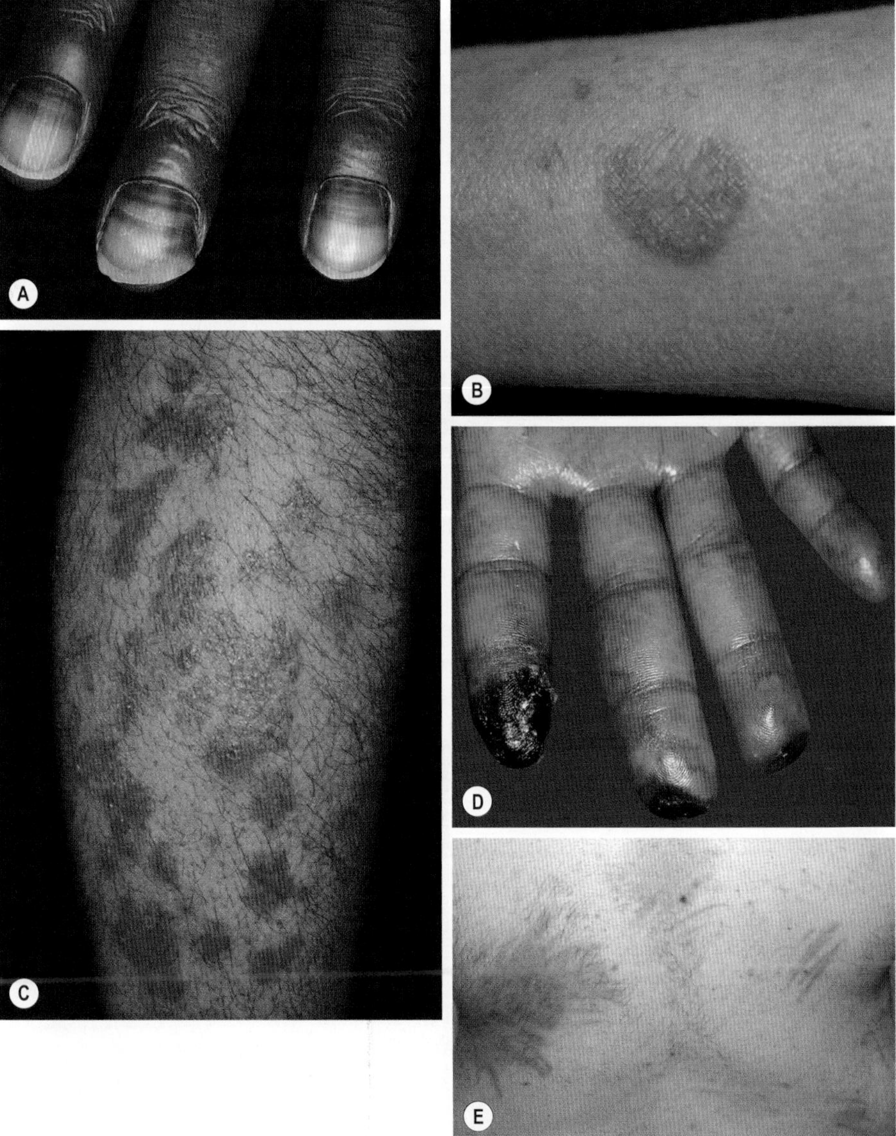

Fig. 17.13 Mucocutaneous side effects of chemotherapeutic agents. A Horizontal melanonychia due to 5-fluorouracil. **B** Inflammation surrounding a seborrheic keratosis in a patient receiving paclitaxel. **C** Neutrophilic eccrine hidradenitis; erythematous plaques on the leg, which may be confused with Sweet syndrome. **D** Raynaud phenomenon and digital necrosis due to systemic bleomycin. **E** Multiple linear (flagellate) erythematous, urticarial plaques in a patient receiving systemic bleomycin. *A, B, Courtesy, Jean L. Bolognia, MD; C, Courtesy, Jean Revuz, MD; D, Courtesy, YDRSC; E, Courtesy, Kalman Watsky, MD.*

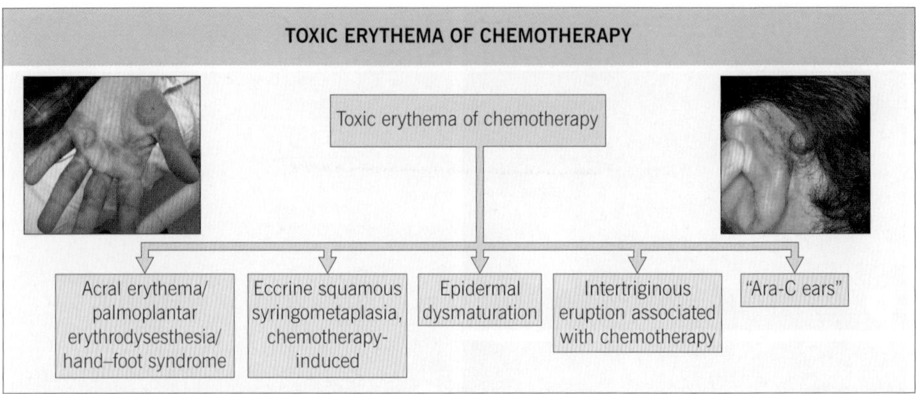

Fig. 17.14 Toxic erythema of chemotherapy (TEC). Use of a number of terms (especially those based on histopathologic findings), including palmoplantar erythrodysesthesia, eccrine squamous syringometaplasia, and epidermal dysmaturation, has created some confusion for clinicians. There is considerable overlap in the appearance of the symmetric erythematous to dusky patches, which can develop edema, erosions, desquamation, or purpura, whether they favor acral sites, intertriginous zones, or the elbows and knees. "Toxic erythema of chemotherapy" has been suggested as an encompassing term that allows simplification. In addition, there is no need to implicate additional diagnoses when lesions are not limited to the hands and feet. Insets: Erythema of the ears due to cytarabine (cytosine arabinoside), sometimes referred to as "Ara-C ears"; the petechiae are due to thrombocytopenia. Dusky edematous plaques of the palm, some of which have developed sterile bullae. *Courtesy, Jean L. Bolognia, MD and Boni Elewski, MD.*

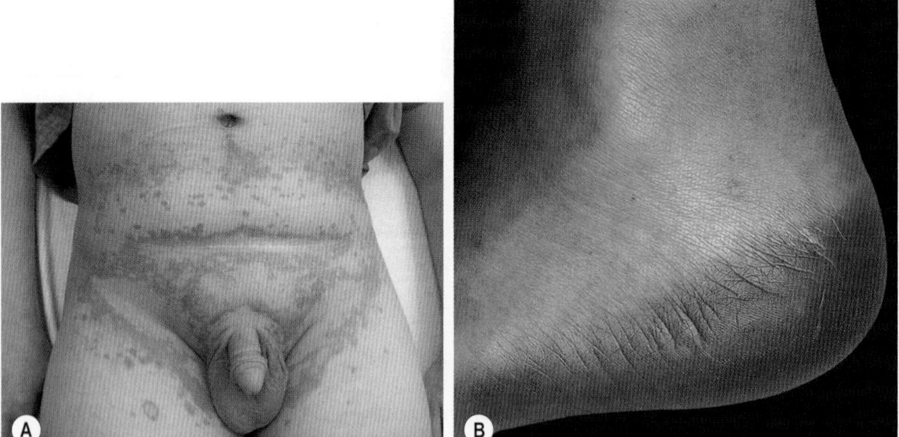

Fig. 17.15 Toxic erythema of chemotherapy. A Symmetric involvement of intertriginous zones and the scrotum. There is central desquamation and some of the lesions have a dusky color. The patient was receiving fludarabine plus intravenous busulfan. **B** Toxic erythema of chemotherapy due to cytarabine, with obvious erythema of the plantar surface. *A, Courtesy, Leonard Kristal, MD; B, Courtesy, Jean L. Bolognia, MD.*

REACTIONS LOCALIZED TO SITES OF INJECTIONS OF MEDICATIONS	
Etanercept	Erythematous plaques, vasculitis, eosinophilic cellulitis
Adalimumab	Erythematous or urticarial plaques
GM-CSF, G-CSF	Pustular reaction, urticarial plaque
Interferon	Vasculopathy with necrosis, development of plaque of psoriasis, lupus-like reaction
Interleukin-2	Lobular panniculitis, granulomas
Anakinra	Erythematous or urticarial plaques
Corticosteroids	Dermal atrophy, lipoatrophy, telangiectasias, deposits, hypopigmentation
Vitamin K	Erythematous plaque, often annular; morpheaform plaque (Texier disease)
Heparin	Necrosis, ecchymosis, erythematous plaques, urticaria
Low-molecular-weight, calcium-containing heparin	Calcinosis cutis
Glatiramer acetate	Fibrosis, panniculitis, lipoatrophy, vasospasm, Nicolau syndrome
Iron	Brown discoloration, hyperpigmentation
Vitamin B_{12}	Pruritus, morpheaform plaque
Enfuvirtide	Erythematous or morpheaform plaque
Bortezomib	Erythematous or urticarial plaque, necrosis
Insulin	Erythema, pruritus, urticaria, induration, lipoatrophy, lipohypertrophy
Desensitization antigens	Subcutaneous sarcoidosis
Hyaluronic acid, silicone	Swelling, granulomatous reaction
	Dermal atrophy, lipoatrophy, telangiectasias, deposits, hypopigmentation
Vaccines*	
Aluminum-containing vaccine	Nodules, foreign body reaction
Thimerosal-containing vaccine	Allergic contact dermatitis
Lipid nanoparticle-encapsulated COVID-19 mRNA-1273 vaccine	Delayed, pruritic erythematous plaque, usually large in diameter, that may or may not recur with second dose

**Localized reactions can also occur, (e.g. pseudocellulitis/excessive limb swelling) as well as generalized reactions, (e.g. anaphylaxis, Sweet syndrome, AGEP, bullous pemphigoid, linear IgA bullous dermatosis, lichenoid eruptions, and erythema multiforme).*

Table 17.11 Reactions localized to sites of injections of medications (in addition to extravasation of those administered intravenously). G-CSF, granulocyte colony-stimulating factor; GM-CSF, granulocyte–macrophage colony-stimulating factor.

18 Purpura and Disorders of Microvascular Occlusion

- Purpura represents visible hemorrhage into the skin or mucous membranes; in contrast to erythema due to vasodilation, it is nonblanching upon application of external pressure.
- Purpura can be *primary*, where hemorrhage is an integral part of lesion formation, or *secondary*, where there is hemorrhage into established lesions due to factors such as venous hypertension, gravity, or thrombocytopenia.
- As purpuric lesions fade, their color evolves from red-purple or blue to brown or yellow-green.
- Primary purpura has a broad differential diagnosis, and it is helpful to categorize purpuric lesions based on their size and morphology.
  - *Petechiae*: ≤3 mm and macular (Table 18.1; Fig. 18.1A)
  - *Ecchymoses*: usually >1 cm and macular with round/oval to slightly irregular borders, and typically have an element of trauma in their pathogenesis (see Table 18.1; Fig. 18.1B); a greater volume of hemorrhage leads to a *hematoma*, which is palpable
  - *Retiform purpura*: reticulated, branching or stellate morphology, which reflects occlusion of the vessels that produce the livedo reticularis pattern (see Ch. 87; Tables 18.2 and 18.3; Figs 18.1C and 18.2–18.9)
  - *Classic "palpable purpura"*: round red-purple papules that are occasionally targetoid, with a component of blanching erythema in early lesions; represents the most common presentation of cutaneous small vessel vasculitis (see Ch. 19; Fig. 18.1D)

CAUSES OF PETECHIAE AND ECCHYMOSIS WITH MINOR TRAUMA
Petechiae (≤3 mm in diameter)
Significant thrombocytopenia (e.g. <20,000/mm^3) • Etiologies include ITP, TTP, DIC, drugs, and bone marrow infiltration/failure **Platelet dysfunction** • Hereditary or acquired (e.g. due to aspirin or NSAIDs) **Etiologies unrelated to platelets** • Increased intravenous pressure, e.g. due to the Valsalva maneuver (coughing, childbirth) or use of a blood pressure cuff (Rumpel–Leede sign) • Trauma (often linear configuration) • Scurvy (perifollicular distribution) • Inflammatory conditions, especially in dependent sites (e.g. pigmented purpuric dermatoses, hypergammaglobulinemic purpura of Waldenström)
Ecchymosis with minor trauma (lesions usually >1 cm in diameter)
Defective coagulation • Etiologies include anticoagulant use, hepatic insufficiency, and vitamin K deficiency **Poor dermal support of blood vessels** • Etiologies include actinic purpura (Fig. 18.1B), corticosteroid use, scurvy, primary systemic amyloidosis, and Ehlers–Danlos syndrome **Thrombocytopenia or platelet dysfunction** (see above)

Table 18.1 Causes of petechiae and ecchymosis with minor trauma. DIC, disseminated intravascular coagulation; ITP, idiopathic thrombocytopenia purpura; TTP, thrombotic thrombocytopenic purpura. *Courtesy, Warren W. Piette, MD.*

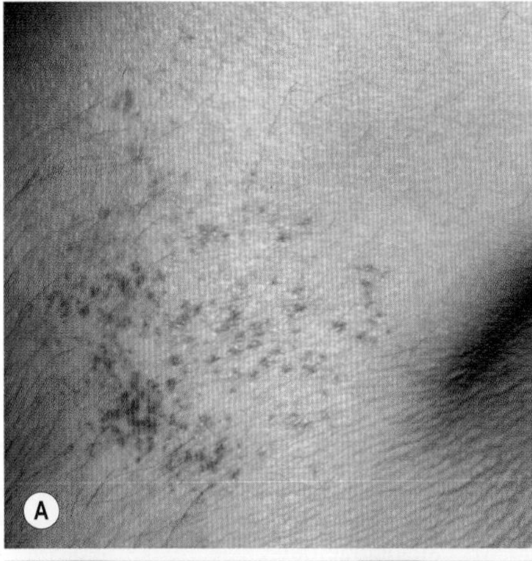

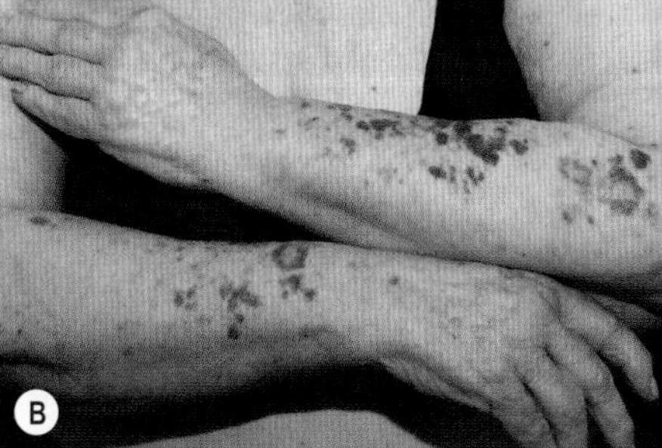

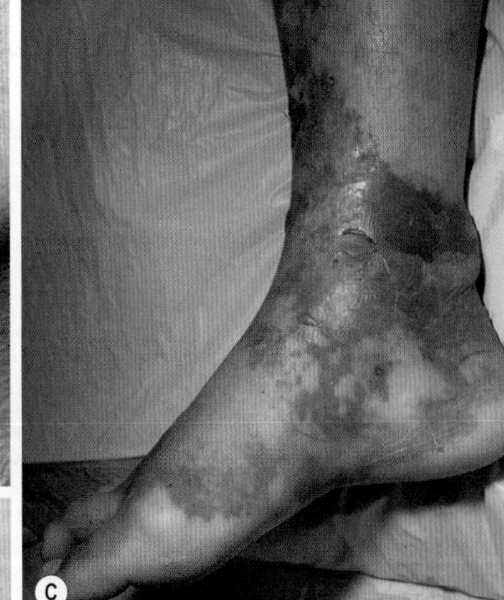

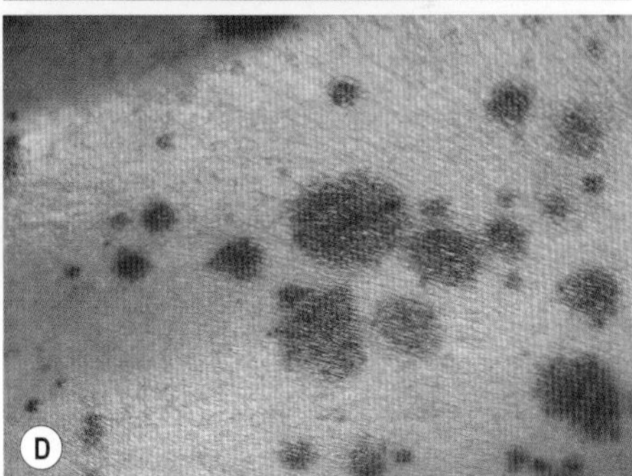

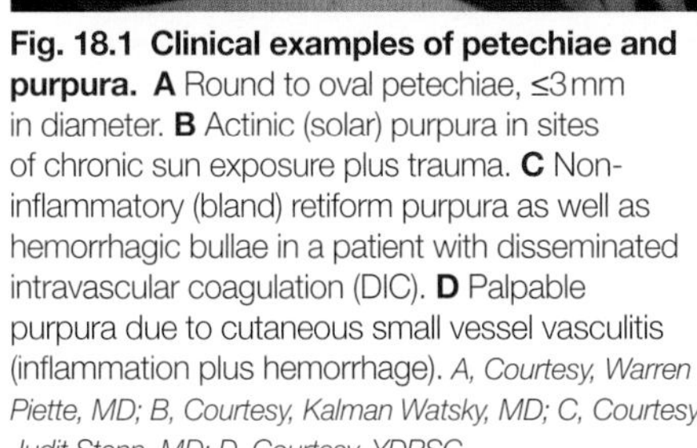

Fig. 18.1 Clinical examples of petechiae and purpura. A Round to oval petechiae, ≤3mm in diameter. **B** Actinic (solar) purpura in sites of chronic sun exposure plus trauma. **C** Non-inflammatory (bland) retiform purpura as well as hemorrhagic bullae in a patient with disseminated intravascular coagulation (DIC). **D** Palpable purpura due to cutaneous small vessel vasculitis (inflammation plus hemorrhage). *A, Courtesy, Warren Piette, MD; B, Courtesy, Kalman Watsky, MD; C, Courtesy, Judit Stenn, MD; D, Courtesy, YDRSC.*

- A biopsy specimen can be helpful in determining the etiology of a purpuric eruption, e.g. whether there is vascular occlusion with minimal inflammation or vasculitis (inflammation and fibrinoid necrosis of vessel walls). Because secondary changes of vasculitis may be seen when an older lesion of microvascular occlusion is sampled, and likewise a late lesion of vasculitis may have minimal residual inflammation, it is preferable to choose a well-developed but relatively early lesion (e.g. 24–48 hours old).

Selected Microvascular Occlusion Syndromes (See Table 18.2)

Antiphospholipid Syndrome (APS)

- Acquired systemic autoimmune disorder characterized by vascular thrombosis and/or pregnancy complications in the presence of elevated levels of antiphospholipid antibodies (Table 18.4).
- Predilection for young to middle-aged women (5:1 female:male ratio in adults) and often associated with systemic lupus erythematosus.

CAUSES OF RETIFORM PURPURA	
Disorder	**Major features**
Microvascular platelet plugs	
Heparin-induced thrombocytopenia (HIT)	• ~1–5% of patients receiving heparin* (IV or SC) develop an Ab that binds to heparin–platelet factor 4 complexes and leads to ↓ platelets ± thrombosis, typically with onset on day 5–10 of therapy* • Retiform purpura can be distant from or at sites of heparin injection (Fig. 18.2)
Thrombocytosis due to myeloproliferative disorders	• Occurs in essential thrombocythemia > polycythemia vera; may be associated with secondary erythromelalgia (see Ch. 87)
Paroxysmal nocturnal hemoglobinuria	• Acquired somatic *PIGA* mutation leads to complement-mediated injury of blood cells, resulting in hemolysis, thrombosis (especially venous), and cytopenias • Other skin findings can include petechiae, hemorrhagic bullae, and leg ulcers • **Rx:** eculizumab to inhibit terminal complement cascade (↑ meningococcemia risk)
Thrombotic thrombocytopenic purpura (TTP) ± hemolytic uremic syndrome (HUS)	• May be *primary* (Ab against or genetic defect in ADAMTS13 protease → reduced cleavage of vWF) or *secondary* (often with HUS, e.g. due to hemorrhagic colitis or drugs) • Petechiae > retiform purpura; also fever, thrombocytopenia, microangiopathic hemolytic anemia, renal dysfunction, and CNS involvement
Cold-related agglutination	
Cryoglobulinemia type I > cryofibrinogenemia†	• Retiform purpura that favors acral sites (Fig. 18.3); see Table 18.3
Altered coagulation	
Antiphospholipid syndrome	• See text and Table 18.4 (Figs 18.4 and 18.5)
Protein C or S deficiency/dysfunction	• *Warfarin necrosis* (protein C – short half-life, so function decreases faster than for procoagulant factors Fig. 18.6): 2–5 days after starting warfarin without heparin, especially if large loading dose; favors sites of abundant fat in women (see Fig. 17.5) • *Sepsis-associated purpura fulminans* (protein C; see Fig. 18.1C) • *Post-infectious purpura fulminans* (Ab blocks protein S): ~2 weeks after streptococcal infection or varicella • *Neonatal purpura fulminans* (homozygous/compound heterozygous protein C > S defect; Fig. 18.7)

Table 18.2 Causes of retiform purpura. *PIGA*, phosphatidylinositol glycan anchor class A; vWF, von Willebrand factor. *Continued*

CAUSES OF RETIFORM PURPURA	
Disorder	**Major features**
"Vascular coagulopathy"	
Livedoid vasculopathy	• Often associated with thrombophilia (Table 18.5); see text (Fig. 18.8)
Degos disease (malignant atrophic papulosis)	• Vaso-occlusive disorder of skin, GI tract, and CNS; favors young adults • Small erythematous papules on trunk and extremities evolve over 2–4 weeks to porcelain white scars with rim of telangiectasias; similar lesions can be seen in antiphospholipid syndrome
Sneddon syndrome – often in setting of antiphospholipid syndrome or adenosine deaminase 2 deficiency (± associated polyarteritis nodosa)	• Triad of widespread livedo reticularis/racemosa ("broken" livedo), labile hypertension, and cerebrovascular disease; favors young women
Embolization and/or crystal deposition	
Cholesterol emboli ("warfarin blue toe syndrome")	• Atherosclerosis (especially in older men) leads to emboli, often triggered by: (1) Arterial/coronary catheterization or thrombolytic therapy (hours–days later) (2) Prolonged anticoagulation (after 1–2 months of treatment) • Retiform purpura of distal leg(s) + more extensive livedo reticularis (Fig. 18.9) • Fever, myalgias, multisystem involvement (e.g. renal, GI, CNS); often peripheral eosinophilia
Other sources of emboli and/or crystal deposition	• Infective endocarditis (acute > subacute**), marantic endocarditis, atrial myxomas, hypereosinophilic syndrome (with intracardiac thrombus‡), systemic oxalosis (e.g. in primary hyperoxaluria), crystalglobulin vasculopathy (associated with monoclonal gammopathy)
Reticulocyte/red blood cell occlusion (e.g. in sickle cell disease or severe malaria)	
Organisms within vessels (usually in immunocompromised patients)	
Ecthyma gangrenosum	• See Ch. 61
Vessel-invasive fungi	• e.g. *Aspergillus*, *Mucor* (see Ch. 64)
Disseminated strongyloidiasis	• "Thumbprint" purpura in periumbilical region
Lucio phenomenon	• Reactional state in lepromatous leprosy, primarily in Mexico and Central America (see Ch. 62)
Other causes	
Vasculitis (usually involving small and medium-sized vessels)	• e.g. ANCA-associated vasculitides, polyarteritis nodosa (see Ch. 19); early lesions often exhibit prominent erythema and induration
Calciphylaxis	• See Ch. 42
Necrotic spider bite reaction	• See Ch. 72
Intravascular lymphoma	• Most often B cell (Fig. 18.10); see Table 97.3

**Less common with low-molecular-weight heparin (≤1%) than unfractionated heparin; a transient decrease in the platelet count can also occur within the first 2 days of heparin therapy due to its direct effects on platelet activation.*
†May be an incidental finding in hospitalized patients; cold agglutinins rarely lead to acrocyanosis or purpura.
***Skin lesions on the hands and feet associated with subacute endocarditis are more likely to be tender red-purple papules due to immune complex deposition ("Osler nodes"),than purpuric macules representing septic emboli ("Janeway lesions"; more common in acute endocarditis).*
‡Cutaneous microthrombi and superficial thrombophlebitis have also been described.

Table 18.2 *Continued* **Causes of retiform purpura.** *Courtesy, Warren W. Piette, MD.*

CLASSIFICATION OF CRYOGLOBULINS				
Type	**Composition**	**Associations**	**Pathophysiology**	**Clinical manifestations**
I	Monoclonal IgM or IgG >> IgA	Plasma cell dyscrasias, lymphoproliferative disorders	Vascular occlusion	Retiform purpura (often acral; Fig. 18.3), gangrene, acrocyanosis, Raynaud phenomenon
II**	Monoclonal IgM* (>IgG*) against polyclonal IgG	HCV, HIV, autoimmune connective tissue diseases, lymphoproliferative disorders	Vasculitis	Palpable purpura, arthralgias, peripheral neuropathy, glomerulonephritis
III**	Polyclonal IgM* against polyclonal IgG			

**Typically have rheumatoid factor activity (i.e. are directed against the Fc portion of IgG).*
***Referred to as "mixed" cryoglobulins.*

Table 18.3 Classification of cryoglobulins. HCV, hepatitis C virus.

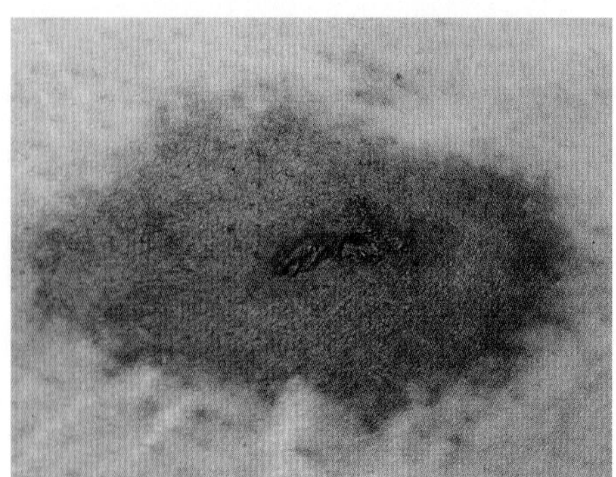

Fig. 18.2 Heparin necrosis at site of subcutaneous heparin injection. Note the branching or retiform pattern of intense hemorrhage and the necrosis in the center of the lesion. *From Robson K, Piette W. Adv Dermatol. 1999;15:153–182, used with permission.*

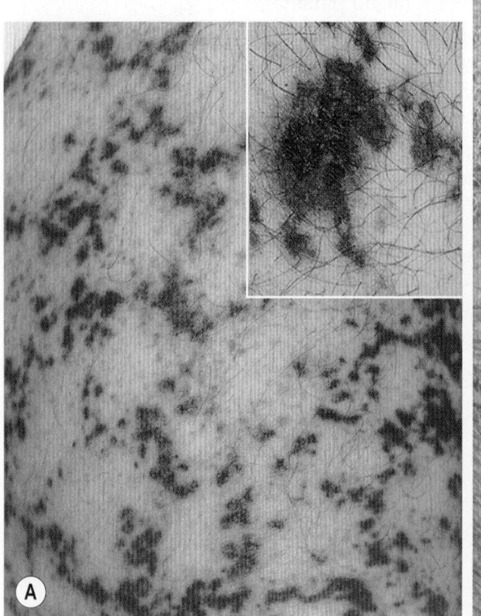

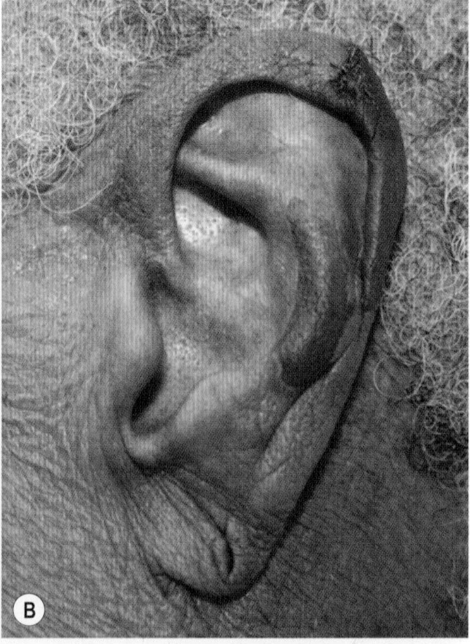

Fig. 18.3 Type I cryoglobulinemia in a patient with multiple myeloma (IgG type). A Note the retiform purpura and the areas of necrosis within the purpuric areas (inset). **B** Lesions favor the helices of the ears as well as the distal extremities and nose. *A, Courtesy, Jean L. Bolognia, MD. B, Courtesy, Jonathan Leventhal, MD.*

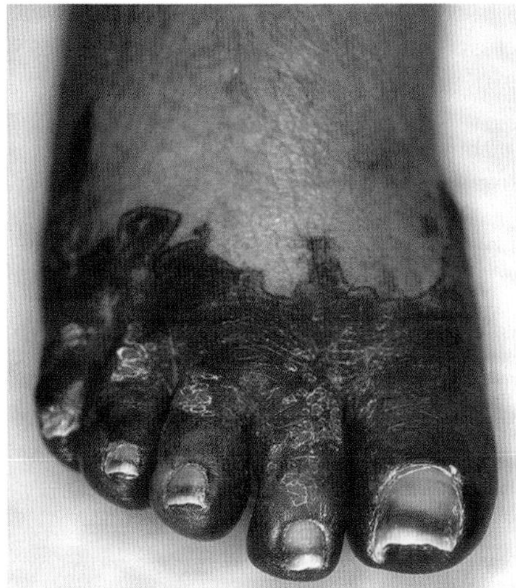

Fig. 18.4 Retiform purpura in antiphospholipid syndrome. Purpura and ischemia of the distal portion of the foot. The purpuric lesions have irregular borders (marked with ink). *Courtesy, Jean L. Bolognia, MD.*

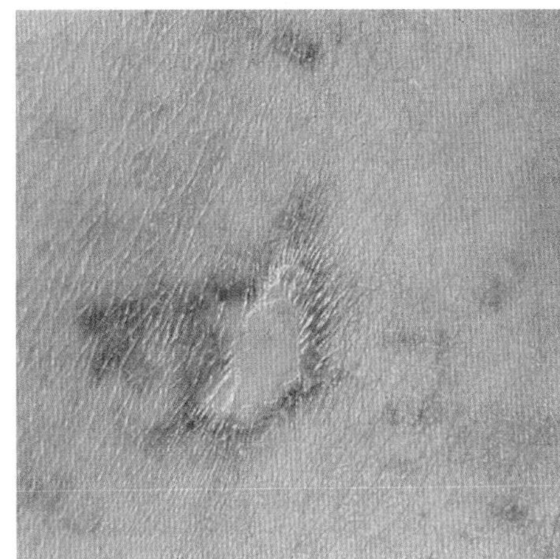

Fig. 18.5 Atrophie blanche-like scarring in antiphospholipid syndrome. This patient had lupus erythematosus. *Courtesy, Warren Piette, MD.*

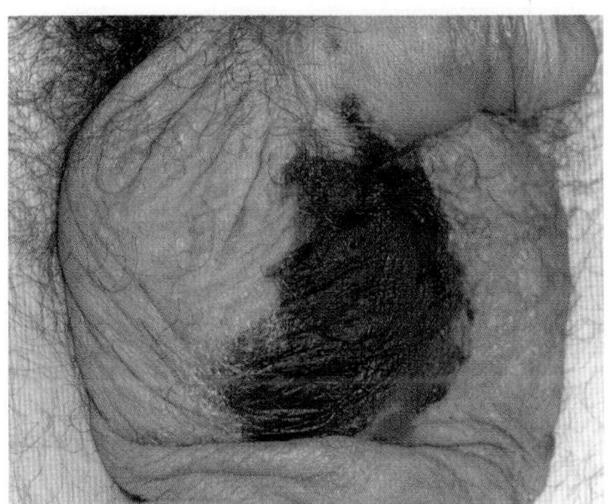

Fig. 18.6 Warfarin (Coumadin®) necrosis. Striking area of retiform purpura and ischemia on the scrotum. *Courtesy, Kenneth Greer, MD.*

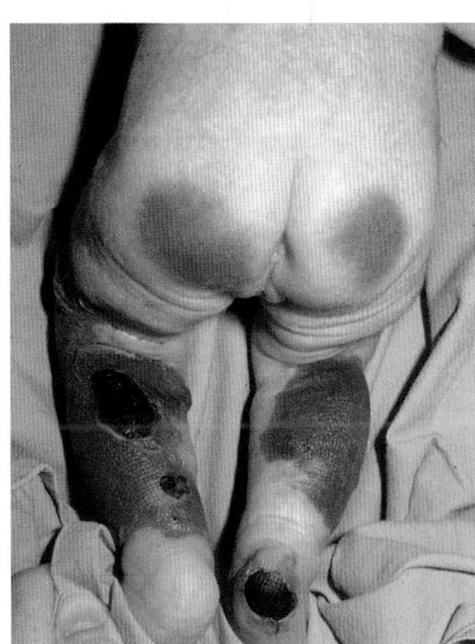

Fig. 18.7 Protein C deficiency in an infant. Large purpuric plaques, with development of bullae and necrotic ulcerations within those on the lower extremities. Note the retiform purpura surrounding the heel ulcer. *Courtesy, Luis Requena, MD.*

- Cutaneous findings can include livedo reticularis, retiform purpura progressing to cutaneous necrosis, leg ulcers, livedoid vasculopathy, Degos-like lesions, nail bed infarcts, superficial thrombophlebitis, and anetoderma (see Figs 18.4 and 18.5).
- Deep venous thrombosis and CNS disease are the most common extracutaneous manifestations; catastrophic APS affecting multiple organ systems together with widespread retiform purpura occasionally occurs.
- **Rx:** anticoagulant and antiplatelet agents; also immunomodulatory agents (e.g. systemic CS, rituximab) for catastrophic APS.

Livedoid Vasculopathy

- Chronic condition that occurs primarily in young to middle-aged women, often with underlying thrombophilia (Table 18.5).

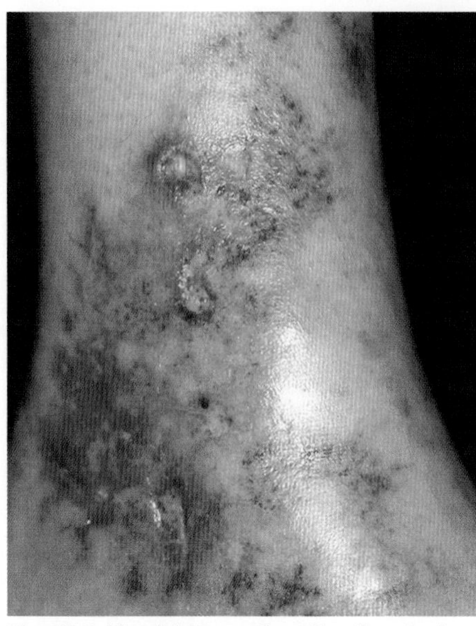

Fig. 18.8 Livedoid vasculopathy. Punched-out ulcers on the ankle as well as multiple stellate purpuric macules. *Courtesy, YDRSC.*

- Recurrent development of hemorrhagic crusts resembling ground pepper and extremely painful, punched-out ulcers on the legs (especially the ankles); frequently arises within a background of retiform purpura ± livedo reticularis (see Fig. 18.8).
- The ulcers heal slowly, forming stellate, ivory-white, atrophic scars bordered by papular telangiectasias and hemosiderin pigmentation; such lesions, referred to as *atrophie blanche*, also occur in other settings such as venous hypertension, antiphospholipid syndrome (see Fig. 18.5), and cutaneous vasculitis.
- **Rx:** anticoagulant, antiplatelet, and fibrinolytic agents (especially if thrombophilia).

Other Purpuric Disorders

Pigmented Purpuric Dermatoses (Capillaritis)

- Group of disorders characterized by clustered petechial hemorrhage due to inflammation affecting capillaries.

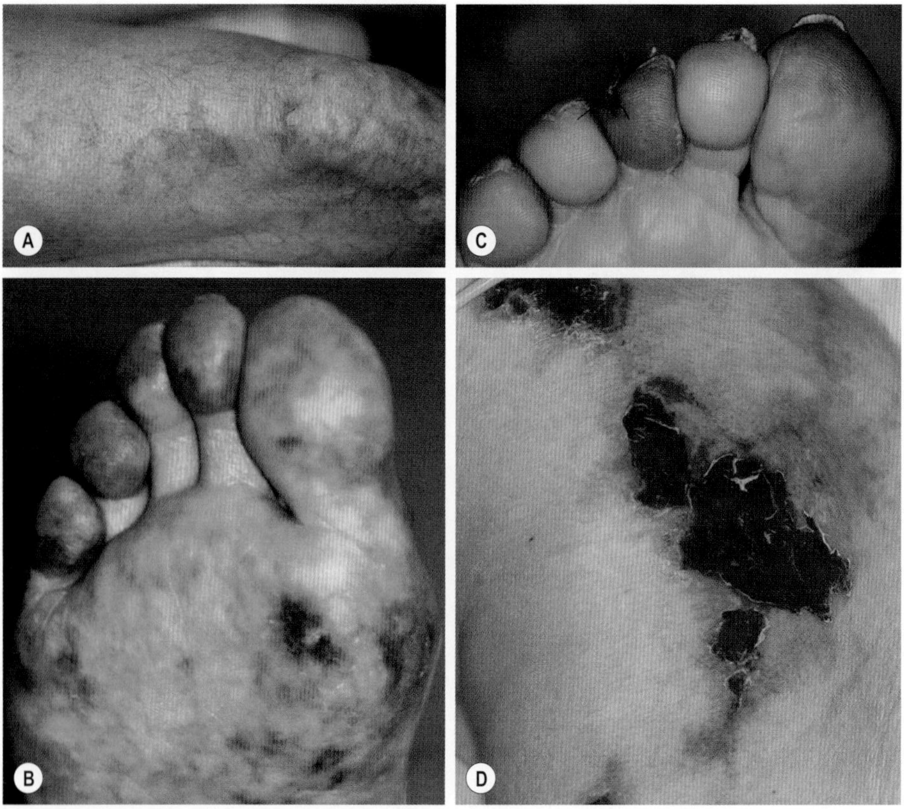

Fig. 18.9 Cholesterol emboli. A Livedo reticularis proximally on the thigh. **B** Both livedo reticularis and retiform purpura distally. **C** Purpura of the digits in "warfarin blue toe syndrome". **D** Several irregularly shaped ulcers with eschars surrounded by retiform purpura. *A, B, Courtesy, Norbert Sepp, MD; C, Courtesy, YDRSC; D, Courtesy, Kalman Watsky, MD.*

ANTIPHOSPHOLIPID ANTIBODY SYNDROME: SAPPORO–SYDNEY CRITERIA
At least one clinical criterion and one laboratory criterion required*
Clinical criteria
1. Vascular thrombosis – One or more objectively confirmed episodes of arterial, venous, or small vessel thrombosis occurring in any tissue or organ 2. Pregnancy morbidity – One or more unexplained deaths of morphologically normal fetuses at or after the 10th week of gestation – *or* – – One or more premature births of morphologically normal neonates at or before the 34th week of gestation because of eclampsia, pre-eclampsia, or placental insufficiency – *or* – – Three or more unexplained consecutive spontaneous abortions before the 10th week of gestation
Laboratory criteria – present on two or more occasions at least 12 weeks apart*
1. Anti-cardiolipin antibodies, IgG or IgM [>40 GPL/MPL *or* >99th percentile as measured by a standardized ELISA] 2. Lupus anticoagulant [detected according to the guidelines of the International Society on Thrombosis and Haemostasis] 3. Anti-β_2-glycoprotein I antibodies, IgG or IgM [>99th percentile as measured by a standardized ELISA]

**Patients who do not meet these criteria may still have antiphospholipid antibody syndrome.*

Table 18.4 Antiphospholipid syndrome: Sapporo–Sydney criteria. GPL, IgG phospholipid units; MPL, IgM phospholipid units. *Adapted from Lim W. Thrombotic risk in the antiphospholipid syndrome Semin Thromb Hemost 2014;40:741–6.*

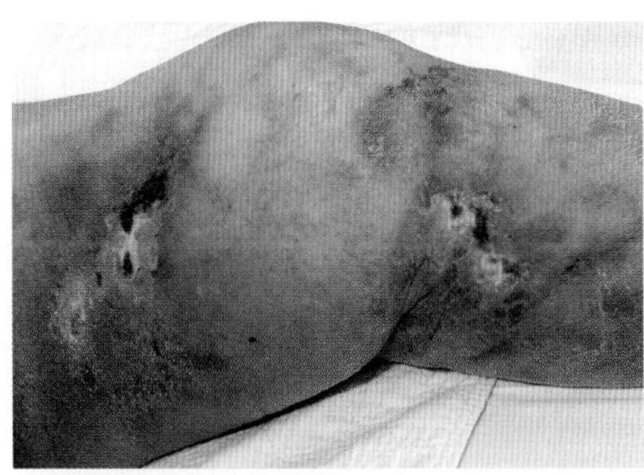

Fig. 18.10 Intravascular B-cell lymphoma. The clinical presentation in this patient was retiform purpura and necrosis with livedo. *Courtesy, Lucinda Buescher, MD.*

- *Schamberg disease:* most common form, occurring in both children and adults; recurrent crops of discrete yellow-brown patches containing pinpoint petechiae ("cayenne pepper") on the lower legs > thighs, buttocks, trunk, and arms (Fig. 18.11A); the yellow-brown color reflects deposits of hemosiderin, derived from extravasated RBCs, within the dermis.
- *Purpura annularis telangiectodes (of Majocchi)*: favors adolescent girls and young women; expanding annular plaques with punctate telangiectasias and petechiae in their borders (Fig. 18.12A).
- *Lichen aureus*: solitary golden to rust-colored or purple-brown patch or thin plaque, typically on the leg overlying a perforator vein.
- Other forms include *pigmented purpuric lichenoid dermatitis* presenting as red-brown papules and *eczematid-like purpura* with scaling and pruritus (Fig. 18.12B); these variants favor the lower legs of men.
- **DDx:** "stasis purpura" presenting as petechiae superimposed on diffuse hemosiderin deposition on the legs (see Fig. 18.11B); purpuric forms of allergic contact dermatitis, drug eruptions or mycosis fungoides; suction-induced purpura (e.g. with cupping), hypergammaglobulinemic purpura of Waldenström, angioma serpiginosum; *for lichenoid variant:* primarily small vessel vasculitis.

EVALUATION FOR THROMBOPHILIA (HYPERCOAGULABILITY)		
Disorder	**~% of population**	**Potential confounding conditions**
Hereditary		
Factor V Leiden (can screen with activated protein C resistance)	5	Warfarin, OCP, pregnancy, ↑ factor VIII levels, lupus anticoagulant
Prothrombin G20210A mutation	3	–
Hyperhomocysteinemia (↑ homocysteine level*)	>5	Deficient folate, B_{12}, or B_6; older age, smoking
Protein C deficiency (↓ activity)	0.3	Warfarin, OCP, pregnancy, liver disease
Protein S deficiency (↓ free antigen level)	≤0.3	Warfarin, OCP, pregnancy, liver disease
Antithrombin III deficiency	0.05	Heparin, liver disease
Excess factor VIII activity	10	Acute-phase response, OCP, pregnancy, old age
Dysfibrinogenemia (↓ fibrinogen activity relative to antigen level; ↑ reptilase time)	–	Liver or renal disease, amyloidosis, malignancy
Excess plasminogen activator inhibitor-1 (PAI-1) activity*	10+	Wide range of normal values
Acquired		
Lupus anticoagulant†	–	Warfarin, heparin
Anticardiolipin antibodies (IgG or IgM)†	–	Various infectious diseases
Anti-β_2-glycoprotein I antibodies (IgG or IgM)†	–	–
Cryoglobulinemia, type I	–	–
Cryofibrinogens	–	Acute-phase response

**May subsequently test for a homozygous* MTHFR *mutation (although hyperhomocysteinemia can also be due to other genes or acquired) or* PAI-1 *4G/5G polymorphism.*
†Antiphospholipid antibodies (see Table 18.4); additional studies may include anti-phosphatidylserine and/or prothrombin antibodies.

Table 18.5 Evaluation for thrombophilia (hypercoagulability). Evaluation for entities in the rows shaded gray is often considered as second tier. The initial laboratory evaluation should also include a CBC with differential and platelet count, examination of a peripheral blood smear, ESR, activated partial thromboplastin time (PTT), and hepatic and renal function panels. Testing for ANCA can be considered for patients with retiform purpura, as ANCA-positive vasculitides occasionally present with minimally inflammatory lesions.

• **Rx:** difficult; topical CS if pruritic, phototherapy.

Hypergammaglobulinemic Purpura of Waldenström

• Recurrent crops of petechiae, purpuric macules, and/or palpable purpura (Fig. 18.13) on the lower extremities, often in young women with an autoimmune connective tissue disease (especially Sjögren syndrome).

• Associated with polyclonal hypergammaglobulinemia, an elevated ESR, rheumatoid factor (IgG or IgA), and anti-SSA/Ro and anti-SSB/La antibodies.

For further information see Chs 22 and 23 from *Dermatology, Fourth Edition*.

For additional online figures visit www.expertconsult.com

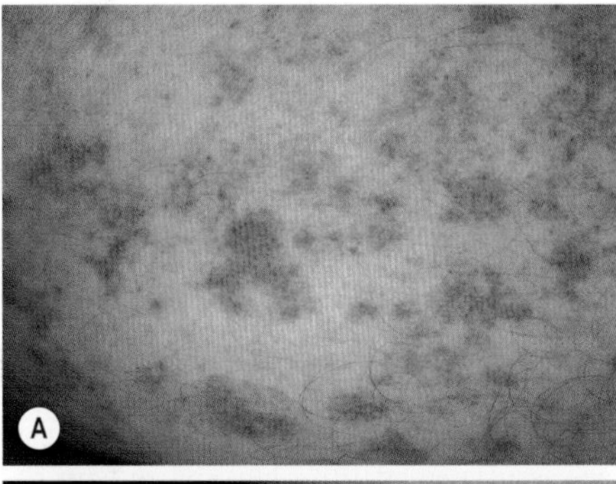

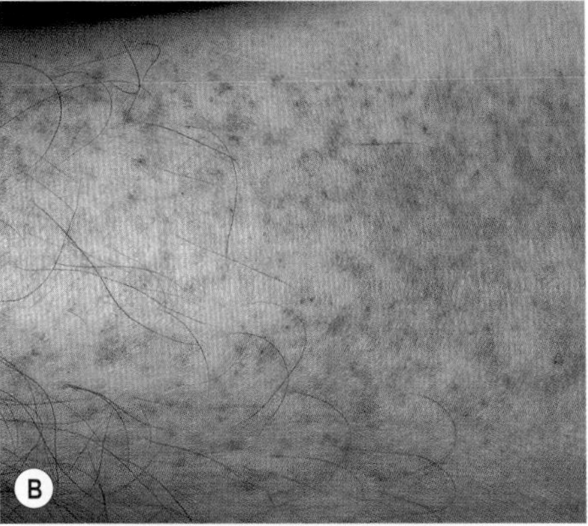

Fig. 18.11 Schamberg disease versus petechiae and hemosiderin secondary to venous hypertension. A Discrete yellow-pink patches with superimposed petechiae in Schamberg disease. **B** Petechiae within a background of more diffuse hemosiderin deposition in the setting of venous hypertension, referred to as "stasis purpura." *A, Courtesy, YDRSC; B, Courtesy, Jean L. Bolognia, MD.*

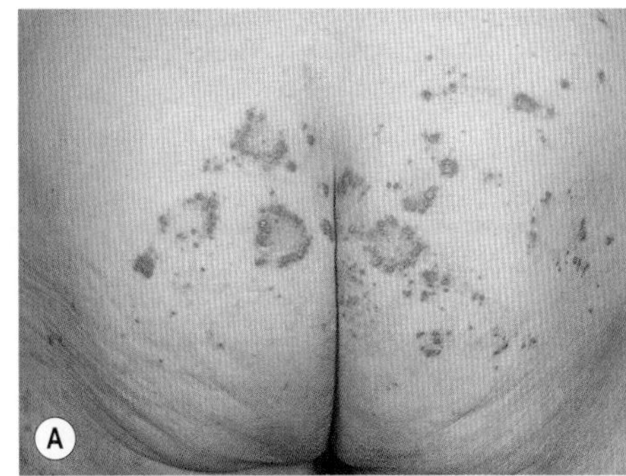

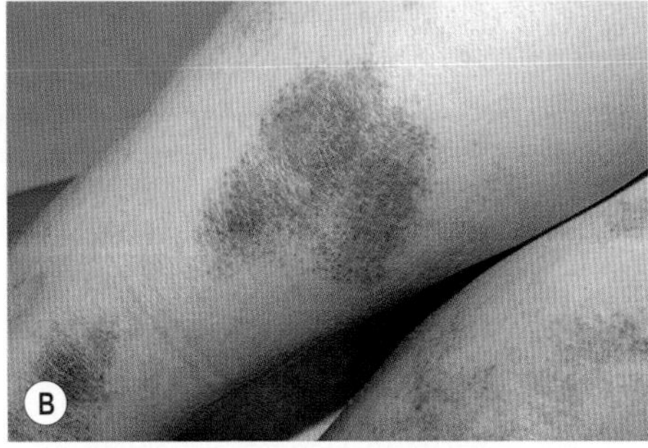

Fig. 18.12 Less common forms of pigmented purpuric eruptions. A Purpura annularis telangiectodes of Majocchi characterized by annular plaques with "cayenne pepper" petechiae in the border. **B** Eczematid-like purpura that typically presents with pruritus. *A, Courtesy, YDRSC; B, Courtesy, Kalman Watsky, MD.*

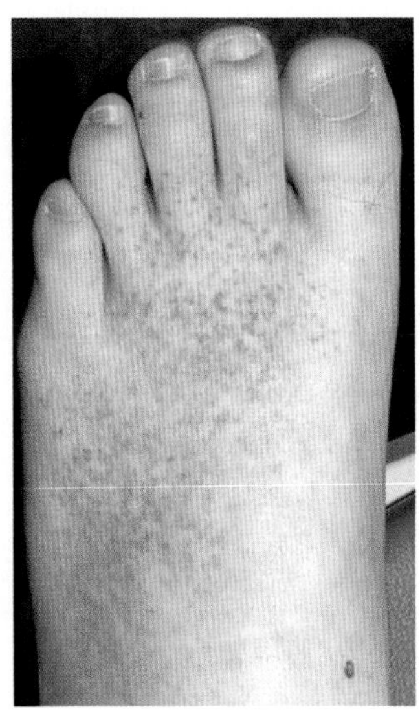

Fig. 18.13 Hypergammaglobulinemic purpura of Waldenström. This young woman with Sjögren syndrome had recurrent crops of petechiae on her lower legs. Note the hemosiderin deposition at sites of older lesions. *Courtesy, Julie V. Schaffer, MD.*

19 Vasculitis

- Vasculitis is characterized by an inflammatory infiltrate that targets blood vessels and leads to destruction of their walls.
- Cutaneous vasculitis can occur in isolation or together with involvement of other organs; in the latter scenario, skin findings may represent important signs of systemic disease.
- Cutaneous vasculitides are classified based on the size of the vessels affected, which determines the morphology of the skin lesions (Table 19.1).
- Other features that assist in categorization include direct immunofluorescence findings (e.g. IgA deposits in Henoch–Schönlein purpura [HSP]), the presence or absence of antineutrophil cytoplasmic antibodies (ANCA), and systemic manifestations (e.g. hematuria, abdominal pain, paresthesias).
- Constitutional symptoms (e.g. fevers, malaise) and arthralgias or arthritis can develop in most forms of vasculitis.
- Favors adults but can occur at any age; HSP accounts for the majority of cases in children.
- The pathogenesis of cutaneous small vessel vasculitis (CSVV) and several other vasculitides (e.g. cryoglobulinemic vasculitis, polyarteritis nodosa) is related to immune complex deposition, which results in complement activation and recruitment of neutrophils; in contrast, neutrophils directly mediate vessel damage in ANCA-associated "pauci-immune" vasculitis.

Cutaneous Small Vessel Vasculitis (CSVV)

- The clinical hallmark of CSVV is palpable purpura – nonblanching red-purple papules that favor dependent sites and areas of trauma (Koebner phenomenon) or pressure (e.g. from tight clothing); however, lesions often begin as partially blanching urticarial papules or purpuric macules, and occasionally other morphologies may be observed (e.g. vesicles or pustules; see Table 19.1, Figs 19.1 and 19.2); frequently asymptomatic but can have associated pruritus, burning, or pain.
- Possible underlying conditions are presented in Figs 19.3 and 19.4.
- Characterized by the histologic finding of *leukocytoclastic vasculitis (LCV)* – transmural infiltration of postcapillary venules by neutrophils that undergo fragmentation (leukocytoclasia), leading to fibrinoid necrosis of the vessel walls (see Fig. 1.14).
- **DDx:** specific CSVV subtypes or systemic vasculitides (see Table 19.1 and below), morbilliform drug eruptions or arthropod bites (with hemorrhage in dependent sites), petechial viral exanthems (see Fig. 68.1), pigmented purpura, erythema multiforme, pityriasis lichenoides, septic emboli.
- Usually resolves within several weeks to months, typically with postinflammatory hyperpigmentation; chronic or recurrent in ~10% of patients, especially if an underlying AI-CTD or cryoglobulinemia.
- **Rx:** eliminate possible triggers, evaluate for systemic involvement (see Fig. 19.15), and provide supportive care (e.g. leg elevation, NSAIDs); for more severe or persistent (e.g. >4 weeks) skin disease, oral dapsone ± colchicine; if rapidly progressive or ulcerating, a 4- to 6-week course of prednisone may be considered.

Henoch–Schönlein Purpura (HSP)

- Form of CSVV characterized by prominent vascular IgA deposition, which is evident via direct immunofluorescence (DIF) of a skin biopsy specimen (see Fig. 23.2); favors children <10 years of age, often presenting 1–2 weeks after an upper respiratory tract infection (URI).
- Urticarial papules evolve into palpable purpura, occasionally progressing to bullous or necrotic lesions (Fig. 19.5); typically involves the buttocks and lower extremities, but may be more widespread.

CLASSIFICATION OF CUTANEOUS VASCULITIS			
Size of predominantly affected vessels	**Types of vessels affected in the skin**	**Forms of cutaneous vasculitis**	**Cutaneous morphologies**
Small	Arterioles, capillaries and venules in *superficial to mid dermis*	**Idiopathic** **Secondary causes** (e.g. drugs, infections, inflammatory disorders; Fig. 19.3) **Henoch–Schönlein purpura** **Urticarial vasculitis** **Acute hemorrhagic edema of infancy** **Erythema elevatum diutinum**	• Palpable purpura (Fig. 19.1) > macular purpura or petechiae • Urticarial, annular or targetoid papules/plaques (Fig. 19.2A,B) • Vesicles, bullae (Fig. 19.2C), pustules
Small ± medium-sized		**Cryoglobulinemic vasculitis** **ANCA-associated vasculitis** • Granulomatosis with polyangiitis • Eosinophilic granulomatosis with polyangiitis • Microscopic polyangiitis **Secondary causes** (e.g. drugs, rheumatoid arthritis; Fig. 19.3)	
Medium-sized	Small arteries and veins in *deep dermis to subcutis*	**Polyarteritis nodosa (PAN)** • Classic (systemic) PAN • Cutaneous PAN	• Livedo racemosa ("broken" livedo reticularis) • Retiform purpura • Subcutaneous nodules • Ulcers, digital necrosis
Large	(*Extracutaneous* named arteries*)	**Temporal arteritis** **Takayasu arteritis**	• Temporal arteritis*: erythema, alopecia, purpura, tender nodules → ulcers on frontotemporal scalp; ulcers on tongue • Takayasu arteritis*: nodules, ulcers

Cutaneous involvement is uncommon.

Table 19.1 Classification of cutaneous vasculitis.

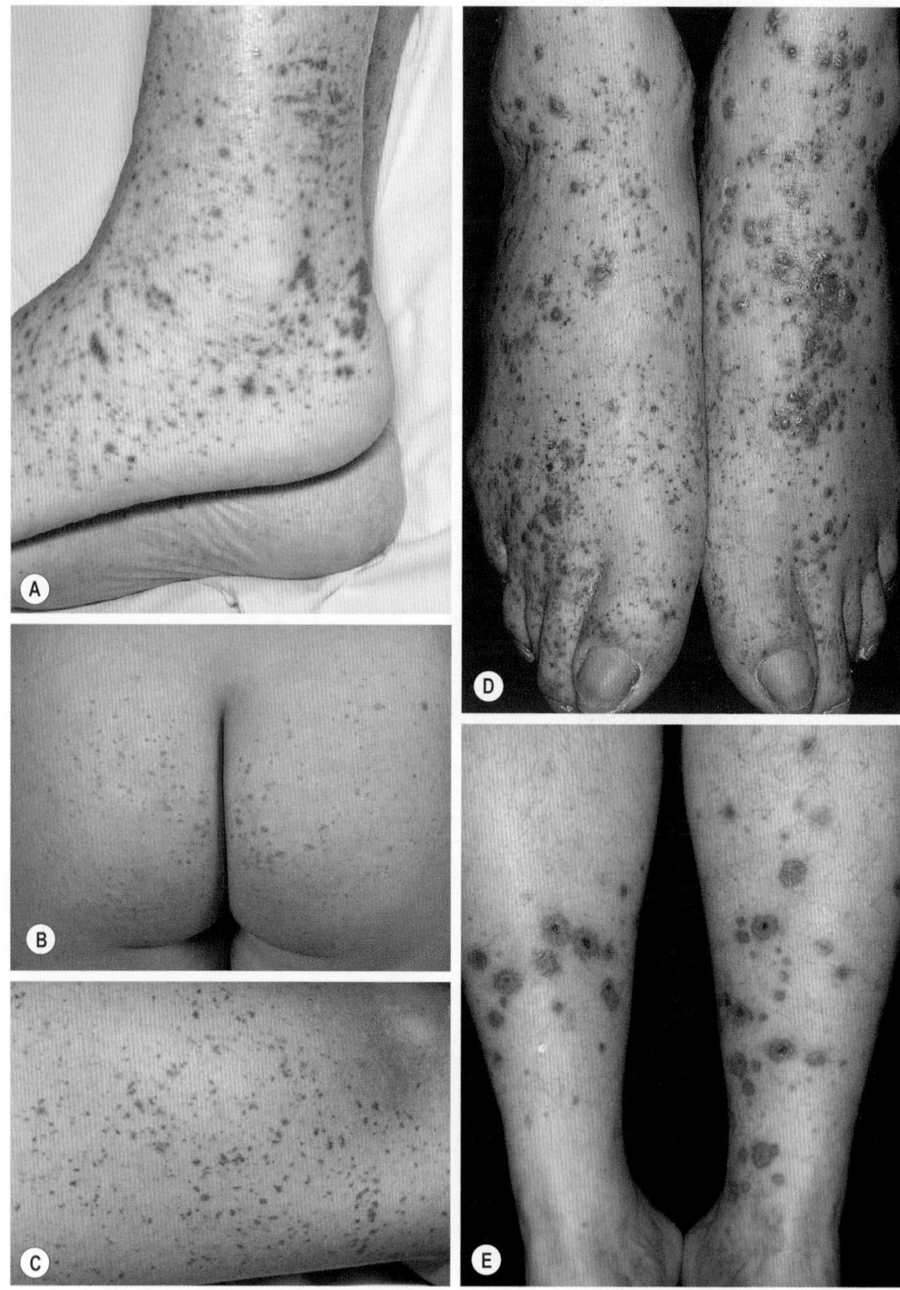

Fig. 19.1 Cutaneous small vessel vasculitis. A Classic presentation of purpuric macules and papules on the distal lower extremities. **B** Early lesions may be erythematous rather than purpuric. **C** Eventually inflammatory lesions can no longer be blanched due to hemorrhage within the dermis. **D** Hemorrhagic vesicles in addition to palpable purpura. **E** Central necrosis with formation of hemorrhagic crusts. *A, C, Courtesy, Kalman Watsky, MD; B, Courtesy, NYU Slide Collection; D, Courtesy, YDRSC; E, Courtesy, Frank Samarin, MD.*

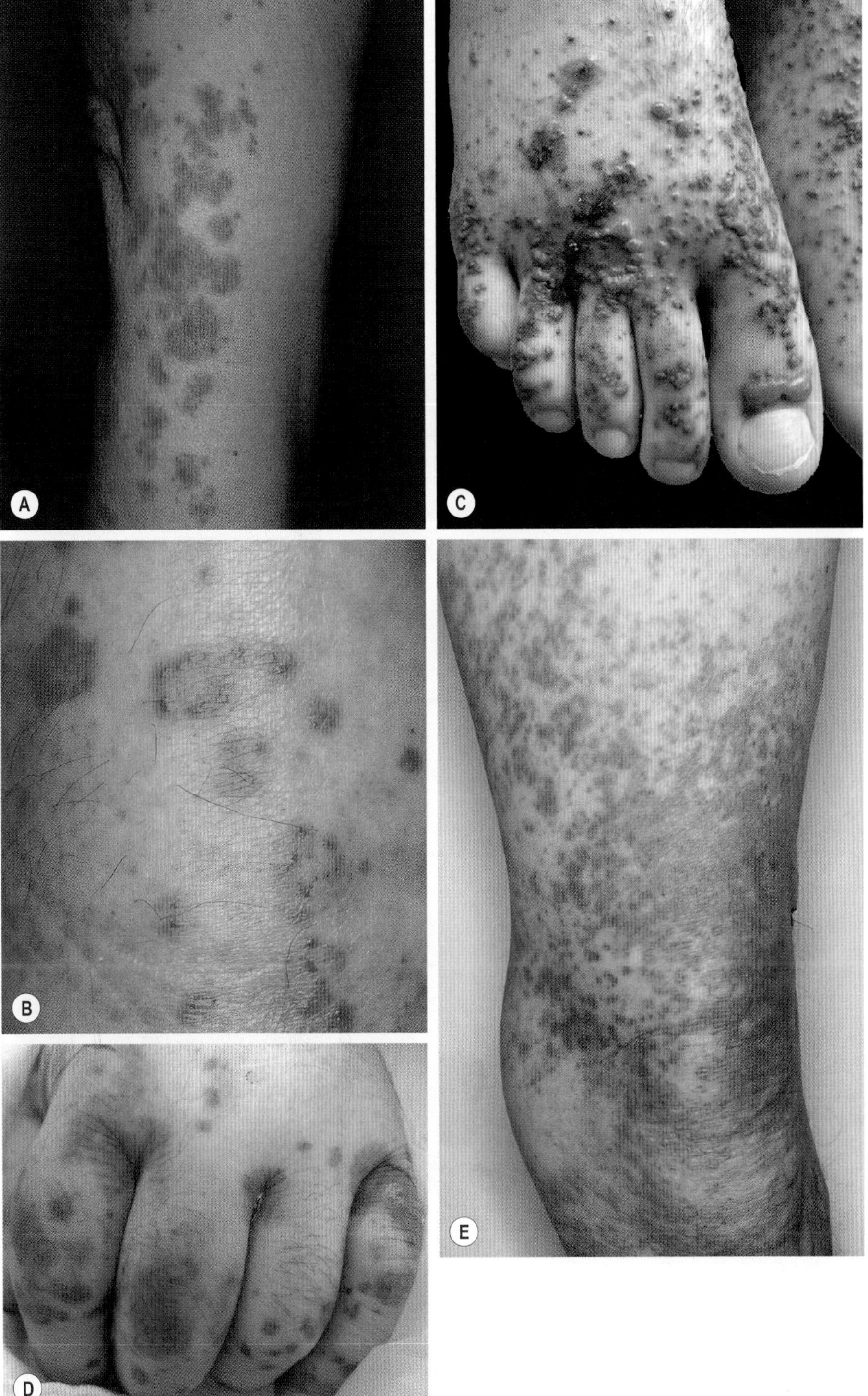

Fig. 19.2 Clinical variants of cutaneous small vessel vasculitis. A Targetoid appearance that can resemble erythema multiforme. **B** Hemorrhagic crusts in annular configuration. **C** Predominantly vesicular lesions on the foot. **D** Lesions limited to the upper extremities. **E** Purpuric macules and papules with areas of confluence resembling a purpuric morbilliform drug eruption. *A, Courtesy, Kalman Watsky, MD; B, Courtesy, YDRSC; C, Courtesy, Karynne O. Duncan, MD; D, Courtesy, Lindy Fox, MD; E, Courtesy, David Wetter, MD, and Jan Dutz, MD.*

ETIOLOGIES OF CUTANEOUS SMALL VESSEL VASCULITIS

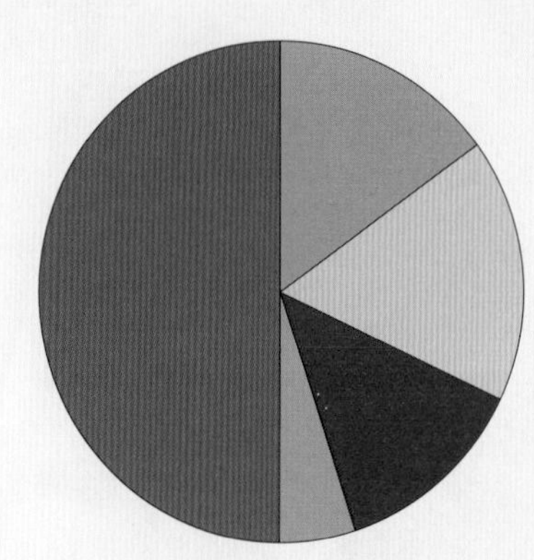

- **Infection** (15–20%)
  e.g. streptococcal or upper respiratory tract infections, hepatitis C>B, leprosy, subacute infective endocarditis
- **Autoimmune connective tissue disease** (15–20%)
  e.g. rheumatoid arthritis, SLE, Sjögren syndrome
- **Drug** (10–15%)
  e.g. penicillins, quinolones, NSAIDs, propylthiouracil*
- **Neoplasm** (5%)
  e.g. plasma cell dyscrasias, myelo- and lymphoproliferative disorders
- **Idiopathic** (45–55%)

*Often associated with antineutrophil cytoplasmic antibodies (ANCA).

Fig. 19.3 Etiologies of cutaneous small vessel vasculitis.

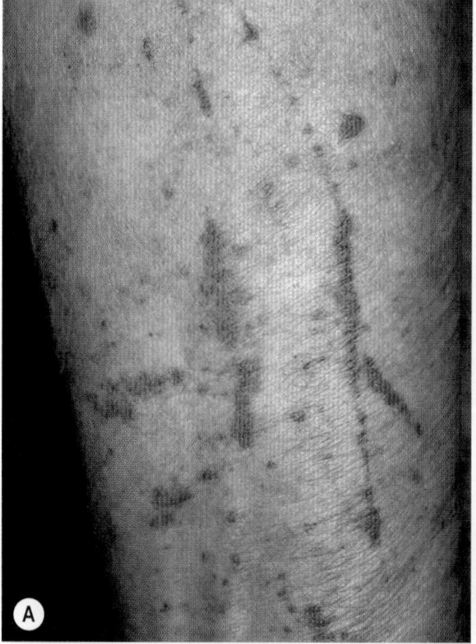

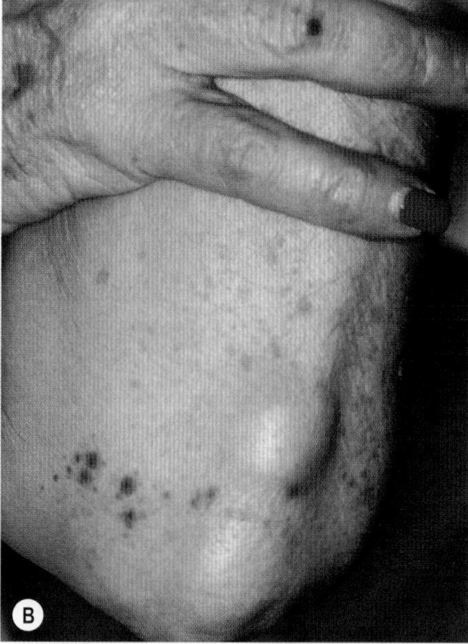

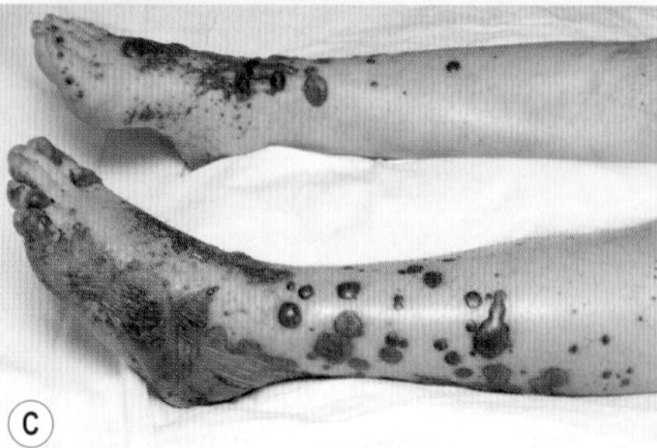

Fig. 19.4 Cutaneous small vessel vasculitis associated with systemic disorders. The underlying diseases were Sjögren syndrome **(A),** rheumatoid arthritis **(B)**, and endocarditis due to *Streptococcus mitis* **(C).** Note the Koebner phenomenon in **(A)** and the rheumatoid nodules in **(B).** *A, B, Courtesy, YDRSC; C, Courtesy, David Wetter, MD, and Jan Dutz, MD.*

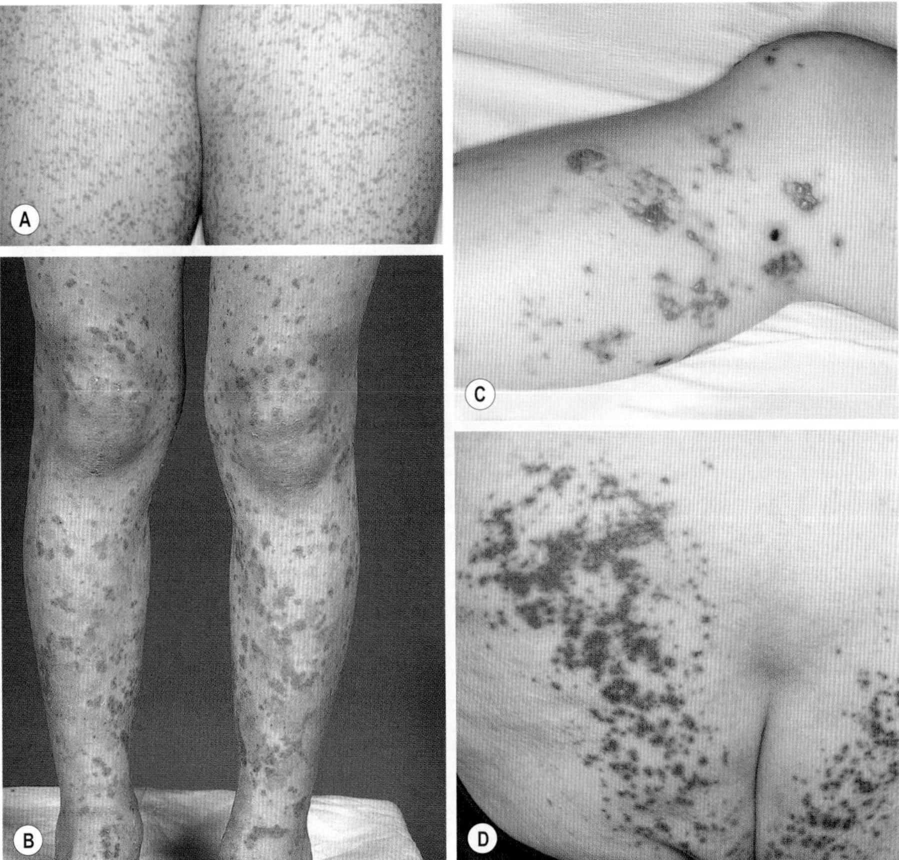

Fig. 19.5 Henoch–Schönlein purpura. A, B Multiple pink, partially blanching papules on the lower extremities. These early lesions are beginning to develop a hemorrhagic component, while sites of previous involvement on the shin are now dull pink patches. **C** Less common vesiculobullous variant. **D** More developed purpuric macules and papules on the buttocks with coalescence into a retiform configuration on the upper left. Inflammatory retiform purpura can be seen in IgA vasculitis. *A, C, D, Courtesy, David Wetter, MD, and Jan Dutz, MD; B, Courtesy, YDRSC.*

- Other manifestations include acral or scrotal edema, arthralgias/arthritis (especially of the knees and ankles; ~75% of children), colicky abdominal pain (~65%; occasionally intussusception), bloody stools (~30%), and microscopic hematuria ± proteinuria (~30–40%; can be delayed up to 3 months).
- Resolves over several weeks to months, with recurrent purpuric eruptions in ~20% and long-term renal impairment in ~2% of children with HSP.
- Adults with HSP are more likely to have necrotic skin lesions, renal involvement, and chronic kidney disease; in adults with unexplained persistent or widespread IgA vasculitis, especially if involving medium-sized vessels, an underlying IgA monoclonal gammopathy or malignancy should be considered.
- **Rx:** as for CSVV above, with monitoring for renal disease and systemic CS therapy as needed for arthritis, abdominal pain, and severe nephritis; however, CS administration does not appear to prevent renal disease or its sequelae.

Acute Hemorrhagic Edema of Infancy

- Uncommon CSVV variant that affects children ≤2 years of age, often following a URI.
- Presents with annular or targetoid purpuric plaques and edema favoring the face, ears, and extremities (Fig. 19.6); patients may be febrile, but extracutaneous involvement is rare and spontaneous resolution occurs within 1–3 weeks.
- **DDx:** urticaria "multiforme" (giant annular urticaria; see Fig. 3.3), serum sickness-like

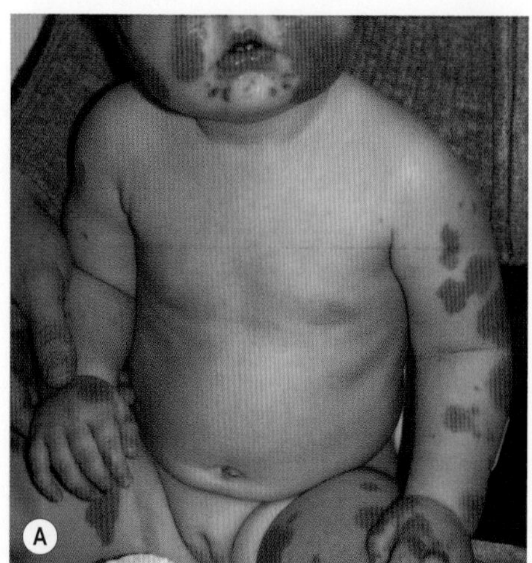

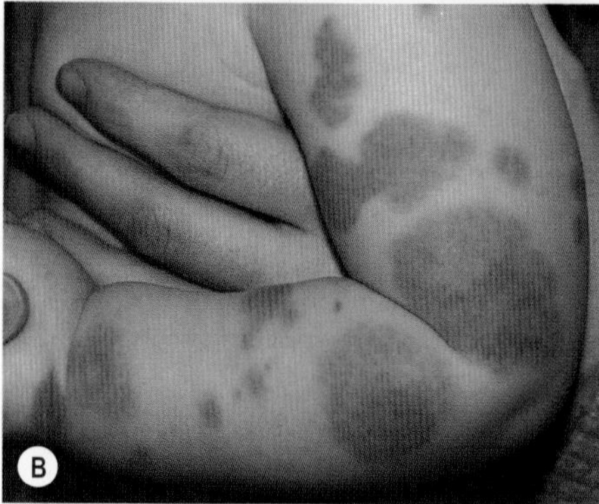

Fig. 19.6 Acute hemorrhagic edema of infancy. Multiple edematous, erythematous plaques on the face and extremities of a toddler. Some of the lesions have begun to become dusky. *Courtesy, Ilona J. Frieden, MD.*

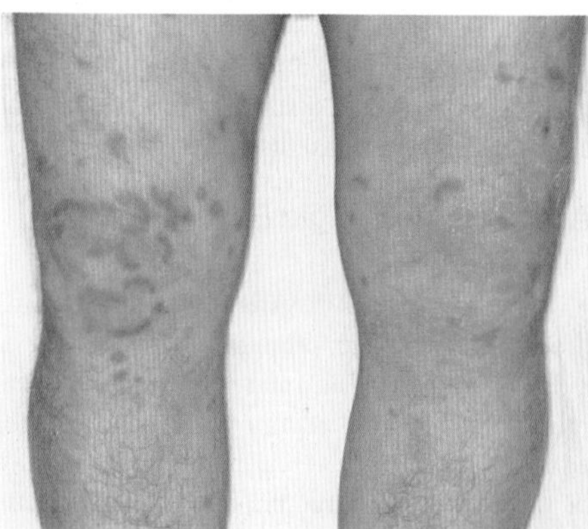

Fig. 19.7 Urticarial vasculitis. Arcuate, dull violet urticarial plaques on the lower extremities. *Courtesy, David Wetter, MD, and Jan Dutz, MD.*

reaction, urticarial vasculitis, Kawasaki disease, erythema multiforme, Sweet syndrome; findings sometimes overlap with HSP.

Urticarial Vasculitis

- Presents with urticarial plaques that have histologic features of LCV (Fig. 19.7); favors middle-aged women, and a hypocomplementemic subset is associated with AI-CTD (especially SLE and Sjögren syndrome).
- In contrast to urticaria, individual lesions last >24 hours, resolve with purpura or hyperpigmentation, and produce burning or pain > pruritus.
- Patients with hypocomplementemic urticarial vasculitis may have arthralgias/arthritis, chronic obstructive pulmonary disease, and involvement of the GI tract, kidneys, or eyes.
- **DDx:** see Table 14.1.

Erythema Elevatum Diutinum

- Chronic form of vasculitis that favors middle-aged to older adults; associated disorders include HIV and other infections (e.g. streptococcal), AI-CTD, and IgA monoclonal gammopathy.
- Presents with persistent violaceous to red-brown plaques on extensor surfaces (e.g. elbows, knees) (Fig. 19.8); patients occasionally have arthralgias or ocular disease, and dapsone therapy is usually effective.

Small and Medium-Sized Vessel Vasculitis

Cryoglobulinemic Vasculitis (see Table 18.3)

- "Mixed" cryoglobulinemia (types II and III) can lead to vasculitis of small ± medium-sized vessels; associated with hepatitis C infection > other infections (e.g. HIV), AI-CTD, and lymphoproliferative disorders.
- Palpable purpura is the most common cutaneous manifestation (Fig. 19.9); other findings can include arthritis/arthralgias, peripheral neuropathy, glomerulonephritis, and hepatitis.
- **Rx:** treatment of associated hepatitis C with direct-acting antivirals (now first-line; e.g. sofosbuvir + ledipasvir or daclatasvir) or interferon + ribavirin; CS or rituximab for severe or refractory systemic disease.

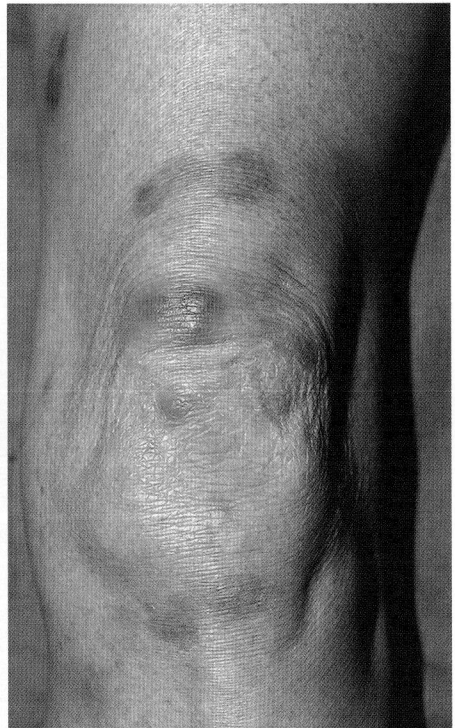

Fig. 19.8 Erythema elevatum diutinum. Erythematous papulonodules on the knee (acute lesions) admixed with resolving lesions. *Courtesy, Kenneth Greer, MD.*

ANCA-Associated Vasculitis

- The features of specific ANCA-associated vasculitides are presented in Table 19.2 and Figs 19.10–19.12.
- Favors middle-aged to older adults, but can occur at any age.
- Requires evaluation for extracutaneous disease (see Fig. 19.15).
- ANCA against various antigens also occur in other diseases (e.g. ulcerative colitis, autoimmune hepatitis); cocaine use can lead to ANCA (typically against myeloperoxidase, proteinase-3, and neutrophil elastase) together with nasal destruction (Table 19.3) or (with levamisole adulteration) more widespread vasculitis or vasculopathy plus neutropenia (see Fig. 75.3).
- **Rx:** induction of remission with systemic CS ± cyclophosphamide or rituximab; maintenance with CS-sparing agents (e.g. methotrexate, azathioprine), trimethoprim–sulfamethoxazole.

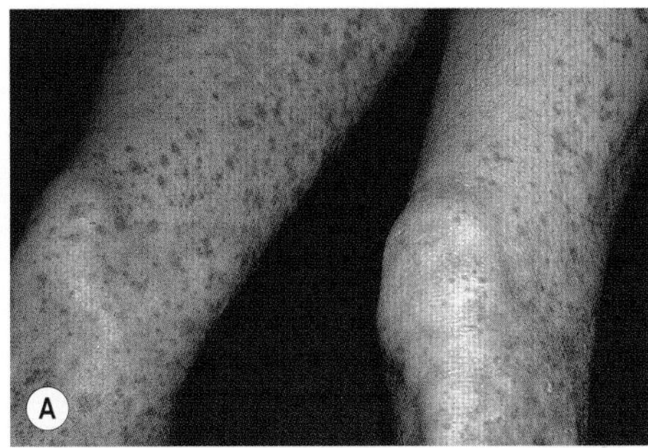

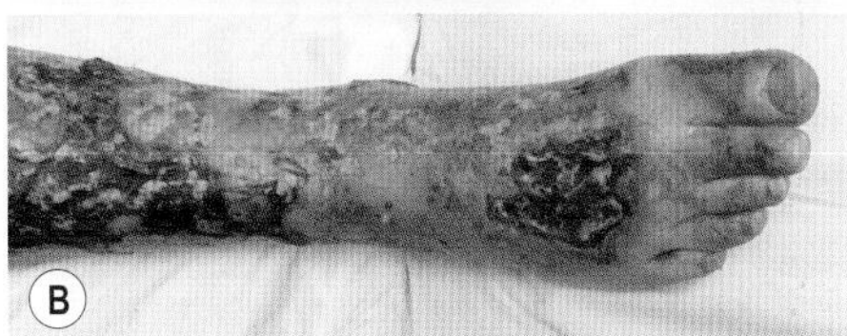

Fig. 19.9 Cutaneous small vessel vasculitis due to mixed cryoglobulinemia. A Palpable purpura represents the most common presentation. **B** Purpuric papules and plaques with central necrosis and ulceration as well as a few vesicles in a patient with type II cryoglobulinemia in the setting of hepatitis C viral infection. The patient also had an elevated rheumatoid factor, decreased C4, and an IgM monoclonal gammopathy. *B, Courtesy, David Wetter, MD, and Jan Dutz, MD.*

Predominantly Medium-Sized Vessel Vasculitis

Polyarteritis Nodosa (PAN): Classic (Systemic) and Cutaneous Variants

- Segmental vasculitis affecting primarily medium-sized vessels, including small arteries in the deep dermis and subcutis.
- Favors middle-aged adults (men > women), but can occur at any age.
- **DDx:** other types of vasculitis; livedoid vasculopathy, antiphospholipid syndrome, and other microvascular occlusion syndromes (see Ch. 18); superficial thrombophlebitis, panniculitis.

CLASSIC (SYSTEMIC) PAN

- Associated with hepatitis B infection in ~10% of patients.
- Approximately 25% of patients have cutaneous manifestations, including livedo racemosa, retiform purpura, palpable purpura (when small vessels are affected), and "punched out" ulcers > subcutaneous nodules and digital infarcts (Fig. 19.13A).

ANCA-ASSOCIATED VASCULITIDES				
Disorder [No. of diagnostic criteria required]	**Predominant ANCA type/antigen**	**Cutaneous and oral findings**	**Extracutaneous manifestations**	**Histologic findings**¶
Granulomatosis with polyangiitis (GPA; Wegener granulomatosis) [2]	C-/PR3 (80–90%*) P-/MPO (~10%)	• Palpable purpura (Fig. 19.10A) • Friable, micropapular gingivae ("strawberry gums"; see Fig. 59.17), oral ulcers (Fig. 19.10B) • PNGD** • Subcutaneous nodules • Pyoderma gangrenosum-like ulcers (Fig. 19.10C)	• **Upper respiratory**: *oral ulcers or purulent/bloody nasal discharge;* septal perforation/saddle nose (Table 19.3); acute hearing loss; chronic sinusitis/otitis/mastoiditis • **Pulmonary**: *nodules, fixed infiltrates or cavities*† • **Renal:** glomerulonephritis, *with hematuria or RBC casts in urine sediment* • **Ocular**: proptosis, scleritis • Less often neurologic, GI, and cardiac involvement	• *Granulomatous inflammation* • Vasculitis of small ± medium-sized vessels
Eosinophilic granulomatosis with polyangiitis (EGPA; Churg–Strauss syndrome)‡ [4]	P-/MPO (~40%) C-/PR3 (~10%)	• Palpable purpura (Fig. 19.11A) • PNGD** (Fig. 19.11B) • Subcutaneous nodules • Urticarial plaques • Livedo racemosa, retiform purpura (Fig. 19.11C), ulcers	• **Upper respiratory**: allergic rhinitis§, nasal polyps§, *sinusitis*† • **Pulmonary**: *asthma*§, *eosinophilic pneumonia*† • **Hematologic**: *peripheral eosinophilia (>10%)*, elevated IgE • **Neurologic**: *mononeuritis multiplex* • **Cardiac**: myo- or pericarditis • Less often renal, GI, and ocular involvement	• *Extravascular eosinophils* • Granulomatous inflammation • Vasculitis of small ± medium-sized vessels
Microscopic polyangiitis [4]	P-/MPO (~60%) C-/PR3 (~30%)	• Palpable purpura (Fig. 19.12) • Erythematous macules, urticarial or purpuric plaques • Livedo racemosa, ulcers, splinter hemorrhages	• **Renal**: glomerulonephritis, *with hematuria or RBC casts in urine sediment* • **Pulmonary**: capillaritis/hemorrhage, *no asthma* • **Neurologic**: mononeuritis multiplex • Less often upper respiratory tract, cardiac, GI, and ocular involvement	• *Vasculitis of small (± medium-sized) vessels* • *No granulomas*

**Approximately 60% in patients with limited/localized disease.*
***Palisaded neutrophilic and granulomatous dermatitis, which typically presents with umbilicated, crusted papulonodules on extensor surfaces (e.g. elbows) or the face (especially in granulomatosis with polyangiitis) (see Ch. 78).*
†Radiographic evidence represents a diagnostic criterion.
‡Occasionally triggered by leukotriene inhibitors and/or rapid discontinuation of CS therapy.
§Usually the initial manifestations.
¶May be observed in biopsies of the skin, mucosa, respiratory tract, kidney, or nerve.

Table 19.2 Antineutrophil cytoplasmic antibody (ANCA)-associated vasculitides. As in other forms of vasculitis, patients often have constitutional symptoms (e.g. fevers, malaise, weight loss), arthralgias, and arthritis. *Classic diagnostic criteria for each disorder (1990 American College of Rheumatology Classification for*

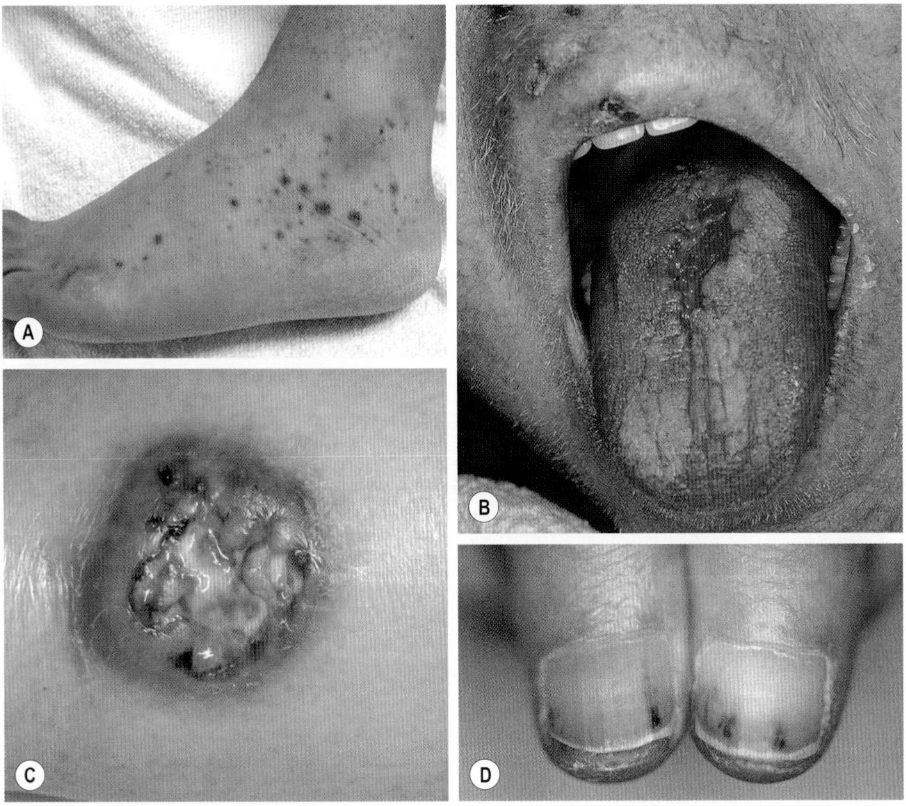

Fig. 19.10 Granulomatosis with polyangiitis (Wegener granulomatosis). A Palpable purpura of the legs due to small vessel vasculitis (leukocytoclastic vasculitis). **B** Ulceration of the tongue**. C** Ulceration on the leg, which may be misdiagnosed as pyoderma gangrenosum. **D** Subungual digital infarcts. *A, B, D, Courtesy, YDRSC; C, Courtesy, David Wetter, MD, and Jan Dutz, MD.*

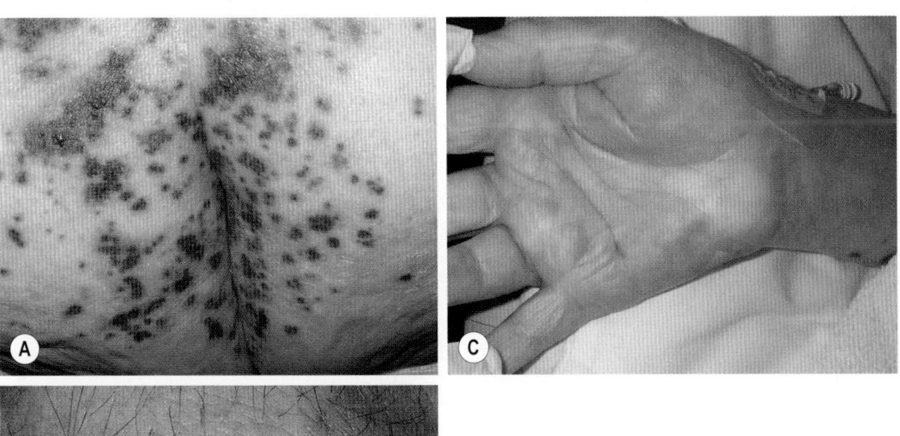

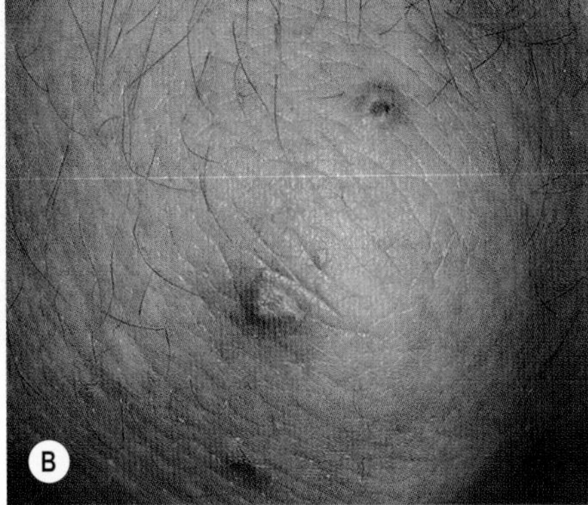

Fig. 19.11 Eosinophilic granulomatosis with polyangiitis (Churg–Strauss syndrome). A Palpable purpura on the buttocks due to small vessel (leukocytoclastic) vasculitis. **B** Palisaded neutrophilic and granulomatous dermatitis presenting with crusted, firm papules on the elbow. **C** Purpuric dermal plaques on the palm due to vasculitis involving a small artery (representing medium-sized vessel). *A, C, Courtesy, Kanade Shinkai, MD, and Lindy P. Fox, MD; B, Courtesy, Kalman Watsky, MD.*

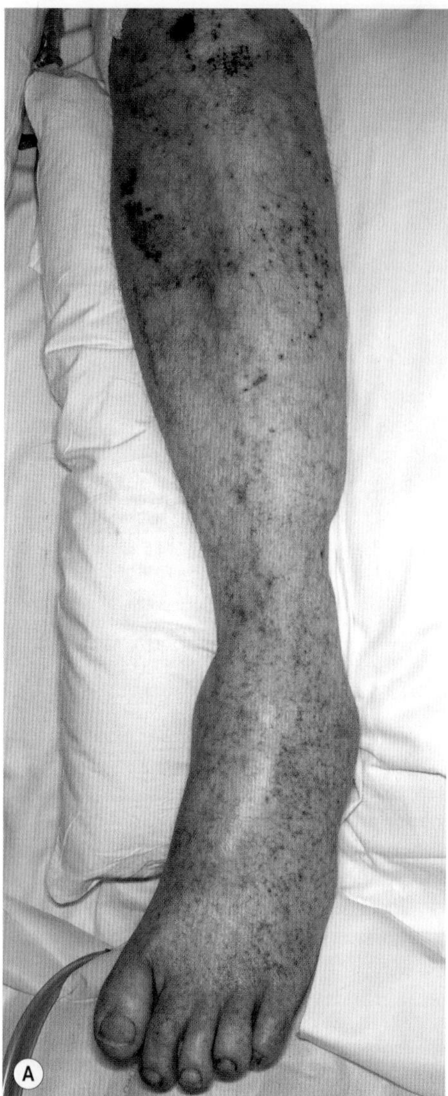

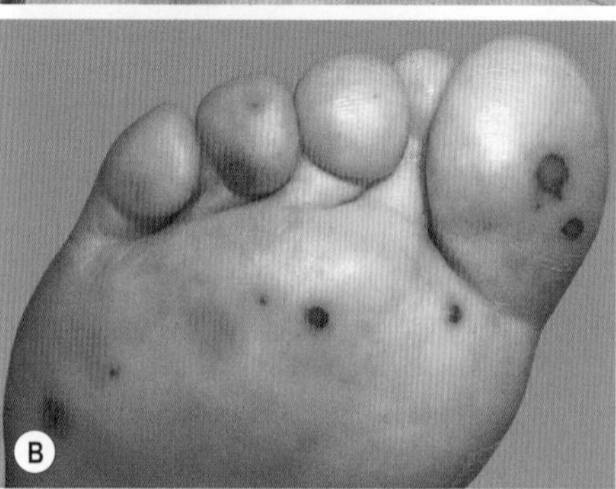

Fig. 19.12 Microscopic polyangiitis. A Petechiae and purpuric macules on the lower extremity; some of the lesions have central hemorrhagic crusts. Histologically, leukocytoclastic vasculitis was seen. **B** Petechiae and multiple purpuric papules with central necrosis on the plantar surface. *A, Courtesy, David Wetter, MD, and Jan Dutz, MD; B, Courtesy, Cora Whitney Hannon, MD, and Robert Swerlick, MD.*

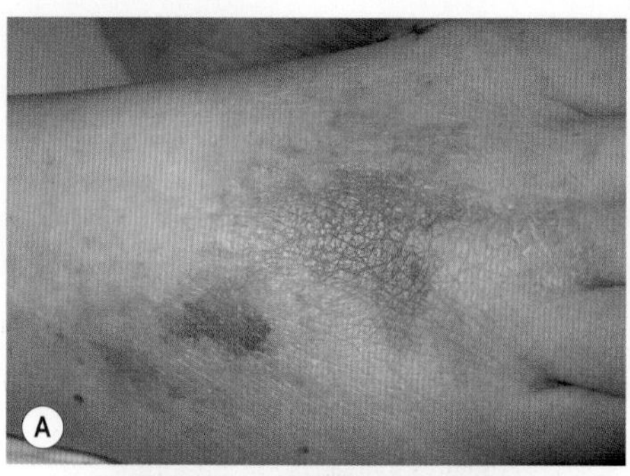

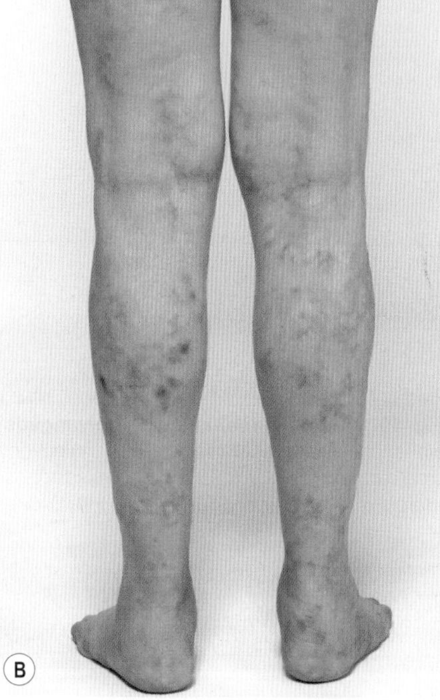

Fig. 19.13 Polyarteritis nodosa (PAN). A Retiform purpura of the dorsal foot in a patient with *systemic* PAN. **B** Livedo racemosa and subcutaneous nodules of the lower extremities in a patient with *cutaneous* PAN. *A, Courtesy, Kanade Shinkai, MD, and Lindy P. Fox, MD; B, Courtesy, David Wetter, MD, and Jan Dutz, MD.*

DIFFERENTIAL DIAGNOSIS OF NASAL DESTRUCTION OR DEFORMITY
Inflammatory disorders
• Granulomatosis with polyangiitis • Relapsing polychondritis • Sarcoidosis
Neoplastic disorders
• Nasal natural killer/T-cell lymphoma (lethal midline granuloma) • Squamous cell and basal cell carcinomas • Neuroblastoma, salivary gland tumors, sarcomas (e.g. rhabdomyosarcoma)
Infectious disorders
• *Bacterial*: rhinoscleroma, glanders, noma, syphilis (late congenital or tertiary), yaws • *Mycobacterial*: leprosy, tuberculosis (lupus vulgaris) • *Fungal*: paracoccidioidomycosis, zygomycosis, aspergillosis • *Parasitic*: mucocutaneous leishmaniasis, acanthamoebiasis, rhinosporidiosis
Other
• Cocaine use (cocaine-induced midline destructive lesion) • Nasal myiasis • Factitious or traumatic

Table 19.3 Differential diagnosis of nasal destruction or deformity.

• Extracutanous manifestations include fevers, weight loss, arthralgias, myalgias, and involvement of arteries supplying the GI tract, kidneys (e.g. renovascular hypertension, *not* glomerulonephritis), nervous system (peripheral > central), heart, and testes.

• **Rx:** systemic CS, treatment of associated hepatitis B; cyclophosphamide for severe or refractory systemic disease.

CUTANEOUS PAN

• Accounts for >30% of childhood PAN and ≤5% of adult PAN.

• May be associated with infections (e.g. streptococcal) or medications (e.g. minocycline – may be P-ANCA+, unlike most forms of PAN); childhood PAN may occur in the setting of adenosine deaminase 2 (ADA2) deficiency, which can also result in early-onset strokes (see Table 37.3).

• Tender subcutaneous nodules favoring the lower extremities, often in a background of livedo racemosa and sometimes following the course of an artery (see Fig. 19.13B); retiform purpura, ulcers, and annular plaques may also be seen.

• Arthralgias, myalgias, and peripheral neuropathy may occur in areas of skin disease; chronic course without systemic progression.

• **Rx:** intralesional or systemic CS, dapsone, methotrexate; TNF inhibitors for ADA2 deficiency.

Diagnostic Approach to Patients with Suspected Cutaneous Vasculitis

• An approach to the evaluation of patients suspected to have vasculitis, including assessment of underlying conditions and systemic manifestations, is presented in Fig. 19.14.

For further information see Ch. 24 from *Dermatology, Fourth Edition*.

For additional online figures and tables visit www.expertconsult.com 

APPROACH TO THE PATIENT WITH SUSPECTED CUTANEOUS VASCULITIS

Patient with suspected cutaneous vasculitis

History and physical examination

- Determine if drug exposure or evidence of an underlying infection; if not, consider an associated inflammatory disorder or malignancy

- Evaluate for extracutaneous signs and symptoms
  - Constitutional: fever, weight loss, fatigue
  - Musculoskeletal: arthralgias, myalgias
  - Renal: hematuria
  - Gastroenterologic: abdominal pain, bloody stools
  - Neurologic: numbness, paresthesias, weakness
  - Cardiopulmonary: shortness of breath, chest pain, cough, hemoptysis
  - Ear/Nose/Throat: sinusitis

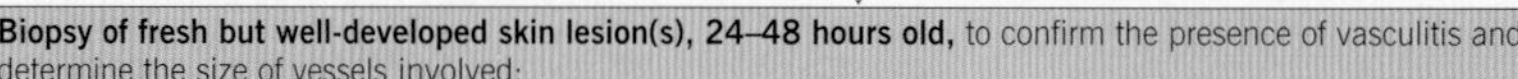

Biopsy of fresh but well-developed skin lesion(s), 24–48 hours old, to confirm the presence of vasculitis and determine the size of vessels involved:

- If suspect small vessel vasculitis (e.g. if palpable purpura): punch biopsies for routine histology and direct immunofluorescence (the latter of a lesion $\leq$ 24 hours old)
- If suspect medium-sized vessel vasculitis: deep incisional biopsy (including subcutaneous tissue) of a nodule (preferred) or retiform purpura > the edge of an ulcer*

Pertinent positives on skin biopsy

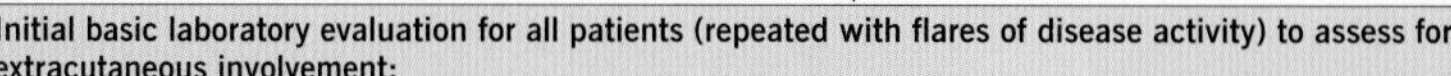

Initial basic laboratory evaluation for all patients (repeated with flares of disease activity) to assess for extracutaneous involvement:

- CBC with differential, platelet count, ESR +/– C-reactive protein
- Hepatic panel, BUN & creatinine, urinalysis, stool guaiac

Additional evaluation for associated diseases and specific vasculitides, depending on clinical suspicion (i.e. chronic or recurrent disease, unclear cause, history and physical examination suggest underlying internal organ involvement or associated systemic disorder):

Infection	• Antistreptolysin O and anti-DNase B titers; hepatitis B/C and HIV serologies; throat, urine or blood culture as indicated
Inflammatory	• Cryoglobulins • ANCAs**
AI-CTD	• Rheumatoid factor, ANA, anti-ENA antibodies (e.g. anti-Ro) • CH50/C3/C4 if suspect urticarial vasculitis (also C1q if low C4)
Malignancy	• Serum & urine protein electrophoresis, serum immunofixation electrophoresis, peripheral blood smear • Age-appropriate screening +/– sign/symptom-directed evaluation for malignancies

Additional evaluation for extracutaneous involvement in systemic vasculitides:

ANCA-associated vasculitis

- Chest X-ray, CT of chest & sinuses
- Depending on the specific condition and clinical findings, consider: electromyogram/nerve conduction studies, echocardiogram/electrocardiogram, and biopsy of the respiratory tract (upper or lower), nerve, kidney or muscle

Classic (systemic) polyarteritis nodosa

- Mesenteric/renal/celiac angiogram
- Consider biopsy of muscle, nerve, kidney or testicles

*Include peripheral rim of inflammation if present; vasculitis underlying an ulcer can occur as a secondary phenomenon and is not diagnostic.

**Indirect immunofluorescence (IIF) followed by confirmation with antigen-specific ELISAs for proteinase-3 (PR3) and myeloperoxidase (MPO).

Fig. 19.14 Approach to the patient with suspected cutaneous vasculitis. ENA, extractable nuclear antigen; ENT, ear, nose, and throat; GU, genitourinary.

Eosinophilic Dermatoses 20

As with the group of disorders known as neutrophilic dermatoses, there is significant overlap in the cutaneous findings of entities where eosinophils play a role – from papular urticaria triggered by arthropod bites to Wells syndrome and hypereosinophilic syndrome (Fig. 20.1; Table 20.1). The exception is granuloma faciale, which has a more specific presentation.

Granuloma Faciale

- Idiopathic disorder characterized by one or more persistent red-brown to violet-brown plaques on the face (Fig. 20.2); prominent follicular openings are often noted and a third of patients have multiple plaques.
- Most commonly occurs in middle-aged adults, and extrafacial involvement is unusual (<10% of patients).
- The clinical diagnosis is confirmed via histopathology where eosinophils, neutrophils, and lymphocytes are seen in the dermis.
- **DDx:** sarcoidosis, foreign body granuloma, granulomatous rosacea, and other entities that lead to persistent red to red-brown plaques of the face (see Fig. 99.2).
- **Rx:** often difficult; intralesional CS, topical calcineurin inhibitors, cryosurgery, vascular lasers.

Exaggerated Insect Bite and Insect Bite-Like Reactions (Eosinophilic Dermatosis Associated with Hematologic Disorders/ Malignancies)

- Lesions may occur at sites of known insect bites but a history of bites may be lacking, hence the term insect bite-like reaction; presents as pruritic, erythematous, edematous papulonodules and vesiculobullae.
- The most common associated systemic disorder is chronic lymphocytic leukemia, but these reactions can also be seen in patients with other lymphoproliferative as well as myeloproliferative disorders (see Table 99.2) and at sites of mosquito bites in those with EBV-associated NK/T-cell lymphoproliferative disorders.

Papuloerythroderma of Ofuji

- Widespread red-brown papules that coalesce into an erythroderma with sparing of skin folds ("deck-chair" sign), often with peripheral eosinophilia; primarily elderly men, frequently Japanese.
- Usually idiopathic, but occasionally there is an underlying lymphoma (especially T-cell) or carcinoma (most commonly gastric).
- **DDx:** other causes of erythroderma (see Ch. 8).

Wells Syndrome (Eosinophilic Cellulitis)

- Recurrent burning, pruritic or painful pink to red plaques that are often edematous, thus resembling infectious cellulitis; over time the lesions may become more infiltrative (Fig. 20.3).
- As the plaques and nodules spontaneously fade over a period of 1–2 months, a residual brown to gray or even green color may be seen.
- Associated symptoms include malaise and occasionally fever; peripheral eosinophilia is common.
- Unknown etiology; the possibility of triggers such as arthropod bites, parasitic infections (e.g. toxocariasis), or an underlying myeloproliferative disorder is a matter of debate.
- Within the dermis, there is a discharge of the granular contents of eosinophils, which then coat collagen fibers and lead to the formation of "flame figures"; the latter can also be seen in other disorders in which there are numerous eosinophils in the skin.

EVALUATION OF ADULT PATIENTS WITH EOSINOPHILIC DERMATOSES

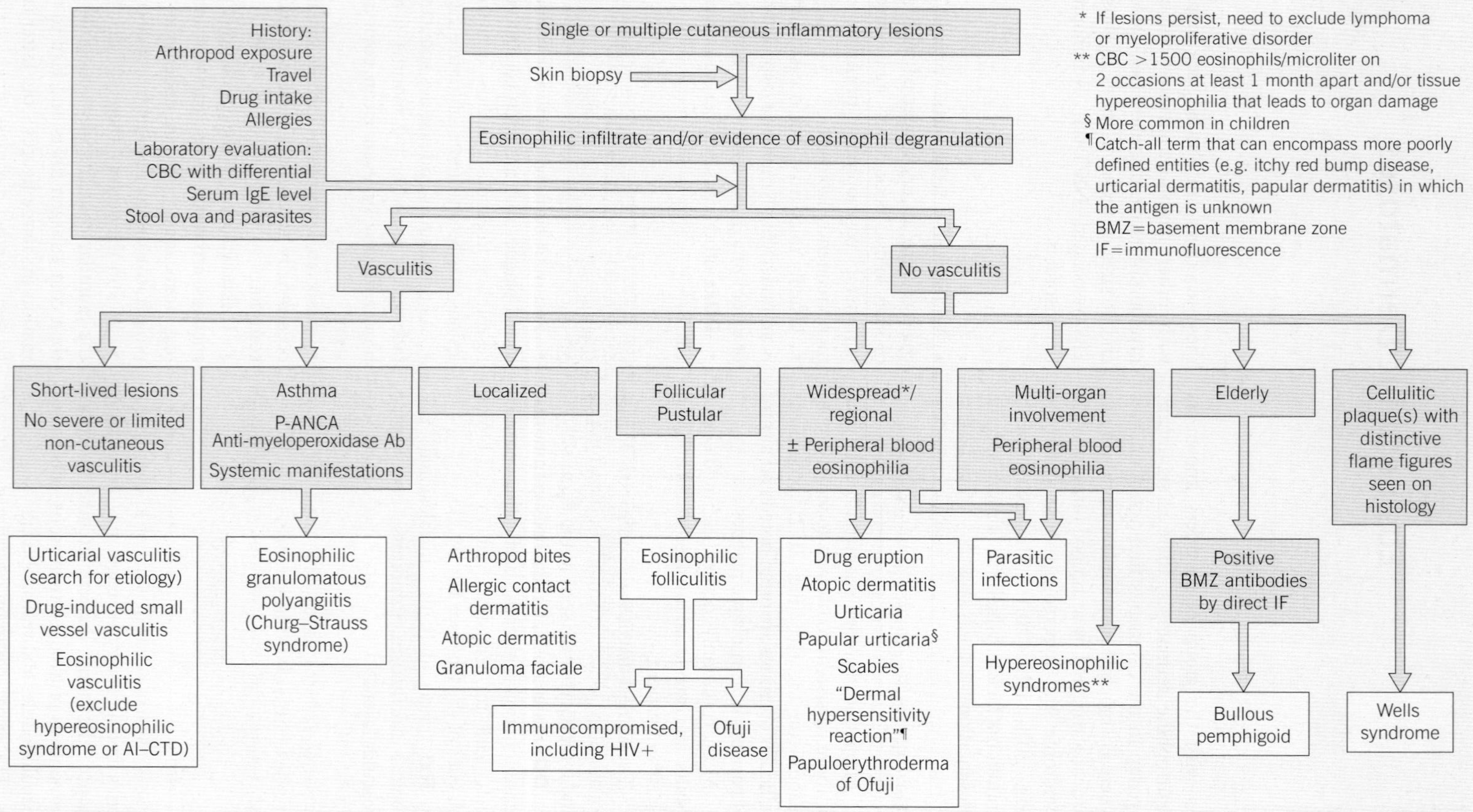

- Single or multiple cutaneous inflammatory lesions
  - Skin biopsy →
- Eosinophilic infiltrate and/or evidence of eosinophil degranulation
  - History: Arthropod exposure; Travel; Drug intake; Allergies. Laboratory evaluation: CBC with differential; Serum IgE level; Stool ova and parasites →
- **Vasculitis**
  - Short-lived lesions; No severe or limited non-cutaneous vasculitis → Urticarial vasculitis (search for etiology); Drug-induced small vessel vasculitis; Eosinophilic vasculitis (exclude hypereosinophilic syndrome or AI–CTD)
  - Asthma; P-ANCA; Anti-myeloperoxidase Ab; Systemic manifestations → Eosinophilic granulomatous polyangiitis (Churg–Strauss syndrome)
- **No vasculitis**
  - Localized → Arthropod bites; Allergic contact dermatitis; Atopic dermatitis; Granuloma faciale
  - Follicular; Pustular → Eosinophilic folliculitis → Immunocompromised, including HIV+ / Ofuji disease
  - Widespread*/regional; ± Peripheral blood eosinophilia → Drug eruption; Atopic dermatitis; Urticaria; Papular urticaria§; Scabies; "Dermal hypersensitivity reaction"¶; Papuloerythroderma of Ofuji; → Parasitic infections
  - Multi-organ involvement; Peripheral blood eosinophilia → Parasitic infections; Hypereosinophilic syndromes**
  - Elderly → Positive BMZ antibodies by direct IF → Bullous pemphigoid
  - Cellulitic plaque(s) with distinctive flame figures seen on histology → Wells syndrome

* If lesions persist, need to exclude lymphoma or myeloproliferative disorder
** CBC >1500 eosinophils/microliter on 2 occasions at least 1 month apart and/or tissue hypereosinophilia that leads to organ damage
§ More common in children
¶ Catch-all term that can encompass more poorly defined entities (e.g. itchy red bump disease, urticarial dermatitis, papular dermatitis) in which the antigen is unknown
BMZ=basement membrane zone
IF=immunofluorescence

OTHER DISORDERS WHERE EOSINOPHILS PLAY A ROLE
• Parasitic infections (e.g. larva migrans, onchocerciasis, gnathostomiasis, strongyloidiasis)
• Seabather's eruption – after ocean swimming, pruritic papules in distribution of swimsuit; due to larvae of either jellyfish (*Linuche unguiculata*) or sea anemones (*Edwardsiella lineata*)
• Pruritic papular eruption of HIV disease – nonfollicular pruritic papules
• Polymorphic eruption of pregnancy (also referred to as PUPPP) – urticarial plaques with involvement of striae and periumbilical sparing; pregnant women (third trimester, postpartum)
• Pemphigoid gestationis – urticarial plaques and vesicles similar to bullous pemphigoid; pregnant women
• Angiolymphoid hyperplasia with eosinophilia (epithelioid hemangioma) – nodules of the head and neck; adults
• Langerhans cell histiocytosis (see Ch. 76)
Limited to neonates or infants
• Erythema toxicum neonatorum – papules and pustules with erythematous flare; neonates
• Incontinentia pigmenti (stages I and II) – linear streaks of vesicles and keratotic papules along the lines of Blaschko
• Infantile eosinophilic folliculitis – recurrent crops of pruritic follicular papules and pustules, primarily of the head and neck

Table 20.1 Other disorders where eosinophils play a role (in addition to those listed in Fig. 20.1). PUPPP, pruritic urticarial papules and plaques of pregnancy.

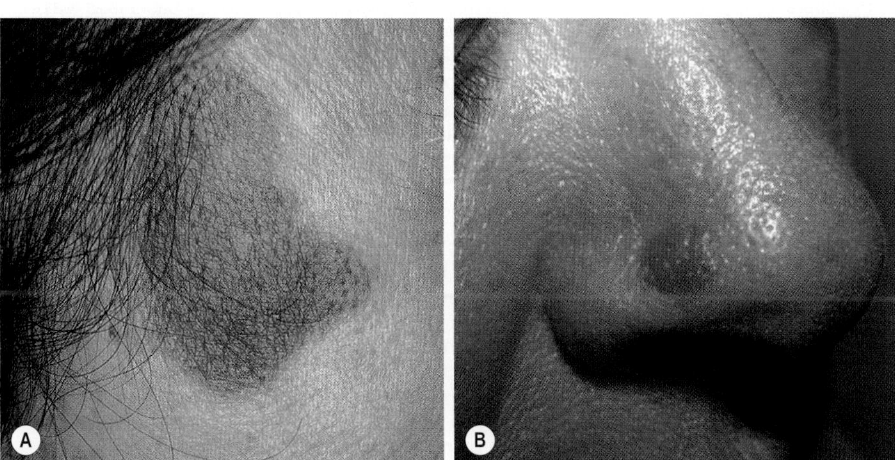

Fig. 20.2 Granuloma faciale. Red-brown plaques on the lateral cheek **(A)** and nose **(B)**. Note the prominent follicular openings. *A, Courtesy, YDRSC; B, Courtesy, Cloyce L. Stetson, MD.*

• **DDx:** infectious cellulitis (edematous lesions), exaggerated arthropod reactions (see above), parasitic infections, and other causes of pseudocellulitis (see Table 61.2).

• **Rx:** systemic CS; occasionally steroid-sparing agents are needed.

Hypereosinophilic Syndrome

• Classically defined as peripheral eosinophilia (>1500 eosinophils/microliter) on two occasions at least one month apart and/or tissue hypereosinophilia leading to multi-organ involvement, but in the absence of an identifiable cause (Table 20.2).

• Divided into major forms: (1) primary (neoplastic) – characterized by specific mutations, in particular the *FIP1L1-PDGFRA* fusion gene, that lead to a clonal proliferation of eosinophils, with a male predominance, and endomyocardial disease; and (2) secondary (reactive) – characterized by a cytokine-driven hypereosinophilia due to an underlying inflammatory or neoplastic disorder (e.g. lymphoma). In the lymphocytic (lymphoid) subtype, clonal T cells produce Th2 cytokines, e.g. IL-5, which activate eosinophils.

• Mucocutaneous lesions are seen in at least 50% of patients and include nonspecific pruritic erythematous papules and nodules, urticaria, angioedema, dermatitis, erythroderma, and in the myeloproliferative form, mouth or anogenital ulcers; thromboses can lead to retiform purpura.

• **DDx:** with the exception of granuloma faciale and eosinophilic folliculitis, the entities outlined in Fig. 20.1; several of the entities in Table 20.1, in particular parasitic infections; hereditary and acquired angioedema; for lymphoproliferative form, cutaneous T-cell lymphoma; if oral ulcers, oral aphthae.

• **Rx:** *FIP1L1-PDGFRA*-positive myeloproliferative form – imatinib, other tyrosine kinase inhibitors (e.g. nilotinib); lymphoproliferative form – systemic CS ± mepolizumab (anti-IL-5 monoclonal antibody).

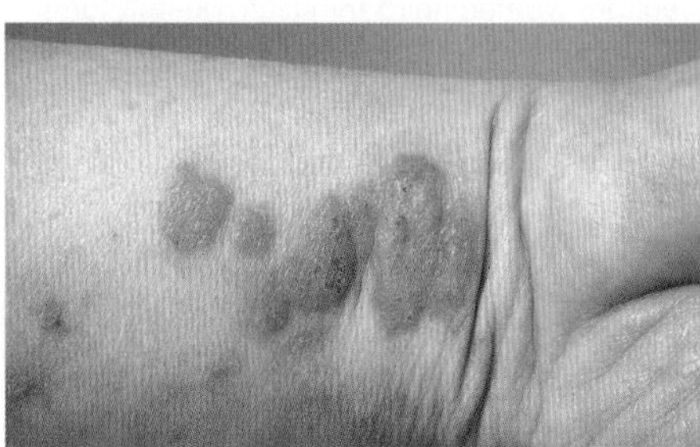

Fig. 20.3 Wells syndrome. Edematous and infiltrated nodules and plaques. *Courtesy, NYUDSC.*

<table>
<tr><th colspan="3">DIAGNOSTIC CRITERIA AND CLASSIFICATION OF HYPEREOSINOPHILIC SYNDROMES (HES)</th></tr>
<tr><td colspan="3">Diagnostic criteria</td></tr>
<tr><td colspan="3">• Peripheral blood eosinophil counts >1500/microliter (1.5 × 10⁹/L) on two occasions at least one month apart and/or major tissue hypereosinophilia (includes marked deposition of eosinophil granule proteins, >20% eosinophils in bone marrow biopsy)
• Organ damage and/or dysfunction attributable to tissue hypereosinophilia
• Exclusion of other disorders or conditions as major reasons for organ damage (e.g. parasitic infection, drug hypersensitivity reaction, primary immunodeficiency [see Ch. 49])</td></tr>
<tr><td colspan="3">Subtypes</td></tr>
<tr><td>Primary (neoplastic) HES</td><td>Secondary (reactive) HES</td><td>Other syndromes†</td></tr>
<tr><td rowspan="3">• Underlying neoplasm of stem cells, myeloid cells or eosinophils
• Eosinophils are considered (or shown) to be clonal*
• Male predominance, endomyocardial disease; mucosal ulcers poor prognostic sign
• Some patients have high serum tryptase and vitamin B12 levels, tissue fibrosis, splenomegaly, and bone marrow biopsies with increased numbers of CD25+ atypical spindle-shaped mast cells (see Table 96.1)</td><td>• Underlying inflammatory or neoplastic disorder
• Hypereosinophilia is cytokine-driven rather than due to clonal proliferation of eosinophils
• In the lymphocytic (lymphoid) subtype, clonal T cells produce Th2 cytokines, e.g. IL-5</td><td rowspan="3">• Episodic angioedema with eosinophilia (EAE; Gleich syndrome)
• Nodules, eosinophilia, rheumatism, dermatitis, and swelling (NERDS) syndrome
• IgG4-related diseases
• Eosinophilic granulomatosis with polyangiitis</td></tr>
<tr><td>Idiopathic HES</td></tr>
<tr><td>• No identified reactive or neoplastic disorder that induces hypereosinophilia</td></tr>
</table>

**FIP1L1-PDGFRA fusion gene and other rarer fusion genes or rearrangements involving PDGFRB or FGR1, which encode platelet-derived growth factor receptor-β and fibroblast growth factor receptor-1, respectively; included patients with eosinophilic leukemia who may have other cytogenetic abnormalities.*
†List is not exhaustive.

Table 20.2 Diagnostic criteria and classification of hypereosinophilic syndromes (HES).

For further information see Ch. 25 from *Dermatology, Fourth Edition*.

For additional online figures visit www.expertconsult.com 

Neutrophilic Dermatoses 21

This group of disorders, in an untreated state, is characterized by infiltrates of neutrophils within the skin. In addition, these dermatoses lack an identifiable infectious etiology, despite the presence of neutrophils (Fig. 21.1). There can be significant overlap in the clinical presentations of the neutrophilic dermatoses; for example, in a patient with acute myelogenous leukemia, bullous pyoderma gangrenosum may be difficult to distinguish from Sweet syndrome. In addition, infiltrates of neutrophils can occur in other organs, particularly the joints, eyes, lungs, and bones. Bone involvement raises the possibility of SAPHO (*s*ynovitis, *a*cne, *p*ustulosis, *h*yperostosis, *o*steitis) syndrome.

Sweet Syndrome (Acute Febrile Neutrophilic Dermatosis)

- Acute onset of erythematous edematous papules and plaques that are tender, but not pruritic; if the edema is intense, the lesions may become bullous and, occasionally, they resemble erysipelas; favored sites are the face, neck, upper trunk, and upper extremities (Fig. 21.2).
- Less commonly, nodules develop due to neutrophilic panniculitis or pustules form within the plaques; a variant occurs on the dorsal aspect of the hands and is referred to as "neutrophilic dermatosis of the dorsal hands" (Fig. 21.3).
- Associated systemic findings include fever, malaise, and arthralgias, and a peripheral leukocytosis is commonly observed (Table 21.1); some patients also develop systemic manifestations, including ocular, pulmonary, and skeletal involvement (Fig. 21.4, Table 21.2).
- Most often seen in adults, with a female:male ratio of 4:1 (except in the case of malignancy-associated disease); may first appear or flare during pregnancy; idiopathic in up to 50% of patients.
- Underlying disorders include: (1) *infections* – upper respiratory tract (e.g. viral, streptococcal) or gastrointestinal (e.g. yersiniosis) > HIV or atypical mycobacteria; (2) *hematologic malignancies* (10–20% of patients), particularly acute myelogenous leukemia (AML) but also myelodysplasia and myeloproliferative disorders; (3) *inflammatory bowel disease*; (4) *autoimmune connective tissue disease*, particularly systemic lupus erythematosus (SLE); (5) *drugs* – G-CSF, all-*trans*-retinoic acid > furosemide, minocycline; and (6) *carcinomas* – genitourinary, breast, colon.
- The vesiculobullous form is more often associated with AML, and in malignancy-associated Sweet syndrome, the lesions tend to be more widespread, including within the oral cavity.
- Histologically, diffuse infiltrates of neutrophils are seen within the dermis and occasionally the subcutaneous fat; leukocytoclastic vasculitis is absent or minimal. The infiltrate may include immature myeloid cells that resemble histiocytes.
- **DDx:** bullous pyoderma gangrenosum, neutrophilic eccrine hidradenitis, erysipelas, erythema multiforme, causes of pseudocellulitis (see Table 61.2), infectious cellulitis, vasculitis (urticarial, small vessel, septic), halogenoderma, autoinflammatory diseases, as well as additional entities in Fig. 21.1.
- There are differing opinions regarding whether the development of a non-bullous neutrophilic dermatosis in the setting of LE is a distinct entity or is simply Sweet syndrome associated with LE.
- **Rx:** usually spontaneously resolves over a few months, but may recur in up to 30% to 50% of patients with idiopathic versus malignancy-associated disease, respectively;

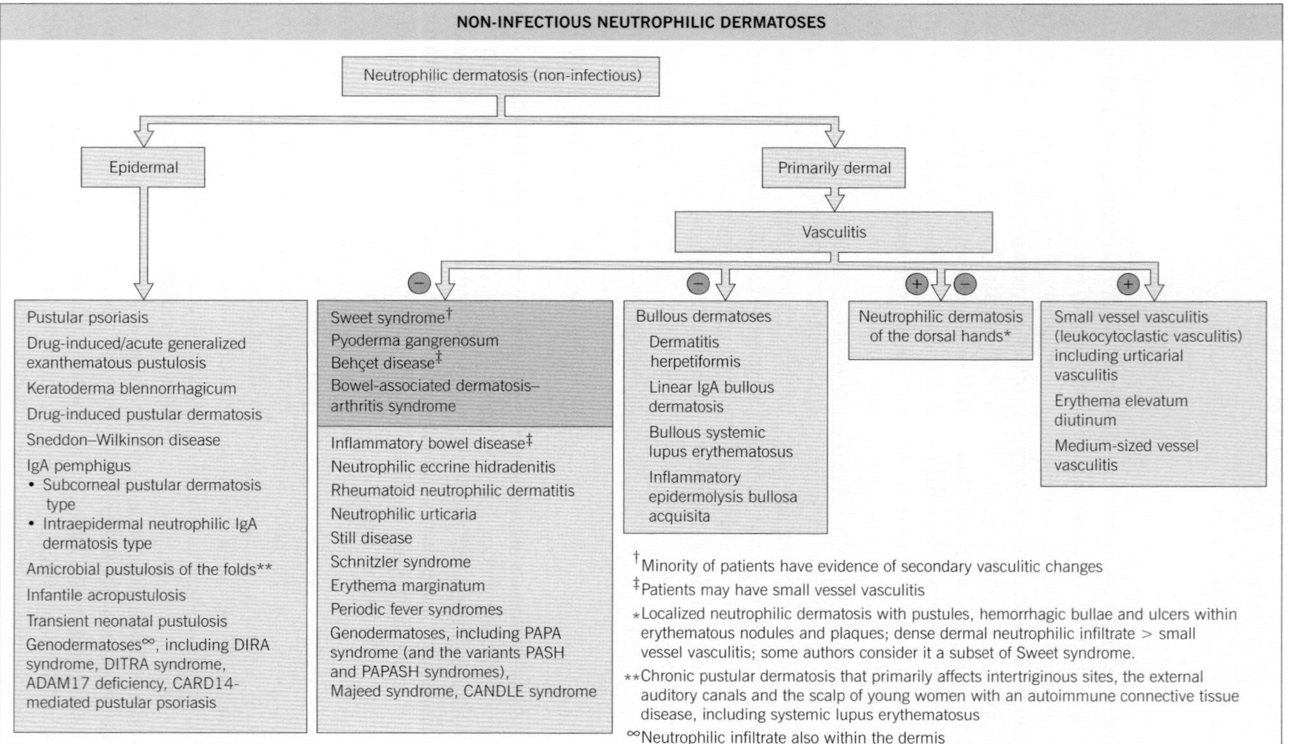

Fig. 21.1 Non-infectious neutrophilic dermatoses. Entities in the darker box are discussed in this chapter. CANDLE, chronic atypical neutrophilic dermatosis with lipodystrophy and elevated temperature; DIRA, deficiency of interleukin-1 receptor antagonist; DITRA, deficiency of the IL-36R antagonist; PAPA, pyogenic arthritis, pyoderma gangrenosum, and acne; PAPASH, pyogenic arthritis, pyoderma gangrenosum, acne, and suppurative hidradenitis; PASH, pyoderma gangrenosum, acne, and suppurative hidradenitis.

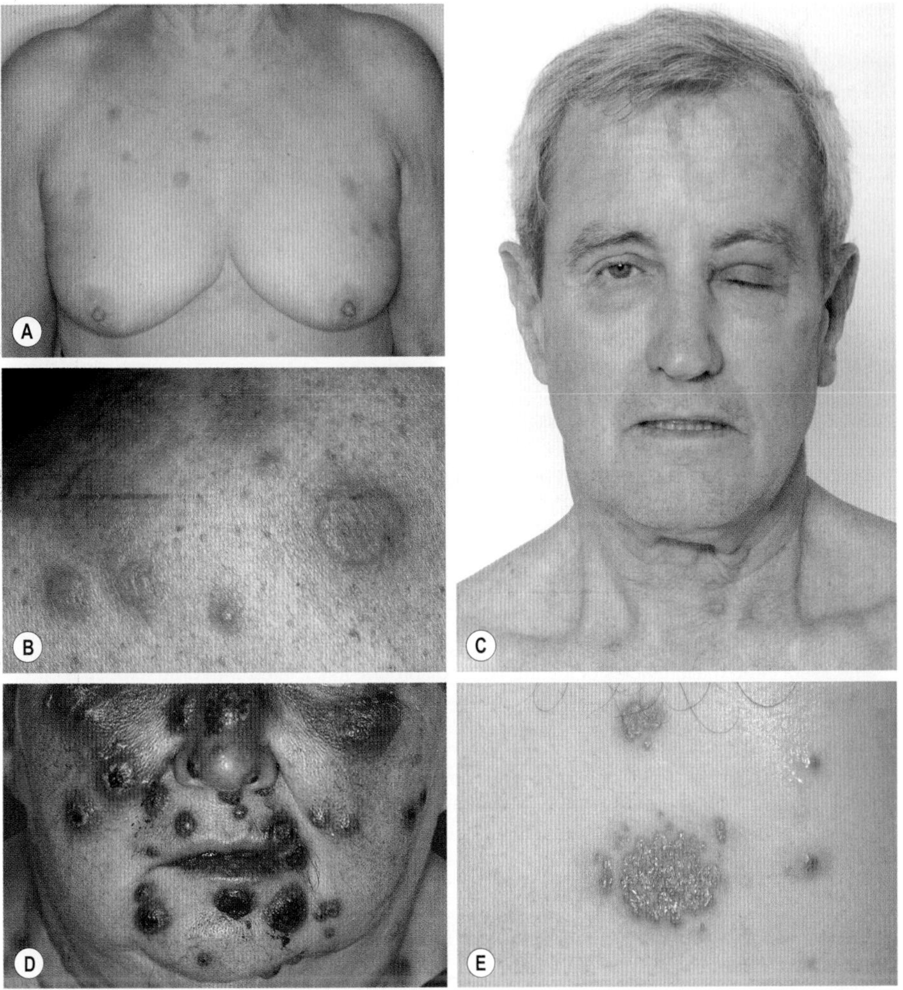

Fig. 21.2 Spectrum of cutaneous findings in Sweet syndrome. **A** Scattered edematous pink papules and plaques on the chest. **B** Markedly edematous plaques on the upper back, some of which are pseudovesicular while others are becoming bullous. **C** The periocular lesion demonstrates how some lesions can mimic cellulitis (pseudocellulitis). This patient also had neutrophilic esophageal ulcerations and subsequently developed colon cancer. **D** Central hemorrhagic crusts within facial plaques. **E** Plaques can also have a pseudomammillated appearance due to the associated edema. *A, C, Courtesy, Mark Davis, MD; B, D, Courtesy, Kalman Watsky, MD; E, Courtesy, Mark Davis, MD.*

antimicrobials for any underlying infection such as streptococcal pharyngitis; for moderate to severe disease, systemic CS (e.g. prednisone 0.5–1 mg/kg/day tapered over several months), dapsone, potassium iodide; for milder disease, ultrapotent topical CS and NSAIDs.

Pyoderma Gangrenosum (PG)

- The most common presentation is a painful, rapidly enlarging ulcer of the lower extremity with a gray-violet, undermined, necrotic border; there is often a peripheral rim of erythema, and the base of the ulcer may be purulent (Fig. 21.5).
- Ulcers can occur at other sites, including the face, upper extremities, and trunk, as well as peristomally (Fig. 21.6); once partially treated, the ulcer may lose some of its characteristic features.
- Lesions can begin as an inflammatory papulopustule (which may be follicular), as a bulla on a violaceous base, or at the site of trauma

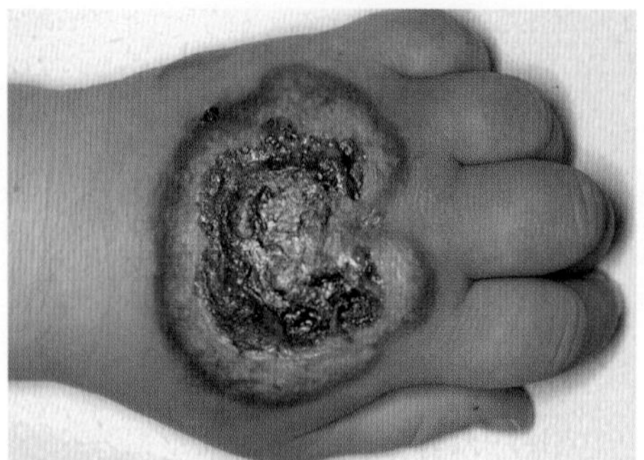

Fig. 21.3 Neutrophilic dermatosis of the dorsal hands. Clinically and histologically, there is overlap with Sweet syndrome and bullous pyoderma gangrenosum. *Courtesy, Mark Davis, MD.*

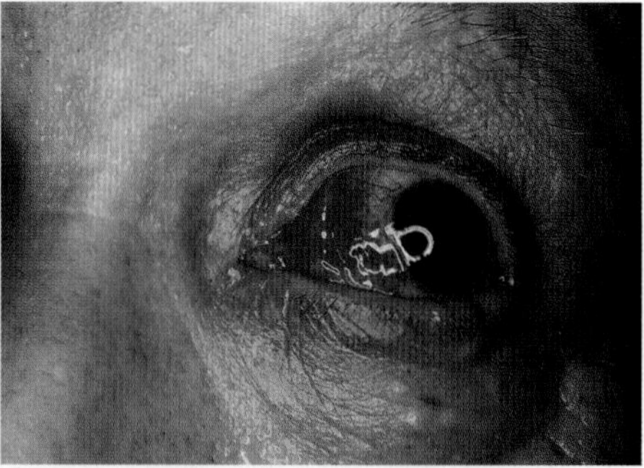

Fig. 21.4 Ocular involvement in Sweet syndrome. Erythema and hemorrhage of the sclera and conjunctiva. *Courtesy, Kalman Watsky, MD.*

CRITERIA FOR THE DIAGNOSIS OF SWEET SYNDROME
Major criteria
1. Abrupt onset of typical cutaneous lesions 2. Histopathology consistent with Sweet syndrome
Minor criteria
1. Preceded by one of the associated infections or vaccinations; accompanied by one of the associated malignancies or inflammatory disorders; associated with drug exposure or pregnancy 2. Presence of fever and constitutional signs and symptoms 3. Leukocytosis 4. Excellent response to systemic corticosteroids

Table 21.1 Criteria for the diagnosis of Sweet syndrome. Both of the major criteria and two of the minor criteria are needed for the diagnosis. *From Su WPD, Liu HNH. Diagnostic criteria for Sweet syndrome. Cutis 1986;37:167–174.*

SYSTEMIC MANIFESTATIONS OF SWEET SYNDROME
Common (≥50%) • Fever • Leukocytosis
Less common (20–50%) • Arthralgias • Arthritis: asymmetric, non-erosive, sterile, favors knees and wrists • Myalgias • Ocular involvement: conjunctivitis, episcleritis, limbal nodules, iridocyclitis
Uncommon • Neutrophilic alveolitis: cough, dyspnea, and pleurisy; radiographic findings include interstitial infiltrates, nodules, pleural effusions • Multifocal sterile osteomyelitis, a subtype of SAPHO syndrome • Renal involvement (e.g. mesangial glomerulonephritis): hematuria, proteinuria, renal insufficiency, acute renal failure
Unusual/rare • Acute myositis • Hepatitis, pancreatitis, ileitis, colitis • Aseptic meningitis, encephalitis, bilateral sensorineural hearing loss • Other: aortitis, oral aphthae, pharyngitis, pharyngeal edema

Table 21.2 Systemic manifestations of Sweet syndrome. SAPHO, synovitis, acne, pustulosis, hyperostosis, osteitis.

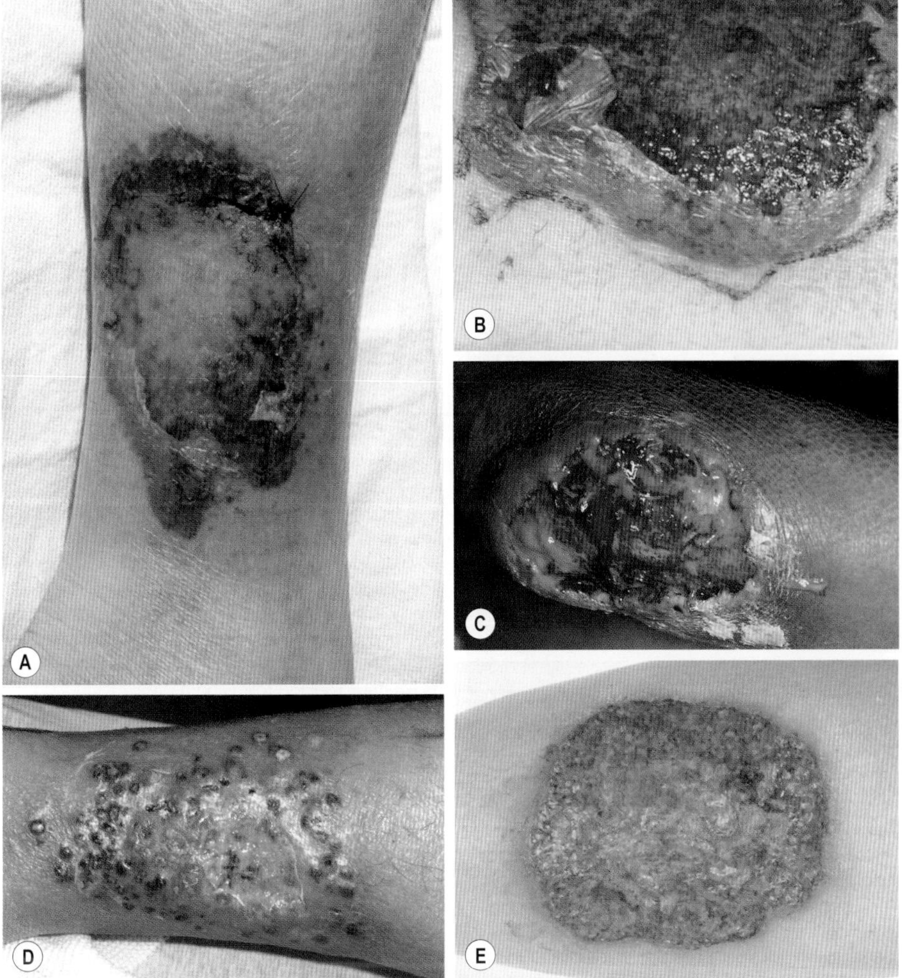

Fig. 21.5 Classic ulcerative pyoderma gangrenosum. A,B The ulcers have an undermined and overhanging violet-gray edge surrounded by a violaceous border; a peripheral erythematous rim is also present in **A**. **C** In addition to an overhanging border, this deep ulceration on the elbow has a purulent base. **D** Central ulceration surrounded by inflammatory papules and pustules. **E** Centrally, there is healing with cribriform (sievelike) scarring. *A, B, E, Courtesy, Mark Davis, MD; C, D, Courtesy, YDRSC.*

(pathergy) (Fig. 21.7); in some patients, especially those with underlying inflammatory bowel disease and/or arthritis, the ulcers may expand more slowly with significant granulation tissue in their bases; healing of PG ulcers often leads to a distinctive cribriform pattern of scarring (Fig. 21.5E).

• There are several clinical variants of PG and they are outlined in Table 21.3; the diagnosis of PG requires clinicopathologic correlation and exclusion of other entities in the **DDx** (Tables 21.4 and 21.5).

• Although idiopathic in up to 50% of patients, the age distribution of PG tends to reflect the major underlying disorders, which are: (1) *inflammatory bowel disease*, either ulcerative colitis or Crohn disease (20–30% of patients); (2) *inflammatory arthritis*, including rheumatoid and seronegative (20%); (3) *plasma cell dyscrasias*, particularly an IgA monoclonal gammopathy (up to 15%); and (4) *other hematologic malignancies*, particularly AML, as well as myelodysplasia, chronic myelogenous leukemia, and hairy cell leukemia; the underlying disorder may be antecedent, coincident, or subsequent.

• PG is included in a few rare syndromes that have various combinations of sterile

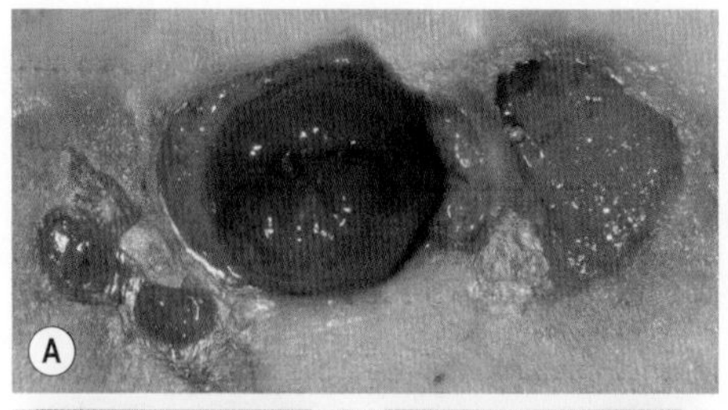

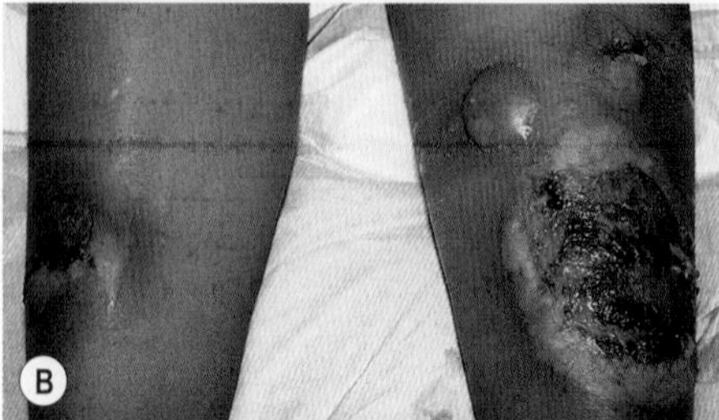

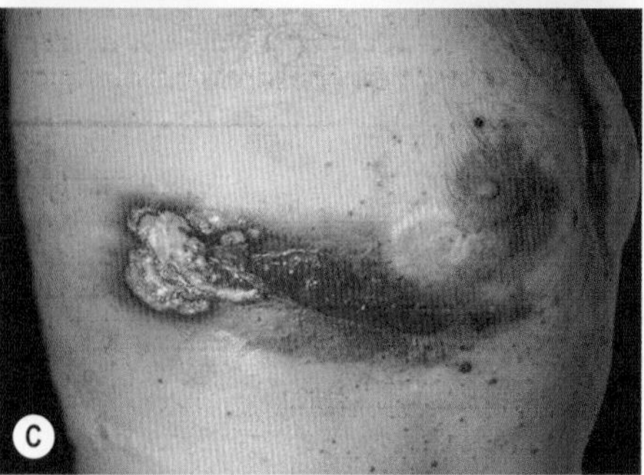

Fig. 21.6 Pyoderma gangrenosum (PG) and underlying disorders – ulcerative colitis and PAPA syndrome. **A** Multiple ulcers surround an ileostomy (following a total proctocolectomy) in a patient with refractory chronic ulcerative colitis. Although peristomal PG occurs most commonly following intestinal resection of inflammatory bowel disease, it can also follow resection of gastrointestinal or bladder carcinoma. **B** Bullous PG in a patient with ulcerative colitis. **C** PG in a patient with PAPA syndrome (pyogenic arthritis, PG, and acne). *A, Courtesy, Mark Davis, MD; B, Courtesy, YDRSC; C, Courtesy, Maria Chanco Turner, MD.*

arthritis, acne, and hidradenitis suppurativa – e.g. PAPA (*p*yogenic sterile *a*rthritis, *P*G and *a*cne; Fig. 21.6C), PASH (*P*G, *a*cne, *s*uppurative *h*idradenitis), and PAPASH (*p*yogenic *a*rthritis, *P*G, *a*cne, *s*uppurative *h*idradenitis) syndromes.

- **DDx** for classic ulcerative PG: in the *untreated state*, it consists primarily of infectious etiologies and vasculitis, but in a *partially treated state* (usually with oral CS), it includes a host of other causes of ulcers, from venous ulcers to lymphoma and SCC to drug-induced (see Fig. 86.1).

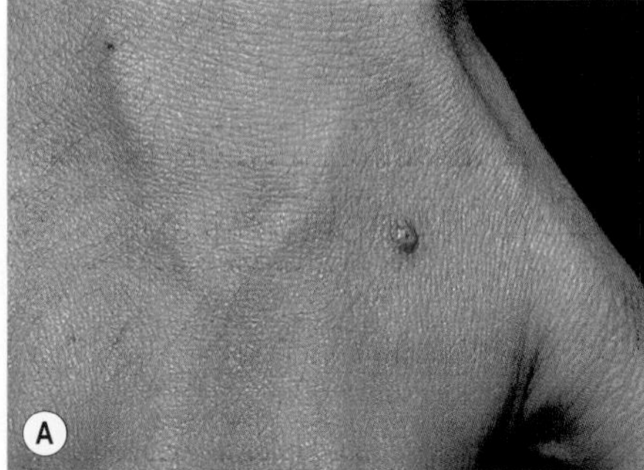

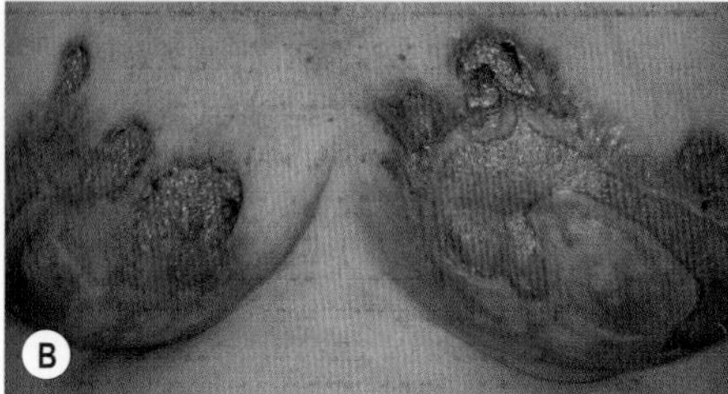

Fig. 21.7 Pyoderma gangrenosum (PG) – early lesion and demonstration of pathergy. **A** The earliest clinical lesion is a pustule with an inflammatory base; this patient had Crohn disease. **B** Postsurgical PG following a breast reduction; multiple debridements had been performed and systemic antibiotics administered because the original diagnosis was soft tissue infection. *A, Courtesy, YDRSC; B, Courtesy, Mark Davis, MD.*

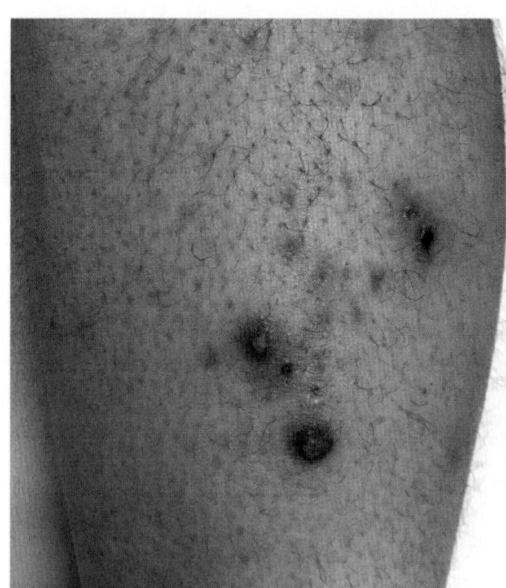

Fig. 21.8 Pyoderma gangrenosum – pustular variant. *Courtesy, Karynne O. Duncan, MD.*

- **Rx:** treatment of the underlying disorder; systemic CS (e.g. prednisone 1 mg/kg/day), intralesional CS into the edge of the ulcer (e.g. triamcinolone 5–10 mg/cc, but initially only a few test sites to confirm no worsening due to pathergy),

CLINICAL VARIANTS OF PYODERMA GANGRENOSUM (PG)
Vesiculobullous (also referred to as atypical or bullous PG)
• Lesions favor the face and upper extremities, especially the dorsal hands • Clinical appearance overlaps with the superficial bullous variant of Sweet syndrome (Fig. 21.6B) • Occurs most commonly in the setting of acute myelogenous leukemia, myelodysplasia, and myeloproliferative disorders such as chronic myelogenous leukemia and when drug-induced (e.g. G-CSF)
Pustular
• Multiple, small, sterile pustules (Fig. 21.8) • Lesions usually regress without scarring, but can evolve into classic PG • Most commonly observed in patients with inflammatory bowel disease • Similar eruption may be seen in patients with Behçet disease or bowel-associated dermatosis–arthritis syndrome
Superficial granulomatous pyoderma
• Localized, superficial vegetative or ulcerative lesion, which favors the trunk and usually follows trauma (e.g. surgery) • Base of ulcer more likely to have granulation, rather than necrotic, tissue • Histologically, a superficial granulomatous response with a less intense neutrophilic infiltrate • Tends to respond to less aggressive anti-inflammatory therapy • Controversy as to whether it is a variant of PG, a separate disorder, or related to granulomatosis with polyangiitis (formerly Wegener granulomatosis)
Pyostomatitis vegetans
• Chronic, vegetative, sterile pyoderma of the labial and buccal mucosa (Fig. 21.9A) • May be associated with vegetative or ulcerative cutaneous PG (Fig. 21.9B) • Seen in patients with inflammatory bowel disease

Table 21.3 Clinical variants of pyoderma gangrenosum (PG). G-CSF, granulocyte colony-stimulating factor.

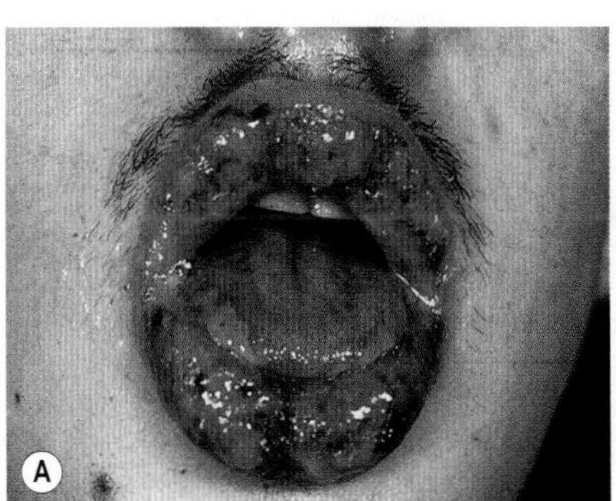

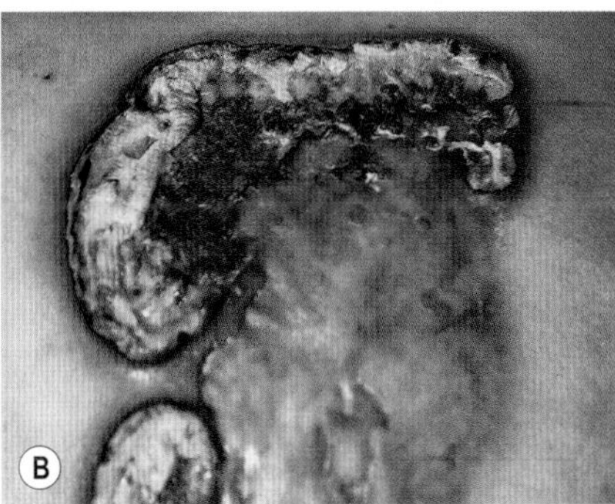

Fig. 21.9 Pyostomatitis vegetans and vegetative pyoderma gangrenosum (PG). A Suppurative pyostomatitis vegetans in a patient with ulcerative colitis. **B** Vegetative form of PG following trauma to the skin. *Courtesy, Samuel L. Moschella, MD.*

CS-impregnated tape when peristomal, pulse CS (1g IV for 3–5 days), cyclosporine, TNF inhibitors; for mild or slowly progressive disease, ultrapotent topical CS, topical tacrolimus, minocycline, dapsone, clofazimine.

Behçet Disease

• A multisystem disease (Table 21.6) whose mucocutaneous features include aphthous orogenital ulcers (Fig. 21.10), sterile pustules (occasionally follicular), and palpable purpura due to small vessel vasculitis, as well as superficial thrombophlebitis and erythema nodosum-like lesions.

• Because the diagnosis is made clinically, there are several sets of criteria, including the one outlined in Table 21.7; there are countries in which the disease is more commonly seen, e.g. Turkey, Japan, and those along the ancient Silk Road; the peak incidence is ages 20–35 years.

- **DDx:** recurrent genital and intraoral HSV (the latter is limited to keratinized/attached mucosa in immunocompetent hosts; see Ch. 59), simple aphthosis, complex aphthosis, inflammatory bowel disease, SLE, pemphigus vulgaris, lichen planus, Marshall syndrome (periodic fever, aphthous stomatitis, pharyngitis, cervical adenitis).
- Features of both Behçet disease and relapsing polychondritis are seen in MAGIC syndrome, which consists of *m*outh *a*nd *g*enital ulcers with *i*nflamed *c*artilage.

DIAGNOSTIC CRITERIA FOR CLASSIC ULCERATIVE PYODERMA GANGRENOSUM – TWO SCHEMES
Major criteria (2004)
1. Rapid[a] progression of a painful,[b] necrolytic *cutaneous ulcer*[c] *with an* irregular, violaceous and *undermined border* (*plus tenderness and peripheral erythema* for 2018 minor criterion [1])*   2. Other causes of cutaneous ulceration have been excluded[d]
Minor criteria (2004)
1. History suggestive of *pathergy*[e] [2] or clinical finding of *cribriform scarring* [3]**   2. Systemic diseases associated with pyoderma gangrenosum[f]   3. Histopathologic findings (sterile dermal **neutrophilia**, ± mixed inflammation, ± lymphocytic vasculitis)   4. Treatment response (rapid response to systemic corticosteroids)[g]

In the 2004 scheme, diagnosis requires both of the major criteria and at least two minor criteria. In the 2018 scheme, diagnosis requires 1 major criterion (neutrophilic infiltrate [in ***bold***]*) and 4 of 8 minor criteria which are in italics and numbered in [ ].*

[a]*Characteristic margin expansion of 1–2 cm per day, or a 50% increase in ulcer size within 1 month.*

[b]*Pain is usually out of proportion to the size of the ulceration.*

[c]*Typically preceded by a papule, pustule, or bulla (plus rapidly leading to an ulceration is 2018 minor criterion [4]).*

**Major difference between 2004 and 2018 schemes is that the latter requires multiple ulcerations with ≥1 on the anterior lower leg [5].*

[d]*Usually necessitates skin biopsy and additional evaluation (see Table 21.5) to exclude other causes; only exclusion of infection is 2018 minor criterion [6].*

[e]*Ulcer development at sites of minor cutaneous trauma (also 2018 minor criterion [2]).*

***Or "wrinkled paper" scar [3].*

[f]*Inflammatory bowel disease, inflammatory arthritis, IgA gammopathy, or underlying malignancy (history of either of the first two disorders is 2018 minor criterion [7]).*

[g]*Generally responds to prednisone (1–2 mg/kg/day) or another corticosteroid at an equivalent dosage, with a 50% decrease in size within 1 month (2018 minor criterion states just decrease [not %] with immunosuppressive therapy [8]).*

Table 21.4 Diagnostic criteria for classic ulcerative pyoderma gangrenosum – two schemes. *From Su WP, et al. Pyoderma gangrenosum: Clinicopathologic correlation and proposed diagnostic criteria. Int J Dermatol 2004;43:790–800; Maverakis E, et al. Diagnostic criteria of ulcerative pyoderma gangrenosum: A Delphi consensus of international experts. JAMA Dermatol 2018;154:461–8.*

EVALUATION OF A PATIENT WITH PRESUMED PYODERMA GANGRENOSUM
1. Thorough history and physical examination; review medications   2. Sterile skin biopsy of *active* skin lesion with sufficient depth (panniculus) and sufficient tissue for special stains and culture (bacterial, mycobacterial, fungal, and viral). Possibility of future additional biopsies for immunofluorescence or PCR studies   3. Gastrointestinal tract studies – stool for occult blood and parasites, colonoscopy, biopsy, radiography, liver function tests, and, if indicated, hepatitis evaluation   4. Hematologic studies – complete blood and platelet count, peripheral blood smear, and, if indicated, bone marrow examination   5. Serologic studies – serum protein electrophoresis, immunofixation electrophoresis, antinuclear antibodies, antiphospholipid antibodies, ANCA antibodies, VDRL   6. Chest X-ray and urinalysis

Table 21.5 Evaluation of a patient with presumed pyoderma gangrenosum.

SYSTEMIC MANIFESTATIONS OF BEHÇET DISEASE	
Ocular (leading cause of morbidity)	**Neurologic**
• Occurs in 90% of patients; favors men, in whom it is more severe • Can be painful and may lead to blindness • Retinal vasculitis (more frequently associated with blindness) • Posterior uveitis (most characteristic ocular finding) • Anterior uveitis, hypopyon • Secondary glaucoma, cataracts • Conjunctivitis, scleritis, keratitis, vitreous hemorrhage, optic neuritis	• Usually appears later during the evolution of the disease • Associated with a poor prognosis • Acute meningoencephalitis that may resolve spontaneously • Cranial nerve palsies • Brain stem lesions that can induce swallowing difficulties, laughter, and crying • Pyramidal or extrapyramidal signs
Joints	**Vascular**
• Approximately 50% of patients develop arthritis • In majority (~80% of patients), duration of attacks is <2 months • Mono- or polyarthritic and non-erosive • Most commonly knees, wrists, and ankles	• Aneurysmal or occlusive arterial disease • Superficial or deep venous thrombosis **Cardiopulmonary** • Coronary arteritis, valvular disease, myocarditis • Recurrent ventricular arrhythmias • Pulmonary artery aneurysms
Gastrointestinal	**Renal**
• Abdominal pain and/or hemorrhage may be difficult to distinguish from IBD • Ulcerations* develop within the small bowel (particularly the ileocecal region) as well as the transverse and ascending colon and esophagus; perforation can occur	• Glomerulonephritis

Resemble anogenital aphthae.

Table 21.6 Systemic manifestations of Behçet disease. IBD, inflammatory bowel disease.

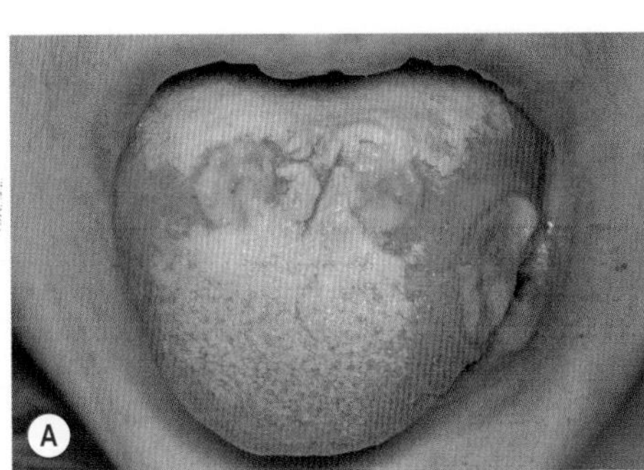

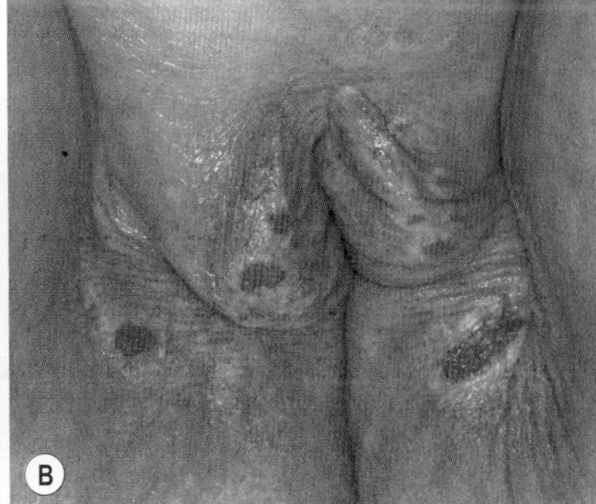

Fig. 21.10 Oral and genital ulcers of Behçet disease. A Three major aphthae on the tongue, which are deeper and larger than minor aphthae but share the presence of a pseudomembrane and associated pain. Oral aphthosis is often the initial symptom of Behçet disease and may flare with the onset of other symptoms. **B** Aphthae of the vulvar and inguinal region. *Courtesy, Mark Davis, MD.*

Bowel-Associated Dermatosis–Arthritis Syndrome (Bowel Bypass Syndrome)

- Although initially described following jejunoileal bypass, this syndrome can develop in association with blind loops of bowel due to surgery or inflammatory bowel disease; presumably, there is overgrowth of bacteria and formation of immune complexes containing bacterial antigens that leads to a serum sickness-like picture.
- Cutaneous lesions include erythematous and purpuric papules and vesiculopustules as well as subcutaneous nodules that are accompanied by polyarthritis and tenosynovitis.

Synovitis, Acne, Pustulosis, Hyperostosis, and Osteitis (SAPHO) Syndrome

- Characterized by aseptic neutrophilic dermatoses plus aseptic osteoarticular involvement, with a subtype referred to as chronic recurrent multifocal osteomyelitis; the latter favors the anterior chest and axial skeleton.
- Associated skin disorders include: (1) the "acne family" – acne fulminans, follicular occlusion tetrad; (2) the "psoriasis family" – palmoplantar pustulosis, pustular psoriasis, psoriasis vulgaris, Sneddon–Wilkinson disease; (3) linear IgA bullous dermatosis; and (4) the neutrophilic dermatoses discussed in this chapter.

INTERNATIONAL STUDY GROUP CRITERIA FOR THE DIAGNOSIS OF BEHÇET DISEASE	
Criteria	**Required features**
Major criterion:	
Recurrent oral ulceration	Aphthous (idiopathic) oral ulceration observed by physician or patient, recurring at least three times in a 12-month period
Plus any two of the following minor criteria:	
Recurrent genital ulceration	Aphthous genital ulceration or scarring, observed by physician or patient
Eye lesions	Anterior or posterior uveitis; cells in the vitreous by slit lamp examination; or retinal vasculitis observed by ophthalmologist
Cutaneous lesions	Erythema nodosum-like lesions observed by physician or patient; papulopustular lesions or pseudofolliculitis; or characteristic acneiform nodules observed by physician in postadolescent patient not on corticosteroids
Pathergy test*	Interpreted at 24–48 hours by physician

**Pathergy test is performed on the flexor forearm by obliquely inserting a 20- to 22-gauge sterile hypodermic needle to a depth of 5 mm ± an intradermal injection of 0.1 ml of normal saline. A positive reaction is defined as the development of a papule or pustule.*

Table 21.7 International study group criteria for the diagnosis of Behçet disease. *From International Study Group for Behçet's disease. Criteria for the diagnosis of Behçet's disease. Lancet 1990;335:1078–1080.*

For further information see Ch. 26 from *Dermatology, Fourth Edition*.

For additional online figures visit www.expertconsult.com 

Pregnancy Dermatoses

22

There are several dermatoses that occur either during pregnancy or immediately postpartum, in particular polymorphic eruption of pregnancy, pemphigoid gestationis, and atopic eruption of pregnancy. Pruritus due to intrahepatic cholestasis of pregnancy leads to nonspecific skin lesions, including excoriations due to scratching. Impetigo herpetiformis simply represents pustular psoriasis occurring during pregnancy, and this may be related to the relative hypocalcemia of pregnancy. Lastly, there are physiologic changes that occur during pregnancy.

Polymorphic Eruption of Pregnancy (PEP; Pruritic Urticarial Papules and Plaques of Pregnancy [PUPPP])

- Relatively common disorder (~1 in 160 deliveries) that begins late in the third trimester or during the immediate postpartum period; occurs primarily in primiparous women, with an increased frequency in those with multigestational pregnancies.
- Pruritic edematous papules and plaques, whose color varies from pink to red-brown depending on skin phototype, that often involve the abdominal striae but spare the umbilicus (Fig. 22.1); the polymorphic presentation includes patches of erythema, targetoid lesions, tiny vesicles, and eczematous plaques (Fig. 22.2).
- Lesions can become widespread, but usually spare the face, palms, and soles; the eruption spontaneously resolves within 4–6 weeks after delivery.
- In general, does not recur with subsequent pregnancies, in contrast to pemphigoid gestationis (PG), and there is no fetal risk.
- **DDx:** PG (may require direct immunofluorescence [DIF] of perilesional skin to distinguish [see Fig. 23.2]), urticarial drug eruption, viral exanthem, allergic contact dermatitis, scabies, erythema multiforme minor.
- **Rx:** topical CS and oral antihistamines usually suffice (Table 22.1); occasionally, severe cases require oral CS (prednisolone preferred during pregnancy because of significant inactivation by placenta, leading to a mother : fetus ratio of 10 : 1).

Pemphigoid Gestationis (PG; Gestational Pemphigoid)

- Unusual pruritic vesiculobullous disorder that has significant clinical and histopathologic overlap with bullous pemphigoid (see Ch. 24).
- Usually develops during the later stages of pregnancy or immediately postpartum and is due to circulating autoantibodies against bullous pemphigoid antigen 180 (BP180) present within the hemidesmosomal component of the basement membrane zone (BMZ).
- In theory, it is related to aberrant expression of MHC class II antigens of paternal origin in the placenta that trigger an autoimmune response to the placental BMZ, followed by cross-reactivity with the BMZ of the skin.
- Lesions often begin on the abdomen, including around and within the umbilicus, but then become more widespread on the trunk as well as the extremities; in addition to vesicles and bullae, edematous urticarial plaques are seen (Fig. 22.3).
- DIF of perilesional skin shows linear deposits of C3 at the BMZ (see Fig. 23.3F).
- Increased risk of small-for-gestational age and premature neonates and ~10% of newborns have mild skin involvement; often flares at the time of delivery and recurs during subsequent pregnancies.
- **DDx:** primarily PEP (but in PEP, patients are usually primiparous, large bullae are rare unless there is marked background edema,

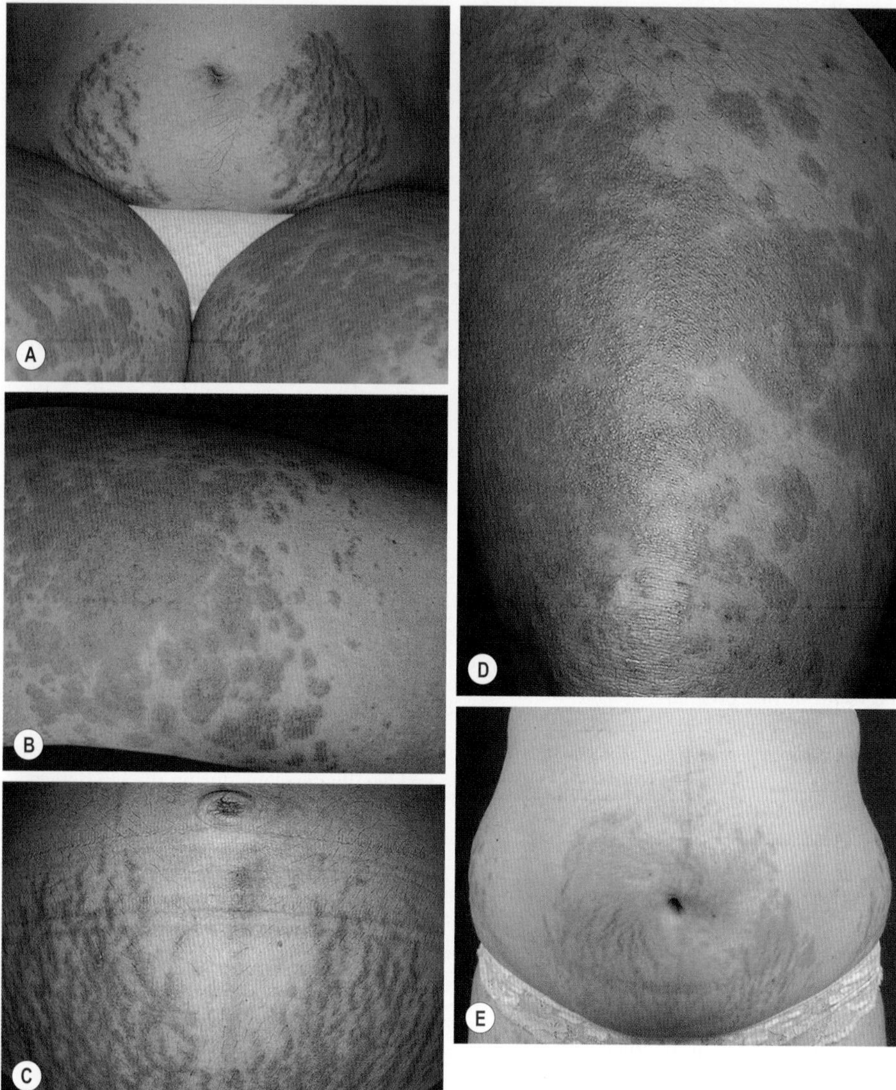

Fig. 22.1 Polymorphic eruption of pregnancy. The edematous urticarial lesions favor the striae **(A, C)** and the upper thighs **(B, D)** and spare the umbilicus. Note the pink color in a woman with skin phototype II versus the red-brown color in a more darkly pigmented patient. **E** Although there is periumbilical involvement, the umbilicus itself is spared and edematous striae point to the diagnosis. *A–D, Courtesy, YDRSC; E, Courtesy, Christina M. Ambros-Rudolph, MD.*

lesions spare the umbilicus, and DIF of perilesional skin is negative) (Fig. 22.4); urticarial drug eruption, allergic contact dermatitis.

- **Rx:** potent topical or oral CS (prednisolone 0.5 mg/kg/day; see Appendix), depending on severity.

Atopic Eruption of Pregnancy

- Pruritic papules and eczematous plaques that usually develop earlier during pregnancy than other disorders described in this chapter (Fig. 22.5).
- Patients have an atopic diathesis, but this eruption is more likely to have its initial presentation during pregnancy and less often it represents a flare of pre-existing atopic dermatitis.
- May be explained by the predominance of a Th2 immune response during pregnancy.
- No maternal or fetal risks, but recurrence during subsequent pregnancies common.

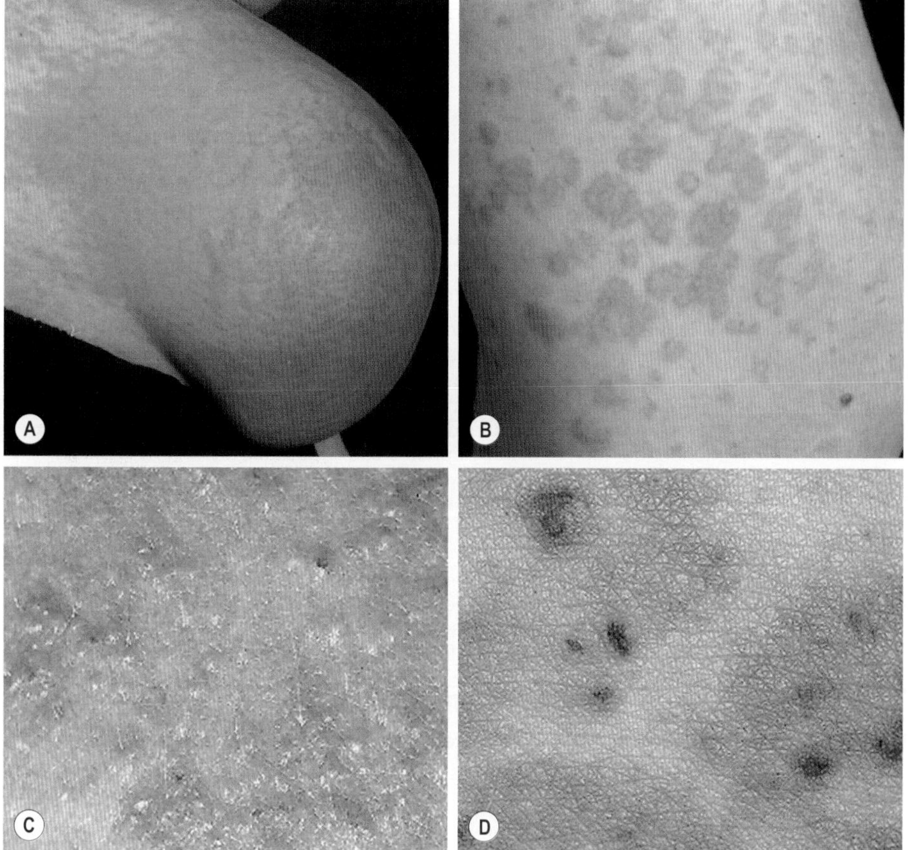

Fig. 22.2 Polymorphic eruption of pregnancy. The clinical spectrum includes: **(A)** macular erythema, which can be widespread; **(B)** targetoid lesions; **(C)** tiny vesicles due to marked epidermal spongiosis or dermal edema; and **(D)** eczematous plaques, especially as lesions age. *A–D, Courtesy, Christina M. Ambros-Rudolph, MD.*

- **DDx:** intrahepatic cholestasis of pregnancy, scabies, allergic contact dermatitis, PEP, drug eruption or viral exanthem (if papular).
- **Rx:** topical CS, oral antihistamines, and other routine therapies for atopic dermatitis (e.g. emollients; oral antibiotics such as cephalexin if secondary bacterial infection; see Ch. 10); NB-UVB phototherapy or oral CS for more severe cases (see Table 22.1).

Intrahepatic Cholestasis of Pregnancy

- Onset usually during the third trimester, related in part to peak in estrogen levels; genetic predisposition with higher incidence in native South Americans; hepatitis C viral infection is also a risk factor.
- Cholestasis leads to elevated serum levels of bile acids and this leads to intense pruritus.
- Cutaneous lesions are nonspecific and vary from excoriations to prurigo nodularis (Fig. 22.6); jaundice occurs in a small minority of patients.
- Important to diagnose because cholestasis of pregnancy is associated with intrapartum fetal distress, prematurity, and stillbirths; in severe cases, vitamin K deficiency may occur, with an increased risk of hemorrhage.
- Diagnosis is based on measurement of total serum bile acids, with elevations typically ranging from 3 to 100 times normal.
- **DDx:** other causes of cholestasis (e.g. primary biliary cholangitis) and hepatitis (e.g. hepatitis B virus, hepatitis C virus), especially if pruritus does not resolve within days of

SPECIAL CONSIDERATIONS FOR CORTICOSTEROID AND ANTIHISTAMINE USE DURING PREGNANCY	
Corticosteroids	
Topical	• Recent large, population-based studies and a Cochrane review have *not* shown an increased risk of malformations, including oral cleft palate, or preterm delivery • Because fetal growth restriction has been reported with extensive use of potent corticosteroids (CS), particularly >300 gm during pregnancy, mild to moderate CS are recommended over potent CS • If potent CS are required, the treatment period should be limited in duration • Can add to risk of developing striae
Systemic	• Prednisolone is the systemic corticosteroid of choice for dermatologic indications as it is largely inactivated in the placenta (mother : fetus = 10 : 1) • During the first trimester, particularly between weeks 8 and 11, there is a possible (debated) slightly increased risk of cleft lip/cleft palate, especially if high doses prescribed and for >10 days; during this same period, a longer duration of therapy appears safe if dosages are <10–15 mg daily • If use is long-term and extends late into gestation, fetal growth should be monitored and the risk of adrenal insufficiency in the newborn should be addressed
Antihistamines	
Systemic	• During the first trimester, the classic sedating agents (e.g. chlorpheniramine, diphenhydramine, clemastine, dimethindene) are preferred because of the preponderance of safety data • If a non-sedating agent is requested, loratadine is the first choice and cetirizine the second choice; both are considered safe throughout pregnancy

Table 22.1 Special considerations for corticosteroid and antihistamine use during pregnancy.

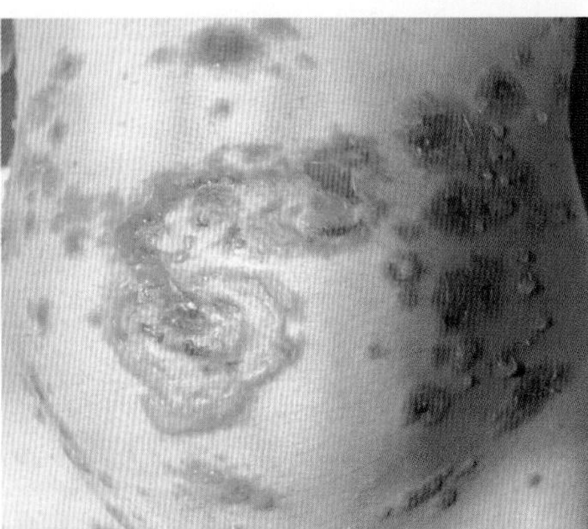

Fig. 22.3 Pemphigoid gestationis. Intact tense bullae arising within areas of edematous erythema as well as erosions due to ruptured bullae. Lesions typically involve the umbilical region. *Courtesy, Christina M. Ambros-Rudolph, MD.*

delivery; scabies, atopic eruption of pregnancy, other causes of primary pruritus (see Fig. 4.2).
• **Rx:** oral ursodeoxycholic acid (300-600 mg twice daily); if elevated prothrombin time, vitamin K injections; alert patient that disorder recurs in at least 50% of subsequent pregnancies.

Physiologic Changes During Pregnancy

These are outlined in Table 22.2.

Autoimmune Progesterone Dermatitis

• Not a specific dermatosis of pregnancy, but may first appear during pregnancy or postpartum.
• Recurrent flares of dermatitis occur during the luteal phase of the menstrual cycle when there is an increase in progesterone levels; pruritus, urticaria, papulovesicles, and erythema multiforme-like lesions can also be seen.
• Urticaria or delayed induration can appear at sites of intradermal injections of progesterone (e.g. 50 mg/ml).

For further information see Ch. 27 from *Dermatology, Fourth Edition*.

For additional online figures and tables, including dermatoses influenced by pregnancy, visit www.expertconsult.com

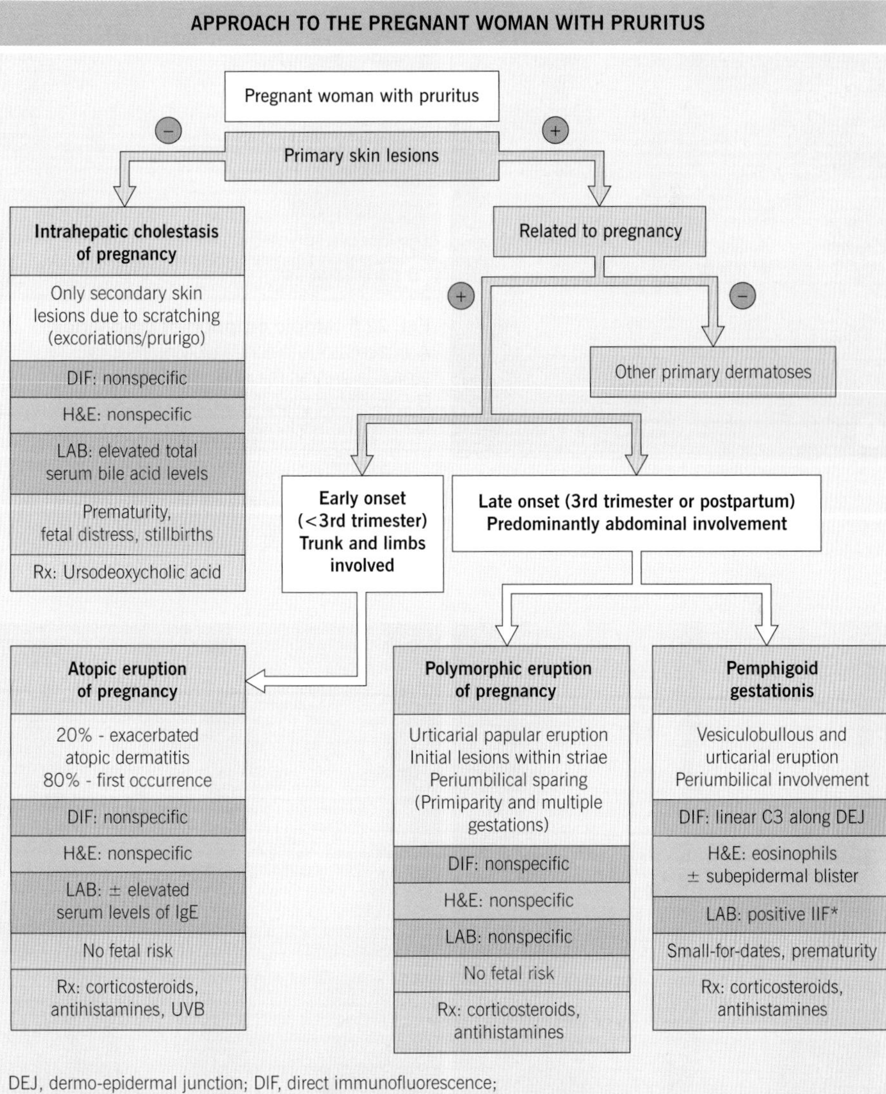

Fig. 22.4 Approach to the pregnant woman with pruritus. Patients with refractory pemphigoid gestationis may benefit from plasmapheresis during pregnancy. Prednisolone is the systemic CS of choice for dermatologic indications during pregnancy as it is largely inactivated in the placenta (mother : fetus ratio = 10 : 1); if use of systemic CS or potent topical CS is long-term during pregnancy, then fetal growth should monitored. During the first trimester, the classic sedating anti-histamines (e.g. chlorpheniramine, diphenhydramine, clemastine) are preferred because of the preponderance of safety data and during the second and third trimesters, if a non-sedating agent is requested, loratidine is the first choice and cetirizine the second choice; both are considered safe. *Courtesy, Christina M. Ambros-Rudolph, MD.*

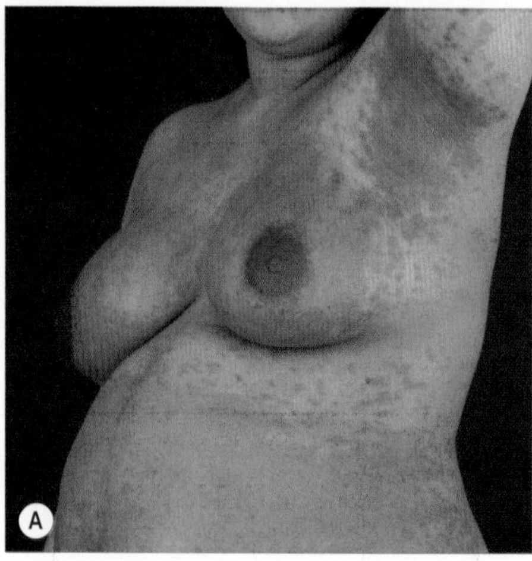

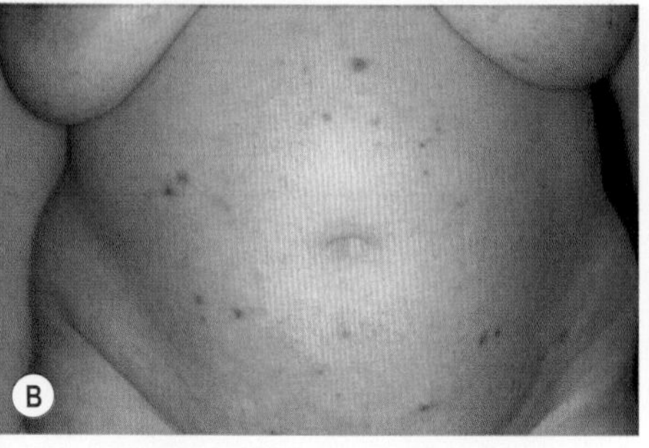

Fig. 22.5 Atopic eruption of pregnancy. **A** Eczematous lesions involving flexural areas as well as the abdomen and breasts. **B** Excoriated papules (prurigo lesions) that favored the abdomen and extremities. The former presentation is seen in approximately two-thirds of patients, whereas the latter is seen in approximately one-third. *Courtesy, Christina M. Ambros-Rudolph, MD.*

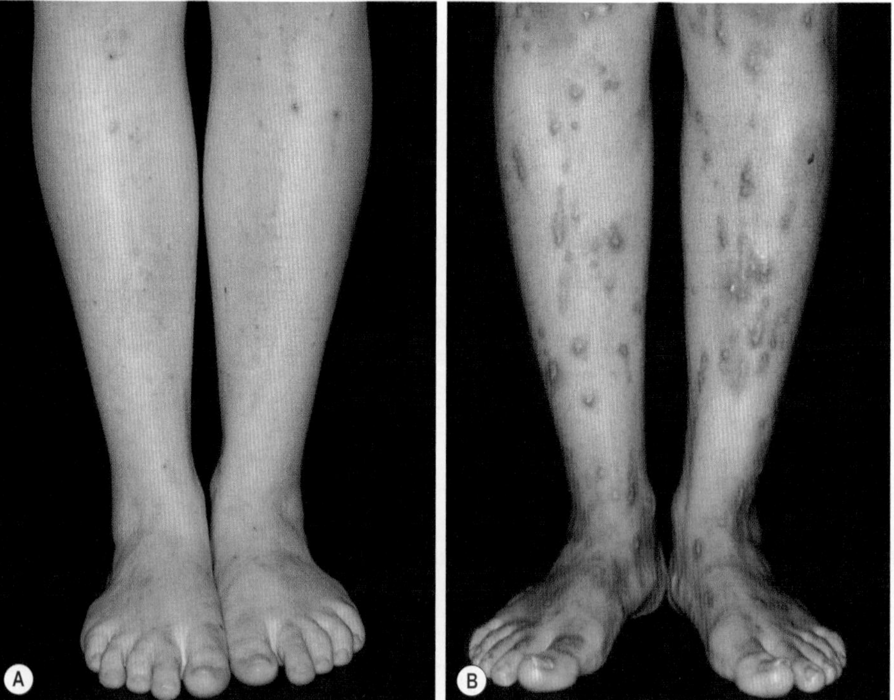

Fig. 22.6 Intrahepatic cholestasis of pregnancy. Marked pruritus leads to secondary skin lesions that vary based on disease duration, from subtle linear excoriations and prurigo simplex early on **(A)** to pronounced prurigo nodularis when the pruritus is longstanding **(B).** *From Ambros-Rudolph CM, Glatz M, Trauner M, Kerl H, Müllegger RR. The importance of serum bile acid level analysis and treatment with ursodeoxycholic acid in intrahepatic cholestasis of pregnancy: A case series from central Europe. Arch. Dermatol. 2007;143:757–762. © (2006) American Medical Association. All rights reserved.*

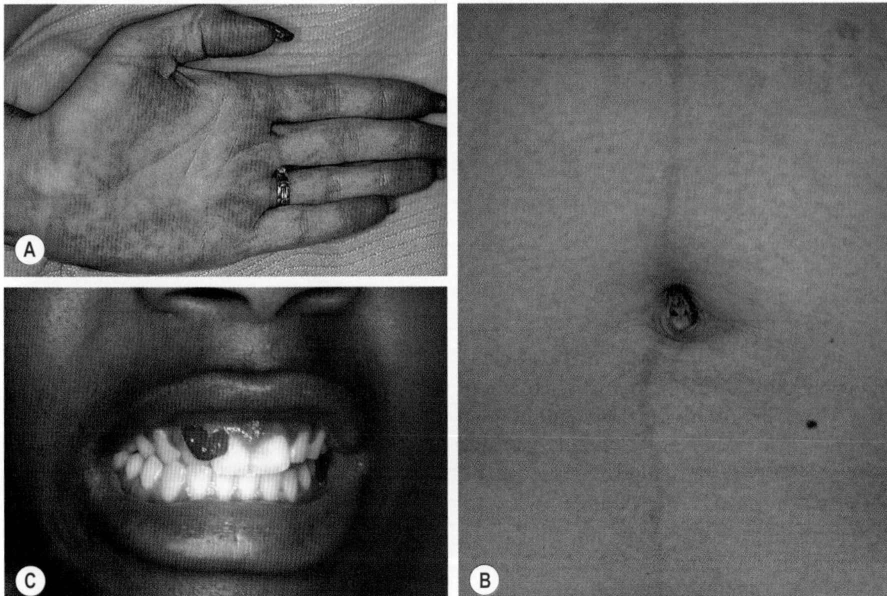

Fig. 22.7 Physiologic changes during pregnancy. A Palmar erythema of pregnancy. **B** Linea nigra. **C** Gingival pyogenic granuloma. *A, C, Courtesy, YDRSC; B, Courtesy, Jean L. Bolognia, MD.*

PHYSIOLOGIC CHANGES DURING PREGNANCY	
Pigmentary	
Hyperpigmentation (e.g. areolae, linea nigra; Fig. 22.7B) Melasma	Hyperpigmentation (up to 90% of patients) and melasma (up to 70% of patients) are presumably of hormonal etiology. Melasma tends to persist postpartum in those with darker skin phototypes
Hair	
Hirsutism Postpartum telogen effluvium Postpartum androgenetic alopecia	Some hirsutism is normal and typically regresses postpartum. Telogen effluvium may last up to 15 months. Postpartum patterned alopecia may or may not revert to normal
Connective tissue	
Striae	Striae gravidarum develop in up to 90% of patients and often resolve. Both hormonal factors and physical stretching of the skin appear to be relevant in their development
Vascular	
Spider angiomas Palmar erythema (Fig. 22.7A) Nonpitting edema Varicosities Vasomotor instability Purpura Gingival hyperemia or hyperplasia Pyogenic granuloma (Fig. 22.7C) Hemorrhoids	Vascular changes result from distention, instability, and new vessel formation. Clinically obvious changes are most pronounced during the third trimester, and most changes regress spontaneously following delivery

Table 22.2 Physiologic changes during pregnancy. Nail changes are nonspecific and include subungual hyperkeratosis, distal onycholysis, transverse grooving, and brittleness. *Adapted from Kroumpouzos G, Cohen LM. Dermatoses of pregnancy. J Am Acad Dermatol. 2001;45:1–19.*

23 Pemphigus

Chapters 23–25 review the major autoimmune bullous diseases (Table 23.1). Because of the overlap in their clinical presentations, histopathologic examination of lesional skin as well as direct immunofluorescence (DIF) of perilesional skin are usually required in order to establish a specific diagnosis (Figs 23.1–23.3). Indirect immunofluorescence (IIF; Fig. 23.2B) and/or ELISA of sera provide additional helpful information; for example, the latter can detect anti-desmoglein 3 (Dsg3) versus anti-Dsg1 antibodies.

Pemphigus is classically divided into three major groups: (1) pemphigus vulgaris, with pemphigus vegetans representing a rare variant; (2) pemphigus foliaceus, with pemphigus erythematosus representing an unusual localized variant, and fogo selvagem, an endemic form; and (3) paraneoplastic pemphigus. Additional subtypes include the two forms of IgA pemphigus and drug-induced pemphigus.

Pemphigus Vulgaris and Pemphigus Vegetans

- Patients have circulating IgG autoantibodies that bind to the cell surface of keratinocytes in the skin and mucous membranes; this binding leads to an inhibition of the function of desmogleins, transmembrane cadherin proteins that are a component of desmosomes and therefore play an important role in cell–cell adhesion.
- In these two disorders, the autoantibodies primarily target Dsg3, which is expressed within the lower portion of the epidermis and is the predominant isoform in mucous membranes; patients with mucosal-dominant disease as well as those with mucocutaneous disease have anti-Dsg3 autoantibodies (the latter group can also have anti-Dsg1 autoantibodies).
- The decrease in cell–cell adhesion leads to the separation of individual keratinocytes from one another (referred to as acantholysis) and the formation of a split within the epidermis or mucosal epithelium, primarily in its lower portion, just above the basal layer (Fig. 23.3B).
- Clinically, almost all patients with pemphigus vulgaris have painful erosions of the oral mucosa and at least half will have flaccid bullae of the skin plus erosions due to their rupture; lesions can be localized or widespread (Fig. 23.4), and there may be involvement of other mucosal surfaces, e.g. conjunctival, nasal, vaginal.
- Additional clinical clues include the development of hemorrhagic crusts of the vermilion lips (Table 23.2) and a positive Nikolsky sign in areas of active disease – the epidermis can be easily moved laterally with rubbing (due to reduction in intercellular adhesion).
- In pemphigus vegetans, vegetative and papillomatous plaques and nodules develop in conjunction with erosions (Fig. 23.5); lesions favor major body folds and pustules can also be seen.
- DIF of perilesional skin demonstrates immunostaining of the cell surface of keratinocytes within the epidermis or mucosa in almost all patients, and the staining may be more predominant in the lower portion of the epithelium (Fig. 23.3C); IIF and ELISA of sera is positive in more than 90% of patients (Fig. 23.2B).
- **DDx:** other forms of pemphigus, bullous pemphigoid, linear IgA bullous dermatosis (LABD), Hailey–Hailey disease; if there is only oral disease, lichen planus, mucous membrane pemphigoid, aphthous stomatitis.
- **Rx:** oral CS, rituximab, steroid-sparing agents (e.g. mycophenolate mofetil, azathioprine, cyclophosphamide), IVIg, plasmapheresis (plus immunosuppression).

CHARACTERISTICS OF MAJOR AUTOIMMUNE BULLOUS DISEASES				
	PV	BP	DH	LABD
Cutaneous lesion	Flaccid vesicles and erosions	Large tense bullae	Grouped papules and small vesicles, often excoriated	Small vesicles and/or large bullae
Distribution	Mucosae; can be widespread	Trunk, extremities, occasionally mucosal surfaces	Extensor surfaces, symmetrical	Similar to DH or BP
Histopathology	Intraepidermal vesicle with acantholysis	Subepidermal bullae with eosinophilic infiltrate	Subepidermal bullae with neutrophilic infiltrate	Subepidermal bullae with neutrophilic infiltrate
Direct IF	Intracellular C3, IgG; occasionally IgA* ("chicken-wire" pattern)	Linear IgG and C3 at BMZ	Granular IgA in dermal papillae	Linear IgA at BMZ, possibly also IgG
Site to biopsy for direct IF	Perilesional	Perilesional	Adjacent normal-appearing skin	Perilesional
Indirect IF	Intracellular IgG (90%)	Linear IgG at BMZ (~70%)	Negative	Linear IgA at BMZ (~70%)
ELISA	Distinguishes anti-Dsg1 vs anti-Dsg3 Ab	Detects anti-BP180 and -BP230 IgG antibodies	Anti-tissue transglutaminase (TG2) & anti-epidermal transglutaminase (TG3) antibodies	n/a
Enteropathy	None	None	>90%	Rare
Dapsone responsiveness	Mild**	Minimal to moderate	Excellent	Good, may also require systemic corticosteroids

*Referred to as IgA pemphigus.
**Greater response if IgA +/or neutrophils.

Table 23.1 Characteristics of major autoimmune bullous diseases. BP, bullous pemphigoid; DH, dermatitis herpetiformis; LABD, linear IgA bullous disease; n/a, not commercially available; PV, pemphigus vulgaris.

Pemphigus Foliaceus, Pemphigus Erythematosus, and Fogo Selvagem

- In pemphigus foliaceus, the circulating autoantibodies are directed solely against Dsg1 (see above) and can be detected in the vast majority of patients by IIF (~85%) or ELISA (~95%); of note, the expression of Dsg1 is greater in the upper epidermis and minimal in the mucosa.
- As a result, acantholysis and *intra*epidermal blister formation occurs within the *upper* layers of the epidermis, usually at the granular layer; by DIF, immunostaining of the cell surface of the keratinocytes is seen in >90% of patients and may be more marked in these upper layers.
- Clinically, the more superficial and fragile nature of the blisters leads to a predominance of erosions with scale-crust rather

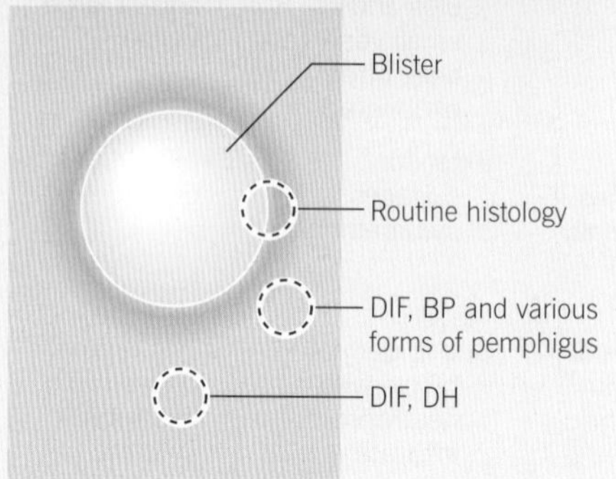

Fig. 23.1 Preferred sites for obtaining biopsy specimens in autoimmune bullous diseases. If the lesion is small enough, the entire vesicle can be removed for routine histopathology. If the lesion is not small, obtaining the edge of a fresh vesicle or bulla plus its inflammatory rim is recommended. For direct immunofluorescence (DIF) in bullous pemphigoid and various forms of pemphigus, perilesional skin is preferred, whereas nearby normal skin is recommended for dermatitis herpetiformis (DH).

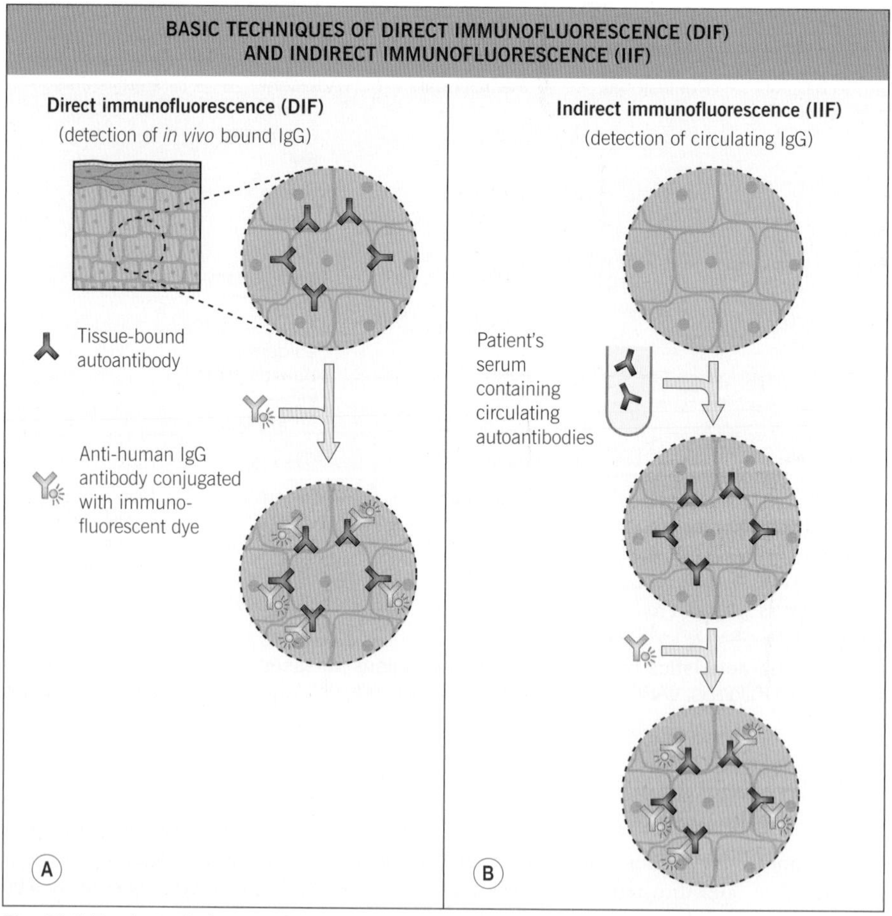

Fig. 23.2 Basic techniques of direct immunofluorescence (DIF) and indirect immunofluorescence (IIF). A DIF is performed on skin biopsy specimens in order to detect *in vivo* (tissue)-bound IgG and other immunodeposits such as C3 (see Fig. 23.1). **B** IIF is performed utilizing patients' sera to detect circulating autoantibodies that bind epithelial antigens. The preferred substrate for IIF is monkey esophagus for pemphigus vulgaris, guinea pig esophagus for pemphigus foliaceus, and human skin for the pemphigoid group and LABD.

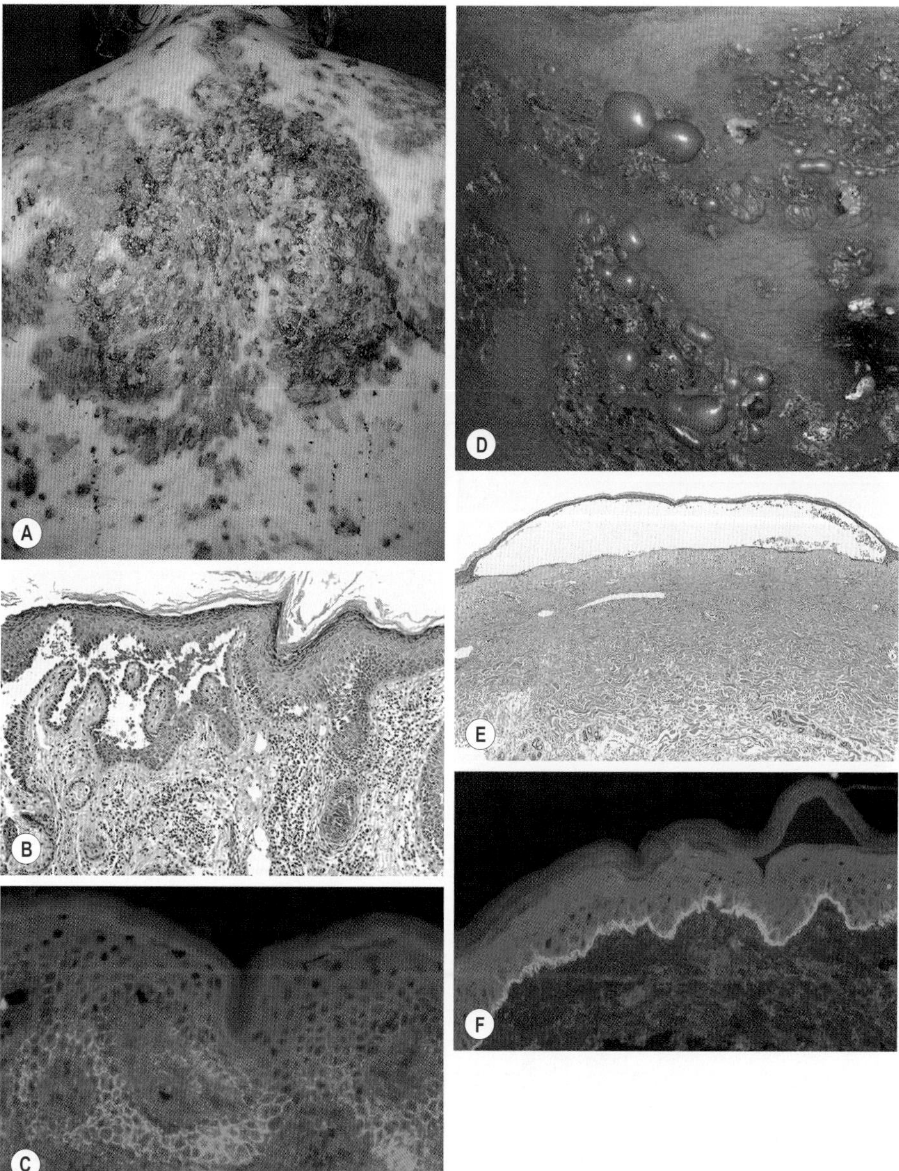

Fig. 23.3 Pemphigus vulgaris (PV) versus bullous pemphigoid (BP). A In PV, fragile blisters are short-lived and rupture easily, leading to crusting and erosions that can become extensive. **B** Acantholysis due to loss of desmosomal function from anti-desmoglein autoantibodies produces an intraepidermal split. Note the retention of hemidesmosomes between the basal cells of the epidermis and the basement membrane leads to a resemblance to tombstones. **C** DIF microscopy (see Fig. 23.2A) demonstrates *in vivo* intercellular deposits of IgG within the lower epidermis in a "chicken wire" pattern. **D** In BP, multiple tense bullae are seen; the contents of the bullae are usually serous, as in this patient. The bullae are longer-lived than in PV, but do eventually rupture, leading to erosions and crusts. **E** A subepidermal separation is seen. The cells within the blister cavity are often eosinophils. **F** DIF microscopy demonstrates linear deposits of C3 at the basement membrane zone; a similar pattern of IgA deposition is seen in linear IgA bullous dermatosis. *A, B, E, Courtesy, Lorenzo Cerroni, MD; C, F, Courtesy, Christine Ko, MD; D, Courtesy, Julie V. Schaffer, MD.*

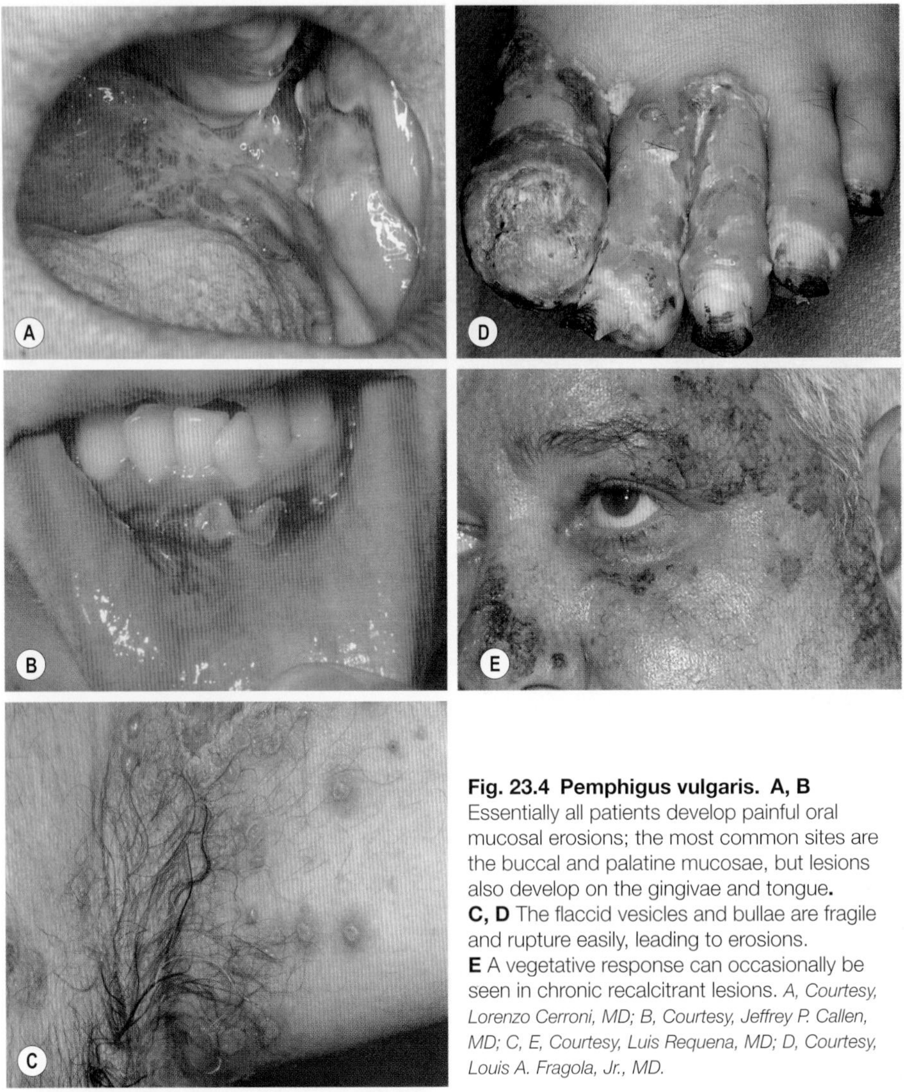

Fig. 23.4 Pemphigus vulgaris. A, B Essentially all patients develop painful oral mucosal erosions; the most common sites are the buccal and palatine mucosae, but lesions also develop on the gingivae and tongue. **C, D** The flaccid vesicles and bullae are fragile and rupture easily, leading to erosions. **E** A vegetative response can occasionally be seen in chronic recalcitrant lesions. *A, Courtesy, Lorenzo Cerroni, MD; B, Courtesy, Jeffrey P. Callen, MD; C, E, Courtesy, Luis Requena, MD; D, Courtesy, Louis A. Fragola, Jr., MD.*

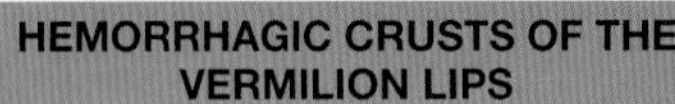

HEMORRHAGIC CRUSTS OF THE VERMILION LIPS
• Herpes simplex
• Herpes zoster
• Pemphigus vulgaris
• Paraneoplastic pemphigus (see Fig. 23.8)
• Stevens–Johnson syndrome/TEN spectrum
• Erythema multiforme major (see Fig. 3.9)

Table 23.2 Hemorrhagic crusts of the vermilion lips.

than bullae (Fig. 23.6); the scale is said to resemble cereal cornflakes; mucosal involvement is absent.

- While lesions favor the scalp, face, and upper trunk, they can become widespread, even leading to an exfoliative erythroderma, or they can be localized to the face (pemphigus erythematosus; Fig. 23.7).
- Fogo selvagem is an endemic form of pemphigus foliaceus seen primarily in rural areas of Brazil and is thought to be related to an immune reaction to antigens introduced by insect bites.
- **DDx:** other forms of pemphigus, impetigo (early limited disease), subacute cutaneous LE, and occasionally psoriasis.
- **Rx:** topical or oral CS, occasionally dapsone; if severe, steroid-sparing agents.

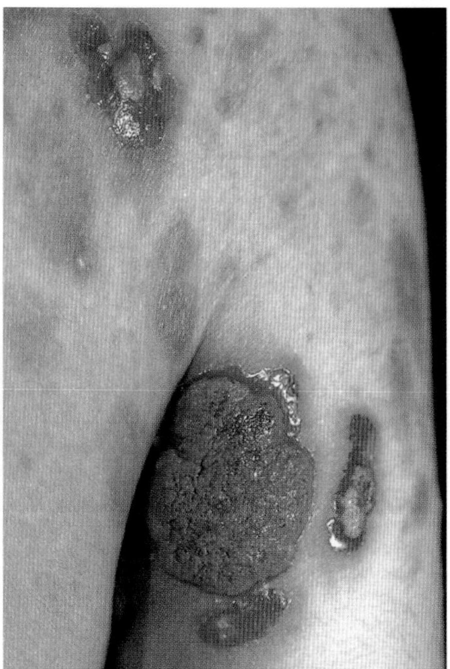

Fig. 23.5 Pemphigus vegetans. Large, thick, vegetating papillomatous plaques arising in conjunction with erosions. Healed lesions have residual postinflammatory hyperpigmentation. *Courtesy, Masayuki Amagai, MD.*

Paraneoplastic Pemphigus

- Develops in patients with an underlying neoplasm, often malignant, and improves slowly following successful treatment of the neoplasm; the most common tumor in children and adolescents is Castleman disease, whereas the most common ones in adults are non-Hodgkin lymphoma and chronic lymphocytic leukemia > Castleman disease and thymomas.
- Cutaneous lesions are variable and they can resemble lichen planus, erythema multiforme, or bullous pemphigoid as well as pemphigus; severe, recalcitrant oral stomatitis is a characteristic feature and conjunctival involvement is common (Fig. 23.8).
- Bronchiolitis obliterans is a serious internal manifestation.
- IgG autoantibodies are directed against at least ten antigens, including desmogleins and plakins; by DIF, there are immunodeposits on the surface of keratinocytes as well as along the basement membrane zone.

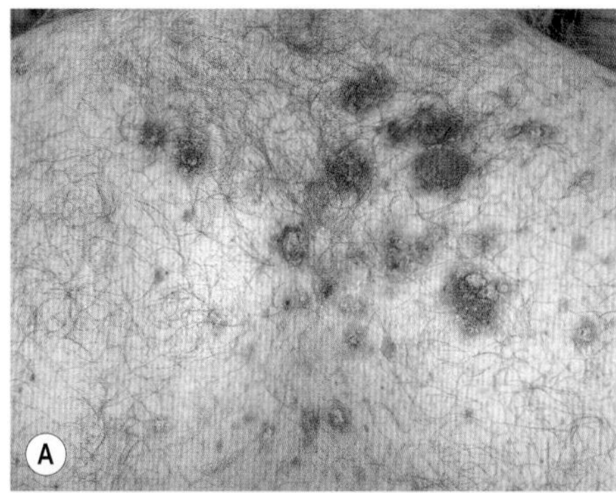

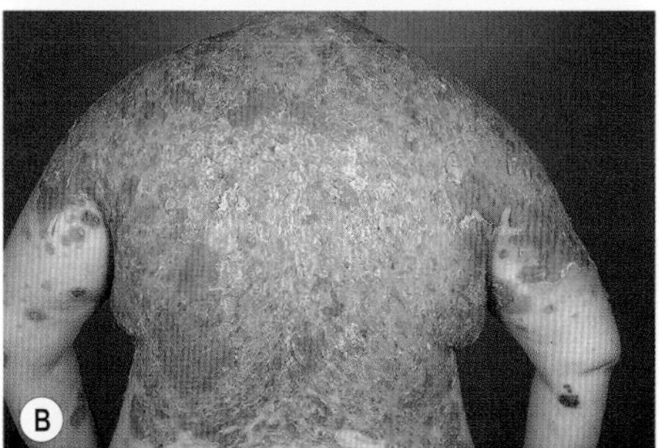

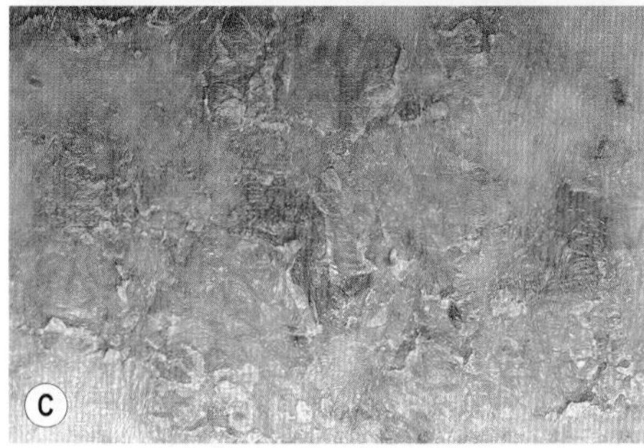

Fig. 23.6 Pemphigus foliaceus. A Several erosions arising on an erythematous base as well as the characteristic scale-crust; the latter can vary in thickness. A common site of involvement is the trunk. **B** As the disease progresses, the lesions become confluent, but because the vesicles are fragile and rupture easily, only erosions with scale-crust are observed. **C** The scales have been likened to cornflakes (cereal). *A, Courtesy, YDRSC; B, C, Courtesy, NYUDSC.*

- In this disorder, the anti-plakin antibodies also bind to simple epithelia such as rat urinary bladder epithelium and this allows distinction from pemphigus vulgaris.
- **DDx:** other forms of pemphigus, mucous membrane pemphigoid, erythema multiforme major, Stevens–Johnson syndrome, lichen planus, GVHD.
- **Rx:** treatment of the underlying neoplasm, but the stomatitis may prove recalcitrant

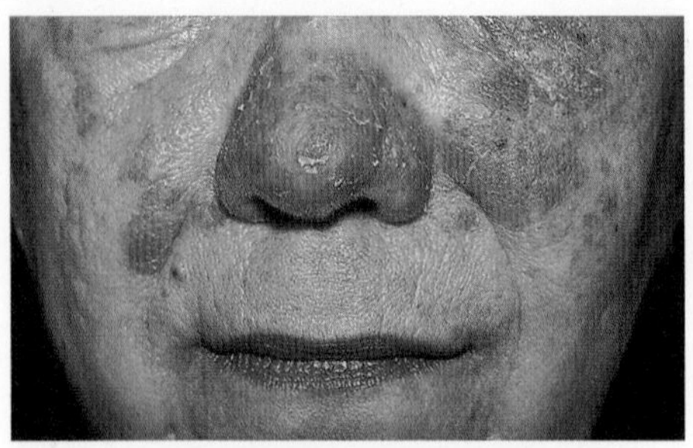

Fig. 23.7 Pemphigus erythematosus. Erythematous plaques with scale-crust and erosions on the nose and malar areas. Initially this disorder was thought to be a combination of pemphigus vulgaris plus lupus erythematosus, but now it is classified as a localized variant of pemphigus foliaceus. *Courtesy, Ronald P. Rapini, MD.*

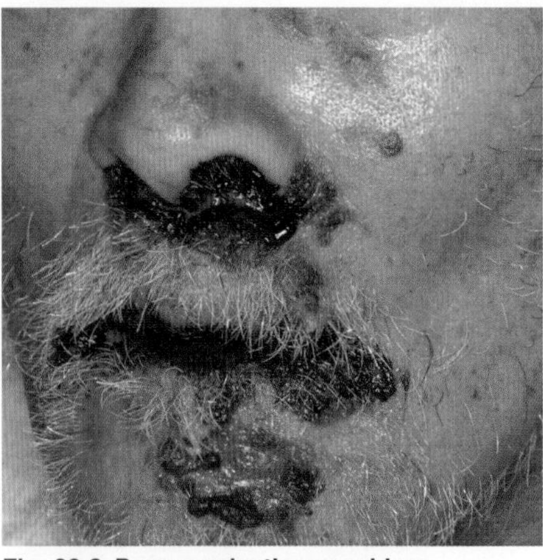

Fig. 23.8 Paraneoplastic pemphigus. Erosions, along with hemorrhagic crusts, can extend onto the vermilion lip and involve the nasal mucosa. The chin lesion resembles pemphigus vulgaris. *Courtesy, Masayuki Amagai, MD.*

despite successful eradication of the associated neoplasm.

IgA Pemphigus

- Two forms of this vesiculopustular eruption exist – subcorneal pustular dermatosis type and intraepidermal neutrophilic type, with the intraepidermal pustules histologically involving the upper versus entire epidermis, respectively.

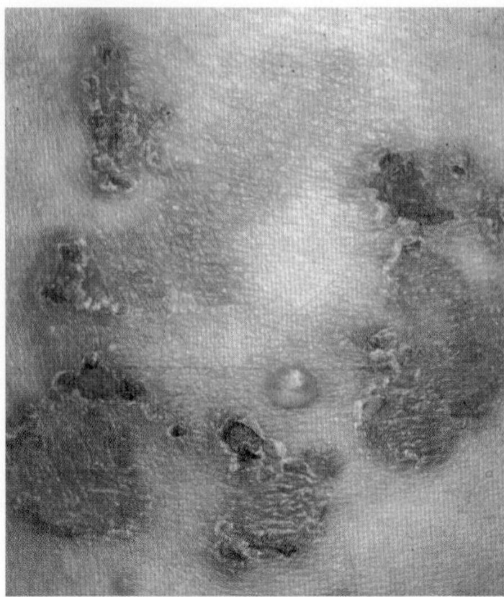

Fig. 23.9 IgA pemphigus – subcorneal pustular dermatosis type. Pustules tend to coalesce to form an annular or figurate pattern with erosions, scale-crust, and postinflammatory hyperpigmentation present centrally. Note the accumulation of the pustular component in the dependent portion of the vesiculopustule. *Courtesy, Masayuki Amagai, MD.*

- Clinically, lesions arise within inflamed or normal skin and assume a figurate arrangement (Fig. 23.9); the most common sites are the axillae and groin.
- By DIF, there is immunostaining of the cell surface of keratinocytes within the epidermis, as in pemphigus vulgaris, but the immunodeposits are IgA rather than IgG.
- **DDx:** Sneddon–Wilkinson disease (negative DIF), pemphigus foliaceus, impetigo (when more limited), LABD, pustular psoriasis.
- **Rx:** dapsone or sulfapyridine and sometimes oral CS.

Drug-Induced Pemphigus

- Occasionally, medications can induce pemphigus vulgaris or pemphigus foliaceus and discontinuation of those drugs can lead to clinical resolution.
- The most common medications are captopril and penicillamine, both of which contain sulfhydryl groups.

For further information see Ch. 29 from *Dermatology, Fourth Edition*.

For additional online figures and tables visit www.expertconsult.com 

Bullous Pemphigoid, Mucous Membrane Pemphigoid, and Epidermolysis Bullosa Acquisita

24

This chapter, in addition to Chapters 23 and 25, covers the autoimmune bullous diseases. The concepts of direct immunofluorescence (DIF) and indirect immunofluorescence (IIF) are reviewed in Chapter 23 (see Fig. 23.2), as are the recommended sites for performing skin biopsies for DIF (see Fig. 23.1).

Bullous Pemphigoid (BP)

- Immunobullous disease due to circulating autoantibodies that bind two components of hemidesmosomes, i.e. structures that provide adhesion between the epidermis and the dermis; the two antigens are collagen XVII (also referred to as BP antigen 2 [BPAG2] or BP180) and BPAG1/BP230 (Fig. 24.1).
- Occurs more commonly in the elderly and can be drug-induced (e.g. furosemide, immune checkpoint inhibitors, dipeptidyl peptidase-IV inhibitors); rarely, lesions are induced by ultraviolet light or radiation therapy.
- Both pruritic fixed urticarial plaques and tense bullae are seen (Figs 24.2–24.4); the latter can develop within normal skin or areas of erythematous skin and their rupture leads to erosions; oral lesions (10–30% of patients) are much less common than in pemphigus vulgaris.
- Pruritus and nonspecific eczematous (see Fig. 24.3B) or papular lesions can precede the more characteristic cutaneous lesions and may be the predominant finding; unusual variants include dyshidrosiform (palms and soles), vegetans (major body folds), and localized (e.g. pretibial in adults; vulvar in children, acral in infants), as well as those that mimic prurigo nodularis and toxic epidermal necrolysis (Fig. 24.5).
- Histologically, a subepidermal bulla plus an infiltrate of eosinophils is seen when

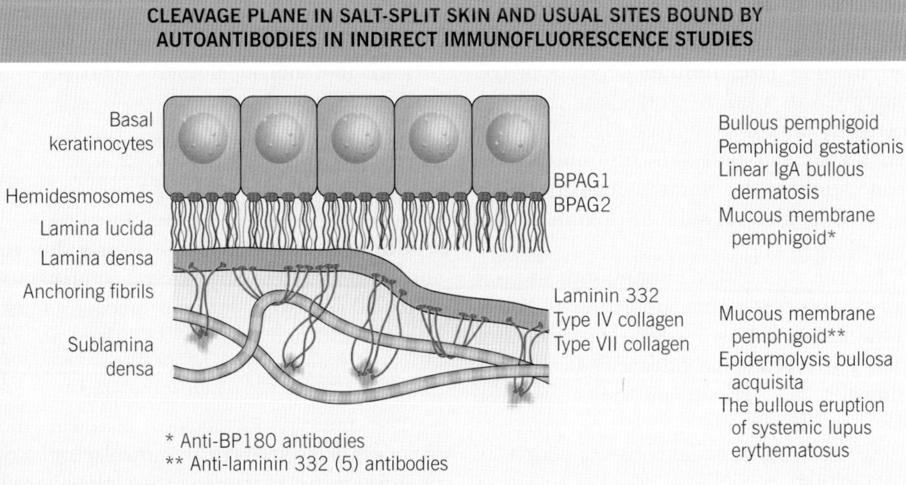

Fig. 24.1 Cleavage plane in salt-split skin and usual sites bound by autoantibodies in indirect immunofluorescence studies. The cleavage plane in 1 M NaCl salt-split skin is in the lower portion of the lamina lucida. Circulating autoantibodies from patients with various subepidermal immunobullous diseases bind to different sites, e.g. the epidermal versus dermal side of the split. *Courtesy, Kim Yancey, MD.*

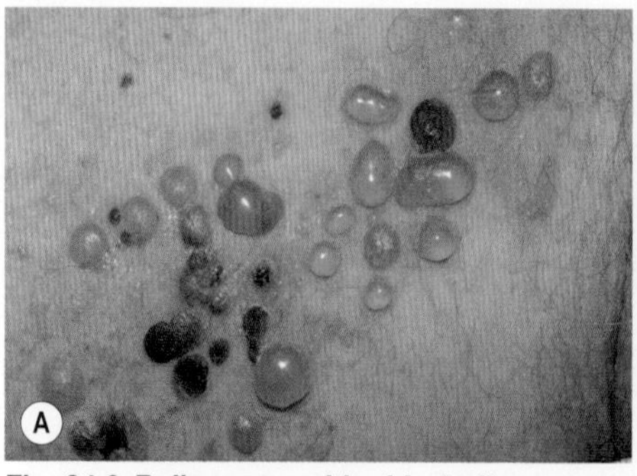
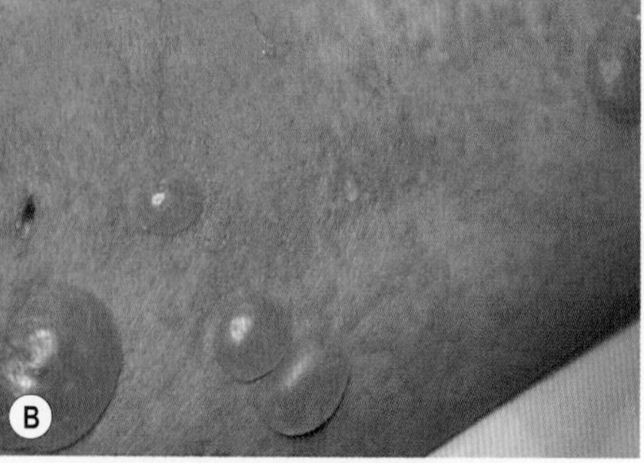

Fig. 24.2 Bullous pemphigoid – bullous presentation. A,B Tense vesicles and bullae vary in size from a few millimeters to several centimeters in diameter and can arise within normal-appearing skin, areas of erythema, or urticarial plaques. The blister fluid may be serous or hemorrhagic. As the bullae age, they become flaccid and rupture, leaving erosions and serous or hemorrhagic crusts. Biopsies of vesiculobullae for routine histology should be obtained from fresh tense blisters. *A, Courtesy, Kalman Watsky, MD; B, Courtesy, YDRSC.*

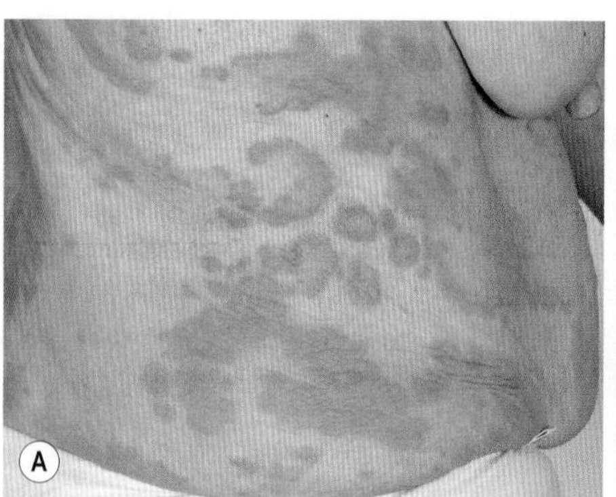
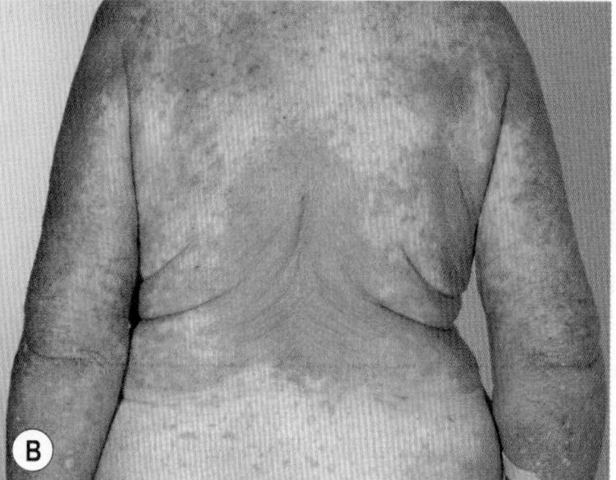

Fig. 24.3 Bullous pemphigoid – urticarial and eczematous presentations. A Multiple firm annular, arciform and polycyclic urticarial plaques. Note the absence of bullae. **B** Large pink eczematous plaques on the trunk and extremities. *Courtesy, Philippe Bernard, MD, and Luca Borradori, MD.*

the lesions are bullous (see Fig. 23.3E); DIF demonstrates immunodeposits of IgG and/or C3 in a linear array along the basement membrane zone (see Fig. 23.3F); in general, by salt-split skin immunofluorescence studies, the immunodeposits are in the roof (epidermal side) of the blister (see Fig. 24.1).

- Both enzyme-linked immunosorbent assay and IIF can detect circulating autoantibodies in the sera in at least 70–80% of patients (see Table 23.1). While the autoantibodies are traditionally IgG, IgE autoantibodies may also play a pathogenic role.
- At least 50% of patients have a peripheral eosinophilia.
- **DDx:** linear IgA bullous dermatosis (LABD), epidermolysis bullosa acquisita (EBA), mucous membrane pemphigoid, various forms of pemphigus, hypersensitivity reactions (including to drugs), primary pruritus, allergic contact dermatitis, scabies, urticaria (but individual lesions transient).
- **Rx:** see Table 24.1.

Mucous Membrane (Cicatricial) Pemphigoid

- Chronic immunobullous disease due to autoantibodies that bind several components of the BMZ of the skin and mucosae, most often BP180 and laminin 332 (laminin 5); although heterogenous in its presentation, a tendency to scarring is typically seen.
- The mucous membranes represent the major site of involvement, in particular conjunctival (erosions, scarring with symblepharon formation, blindness) and oral mucosae (persistent erosions of the buccal and palatal mucosae, desquamative gingivitis) (Figs 24.6 and 24.7).
- Additional sites of involvement are the nasopharynx, larynx, and esophagus; a few

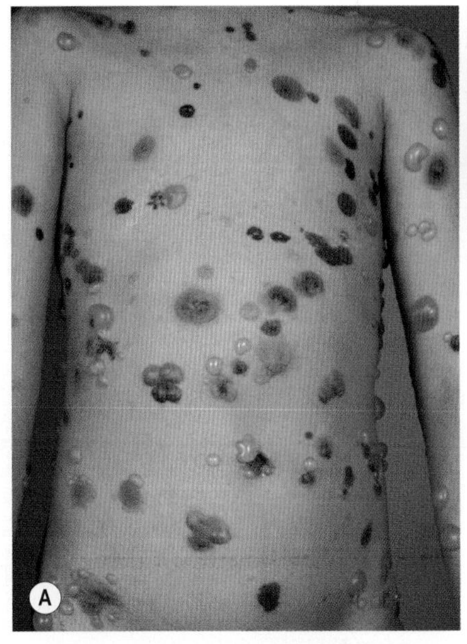

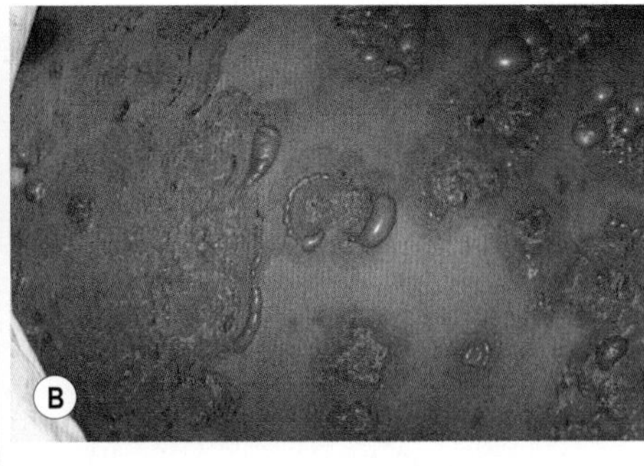

Fig. 24.4 Childhood bullous pemphigoid. **A** Generalized bullae, both tense (fresh) and flaccid (old with re-epithelialization), as well as erosions with hemorrhagic crusts. **B** Tense vesicles and bullae in an annular or figurate array at the edge of expanding lesions, a presentation that might be diagnosed clinically as linear IgA bullous dermatosis. *A, Courtesy, NYUDSC; B, Courtesy, Julie V. Schaffer, MD.*

THERAPEUTIC LADDER FOR BULLOUS PEMPHIGOID
Mild and/or localized disease
First-line • Superpotent topical corticosteroids (1*)
Second-line • Oral corticosteroids (1) • Minocycline, doxycycline, or tetracycline, alone or in combination with nicotinamide (1) • Erythromycin, penicillins (3) • Dapsone, sulfonamides (3) • Topical immunomodulators (e.g. tacrolimus) (3)
Extensive/persistent cutaneous disease
First-line, as primary treatment • Superpotent topical corticosteroids (1*) • Oral corticosteroids† (1)‡
Second-line, or as adjunctive therapy • Azathioprine (2) • Mycophenolate mofetil (2) • Methotrexate§ (2) • Rituximab (2) • Omalizumab (3) • Cyclophosphamide (3) • IVIg (3) • Plasma exchange (2) • Chlorambucil (3)

Key to evidence-based support: (1) prospective controlled trial; (2) retrospective study or large case series; (3) small case series or individual case reports. Note: Superpotent topical corticosteroids should be considered in any patient and may be combined with a systemic therapy.
**Validated.*
†Prednisone doses of at least 0.5–0.75 mg/kg/day seem to be necessary to control extensive disease but increase serious side effects, including mortality.
‡Validated for prednisone.
§In elderly patients, low-dose regimen (2.5–10 mg/week) can be effective.

Table 24.1 Therapeutic ladder for bullous pemphigoid.

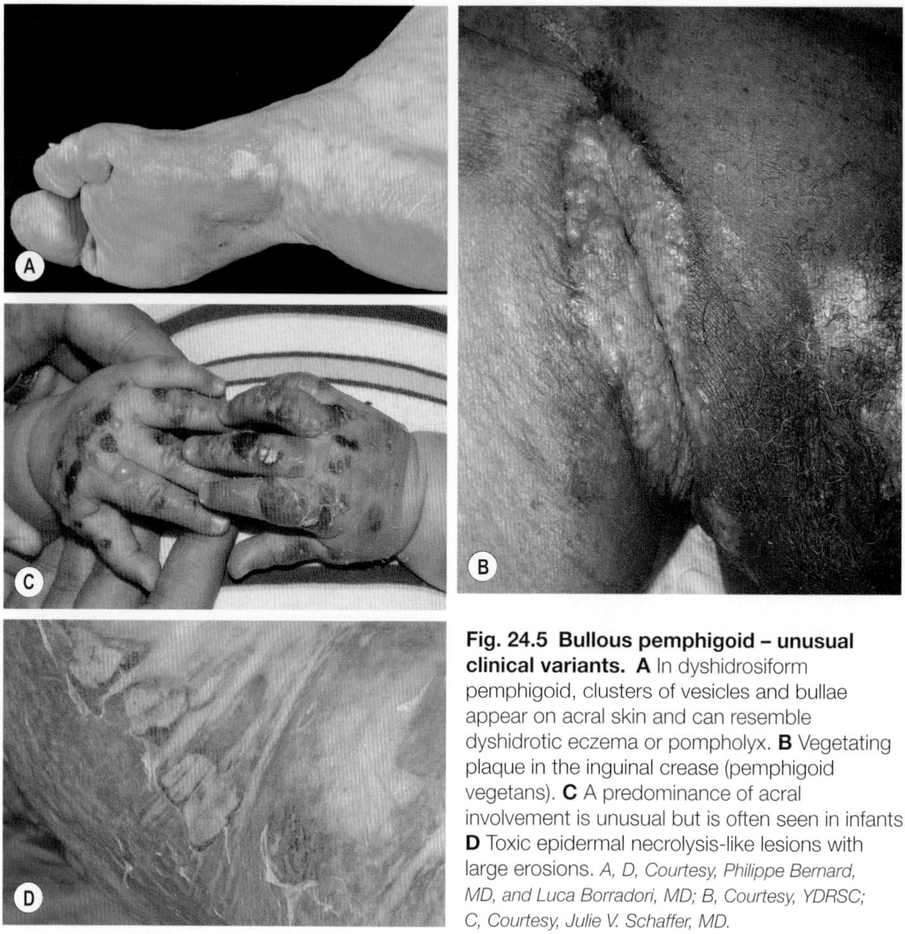

Fig. 24.5 Bullous pemphigoid – unusual clinical variants. **A** In dyshidrosiform pemphigoid, clusters of vesicles and bullae appear on acral skin and can resemble dyshidrotic eczema or pompholyx. **B** Vegetating plaque in the inguinal crease (pemphigoid vegetans). **C** A predominance of acral involvement is unusual but is often seen in infants. **D** Toxic epidermal necrolysis-like lesions with large erosions. *A, D, Courtesy, Philippe Bernard, MD, and Luca Borradori, MD; B, Courtesy, YDRSC; C, Courtesy, Julie V. Schaffer, MD.*

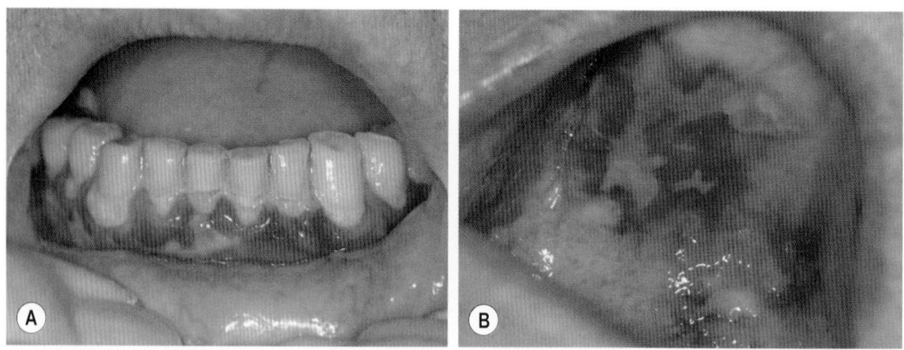

Fig. 24.6 Mucous membrane (cicatricial) pemphigoid – mucosal involvement. **A** Desquamative gingivitis with erythema and erosions of the gingival margins. Note the sloughing of the mucosa with shaggy margins. **B** Chronic erosions on the hard palate with irregular borders. Sloughing of mucosa is seen superiorly. *Courtesy, Philippe Bernard, MD, and Luca Borradori, MD.*

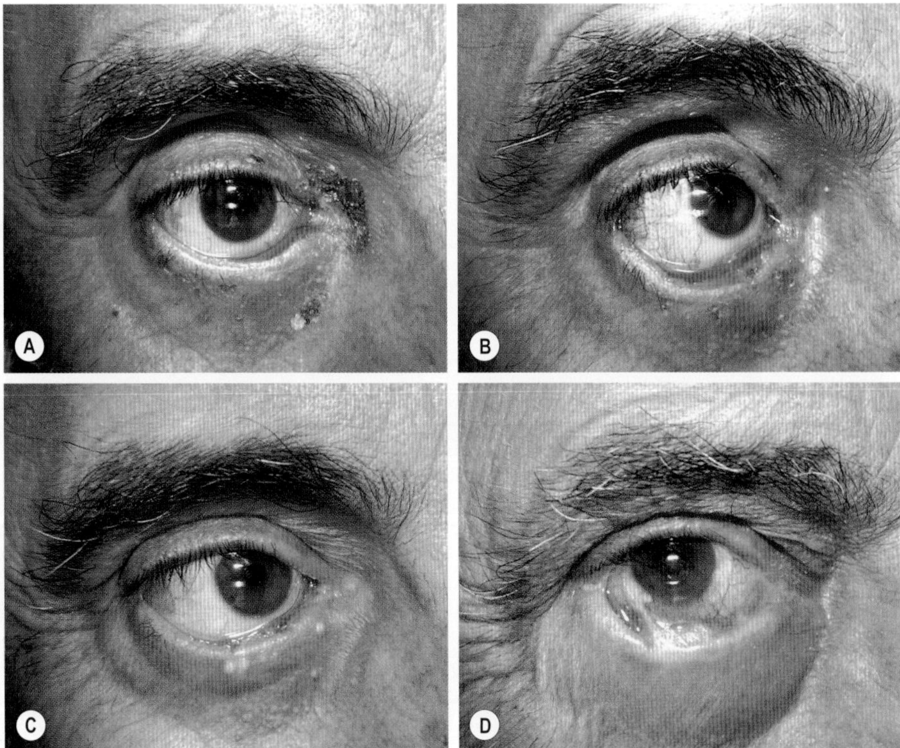

Fig. 24.7 Mucous membrane (cicatricial) pemphigoid progression. **A** Erosion and erythema of the lower medial eyelid margin plus scale-crust of the inner canthus and lower eyelid. **B** Three months later, ectropion and thickening of the lower eyelid in addition to erosions of the palpebral conjunctiva. **C** Six months later, smaller erosions but scarring and milia formation. **D** Seven years later, further scarring with significant shortening of the inferior fornix due to symblepharon. *Courtesy, Louis A. Fragola, Jr., MD.*

authors have suggested that patients with anti-laminin 332 immunodeposits have an increased risk of internal malignancy.

• Cutaneous lesions are seen in a quarter of patients and favor the head and neck region and upper trunk; erythematous plaques that develop vesicles, erosions, and scarring are characteristic (Fig. 24.8).

• Histopathologic and DIF features are similar to BP, but there is usually a sparser infiltrate and fewer eosinophils plus fibrosis may be present; DIF positivity (IgG and/or C3 >> IgA) is greater for mucosa (50–90%) than for skin; circulating autoantibodies are detected by IIF in a minority of patients (20–30%).

• **DDx:** pemphigus vulgaris, occasionally paraneoplastic pemphigus, BP, EBA, and LABD; if limited to oral mucosa, lichen planus or pemphigus vulgaris (see Fig. 59.7); if limited to scalp, consider other causes of scarring alopecia.

• **Rx:** potent topical or intralesional CS, dapsone, cyclophosphamide (severe or progressive ocular disease), alone or in combination with systemic CS, and rituximab.

Epidermolysis Bullosa Acquisita (EBA)

• Autoimmune bullous disease due to autoantibodies that bind to collagen VII; the latter forms anchoring fibrils within the upper dermis and they play an important role in adhesion of the epidermis to the dermis (see Fig. 24.1).

• Two major clinical forms: (1) mechanobullous, which resembles the genetic disorder epidermolysis bullosa; and (2) inflammatory, which resembles bullous pemphigoid (Fig. 24.9).

• In the more common mechanobullous form, bullae arise in sites of friction and are followed by erosions, scarring, and milia formation (Fig. 24.10); oral lesions can also be seen (Fig. 24.11).

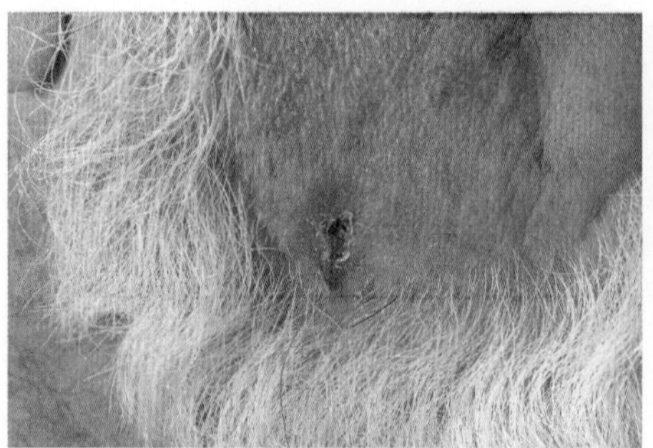

Fig. 24.8 Mucous membrane (cicatricial) pemphigoid – Brunsting–Perry variant. Crusted erosion on the lower cheek within an oval area of inflammation and scar. *Courtesy, Philippe Bernard, MD, and Luca Borradori, MD.*

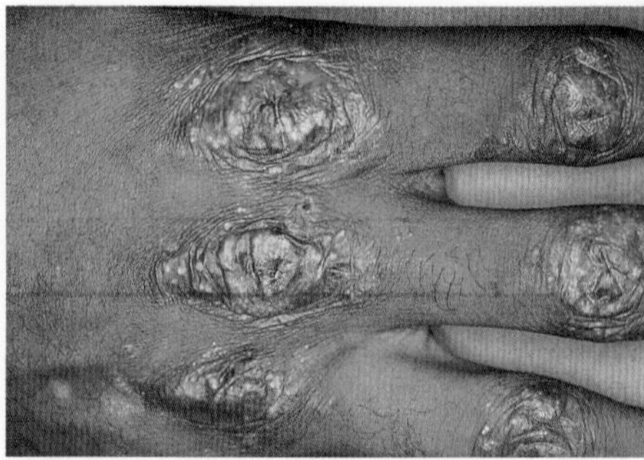

Fig. 24.10 Epidermolysis bullosa acquisita – mechanobullous presentation. Milia and scarring that favor sites of trauma overlying joints, in association with skin fragility. Note the resemblance to dystrophic epidermolysis bullosa. *Courtesy, YDRSC.*

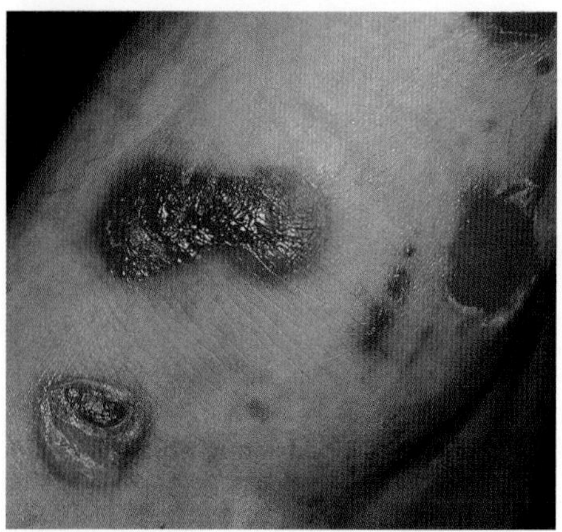

Fig. 24.9 Epidermolysis bullosa acquisita – inflammatory bullous pemphigoid-like presentation. Bullous and erosive lesions in a patient with multiple myeloma. *Courtesy, Philippe Bernard, MD, and Luca Borradori, MD.*

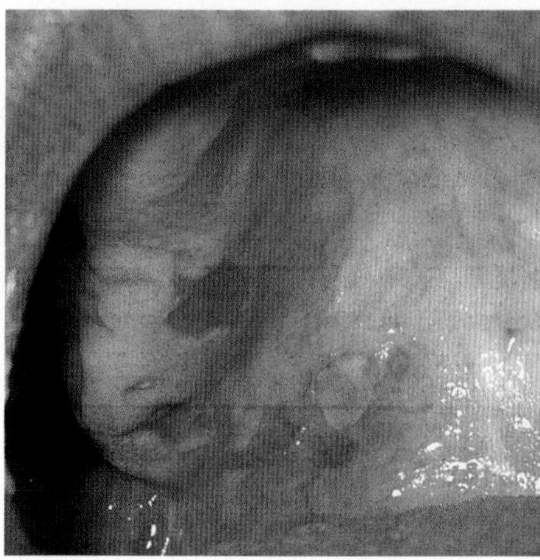

Fig. 24.11 Epidermolysis bullosa acquisita – oral lesions. Multiple erosions of the palate reminiscent of mucous membrane pemphigoid. *Courtesy, Catherine Prost, MD.*

- Associated systemic disorders include inflammatory bowel disease, in particular Crohn disease, and plasma cell dyscrasias.
- Histopathologic and DIF features are similar to BP, but there is usually a sparser infiltrate and fewer eosinophils in the mechanobullous form; DIF studies demonstrate linear IgG > C3 or IgA at the basement membrane zone; circulating autoantibodies are detected in ~50% of patients and by salt-split skin immunofluorescence studies, the immunodeposits are in the floor (dermal side) of the blister (see Fig. 24.1).
- **DDx:** inherited forms of epidermolysis bullosa, porphyria cutanea tarda (and other rare variants of porphyria), pseudoporphyria, bullous pemphigoid, LABD, mucous membrane pemphigoid, bullous systemic lupus erythematosus (also autoantibodies against collagen VII).
- **Rx:** difficult to treat; potent topical CS, oral CS, steroid-sparing agents (e.g. mycophenolate mofetil), dapsone, rituximab.

For further information see Chs 28 and 30 from *Dermatology, Fourth Edition*.

For additional online figures visit www.expertconsult.com 

Dermatitis Herpetiformis and Linear IgA Bullous Dermatosis

25

This is the third chapter, along with Chapters 23 and 24, that deals with autoimmune bullous diseases (see Table 23.1).

Dermatitis Herpetiformis (DH)

- Autoimmune bullous disease that is a cutaneous manifestation of celiac disease, with >90% of patients having histologic evidence of some degree of gluten-sensitive enteropathy; ~20% of patients with DH have symptomatic celiac disease.
- In predisposed individuals (e.g. those with HLA-DQ2), IgA antibodies form against gliadin cross-linked to *tissue* transglutaminase (TG2); the presumed autoantigen in the skin is *epidermal* transglutaminase (TG3; Fig. 25.1).
- Primary lesions consist of pruritic vesicles on an erythematous base and edematous erythematous papules that are often grouped (i.e. herpetiform); however, due to scratching, only excoriated papules and hemorrhagic crusts may be present (Fig. 25.2).
- Favored sites of involvement are the elbows, extensor forearms, knees, posterior neck, and presacral/buttock region, with lesions in a symmetric distribution pattern.
- Histologically, collections of neutrophils are seen within the dermal papillae of involved skin (Fig. 25.3A); by direct immunofluorescence (DIF; see Fig. 23.2), *granular* deposits of IgA are detected within dermal papillae of adjacent, normal-appearing skin in at least 90% of patients (see Fig. 23.1; Fig. 25.3B).
- Patients have circulating anti-tissue transglutaminase and anti-endomysial antibodies, with the level of the latter correlating with degree of enteropathy (Fig. 25.4); they can also develop other autoimmune disorders, in particular Hashimoto thyroiditis.
- **DDx:** linear IgA bullous dermatosis, bullous pemphigoid, prurigo simplex, and bullous systemic LE; crusted lesions of the elbows are also seen in patients with granulomatosis with polyangiitis and eosinophilic granulomatosis with polyangiitis.
- **Rx:** gluten-free diet (also reduces risk of enteropathy-associated T-cell lymphoma), dapsone (initially 25–50 mg per day after screening for glucose-6-phosphate dehydrogenase [G6PD] deficiency; average dose on a normal diet is 100 mg), and sulfapyridine; improvement of pruritus within a few days of instituting dapsone supports the diagnosis of DH.

Linear IgA Bullous Dermatosis (LABD)

- Autoimmune bullous disease that occurs in both children and adults and can be drug-induced (Table 25.1); in children, it is sometimes referred to as 'chronic bullous disease of childhood'.
- Vesicles and bullae arise on the trunk and extremities and in children often favor the lower trunk and groin; lesions can assume a figurate arrangement and have been likened to a crown of jewels (Figs 25.5–25.7).
- Spontaneous remission in children, usually after 2–4 years; ~50% of adults have a spontaneous remission.
- Histologically, a subepidermal bulla is accompanied by an infiltrate of neutrophils; by DIF, *linear* deposits of IgA are detected at the basement membrane zone of perilesional skin (see Figs 23.1 and 23.2).
- By indirect immunofluorescence (IIF), circulating IgA autoantibodies are detected in ~70% of patients with LABD (see Fig. 23.2); the autoantigen in LABD is a cleavage product of one of the two autoantigens of bullous pemphigoid (BP180; see Ch. 24).
- **DDx:** bullous pemphigoid (linear deposits of IgG), DH (granular deposits of IgA), and mucous membrane (cicatricial) pemphigoid;

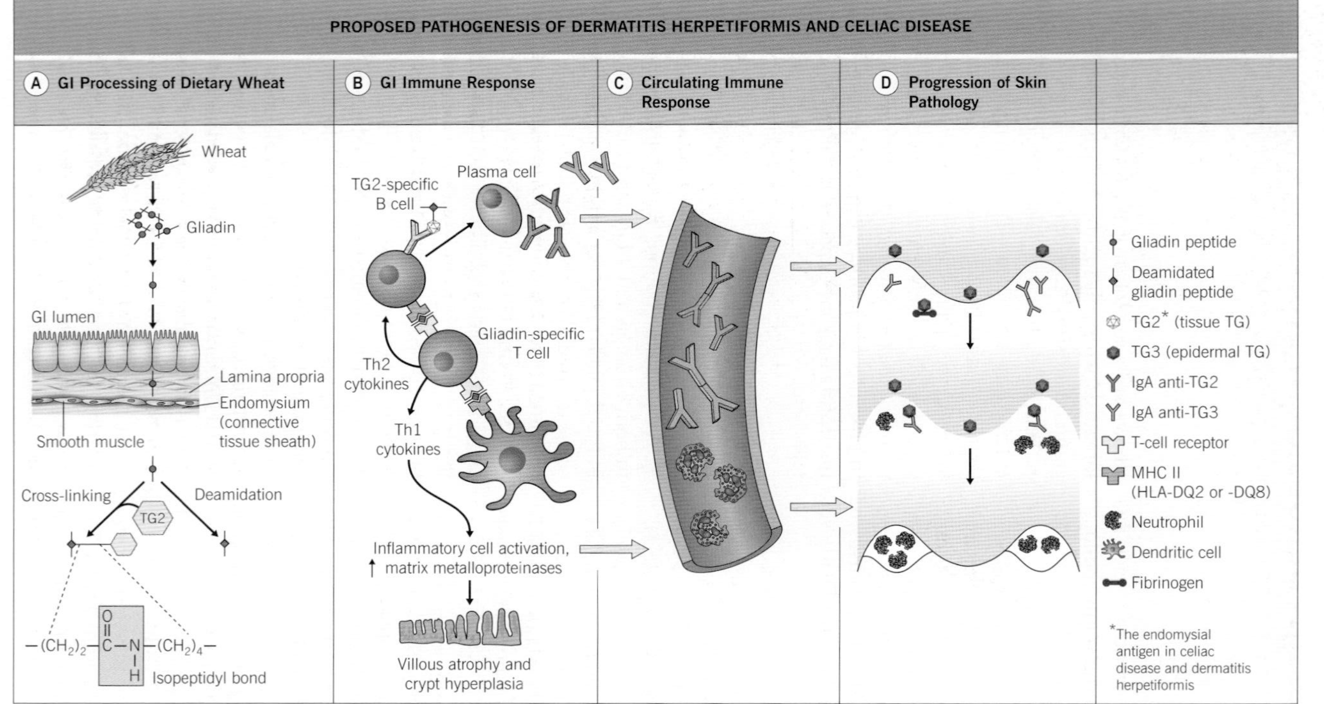

Fig. 25.1 Proposed pathogenesis of dermatitis herpetiformis and celiac disease. **A** Dietary wheat, barley, or rye is processed by digestive enzymes into antigenic gliadin peptides, which are transported intact across the mucosal epithelium. Within the lamina propria, tissue transglutaminase (TG2): (1) deamidates glutamine residues within gliadin peptides to glutamic acid; and (2) becomes covalently cross-linked to gliadin peptides via isopeptidyl bonds (formed between gliadin and TG2 lysine residues). **B** $CD4^+$ T cells in the lamina propria recognize deamidated gliadin peptides presented by HLA-DQ2 or -DQ8 molecules on antigen-presenting cells, resulting in the production of Th1 cytokines and matrix metalloproteinases that cause mucosal epithelial cell damage and tissue remodeling. In addition, TG2-specific B cells take up TG2–gliadin complexes and present gliadin peptides to gliadin-specific helper T cells, which stimulate the B cells to produce IgA anti-TG2. **C** Over time, IgA directed against TG3 (IgA anti-TG3) forms as a result of epitope spreading and both IgA anti-TG2 and IgA anti-TG3 circulate in the bloodstream. **D** When IgA anti-TG3 antibodies reach the dermis, they complex with TG3 antigens which have been produced by keratinocytes (epidermal TG) and then have diffused into the dermis. That is, IgA/TG3 immune complexes are formed *locally* within the papillary dermis. This leads to

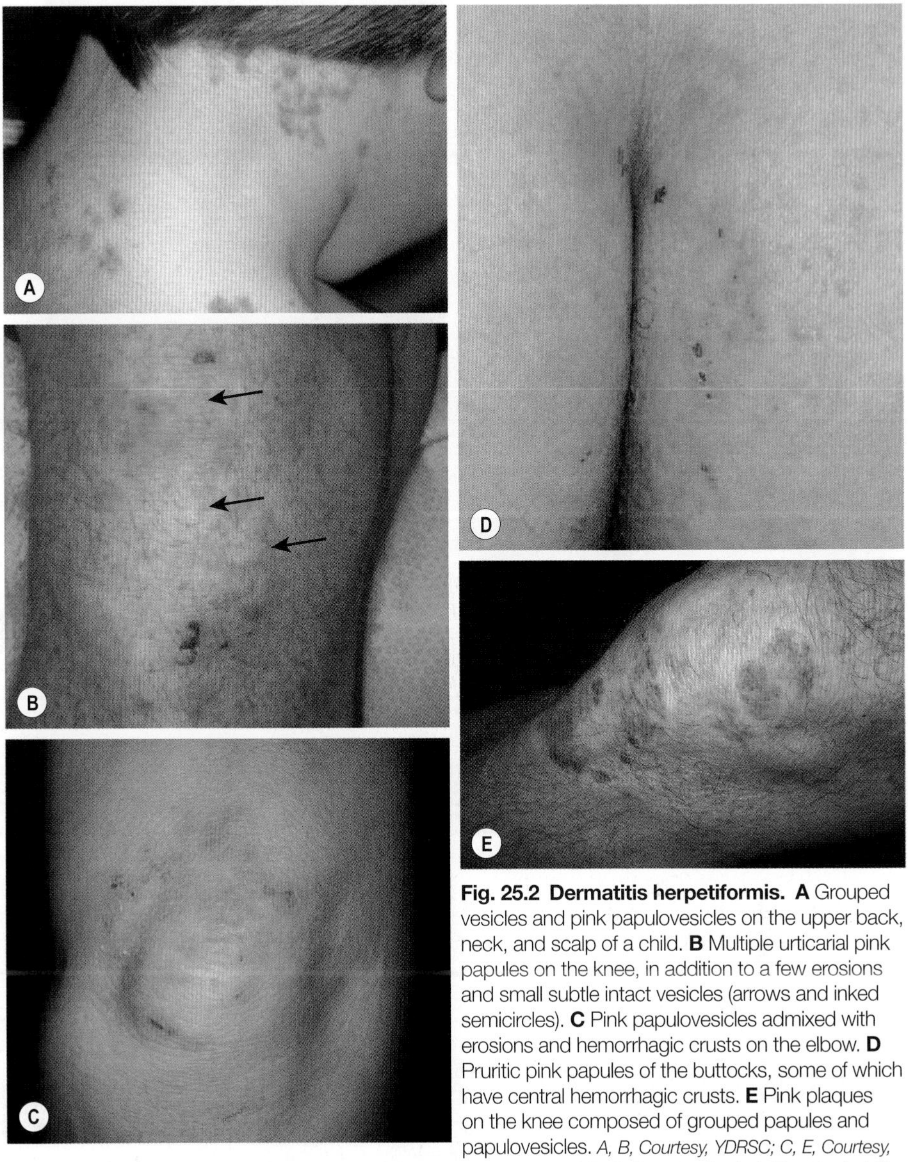

Fig. 25.2 Dermatitis herpetiformis. A Grouped vesicles and pink papulovesicles on the upper back, neck, and scalp of a child. **B** Multiple urticarial pink papules on the knee, in addition to a few erosions and small subtle intact vesicles (arrows and inked semicircles). **C** Pink papulovesicles admixed with erosions and hemorrhagic crusts on the elbow. **D** Pruritic pink papules of the buttocks, some of which have central hemorrhagic crusts. **E** Pink plaques on the knee composed of grouped papules and papulovesicles. *A, B, Courtesy, YDRSC; C, E, Courtesy, Thomas Horn, MD; D, Courtesy, Louis A. Fragola, Jr., MD.*

for vancomycin-induced LABD, toxic epidermal necrolysis.

- Important to review medications and withdraw possible culprits before instituting systemic therapy.
- **Rx:** dapsone (often higher doses than for DH) or sulfapyridine, occasionally requiring the addition of prednisone; antibiotics (e.g. dicloxacillin, doxycycline, erythromycin) can be tried initially.

For further information see Ch. 31 from *Dermatology, Fourth Edition*.

For additional online figures and tables, including side effects of dapsone, visit www.expertconsult.com 

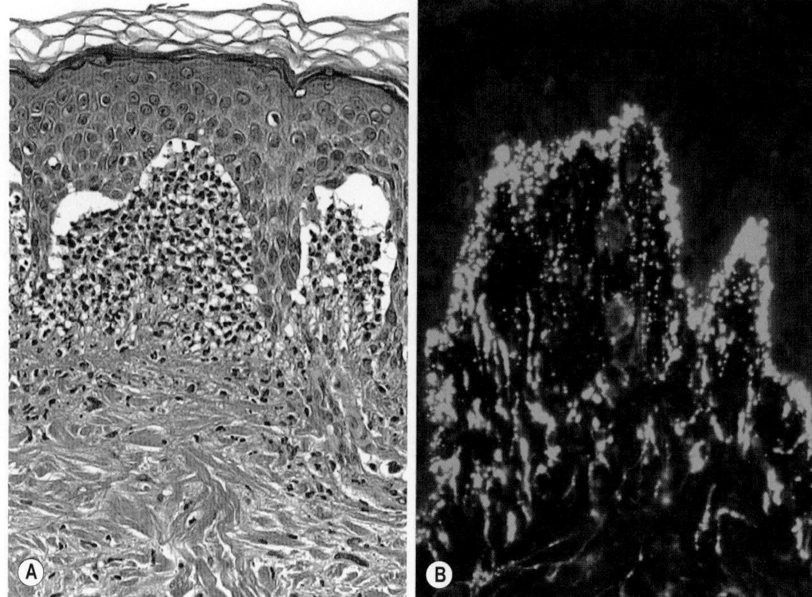

Fig. 25.3 Dermatitis herpetiformis – histopathologic features and direct immunofluorescence (DIF). A Subepidermal clefts beneath which are collections of neutrophils within dermal papillae. Scattered eosinophils are also present. **B** Granular and fibrillar IgA deposition along the dermal–epidermal junction of normal-appearing skin adjacent to a lesion. *A, Courtesy, Lorenzo Cerroni, MD. B, Courtesy, Kristen Leiferman, MD.*

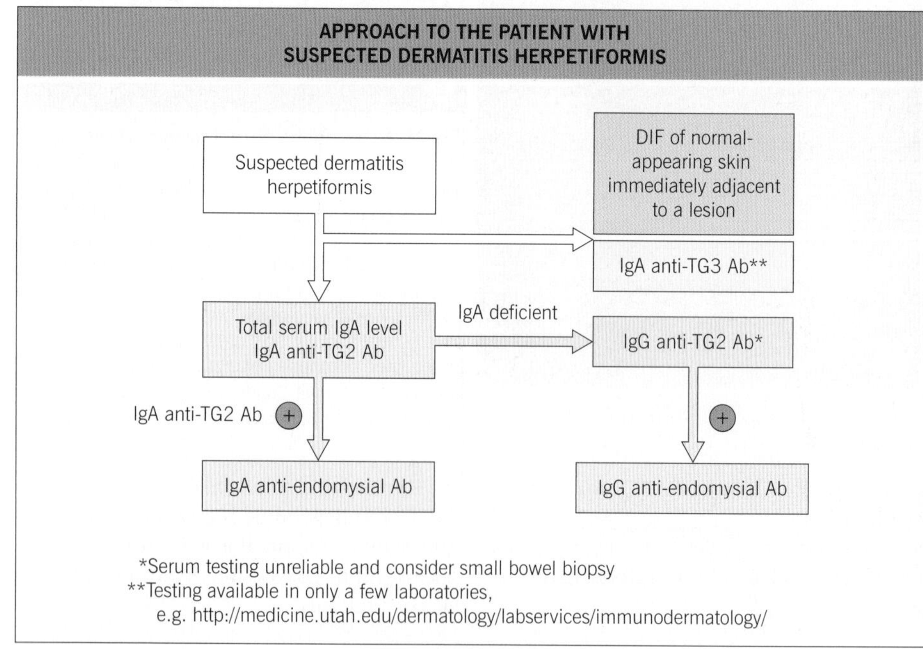

Fig. 25.4 Approach to the patient with suspected dermatitis herpetiformis. IgA anti-TG2 and anti-endomysial antibodies can be monitored over time to assess compliance with a gluten-free diet. Because the anti-endomysial antibody assay is based upon analysis of indirect immunofluorescence, it is more expensive than the IgA anti-TG2 antibody assay. Anti-deamidated gliadin peptide IgA/IgG testing may have utility for individuals with IgA deficiency or weakly positive anti-TG2 IgA. DIF, direct immunofluorescence; TG2, tissue transglutaminase; TG3, epidermal transglutaminase. *Courtesy, John J. Zone, MD.*

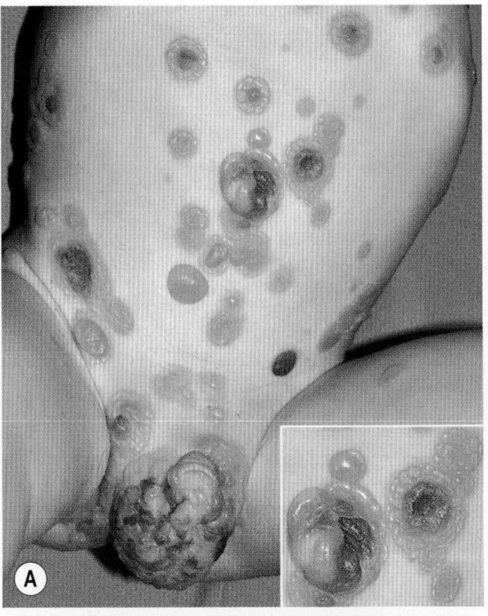

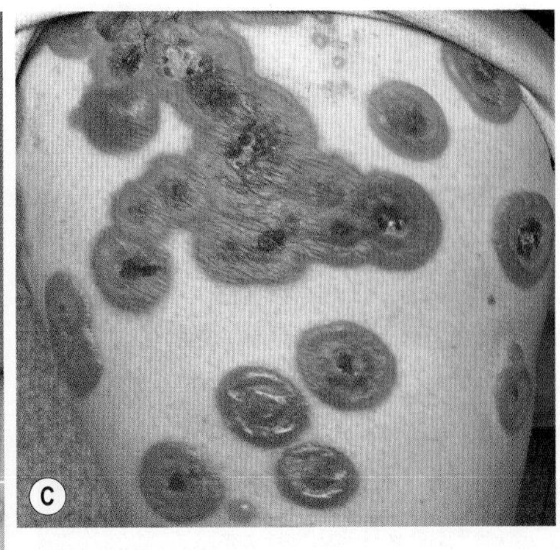

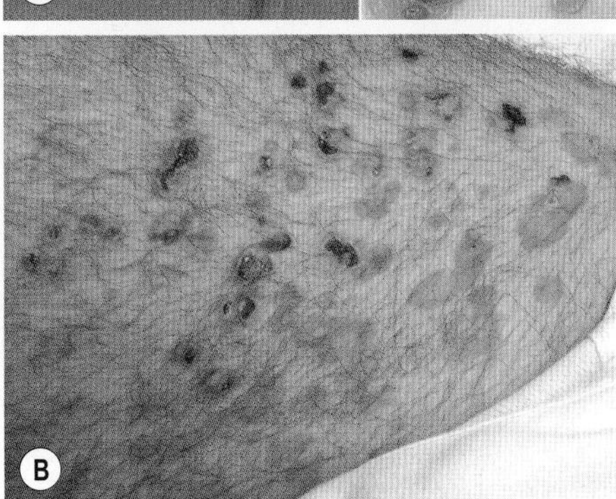

Fig. 25.5 Linear IgA bullous dermatosis. **A** Characteristic findings in this child include the annular array of bullae (inset) and involvement of the genital region. There are also tense bullae arising on normal-appearing skin with either clear or hemorrhagic fluid and annular bullae with central crusting. **B** Annular and herpetiform vesicles arising on an inflammatory base. Annular pink plaques are also present. **C** Striking annular vesiculobullous lesions on the thigh with central erosions and crusting. A figurate outline is seen in the area of coalescence. *A, Courtesy, Antonio Torrelo, MD; B, Courtesy, Jeffrey P. Callen, MD; Courtesy, John J. Zone, MD.*

DRUG-INDUCED LINEAR IgA BULLOUS DERMATOSIS
Common
• Vancomycin*
Less common
• Penicillins • Cephalosporins • Captopril > other ACE inhibitors • NSAIDs: diclofenac, naproxen, oxaprozin, piroxicam
Uncommon
• Phenytoin • Sulfonamide antibiotics: sulfamethoxazole, sulfisoxazole

Based on case reports, additional drugs have been implicated and they are listed in Table 31.5 of Dermatology, Fourth Edition.

Unusual variants include toxic epidermal necrolysis-like and morbilliform.

Table 25.1 Drug-induced linear IgA bullous dermatosis. ACE, angiotensin-converting enzyme.

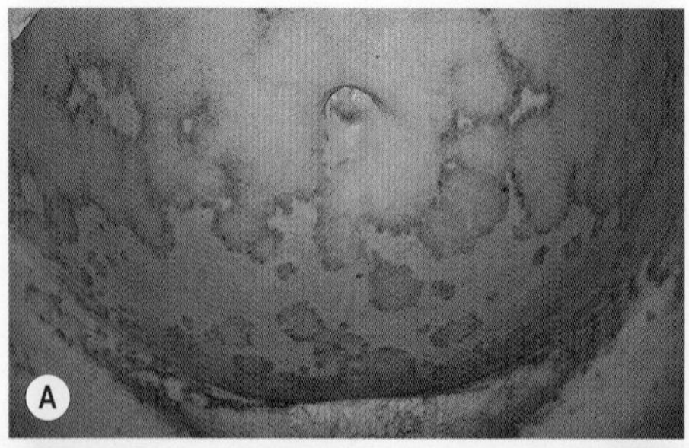

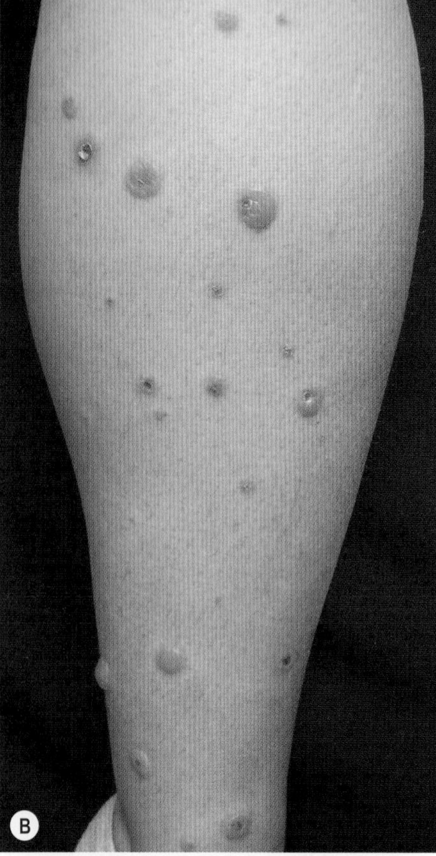

Fig. 25.6 Linear IgA bullous dermatosis. **A** Annular and polycyclic erythematous plaques of the trunk. **B** Vesicles and bullae arising within normal-appearing skin as well as scattered annular lesions. *A, Courtesy, John J. Zone, MD; B, Courtesy, Jeffrey P. Callen, MD.*

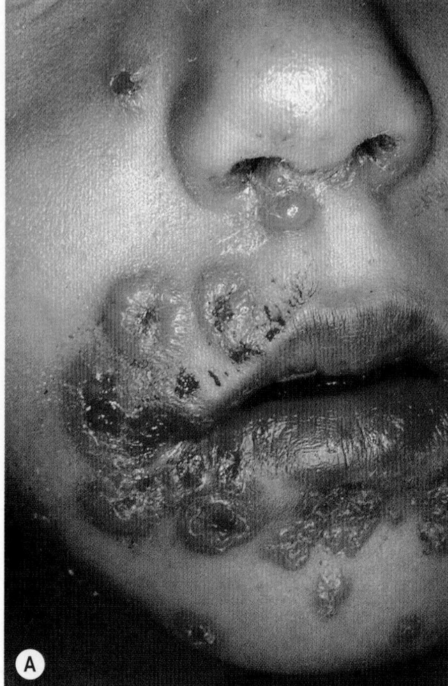

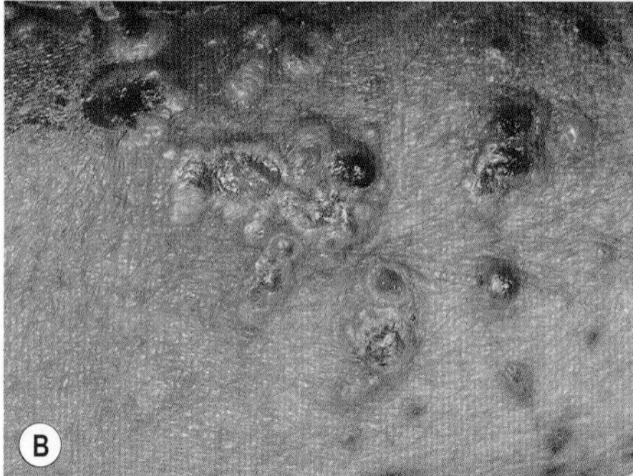

Fig. 25.7 Linear IgA bullous dermatosis. **A** Annular and herpetiform vesiculobullae on the face of a child. **B** Vancomycin-induced variant with a similar arrangement of vesiculopustules. Note the central hemorrhagic crusts in both patients. *Courtesy, YDRSC.*

Epidermolysis Bullosa 26

• Epidermolysis bullosa (EB) is a group of genetic disorders characterized by mechanical fragility of the skin that leads to blister formation with minor trauma or friction.
• Inherited EB is traditionally divided into three major categories – EB simplex (EBS), junctional EB (JEB), and dystrophic EB (DEB) – that differ in the ultrastructural site of blister formation (Fig. 26.1).
• The overall incidence is approximately 1 in 50,000 births, with EBS representing the most common form.
• Mutations in the genes encoding at least 20 structural proteins of the skin can result in EB, with variable clinical phenotypes, ultrastructural findings, and inheritance patterns.
• The major subtypes of EB and Kindler syndrome (now classified as a fourth form of EB) are summarized in Table 26.1.
• Fig. 26.2 presents an approach to the laboratory diagnosis of EB via genetic analysis with a massively parallel (next-generation) sequencing panel as well as traditional methods utilizing immunofluorescence antigenic mapping and/or electron microscopy on a punch biopsy specimen from a freshly induced blister.

Clinical Features of EB

• The severity and distribution of blistering vary depending on the EB subtype (see Table 26.1), the patient's age (e.g. improving over time, especially for EBS), and environmental factors (e.g. sweating, friction).
• Scarring (usually atrophic), milia, and nail dystrophy may develop in any subtype of EB, but they are most common in DEB (Fig. 26.9; see Figs 26.6 and 26.7).
• The molecular defects in EB can also affect other organs/tissues with an epithelial surface, such as the oral mucosa, eye, and gastrointestinal and genitourinary tracts (see Table 26.1).
• **DDx:** sucking blisters and other genetic (e.g. epidermolytic ichthyosis), infectious (e.g. bullous impetigo, staphylococcal scalded skin syndrome) or autoimmune blistering disorders of infancy (see Ch. 28).

Management of EB

• Management focuses on minimizing mechanical trauma, providing wound care, and preventing infection. Protective dressings/padding, soft clothing, and bathing/soaking with dilute sodium hypochlorite (0.5 cup household bleach in full standard bathtub) or 0.25% acetic acid (1 : 20 white vinegar : water) can be helpful.
• Adhesives should be avoided and only nonadherent/"low-tack" dressing materials applied to EB skin, e.g. petrolatum-impregnated gauze (adding extra petrolatum to prevent sticking) and soft silicone dressings (e.g. Mepitel®, Mepilex®), followed by rolled gauze.
• Lancing and draining blisters with placement of a small window can relieve pressure and promote healing; antibiotics should be used judiciously, avoiding chronic treatment with topical mupirocin or oral antibiotics.
• A multidisciplinary approach is helpful, especially for more severe forms of EB, with attention to oral/dental care, growth, nutritional status, and other potential complications.
• Older children and adults with recessive DEB require periodic total-body skin examinations, with biopsy of nonhealing ulcers to exclude SCC.

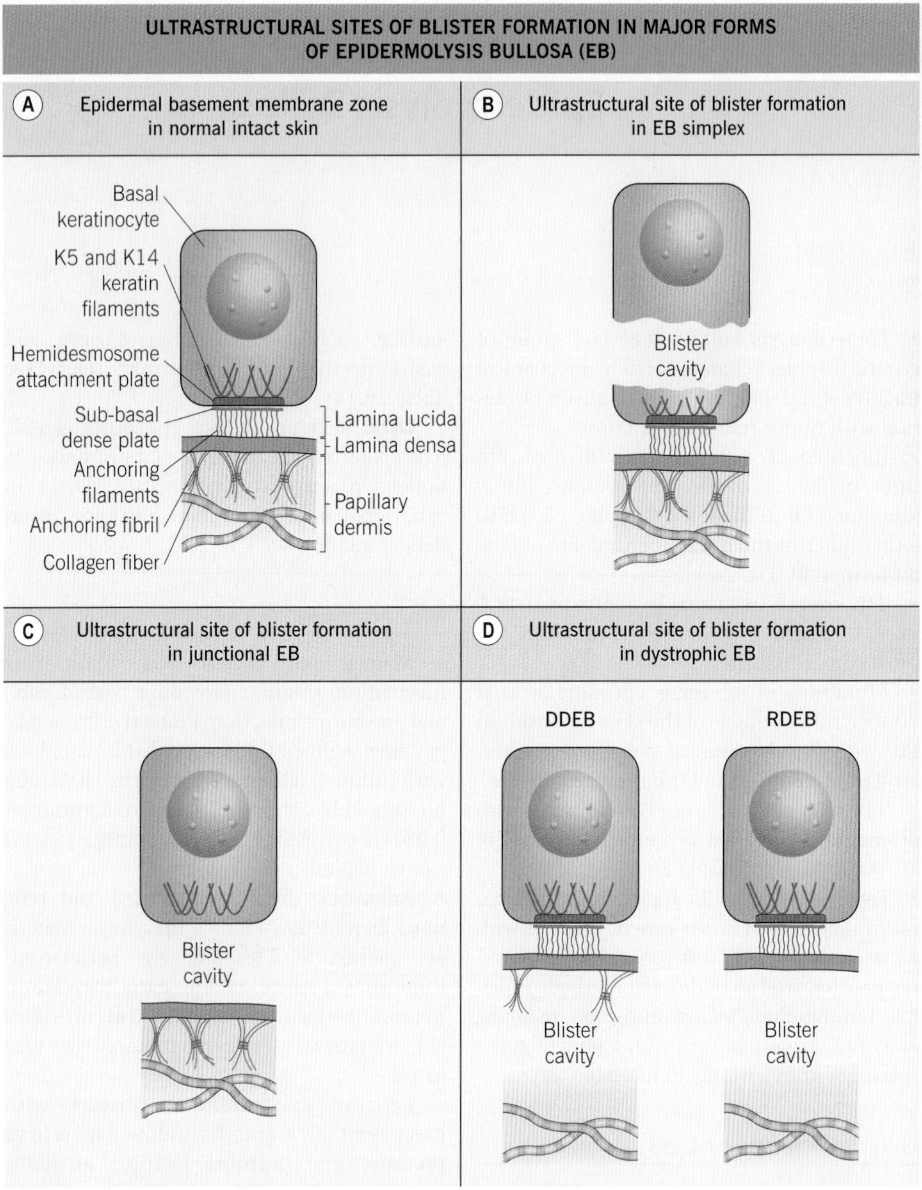

ULTRASTRUCTURAL SITES OF BLISTER FORMATION IN MAJOR FORMS OF EPIDERMOLYSIS BULLOSA (EB)

(A) Epidermal basement membrane zone in normal intact skin

Basal keratinocyte
K5 and K14 keratin filaments
Hemidesmosome attachment plate
Sub-basal dense plate
Anchoring filaments
Anchoring fibril
Collagen fiber
Lamina lucida
Lamina densa
Papillary dermis

(B) Ultrastructural site of blister formation in EB simplex

Blister cavity

(C) Ultrastructural site of blister formation in junctional EB

Blister cavity

(D) Ultrastructural site of blister formation in dystrophic EB

DDEB
RDEB
Blister cavity
Blister cavity

Fig. 26.1 Ultrastructural sites of blister formation in major forms of epidermolysis bullosa (EB). A In intact skin, the ultrastructural regions of the epidermal basement membrane zone consist of (1) basal keratinocytes and the hemidesmosomal plaque; (2) the lamina lucida; (3) the lamina densa; (4) the upper papillary dermis. **B** In EB simplex (EBS), blisters arise within the lower portion of basal keratinocytes. **C** In junctional EB (JEB), blisters form within the lamina lucida. **D** In dystrophic EB (DEB), blisters develop below the lamina densa. Anchoring fibrils are reduced in number in dominant DEB (DDEB) and absent or rudimentary in recessive DEB (RDEB). K5, keratin 5; K14, keratin 14.

MAJOR EPIDERMOLYSIS BULLOSA (EB) SUBTYPES		
Subtype	**Defective proteins (inheritance)**	**Features and complications**
EB simplex (EBS)		
EBS, localized (formerly Weber–Cockayne)	Keratins 5 and 14 (AD)	• Primarily affects palms/soles (Fig. 26.3)
EBS, severe (formerly Dowling–Meara)		• Arcuate/figurate array of blisters (Fig. 26.4A) • PPK (Fig. 26.4B)
EBS, intermediate		• Often worse in early childhood (Fig. 26.4C)
EBS with muscular dystrophy	Plectin (AR)	• Onset of muscular dystrophy may be delayed until adolescence/early adulthood
Junctional EB (JEB)*		
JEB, severe (formerly Herlitz)	Laminin-332 (AR)	• Exuberant granulation tissue (Fig. 26.5) • Often death during infancy from FTT, tracheolaryngeal involvement, and/or sepsis • Systemic complications similar to RDEB-severe in survivors
JEB, intermediate	Laminin-332, type XVII collagen/ BPAG2 (AR)	• Large, irregularly shaped, darkly pigmented nevi ("EB nevi")†
JEB with pyloric atresia	$\alpha_6\beta_4$ integrin (AR)	• Born with pyloric atresia
Dystrophic EB (DEB)		
Dominant DEB, localized or intermediate	Type VII collagen (AD)	• Prominent scarring, milia, and nail dystrophy (Fig. 26.6)
Recessive DEB, severe (formerly Hallopeau–Siemens)	Type VII collagen (AR)	• Pseudosyndactyly (mitten deformity) of hands/feet (Fig. 26.7A) and osteoporosis develop over time • Microstomia, excessive dental caries • Corneal ulcers/scarring, esophageal and urethral strictures, constipation, anemia, FTT, cardiomyopathy, renal failure • >50% risk of cutaneous SCC (Fig. 26.7B) by age 30 years†; represents leading cause of death
Recessive DEB, other subtypes		• Include intermediate, inversa, and localized forms
Other		
Kindler EB (Kindler syndrome)	Kindlin-1‡ (AR)	• Acral blistering, primarily during infancy; ± webbing of fingers/toes (Fig. 26.8A, B), PPK • Photosensitivity that decreases with age • Progressive poikiloderma (Fig. 26.8C), "cigarette paper" atrophy (Fig. 26.8B) • Gingivitis, colitis, stenoses, ectropion

**Dental enamel hypoplasia occurs in all forms of JEB.*

†"EB nevi" occasionally occur in other EB subtypes, and patients with severe RDEB have an increased risk of melanoma.

‡Mediates anchorage between the actin cytoskeleton and the extracellular matrix via focal adhesions.

Table 26.1 Major epidermolysis bullosa (EB) subtypes. Other erosive skin fragility disorders due to desmosomal defects (e.g. plakophilin deficiency) feature intraepidermal blistering (with acantholysis in skin biopsy specimens), PPK, nail dystrophy, and hypotrichosis. AD, autosomal dominant; AR, autosomal recessive; BPAG, bullous pemphigoid antigen; FTT, failure to thrive; PPK, palmoplantar keratoderma.

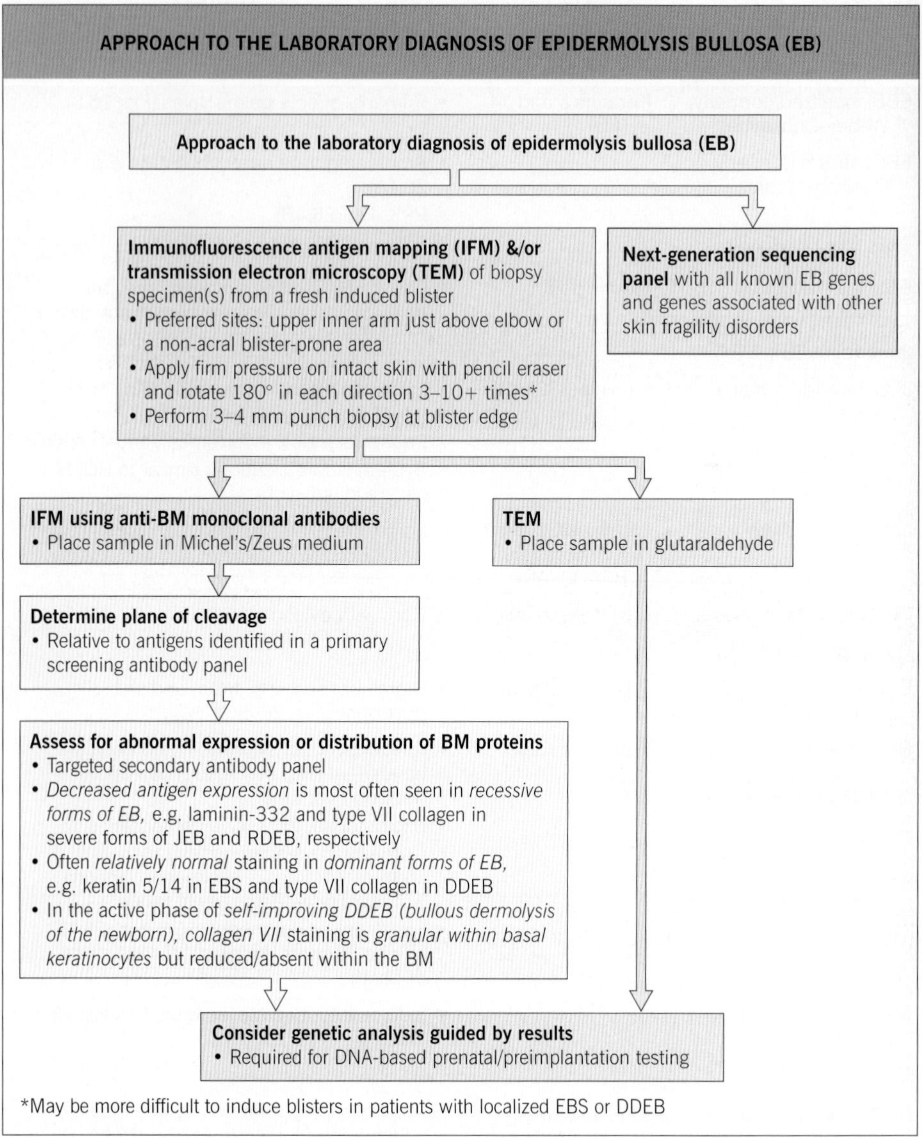

APPROACH TO THE LABORATORY DIAGNOSIS OF EPIDERMOLYSIS BULLOSA (EB)

Approach to the laboratory diagnosis of epidermolysis bullosa (EB)

→ **Immunofluorescence antigen mapping (IFM) &/or transmission electron microscopy (TEM)** of biopsy specimen(s) from a fresh induced blister
- Preferred sites: upper inner arm just above elbow or a non-acral blister-prone area
- Apply firm pressure on intact skin with pencil eraser and rotate 180° in each direction 3–10+ times*
- Perform 3–4 mm punch biopsy at blister edge

→ **Next-generation sequencing panel** with all known EB genes and genes associated with other skin fragility disorders

From IFM/TEM:

→ **IFM using anti-BM monoclonal antibodies**
- Place sample in Michel's/Zeus medium

→ **Determine plane of cleavage**
- Relative to antigens identified in a primary screening antibody panel

→ **Assess for abnormal expression or distribution of BM proteins**
- Targeted secondary antibody panel
- *Decreased antigen expression* is most often seen in *recessive forms of EB,* e.g. laminin-332 and type VII collagen in severe forms of JEB and RDEB, respectively
- Often *relatively normal* staining in *dominant forms of EB,* e.g. keratin 5/14 in EBS and type VII collagen in DDEB
- In the active phase of *self-improving DDEB (bullous dermolysis of the newborn), collagen VII* staining is *granular within basal keratinocytes* but reduced/absent within the BM

→ **TEM**
- Place sample in glutaraldehyde

→ **Consider genetic analysis guided by results**
- Required for DNA-based prenatal/preimplantation testing

*May be more difficult to induce blisters in patients with localized EBS or DDEB

Fig. 26.2 Approach to the laboratory diagnosis of epidermolysis bullosa (EB). BM, basement membrane; DDEB, dominant dystrophic EB; EBS, EB simplex; JEB, junctional EB; RDEB, recessive dystrophic EB.

- Novel topical treatments (e.g. the interleukin-1β inhibitor diacerein and a betulin-based oleogel) as well as cell-based (e.g. hematopoietic stem cell transplantation) and gene therapies, including nuclease-based targeted gene editing techniques (e.g. CRISPR-Cas9 systems), are under investigation for EB patients.
- Physicians and families can obtain helpful information from websites such as www.debra.org and www.debra-international.org.

For further information see Ch. 32 from *Dermatology, Fourth Edition*.

For additional online figures visit www.expertconsult.com 

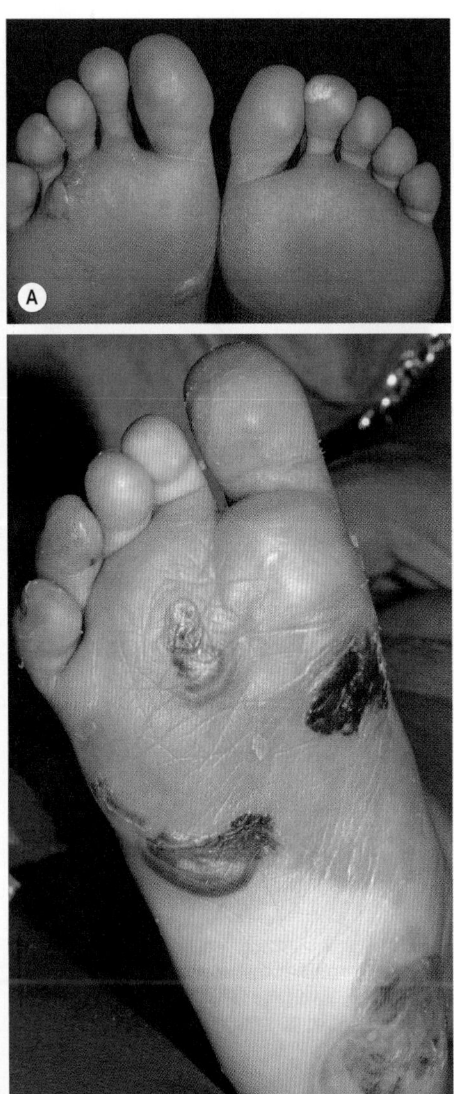

Fig. 26.3 Localized epidermolysis bullosa simplex. A, B Bullae arising on the toes and plantar surfaces at sites of lateral or rotary traction. The majority of blisters occur in acral sites. *A, Courtesy, YDRSC; B, Courtesy, Julie V. Schaffer, MD.*

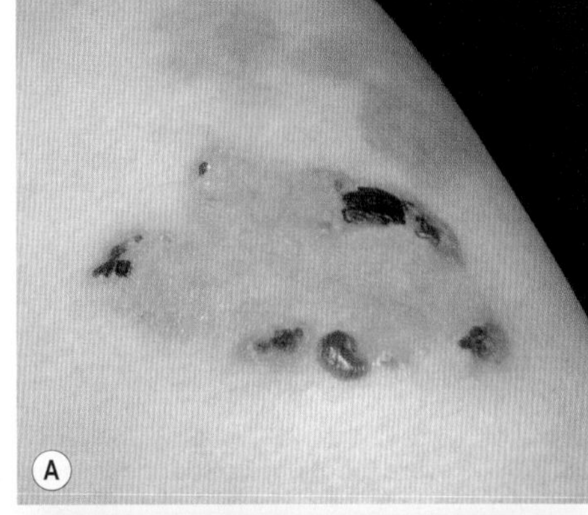

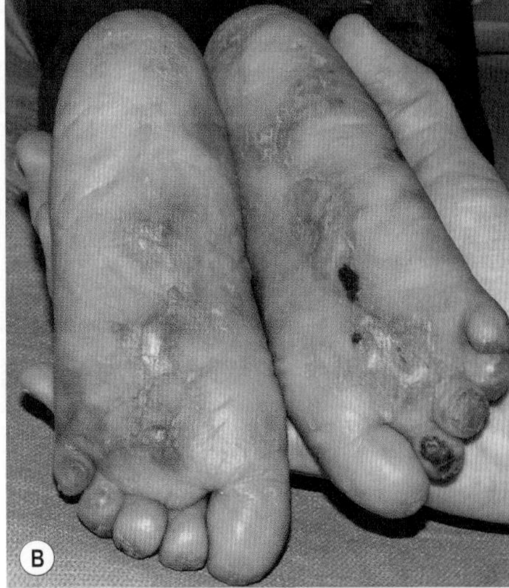

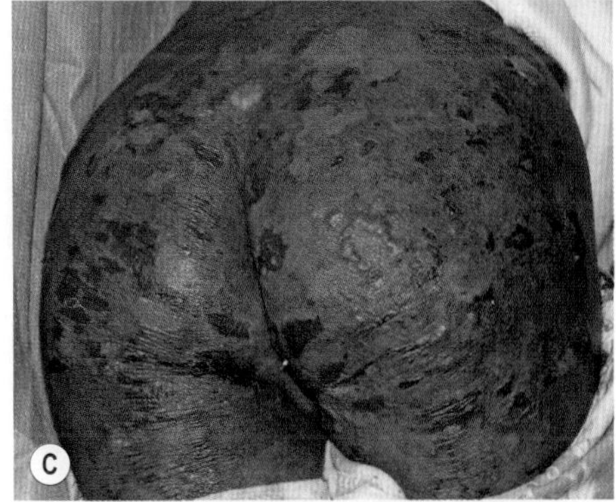

Fig. 26.4 Severe forms of epidermolysis bullosa simplex (EBS). A Arcuate array of vesicles in a child. **B** Blistering in association with focal keratoderma on the soles. **C** Widespread blistering in a toddler. *Courtesy, Julie V. Schaffer, MD.*

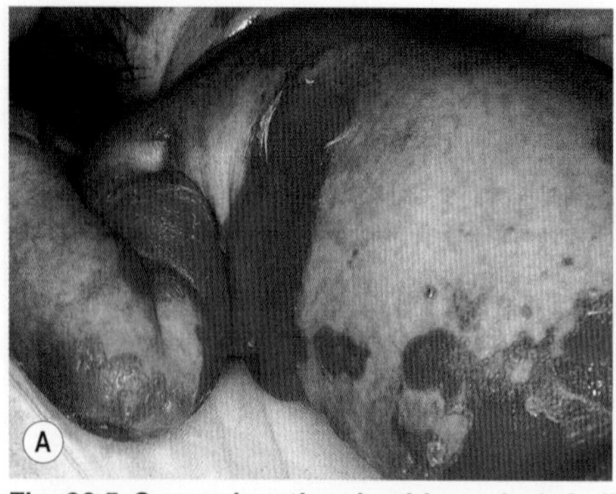

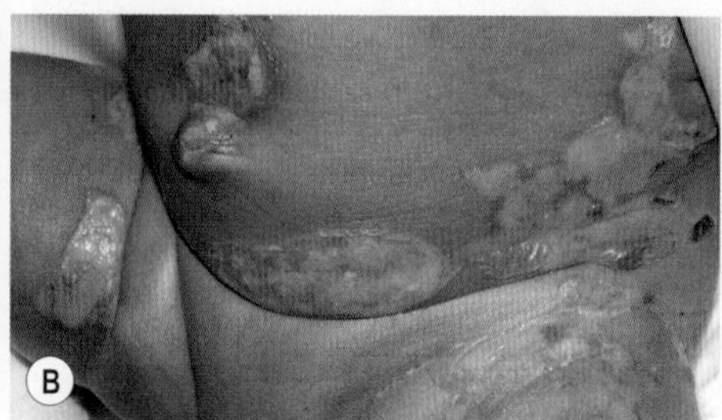

Fig. 26.5 Severe junctional epidermolysis bullosa. A Blisters on the elbow and large areas of denuded skin; note the bright red color in the axilla and groin. **B** Blisters and large erosions on the abdomen of an infant. *A, Courtesy, YDRSC; B, Courtesy, Julie V. Schaffer, MD.*

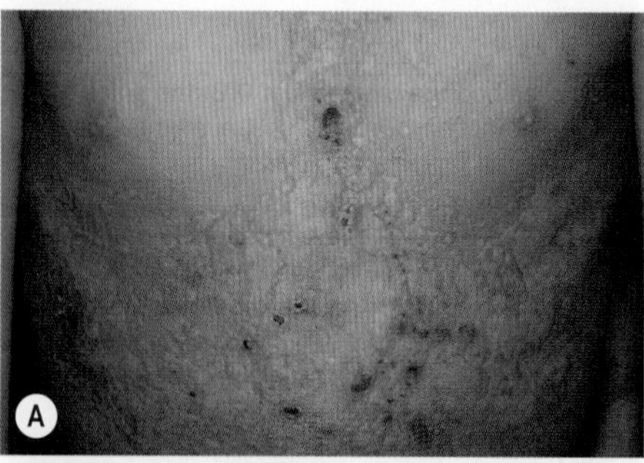

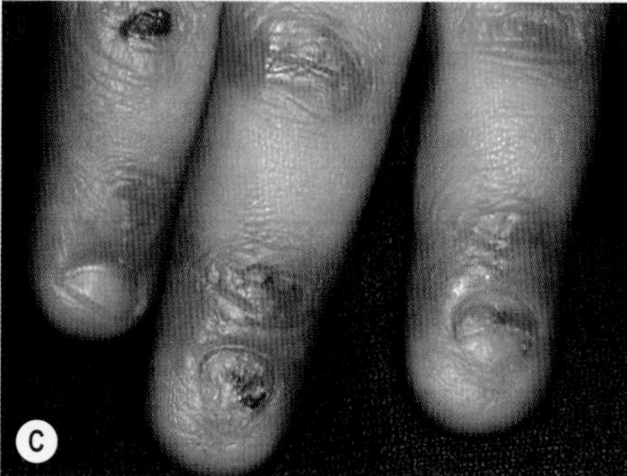

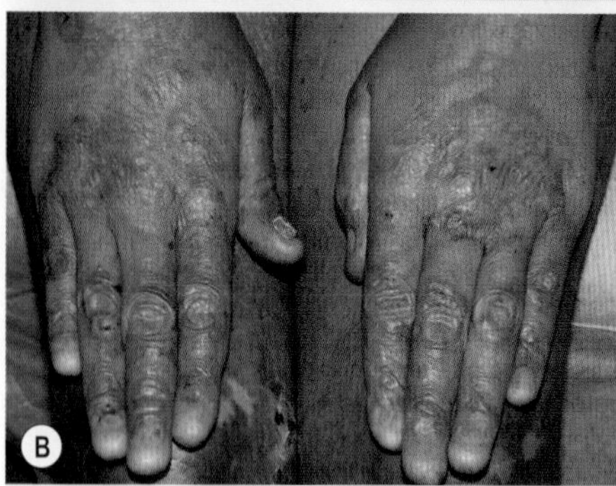

Fig. 26.6 Dominant dystrophic epidermolysis bullosa. Prominent scarring on the chest **(A)** and hands **(B)** as well as milia and loss of the fingernails **(B)** in a teenage boy. **C** Erosions, scarring, and milia on the fingers with partial loss of the nails. *A, C, Courtesy, YDRSC; B, Courtesy, Julie V. Schaffer, MD.*

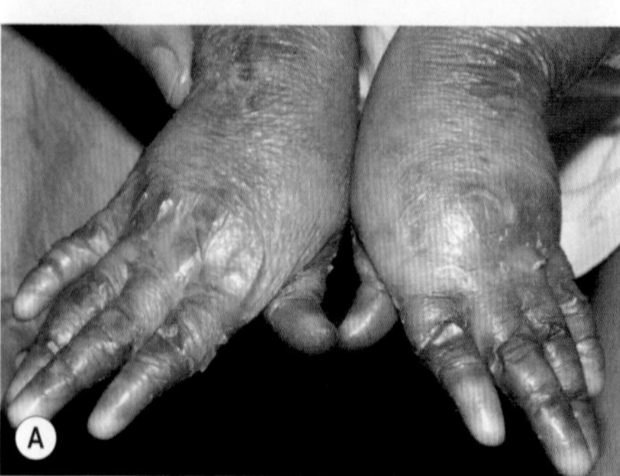

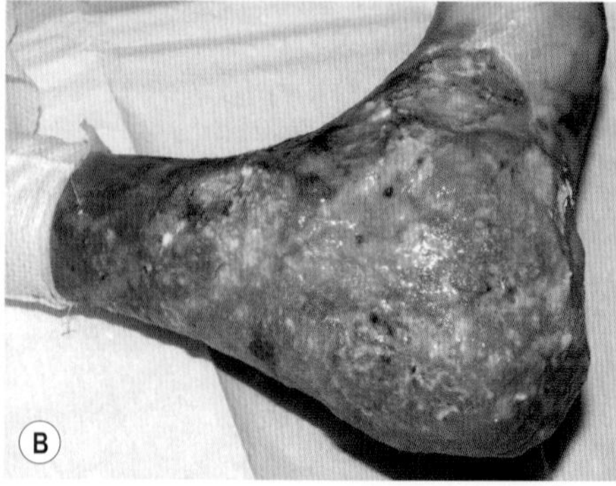

Fig. 26.7 Severe recessive dystrophic epidermolysis bullosa. A Early proximal interdigital web formation together with atrophic scarring and loss of nails in a 5-year-old girl. **B** Large squamous cell carcinoma in a 21-year-old man. *Courtesy, Julie V. Schaffer, MD.*

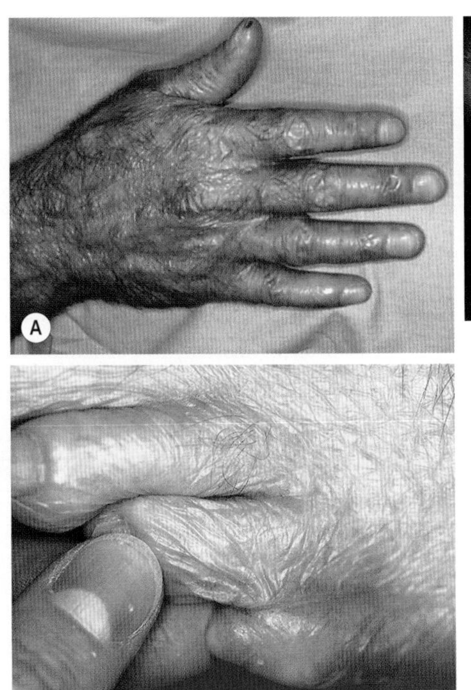

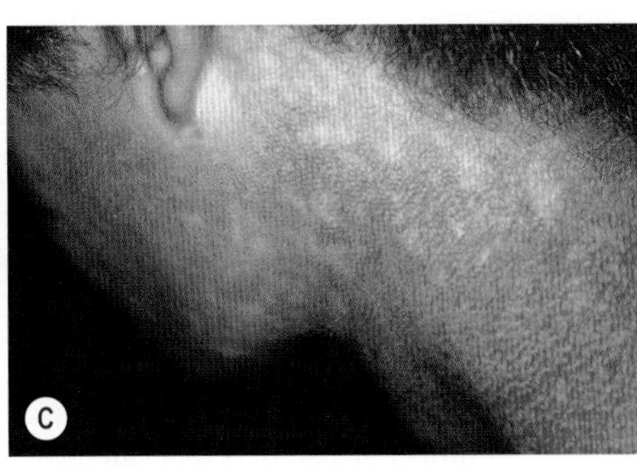

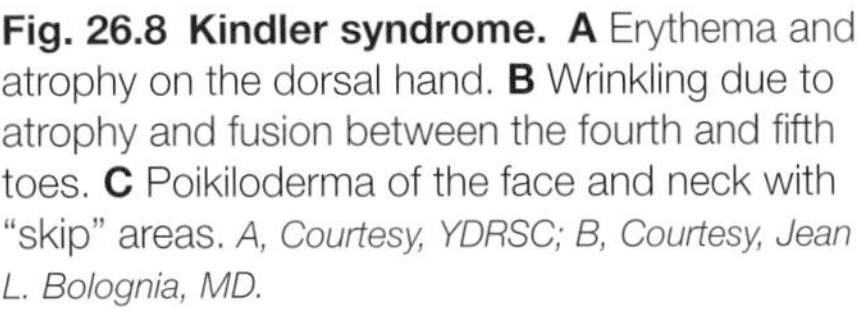

Fig. 26.8 Kindler syndrome. A Erythema and atrophy on the dorsal hand. **B** Wrinkling due to atrophy and fusion between the fourth and fifth toes. **C** Poikiloderma of the face and neck with "skip" areas. *A, Courtesy, YDRSC; B, Courtesy, Jean L. Bolognia, MD.*

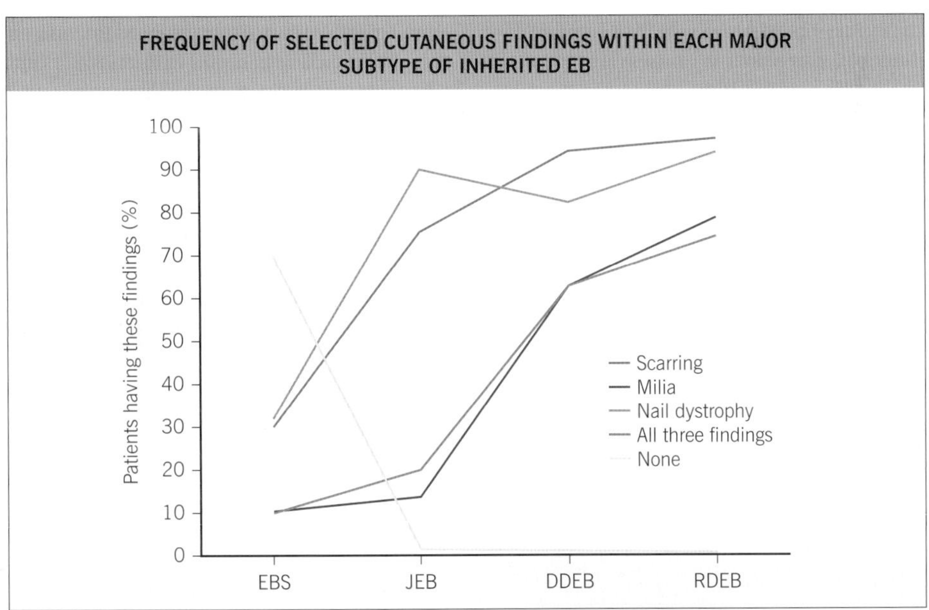

Fig. 26.9 Frequency of selected cutaneous findings within each major subtype of inherited epidermolysis bullosa (EB). Note the increasing frequency from localized EB simplex (EBS) to recessive dystrophic EB (RDEB). JEB, junctional EB; DDEB, dominant dystrophic EB.

27 Other Vesiculobullous Diseases

There are a number of disorders that can present with vesicles and bullae, including exaggerated insect bite reactions (Fig. 27.1; see Ch. 20), autoimmune and inherited blistering diseases (see Chs 23–26), porphyrias (see Ch. 41), the Stevens–Johnson syndrome–toxic epidermal necrolysis spectrum (see Ch. 16), and phototoxicity, from sunburn to phototoxic drug reactions (e.g. due to doxycycline). Even cutaneous small vessel vasculitis can become bullous (Fig. 27.2). This chapter examines a miscellaneous group of disorders, several of which favor the lower extremities, whereas Chapter 28 reviews vesiculobullous diseases in newborns and infants.

Friction Blisters

- Most commonly develop on the heels, soles, and palms; the blister develops within the epidermis, contains clear or hemorrhagic fluid ("blood blister"), and heals spontaneously without scarring.
- Due to repeated friction (e.g. prolonged walking in ill-fitting shoes) and repetitive actions (e.g. raking leaves).

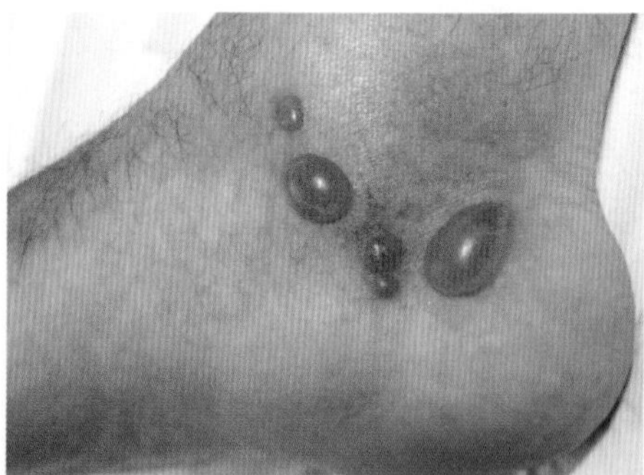

Fig. 27.1 Bullous insect bite reactions. The sterile blister fluid is serous and the ankle is a common site. *Courtesy, Luis Requena, MD.*

- **DDx:** if exaggerated response, can consider inherited blistering disease, in particular the localized form of epidermolysis bullosa simplex (see Ch. 26).
- **Rx:** if significant fluid accumulation, drainage of fluid can relieve pressure; the roof of the blister should be left in place to act as a "natural Band-Aid®"; secondary soft tissue infection is unusual in immunocompetent individuals.

Edema Bullae (Edema Blisters)

- The bullae are bland (i.e. non-inflammatory), initially tense, and may reach several centimeters in diameter; they arise within areas of significant edema and contain sterile, usually clear but occasionally blood-tinged, fluid.
- The most common location is the distal lower extremities, often in the setting of an acute exacerbation of chronic edema in an elderly patient; in patients with anasarca and those who are bedridden, the distribution can be more widespread (Fig. 27.3).
- **DDx:** bullosis diabeticorum and bullous pemphigoid, including the variant localized to the lower extremities; if there is surrounding erythema, warmth and tenderness, then bullous cellulitis needs to be excluded.
- **Rx:** as bullae resolve in concert with the edema, only drainage of larger bullae needs to be considered (see section below).

Bullosis Diabeticorum (Diabetic Bullae)

- In patients with diabetes mellitus, tense bland bullae arise rather suddenly within normal-appearing skin; the diameter varies from 0.5 to several centimeters (Fig. 27.4); the blister fluid is sterile and clear, but may be more viscous than that of friction or edema blisters.

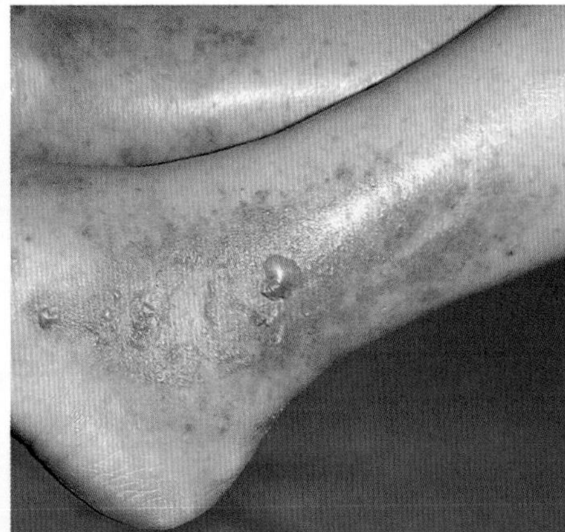

Fig. 27.2 Bullous variant of cutaneous small vessel vasculitis. There is a background of purpuric papules and plaques. *Courtesy, Jeffrey P. Callen, MD.*

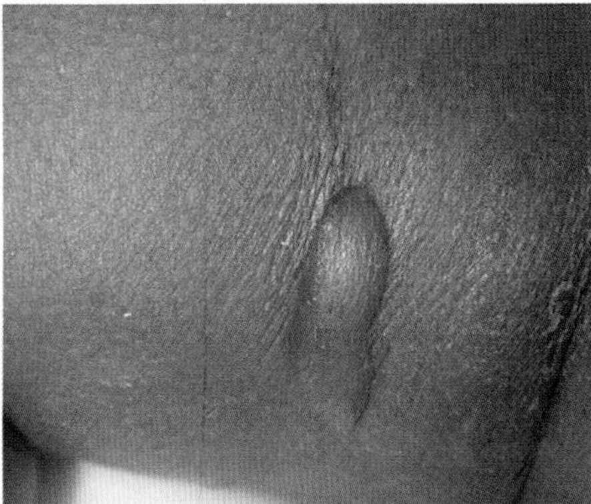

Fig. 27.3 Edema bullae on the thigh of an infant. The bullae are tense and are surrounded by edema. Desquamation from a ruptured bulla is also seen. *Courtesy, YDRSC.*

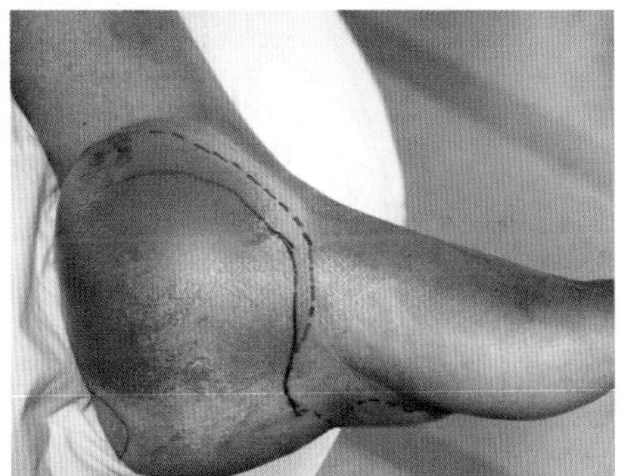

Fig. 27.4 Bullosis diabeticorum. A large, tense bulla overlying the medial malleolus. Note the absence of erythema or edema in the surrounding skin. *Courtesy, YDRSC.*

- Most commonly develops on the distal extremities (lower > upper) of adults and may be accompanied by peripheral neuropathy.
- **DDx:** bullous pemphigoid, epidermolysis bullosa acquisita, porphyria cutanea tarda, pseudoporphyria, bullous impetigo, and if significant edema, edema bullae; given the increased risk of soft tissue infections in diabetics, the possibility of bullous cellulitis needs to be excluded if there is surrounding erythema.
- **Rx:** placing a small window in a dependent location in the roof of the blister allows for both drainage and preservation of the blister roof; no further treatment is required for uncomplicated lesions, as they spontaneously heal over 3–6 weeks.

Delayed Postburn/Postgraft Blisters

- Tense vesicles or bullae may develop within areas of previous thermal burns as well as within recipient or donor skin graft sites; occur weeks to months after initial injury has healed.
- Possible explanation is enhanced fragility due to a less mature basement membrane zone within the healing wound.
- **DDx:** limited given specific distribution, but includes ischemia within graft recipient sites, herpetic infections, bullous impetigo, and occasionally autoimmune bullous diseases (locus minoris resistentiae phenomenon).
- **Rx:** supportive as lesions heal spontaneously, but can recur.

Coma Bullae (Coma Blisters)

- Tense cutaneous vesicles and bullae can appear within 2 or 3 days of prolonged pressure secondary to immobilization (Figs 27.5 and 27.6); there is often preceding blanchable erythema.
- The bullae develop at sites of maximum pressure and therefore often develop in the skin overlying joints or bony prominences.
- The prolonged pressure may occur in the setting of a coma, whose cause can vary from drug-induced to metabolic (e.g. hepatic encephalopathy); immobility can also result from neurologic disorders, especially cerebral vascular accidents.

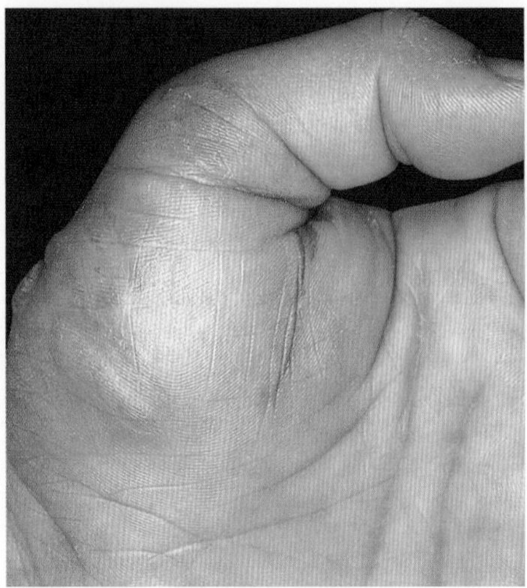

Fig. 27.5 Coma bullae. Blisters developed in an area of pressure in a previously comatose patient. *Courtesy, José M. Mascaró Jr., MD.*

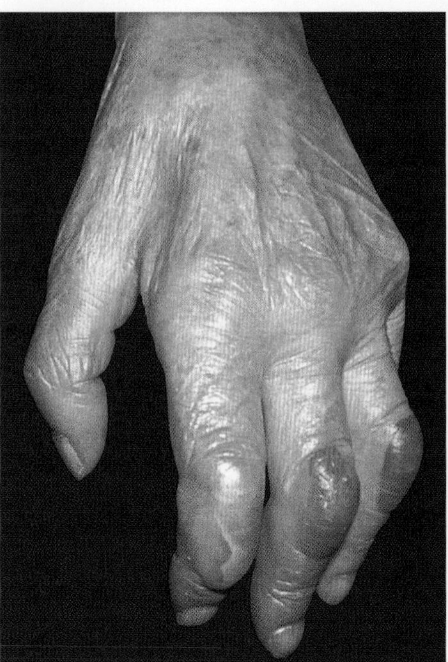

Fig. 27.6 Neurologic blisters. Tense blisters on the dorsal aspect of the fingers on the hemiplegic side of a patient with a previous cerebrovascular accident. *Courtesy, José M. Mascaró Jr., MD.*

- Characteristic histopathologic finding of necrosis of eccrine sweat glands, presumably secondary to local hypoxia.
- **DDx:** usually limited if history of immobilization obtained and distribution pattern limited to pressure points appreciated.
- **Rx:** supportive as lesions heal over 1 or 2 weeks; prevention requires frequent repositioning of the patient.

For further information see Ch. 33 from *Dermatology, Fourth Edition*.

For additional online figures visit www.expertconsult.com 

Vesiculopustular and Erosive Disorders in Newborns and Infants

28

This chapter covers classic transient neonatal eruptions as well as several infectious diseases and other disorders that present with vesiculopustules in the neonatal period or early infancy. Table 28.1 provides a more complete differential diagnosis of vesiculopustules, bullae, erosions, and ulcerations in neonates.

Common Transient Conditions

Erythema Toxicum Neonatorum ("e tox")

- Affects approximately half of full-term neonates; less common in premature infants.
- Typically appears 1–2 days after delivery and lasts up to 2 weeks, with individual lesions resolving within 1 day; occasionally present at birth, and rarely develops as late as 1 to 2 weeks of age.
- Various combinations of erythematous macules, wheals, and small (≤2 mm) papules, pustules, and vesicles surrounded by a larger erythematous flare (Fig. 28.1); lesions may be grouped at sites of mechanical irritation.
- Often begins on the face and progresses to the trunk, buttocks, and proximal extremities; usually spares the palms and soles.
- Wright or Giemsa stain of pustular contents shows numerous eosinophils.
- **Rx:** none.

Transient Neonatal Pustular Melanosis

- Affects up to 5% of full-term neonates with darkly pigmented skin; less common in Caucasian newborns. May exist on a spectrum with erythema toxicum neonatorum.
- Lesions are almost always present at birth.
- Three stages, any of which may be present at a given time (Fig. 28.2).
  - 2- to 10-mm superficial vesiculopustules with little or no surrounding erythema
  - Collarettes of scale at sites of ruptured vesiculopustules
  - Residual brown macules representing postinflammatory hyperpigmentation, which may persist for several months
- Any region can be affected, but favors the forehead, chin, neck, lower back, and shins.
- Wright or Giemsa stain of pustular contents shows neutrophils > eosinophils.
- **Rx:** none.

Miliaria (Heat Rash)

- Common condition in newborns, especially with overheating related to excessive swaddling, warming in an incubator, fever, occlusive dressings, and hot climates.
- Caused by blockage of eccrine sweat ducts.
- Miliaria crystallina.
  - Small clear vesicles (likened to "dew drops") without surrounding erythema (Fig. 28.3A); they are fragile and therefore short-lived
  - Most often on the forehead, upper trunk, and arms
- Miliaria rubra.
  - Usually develops at ≥1 week of age
  - Small erythematous papules, sometimes with a tiny central pustule or vesicle (Fig. 28.3B see Fig. 32.7C)
  - Favors the neck, upper trunk, and occluded areas
- **Rx:** avoid overheating and occlusion; bathing with lukewarm water.

Neonatal Cephalic Pustulosis (Neonatal Acne)

- Affects ~20% of newborns.
- Onset usually within the first 2–3 weeks of life, with spontaneous resolution by 3 months of age.
- Papulopustular eruption on the face (cheeks > forehead, chin, eyelids) (Fig. 28.4) > neck, upper chest, and scalp.

DIFFERENTIAL DIAGNOSIS OF NEONATAL VESICULOPUSTULES, BULLAE, EROSIONS, AND ULCERS
Vesiculopustular eruptions
Infectious diseases and infestations
• Bacterial (see Ch. 61): bullous impetigo; group A>B streptococcal or *Listeria* infection • Candidiasis (congenital or neonatal) • Viral (see Ch. 67): HSV infection, neonatal varicella, herpes zoster (age ≥2 weeks) • Scabies (age ≥3–4 weeks) (see Ch. 71)
Common transient conditions
• Erythema toxicum neonatorum, transient neonatal pustular melanosis • Miliaria crystallina and rubra • Neonatal cephalic pustulosis
Uncommon and rare non-infectious diseases
• Acropustulosis of infancy, eosinophilic pustular folliculitis of infancy • Incontinentia pigmenti • Congenital Langerhans cell histiocytosis (Fig. 28.11) (see Ch.76) • Neonatal papulopustular eruption of autosomal dominant hyper-IgE syndrome (see Ch. 49), neutrophilic and granulomatous dermatitis associated with primary immunodeficiencies • Vesiculopustular eruption* of transient myeloproliferative disorder in Down syndrome • Pustular psoriasis (see Ch. 6), deficiency of the interleukin-1 receptor antagonist (DIRA; see Ch. 37) • Erosive pustular dermatosis of the scalp (more common in older adults)
Bullae, erosions, and ulcers
Infectious diseases
• Bacterial (see Ch. 61): staphylococcal scalded skin syndrome (Fig. 28.12), *Pseudomonas* infection (including noma neonatorum)†, congenital syphilis • Fungal** (see Ch. 64): aspergillosis, zygomycosis • Intrauterine HSV infection, congenital varicella (see Ch. 67)
Conditions with exogenous causes
• Sucking blister, perinatal/iatrogenic injury, irritant contact dermatitis (see Ch. 12)
Uncommon and rare non-infectious diseases
• Mastocytosis (Fig. 28.13; see Ch. 96), ulcerated infantile hemangioma (see Ch. 85) • Aplasia cutis congenita (Fig. 28.14; see Ch. 53) • Genodermatoses, especially epidermolysis bullosa (see Ch. 26) and epidermolytic ichthyosis (Fig. 28.15; see Ch. 46) • Zinc deficiency, acquired or inherited (acrodermatitis enteropathica; see Ch. 43) • Autoimmune bullous diseases (often due to maternal antibodies; see Chs 22–25) • Maternofetal or transfusion-associated GVHD in infants with SCID (see Ch. 49) • Congenital erosive and vesicular dermatosis • Nutritional dermatitis (see Fig. 43.4)

**Favors the cheeks.*

***Evolves into necrotic ulcers; risk factors include prematurity and occlusion; "invasive fungal dermatitis" in very-low-birth-weight premature neonates can be caused by* Aspergillus *or* Trichosporon *as well as* Candida *spp.; biopsy for tissue culture and histopathology can aid in the diagnosis.*

†Evolves into necrotic ulcers that favor the groin; risk factors include prematurity, immunodeficiency, and (especially for noma) malnutrition.

Table 28.1 Differential diagnosis of neonatal vesiculopustules, bullae, erosions, and ulcers. This list is not exhaustive, as other rare diseases such as ankyloblepharon–ectodermal dysplasia–clefting (AEC) syndrome and congenital Behçet disease can have vesiculopustular and erosive presentations. SCID, severe combined immunodeficiency.

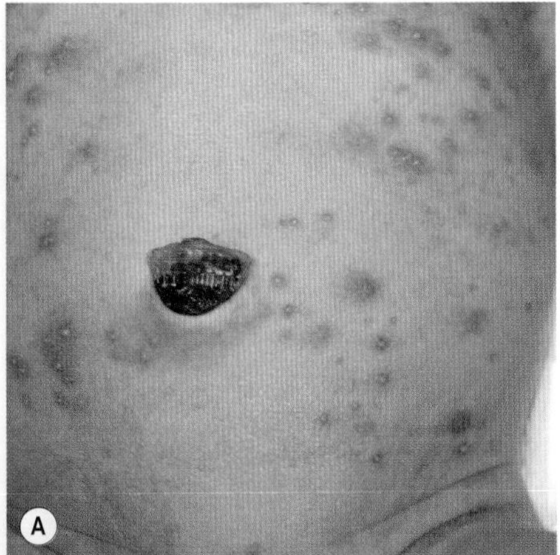

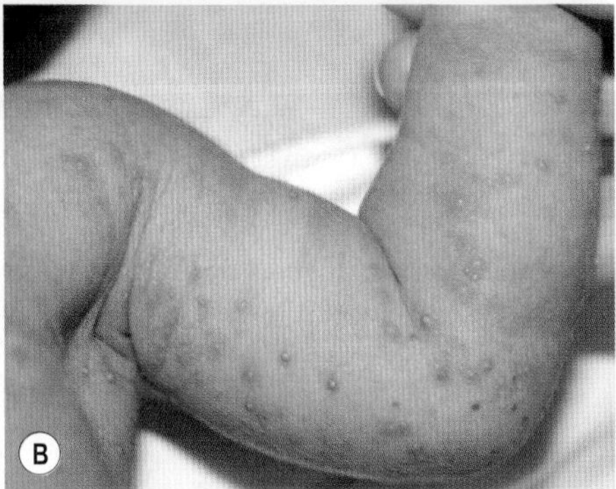

Fig. 28.1 Erythema toxicum neonatorum. Scattered papulovesicles and pustules with an erythematous flare on the abdomen (**A**) and upper extremity (**B**). *Courtesy, Deborah S. Goddard, MD, Amy E. Gilliam, MD, and Ilona J. Frieden, MD.*

- An absence of comedones in neonatal cephalic pustulosis distinguishes it from infantile acne, which typically develops at 3–12 months of age and is more persistent (see Ch. 29).
- May represent an inflammatory response to *Malassezia* spp., a normal component of the skin microbiome that may also trigger seborrheic dermatitis.
- **Rx:** usually not required; topical imidazole (e.g. ketoconazole cream) or hydrocortisone may be helpful.

Sucking Blister

- Caused by habitual sucking of the affected area *in utero*, and resolves spontaneously within days to weeks of birth.
- Intact bulla, erosion, callus, or ulceration on a non-inflamed base (Fig. 28.5A).
- Common sites include the radial forearm, wrist, hand, and fingers.

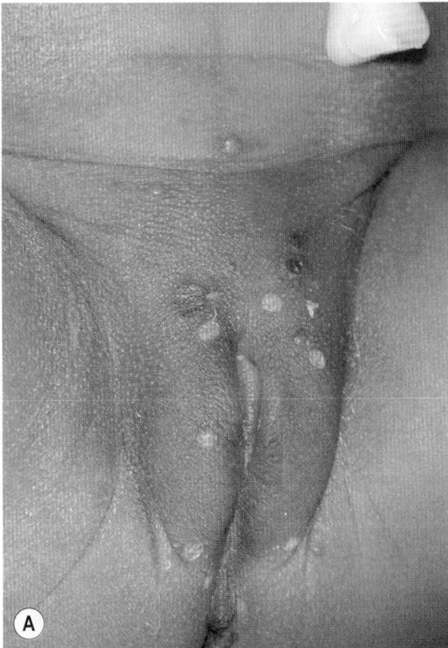

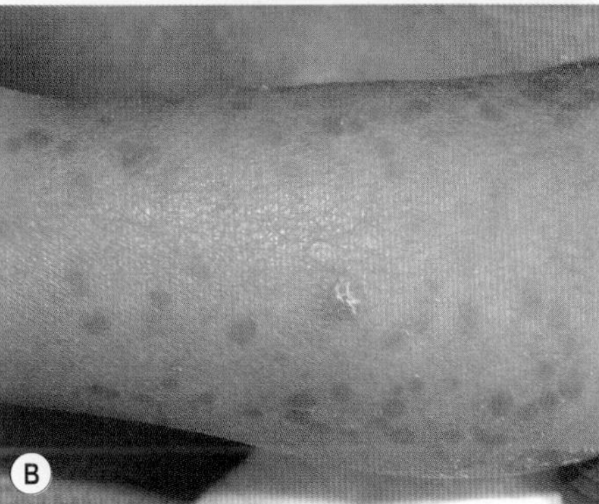

Fig. 28.2 Transient neonatal pustular melanosis in an African-American neonate. A One hour after birth, flaccid vesiculopustules and superficial erosions with minimal surrounding erythema are present in the groin. **B** On the 8th day of life, hyperpigmented macules and a few collarettes of scale are evident on the lower leg. *Courtesy, YDRSC.*

Infectious Diseases

Cutaneous Candidiasis

- *Congenital* candidiasis.
  - Uncommon condition that is acquired *in utero*; risk factors include maternal vaginal candidiasis, a foreign body in the uterus or cervix, and prematurity
  - Evident at birth or during the first week of life
  - Findings range from erythematous papules and pustules with fine scaling

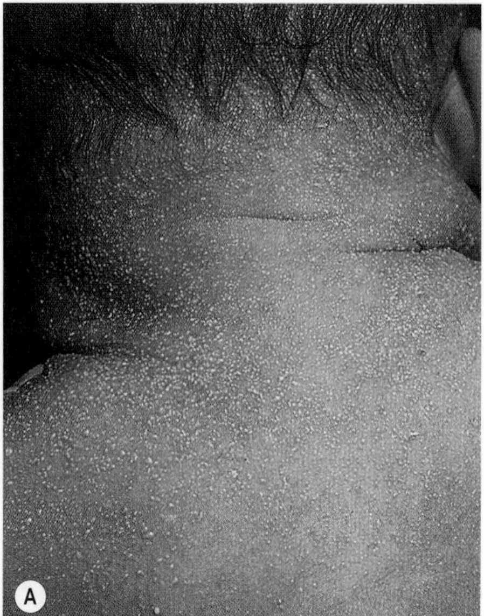

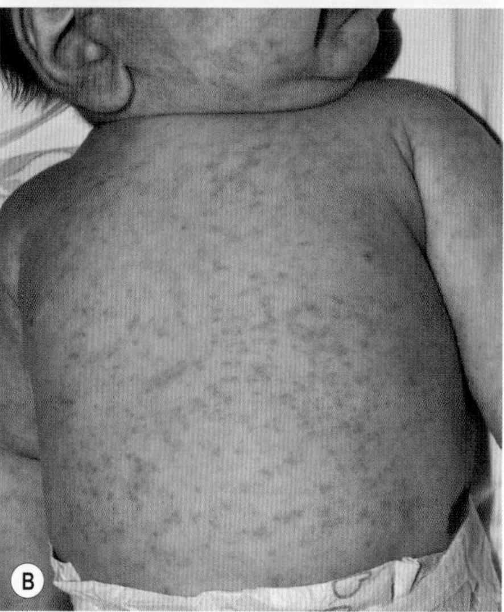

Fig. 28.3 Miliaria. A Tiny, superficial vesicles, seen on the back and neck of this newborn, are characteristic of miliaria crystallina. **B** Widespread miliaria rubra with numerous small papules and pustules. *A, From Eichenfield LF, Frieden IJ, Esterly NB, et al (Eds).* Textbook of Neonatal Dermatology. *© 2001 Saunders. B, Courtesy, Antonio Torrelo, MD.*

in full-term neonates to an *"invasive fungal dermatitis"* presenting as diffuse, "burn-like" erythema and erosions in premature infants with a very low birth weight (often <1000 g; Fig. 28.6A, B)

- Often widespread involvement on the face, trunk, and extremities; the palms, soles, and nails (yellow discoloration,

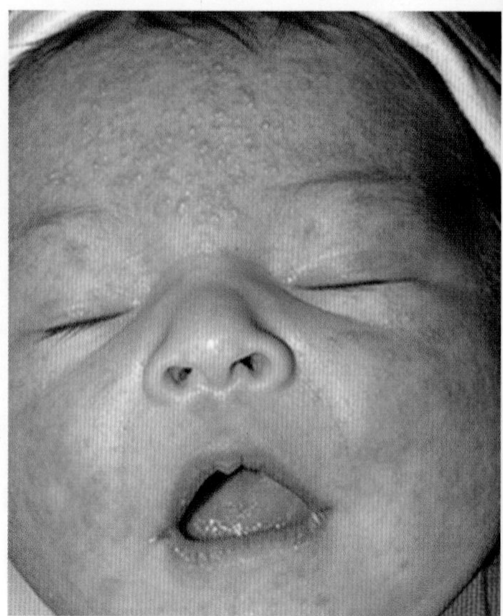

Fig. 28.4 Neonatal cephalic pustulosis. Papulopustules on the forehead and cheeks of a 3-week-old infant. *Courtesy, Julie V. Schaffer, MD.*

transverse ridging) are frequently affected, but the diaper area and oral mucosa are typically spared

- **Dx:** budding yeast and pseudohyphae are seen in a potassium hydroxide preparation of skin scrapings, and culture grows *Candida* spp. (usually *C. albicans*)
- **Rx:** premature infants (especially if <1500 g) are at high risk for disseminated candidiasis and require systemic antifungal agents, as do full-term neonates with extracutaneous involvement (e.g. pneumonia); most full-term neonates have skin-limited disease that can be treated with topical antifungals (e.g. an imidazole cream)

• *Neonatal* candidiasis (see Ch. 64).
  - Common condition that presents at ≥1 week of age as intense erythema with desquamation and satellite papulopustules, favoring the diaper area > other intertriginous sites (see Fig. 13.4); patients may also have oral thrush
  - **Rx:** topical imidazole or nystatin

Staphylococcal Infections – Pyoderma and Bullous Impetigo (See Ch. 61)

• Presents as early as a few days of age with pustules, flaccid vesicles or bullae evolving to superficial shiny red erosions with collarettes of scale, and occasionally furuncles.

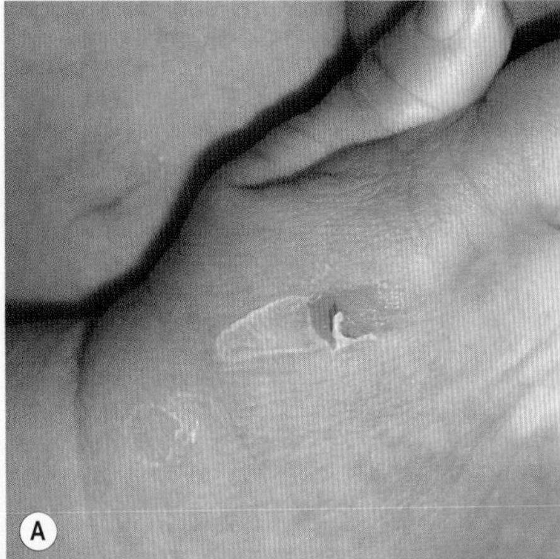

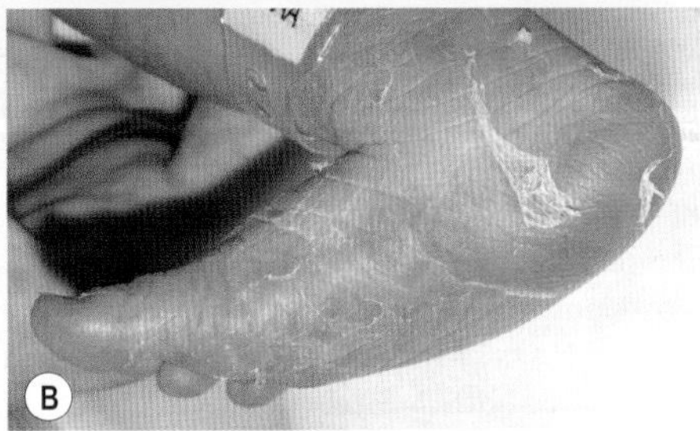

Fig. 28.5 Physiologic skin findings in neonates. A Sucking blister. **B** Post-term desquamation is often most evident acrally. *A, Courtesy, Ana Martín, MD. B, Courtesy, Julie V. Schaffer, MD.*

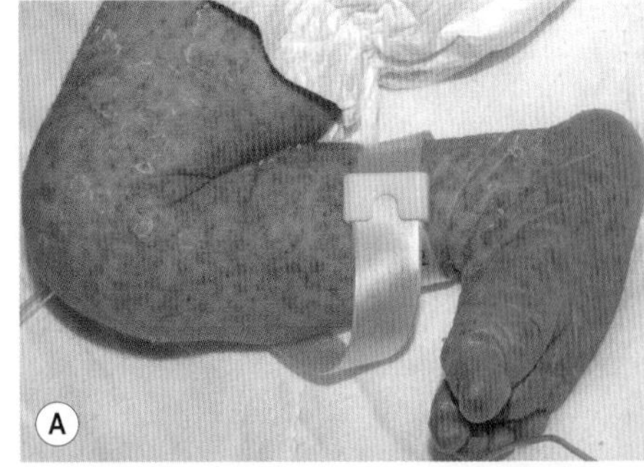

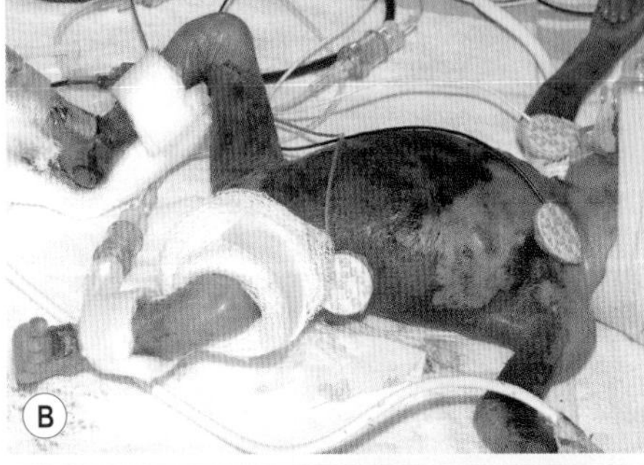

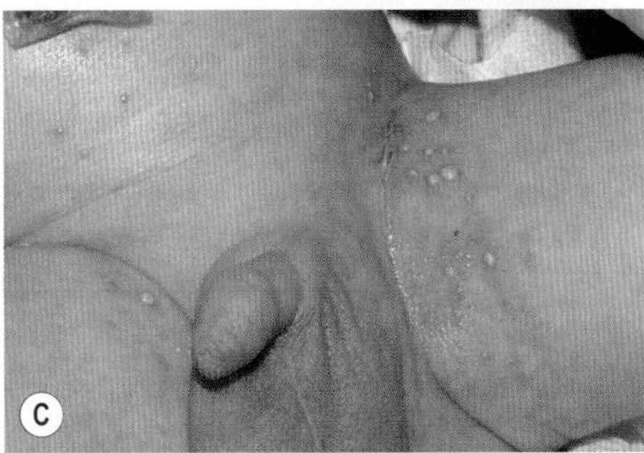

Fig. 28.6 Congenital candidiasis and bullous impetigo. A Numerous pink papules admixed with small superficial pustules and desquamation due to congenital candidiasis in a full-term neonate. Note the plantar involvement. **B** Widespread "burn-like" erosions due to congenital candidiasis in a premature neonate born at 24 weeks' gestation. This presentation is associated with a high risk of systemic involvement. **C** Multiple discrete superficial pustules with surrounding erythema in the diaper area of a 4-day-old boy due to infection with *Staphylococcus aureus*. *Courtesy, Julie V. Schaffer, MD.*

- Favors the diaper area and other intertriginous sites (Fig. 28.6C; see Fig. 13.4).
- **Dx:** Gram stain shows Gram-positive cocci in clusters, and culture grows *Staphylococcus aureus*.
- **Rx:** topical antibiotic (e.g. mupirocin) for uncomplicated localized pustulosis or bullous impetigo; systemic anti-staphylococcal antibiotic if more extensive or deeper involvement, using an intravenous agent, e.g. vancomycin, if the patient is toxic-appearing.

Neonatal Herpes Simplex Virus (HSV) Infection (See Ch. 67)

- Risk of transmission is highest (30–50%) for a mother with her first episode of genital HSV infection (which may be asymptomatic) near the time of delivery and low (<1–3%) for recurrent genital herpes.
- Onset from birth to 2 weeks, but usually ≥5 days of age.
- Localized (favoring the scalp and trunk) or disseminated vesicles, pustules, and crusts; lesions are often grouped and may progress to bullae and erosions with scalloped borders (Fig. 28.7).
- Involvement of the oral mucosa, eye, CNS, and other internal organs can occur.
- **Rx:** intravenous acyclovir.

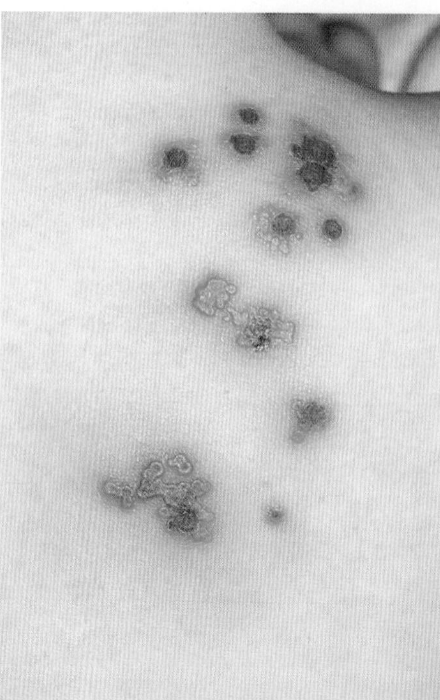

Fig. 28.7 Neonatal HSV infection. Note the clustering of the vesicles on an erythematous base. *Courtesy, Julie V. Schaffer, MD.*

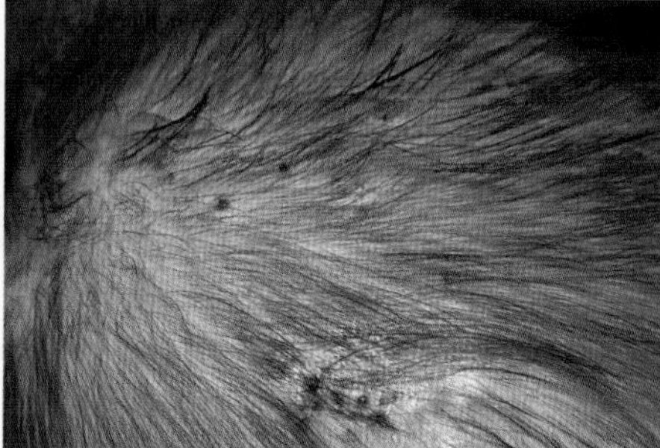

Fig. 28.8 Eosinophilic pustular folliculitis of infancy. Crusted papules and pustules on the scalp of a 1-year-old boy. *Courtesy, Deborah S. Goddard, MD, Amy E. Gilliam, MD, and Ilona J. Frieden, MD.*

Uncommon Conditions

Eosinophilic Pustular Folliculitis of Infancy

- Onset often in the first few months of life, with cyclical recurrences for several months to years.
- Pruritic perifollicular pustules and crusts favoring the scalp (Fig. 28.8) and forehead.
- **DDx:** Erythema toxicum neonatorum (in neonates), bacterial folliculitis, tinea capitis, scabies, arthropod bite reactions.
- **Rx:** potent topical CS (intermittently for flares), oral antihistamines.

Acropustulosis of Infancy (Infantile Acropustulosis)

- Favors darkly pigmented male infants, sometimes representing a persistent hypersensitivity reaction following successful scabies treatment.
- Onset usually between 3 and 6 months of age; occasionally develops in newborns.
- Pruritic vesicles and pustules on the hands and feet (including palms/soles) (Fig. 28.9) > wrists and ankles.
- Outbreaks last 1–2 weeks, with cyclical recurrences until 2–3 years of age.
- **DDx:** scabies.
- **Rx:** potent topical CS (intermittently for flares), oral antihistamines.

Incontinentia Pigmenti (IP) (See Ch. 51)

- Multisystem X-linked disorder caused by mutations in the *NEMO* gene (NF-κB essential modulator); usually lethal in male fetuses.
- Typically presents in the first 2 weeks of life with vesicles on an inflammatory base in linear streaks that favor the extremities (Fig. 28.10); in subsequent weeks, verrucous streaks may develop, followed by more widespread linear and whorled grayish-brown hyperpigmentation.
- Extracutaneous findings in neonates with IP can include peripheral eosinophilia, leukocytosis, seizures, and retinal vascular abnormalities.

For further information see Ch. 34 from *Dermatology, Fourth Edition*.

For additional online figures visit www.expertconsult.com 

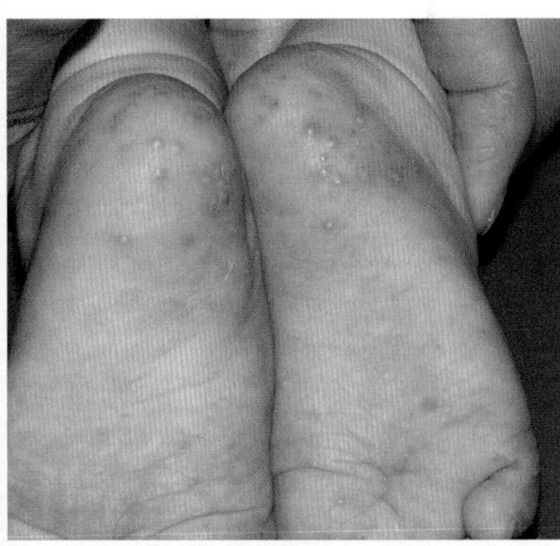

Fig. 28.9 Acropustulosis of infancy. Multiple vesiculopustules with an erythematous base on the heels of an infant. *Courtesy, Julie V. Schaffer, MD.*

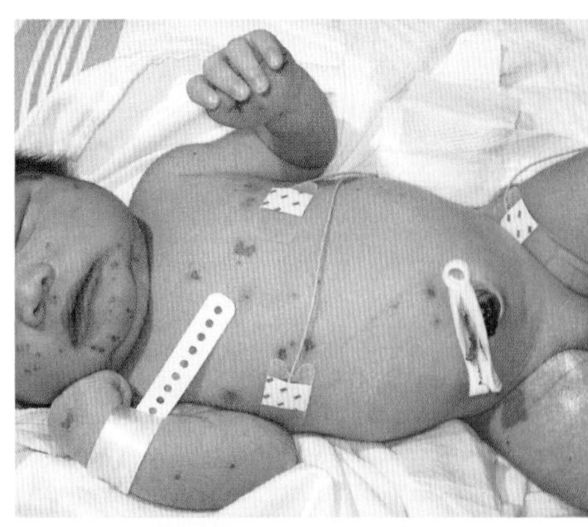

Fig. 28.11 Congenital Langerhans cell histiocytosis. Numerous erosions with crusting on the face and trunk of a newborn. *Courtesy, Deborah S. Goddard, MD, Amy E. Gilliam, MD, and Ilona J. Frieden, MD.*

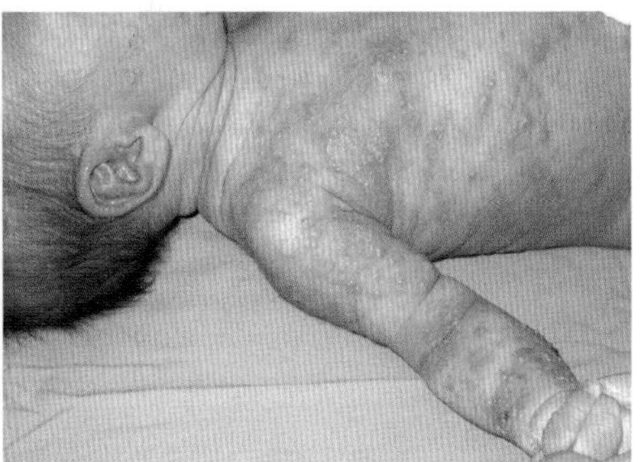

Fig. 28.10 Incontinentia pigmenti stage 1. Vesicles and erythema in a linear and whorled configuration on the trunk, arm, and ear of a female neonate. *Courtesy, Luis Requena, MD.*

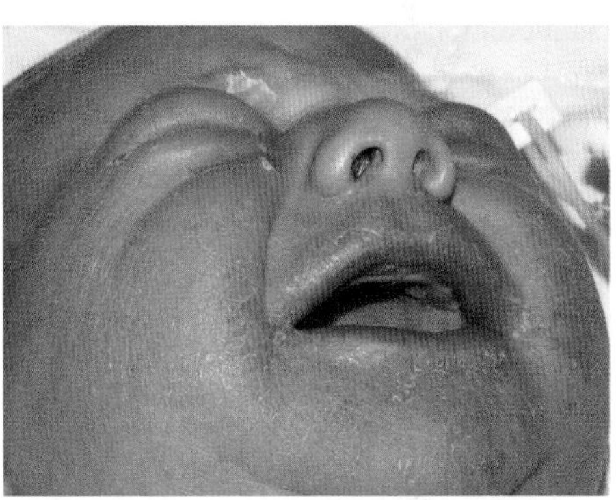

Fig. 28.12 Staphylococcal scalded skin syndrome. Perioral and periorbital erythema and scale-crust in a neonate due to exfoliative toxins. *Courtesy, Julie V. Schaffer, MD.*

29 Acne Vulgaris

• Common pilosebaceous disorder that occurs in ~85% of individuals 12–24 years of age and 15–35% of adults (especially women) in their 30s–40s. Preadolescent acne affecting children between 7 and 11 years of age has also become more common due to the trend for earlier onset of puberty.

• Clinical presentations range from mild comedones to severe, explosive eruptions of suppurative nodules associated with systemic manifestations.

• May result in scarring and psychosocial repercussions such as anxiety, depression, and social withdrawal.

• A tendency to develop moderate to severe acne can run in families.

• Multiple factors affecting the pilosebaceous unit contribute to acne pathogenesis (Fig. 29.1), a process that typically begins when androgen production increases at adrenarche.

• The relationship between diet and acne is controversial, with some evidence of possible associations with milk intake (especially skim milk), whey protein supplements, and a high glycemic index diet.

Clinical Features and Variants of Acne

• Favors the face and upper trunk, sites with well-developed sebaceous glands.

- Non-inflammatory acne
  - *Closed comedones (whiteheads)* are small (~1 mm), skin-colored papules without an obvious follicular opening (Fig. 29.2)
  - *Open comedones (blackheads)* have a dilated follicular opening filled with a keratin plug, which has a black color due to oxidized lipids and melanin (Figs 29.2 and 29.3A)
- Inflammatory acne
  - Erythematous papules and pustules (Fig. 29.3A,B)
  - Nodules and pseudocysts filled with pus or serosanguinous fluid; may coalesce and form sinus tracts (Fig. 29.3B,C)
  - *Acne conglobata* (severe nodulocystic acne) is classified in the follicular occlusion tetrad along with dissecting cellulitis of the scalp, hidradenitis suppurativa, and pilonidal cysts (see Ch. 31); it is also a part of syndromes such as *p*yogenic *a*rthritis, *p*yoderma gangrenosum, and *a*cne conglobata (PAPA); *p*yoderma gangrenosum, *a*cne, and *s*uppurative *h*idradenitis (PASH); and *p*yoderma gangrenosum, *a*cne, *p*soriasis, *a*rthritis, and *s*uppurative *h*idradenitis (PAPASH)

• Inflammatory acne commonly results in postinflammatory hyperpigmentation, especially in patients with darker skin, which fades slowly over time (Fig. 29.4A); nodulocystic acne (and less frequently other inflammatory > comedonal forms) often leads to pitted (Fig. 29.4B) or hypertrophic scars (the latter especially on the trunk; see Fig. 81.4).

Post-Adolescent Acne

• Age >25 years; favors women and may be associated with psychological stress.

• Tends to flare in the week prior to menstruation; up to one-third of these women have hyperandrogenism.

• Typically features papulonodules on the lower face, jawline, and neck.

Acne Excoriée

• Favors teenage girls and young women.

• Habitual picking at comedones and inflammatory papules, resulting in crusted erosions (often linear/angular) and potential scarring (see Fig. 5.4).

• Some patients have an underlying obsessive–compulsive or anxiety disorder.

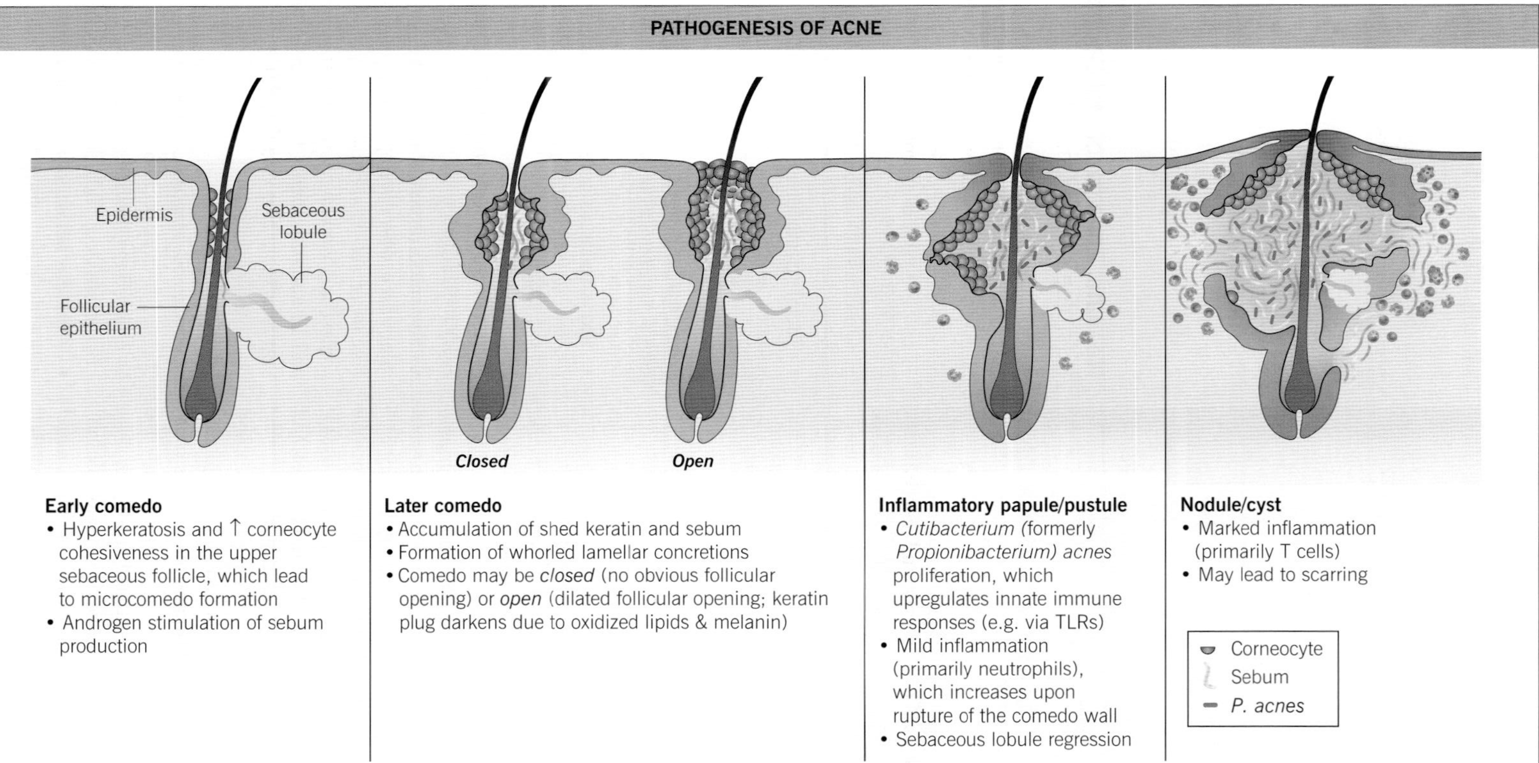

Fig. 29.1 Pathogenesis of acne. TLRs, toll-like receptors.

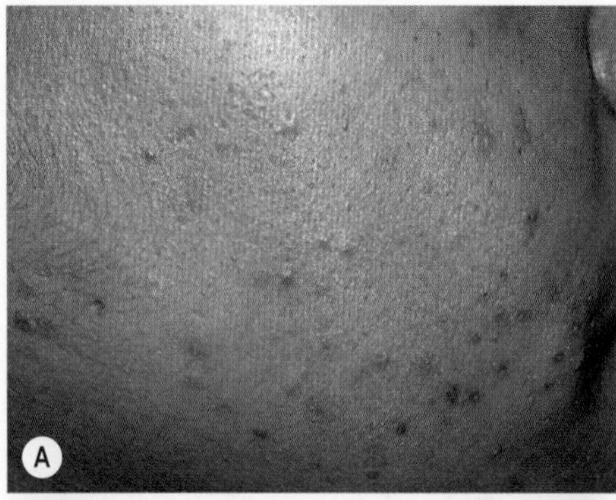

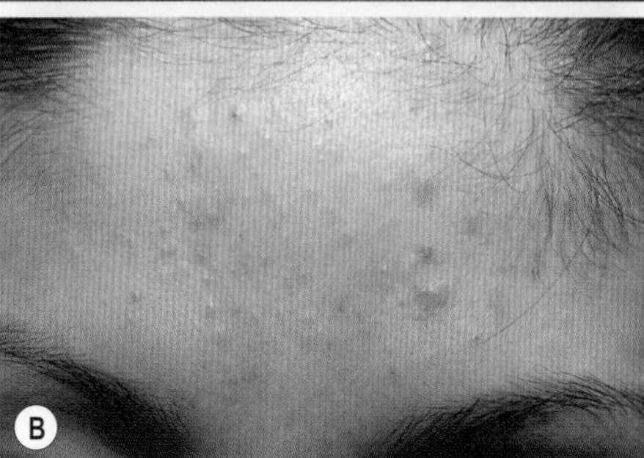

Fig. 29.2 Comedonal acne vulgaris. On the cheek (**A**) and forehead (**B**), there are open and closed comedones as well as postinflammatory hyperpigmentation (**A**) and inflammatory papules (**B**). *A, Courtesy, Andrew Zaenglein, MD, and Diane Thiboutot, MD; B, Courtesy, Kalman Watsky, MD.*

Acne Fulminans

- Favors boys 13 to 16 years of age.
- Sudden development of numerous, markedly inflamed nodular lesions on the face, trunk, and upper arms.
- Coalescence into painful, oozing, friable plaques with hemorrhagic crusting, erosion/ulceration, and eventual scarring (Fig. 29.5).
- Systemic manifestations may include fever, malaise, myalgias, arthralgias, osteolytic bone lesions (most often of clavicles and sternum), and hepatosplenomegaly.
- Laboratory findings: leukocytosis and increased ESR/CRP > anemia and proteinuria.
- **DDx:** an acne fulminans-like flare is occasionally triggered by isotretinoin therapy for acne (especially when initiated at a higher dose and in younger teenage boys), and acne fulminans can be associated with *s*ynovitis, *a*cne, *p*ustulosis, *h*yperostosis, and *o*steitis (SAPHO) syndrome (see Ch. 21).
- **Rx:** prednisone 0.5–1 mg/kg/day as monotherapy for 2–6 weeks (until inflammation subsides), followed by addition of low-dose isotretinoin (e.g. 0.1 mg/kg/day) for ~4 weeks, and then a prednisone taper and slow increase of the isotretinoin dose over 1–2 months.

Solid Facial Edema (Morbihan Disease)

- Woody induration ± erythema of the central face in the setting of chronic inflammation due to acne vulgaris or rosacea (Fig. 29.6).
- **Rx:** isotretinoin (may require an extended course).

Neonatal Acne (Neonatal Cephalic Pustulosis) (see Ch. 28)

- Age 2 weeks to 3 months.
- Facial papulopustular eruption thought to be triggered by *Malassezia* spp.; comedones are *not* present (see Fig. 28.4).

Infantile Acne

- Onset usually at 2–12 months of age; favors boys.
- Facial comedones, papulopustules, and nodules as in classic acne (Fig. 29.7); may result in scarring.
- Reflects physiologic elevation of androgen levels in infants 6–12 months of age (especially boys); patients often have a family history of severe acne.
- **Rx:** similar to adolescent acne; typically resolves within 6–18 months, becoming quiescent until puberty.

Acne Associated with Endocrinologic Abnormalities

- Hyperandrogenism should be suspected in children who develop acne between 2 and 7 years of age (*mid-childhood acne*), in older adolescents/women with irregular menses, and in female patients with signs of virilization (see Table 29.1 and Ch. 57).

Contact Acne

- *Acne mechanica*: comedogenesis due to chronic friction/occlusion from objects such as chin straps, helmets, collars, and musical instruments (e.g. "fiddler's neck" in a violinist).
- *Acne cosmetica*, *pomade acne*, and *occupational acne*: comedogenesis caused by exposure to follicle-occluding substances in

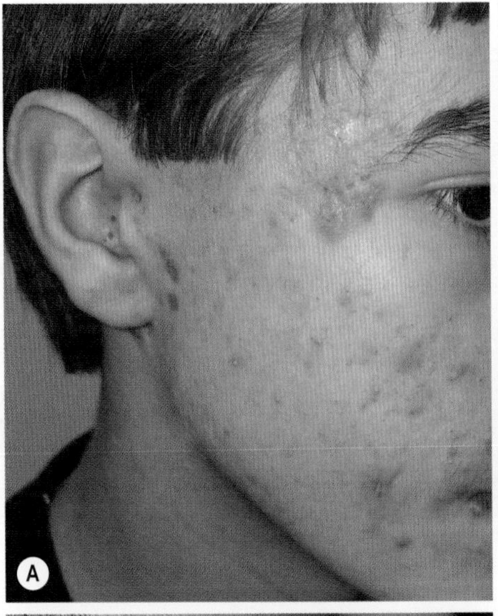

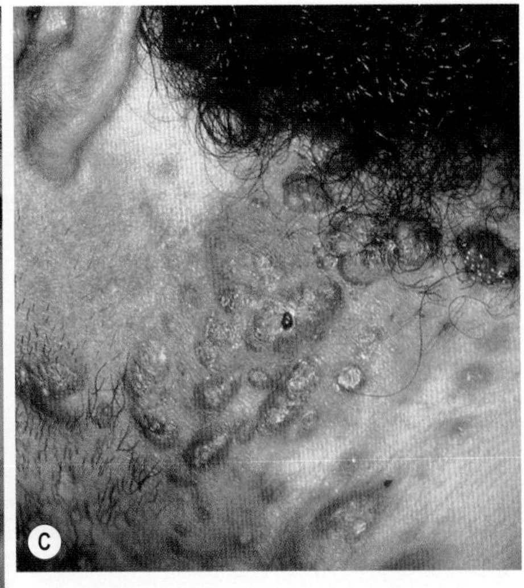

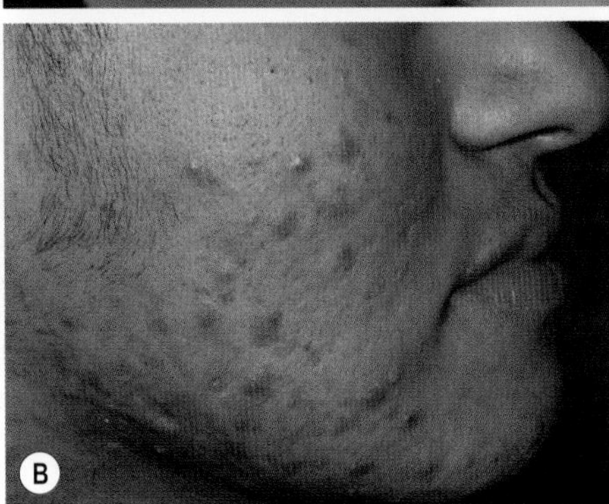

Fig. 29.3 Inflammatory acne vulgaris. **A** Inflammatory papules and pustules as well as both open and closed comedones are evident. Note the nodular lesion on the temple, scarring in the preauricular area, and open comedones in the concha of the ear. **B** Multiple papulopustules and papulonodules on the cheek with a sinus tract, linear scarring and depressions along the jawline. **C** Severe nodulocystic acne. This form is best treated with low doses of isotretinoin initially (± a preceding course of oral antibiotics) to avoid precipitating a flare. *A, Courtesy, Andrew Zaenglein, MD, and Diane Thiboutot, MD; B, Courtesy, Julie V. Schaffer, MD; C, Courtesy, YDRSC.*

cosmetics, hair products (favoring forehead and temples), and materials used in the workplace (e.g. cutting oils, coal tar derivatives).

Chloracne

- Results from exposure (usually occupational) to halogenated aromatic hydrocarbons (e.g. polychlorinated dibenzodioxins and dibenzofurans) in agents such as herbicides and insecticides.
- Comedones and cystic papulonodules develop within 2 months of exposure, favoring malar and retroauricular areas of the face (see Fig. 12.19) as well as the axillae and scrotum; often persists for years.

Drug-Induced Acne and Acneiform Eruptions

- Systemic CS can trigger an eruption of monomorphous follicular papulopustules favoring the upper trunk (Fig. 29.8).
- Acneiform eruptions represent a frequent side effect of epidermal growth factor receptor (EGFR) inhibitors (e.g. cetuximab, erlotinib) used to treat solid tumors; patients present with follicular pustules and papules on the face, scalp, and upper trunk, usually 1–3 weeks after beginning treatment, which may correlate with a therapeutic response (Fig. 29.9; see Fig. 17.16 and Table 17.9).
- Other common causes of drug-induced acne include anabolic steroids, bromides (found in sedatives and cold remedies), iodides (found in contrast dyes and supplements), isoniazid (Fig. 29.10), lithium, phenytoin, and progestins.

Acne Associated with a Syndrome

- Examples include Apert, PAPA, PASH, PAPASH, and SAPHO (see Ch. 21) syndromes.

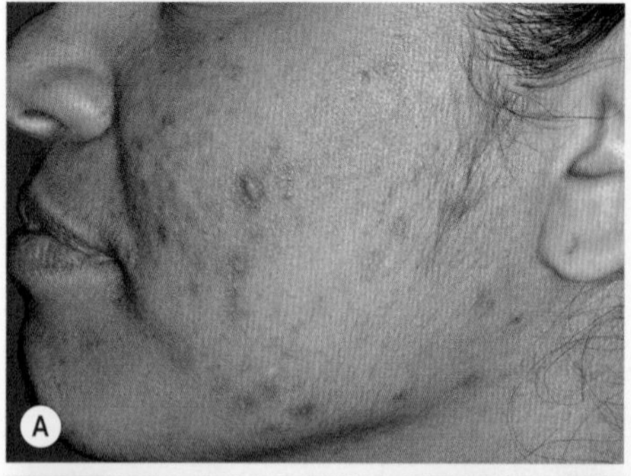

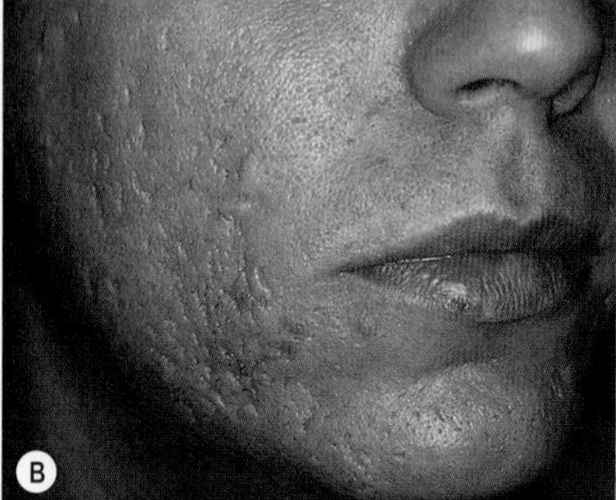

Fig. 29.4 Sequelae of acne. A Postinflammatory hyperpigmentation. Such pigmentary changes are most common in patients with darker skin colors. **B** "Ice-pick" scarring secondary to nodulocystic acne. *A, Courtesy, Andrew Zaenglein, MD, and Diane Thiboutot, MD; B, Courtesy, YDRSC.*

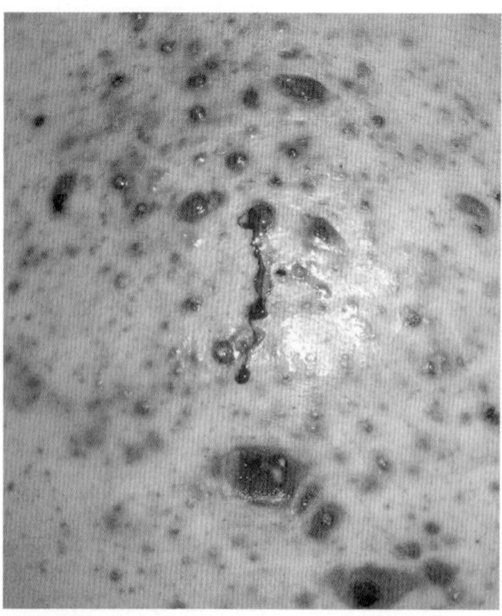

Fig. 29.5 Acne fulminans. Inflamed, friable papulopustules and plaques with erosions, oozing, and formation of granulation tissue. *Courtesy, Julie V. Schaffer, MD.*

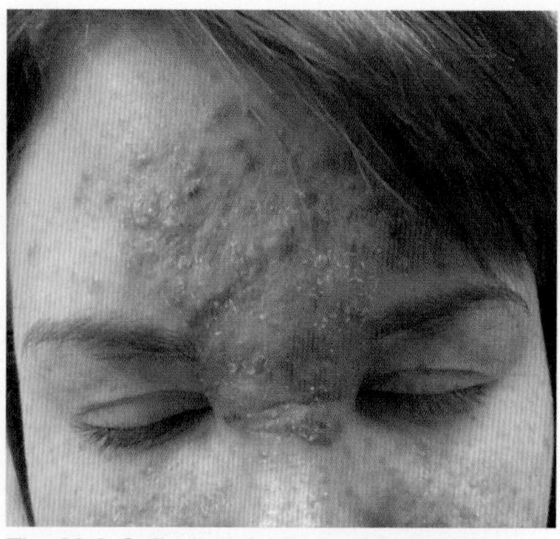

Fig. 29.6 Solid facial edema due to acne vulgaris. There is soft tissue swelling in the central portion of the face. *Courtesy, Boni Elewski, MD.*

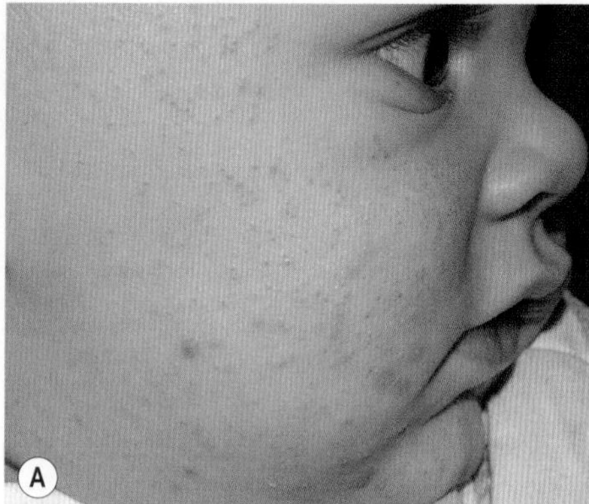

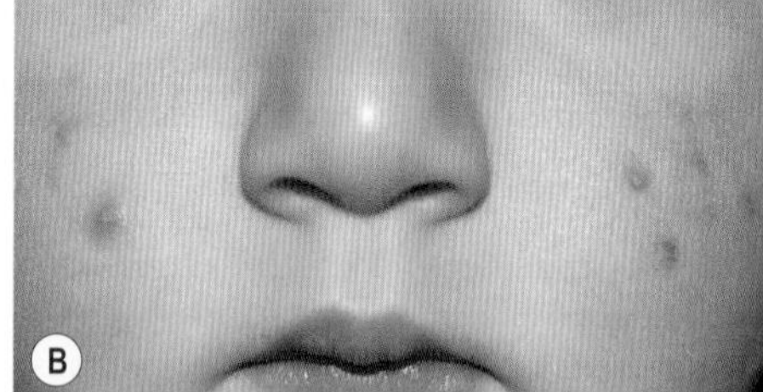

Fig. 29.7 Infantile acne. Presentations can range from numerous open comedones (**A**) to primarily papulopustules (**B**). *A, Courtesy, Julie V. Schaffer, MD; B, Courtesy, Kalman Watsky, MD.*

HISTORY AND PHYSICAL EXAMINATION OF THE ACNE PATIENT	
History	**Physical examination**
• Sex • Age* • Degree of motivation for treatment • Lifestyle/hobbies, occupation • Current and previous acne treatments • Use of cosmetics, sunscreens, cleansers, moisturizers • Menstrual history* and oral contraceptive use • Medications (see text on drug-induced acne) • Other medical conditions • Family history of acne, polycystic ovary syndrome, and inflammatory disease	• Skin type (e.g. oily vs dry) • Skin color/phototype • Distribution of acne – Face (e.g. "T-zone," cheeks, jawline) – Neck, chest, back, upper arms • Overall degree of involvement (mild, moderate, or severe) • Lesion morphology – Comedones – Inflammatory papules and pustules – Nodules and cysts, sinus tracts • Postinflammatory pigmentary changes • Scarring (e.g. pitted, hypertrophic, atrophic) • Signs of virilization* (in female patients) – Hirsutism, androgenetic alopecia – Deep voice, muscular habitus, clitoromegaly

**Evaluation often includes serum levels of testosterone (total and free), DHEAS, and 17-hydroxyprogesterone (see Fig. 57.10) as well as hand/wrist x-rays to evaluate bone age in prepubertal children.*

Table 29.1 History and physical examination of the acne patient.

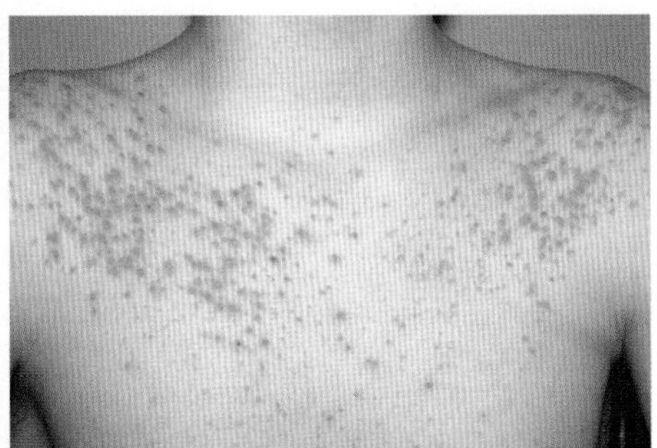

Fig. 29.8 Acneiform eruption secondary to systemic corticosteroid therapy. Abrupt eruption of monomorphous follicular papules and pustules on the chest. *Courtesy, Andrew Zaenglein, MD, and Diane Thiboutot, MD.*

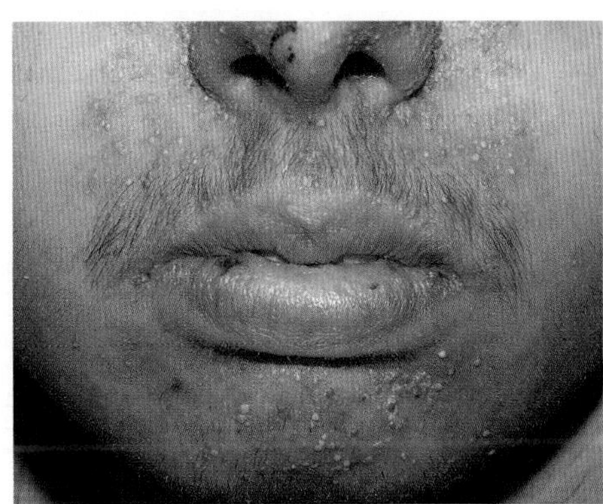

Fig. 29.9 Acneiform eruptions due to epidermal growth factor receptor inhibitors. Numerous monomorphous follicular pustules and crusted papules on the face of an adolescent boy treated with erlotinib. *Courtesy, Julie V. Schaffer, MD.*

Evaluation and Treatment of Acne

- Table 29.1 lists key components in the history and physical examination of an acne patient.
- **DDx:** presented in Table 29.2.
- **Rx:** outlined in Tables 29.3 and 29.4.
- Once active acne has been successfully treated, intralesional CS (for hypertrophic scars) or surgical modalities (e.g. fractional or traditional laser resurfacing, dermabrasion, fillers) can be used for residual scarring if needed.

For further information see Ch. 36 from *Dermatology, Fourth Edition*.

For additional online figures visit www.expertconsult.com 

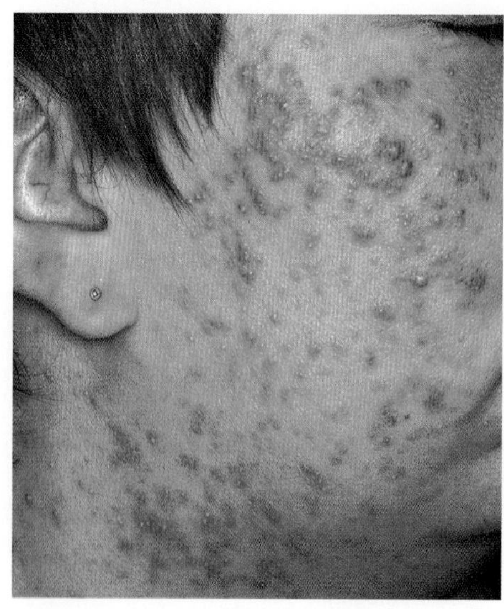

Fig. 29.10 Drug-induced acne due to isoniazid. *Courtesy, Kalman Watsky, MD.*

DIFFERENTIAL DIAGNOSIS OF ACNE VULGARIS
Comedonal acne
• Contact acne, chloracne, drug-induced acne • "Pseudoacne" of the transverse nasal crease (in prepubertal children; Fig. 29.11A)
Closed comedones
• Milia, sebaceous hyperplasia, adnexal neoplasms (e.g. syringomas, fibrofolliculomas), osteoma cutis, colloid milia • Eruptive vellus hair cysts or steatocystomas (for truncal lesions)
Open comedones
• Childhood flexural comedones (double-orifice; axilla > groin), dilated pore of Winer (solitary lesion) • Trichostasis spinulosa (Fig. 29.11B), trichofolliculoma (solitary lesion) • Favre–Racouchot disease (in photoaged skin), radiation-induced comedones • Nevus comedonicus, basaloid follicular hamartoma, familial dyskeratotic comedones, Dowling–Degos disease • Follicular spines (e.g. drug-induced [e.g. BRAF inhibitors] and in trichodysplasia spinulosa, multiple myeloma, and HIV-associated follicular syndrome)
Inflammatory acne
• Rosacea, periorificial dermatitis, idiopathic facial aseptic granuloma (solitary nodule in young children) • Folliculitis: normal flora, staphylococcal, *Pityrosporum*, Gram-negative, eosinophilic, *Demodex* • Drug-induced acne/acneiform eruptions, neutrophilic dermatoses • Pseudofolliculitis barbae, acne keloidalis nuchae • Keratosis pilaris, angiofibromas, follicular mucinosis (Fig. 29.11C) • Tinea faciei, molluscum contagiosum (inflamed lesions), trichodysplasia spinulosa

Table 29.2 Differential diagnosis of acne vulgaris. Folliculotropic mycosis fungoides can mimic comedonal or inflammatory acne.

TREATMENT OF ACNE VULGARIS
Topical retinoids (comedolytic > anti-inflammatory effects): tretinoin*, adapalene, tazarotene*, trafarotene • Response requires 3–4 weeks (sometimes preceded by pustular flare); use a small amount and treat all acne-prone areas • Initial use of lower concentration and/or alternate-night application can minimize irritation **Topical antimicrobials**: benzoyl peroxide (BPO)** and/or antibiotic (e.g. clindamycin†, erythromycin†, minocycline, sodium sulfacetamide/sulfur) **Oral antibiotics**: *first-line* – tetracycline derivatives (doxycycline, minocycline, sarecycline); *alt.* – azithromycin, trimethoprim–sulfamethoxazole • Often used for 3–6 months; tetracyclines are avoided in children <8 years of age (although use for ≤21 days is acceptable) and pregnant women **OCPs**: FDA-approved for acne – Ortho Tri-Cyclen® (EE 35 mcg, norgestimate 180/215/250 mcg), Yaz®/Loryna®/Nikki®/Melamisa®/Lo-Zumandimine® (EE 20 mcg, drospirenone 3000 mcg), Estrostep® (EE 20/30/35 mcg, norethindrone 1000 mcg) **Antiandrogens**: spironolactone (50–200 mg/day) **Oral isotretinoin§**: typically 0.5–1 mg/kg/day (lower initially, especially if acne fulminans) × 4–6 months (cumulative dose 120–150+ mg/kg)

	Mild acne		**Moderate acne**	**Severe acne (e.g. conglobata, fulminans)**
	Comedonal	**Mostly inflammatory**		
First-line	• Topical retinoid	• Topical antimicrobial‡ + topical retinoid	• Oral antibiotic + topical retinoid ± BPO	• Oral isotretinoin (+ oral CS for acne fulminans)
Second-line	• Alt. topical retinoid • Azelaic acid • Salicylic acid • Clascoterone	• Alt. topical retinoid + antimicrobial • Azelaic acid • Topical dapsone • Clascoterone	• Alt. oral antibiotic + alt. topical retinoid ± BPO/azelaic acid • Oral isotretinoin (if nodular, scarring or recalcitrant)	• Oral dapsone • High-dose oral antibiotic + topical retinoid + BPO
Options for female patients			• OCP/ oral antiandrogen	• OCP/ oral antiandrogen
Procedural options	• Comedo extraction		• Comedo extraction • Intralesional CS (2–5 mg/ml triamcinolone)	• Intralesional CS (2–5 mg/ml triamcinolone)
Refractory to treatment		Exclude Gram-negative folliculitis (see Ch. 31)		
			• Female patient: exclude adrenal or ovarian dysfunction • Exclude use of anabolic steroid or other acne-exacerbating drugs	
Maintenance	• Topical retinoid	• Topical retinoid ± BPO	• Topical retinoid ± BPO	

**Standard tretinoin is photolabile and inactivated by BPO (so generally applied at night, separately from BPO); tazarotene is the most irritating of the topical retinoids and is contraindicated during pregnancy.*
***Can bleach clothing/bedding and cause contact dermatitis (irritant > allergic); unlike topical antibiotics, bacterial resistance does not occur.*
†Increased effectiveness when used in conjunction with BPO or a retinoid.
§Severe teratogenicity; in the United States, prescribers and patients must register in a risk management program (iPLEDGE™) that requires monthly visits. The most common side effects are cheilitis > mucosal dryness (ocular, nasal) and xerosis (Fig. 29.12).
‡BPO ± a topical antibiotic may also be used as monotherapy, especially as an initial treatment in a younger patient.

Table 29.3 Treatment of acne vulgaris. Lack of response should prompt consideration of non-adherence and alternative diagnoses. In general, monotherapy with a topical or oral antibiotic should be avoided. Laser (e.g. 1450-nm diode), light (e.g. blue, intense pulsed), or photodynamic therapies may be of benefit to some patients but are not first-line, and superficial chemical peels (e.g. 20–30% salicylic acid, 30–50% glycolic acid) are occasionally useful to reduce comedones. Alt, alternative; EE, ethinyl estradiol; OCP, oral contraceptive pill.

TIPS FOR TOPICAL ACNE THERAPY	
Improve adherence – often compromised due to patients having busy schedules or quitting when the response is not rapid	• Simplify the regimen: once daily when possible; consider combination products (e.g. benzoyl peroxide + adapalene or clindamycin; tretinoin + clindamycin), especially in less motivated adolescents • Inform patients that it will take 6–8 weeks of treatment for substantial improvement • Ask specifically about adherence: "Out of 7 nights, how many times do you apply the medication?"
Educate on proper use	• In general, topical medications (especially retinoids) should be used to the entire acne-prone region rather than as "spot treatment" of individual lesions • Provide instructions on where to apply the medication and how much to use
Minimize irritation – most common in adolescents with atopic dermatitis and adults	• Note that using too much medication or applying it too frequently can increase irritation • Devise a gradual initial approach to improve tolerance in patients with sensitive skin; for example, a single agent may be used for the first 2–3 weeks (starting every other day for retinoids), followed by slow introduction of a second medication (e.g. transitioning from alternate days to daily) • Advise to avoid harsh scrubs and other irritating agents (e.g. toners, acne products that are not part of the regimen) • Suggest use of a non-comedogenic sensitive skin moisturizer if dryness occurs
Avoid exacerbation	• Review all skin care products and cosmetics; having patients bring everything that they apply to their face to a visit may help to determine the source of problems • Advise non-comedogenic products (e.g. moisturizers, sunscreens, make-up) and to avoid having oily hair or using pomades that may contribute to acne • Instruct patients not to pick or manipulate lesions
Reinforce the plan – patients often forget what is recommended and are bombarded by advertising and false information about acne	• Provide a written handout with your specific instructions • Recommend additional reliable educational resources about acne and its treatment, e.g.: www.aad.org/public/diseases/acne www.webmd.com/skin-problems-and-treatments/acne/default.htm

Table 29.4 Tips for topical acne therapy.

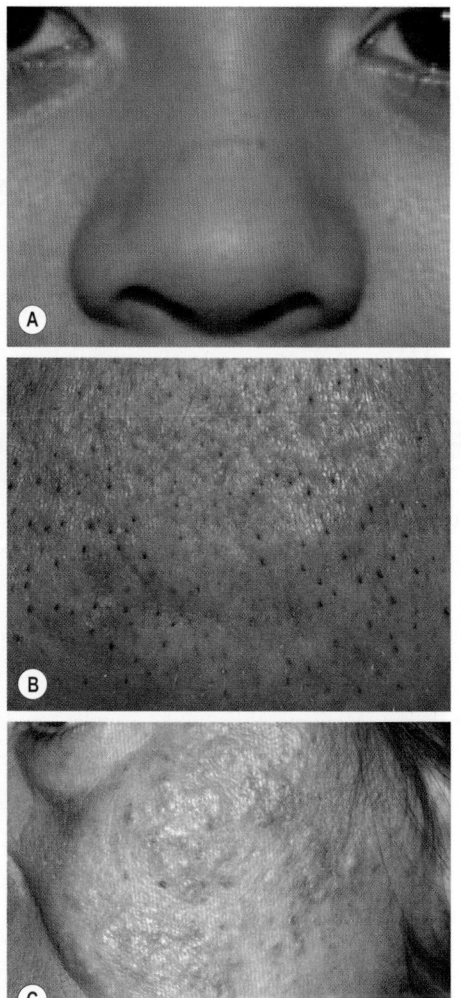

Fig. 29.11 Disorders in the differential diagnosis of comedonal acne vulgaris. A "Pseudoacne" of the transverse nasal crease in a young child. Note the milia and comedones located along this anatomical demarcation line. **B** Trichostasis spinulosa. Multiple vellus hairs and keratinous debris are found within the dilated follicular orifices. **C** Acneiform follicular mucinosis on the cheek of a woman. *A, Courtesy, Julie V. Schaffer, MD; B, Courtesy, Judit Stenn, MD; C, Courtesy, Lorenzo Cerroni, MD.*

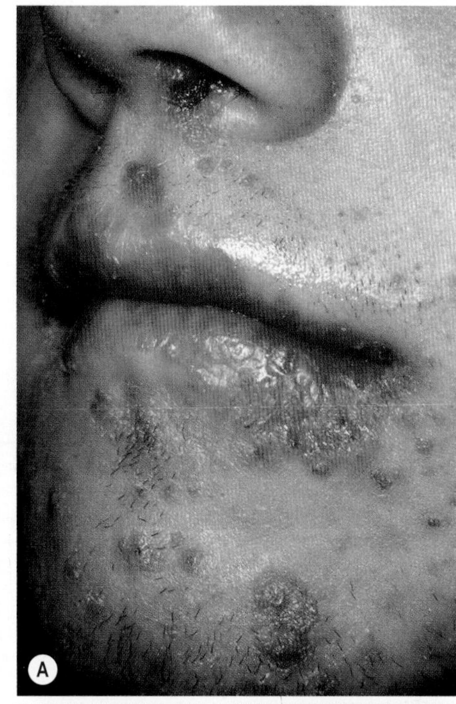

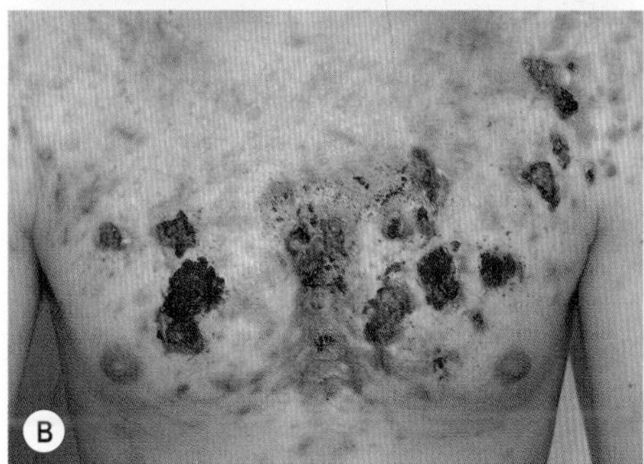

Fig. 29.12 Cutaneous complications of isotretinoin therapy. A Multiple serous crusts are evident. Dryness and fragility of the skin, lips, and nasal mucosa in patients treated with isotretinoin increase susceptibility to staphylococcal infections. **B** Pyogenic granuloma-like healing on the chest of an adolescent boy receiving his third month of isotretinoin therapy. *Courtesy, Andrew Zaenglein, MD, and Diane Thiboutot, MD.*

30 Rosacea and Periorificial Dermatitis

Epidemiology

- Seen in all skin types, but considerably more common in patients with skin phototypes I–II.
- Onset generally in the 4th decade of life.

Clinical Features

- Highly variable degree of severity, from a few papulopustules to extreme distortion of the nose.
- Lesions typically develop on the face, especially its central portion; uncommonly other sites such as the scalp and chest are involved.
- Etiology is multifactorial, including vascular hyperreactivity, alterations in innate immunity, e.g. cathelicidins, and *Demodex* plus its commensal bacteria. There is some evidence to suggest association of rosacea with cardiovascular disorders.
- Table 30.1 lists diagnostic phenotypes and features of rosacea (Figs 30.1–30.5) and their characteristics.

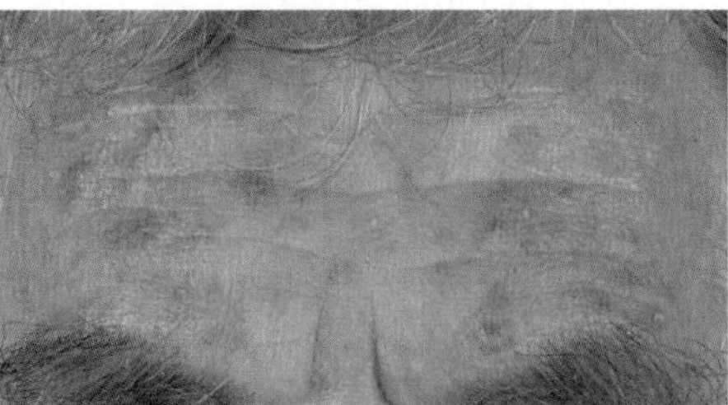

Fig. 30.1 Rosacea. Moderate papulopustular rosacea of the forehead. Note the superficial nature of the inflammatory lesions. *Courtesy, Frank C. Powell, MD.*

- Variants include granulomatous rosacea and periorificial dermatitis
  - Granulomatous rosacea
    - Red to red-brown papules secondary to granulomatous inflammation (Fig. 30.6)
  - Periorificial dermatitis
    - Originally referred to as perioral dermatitis but lesions can surround other orifices, hence the term periorificial
    - Affects children and adults
    - Lesions around the mouth and nose > eyes
    - Monomorphic pink papules and fine pustules (Figs 30.7 and 30.8) admixed with eczematous patches and thin plaques, sometimes with fine scale
    - Lesions recur over weeks to months
    - May initially improve with topical CS but ultimately this treatment leads to exacerbation and should not be used
    - If topical CS are an exacerbating factor, taper strength of CS over a period of weeks or substitute topical calcineurin inhibitors in order to reduce rebound
  - Mid-facial edema
    - Erythematous, firm, non-pitting, painless swelling of the mid-face (Fig. 30.9)
  - Rosacea fulminans
    - Acute facial plaque studded with pustules
- **DDx**: Table 30.2.
- **Rx**: Tables 30.3 and 30.4.

For further information see Ch. 37 from *Dermatology, Fourth Edition*.

For additional online figures visit www.expertconsult.com 

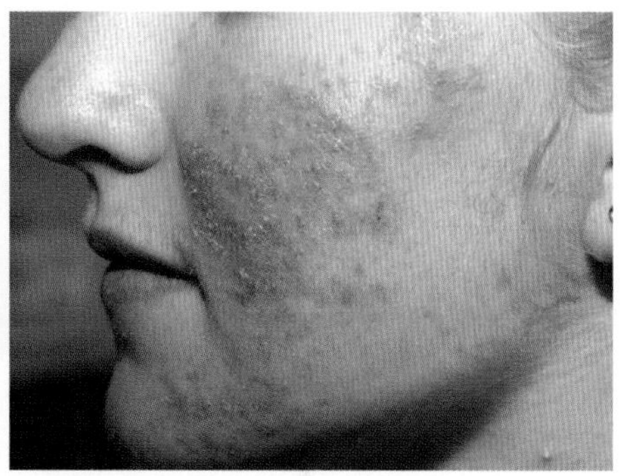

Fig. 30.2 Rosacea dermatitis. When there is more severe disease, scaling and superficial crusting may be seen as on the cheek of this woman. *Courtesy, Kalman Watsky, MD.*

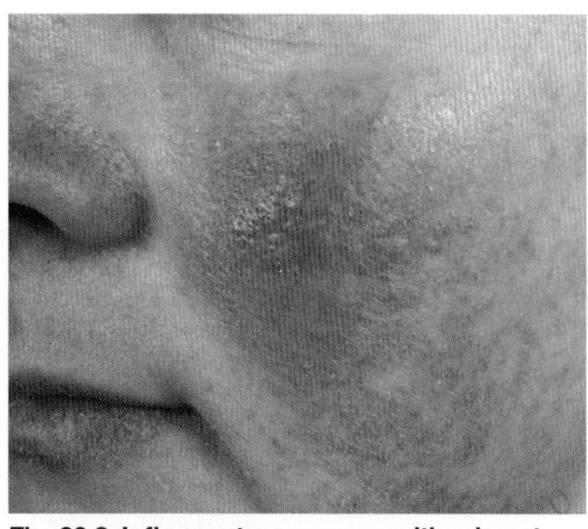

Fig. 30.3 Inflammatory rosacea with edematous changes. An intensely erythematous plaque is present on the medial aspect of the cheek. This may improve once the underlying inflammation is treated appropriately. *Courtesy, Frank C. Powell, MD.*

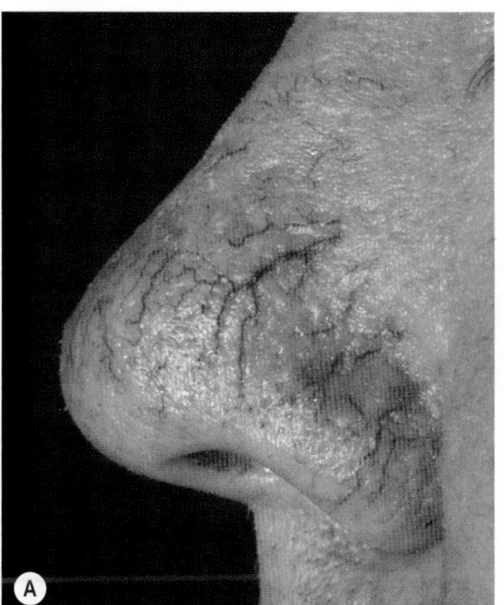

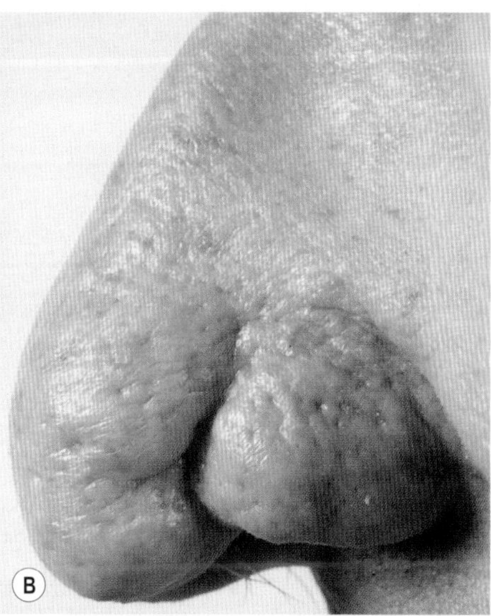

Fig. 30.4 Rhinophyma – early versus advanced disease. A Tortuous, telangiectatic vessels on the distal aspect of the nose contribute to its hyperemic appearance; this hyperemia may predispose to the subsequent hypertrophic changes of rhinophyma. Note the early sign of dilated follicles. **B** Distortion of nasal tissue due to tissue hypertrophy. Electrosurgery or laser therapy can be used to debulk and resculpt this nose. *Courtesy, Frank C. Powell, MD.*

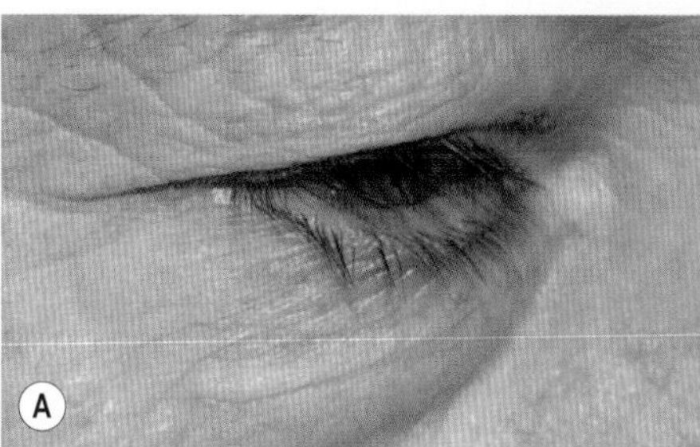

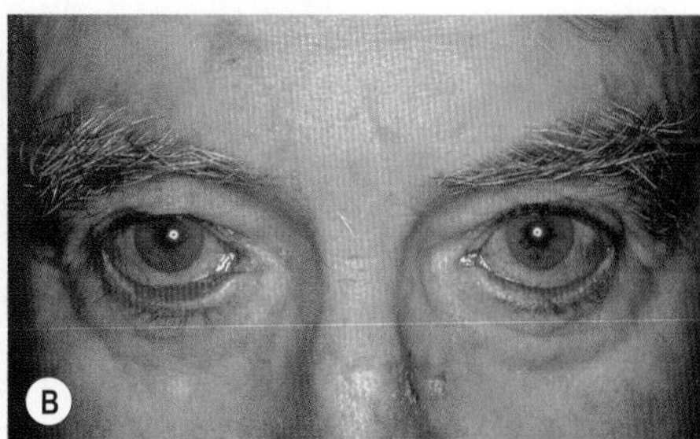

Fig. 30.5 Ocular rosacea. A Erythema of the mucosal portion of the lower eyelid and ectropion. **B** Marked injection of the conjunctivae, leading to the appearance of red eyes. Ectropion is also present. *A, Courtesy, Kalman Watsky, MD; B, Courtesy, YDRSC.*

TYPES OF ROSACEA		
Types		**Major features (presence of 2 or more are diagnostic)**
A Fixed centrofacial erythema in a characteristic pattern that may periodically intensify		
Erythemato-telangiectatic (neurovascular)	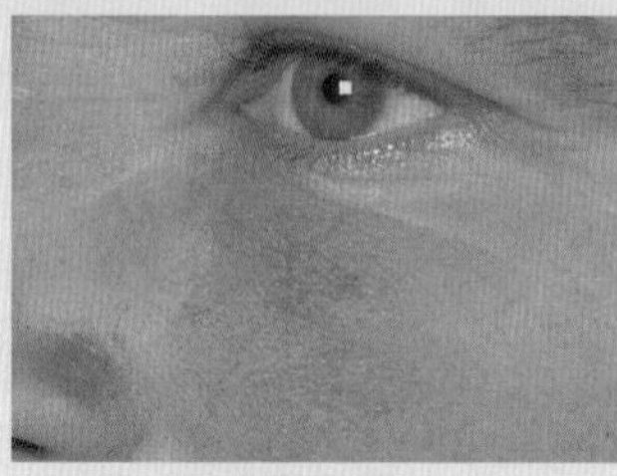	1. Recurrent flushing/blushing, may eventuate in fixed central facial erythema 2. Telangiectasias
Papulopustular (inflammatory)	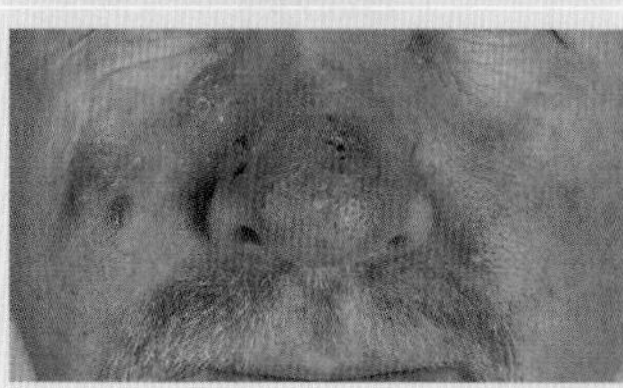	3. Intermittent pink to red papules and inflammatory pustules (Fig. 30.1)
B Phymatous		
	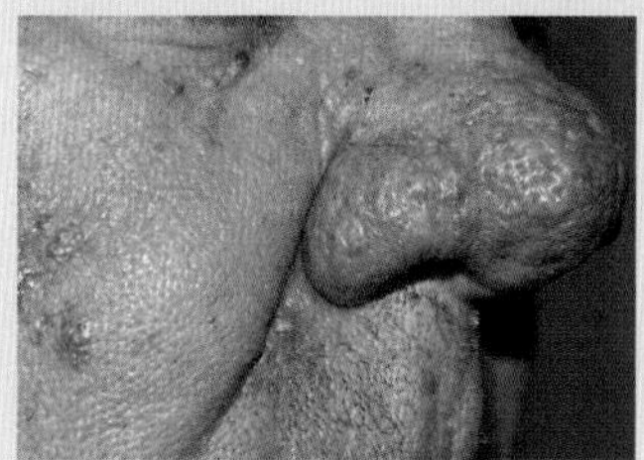	Hypertrophy and irregular (lumpy) thickening of nose (Fig. 30.4) >> forehead, cheeks, chin, or ears
Ocular		
Symptoms Burning, stinging, pruritus, foreign-body sensation in the eye, photophobia, dryness, blurry vision	**Signs** Blepharitis, conical dandruff or "honey crust" on eyelashes, periorbital edema, recurrent "styes" (chalazia or hordeola), irregularity of lid margin, ectropion (see Fig. 30.5), rapid tear breakup time 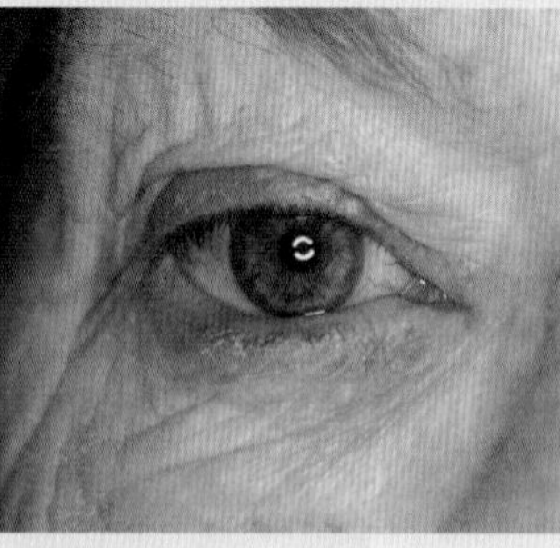	4. Lid margin telangiectasia 5. Interpalpebral conjunctival injection (Fig. 30.5B) *On slit-lamp examination* 6. Spade-shaped infiltrates in the cornea 7. Scleritis and sclerokeratitis

Table 30.1 Types of rosacea. A diagnosis of rosacea can be based on cutaneous presentations in **A** or **B** OR the presence of 2 or more major features. Some patients also have seborrheic dermatitis and/or actinic damage. Edema of the facial skin can also develop.

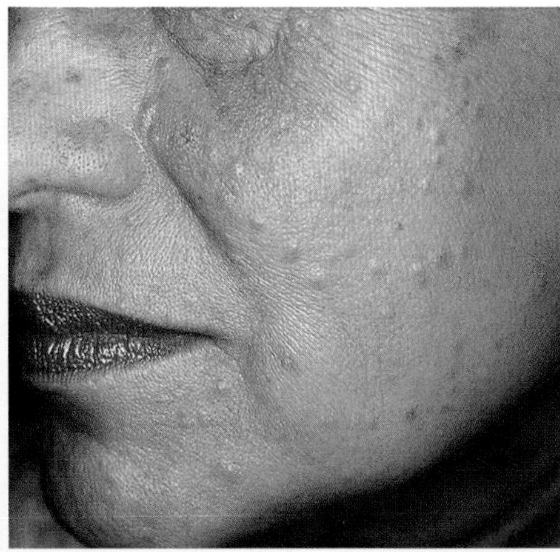

Fig. 30.6 Granulomatous rosacea. Discrete skin-colored to brown papules scattered on the face. *Courtesy, Frank C. Powell, MD.*

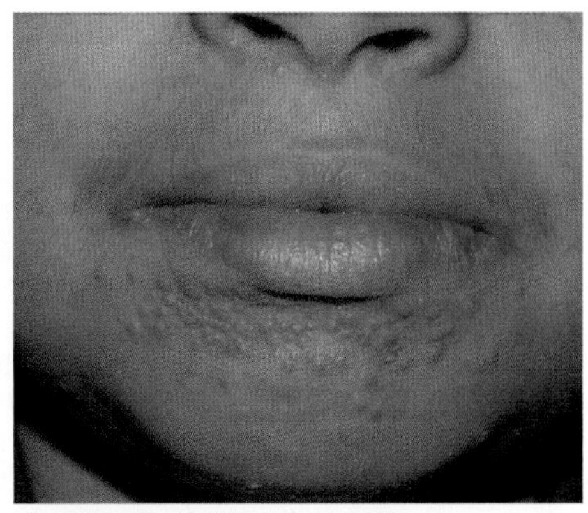

Fig. 30.7 Periorificial dermatitis, granulomatous form. Discrete dull pink-red papules around the mouth and nose. While periorificial dermatitis is often misdiagnosed as eczema, this more granulomatous form may be misdiagnosed as sarcoidosis if a biopsy has been performed. *Courtesy, Julie V. Schaffer, MD.*

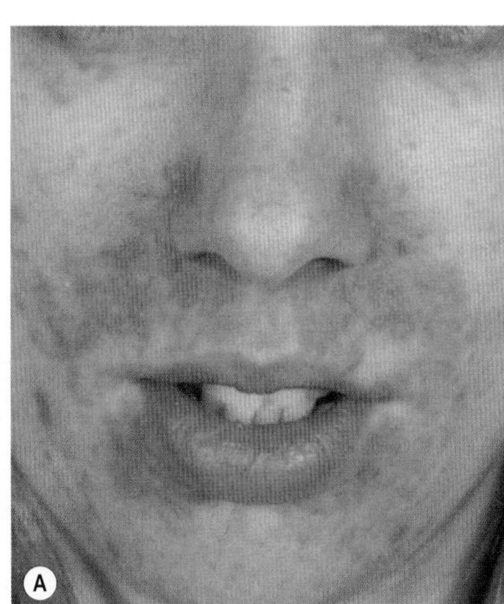

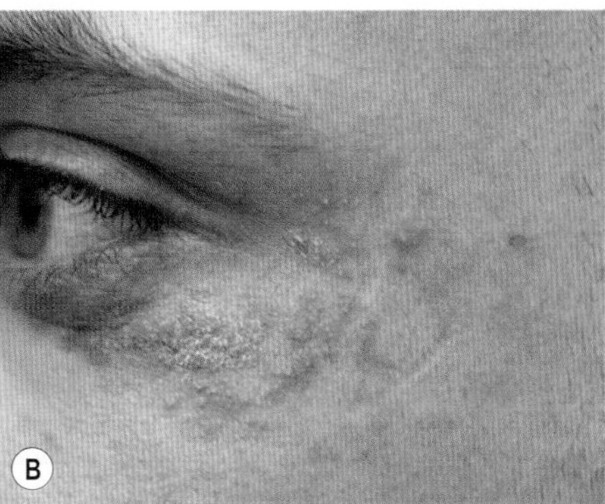

Fig. 30.8 Periorificial dermatitis (often referred to as perioral dermatitis). A, B Pink papules, patches and thin plaques as well as pinpoint superficial pustules around orifices, i.e. in a perioral, perinasal, and/or periorbital distribution pattern. In contrast to papulopustular rosacea, the papules are usually at the same stage of evolution. *A, Courtesy, Frank C. Powell, MD; B, Courtesy, Kalman Watsky, MD.*

DIFFERENTIAL DIAGNOSIS OF ROSACEA	
Disease	**Distinguishing feature(s) from rosacea**
Erythematotelangiectatic rosacea	
Actinic damage	May be difficult to distinguish because this also leads to telangiectasias and erythema, and some patients have both disorders
Seborrheic dermatitis	Erythema with greasy scale in nasolabial folds, ear canals, eyebrows, and scalp
Keratosis pilaris rubra	• Usually presents during adolescence • Background erythema of the lateral cheeks with superimposed tiny follicular papules
Erythromelanosis follicularis faciei	Pink to red-brown patches with multiple pinpoint follicular white papules on the lateral cheeks
Acute cutaneous lupus erythematosus	• Absence of inflammatory papulopustules and ocular changes • At least 75–80% of patients have systemic signs/symptoms • Often more well-demarcated edematous plaques
Flushing (idiopathic or secondary)	• Intermittent erythema and warmth • Flushing in patients with rosacea is usually limited to the face • Consider other common etiologies (e.g. menopause, anxiety disorder) or a tumor-related phenomenon (carcinoid syndrome, occult pheochromocytoma, mastocytosis) when additional anatomic sites are involved or there are associated symptoms such as tachycardia and sweating
Papulopustular rosacea	
Acne (vulgaris)	Onset at a younger age
	Comedones, both open and closed
	Cysts
	Greater involvement of the upper trunk
Demodicosis (*Demodex* folliculitis)	Patients often immunosuppressed (HIV infection, leukemia)
	Daily cleansing of face with mild soaps, sulfacetamide washes Responds to topical permethrin ± oral ivermectin
Steroid-induced rosacea	Clinical overlap with periorificial dermatitis (see above) (Fig. 30.11)
Papulopustular eruption due targeted inhibitors (e.g. epidermal growth factor receptor [EGFR] inhibitor)	More abrupt onset after starting the targeted inhibitor (Fig. 30.10) May also involve the scalp, neck, and trunk
Ocular rosacea	
Seborrheic dermatitis	Involvement beyond the eyelid margin; may be accentuated in the eyelid creases
Drug-induced ocular rosacea	Eyedrops used to treat other ocular disorders, e.g. glaucoma

Table 30.2 Differential diagnosis of rosacea.

MEDICAL AND SURGICAL THERAPIES FOR ROSACEA AND PERIORIFICIAL DERMATITIS	
Papulopustular rosacea	**Periorificial dermatitis**
Topical agents – mild disease, adjunct to oral therapy or maintenance after oral therapy (daily to BID) • Metronidazole (0.75–1%) • Sodium sulfacetamide wash • Azelaic acid (15%) • Ivermectin (1%) • Benzoyl peroxide (5%)/clindamycin (1%) • Clindamycin (1%) • Erythromycin (2%)	**Adults** Similar to papulopustular rosacea, but often unresponsive to topicals and a 4- to 8-week course of oral antibiotics is required **Children** • Topical metronidazole (0.75–1%) • Oral antibiotic for 4–8 weeks Azithromycin 5–10 mg/kg TIW *-or-* Erythromycin 15–25 mg/kg BID *-or-* Doxycycline/minocycline (see to the left) if age >8 years
Oral medications (discontinue or taper to lowest effective dose) • Initially: Doxycycline 20 to 100 mg orally BID *-or-* Tetracycline 500 mg orally BID *-or-* Minocycline 100 mg orally BID *-or-* Doxycycline 40 mg orally daily* • After 4–8 weeks: Decrease dose by ½ or to once daily • Long term: Topicals ± doxycycline 20–50 mg TIW • If very severe: Isotretinoin 10–40 mg orally daily for several months	**Erythematotelangiectatic rosacea** • Laser (e.g. PDL, KTP) or intense pulsed light therapy • Use of topical vasoconstrictors (e.g. brimonidine, oxymetazoline HCl) **Ocular rosacea** • Warm compresses • Gentle digital massage with baby shampoo or 50% tea tree oil scrubs • Low-dose doxycycline • Ophthalmology consultation **Phymatous rosacea** • Surgical excision • Electrosurgery (Fig. 30.12)

Sub-antimicrobial dose.

Table 30.3 Medical and surgical therapies for rosacea and periorificial dermatitis. KTP, potassium titanyl phosphate laser; PDL, pulsed dye laser; TIW, three times per week.

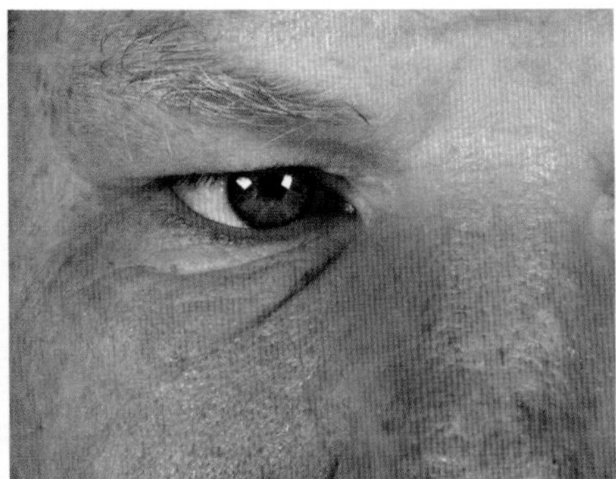

Fig. 30.9 Facial edema secondary to rosacea (Morbihan disease). Erythematous, firm, non-pitting, non-painful swelling of the upper face. Areas of greatest involvement have acquired a "peau d'orange" appearance. *Courtesy, Frank C. Powell, MD.*

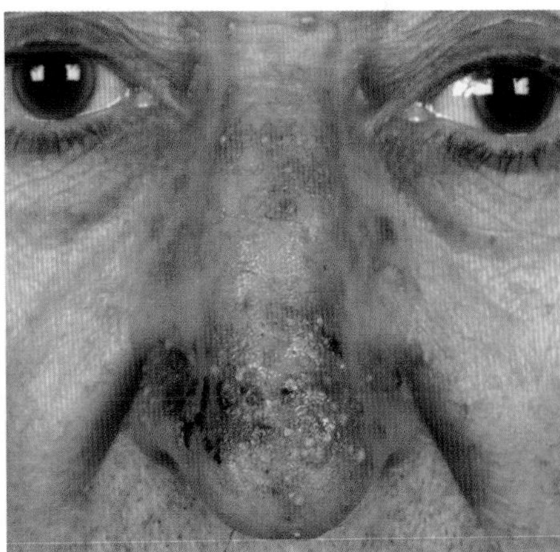

Fig. 30.10 Papulopustular eruption due to an epidermal growth factor receptor (EGFR) inhibitor. There is resemblance to rosacea but the onset is more abrupt. *Courtesy, Frank C. Powell, MD.*

GENERAL RECOMMENDATIONS FOR FACIAL SKIN CARE AND EDUCATION IN PATIENTS WITH ROSACEA
Facial skin care
• Wash with lukewarm water and use soap-free cleansers that are pH balanced • Cleansers are applied gently with fingertips • Use sunscreens with both UVA and UVB protection and an SPF ≥30 • Sun-blocking creams containing the physical barriers titanium dioxide and/or zinc oxide are usually well tolerated • Use cosmetics and sunscreens that contain protective silicones • Water-soluble facial powder containing inert green pigment helps to neutralize the perception of erythema • Moisturizers containing humectants (e.g. glycerin) and occlusives (e.g. petrolatum) help to repair the epidermal barrier • Avoid astringents, toners, and abrasive exfoliators • Avoid cosmetics that contain alcohol, menthols, camphor, witch hazel, fragrance, peppermint, and eucalyptus oil • Avoid waterproof cosmetics and heavy foundations that are difficult to remove without irritating solvents or physical scrubbing • Avoid procedures such as glycolic peels or dermabrasion
Patient education
• Reassure the patient about the benign nature of the disorder and the rarity of rhinophyma, particularly in women • Emphasize the chronicity of the disease and the likelihood of exacerbations • Direct patients to information websites such as those of the National Rosacea Society (http://www.rosacea.org) or the American Academy of Dermatology (http://www.aad.org) • Advise to avoid recognized triggers • Explain the importance of compliance with topical regimens • Educate on the importance of sun avoidance

Table 30.4 General recommendations for facial skin care and education in patients with rosacea. *Adapted from Powell FC. Rosacea. N Engl J Med 2005;352:793–803; Pelle MT, Crawford GH, James WD. Rosacea: II. Therapy. J Am Acad Dermatol 2004;51:499–512; and Del Rosso JQ, Baum EW. Comprehensive medical management of rosacea: An interim study report and literature review. J Clin Aesthet Dermatol 2008;1:20–25.*

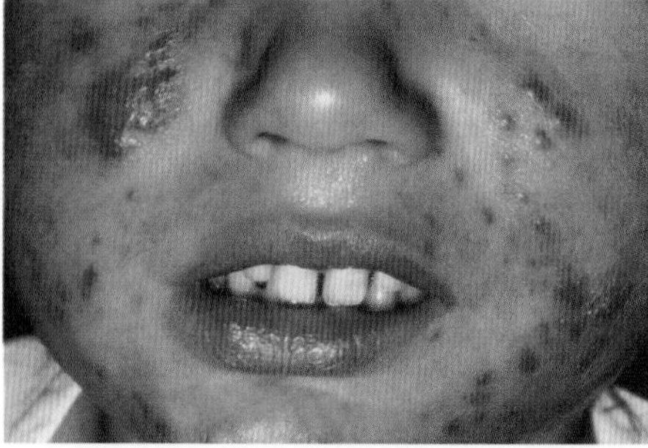

Fig. 30.11 Steroid rosacea. Severe disease in a child with confluence of erythematous papulopustules. *Courtesy, YDRSC.*

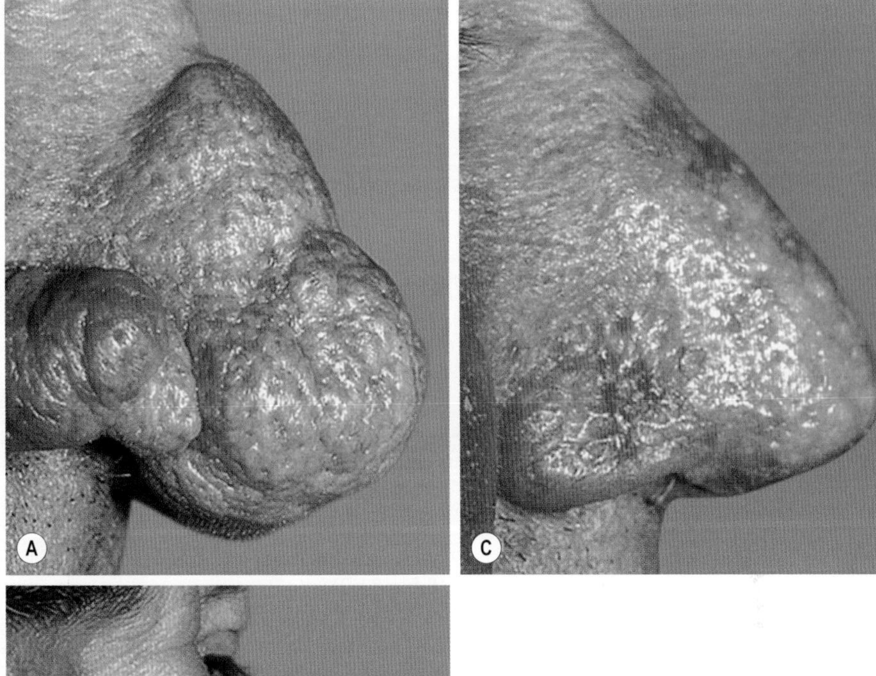

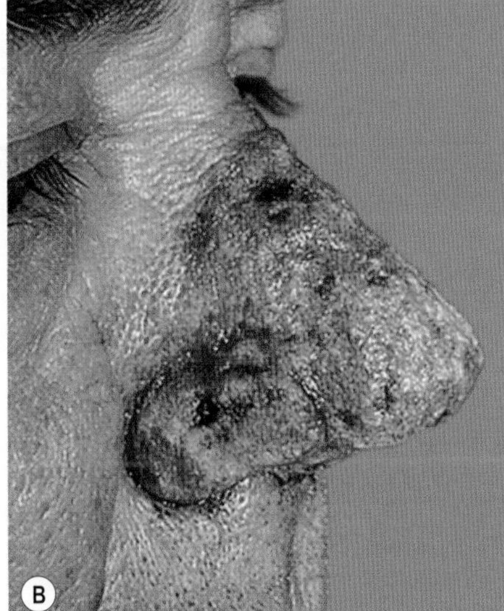

Fig. 30.12 Rhinophyma. A Moderately severe rhinophyma in a middle-aged man. **B** Immediately after electrosurgical planing of excess sebaceous glands. Care is taken to perform subtotal removal as very aggressive therapy can result in significant scarring and possible deformity caused by scar contracture. **C** Four weeks later, healing with good cosmetic outcome is noted. During healing, the wound is kept moist with an ointment and semi-occlusive dressings. *Courtesy, Sheldon V. Pollack, MD.*

31 Folliculitis

• The folliculitides are divided into superficial and deep forms (Table 31.1).

• Follicular papules and pustules can be distinguished from non-follicular lesions by the presence of a hair piercing the lesion in the former; if hair shafts are not apparent, then determining if the lesions correspond to the spatial pattern of hair follicles can aid in diagnosis.

Superficial Folliculitis

• Common; characterized by follicular papules or pustules that are often on an erythematous base.

• Often pruritic, sometimes painful.

• Favors areas with terminal hairs, such as the scalp and beard; also common on the trunk, buttocks, and thighs > axillae and groin.

• The most common type is culture-negative/normal flora, followed by bacterial folliculitis caused by *Staphylococcus aureus*.

• Multiple, less common etiologies (Table 31.1), require a systematic approach for adequate diagnosis and treatment (Fig. 31.1; Table 31.2).

• **DDx:** acne vulgaris, pseudofolliculitis barbae, rosacea; Grover disease in adults; pustular miliaria in children.

CLASSIFICATION OF THE FOLLICULITIDES	
Superficial folliculitides	**Deep folliculitides**
Infectious • Bacterial 1. *Staphylococcus aureus* (Fig. 31.2) 2. Gram-negative bacilli 3. Hot tub folliculitis (Fig. 31.3) • Fungal 1. Dermatophyte (Fig. 31.4A) 2. *Malassezia* spp. (*Pityrosporum*) 3. *Candida* spp. • Viral 1. Herpes simplex (Fig. 31.4B) 2. Varicella zoster • Other 1. *Demodex* (Fig. 31.4C, D) **Non-infectious** • Culture-negative/normal flora (Fig. 31.5) • Irritant • Drug-induced • Eosinophilic (Fig. 31.6) 1. Eosinophilic pustular folliculitis (Ofuji disease) 2. Immunosuppression (or HIV)-associated eosinophilic pustular folliculitis 3. Eosinophilic pustular folliculitis of infancy • Disseminate and recurrent infundibulofolliculitis	• Furuncles • Sycosis (Table 31.3) 1. Barbae (Fig. 31.2B) 2. Lupoid 3. Mycotic (Fig. 31.7) 4. Herpetic • Pseudofollicultis barbae • Acne keloidalis • Hidradenitis suppurativa*

**Part of the follicular occlusion tetrad, which also includes acne conglobata (see Ch. 29), dissecting cellulitis of the scalp (see Ch. 56), and pilonidal sinus/cyst (see Ch. 90).*

Table 31.1 Classification of the folliculitides.

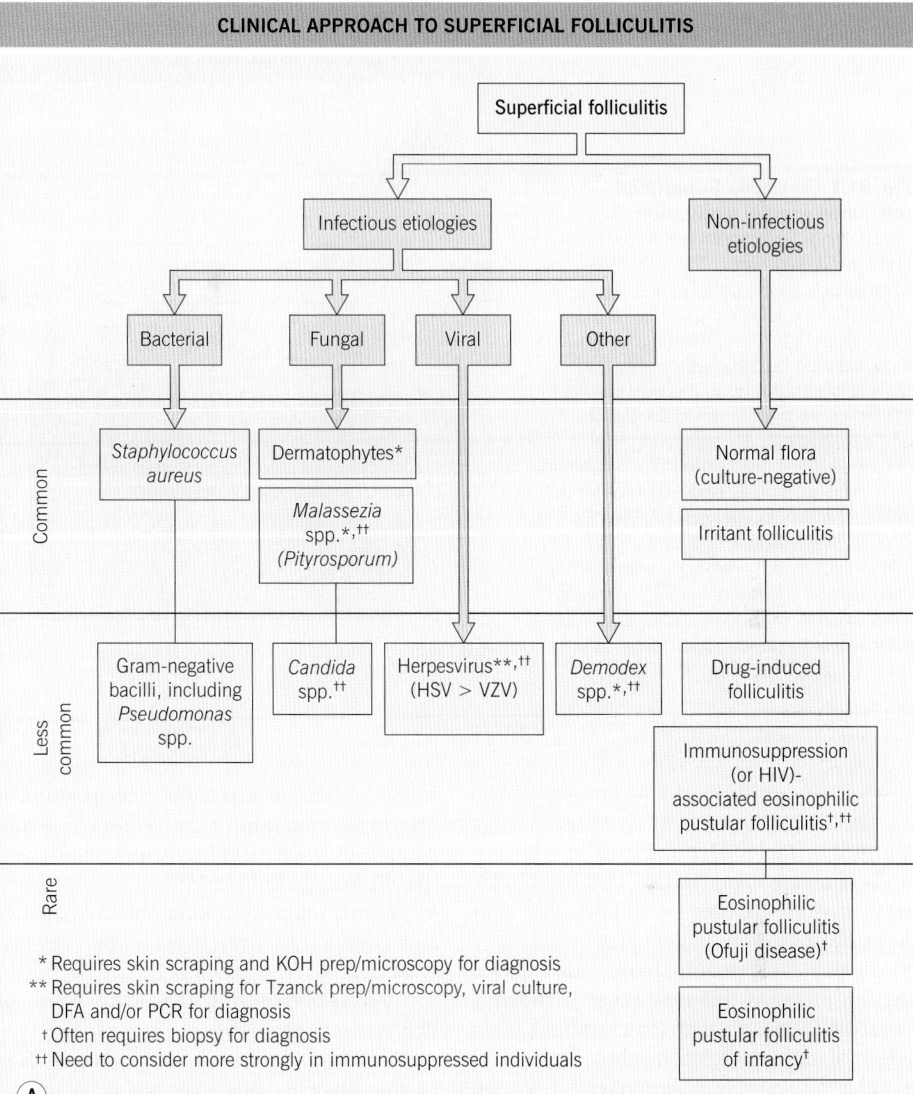

Fig. 31.1 Superficial folliculitis – clinical approach. A Edematous lesions of folliculitis are most suggestive of eosinophilic folliculitis, *Demodex* folliculitis, and *Pseudomonas* "hot tub" folliculitis. *Continued*

Fig. 31.1 *Continued* **Superficial folliculitis – initial evaluation. B** If considering dermatophytes, *Malassezia* spp., or *Candida* spp., then obtain scrapings from the peripheral scale and the roof of the follicular pustule for KOH (potassium hydroxide) microscopy (1). If considering bacterial etiologies, and depending on the host, the pustular fluid should be sent for Gram stain, culture, and sensitivity (2). If considering viral etiologies, the base of the unroofed lesion should be vigorously scraped in order to collect the viral-laden keratinocytes for Tzanck prep/microscopy, viral culture, DFA (direct fluorescent antibody), and/or PCR (polymerase chain reaction) (3). Likewise, if considering *Demodex* folliculitis, scrape the base of the lesion vigorously for KOH microscopy (3) (see Fig. 31.4D).

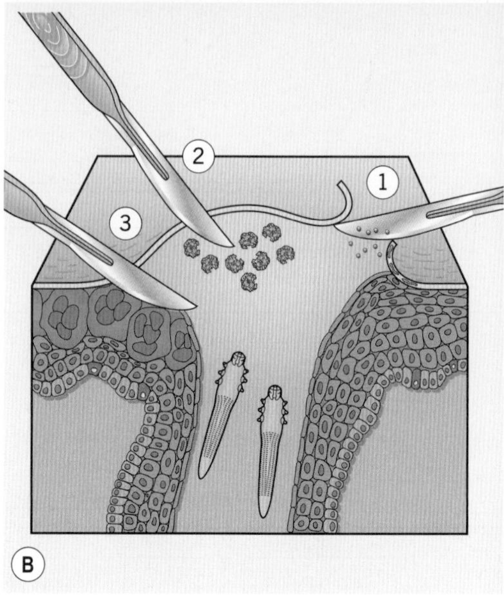

Deep Folliculitis

- The major forms of deep folliculitis are outlined in Tables 31.1 and 31.3.
- Lesions are characterized by firm, tender, erythematous papules or nodules that may measure up to 2 cm in diameter.
- Should avoid manipulating (i.e. squeezing) furuncles as this may cause bacteremia or seeding of heart valves (endocarditis), brain (abscess), or bones (osteomyelitis).
- The "follicular occlusion tetrad" is a term that was coined for the common association of acne conglobata, hidradenitis suppurativa, dissecting cellulitis of the scalp, and pilonidal sinus/cyst; also called "acne inversa."

Pseudofolliculitis Barbae (PFB)

- A common, chronic inflammatory disorder occurring most often in the beard area of men who shave.
- Favors males > females; African-Americans, and others with darkly pigmented skin and tightly curled hair.
- The proposed etiology is tightly curled hairs that curve back into the skin when shaved (Fig. 31.8).
- Also, there is a genetic predisposition if carrying a mutation in the 1A α-helical subdomain of the hair follicle companion layer-specific keratin K6hf (K75).
- Lesions range from inflammatory papules and pustules to firm papules and keloidal scars (Fig. 31.9).
- Intervention during the acute phase of PFB is essential.
- **Rx:** while the easiest way to cure PFB is to stop shaving, this may not be practical; laser hair removal systems that are skin-color appropriate offer the best option for a more permanent solution.
- In addition, shaving techniques can be optimized (Table 31.4) and other treatments may provide some control (Table 31.5).

Acne Keloidalis

- Begins as a chronic folliculitis of the posterior neck and occipital scalp; with time, keloidal papules and plaques develop (Fig. 31.10).
- Seen almost exclusively in males of African descent.
- Lesions are usually pruritic and sometimes painful and disfiguring.

CLINICAL FEATURES AND TREATMENT OF SELECTED SUPERFICIAL FOLLICULITIDES		
Type	**Clinical features**	**Therapy**
Infectious folliculitides		
Bacterial		
Staphylococcus aureus folliculitis		
• Most common infectious folliculitis • Increased risk with diabetes, atopic dermatitis, hot and humid weather, occlusion, waxing/plucking/shaving hair, use of topical CS	• Follicular pustules or papules on erythematous base (Fig. 31.2) • Favors face, trunk, axillae, buttocks • If no pustules present, clue to diagnosis may be a superimposed collarette of scale	**Localized** • Topical mupirocin 2% ointment TID for 7–10 days **Widespread or recurrent** • Weekly–twice weekly washes (e.g. benzoyl peroxide, chlorhexidine, bleach baths*) • Treat chronic *S. aureus* nasal carriage • Culture-guided oral antibiotics
Gram-negative folliculitis		
• Due to *Klebsiella, Enterobacter*, and *Proteus* spp. • Typically seen in acne patients receiving long-term antibiotics • Also seen in adult men with oily skin	• Pustules in the T-zone and perinasal regions of face	• Topical gentamicin or benzoyl peroxide • Systemic quinolones **Severe or recurrent** • Isotretinoin 0.5–1 mg/kg/day for up to 16 weeks
Hot tub folliculitis		
• Due to *Pseudomonas aeruginosa* in the setting of hot tub/whirlpool use 12–48 hours prior to onset	• Edematous pink-red follicular papules and pustules • Favors trunk (Fig. 31.3); often pruritic • Usually self-limited in immunocompetent host • More serious in immunocompromised	• Maintenance of hot tub/whirlpool to ensure adequate chlorine levels **Severe or immunocompromised host** • Oral quinolones for 1–2 weeks

Table 31.2 Clinical features and treatment of selected superficial folliculitides. *Continued*

CLINICAL FEATURES AND TREATMENT OF SELECTED SUPERFICIAL FOLLICULITIDES		
Type	**Clinical features**	**Therapy**
Fungal		
Dermatophyte folliculitis		
• Tinea barbae in beard area (*Trichophyton mentagrophytes* or *T. verrucosum*); classically occurs in farmworkers • Majocchi granuloma (usually due to *T. rubrum*); classically occurs on the legs of women who shave; additional risk factors include immunosuppression, occlusion, and the use of potent topical CS	• Inflammatory follicular papules and pustules in beard area; crusts; loosened hairs • Follicular pustules, papules, or nodules, most often on lower legs (Fig. 31.4A)	• Topical antifungals often ineffective • Terbinafine, 250 mg/day PO for 2–3 weeks • Micronized or ultramicronized griseofulvin, 500–1000 mg/day or 500–750 mg/day PO, respectively, for 4–6 weeks • Itraconazole, 200 mg PO twice daily for 1 week per month, for 2 pulses
Malassezia (Pityrosporum) folliculitis		
• Caused by *Malassezia* spp. • Typically seen in young adults • Inciting factors include warm weather, occlusion, excessive sebum production, antibiotic therapy, iatrogenic immunosuppression	• Pruritic follicular pustules and papules • Favors chest, back, shoulders • Abundant yeast forms on KOH microscopy	**Topicals** • Antifungals (e.g. ketoconazole cream) • Selenium sulfide or antifungal shampoos **Systemic** • Fluconazole 100–200 mg/day PO for 3 weeks or 200–300 mg once weekly for 1–2 months • Itraconazole 200 mg/day PO for 1–3 weeks
Candida folliculitis		
• Seen primarily in diabetics • Also in immunocompromised hosts and patients on antibiotic or CS therapy • Common in hospitalized or bedridden, febrile patients on the back	• Pruritic follicular pustules on erythematous base • Favors warm, moist and occluded environments, such as intertriginous areas • Often present as satellite pustules surrounding areas of intertriginous candidiasis • Facial lesions may mimic tinea barbae	• Prevent skin-to-skin contact in intertriginous areas • If possible, discontinue antibiotics or CS therapy **Mild** • Topical antifungals **Severe or recalcitrant** • Fluconazole 100 mg/day PO × 1 week, then every other day × 1 month

Table 31.2 *Continued* **Clinical features and treatment of selected superficial folliculitides.** *Continued*

CLINICAL FEATURES AND TREATMENT OF SELECTED SUPERFICIAL FOLLICULITIDES

Type	Clinical features	Therapy
Viral		
Herpes simplex folliculitis		
• **Immunocompetent host:** most common scenarios are occurrence on the face of men or pubic area of women (with histories of recurrent HSV infections) who shave with blade razors • **Immunocompromised host:** widespread or unusual presentations seen; consider VZV when submitting specimens for culture, DFA, and/or PCR	• Rapid development of individual and grouped follicular pustules and vesicles on an erythematous base (Fig. 31.4B) • Multinucleated giant cells seen on Tzanck smear	• Acyclovir 200 mg PO 5 times per day for 5–10 days • Famciclovir 500 mg PO 3 times per day for 5–10 days • Valacyclovir 500 mg PO 3 times per day for 5–10 days
Other		
Demodex folliculitis		
• May be associated with immune suppression • Sometimes associated with flares of rosacea	• Erythematous follicular papules and pustules on the face, often within a background of diffuse erythema (Fig. 31.4C) • Skin scrapings under microscopy reveal numerous *Demodex* mites (Fig. 31.4D)	• Topical 1% ivermectin cream, 5% permethrin cream • Systemic single dose of ivermectin 200 mcg/kg PO • Prevention with daily cleansing using a medicated wash, e.g. sulfacetamide
Non-infectious folliculitides		
Culture-negative/normal flora folliculitis		
• The most common of all the folliculitides	• May look like *S. aureus* folliculitis clinically but cultures reveal no growth or only normal flora • Favors trunk and scalp (Fig. 31.5) • Often pruritic	• Topical benzoyl peroxide • Topical antibiotics (e.g. clindamycin) • Oral antibiotics (e.g. doxycycline, tetracycline) used primarily for their anti-inflammatory effects
Irritant folliculitis		
• Usually occurs following the application of a topical medication or ointment (e.g. tar preparations) • May be seen on thighs from rubbing of denim jeans	• Follicular pustules in the sites of application or rubbing • Favors areas with terminal hairs	• Stop inciting agent • Apply topical medications in the same direction as hair growth • Topical mid-potency CS lotion or cream

Table 31.2 *Continued* **Clinical features and treatment of selected superficial folliculitides.** *Continued*

CLINICAL FEATURES AND TREATMENT OF SELECTED SUPERFICIAL FOLLICULITIDES		
Type	**Clinical features**	**Therapy**
Drug-induced folliculitis		
• Most common in acne-prone patients and age groups • Can develop within 2 weeks of starting the culprit agent • Risk is proportional to the dose and duration of therapy • Common culprits: CS, androgenic hormones, EGFR inhibitors, MEK inhibitors, sirolimus, iodides, bromides, lithium, isoniazid, anti-convulsants	• Acute eruption of monomorphic erythematous follicular papules and pustules • Favors trunk, shoulders, and upper arms • Multiple papulopustules of the face and scalp, sometimes admixed with scale-crust (see Fig. 17.16) • Unlike acne vulgaris, typically no comedones	• Stop culprit medication, if possible **Topicals** • Benzoyl peroxide, clindamycin, erythromycin, or retinoids **Systemic** • Tetracycline, doxycycline, minocycline
Eosinophilic folliculitis		
Eosinophilic pustular folliculitis (Ofuji disease)		
• Most reported cases from Japan • Not associated with systemic disease	• Recurrent episodes of follicular papulopustules; erythematous patches and plaques with super-imposed coalescent pustules; and later central clearing which leads to figurate lesions • Favors face, upper extremities, and trunk; occasionally palms and soles • Pruritus often severe • Lesions last 7–10 days • Spontaneous resolution with relapse is the norm	• Topical antipruritics, oral antihistamines, and topical CS for relief of pruritus **First-line** • Oral indomethacin 50 mg/day PO **Second-line** • UVB phototherapy • Oral minocycline, dapsone, CS, or colchicine
Immunosuppression (or HIV)-associated eosinophilic folliculitis		
• Correlates with a low CD4 count (<300/mm^3) • Also reported in other immunosuppressed individuals, such as those with lymphoma, leukemias, and stem cell transplant recipients • Can be part of the *i*mmune *r*econstitution *i*nflammatory *s*yndrome (IRIS)	• Chronic, persistent pruritic follicular papules; perhaps no pustules (Fig. 31.6) • Favors the face, scalp, and upper trunk • Intense pruritus	• Clinical improvement occurs with elevation of CD4 count via ART • Topical and oral antipruritics and CS often inadequate • UVB phototherapy can be helpful for pruritus • Additional: topical tacrolimus, permethrin; oral antibiotics, itraconazole, isotretinoin

**Bleach bath involves mixing ¼ cup of household bleach into a half-filled, regular-sized bathtub.*

- Often there is patchy alopecia or complete hair loss; occasionally there are subcutaneous abscesses with malodorous draining sinuses.
- The sooner this condition is treated, the less likely it will become disfiguring.
- **Rx:** outlined in Table 31.6.
- Prevention is important, and patients should avoid mechanical irritation of the posterior hairline.

Hidradenitis Suppurativa

- An inflammatory disorder originating from the hair follicle that targets the apocrine gland-bearing skin sites, particularly the axillae and anogenital region.
- A chronic condition characterized by recurrent "boils" and draining sinus tracts with subsequent scarring.
- Favors females > males and persons of African descent; onset at or soon after puberty.
- **Initially** inflammatory nodules and sterile abscesses arise in the axillae, groin, perianal, and/or inframammary areas; often very painful (Fig. 31.11A, B).
- **With time** sinus tracts (Fig. 31.11B, C) and hypertrophic scars develop (Fig. 31.11D); chronic, malodorous drainage also occurs.
- **Complications** may include anemia of chronic disease, secondary amyloidosis, lymphedema, fistulas, arthropathy, and the rare development of SCCs within the chronic scars.
- **DDx:** staphylococcal furunculosis, Crohn disease, granuloma inguinale, mycetoma, and scrofuloderma (a form of tuberculous lymphadenitis with cutaneous extension).
- **Rx:** difficult to treat and no one perfect treatment exists; a therapeutic approach, based on disease severity is outlined in Table 31.7.
- Avoid incision and drainage, as may lead to further scarring and sinus tract formation.
- In general, medical treatment is recommended in early stages; surgical treatment should be performed as early as possible once abscesses, fistulas, sinus tracts, and scars develop.

For information on the following follicular disorders, refer to the associated chapters: lichen spinulosus (Ch. 9), trichostasis spinulosa (Ch. 29), erythromelanosis follicularis faciei (Ch. 30), phrynoderma (Ch. 43), viral-associated trichodysplasia (Ch. 68), and keratosis pilaris atrophicans (Ch. 82)

For further information see Ch. 38 from *Dermatology, Fourth Edition*.

For additional online figures visit www.expertconsult.com 

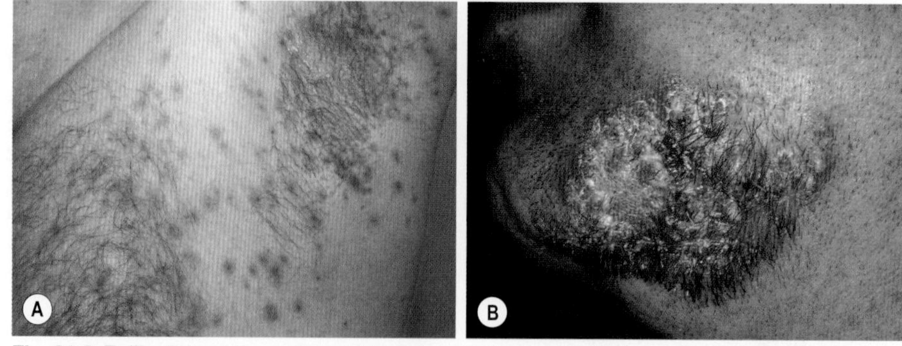

Fig. 31.2 Folliculitis of the axilla and beard area due to *Staphylococcus aureus*. A Numerous follicular pustules with an erythematous rim emanating from the axillary vault. **B** Discrete papulopustules are seen posteriorly, while centrally there is deeper involvement with plaque formation (sycosis barbae). *A, Courtesy, Kalman Watsky; B, Courtesy, YDRSC.*

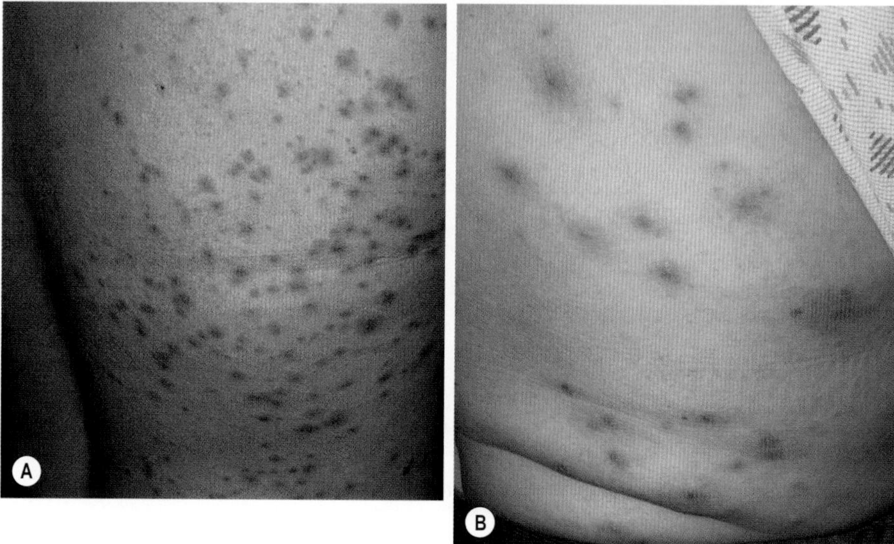

Fig. 31.3 *Pseudomonas* "hot tub" folliculitis. A, B Edematous follicular papules on the flank that began to develop 2–3 days following the use of a hot tub. The number and size can vary. *A, Courtesy, YDRSC; B, Courtesy, Kalman Watsky, MD.*

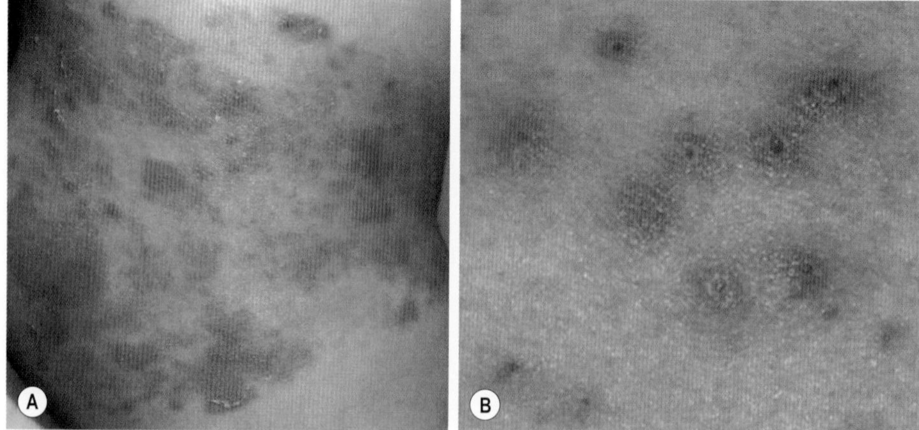

Fig. 31.4 Folliculitis – fungal, viral, and ectoparasitic. A Firm follicular papules of dermatophyte folliculitis (Majocchi granuloma) in the setting of extensive tinea corporis. **B** Follicular herpes simplex viral infection in an immunocompromised host. *A, Courtesy, Amy McMichael, MD; B, Courtesy, Karynne O. Duncan, MD.* *Continued*

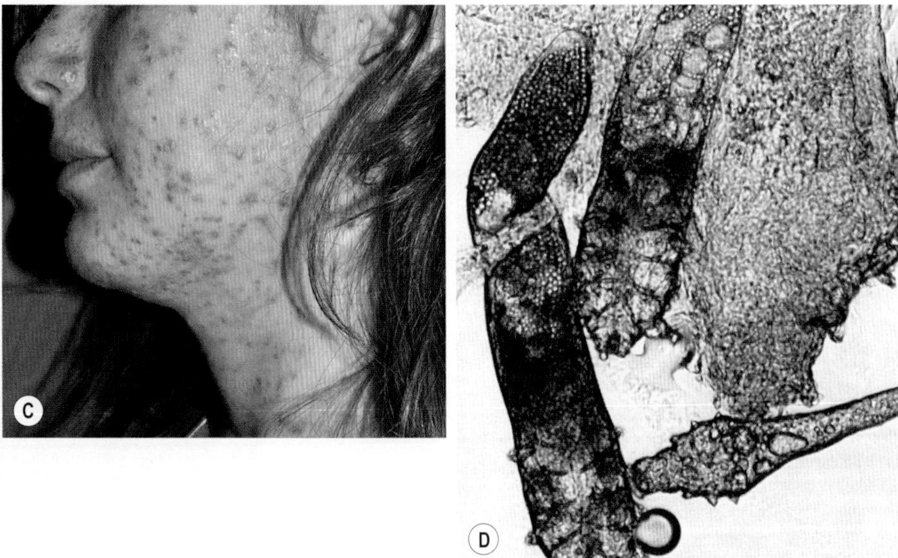

Fig. 31.4 *Continued* **Folliculitis – fungal, viral, and ectoparasitic. C** Numerous papules and papulopustules of *Demodex* folliculitis on the face and neck; note the edematous nature of several of the lesions. **D** Microscopic findings of follicular contents obtained via scraping of *Demodex* folliculitis. *C, Courtesy, Angela Hernandez-Martin, MD; D, Courtesy, YDRSC.*

FORMS OF SYCOSIS	
Type	**Characteristics**
Barbae	• Bacterial folliculitis of the beard and/or mustache areas, usually caused by *Staphylococcus aureus* (see Fig. 31.2B) • Deep-seated, edematous, perifollicular papules and pustules that may coalesce to form plaques studded with pustules and crusts • Subacute to chronic course with frequent relapses
Lupoid	• Scarring form of deep folliculitis, typically affecting the beard area; may be caused by *S. aureus* (although cultures often fail to reveal pathogenic organisms) • Peripheral extension of perifollicular papules and pustules with central atrophic scarring/cicatricial alopecia; granulomatous inflammation can lead to an appearance reminiscent of lupus vulgaris • Chronic course, refractory to treatment
Mycotic	• Dermatophyte folliculitis of the beard area (most often the chin), usually caused by zoophilic organisms • Inflammatory perifollicular papules and pustules coalesce to form nodules and plaques with purulent discharge from patulous follicles, crusting, and loose hairs that can be painlessly removed (Fig. 31.7)
Herpetic	• See Table 31.2

Table 31.3 Forms of sycosis. Sycosis is defined as chronic inflammation of hair follicles, especially of the beard.

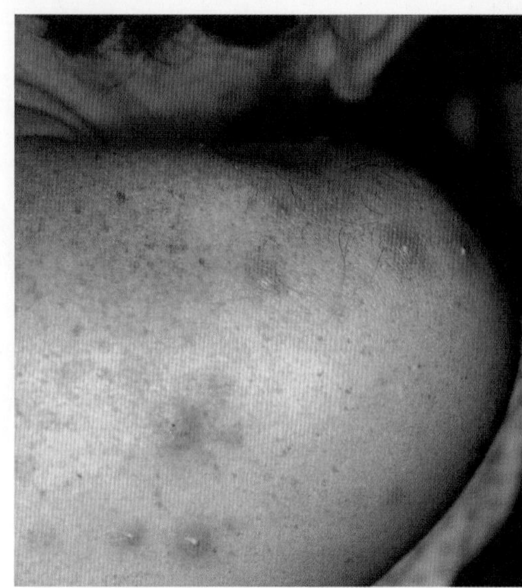

Fig. 31.5 Folliculitis (culture-negative). Follicular pustules with an erythematous rim are present on the upper back. The differential diagnosis is primarily folliculitis due to *Staphylococcus aureus* and acne. *Courtesy, YDRSC.*

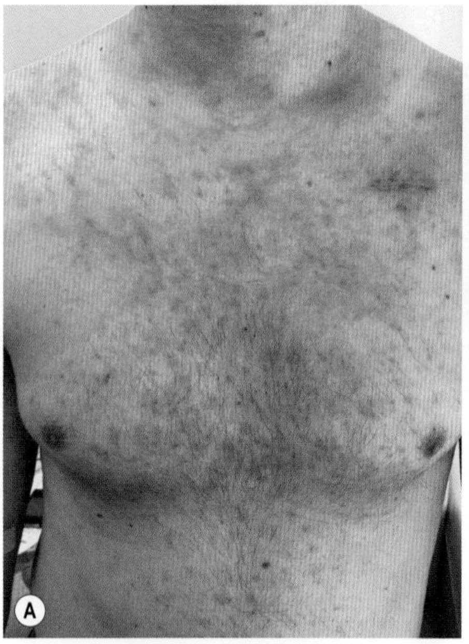

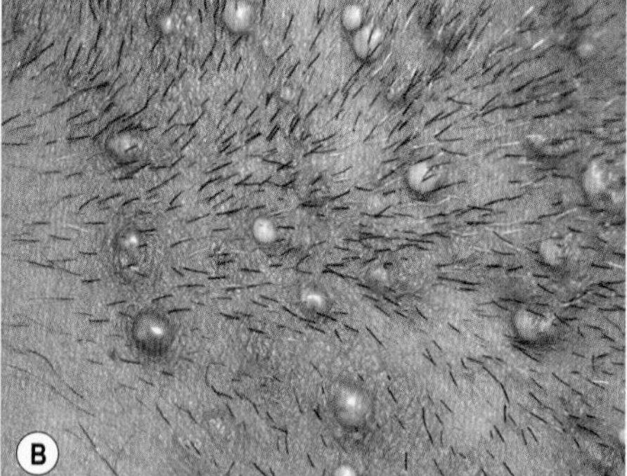

Fig. 31.6 Immunosuppression-associated eosinophilic folliculitis. A Multiple follicular papules on the anterior trunk in a patient who had received an allogeneic hematopoietic stem cell transplant. Note the edematous nature of some of the lesions. Very few pustules were present. **B** In some patients, multiple follicular pustules are seen. *A, Courtesy, Dennis Cooper, MD; B, Courtesy, Luis Requena, MD.*

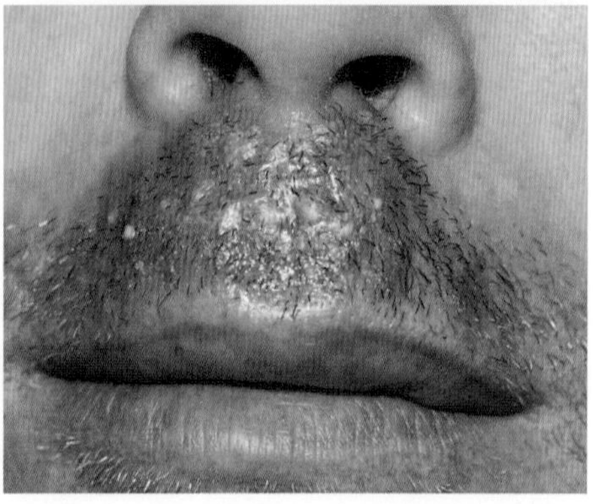

Fig. 31.7 Mycotic sycosis. Firm plaque of the upper cutaneous lip studded with multiple pustules due to a zoophilic dermatophyte. *Courtesy, Kalman Watsky, MD.*

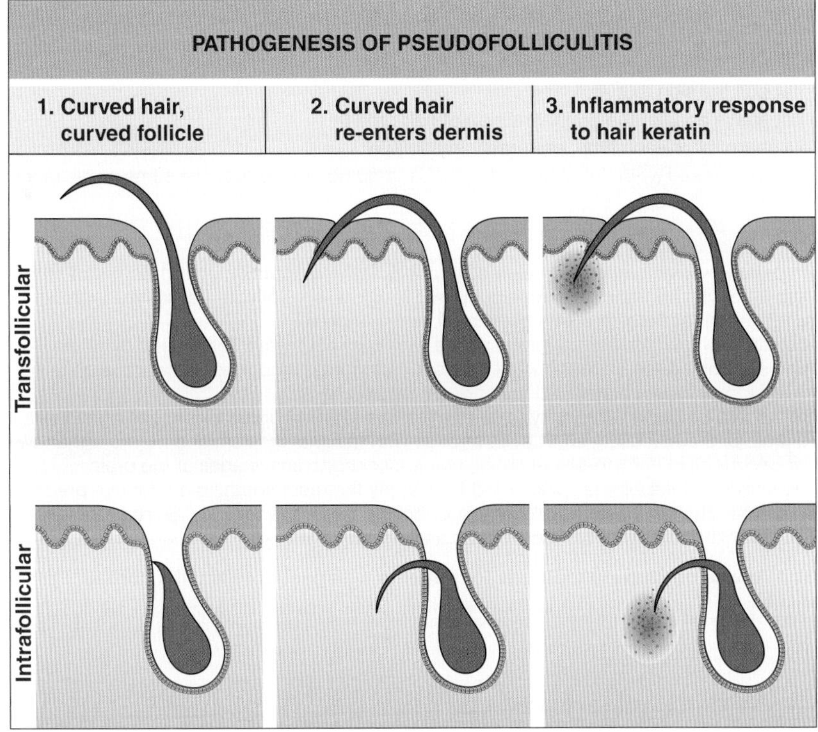

Fig. 31.8 Pathogenesis of pseudofolliculitis. *Courtesy, M.A. Abdallah, MD.*

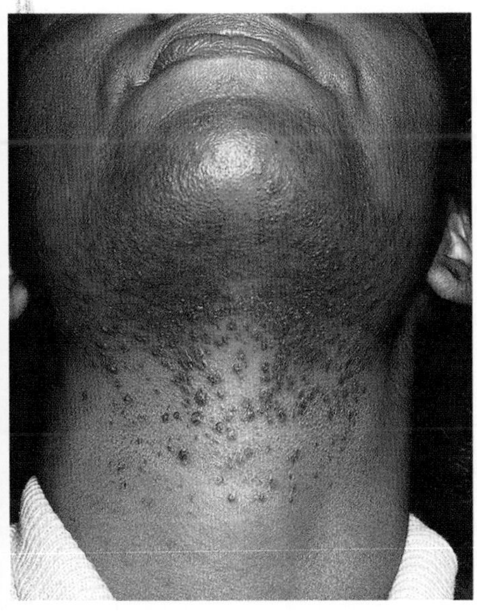

Fig. 31.9 Pseudofolliculitis barbae. Multiple firm hyperpigmented papules on the lower face and neck (beard distribution). *Courtesy, A. Paul Kelly, MD.*

ADVICE ON SHAVING METHODS FOR PATIENTS WITH PSEUDOFOLLICULITIS BARBAE
Important points
• Do not pull the skin taut • Do not shave against the grain/direction of hair growth • Use a sharp razor each time, preferably multiblade • Take short strokes (with the grain of the hair) and do not shave over the same areas more than twice
Method
1. Remove pre-existing hairs with electric clippers, leaving approximately 1–2 mm of stubble 2. Wash area with non-abrasive acne soap and rough wash cloth; in areas with "ingrown hairs," gentle massaging with a soft toothbrush may help 3. Rinse area with water, then compress face with warm tap water for several minutes 4. Using shaving cream of your choice, massage moderate amount of lather on area to be shaved (do not allow lather to dry; if it does, reapply it) 5. Use a sharp blade (whichever type seems to cut best but not too close) and shave with the grain of the hair using short even strokes with minimal tension (and no more than twice over one area); in hard-to-shave areas, you may need to shave against the grain 6. After shaving, rinse with tap water and then apply the most soothing aftershave preparation of your choice. If significant burning or itching ensues, a topical CS cream or lotion (1–2.5% hydrocortisone) can be used as an alternative aftershave preparation

Table 31.4 Advice on shaving methods for patients with pseudofolliculitis barbae. *Courtesy, A. Paul Kelly, MD.*

THERAPEUTIC APPROACH TO PSEUDOFOLLICULITIS BARBAE	
Shaving	• Mild to moderate disease: continue shaving daily, but follow guidelines in Table 31.4 • Severe disease: discontinue shaving until all inflammatory lesions have cleared and all "ingrown hairs" are released; during this period, the patient can trim beard to a minimum length of 0.5 cm using scissors or electric clippers
Compresses and release of ingrowing hairs	• Warm tap water, saline, or Burow's solution (aluminum acetate) compresses for 10 minutes three times daily to soothe lesions, remove any crusts, reduce drainage secondary to inflammation and/or excoriations, and soften the epidermis to allow easier release of "ingrown hairs"
Topical therapy	• Low-potency topical CS lotion and/or topical clindamycin should be applied after compresses and freeing of embedded hairs
Secondary bacterial infection	• Appropriate systemic antibiotic should be prescribed, based upon bacterial cultures
Recalcitrant disease	• Prednisone (45–60 mg) or its equivalent every morning for 7–10 days may be necessary • Topical eflornithine cream twice daily may be helpful* • Laser hair removal (utilizing appropriate laser for skin color) with goal of permanent hair reduction

**Based upon case series.*

Table 31.5 Therapeutic approach to pseudofolliculitis barbae. *Courtesy, A. Paul Kelly, MD.*

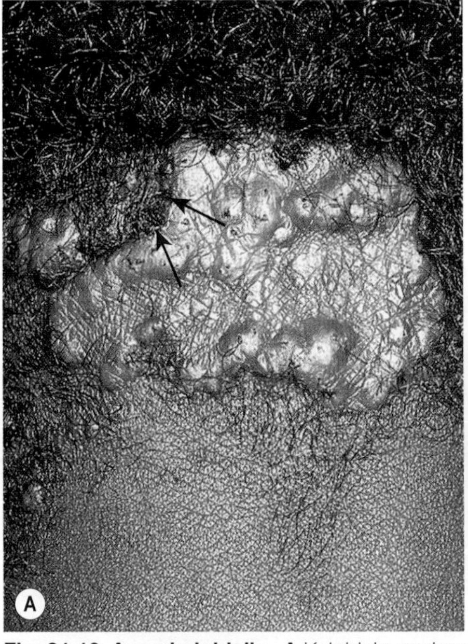

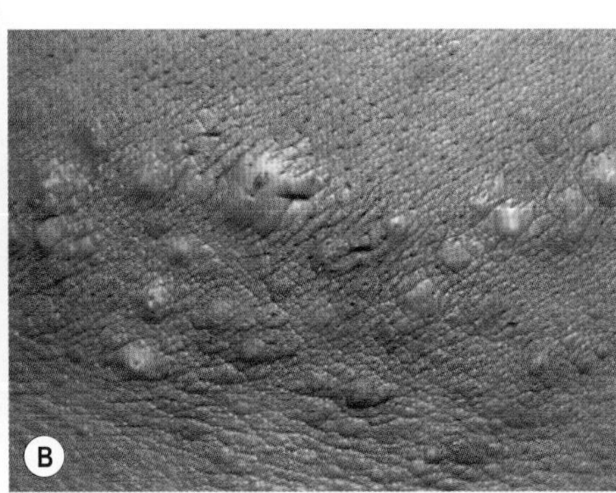

Fig. 31.10 Acne keloidalis. A Keloidal papulonodules and a large plaque of the occipital scalp, associated with scarring alopecia. Note the tufts of hair at the superior border of the scar (arrows). **B** A close-up view, showing an admixture of follicular papules, crusted papules, and firm fibrotic hyperpigmented papules on the posterior neck and occipital scalp. There is associated alopecia. *A, Courtesy, A. Paul Kelly, MD; B, Courtesy, A. Paul Kelly, MD, and Amy McMichael, MD.*

THERAPEUTIC OPTIONS FOR ACNE KELOIDALIS	
Non-inflamed papules and plaques	Mixture of tretinoin gel and potent CS gel twice daily
Inflamed lesions with pustules	Bacterial culture and appropriate systemic antibiotic or a course of oral isotretinoin
Small keloidal papules	Intralesional CS (e.g. triamcinolone acetonide 5–20 mg/ml) Punch excision to below level of hair follicles
	Close primarily or allow to heal secondarily Laser hair removal for permanent hair reduction
Plaques ≤1.5 cm in vertical diameter	Excise and close primarily
Larger plaques and nodules (>1.5 cm in vertical diameter)	Excise with horizontal ellipse
	Extend excision below posterior hairline and include fascia or deep subcutaneous tissue
	Allow to heal by second intention
	Do not inject CS into postoperative site
	Laser excision and cryosurgery are sometimes successful
Postoperative care	Topical imiquimod daily for 6 weeks (8 weeks every other day if irritation)
Maintenance	Tretinoin–CS gel mixture, intermittent intralesional CS and/or oral or topical antibiotics (when needed)

Table 31.6 Therapeutic options for acne keloidalis. *Courtesy, A. Paul Kelly, MD.*

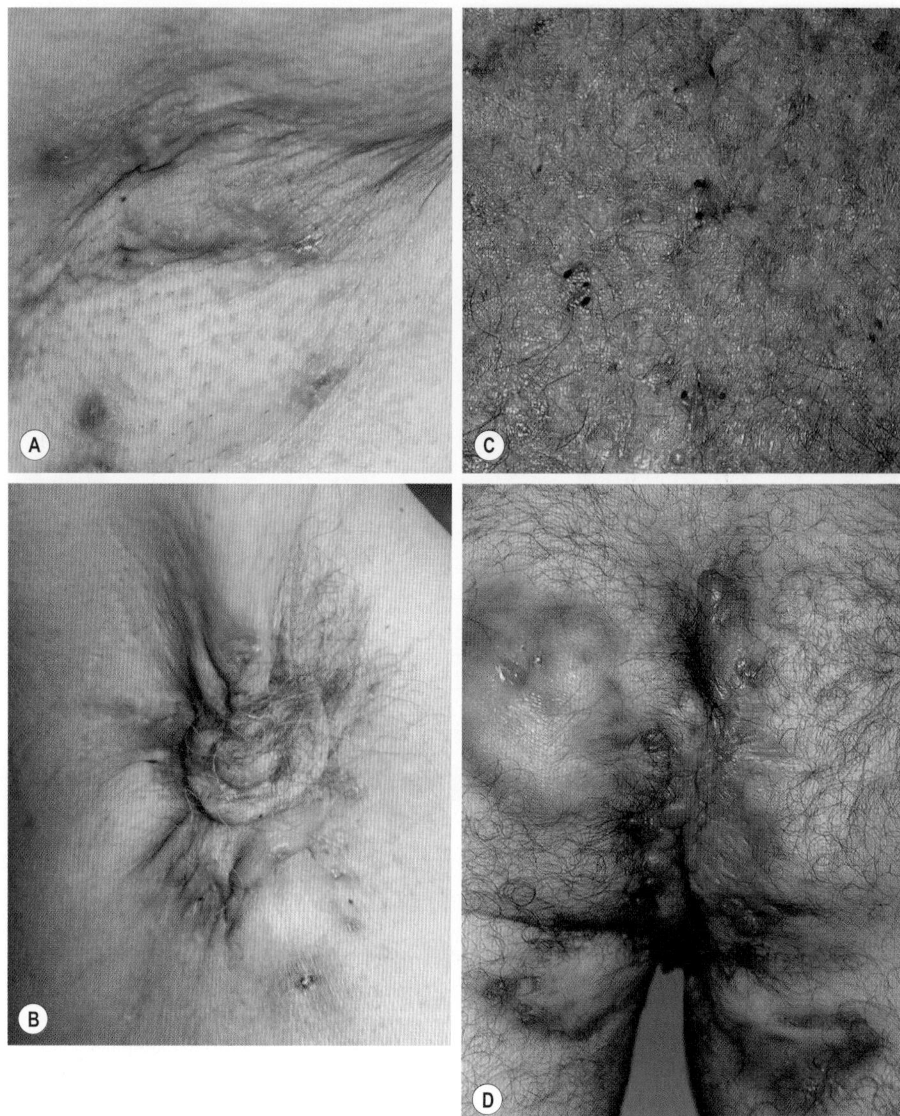

Fig. 31.11 Hidradenitis suppurativa. A, B Papulopustules, nodules, sinus tracts, and scarring in the axilla (Hurley stage II **[A]** and III **[B]**). **C** Superficial sinus tracts that serve as a clue to the diagnosis, even in the absence of active disease. **D** Severe disease (Hurley stage III) with inflammatory nodules, hypertrophic scarring, draining fistulae, and sinus tract formation of the perianal region, buttocks, and upper thighs. This is the type of patient who is at risk for the development of squamous cell carcinoma and secondary amyloidosis. *A, Courtesy, Kalman Watsky, MD; B, Courtesy, Marco Romanelli, MD; C, D, Courtesy, YDRSC.*

HIDRADENITIS SUPPURATIVA (HS) – GRADING SYSTEMS AND THERAPEUTIC LADDER	
Hurley staging system	
Stage I – one or more abscesses with no sinus tract or scar formation Stage II – one or more widely separated recurrent abscesses, with sinus tract and scar formation Stage III – multiple interconnected sinus tracts and abscesses throughout an affected region; more extensive scarring	
Other grading/scoring systems	
1. **Sartorius grading system** (based upon anatomical regions, types of lesions, and distance between lesions) 2. **Modified Sartorius score** (more detailed, requiring measurements and precise counting of lesions) 3. **HS-PGA** (categorizes patients into clear, minimal, mild, moderate, severe, or very severe disease) 4. HS clinical response (HiSCR) score (a binary scoring system for patients with 3 or more abscesses or inflammatory nodules)	
Therapeutic ladder	
Indication	Therapeutic interventions
General measures	• If obese or overweight, weight reduction • Reduce friction and moisture via loose undergarments, absorbent powders, and topical aluminum chloride • Antiseptic soaps (e.g. chlorhexidine) • Smoking cessation
Hurley Stage I	• Intralesional triamcinolone (5–10 mg/ml) injections into early inflammatory lesions • Topical clindamycin • Eradication of *S. aureus* carriage with topical mupirocin in nose, axillae, umbilicus, and perianal regions • Oral antibiotics tailored to results of bacterial cultures from pustular discharge or abscess contents • Oral antibiotic therapy (alone or in combination) for its anti-inflammatory effect (rifampin + clindamycin*, tetracycline, doxycycline, minocycline, dapsone, trimethoprim–sulfamethoxazole) • Oral anti-androgen therapy (e.g. oral contraceptives, spironolactone, finasteride [for males])
Hurley Stage II (see Fig. 31.11A)	• Oral antibiotic therapy (see Stage I) • Acitretin • Systemic immunosuppressive agents including adalimumab^, infliximab, and cyclosporine Surgical treatments† • Limited local excisions with second intention healing • CO_2 laser ablation with second intention healing • Nd:YAG laser treatments, at least 3–4 monthly sessions
Hurley Stage III (see Fig. 31.11B, D)	Medical treatments outlined for Stages I and II Surgical treatments† • Early wide surgical excision of involved areas • CO_2 laser ablation with second intention healing

**There is the most evidence of effectiveness for this combination of antibiotics, each dosed at 300 mg twice a day; note that rifampin may turn body secretions orange in color.*
^FDA-approved dosing regimen: 160 mg (four 40 mg injections) on Day 1 -or- 80 mg daily on Days 1 and 2 followed by 80 mg on Day 15 then 40 mg on Day 29 and weekly thereafter.
†Incision and drainage is discouraged given high rate of recurrence.

Table 31.7 Hidradenitis suppurativa (HS) – grading systems and therapeutic ladder. For further information see Ch. 38 from *Dermatology, Fourth Edition*. PGA, physician global assessment.

32 Disorders of Eccrine and Apocrine Glands

Eccrine and apocrine glands represent the two major types of sweat glands (see Fig. 91.1).

Eccrine Glands

- Functional from birth and activated by thermal stimuli via the hypothalamic sweat center; while their major function is thermoregulation by evaporative heat loss, they are also activated by emotional stimuli.
- Innervated by sympathetic fibers that have acetylcholine as their major neurotransmitter.
- Generalized distribution, with greatest concentration on the palms and soles.
- The eccrine duct opens directly onto the skin surface, and the excretory product is a clear hypotonic fluid that is mostly water but also contains NaCl.

Apocrine Glands

- Unclear function in humans; functional development requires androgens.
- More limited distribution – primarily axillae, nipples/areolae, and umbilical and anogenital regions; modified apocrine glands are found in the external auditory canals and eyelid margins.
- The apocrine duct drains into the superficial portion of the hair follicle (see Fig. 91.1).
- "Decapitation" of apocrine gland cells produces an odorless and viscous fluid; however, its degradation by flora on the skin surface can lead to an odor.

Hyperhidrosis

- Excessive production of eccrine sweat is usually due to *primary cortical* (emotional) hyperhidrosis and the favored sites are the axillae or palms and soles (Fig. 32.1) > the face (Fig. 32.2); involvement is bilateral and symmetric (Fig. 32.3).
- *Secondary cortical* hyperhidrosis is associated with genodermatoses, including palmoplantar keratodermas and epidermolysis bullosa simplex; associated odor reflects maceration and degradation of keratin by bacteria.

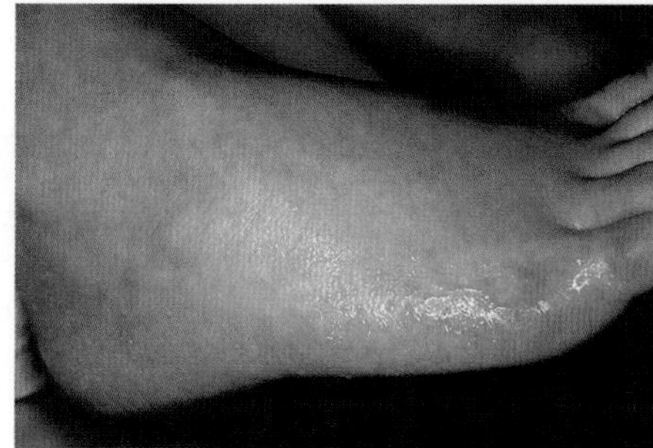

Fig. 32.1 Volar hyperhidrosis (primary cortical). The palmoplantar skin displays excessive eccrine sweat production, including the portions that extend onto the sides of the hands, feet, and digits. Its onset is during childhood as opposed to axillary hyperhidrosis, which has its onset around puberty. *Courtesy, Jean L. Bolognia, MD.*

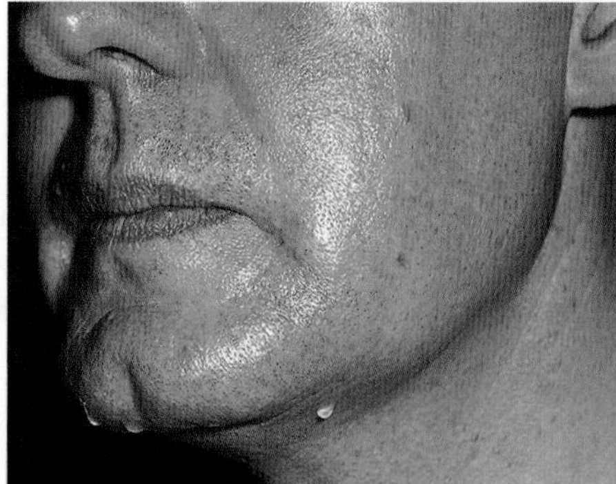

Fig. 32.2 Primary cortical (emotional) hyperhidrosis involving the face. Sweat droplets are evident on the upper cutaneous lip, jawline, and chin. *Reproduced from Hurley HJ. Hyperhidrosis. Curr Opin Dermatol. 1997;4:105–114. Philadelphia: Rapid Science Publishers.*

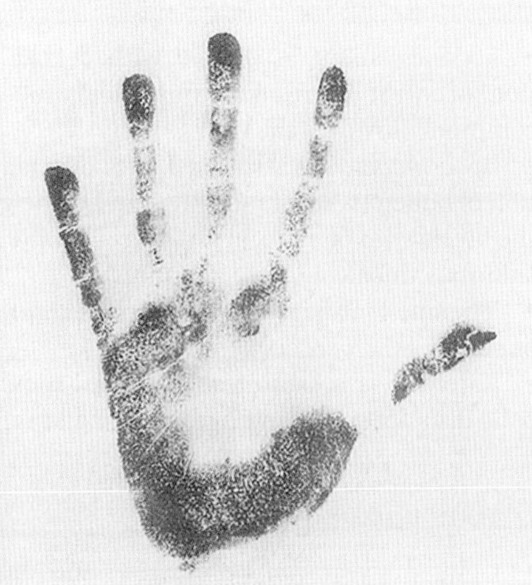

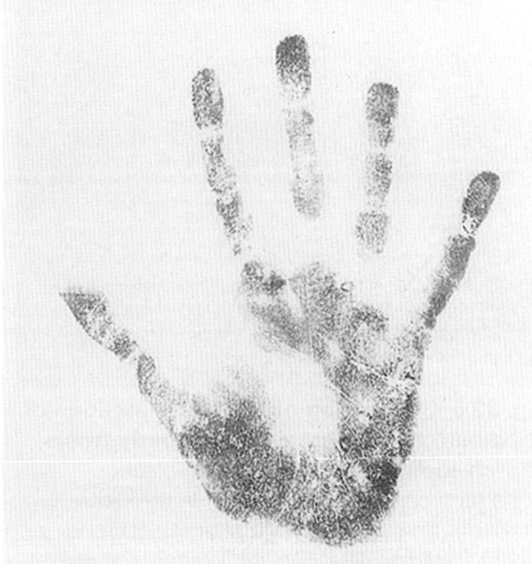

Fig. 32.3 Palmar hyperhidrosis as assessed by the semiquantitative starch paper–iodine technique. Sweating can also be demonstrated directly on palmar skin by the starch–iodine technique, as shown in Figs 32.4 and 32.5. *Courtesy, Harry Hurley, MD.*

CAUSES OF SECONDARY HYPOTHALAMIC HYPERHIDROSIS
• **Infections**, e.g. acute febrile bacterial and viral infections (defervescence), malaria
• **Neoplasms**, e.g. lymphoma (B symptom), pheochromocytoma
• **Endocrinologic disorders**, e.g. hypoestrogenemia of menopause, hyperthyroidism
• **Vasomotor disorders**, e.g. cold injury, Raynaud phenomenon, RSD
• **Neurologic diseases**, e.g. CNS tumors, CVAs (contralateral)
• **Drugs and toxins**, e.g. opioid withdrawal, alcohol withdrawal, combination of drugs that result in the serotonin syndrome (MAOI plus tricyclic or SSRI antidepressant)
• **Miscellaneous**, e.g. compensatory in the setting of a sympathectomy, extensive miliaria or diabetes mellitus

Table 32.1 Causes of secondary hypothalamic hyperhidrosis. CVA, cerebrovascular accident; MAOI, monoamine oxidase inhibitor; RSD, reflex sympathetic dystrophy, also referred to as complex regional pain syndrome. Linezolid is an MAOI.

- *Secondary hypothalamic* (thermoregulatory) hyperhidrosis can be due to a number of systemic diseases, from infections to neoplasms (Table 32.1).
- *Secondary medullary* (gustatory) hyperhidrosis can be physiologic as exemplified by the facial sweating that occurs with spicy foods, or pathologic as occurs in Frey syndrome (Fig. 32.4); in the former, taste receptors send afferent impulses, whereas in the latter, disrupted nerves for sweat aberrantly connect with nerves for salivation.
- Injuries or diseases affecting the spinal cord can result in segmental hyperhidrosis.
- In addition to embarrassment, hyperhidrosis can lead to overhydration of the skin and a higher risk of bacterial and fungal infections.

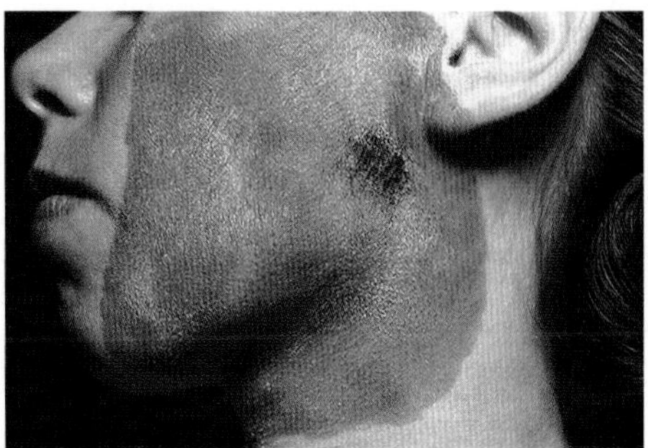

Fig. 32.4 Gustatory sweating in the auriculotemporal (Frey) syndrome, as a consequence of parotid surgery. The blue-black area represents sweating (starch–iodine technique). Salivary stimulation induced this sweating response. *Reproduced from Hurley HJ. Hyperhidrosis. Curr Opin Dermatol. 1997;4:105–114. Philadelphia: Rapid Science Publishers.*

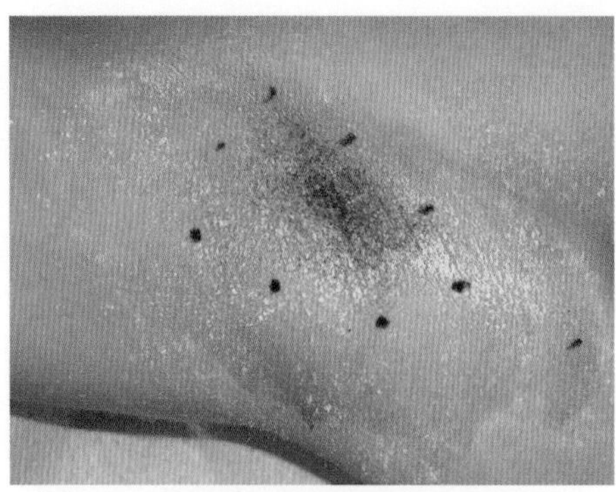

Fig. 32.5 Delineation of area for injections of botulinum toxin A for axillary hyperhidrosis (starch–iodine technique). Blue-black areas represent foci of sweating. In the case of onabotulinumtoxin A, a total of 50–100 U is injected, utilizing 10–15 injection sites. *Courtesy, Alastair Carruthers, MD, and Jean Carruthers, MD.*

- Sweating only during waking hours points to primary cortical (emotional) hyperhidrosis; after consideration of possible underlying etiologies, topical antiperspirants containing aluminum chloride (e.g. Certain Dri®) or aluminum chloride hexahydrate (e.g. Xerac™ AC [6.25%], Drysol® [20%]) can be applied at bedtime, and if necessary, initially preceded by oral glycopyrrolate or oxybutynin. A glycopyrronium-containing cloth can also be applied daily.
- Injection of botulinum toxin type A every ~6 months is very effective for primary cortical (emotional) hyperhidrosis (Fig. 32.5); tap water iontophoresis is less effective.

Hypohidrosis (and Anhidrosis)

- There are multiple etiologies of hypohidrosis and anhidrosis including the following:
  - A side effect of medications with anticholinergic properties (e.g. atropine, tricyclic antidepressants, glycopyrrolate)
  - Manifestation of inherited disorders, in particular ectodermal dysplasias (see Ch. 52), as well as acquired disorders such as Sjögren syndrome
  - Neurologic disorders, from tumors or infarcts of the hypothalamus, pons or medulla to peripheral neuropathies
  - Rarely, and primarily in Asians, due to acquired idiopathic generalized anhidrosis
- Increased risk of developing hyperthermia.
- Evaluation includes colorimetric testing (see Fig. 32.5) and biopsy of affected skin.

Bromhidrosis (Foul-Smelling Sweat)

- *Eccrine* variant associated with degradation of sweat by resident microflora; most commonly involves the feet.
- *Apocrine* variant associated with degradation of odiferous substances by skin flora (e.g. the breakdown of a precursor molecule into a sulfurous thioalcohol by *S. hominis*)
- The smell can be rancid (*Corynebacterium*) or sweaty (*Micrococcus*).
- Rarely, it is a sign of an inherited metabolic disorder, e.g. maple syrup urine disease.

Chromhidrosis

- Colored sweat can be *intrinsic* and due to the lipofuscin content of apocrine sweat (yellow, green, black) or *extrinsic* and due to staining of sweat by clothing or chromogenic bacteria (e.g. *Corynebacterium*) or fungi.

Sweat Retention Disorders

Miliaria

- Excessive sweating leads to maceration and blockage of eccrine ducts; can be exacerbated by occlusion, e.g. clothing, athletic equipment, prolonged bed rest.
- Classically divided into three major types: (1) *crystallina* – tiny, superficial, short-lived, clear vesicles (Fig. 32.6; see Fig. 28.3A); (2) *rubra* (prickly heat) – pruritic erythematous papulovesicles and occasionally pustules that favor the upper trunk (Fig. 32.7); and (3) *profunda* – white papules due to excessive sweating in a hot climate (rare); these three forms reflect ductal occlusion within the stratum corneum, mid-epidermis, and dermal–epidermal junction, respectively.
- If extensive, decrease in eccrine function can give rise to hyperpyrexia.
- **DDx:** miliaria rubra needs to be distinguished from folliculitis, Grover disease, neutrophilic eccrine hidradenitis, and cutaneous candidiasis.
- **Rx:** cool environment.

Fox–Fordyce Disease (Apocrine Miliaria)

- Occlusion then rupture of apocrine sweat gland ducts in the axillae > anogenital or periareolar region > periumbilical or presternal area; seen primarily in women ages 15–35 years.

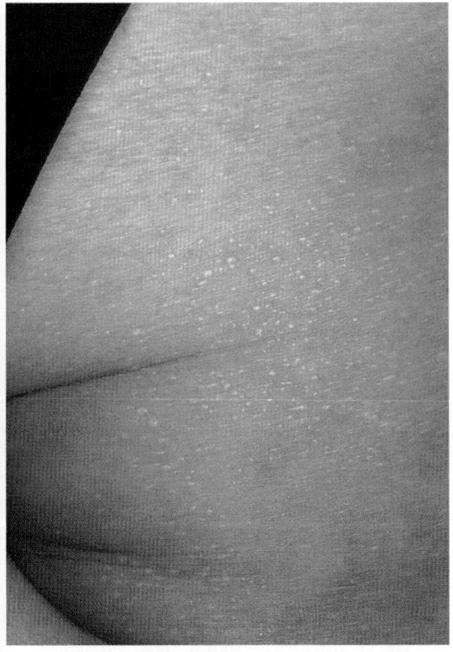

Fig. 32.6 Miliaria crystallina. Multiple small superficial vesicles with clear fluid. *Courtesy, YDRSC.*

- Multiple skin-colored papules that are follicular, dome-shaped, and often pruritic (Fig. 32.8).
- May improve with oral contraceptive pills (OCPs) or pregnancy.
- **Rx:** topical CS or calcineurin inhibitors and OCPs.

Grover Disease

- Grover disease (transient acantholytic dermatosis) is covered in Ch. 73.

Hidradenitis

Neutrophilic Eccrine Hidradenitis

- Most commonly related to administration of chemotherapy (e.g. cytarabine) and is thought to result from excretion of the drug(s) into the eccrine sweat, leading to a toxic insult.
- Erythematous papules and plaques that may have clinical overlap with Sweet syndrome (Fig. 32.9).

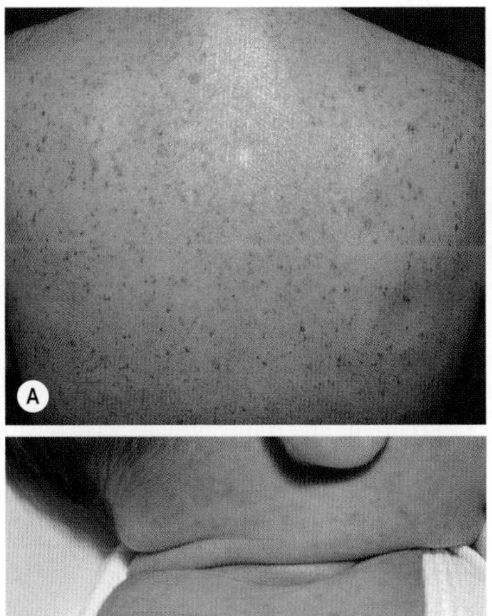

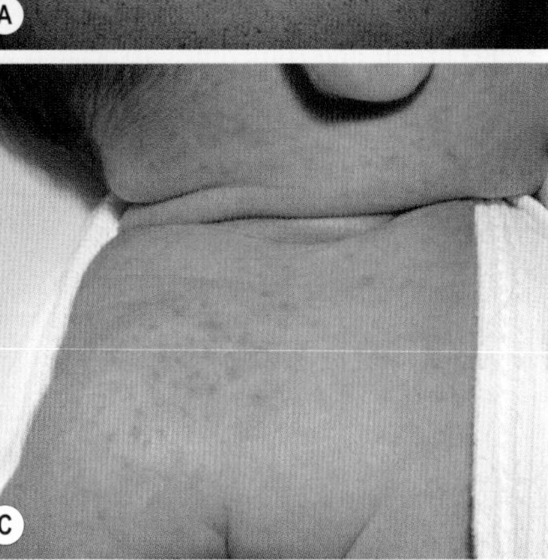

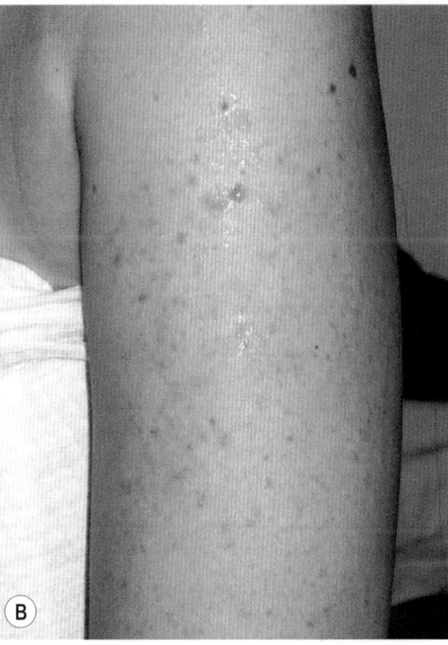

Fig. 32.7 Miliaria rubra. Multiple erythematous nonfollicular papules and papulovesicles on the back (**A**) and arm (**B**) of two adults and the upper trunk and neck of a neonate (**C**). Note that several of the lesions in the neonate have become pustular. *A, Courtesy, YDRSC; B, Courtesy, Jennifer Powers, MD; C, Courtesy, Julie V. Schaffer, MD.*

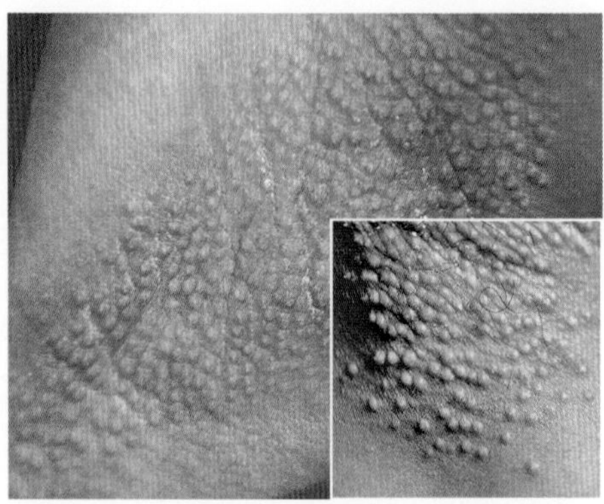

Fig. 32.8 Fox–Fordyce disease. Monomorphic skin-colored papules in the axillary vault. The dome shape is appreciated in the inset. *Courtesy, YDRSC.*

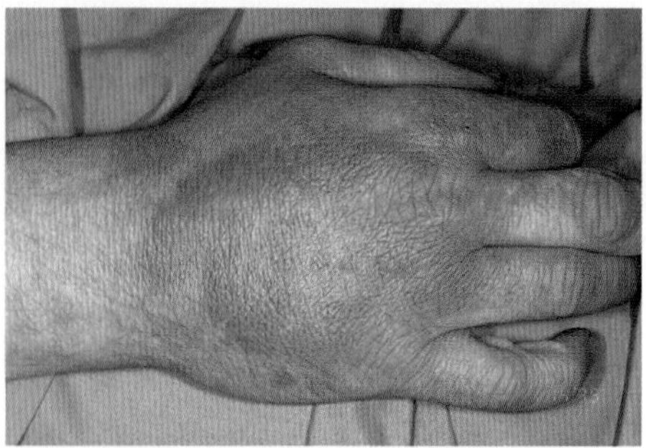

Fig. 32.9 Neutrophilic eccrine hidradenitis. Pink annular plaque on the dorsal hand. *Courtesy, Jeffrey P. Callen, MD.*

- **Rx:** spontaneously resolves but sometimes a short course of systemic CS is prescribed once an infectious process such as cellulitis or septic emboli is excluded.

Idiopathic Palmoplantar Hidradenitis

- Occurs following vigorous physical activity, primarily in healthy children.
- Thought to be precipitated by rupture of eccrine glands.
- Erythematous, tender nodules appear suddenly, most often on the soles (Fig. 32.10), and then spontaneously resolve over days to weeks.

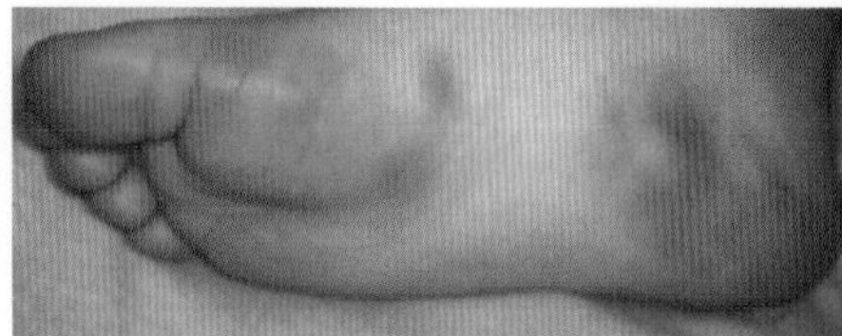

Fig. 32.10 Idiopathic palmoplantar hidradenitits. Tender erythematous papules and nodules on the plantar surface. *Courtesy, Michael L. Smith, MD.*

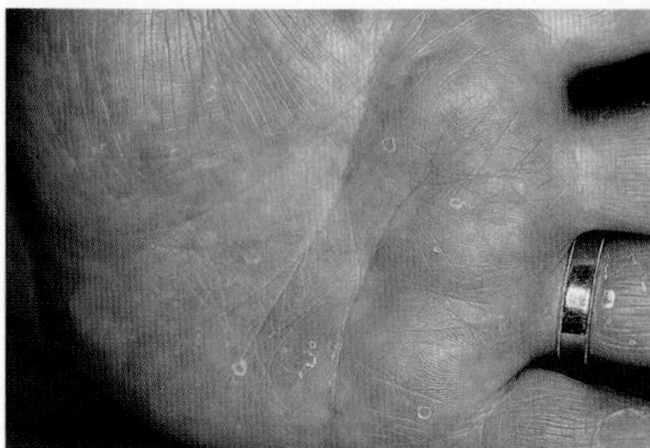

Fig. 32.11 Keratolyis exfoliativa. Small annular collarettes of scale on the palm. *Courtesy, Jean L. Bolognia, MD.*

- **DDx:** *Pseudomonas* hot-foot syndrome, pernio, symmetric lividity of the soles, delayed pressure urticaria.

Other

Keratolysis Exfoliativa

- Common disorder in healthy individuals; affects the palms >> soles.
- Multiple annular and semi-annular collarettes of white scale that usually measure <5 mm, but may be larger (Fig. 32.11); no preceding vesicles or inflammation clinically.
- Recurrent and sometimes associated with hyperhidrosis.
- **Rx:** nonspecific; effectiveness of topical agents, e.g. 12% ammonium lactate, 20% urea, is limited.

For further information see Chs 35 and 39 from *Dermatology, Fourth Edition*.

For additional online figures visit www.expertconsult.com 

Lupus Erythematosus 33

General

- A multisystem AI-CTD disorder that prominently affects the skin.
- Broadly divided into systemic lupus erythematosus (SLE), cutaneous lupus erythematosus (CLE), and drug-induced lupus erythematosus (DI-LE) (Fig. 33.1).
- CLE is further classified into *specific* and *nonspecific* skin lesions, based on the histopathologic presence (*specific*) or absence (*nonspecific*, Table 33.1) of an "interface dermatitis"; however, this is not a perfect classification scheme because some specific entities (e.g. LE tumidus, lupus panniculitis) do not demonstrate an "interface dermatitis" and other, non-lupus entities may display an "interface dermatitis" on histopathology (e.g. dermatomyositis).
- Classically, the three major forms of *specific* skin lesions are chronic cutaneous LE (CCLE), subacute cutaneous LE (SCLE), and acute cutaneous LE (ACLE), with CCLE being subdivided into four different entities (see Fig. 33.1 and Fig. 33.2).
- Cutaneous lesions may be the sole manifestation of LE or they may be associated with systemic disease (SLE), either concurrently or sequentially.
- For all types of LE: women > men; African Americans or Black Africans > other populations; onset typically post-puberty to middle age.
- Histopathologic examination of cutaneous lesions often plays an important role in establishing the diagnosis of CLE; direct immunofluorescence of lesional skin can be helpful in distinguishing CLE from other disorders, in particular lichen planus; accurate subtyping requires clinicopathologic correlation.
- Once a diagnosis of CLE is made, initial and longitudinal evaluation for systemic manifestations of SLE is recommended (Tables 33.2–33.3).
- Before making a definitive diagnosis of cutaneous lupus, it is necessary to exclude a drug-induced etiology (Tables 33.4–33.5).
- Treatment options for the various subtypes of CLE are fairly similar (Table 33.6).

Drug-Induced Lupus Erythematosus

- There are two major forms: *drug-induced SLE (DI-SLE)* and *drug-induced SCLE (DI-SCLE)*; skin lesions are indistinguishable from classic, non-drug-related LE (Table 33.4).
- Attention should be given to those medications that were initiated within weeks to 9 months prior to the onset of the eruption (see Tables 33.4–33.5).
- Usually resolves upon discontinuation of the responsible medication along with sun protection and topical therapy; occasionally a patient will require systemic therapy for persistent disease.

Cutaneous Lupus Erythematosus: Specific Lesions

Chronic Cutaneous Lupus Erythematosus (CCLE)

DISCOID LUPUS ERYTHEMATOSUS (DLE)

- Most common skin manifestation of LE; the terms CCLE and DLE are often used interchangeably, but CCLE encompasses four entities (see Fig. 33.1).
- Overall, ~5–10% of patients will go on to develop SLE; DLE can also be a presenting manifestation of SLE.
- Three clinical variants of DLE are recognized:

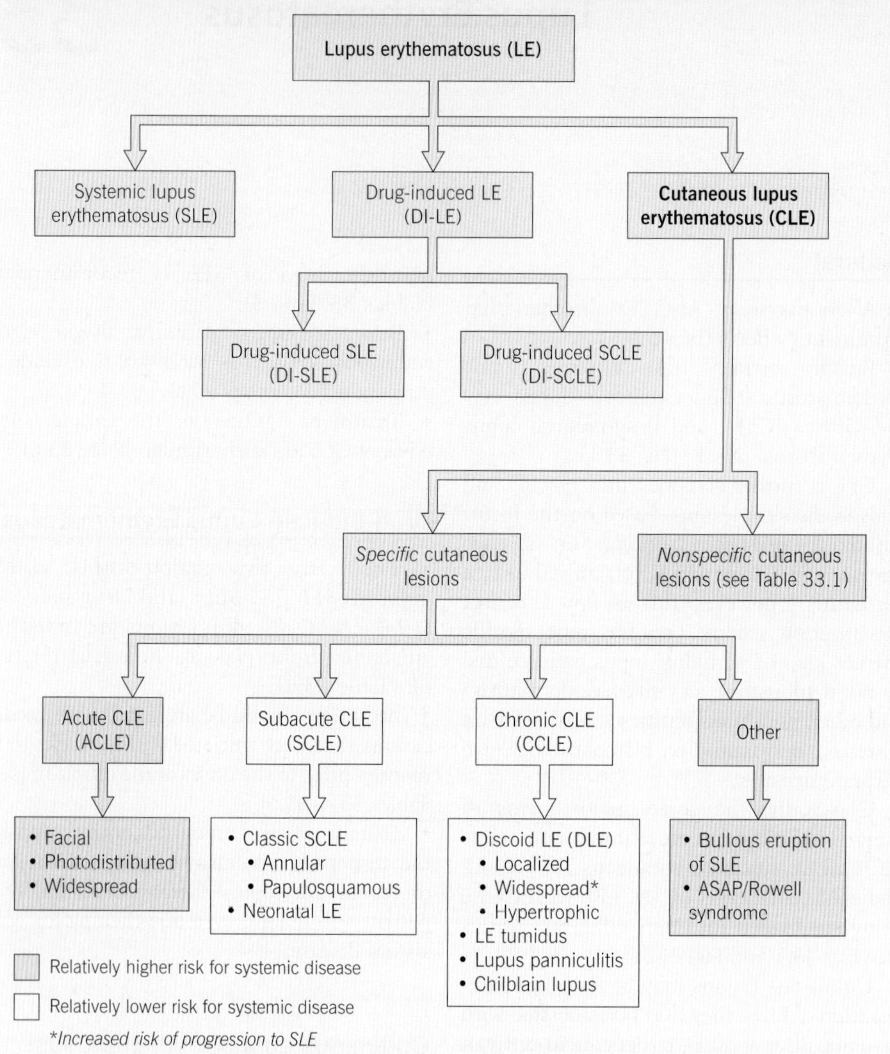

Fig. 33.1 Spectrum of lupus erythematosus (LE) and classification of cutaneous LE. The classification of cutaneous LE is based upon the classification system originally proposed by Gilliam and Sontheimer (Gilliam JN, Sontheimer RD. Distinctive cutaneous subsets in the spectrum of lupus erythematosus. J Am Acad Dermatol 1981; 4:471–5). ASAP, acute syndrome of apoptotic pan-epidermolysis.

- *Localized:* Most common; involves the head and neck region; ≤5% risk of progression to SLE
- *Widespread:* Lesions extend beyond the head and neck region to involve the extremities and/or trunk; up to 20% of patients can progress to SLE
- *Hypertrophic:* Unusual variant; favors extensor arms > face, upper trunk (Fig. 33.3H); thick scale overlying or at periphery of DLE lesions; may resemble hypertrophic actinic keratoses, SCC, hypertrophic lichen planus, or prurigo nodularis

• Occasionally can involve mucosal surfaces, palms and soles (see Fig. 33.3F,G).

• May occur in sun-exposed or sun-protected sites (e.g. scalp).

CUTANEOUS FINDINGS (NONSPECIFIC) THAT SUGGEST THE DIAGNOSIS OF SYSTEMIC LUPUS ERYTHEMATOSUS
Vascular lesions
• Vasculitis – Urticarial vasculitis – Small vessel vasculitis – Polyarteritis nodosa-like lesions • Vasculopathy – Raynaud phenomenon – Livedo reticularis – Nailfold telangiectasias and erythema – Palmar erythema – Livedoid vasculopathy • Cutaneous signs of antiphospholipid syndrome – Livedo reticularis (more widespread and persistent) – Multiple subungual splinter hemorrhages – Digital gangrene and cutaneous necrosis – Superficial thrombophlebitis – Degos-like lesions – Atrophie blanche-like lesions – Anetoderma
Other
• Alopecia – "Lupus hair," diffuse and nonscarring – Telogen effluvium • Papulonodular mucinosis • Sweet syndrome–like neutrophilic dermatosis

Table 33.1 Cutaneous findings (nonspecific) that suggest the diagnosis of systemic lupus erythematosus. These cutaneous lesions are associated with LE but are not specific to LE itself. The presence of nonspecific LE skin lesions raises the possibility of SLE and may signify more significant internal disease. The presence of these nonspecific lesions should prompt an evaluation for SLE (see Tables 33.2 and 33.3).

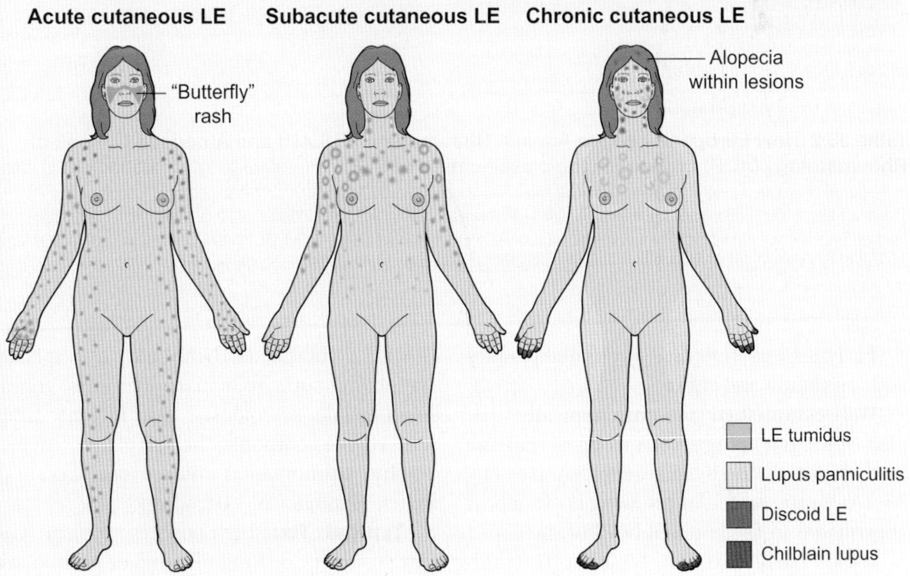

Fig. 33.2 Characteristic sites of involvement for the three major forms of cutaneous lupus erythematosus (LE).

NEW EULAR/ACR CRITERIA FOR THE CLASSIFICATION OF SLE

Clinical domains	Points
Constitutional domain	
Fever	2
Cutaneous domain	
Non-scarring alopecia	2
Oral ulcers	2
Subacute cutaneous or discoid lupus	4
Acute cutaneous lupus	6
Arthritis domain	
Synovitis in at least two joints or tenderness in at least two joints, and at least 30 min of morning stiffness	6
Neurologic domain	
Delirium	2
Psychosis	3
Seizure	5
Serositis domain	
Pleural or pericardial effusion	5
Acute pericarditis	6
Hematologic domain	
Leukopenia	3
Thrombocytopenia	4
Autoimmune hemolysis	4
Renal domain	
Proteinuria >0.5 gm/24 hr	4
Class II or V lupus nephritis	8
Class III or IV lupus nephritis	**10**

Immunologic domains	Points
Antiphospholipid antibody domain	
Anticardiolipin IgG >40 GPL or anti β2GP1 IgG >40 units or lupus anticoagulant	2
Complement proteins domain	
Low C3 or low C4	3
Low C3 and low C4	4
Highly specific antibodies domain	
Anti-dsDNA antibody	6
Anti-Smith antibody	6

All patients classified as having SLE must have a serum titer of antinuclear antibody of at least 1:80 on human epithelial-2 positive cells or an equivalent positive test. In addition, a patient must tally at least 10 points from these criteria. A criterion is not counted if it has a more likely explanation than SLE. Occurrence of the criterion only once is sufficient to tally the relevant points, and the time when a patient is positive for one criterion need not overlap with the time when the patient is positive for other criteria. SLE classification requires points from at least one clinical domain, and *if a patient is positive for more than one criterion in a domain, only the criterion with the highest point value counts.*

Please refer to online Tables 33.2 and 33.3 for 1) The 1997 Update of the 1982 American College of Rheumatology revised criteria for classification of systemic lupus erythematosus and 2) The 2012 Systemic Lupus International Collaborating Clinics classification criteria for SLE, respectively.

Table 33.2 New European League Against Rheumatism (EULAR) and American College of Rheumatology (ACR) criteria for the classification of SLE. GPL refers to IgG Phospholipid Units; anti–β2GP1, anti–β2–glycoprotein 1; dsDNA, double-stranded DNA. *From Aringer M, Costenbader K, Daikh D, et al. 2019 European League Against Rheumatism/American College of Rheumatology classification criteria for systemic lupus erythematosus. Arthritis Rheumatol 2019; 71(9):1400–12. Copyright © 2019 American College of Rheumatology. Adapted with permission of John Wiley & Sons Inc.*

- **Early lesions:** inflamed, indurated plaques with erythema and scale.
- **Well-established lesions:** typically display follicular plugging, atrophy, scarring (and alopecia), and dyspigmentation (see Fig. 33.3A–E); the follicular plugging is often best appreciated in the conchal bowl of the ear.
- **DDx: Early lesions:** lymphocytic infiltrate of Jessner, polymorphic light eruption (PMLE), cutaneous lymphoid hyperplasia, lymphoma cutis, follicular mucinosis, granuloma faciale, sarcoidosis; **Late lesions:** tinea (e.g. capitis, corporis), lichen planus (hypertrophic, palmoplantar and mucosal variants), lichen planopilaris, sarcoidosis.
- **Typical Rx:** high-potency topical CS, intralesional CS (5 mg/ml), and/or antimalarials (see Table 33.6).

EVALUATION FOR SYSTEMIC LUPUS ERYTHEMATOSUS
History and review of systems
Physical examination
• Specific cutaneous lesions (see Fig. 33.1) • Nonspecific cutaneous lesions (see Table 33.1) • Lymphadenopathy, arthritis, friction rubs
Laboratory tests
• ANA with profile (anti-dsDNA, -Sm) • Urinalysis • CBC with differential, platelet count • Chemistries (BUN, Cr) and LFTs • ESR, CRP • Complement levels (C3, C4) • Antiphospholipid antibodies

Table 33.3 Evaluation for systemic lupus erythematosus. ds, double-stranded; Sm, Smith.

CLASSIC DISTINCTIONS BETWEEN DRUG-INDUCED SUBACUTE CUTANEOUS LUPUS ERYTHEMATOSUS (DI-SCLE) AND DRUG-INDUCED SYSTEMIC LUPUS ERYTHEMATOSUS (DI-SLE)				
Disease	**Most commonly associated medications**	**Cutaneous findings**	**Systemic findings**	**Associated autoantibodies**
DI-SCLE	• See Table 33.5	• Identical to SCLE	• **Typically no systemic symptoms** • Occasionally arthralgias	• Anti-SSA/Ro • Anti-SSB/La
DI-SLE	• TNF inhibitors*, minocycline, hydralazine, procainamide, isoniazid, quinidine, methyldopa, chlorpromazine, interferons	• **Typically no skin findings** • Occasionally malar or photodistributed erythema	• Constitutional symptoms such as fever, weight loss, myalgia • Serositis (e.g. arthritis, pericarditis, pleuritis)	• Anti-histone** • Anti-dsDNA (reported with TNF inhibitors)

**TNF inhibitors have been associated with both DI-SCLE and DI-SLE (as well as drug-induced discoid lupus erythematosus).*
***Anti-histone antibodies are not specific for DI-SLE as they are commonly found in patients with classic SLE, as well as in other autoimmune connective tissue diseases.*

Table 33.4 Classic distinctions between drug-induced SCLE (DI-SCLE) and drug-induced SLE (DI-SLE).

LUPUS ERYTHEMATOSUS (LE) TUMIDUS

- LE tumidus is an entity that overlaps with lymphocytic infiltrate of Jessner and reticular erythematous mucinosis (REM); there is debate as to whether it is a distinct entity or whether it should be considered a specific type of lupus.
- Photo-induced, but often this is not appreciated because of the delay of 1–2 weeks between UVR exposure and onset of the eruption.
- Most common on the face and upper trunk; reportedly <1% of patients eventually develop SLE.
- Lesions characterized by erythema, induration, and often central clearing (Fig. 33.4); scale, follicular plugging, scarring, and atrophy are absent.
- **DDx:** lymphocytic infiltrate of Jessner, PMLE, REM (chest lesions), papulonodular mucinosis, cutaneous lymphoid hyperplasia.

MEDICATIONS ASSOCIATED WITH DRUG-INDUCED SUBACUTE CUTANEOUS LUPUS ERYTHEMATOSUS (DI-SCLE)
More common/higher risk*
Terbinafine **Thiazide diuretics** (e.g. hydrochlorothiazide) TNF inhibitors** Proton pump inhibitors (e.g. lansoprazole, pantoprazole, omeprazole, esomeprazole**) Calcium channel blockers (e.g. diltiazem, nifedipine, verapamil) Anti-epileptics (e.g. carbamazepine, phenytoin) Taxanes (e.g. docetaxel, paclitaxel) Thrombocyte inhibitors (e.g. ticlopidine) Anti-PD1 and anti-PD-L1 immunotherapy (nivolumab, pembrolizumab)
Less common*
ACE inhibitors (e.g. captopril, enalapril, lisinopril) β-blockers Doxorubicin Interferon-α and -β Leflunomide Ranitidine HMG-CoA reductase inhibitors ("statins") Capecitabine**
**Medications are classified as being more common or having a higher risk if there were >10 cases reported in the literature as of 2020 or the relative risk was ≥2.0. Medications are classified as being less common if there have been 3–10 cases reported and the relative risk was <2.0.* ***Have also been associated with drug-induced discoid lupus erythematosus as well as drug-induced SLE (TNF inhibitors).*

Table 33.5 Medications associated with drug-induced subacute cutaneous lupus erythematosus (DI-SCLE). Most common drugs are in bold. ACE, angiotensin converting enzyme.

LUPUS PANNICULITIS (SEE CH. 83)

- Initially characterized by intense inflammation in the subcutaneous fat; eventuates into lipoatrophy.
- The most common sites of involvement are the face, upper outer arms, upper trunk, breasts, buttocks, and thighs, with the majority representing sites of abundant fat (Fig. 33.5).
- Sometimes overlying DLE lesions are seen (termed "lupus profundus").

CHILBLAIN LUPUS (SLE PERNIO)

- Typically presents with erythematous to dusky purple papulonodules and plaques on the toes, fingers > nose, elbows, knees, and lower legs (Fig. 33.6).
- Lesions are triggered or exacerbated by cold temperatures, often in combination with damp conditions.
- With time, some lesions may progress to resemble DLE both clinically and histopathologically.
- **DDx:** idiopathic chilblains (following exclusion of SLE), familial chilblain lupus (*TREX1* or *SAMHD1* mutations), other cold-induced syndromes (see Ch. 74).
- Up to 20% of patients may go on to develop SLE.

Subacute Cutaneous Lupus Erythematosus (SCLE)

- Characterized by non-scarring, annular, or papulosquamous eruptions in photodistributed sites (Fig. 33.7).
- Favors the upper trunk and upper outer arms > lateral neck, forearms, hands (see Fig. 33.7).
- Interestingly, often spares the mid-face
- Two common clinical presentations are recognized:
  - *Annular*: raised erythematous borders with central clearing (see Fig. 33.7B, C)
  - *Papulosquamous*: psoriasiform or eczematous appearance (see Fig. 33.7A)
- Long-term residual changes include dyspigmentation (most often hypo- to depigmentation).
- Approximately 10–15% of patients may over time develop SLE.

SUGGESTED THERAPIES FOR CUTANEOUS LUPUS ERYTHEMATOSUS (CLE)
General measures for all patients
• Sun protective measures* • Avoid potentially photosensitizing medications • Stop smoking • Oral vitamin D_3 supplementation, guided by serum vitamin D_3 levels
Localized treatment options
• Topical and intralesional CS • Topical calcineurin inhibitors (facial lesions) • Topical retinoids (perhaps helpful in hypertrophic DLE) • Topical imiquimod 5% (anecdotal)
Systemic treatment options
First-line (antimalarials**) • Hydroxychloroquine (*Adult*: 200 mg daily – twice daily, up to 5.0 mg/kg actual body weight/day or 400 mg/day (whichever is lower); *Children*: ≤5.0 mg/kg actual body weight/day up to a maximum of 400 mg/day) • Chloroquine (*Adult*: 125–250 mg/day, up to 2.3 mg/kg actual body weight/day; *Children*: ≤2.3 mg/kg actual body weight/day) • Quinacrine*** (in case of retinopathy) (*Adult* and *Children*: 100 mg/day) **Second-line** (these agents may be combined with antimalarials or used alone) • Methotrexate (7.5–25 mg/week, orally, IM, SC) • Mycophenolate mofetil (1000–2000 mg/day) • Oral retinoids† (e.g. acitretin, isotretinoin) • Dapsone‡ (primarily for bullous eruption of SLE; 50–150 mg/day) • Thalidomide† (50–100 mg/day for clearing and, if necessary, 25–50 mg/day – twice weekly for maintenance) • Sulfasalazine • Lenalidomide **Third-line** (refractory cases) • Azathioprine • IVIg (costly) • Belimumab (not as effective in African-Americans) • Rituximab (best for SLE with severe active CLE) **Life-threatening or severe inflammatory cutaneous disease** (e.g. ASAP/Rowell syndrome) • Systemic CS
**Broad-spectrum sunscreen, sun avoidance, sun-protective clothing.* ***Delayed onset of action (4–8 weeks); earlier institution may stave off progression of CLE to SLE; recommended monitoring includes baseline and every 6 month CBC, LFTs, BUN/Cr; and baseline/serial eye examinations.* ****Quinacrine can be added, as combination therapy, to either hydroxychloroquine or chloroquine.* *†Risk of teratogenicity; best if used concurrently with antimalarials, as the latter may reduce risk of thrombosis.* *‡Exclude glucose-6-phosphate dehydrogenase deficiency.*

Table 33.6 Suggested therapies for cutaneous lupus erythematosus (CLE). All patients should be counseled about daily sun protection, as both UVA and UVB can trigger flares of CLE and may even lead to exacerbations of systemic symptoms. Topical therapy is indicated in local disease and as an adjunct to systemic therapy in severe and widespread CLE. Systemic therapy is indicated when skin lesions are widespread, disfiguring, scarring, or refractory to topical agents, or when extracutaneous manifestations are present, e.g. arthritis. ASAP, acute syndrome of apoptotic pan-epidermolysis; DLE, discoid lupus erythematosus.

• Depending on the laboratory, ~70% of patients have associated anti-SSA/Ro antibodies.

• Roughly 50% of patients fulfill ≥4 American College of Rheumatology (ACR) criteria for SLE (see Table 33.2), but they rarely develop serious systemic involvement; arthralgias most common.

•**DDx: Annular variant:** dermatophytosis, granuloma annulare, erythema annulare centrifugum, or other annular erythemas (see Ch. 15);

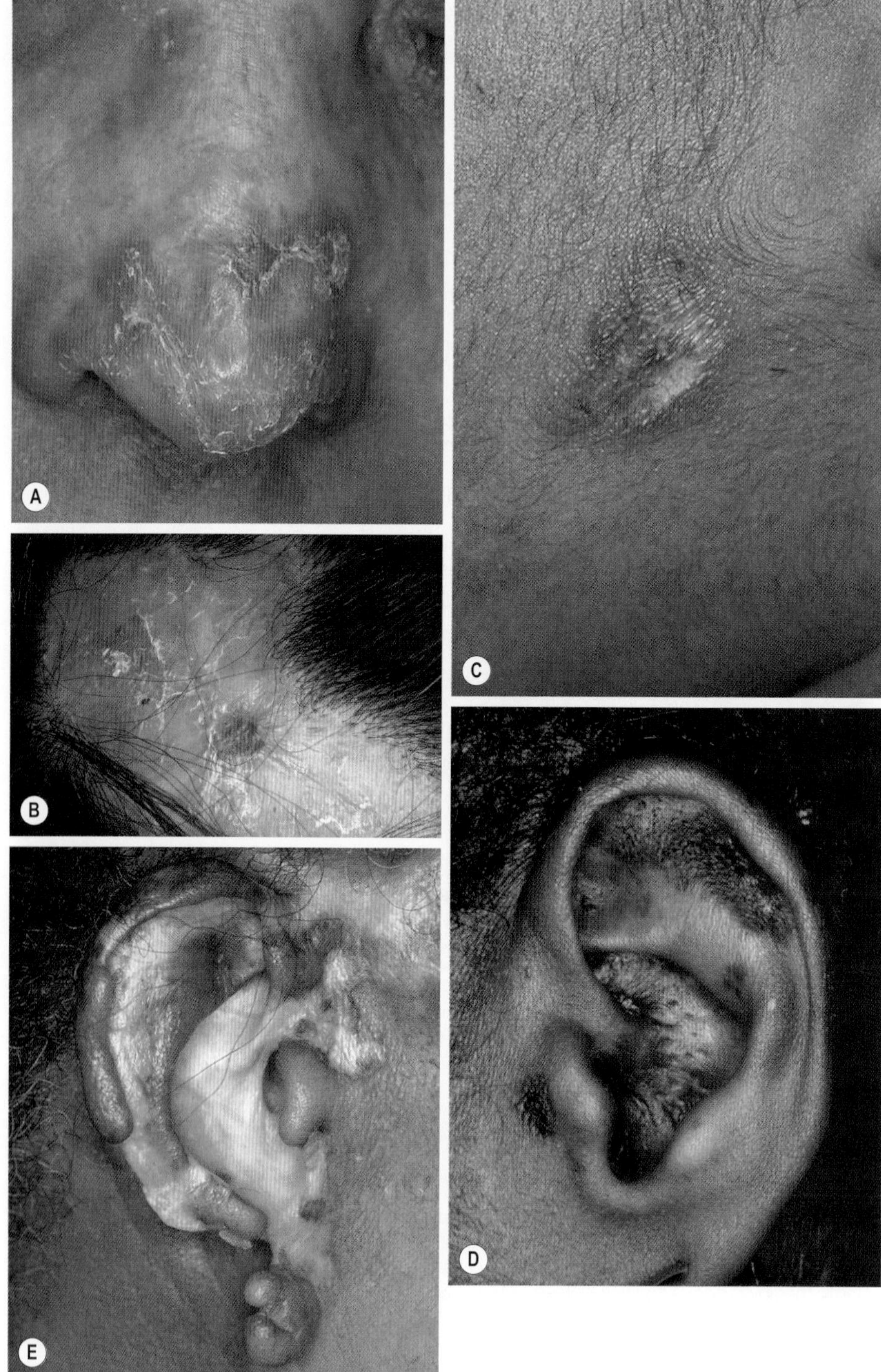

Fig. 33.3 Various presentations of discoid lesions of lupus erythematosus (DLE). Lesions, which favor the head and neck region may show erythema, scaling, atrophy, and dyspigmentation in addition to scarring (and alopecia) **(A–D).** The scarring process may be destructive **(E)**. *Continued*

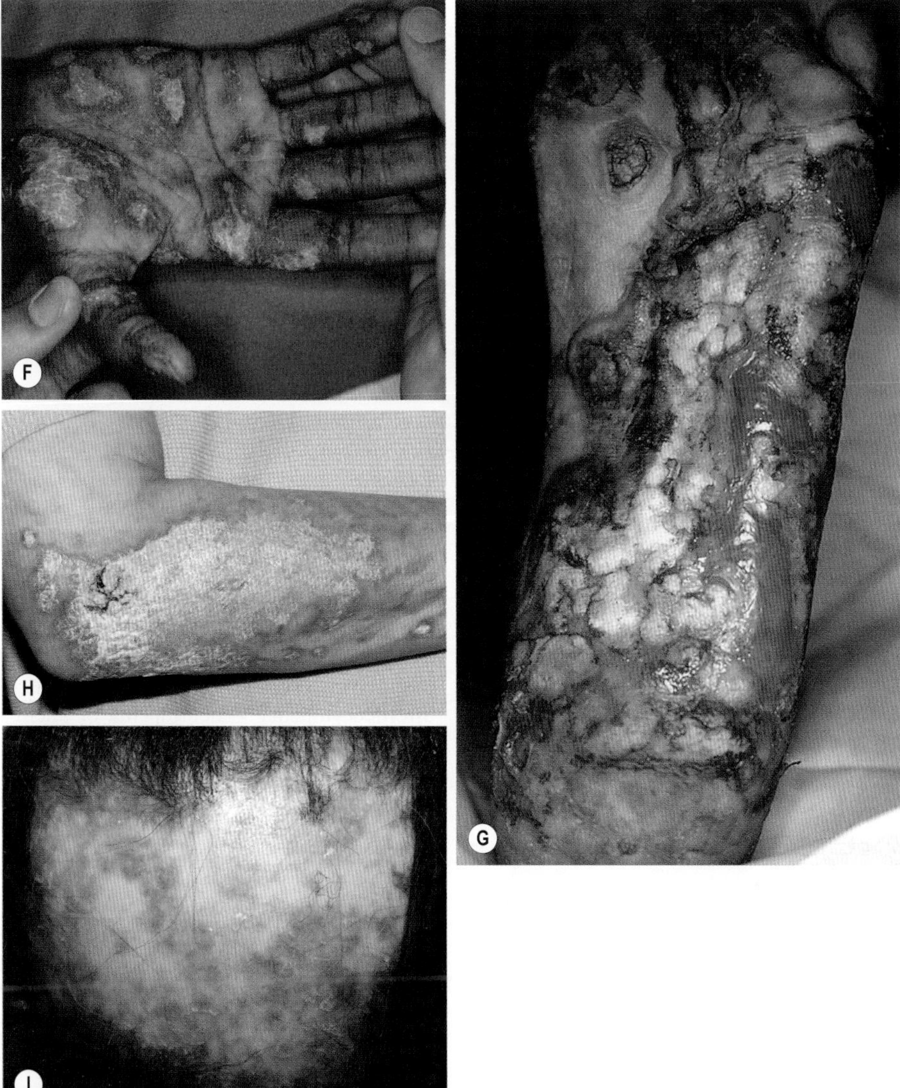

Fig. 33.3 *Continued* **Various presentations of discoid lesions of lupus erythematosus (DLE).** Less common sites include the palms and soles, where lesions can be keratotic or ulcerative **(F, G),** as seen in lichen planus. The latter patient had systemic lupus erythematosus and responded well to isotretinoin. **H** Occasionally, hypertrophic lesions develop within significant hyperkeratosis. **I** Discoid lupus lesions with dyspigmentation and scarring alopecia. Hypopigmentation often develops centrally with areas of hyperpigmentation at the periphery. Note the plugging of follicular openings at 12 o'clock. *A, B, D–G, Courtesy, YDRSC; C, I, Courtesy, Kalman Watsky, MD; H, Courtesy, Julie V. Schaffer, MD.*

papulosquamous variant: photo-lichenoid drug reaction (e.g. HCTZ, antimalarials), psoriasis, photo-exacerbated eczema, GVHD, lichen planus, PMLE, pemphigus foliaceus.

- Before a diagnosis of classic SCLE can be made, exclude the possibility of DI-SCLE (see Table 33.4).

NEONATAL LUPUS ERYTHEMATOSUS (NLE)

- Occurs in infants whose mothers have anti-SSA/Ro autoantibodies that are passively transferred to the fetus.
- These infants primarily have anti-SSA/Ro antibodies (>98%), but they may also have anti-SSB/La or anti-U1RNP antibodies.

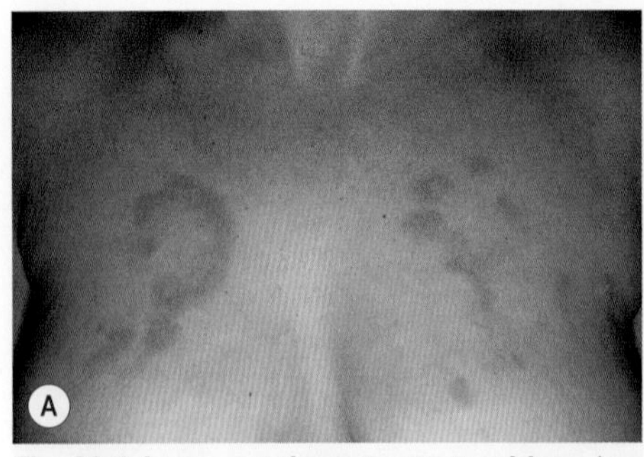

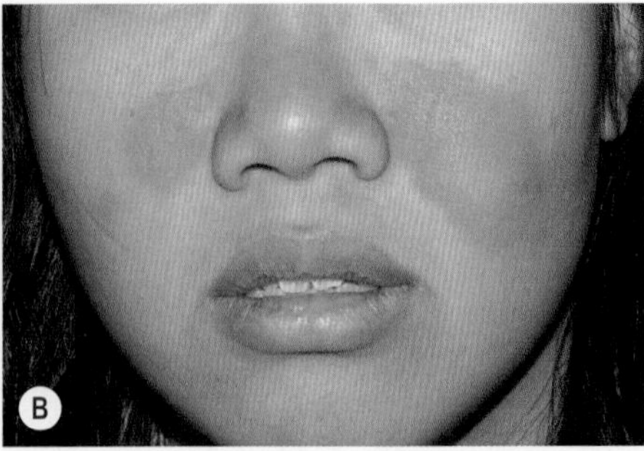

Fig. 33.4 Lupus erythematosus tumidus. Annular pink plaques on the chest **(A)** and pink-violet plaques on the face **(B).** None of the lesions have epidermal change. *A, Courtesy, YDRSC; B, Courtesy, Julie V. Schaffer, MD.*

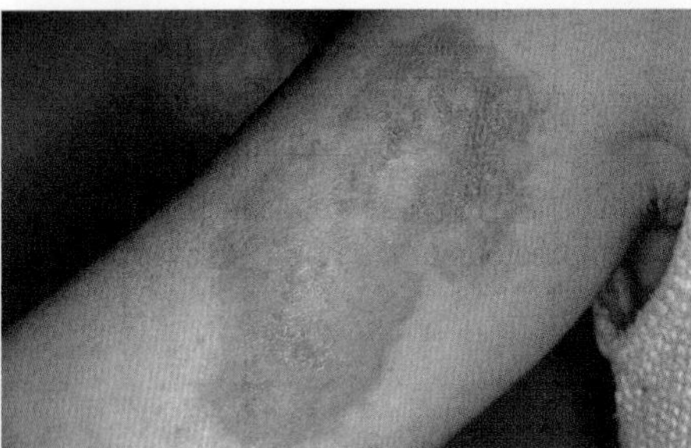

Fig. 33.5 Lupus panniculitis. Erythematous plaque on the upper arm. The lesions may resolve with lipoatrophy. *Courtesy, YDRSC.*

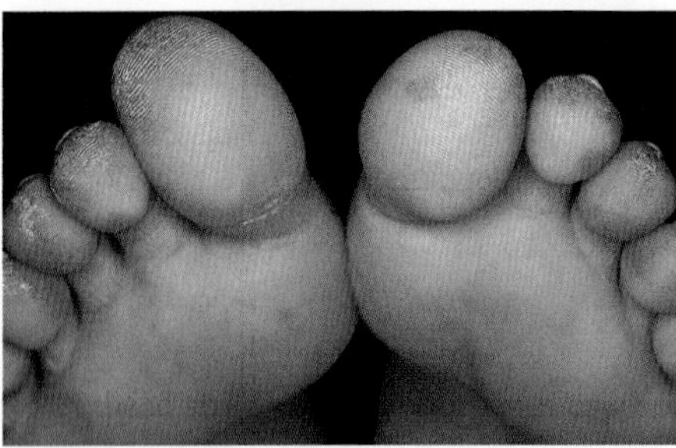

Fig. 33.6 Chilblain lupus. Violaceous plaques, some with scale, on toes. If there is a family history of this disorder, the possibility of mutations in *TREX1*, which encodes a DNA exonuclease, or *SAMHD1*, which encodes a host restriction nuclease that plays a role in the innate immune response, can be considered. *Courtesy, YDRSC.*

- Approximately 1–5% of mothers with anti-SSA/Ro antibodies will have infants with NLE, with risk increasing to 10–25% with subsequent pregnancies.
- Cutaneous lesions are similar to adult SCLE but favor the face and periorbital areas and may be atrophic (Fig. 33.8).
- Photosensitivity is common, but sun exposure is not necessary for lesion formation.
- New lesions typically cease to develop by 6–9 months of age, i.e. once the antibodies are cleared; however, there may be residual changes such as dyspigmentation and telangiectasias.
- The most common internal manifestations are: (1) congenital heart block (± associated cardiomyopathy); (2) hepatobiliary disease; (3) thrombocytopenia > neutropenia or anemia; (4) macrocephaly or skeletal dysplasia.
- Heart block, if it is going to occur, is almost always present at birth and a pacemaker is often required.
- If skin signs of NLE are present, an evaluation, including physical examination, ECG, echocardiogram, CBC, and LFTs is indicated; the latter laboratory tests should be repeated periodically over the first 6 months of life.

Acute Cutaneous Lupus Erythematosus (ACLE)

- The CLE variant most closely associated with SLE and if diagnosed the patient should be evaluated for internal disease.
- Three clinical presentations are recognized:
  - *Facial (malar)*: the classic "butterfly" eruption, presenting with symmetric erythematous patches or more infiltrated plaques over the nasal bridge and cheeks; spares nasolabial folds (Fig. 33.9A–C)
  - *Photodistributed*: exanthematous to urticarial eruption involving primarily UV-exposed skin, e.g. upper chest, extensor arms (Fig. 33.9D), dorsal hands (with sparing of the knuckles)
  - *Widespread*: extends beyond photodistributed sites

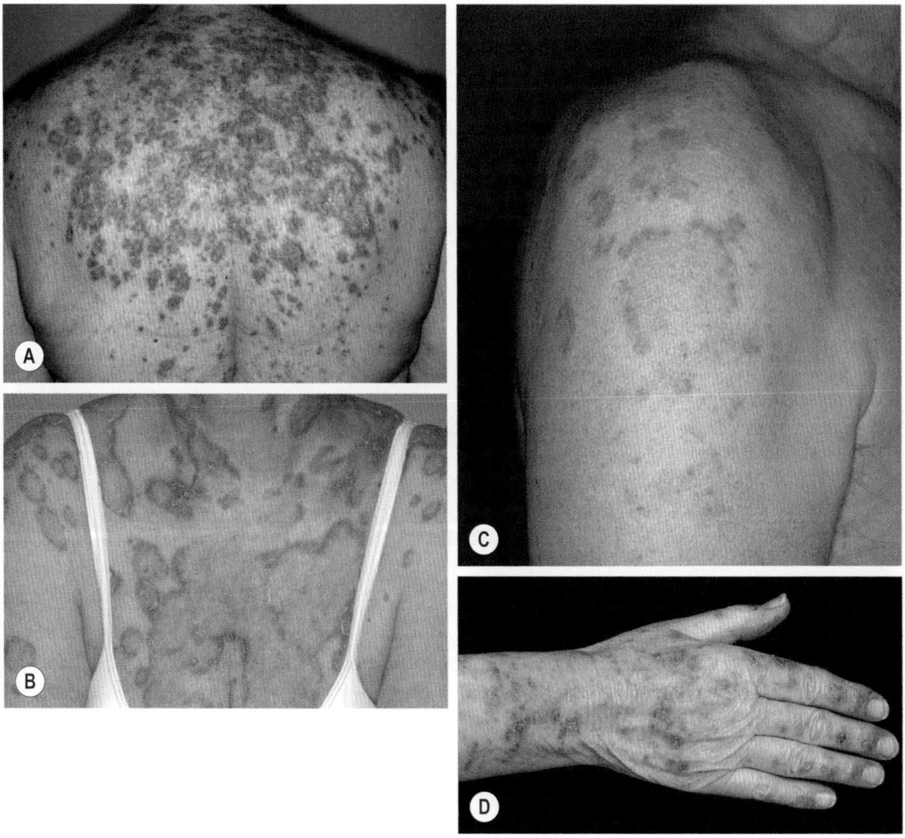

Fig. 33.7 Subacute cutaneous lupus erythematosus (SCLE). A Numerous erythematous annular plaques on the back, some of which have associated white scale. **B** Lesions are most commonly seen on the upper trunk and sun-exposed aspects of the upper extremities. The margins of the annular lesions may have scale-crust (**B**) or be composed of multiple papules (**C**). **D** Note the peripheral scale and relative sparing of the proximal interphalangeal joints. *A, Courtesy, Kathryn Schwarzenberger, MD; B, Courtesy, Lela Lee, MD and Victoria Werth, MD; C, Courtesy, YDRSC; D, Courtesy, Lorenzo Cerroni, MD.*

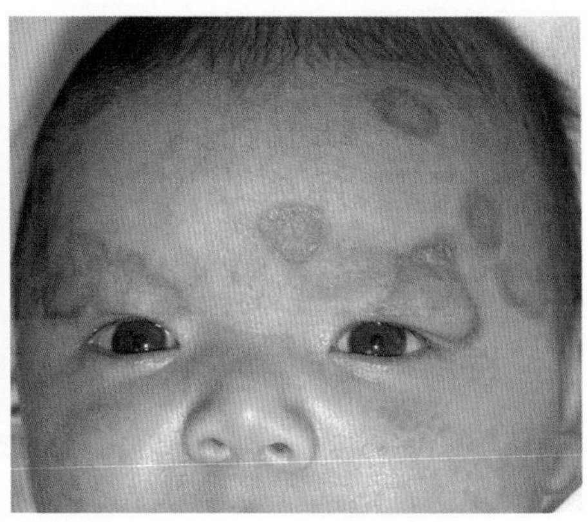

Fig. 33.8 Neonatal lupus erythematosus (NLE). Annular erythematous plaques on the forehead and scalp. Note the resemblance to the annular form of subacute cutaneous lupus erythematosus. *Courtesy, Julie V. Schaffer, MD.*

- A particular patient's ACLE clinical presentation will often repeat itself with subsequent flares, representing a "signature" pattern.
- Lesions typically respond to systemic CS and resolve without scarring; may leave residual dyspigmentation.
- **DDx: Facial:** seborrheic dermatitis, rosacea, sunburn, perioral dermatitis, tinea faciei, cellulitis/erysipelas, contact dermatitis; **Photodistributed**: drug-induced photosensitivity, dermatomyositis; **Widespread**: exanthem (viral or drug-induced).

Other

BULLOUS ERUPTION OF SLE

- Clinically presents as blisters (ranging from tiny vesicles to large tense bullae) on an erythematous base, typically involving the

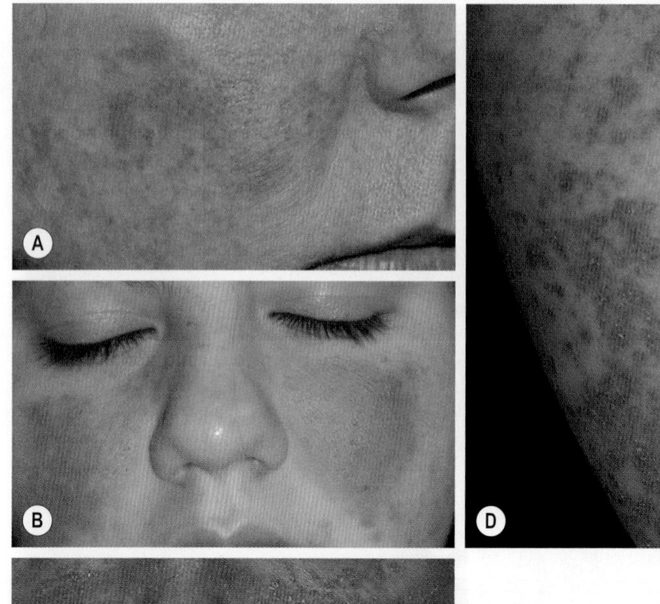

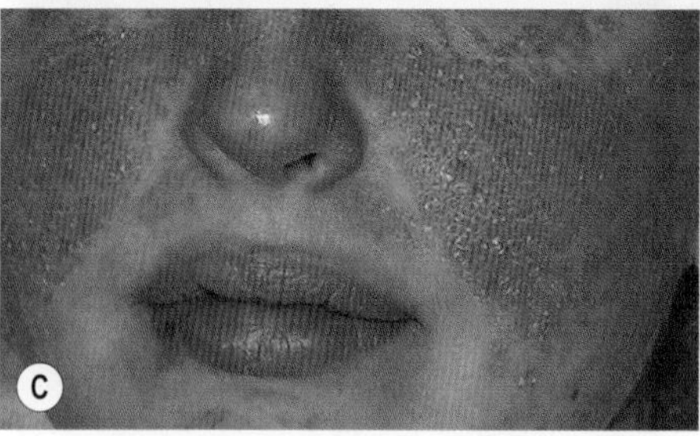

Fig. 33.9 Acute cutaneous lupus erythematosus (ACLE). The facial erythema, often referred to as a "butterfly rash," may be variable **(A),** edematous **(B),** or have associated scale **(C).** The presence of small erosions can aid in the clinical differential diagnosis. This patient **(D)** had ACLE lesions on the arms as well as the face. *A, Courtesy, Kalman Watsky, MD; B–D, Courtesy, Lela Lee, MD.*

face, neck, upper trunk, proximal extremities, and mucosal surfaces; seen in patients with underlying SLE (Fig. 33.10).

- Autoantibodies against type VII collagen are present.
- **DDx: Clinical:** autoimmune blistering diseases, contact dermatitis, acute syndrome of apoptotic pan-epidermolysis (ASAP); **Histopathological**: dermatitis herpetiformis.

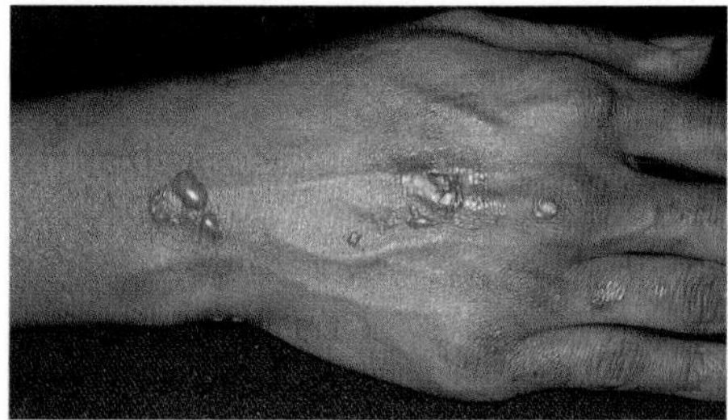

Fig. 33.10 Bullous eruption of systemic lupus erythematosus. Vesicles and bullae due to autoantibodies against type VII collagen can develop in patients with systemic disease. *Courtesy, YDRSC.*

ACUTE SYNDROME OF APOPTOTIC PAN-EPIDERMOLYSIS (ASAP)/ROWELL SYNDROME

- The term *ASAP* embraces various entities in which there is acute and widespread epidermal cleavage resulting from hyperacute apoptotic injury of the epidermis from various causes (e.g. drug-induced toxic epidermal necrolysis [TEN], TEN-like GVHD, and TEN-like ACLE).
- Rowell syndrome and TEN-like ACLE are thought to occur along a spectrum of ASAP, with the former representing a less severe erythema multiforme major-like presentation in the setting of lupus and the latter a potentially

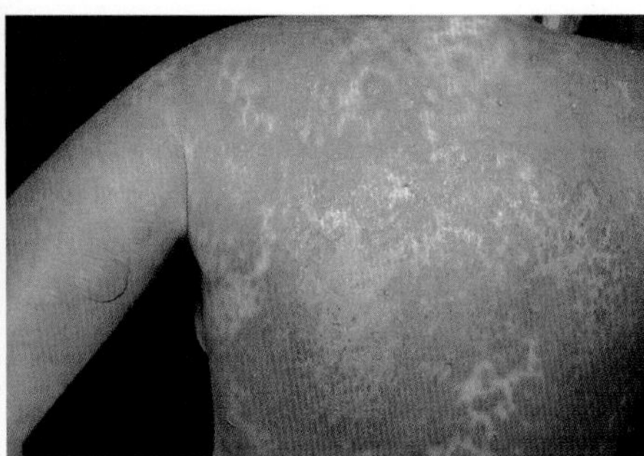

Fig. 33.11 Acute syndrome of apoptotic pan-epidermolysis (ASAP). One form of ASAP is a potentially life-threatening TEN-like presentation in the setting of ACLE. *Courtesy, YDRSC.*

life-threatening TEN-like presentation in the setting of ACLE (Fig. 33.11).
- This spectrum of cutaneous findings may occur *de novo* or in the setting of rebound ACLE or SCLE; significant internal organ involvement (e.g. kidney and CNS) is common.

Cutaneous Lupus Erythematosus: Nonspecific Lesions

- A variety of cutaneous lesions not entirely specific to LE may be seen, signaling not only internal organ involvement (SLE) but also increased systemic disease activity (see Table 33.1).

VASCULAR LESIONS AND THE ANTIPHOSPHOLIPID SYNDROME (APS)

- Vascular lesions and APS are common in patients with LE, especially those with SLE (see Table 33.1).
- Approximately one-third of APS cases occur in the setting of lupus (see Ch. 18); compared to primary APS, these patients are more likely to have arthritis, livedo reticularis (LR), and cytopenias.
- Patients with LE and APS may benefit from antimalarial therapy.

Systemic Lupus Erythematosus (SLE)

- The organ systems most commonly involved are the joints, skin, hematologic, lungs, kidneys, and CNS, which in large part are reflected in the ACR criteria for SLE diagnosis (see Table 33.2); however, this list is not exhaustive and clinical judgment is required.
- In individual patients it is often only one or a few organs that are significantly affected.
- ACLE is the specific CLE variant most closely associated with SLE, but patients with any type of CLE may develop internal involvement (SLE).
- Indicators of an increased risk for SLE in patients presenting with CLE include fever, weight loss, fatigue, myalgia, lymphadenopathy, and *nonspecific* skin findings (see Table 33.1).
- The basic evaluation for SLE is highlighted in Table 33.3, and it is important to exclude drug-induced SLE (see Table 33.4).
- A negative ANA is helpful because it is highly unlikely that a patient with a negative ANA has SLE.
- A positive ANA is less helpful, as it may occur in normal individuals (usually at low titers) and in patients with CLE.
- Specific antibodies to SLE include dsDNA and Sm.

For further information see Ch. 41 from *Dermatology, Fourth Edition*.

For additional online figures and tables visit www.expertconsult.com 

34 Dermatomyositis

Dermatomyositis is an autoimmune connective tissue disease (AI-CTD) that may overlap with other AI-CTDs. It may be triggered by outside factors, most commonly malignancy (e.g. breast cancer, ovarian cancer) and occasionally drugs (e.g. "statins," hydroxyurea, checkpoint inhibitors) or rarely infectious agents (e.g. picornavirus).

- Bimodal age distribution (juvenile – mean 8 years of age; adult – mean 52 years of age); female predominance.
- Often clinical and laboratory evidence of proximal inflammatory myopathy (the term polymyositis is used when the disease affects only muscles; Table 34.1); patients may report difficulty combing hair or rising from a sitting position.
- Pathogeneses of dermatomyositis and polymyositis are different (humoral immunity versus cell-mediated immunity, respectively).
- May affect the skin only (amyopathic dermatomyositis, formerly termed dermatomyositis sine myositis; see Table 34.1); Fig. 34.1 outlines an approach to the diagnosis of this form of dermatomyositis.

REVISED CLASSIFICATION SYSTEM FOR THE IDIOPATHIC INFLAMMATORY DERMATOMYOPATHIES
This classification scheme recognizes, with equal weighting, the cutaneous and muscle manifestations of this group of disorders.
Dermatomyositis (DM)
Adult-onset
Classic DM
Classic DM with malignancy*
Classic DM as part of an overlapping connective tissue disorder**
Clinically amyopathic DM†
Amyopathic DM
Hypomyopathic DM
Juvenile-onset
Classic DM
Clinically amyopathic DM†
Amyopathic DM
Hypomyopathic DM
Polymyositis
Isolated polymyositis
Polymyositis as part of an overlapping connective tissue disorder
Inclusion body myositis
*In up to 25% of adults; ovarian, colon, breast, lung, gastric, pancreatic carcinomas (nasopharyngeal in Southeast Asian populations), and lymphoma; risk decreases to normal after 2–5 years.
**Systemic sclerosis > SLE, Sjögren syndrome, rheumatoid arthritis.
†Provisional = cutaneous findings without muscle weakness and with normal muscle enzymes for >6 months; confirmed = for 24 months.

Table 34.1 Revised classification system for the idiopathic inflammatory dermatomyopathies. *Adapted from Sontheimer RD. Would a new name hasten the acceptance of amyopathic dermatomyositis (dermatomyositis sine myositis) as a distinctive subset within the idiopathic inflammatory dermatomyopathies spectrum of clinical illness? J Am Acad Dermatol 2002;46:626–36.*

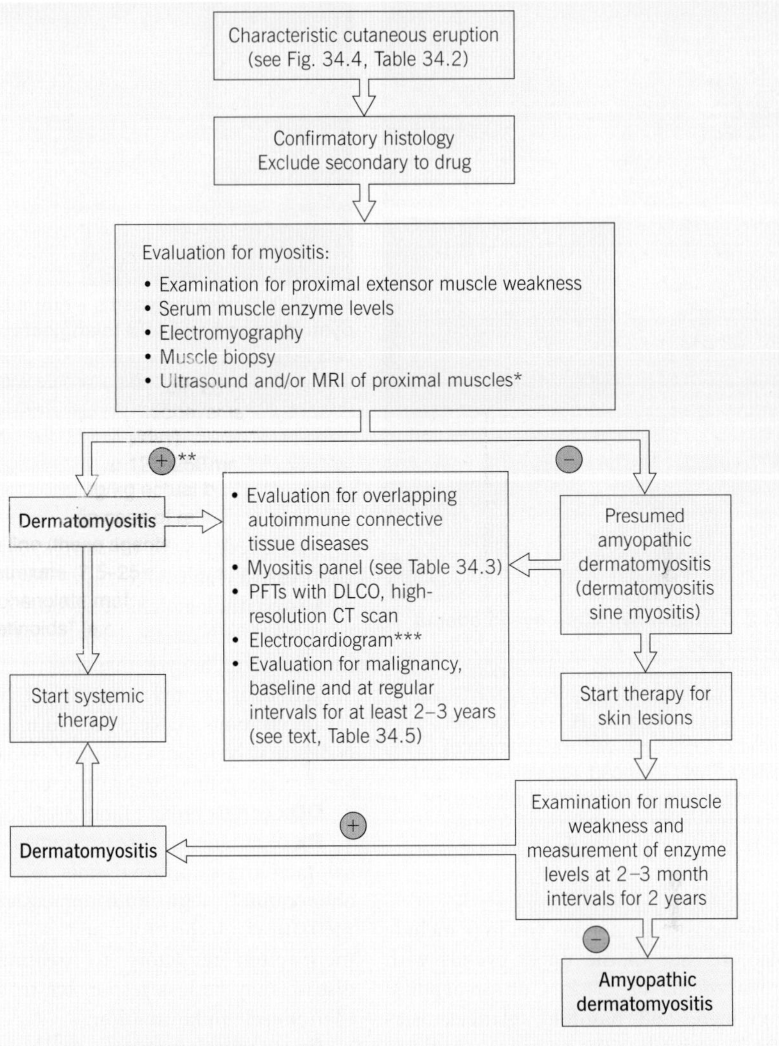

Fig. 34.1 Approach to adult dermatomyositis. The approach for children is similar but without the malignancy evaluation. Some authors classify patients with no evidence of myositis for 6 months after the onset of skin disease as having amyopathic dermatomyositis, but such individuals may go on to develop muscle disease. If planning administration of chronic systemic CS, a baseline DEXA bone density scan is recommended. DLCO, diffusing capacity of the lung for carbon monoxide; PFTs, pulmonary function tests.

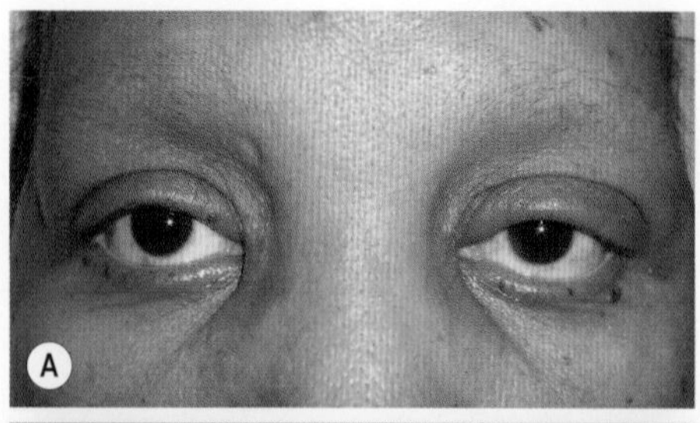

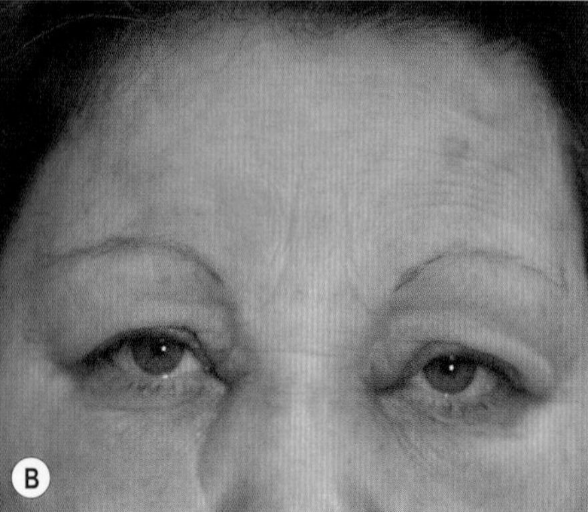

Fig. 34.2 Dermatomyositis – eyelid edema and heliotrope sign. A Inflammation of the upper eyelids can be more subtle in darkly pigmented skin; note involvement of the lateral nasal root and the cheeks. **B** The characteristic pink-violet color is seen with involvement of the hairline, lower forehead, upper eyelids, and cheeks; the edema is striking and involves the nasal root as well as the eyelids. *A, Courtesy, YDRSC; B, Courtesy, Jean L. Bolognia, MD.*

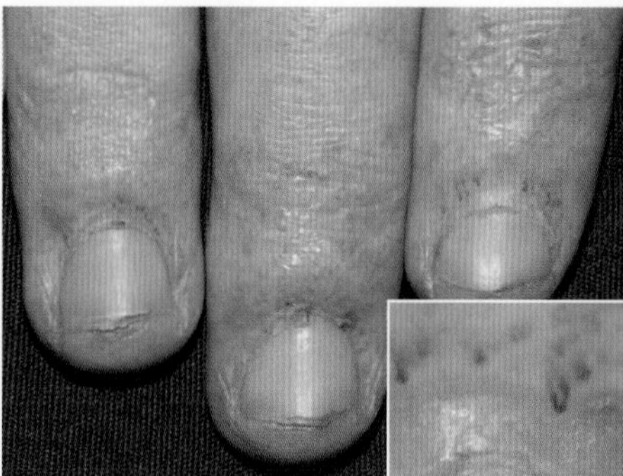

Fig. 34.3 Dermatomyositis – cuticular dystrophy and nail-fold telangiectasias. The cuticles are "ragged" and within the proximal nail fold, dilated capillary loops alternate with vessel dropout (inset). Atrophy, telangiectasias, and hypopigmentation are present on the fingers. *Courtesy, Julie V. Schaffer, MD.*

- Characteristic cutaneous findings include a violaceous hue of the upper eyelids with periorbital edema (Fig. 34.2), Gottron papules/Gottron sign, and nail-fold telangiectasias (Fig. 34.3), as well as the cutaneous findings outlined in Table 34.2 and represented in Fig. 34.4A; these may precede systemic manifestations (Fig. 34.4B).
- Interstitial lung disease affects 15–30% of patients, and baseline pulmonary function tests that include the CO diffusion coefficient are recommended; high-resolution CT may be required to detect involvement.
- May overlap with other AI-CTDs (1 in 5 adult cases) (Table 34.1).
- Histopathologic changes: skin – interface dermatitis with mucin deposits in the dermis; muscle – lymphocytic myositis.
- Various associated autoantibodies with clinical implications (Table 34.3); antinuclear antibodies may be negative as many autoantibodies are directed against cytoplasmic antigens.
- **DDx** can be broad (Table 34.4).
- **Rx** of cutaneous disease: topical CS, topical tacrolimus, antimalarials (e.g. hydroxychloroquine), immunosuppressives (e.g. methotrexate); pruritus and scalp involvement often refractory to treatment; skin disease may be less responsive to treatment than muscle inflammation.
- **Rx** of muscle/systemic involvement (Fig. 34.5): systemic CS (e.g. prednisone 1 mg/kg/day with slow taper) ± other immunosuppressive drugs (e.g. methotrexate); for severe cases, consider IVIg or JAK inhibitors.
- In classic dermatomyositis with malignancy (Table 34.5), cutaneous findings may improve gradually over time in the setting of a treatment-responsive tumor.

For further information see Ch. 42 from *Dermatology, Fourth Edition*.

For additional online figures visit www.expertconsult.com 

CUTANEOUS MANIFESTATIONS OF DERMATOMYOSITIS
Distribution of common cutaneous features (Figs 34.6–34.11)
Sun-exposed sites
May resemble a photodrug eruption
Pink-violet color and/or telangiectasias (e.g. face (Fig. 34.6); V of the chest/upper back, referred to as the "shawl sign" (Fig. 34.7)) Poikiloderma with hyperpigmentation, hypopigmentation, and atrophy in addition to telangiectasias
Extensor surfaces of hands (knuckles), elbows, and knees
May resemble psoriasis
Violaceous discoloration over joints (knuckles, knees, elbows), referred to as Gottron sign (Fig. 34.10) Over time, flat-topped papules develop on the knuckles (Gottron papules; (Fig. 34.11), and they may become atrophic
Scalp
May resemble seborrheic dermatitis
Scaly, pink patches (Fig. 34.12) Very pruritic Posterior > anterior scalp
Periocular
May resemble an airborne contact dermatitis
Pink-violet discoloration of the upper eyelids (heliotrope rash) (Fig. 34.2) Periocular edema that may be severe These findings can be subtle and wax and wane
Nail folds
Dilated capillary loops alternating with dropout of capillaries (Fig. 34.3) Ragged cuticles
Additional cutaneous features
Calcinosis cutis
More common in juvenile-onset dermatomyositis (Fig. 34.13) Associated with delay in Rx or Rx-resistant disease Hard, irregular nodules or plaques that can become extensive; may discharge chalky material
Pruritus
Raynaud phenomenon
Less common mucocutaneous features
When disease is severe, there may be erosions or ulcerations (Fig. 34.14) as well as anasarca Pink-violet patches of the lateral thighs (holster sign) Flagellate erythema (Fig. 34.14) Panniculitis/lipoatrophy (more common in children) Gingival telangiectasias

Table 34.2 Cutaneous manifestations of dermatomyositis. For a schematic representation of the cutaneous features, see Fig. 34.4A.

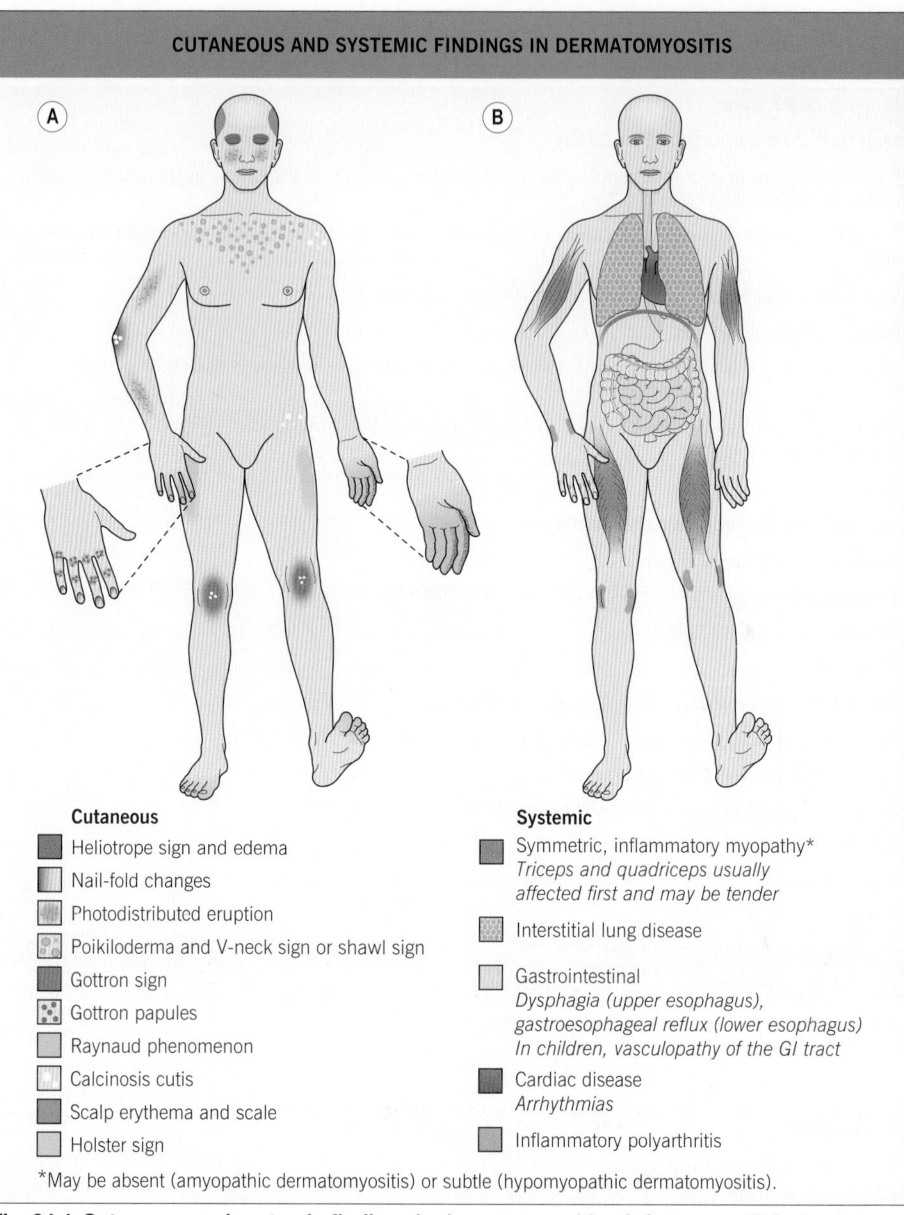

Fig. 34.4 Cutaneous and systemic findings in dermatomyositis. A Cutaneous. **B** Systemic. Nail-fold changes include dilated capillary loops, capillary dropout, cuticular hypertrophy, and ragged cuticles.

AUTOANTIBODIES ASSOCIATED WITH DERMATOMYOSITIS (DM) AND THEIR CLINICAL RELEVANCE	
Autoantibody	**Clinical relevance**
Anti-**aminoacyl**-tRNA synthetases: • Anti-Jo1 (**histidyl**) • Anti-PL-7 (**threonyl**) • Anti-PL-12 (**alanyl**) • Anti-EJ (**glycyl**) • Anti-OJ (**isoleucyl**)	• Antisynthetase syndrome (fever, polyarthritis, "mechanic's hands," Raynaud phenomenon, interstitial lung disease) • Present in up to 20% of adult patients
Anti-Mi-2	• Adult and juvenile DM • Hallmark is cutaneous disease; milder muscle disease • Good response to treatment • Present in up to 10–15% of patients
Anti-SRP	• Acute onset necrotizing myopathy • Often cardiac involvement • May be refractory to treatment
Anti-TIF1-γ (p155)	• Cancer-associated myositis in adult DM • Extensive cutaneous disease in adult and juvenile DM • Palmar hyperkeratotic papules, psoriasiform lesions, red-on-white telangiectatic patches, ovoid palatal patch
Anti-MDA5 (CADM-140)	• Clinically amyopathic DM (CADM) • Characteristic mucocutaneous findings, including tender palmar papules, ulcerations on the knuckles/elbows, oral/gum pain, diffuse alopecia • Rapidly progressive interstitial lung disease (ILD)
Anti-NXP-2 (p140)	• Cancer-associated myositis in adult DM • Adult and juvenile DM with calcinosis • Peripheral edema, myalgia, dysphagia, mild skin disease
Anti-SAE *(not yet available for commercial testing)*	• Adult DM • May present with CADM first • ILD uncommon

Table 34.3 Autoantibodies associated with dermatomyositis (DM) and their clinical relevance. MDA5, melanoma differentiation-associated protein 5; Mi-2, a DNA helicase; NXP-2, nuclear matrix protein; SAE, small ubiquitin-like modifier-activating enzyme; SRP, signal recognition particle; TIF1, transcriptional intermediary factor 1.

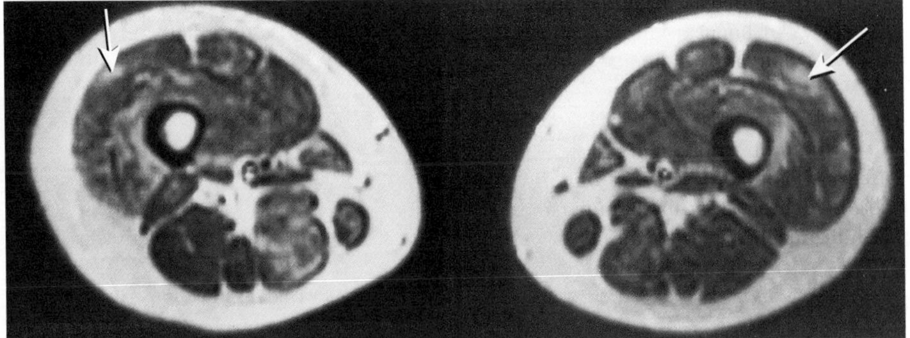

Fig. 34.5 T2-weighted MR images of the proximal thigh in a patient with dermatomyositis. Note the increased signal intensity, primarily in the extensor muscles (white color, arrows). The increased signal correlates with inflammation.

DIFFERENTIAL DIAGNOSIS OF DERMATOMYOSITIS
Systemic lupus erythematosus
Physician might notice the nail-fold telangiectasias and photodistributed poikiloderma but miss the muscle weakness, heliotrope rash, extensor distribution, pruritus, and the violaceous hue (true lupus erythematosus might be present in the setting of an overlap syndrome)
Psoriasis
Involvement of elbows and knees with papulosquamous lesions can lead to misdiagnosis
Airborne or allergic contact dermatitis
Eyelid edema can be marked in dermatomyositis; look for additional sites of dermatitis
Photodrug eruption
Photodistribution
Cutaneous T-cell lymphoma
The poikiloderma often begins in intertriginous zones rather than on the scalp, face, and extensor surfaces
Atopic dermatitis
Usually in children, where the physician focuses on the pruritus and secondary lichenification
Systemic sclerosis (scleroderma)
The nail-fold telangiectasias are similar in appearance, but the dyspigmentation is quite different; edema of the hands is an early sign (true systemic sclerosis may be present in the setting of an overlap syndrome)
Trichinosis
Patients have painful muscles and periorbital edema, but not other features
Photodistributed form of multicentric reticulohistiocytosis (rare)
Firm papules have distinct histologic features

Table 34.4 Differential diagnosis of dermatomyositis.

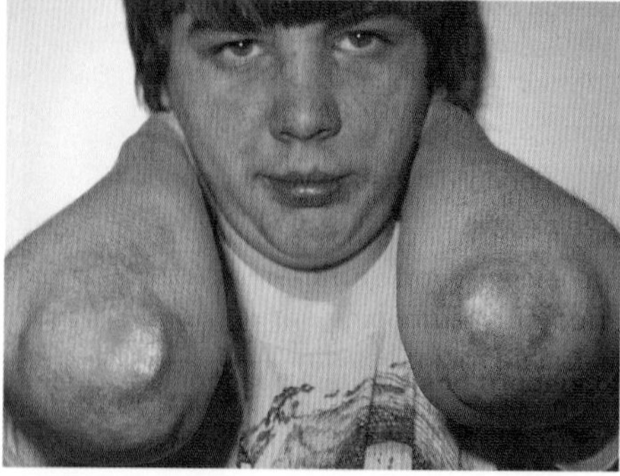

Fig. 34.6 Dermatomyositis. Misdiagnoses include psoriasis and acute cutaneous lupus erythematosus. *Courtesy, Joseph L. Jorizzo, MD.*

SUGGESTED MALIGNANCY SCREENING TESTS FOR ADULTS WITH DERMATOMYOSITIS
• Urinalysis • Stool occult blood testing • Serum prostate-specific antigen (PSA) in men • Serum CA125 (women) • Mammogram and transvaginal pelvic ultrasound (women) • CT of chest, abdomen, and pelvis • Colonoscopy (if age-appropriate, iron deficiency anemia, occult blood in stool, or symptoms) • Upper endoscopy (if colonoscopy negative in the setting of iron deficiency anemia, occult blood in stool, or symptoms) • Serum protein and immunofixation electrophoresis

Table 34.5 Suggested malignancy screening tests for adults with dermatomyositis. Screening should be performed at the time of diagnosis and annually for a minimum of 3 years thereafter; history and physical examination can be performed more frequently.

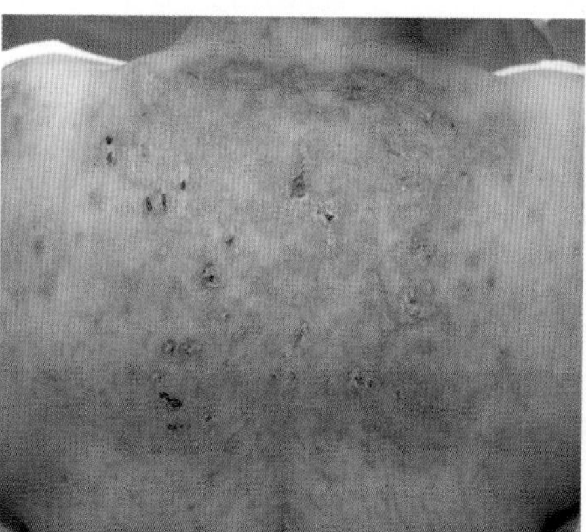

Fig. 34.7 Dermatomyositis – involvement of the upper back. The pink-violet plaques, some with associated scale, were very pruritic, as evidenced by multiple excoriations. Linear streaks of erythema are also seen. *Courtesy, Jean L. Bolognia, MD.*

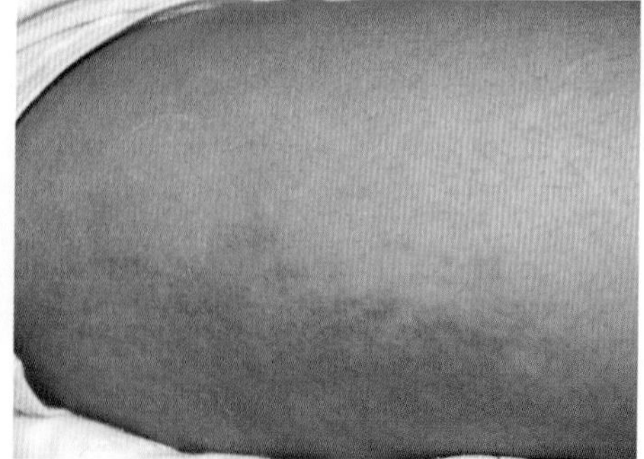

Fig. 34.8 Dermatomyositis, holster sign. Poikiloderma of the lateral thigh. *Courtesy, Sara Perkins, MD.*

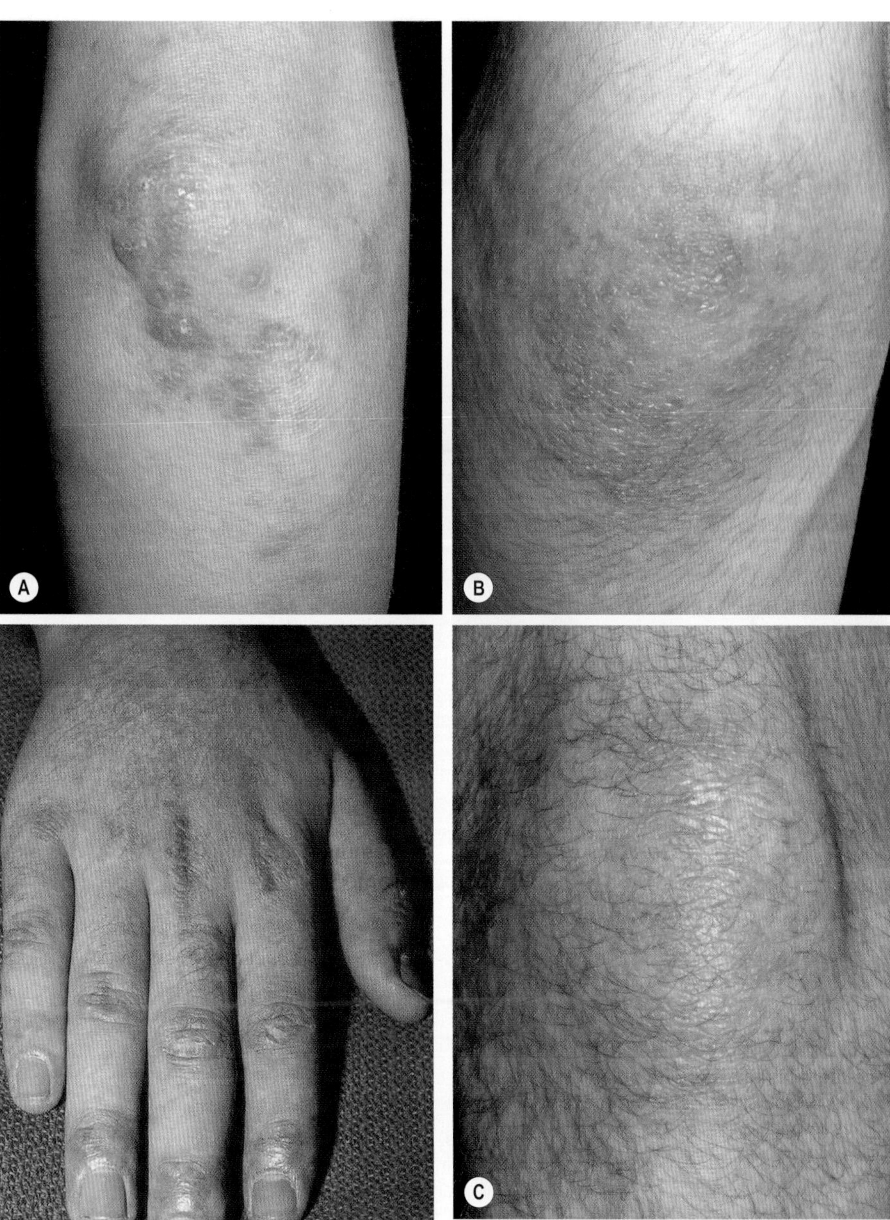

Fig. 34.9 Gottron sign with violaceous poikiloderma over the knuckles.

Fig. 34.10 Dermatomyositis – Gottron sign. Pink-violet papules (**A**) and thin pink plaques (**B**) of the elbows and knee (**C**). Some of the papules on the elbow are flat-topped (lichenoid) and others have white scale. The presence of plaques on the elbows and knees can lead to the misdiagnosis of psoriasis. *A, Courtesy, Ruth Ann Vleugels, MD; B, C, Courtesy, Julie V. Schaffer, MD.*

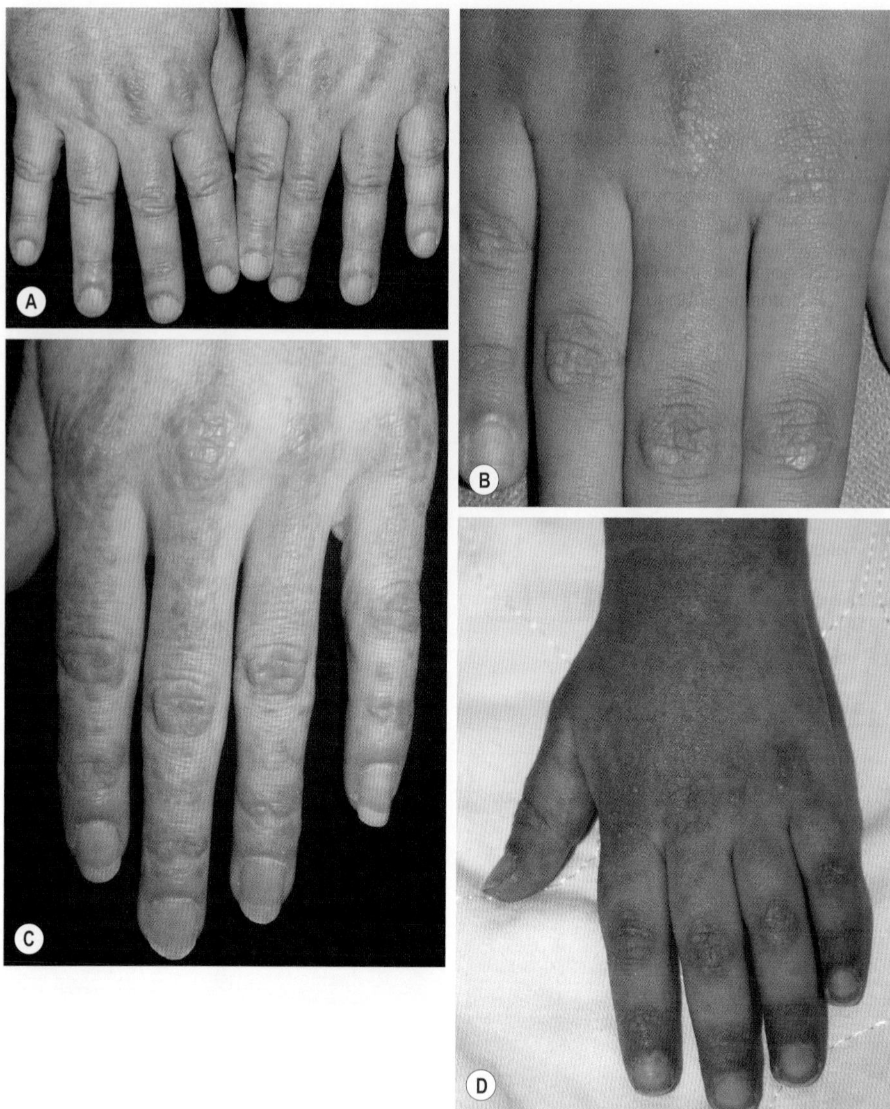

Fig. 34.11 Dermatomyositis – Gottron papules. A Only a few Gottron papules are present, but there is definite accentuation of the pink-violet inflammation over the metacarpophalangeal (MCP) joints and proximal and distal interphalangeal (PIP, DIP) joints as well as the proximal nail folds. Note the ragged cuticles. **B** The flat-topped (lichenoid) papules overlying the DIP, PIP, and MCP joints (knuckles) are subtle and were misdiagnosed as verrucae vulgares in this child. **C** More obvious disease in which the multiple pink-violet lichenoid papules are coalescing and there is some involvement of the interphalangeal skin. **D** Flat-topped (lichenoid) papules over the knuckles, ragged cuticles, and poikiloderma of the dorsal hand. *A, Courtesy, Kalman Watsky, MD; B, C, Courtesy, Julie V. Schaffer, MD; D, Courtesy, Sara Perkins, MD.*

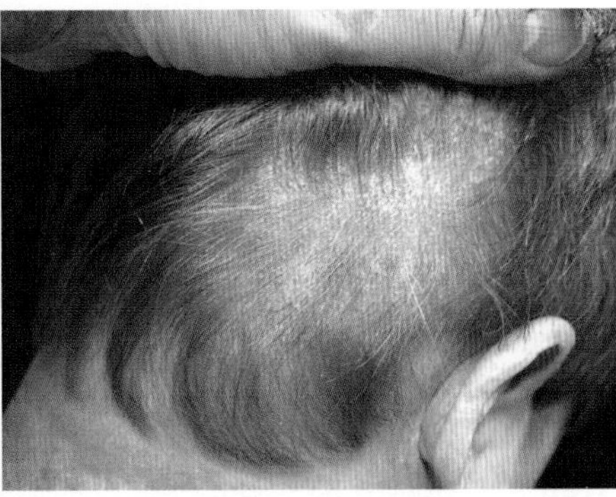

Fig. 34.12 Seborrheic-like dermatitis due to dermatomyositis. This patient presented with severe pruritus of the scalp. In addition to the scalp involvement, she had Gottron papules and a photodistributed poikiloderma. *Courtesy, Jeffrey P. Callen, MD.*

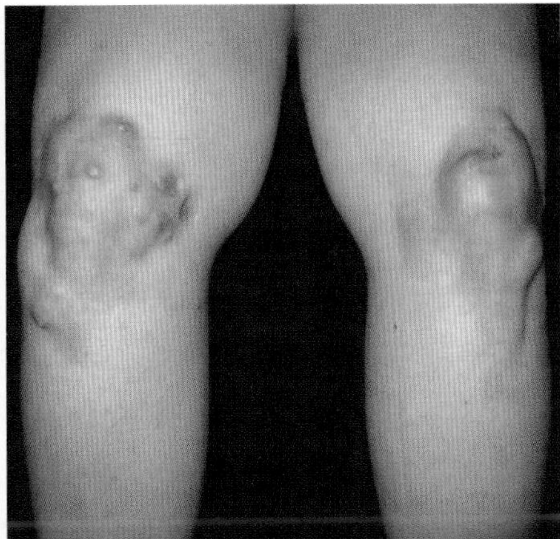

Fig. 34.13 Juvenile dermatomyositis – calcinosis cutis. The nodules favor the extensor surface of the knees and result in a decrease in joint mobility.

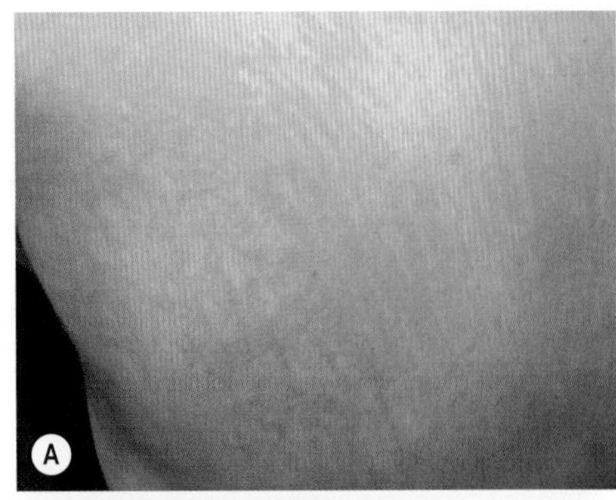

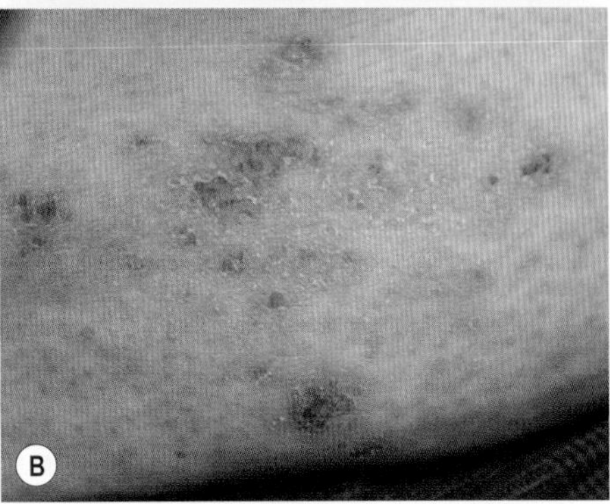

Fig. 34.14 Dermatomyositis – less common presentations. A Flagellate erythema of the posterior trunk. **B** Secondary changes include scale, erosions, and serous as well as hemorrhagic crusts. *A, Courtesy, Ruth Ann Vleugels, MD; B, Courtesy, YDRSC.*

35 Systemic Sclerosis and Sclerodermoid Disorders

• The spectrum of sclerosing skin disorders is outlined in Fig. 35.1.

Systemic Sclerosis (SSc, Scleroderma)

• An uncommon autoimmune connective tissue disease (AI-CTD) that affects the skin, blood vessels, and various internal organs (e.g. kidney, lung, gastrointestinal tract, heart).

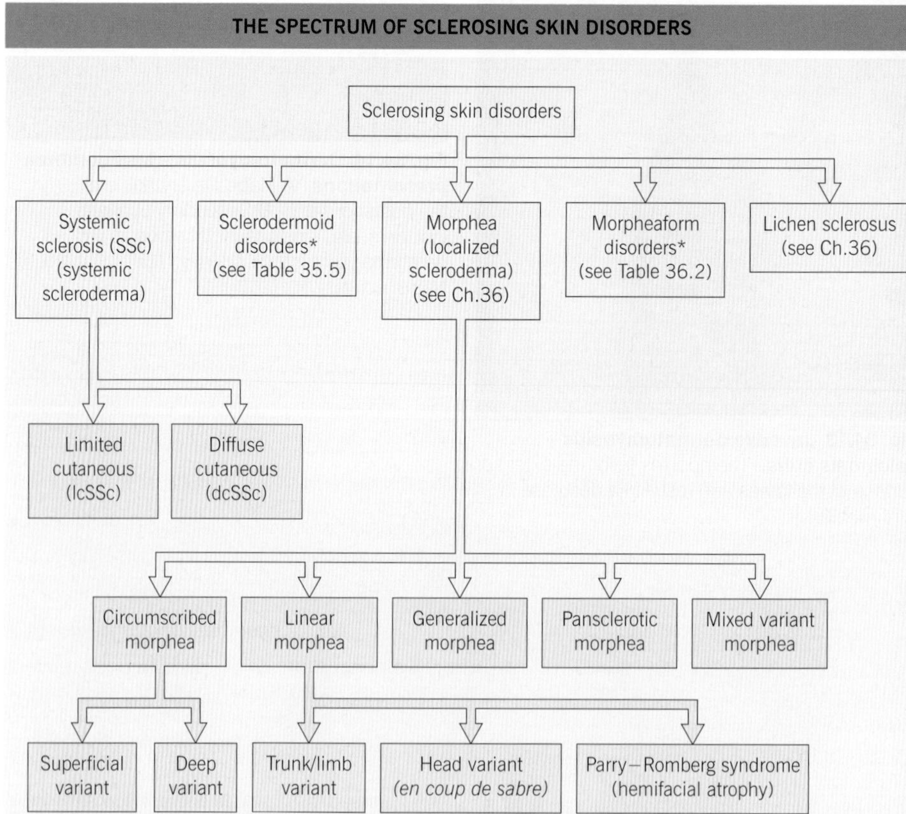

Fig. 35.1 The spectrum of sclerosing skin disorders.

ACR/EULAR CRITERIA FOR THE CLASSIFICATION OF SYSTEMIC SCLEROSIS		
Item	**Sub-item**	**Weight/score**
Skin thickening of the fingers of both hands extending proximal to the MCP joints (*sufficient criterion*)	–	9
Skin thickening of the fingers	Puffy fingers - *or* - sclerodactyly	2 4
Fingertip lesion	Digital tip ulcers - *or* - pitting scars	2 3
Telangiectasias	–	2
Abnormal nail-fold capillaries	–	2
Pulmonary arterial hypertension - *or* - interstitial lung disease		2 2
Raynaud phenomenon	–	3
SSc-related autoantibodies	Anti-centromere Anti-topoisomerase I Anti-RNA polymerase III	3

Table 35.1 2013 American College of Rheumatology (ACR)/European League Against Rheumatism (EULAR) criteria for the classification of systemic sclerosis (SSc). The total score is determined by adding the maximum weight (score) in each category. Patients with a total score of ≥9 are classified as having *definite* SSc. *From Van den Hoogen F, Khanna D, Fransen J, et al. 2013 classification criteria for systemic sclerosis. Arthritis Rheum 2013;65:2737–47.*

- Etiology is unknown but pathogenesis involves vascular dysfunction, immune activation with autoantibody production, and tissue sclerosis.
- Seen more frequently in women; onset is typically in the 3rd to 4th decades of life; diffuse cutaneous SSc is more frequently seen in African-Americans.
- The criteria for the classification/diagnosis of SSc were updated in 2013 (Table 35.1).
- There are two *major* clinical subtypes of SSc, based upon the amount of skin sclerosis (Fig. 35.2): *limited cutaneous SSc (lcSSc)* and *diffuse cutaneous SSc (dcSSc)*.
- LcSSc is characterized by skin sclerosis involving the distal extremities and face; whereas in dcSSc, the distal and proximal extremities, trunk, and face are involved; internal organ involvement can be seen in both subtypes.
- LcSSc and dcSSc can also occur in conjunction with other AI-CTDs (called "overlap syndrome"), most notably polymyositis and SLE.
- Raynaud phenomenon is present in almost all SSc patients and is often the earliest presenting feature (Table 35.2; Figs 35.3–35.5).
- Mat telangiectasias (Fig. 35.6), proximal nail-fold capillary abnormalities, and cutaneous ulcerations (Fig. 35.7) are present in both lcSSc and dcSSc subtypes and are important clues to the Dx; additional common cutaneous findings are outlined in Table 35.2.
- Patients often have a characteristic facies with microstomia, retraction of the lips, perioral furrows, and a beaked nose; three types of dyspigmentation can also be seen, including diffuse hyperpigmentation and leukoderma of SSc (Fig. 35.8).
- Internal organ involvement is seen in both lcSSc and dcSSc (Table 35.3), but patients with dcSSc are at increased risk for more clinically severe extracutaneous disease and overall worse outcomes.
- Most patients (>95%) with SSc are ANA (+); antinuclear autoantibodies unique to SSc, in particular anti-centromere, anti-topoisomerase I, and anti-RNA polymerase III,

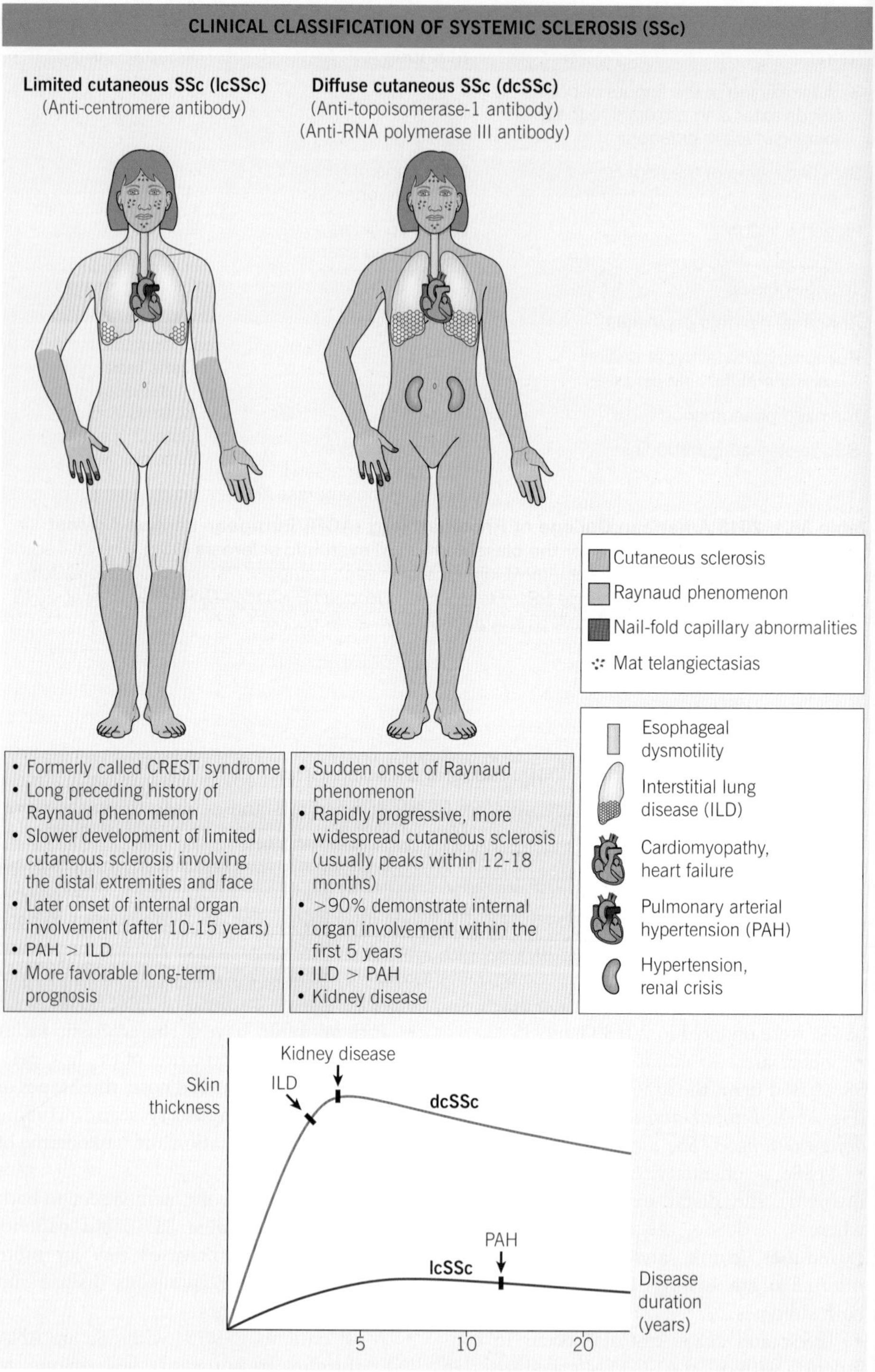

CLINICAL CLASSIFICATION OF SYSTEMIC SCLEROSIS (SSc)

Limited cutaneous SSc (lcSSc)	Diffuse cutaneous SSc (dcSSc)
• Formerly called CREST syndrome • Long preceding history of Raynaud phenomenon • Slower development of limited cutaneous sclerosis involving the distal extremities and face • Later onset of internal organ involvement (after 10-15 years) • PAH > ILD • More favorable long-term prognosis	• Sudden onset of Raynaud phenomenon • Rapidly progressive, more widespread cutaneous sclerosis (usually peaks within 12-18 months) • >90% demonstrate internal organ involvement within the first 5 years • ILD > PAH • Kidney disease

Fig. 35.2 Clinical classification of systemic sclerosis (SSc). In addition to the two major clinical subsets shown here, two others are recognized: *systemic sclerosis sine scleroderma (ssSSc)*, considered a subset of lcSSc, in which cutaneous sclerosis is absent, but the presence of internal organ involvement, Raynaud phenomenon, nail-fold capillary abnormalities, and positive serologies are present; and overlap syndrome, in which either lcSSc or dcSSc coexists with another AI-CTD, e.g. polymyositis or SLE. CREST, *c*alcinosis, *R*aynaud phenomenon, *e*sophageal dysmotility, *s*clerodactyly, *t*elangiectasias.

CUTANEOUS FEATURES OF SYSTEMIC SCLEROSIS – POSSIBLE TREATMENTS	
Cutaneous feature	**Possible treatment options**
Cutaneous sclerosis (Figs 35.3 and 35.5)	• Topical therapies • UV phototherapy • D-penicillamine* • Minocycline** • Methotrexate (if no ILD)† • Mycophenolate mofetil (when ILD)
Raynaud phenomenon (Fig. 35.9) (Tables 35.6 and 35.7)	**First-line** • Cold avoidance • Hand and feet warming packets • Discontinue all tobacco products **Second-line** • Calcium channel blockers (e.g. nifedipine SR 30 mg daily–BID, amlodipine 2.5–10 mg daily) **Third-line** (especially when accompanied by ulceration) • Phosphodiesterase type 5 inhibitors (e.g. sildenafil, tadalafil) • α-Adrenergic blockers (e.g. prazosin) • Angiotensin II receptor blockers (e.g. losartan) • Endothelin receptor antagonists (e.g. bosentan) **Fourth-line** • Serotonin reuptake inhibitors (e.g. fluoxetine)
Cutaneous ulcers (Figs 35.5B and 35.7)	• Avoid excessive debridement • Moist, nonadherent dressings • Therapies listed above for Raynaud phenomenon • Low-dose aspirin or clopidogrel • IV prostanoid (e.g. epoprostenol)
Calcinosis cutis (Fig. 35.4) (see Ch. 42)	• Low-dose warfarin • Calcium channel blockers • Sodium thiosulfate
Mat telangiectasias (Fig. 35.6)	• Lasers appropriate for vascular lesions

**Nowadays used infrequently.*
***Minimal effect.*
†Methotrexate-induced pneumonitis may complicate SSc-ILD picture.

Table 35.2 Cutaneous features of systemic sclerosis – possible treatments. ILD, interstitial lung disease; SR, slow release.

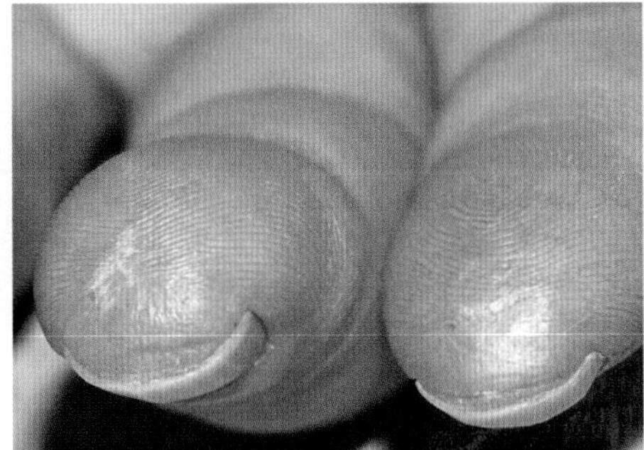

Fig. 35.3 Pitted scars of the digital pulp in a patient with systemic sclerosis. *Courtesy, Kalman Watsky, MD.*

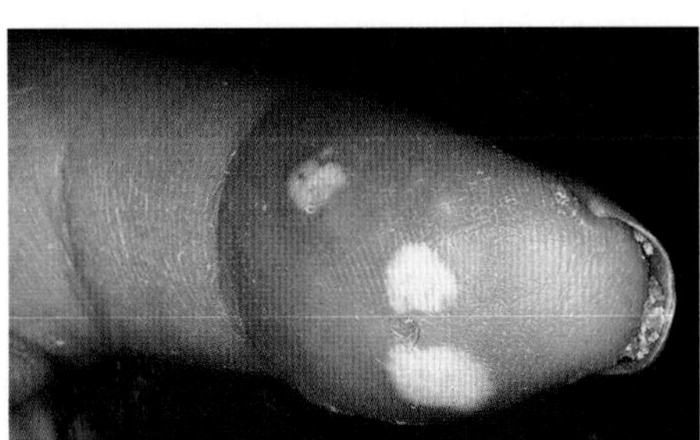

Fig. 35.4 Calcinosis cutis of the finger in a patient with systemic sclerosis. *Courtesy, YDRSC.*

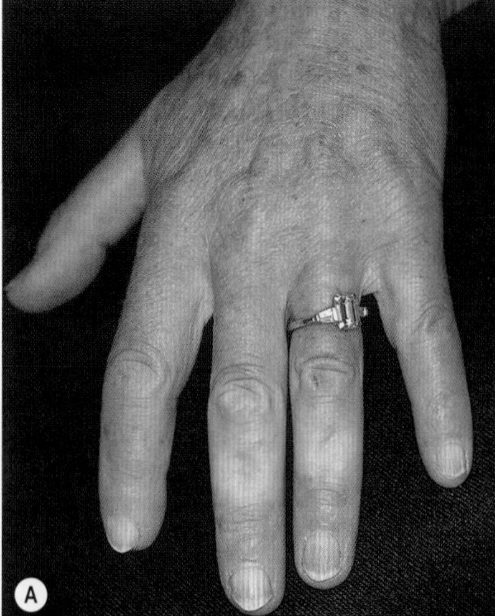

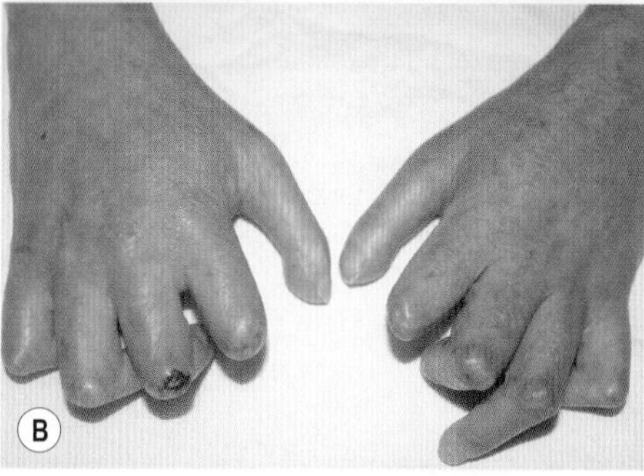

Fig. 35.5 Early versus late stages of systemic sclerosis (SSc) involving the hands. A Early edematous phase of SSc (note the demonstration of pitting edema on two of the digits). **B** Late stage of dcSSc with fixed flexion contractures, sclerodactyly, and digital ulceration overlying the third proximal interphalangeal joint. *A, Courtesy, Jean L. Bolognia, MD; B, Courtesy, M. Kari Connolly, MD.*

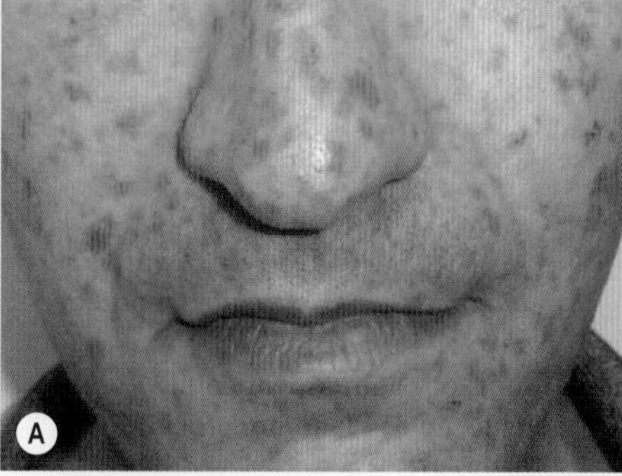

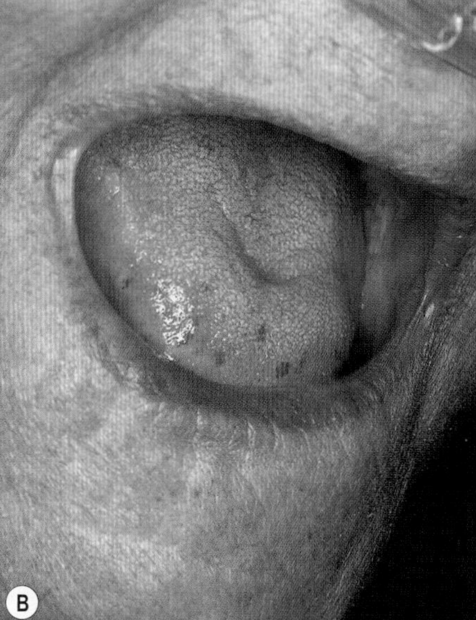

Fig. 35.6 Mat (squared-off) telangiectasias in systemic sclerosis (SSc). The first patient **(A)** had limited cutaneous systemic sclerosis (lcSSc) while the second patient **(B)** presented with diffuse hyperpigmentation and interstitial lung disease. *A, Courtesy, M. Kari Connolly, MD; B, Courtesy, Jean L. Bolognia, MD.*

are useful for diagnostic and prognostic purposes (Table 35.4).

- There are three phases of cutaneous disease:
  - (1) **Early edematous phase**, featuring puffy hands and pitting edema of the digits (see Fig. 35.5A)
  - (2) **Indurated phase**, characterized by hardening of the skin with taut and shiny appearance (see Fig. 35.5B)
  - (3) **Atrophic phase**, with potential/gradual softening of the skin
- The degree of skin sclerosis does not predict the degree of internal organ involvement, and survival is dependent on the type and degree of internal organ involvement.
- Pulmonary disease (interstitial lung disease [ILD] > pulmonary arterial hypertension [PAH]) is the most common cause of mortality.
- All SSc patients should be screened and periodically monitored for internal organ involvement, especially lung and renal disease (Table 35.3).

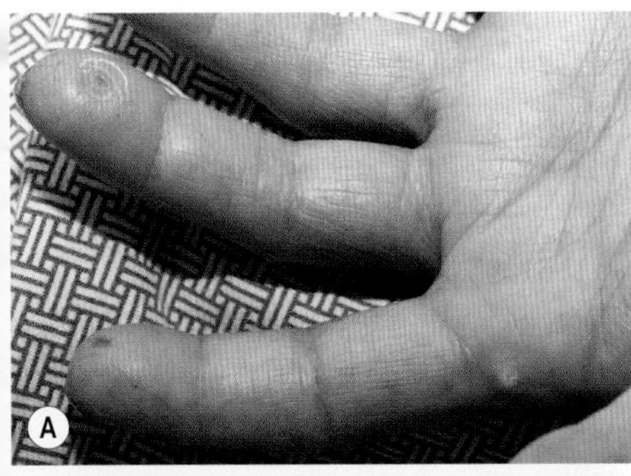

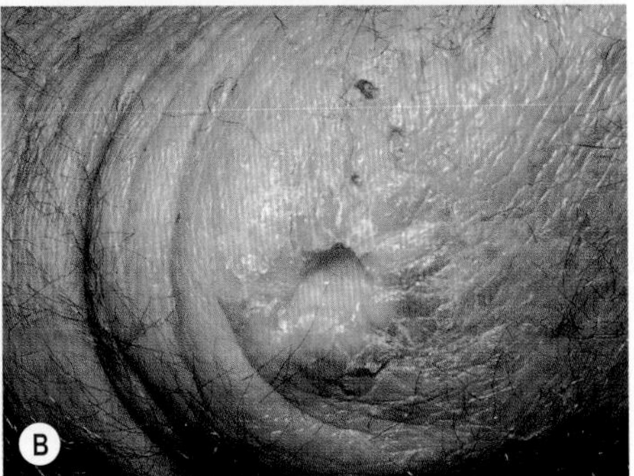

Fig. 35.7 Cutaneous ulcerations in systemic sclerosis (SSc). Ulcers favor the digits (**A**) and sites of trauma, such as the elbow (**B**). Note the calcinosis cutis at the base of the forefinger and the pterygium inversum unguis of the third finger. *A, Courtesy, Kalman Watsky, MD; B, Courtesy, Joyce Rico, MD.*

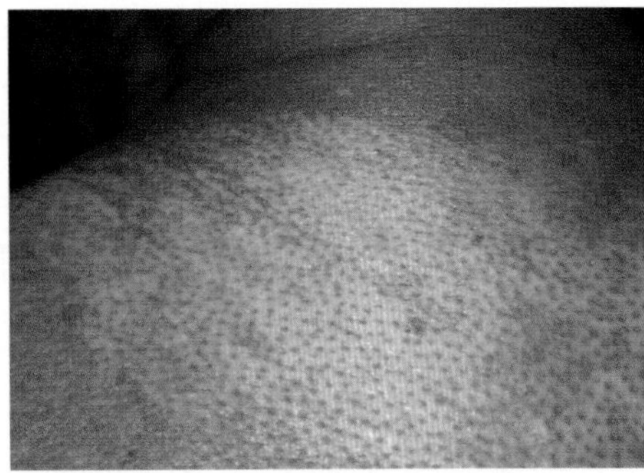

Fig 35.8 The "salt and pepper" sign. Leukoderma with retention of perifollicular pigmentation in a patient with systemic sclerosis. *Courtesy, Joyce Rico, MD.*

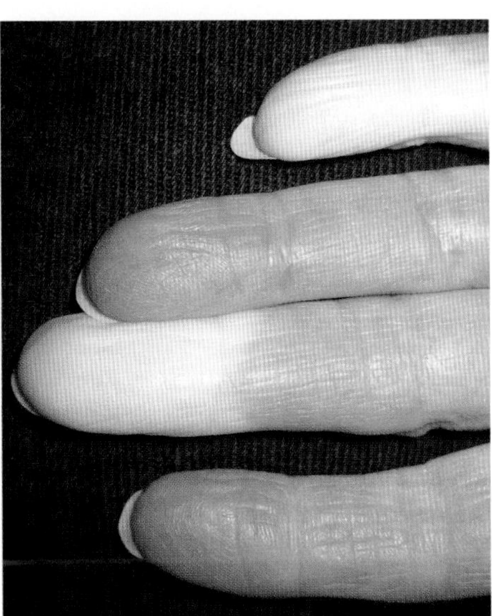

Fig. 35.9 Raynaud phenomenon in a patient with early systemic sclerosis (SSc). There is obvious blanching of two fingers, as well as violaceous hue of the forefinger. *Courtesy, Jeffrey P. Callen, MD.*

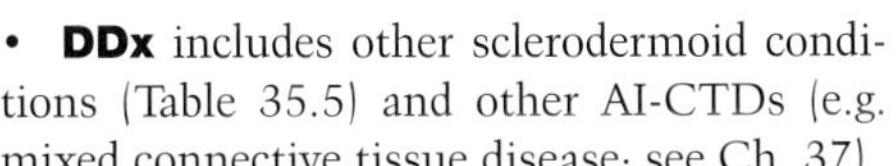

- **DDx** includes other sclerodermoid conditions (Table 35.5) and other AI-CTDs (e.g. mixed connective tissue disease; see Ch. 37).
- Recommendations for the initial evaluation of all patients with suspected SSc are presented in Table 35.3.
- **Rx** options for various cutaneous and extracutaneous features of SSc are outlined in Tables 35.2 and 35.3.

Raynaud Phenomenon

- Characterized by episodic vasospasm of the digital arteries, resulting in white, blue, and red discoloration of the fingers and toes secondary to cold stimuli (Fig. 35.9).
- Occurs in two settings: *primary* Raynaud phenomenon (Raynaud disease) and *secondary* Raynaud phenomenon (Table 35.6).
- *Primary* Raynaud phenomenon is common, affecting 3–5% of the population and typically develops in adolescent girls and young women (median age at onset, ~14 years) and is not associated with any underlying medical issues.
- *Secondary* Raynaud phenomenon is uncommon and is associated with an underlying medical problem, including SSc (Table 35.7).
- An approach to differentiating primary from secondary Raynaud phenomenon is presented in Fig. 35.10.
- **Rx:** Table 35.2.

INTERNAL ORGAN INVOLVEMENT IN SYSTEMIC SCLEROSIS – SCREENING AND TREATMENT OPTIONS		
Internal organ	**Screening tools***	**Treatment options**
Lung*		
• Interstitial lung disease (ILD)	• **PFTs (DLCO, spirometry, and lung volumes)** • **High-resolution CT** • Bronchoalveolar lavage and lung biopsy	• Immunosuppression (e.g. mycophenolate mofetil, cyclophosphamide, rituximab) • Nintedanib**, tocilizumab** • Lung transplantation
• Pulmonary arterial hypertension (PAH)	• **Transthoracic echocardiography** • **Serum *N*-Tpro-BNP level** • Right heart catheterization	• Oxygen • Anticoagulation • Endothelin receptor antagonists (e.g. bosentan) • Phosphodiesterase inhibitors (e.g. tadalafil) • Prostaglandins (e.g. epoprostenol) • Prostacyclin analogues (e.g. treprostinil) • Prostacyclin receptor agonists (e.g. selexipag) • Soluble guanylate cyclase stimulators (e.g. riociguat) • Lung transplantation
Kidney		
• Renal crisis • Hypertension	• **Close monitoring of blood pressure** • **BUN/Cr** • **Urinalysis**	• ACE inhibitors instituted early for treatment but not helpful for prevention
Heart		
• Fibrosis/restrictive cardiomyopathy • Heart failure secondary to PAH	• Echocardiography	• ACE inhibitors
Gastrointestinal tract		
• Esophageal dysmotility • Small bowel involvement	• Barium swallow with small bowel follow through • Manometry • Endoscopy	• Proton pump inhibitors • Promotility agents (e.g. ondansetron)

**Patients are typically asymptomatic in the early stages of ILD and PAH, which is when the diagnosis should be made and treatment instituted; cough, dyspnea on exertion, and shortness of breath are typical later-onset symptoms.*
***FDA-approved for SSc-ILD.*

Table 35.3 Internal organ involvement in systemic sclerosis – screening and treatment options. Items in bold signify those screening tests that are recommended at baseline in all newly diagnosed patients. In addition, autologous hematopoietic stem cell transplantation should be considered for patients with rapidly progressive SSc who are at risk of organ failure. ACE, angiotensin converting enzyme; DLCO, diffusing capacity of the lung for carbon monoxide; *N*-Tpro-BNP, *N*-terminal pro b-type natriuretic peptide; PFTs, pulmonary function tests.

SYSTEMIC SCLEROSIS (SSc) AUTOANTIBODY PROFILE AND THE MORE FREQUENTLY ASSOCIATED CLINICAL PRESENTATIONS	
SSc autoantibody	**Clinical features**
Limited skin sclerosis	
Anti-centromere*	• Increased risk isolated PAH > ILD • Esophageal involvement • Small intestinal involvement with malabsorption
Anti-Th/To	• Frequent in patients with ssSSc • More severe internal organ involvement (ILD, PAH)
Anti-U11/U12 RNP**	• Greatest risk for developing ILD, which is often severe and rapidly progressive
Diffuse skin sclerosis	
Anti-topoisomerase-I* (*formerly Scl-70*)	• Increased risk ILD >PAH • Poor prognosis
Anti-RNA polymerase III*	• Most severe diffuse skin sclerosis; rapidly progressive • Greatest risk for renal crisis • Gastric antral vascular ectasia (GAVE) • Increased risk of internal malignancy (especially breast cancer)
Anti-U3 RNP	• More frequent in African-Americans • Non-inflammatory skeletal myopathy • Early, often severe internal organ involvement (e.g. PAH, cardiomyopathy, small bowel involvement with malabsorption)
Overlap syndromes	
Anti-PM/Scl	• Polymyositis – SSc overlap • Acute-onset inflammatory myositis • Less serious internal organ involvement • Usually better prognosis because responsive to oral CS
Anti-U1RNP†	• MCTD • Increased risk ILD and PAH • Usually better prognosis because responsive to oral CS
Anti-Ku	• Myositis and arthritis • Increased risk of ILD
Anti-RuvBL1/2**	• Combination of diffuse skin sclerosis + myositis

**The most frequently identified autoantibodies in SSc and currently used as criteria for classification/diagnosis (see Table 35.1).*
***Testing is currently not commercially available.*
†The U1RNP antibody is specific for MCTD, which is often considered a distinct clinical entity (see Ch. 37).

Table 35.4 Systemic sclerosis (SSc) autoantibody profile and the more frequently associated clinical presentations. Over 95% of SSc patients will have a (+) ANA. The value of a (+) ANA lies in the subsequent identification of the patient's SSc-specific autoantibody. More than 90% will have one of ten SSc autoantibodies; rarely (~2–3%) will a patient have more than one SSc autoantibody. The ten autoantibodies are mostly mutually exclusive and tend not to change with time. These autoantibodies are rarely found in patients with other AI-CTDs, unless features of SSc are also present. ILD, interstitial lung disease or pulmonary fibrosis; MCTD, mixed connective tissue disease; PAH, pulmonary arterial hypertension; ssSSc, systemic sclerosis sine scleroderma.

DIFFERENTIAL DIAGNOSIS OF SCLERODERMOID CONDITIONS	
Mucinoses	**Neurologic**
• Scleredema • Scleromyxedema	• Complex regional pain syndrome* • Spinal cord injury
Immunologic	**Toxin-mediated**
• Chronic scleroderma-like GVHD* • Eosinophilic fasciitis • Generalized morphea* • Fibroblastic rheumatism • Overlap syndromes	• Nephrogenic systemic fibrosis* • Eosinophilia-myalgia syndrome (historic) • Toxic oil syndrome* (historic) • Silicosis
Paraneoplastic	**Drug- or chemical-induced**
• POEMS syndrome • Amyloidosis (primary systemic)** • Carcinoid syndrome • Paraneoplastic scleroderma-like syndrome	• Bleomycin* • Taxanes • Vinyl chloride, chlorinated hydrocarbons*
Neoplastic	**Venous insufficiency**
• Carcinoma *en cuirasse**	• Lipodermatosclerosis*
Metabolic	**Other**
• Diabetic cheiroarthropathy • Porphyria cutanea tarda*,†	• Restrictive dermopathy§ • Stiff skin syndrome*

**Can overlap with morpheaform disorders, which are listed in Table 36.2.*
***Primary cutaneous amyloidosis can also occur in patients with systemic sclerosis and generalized morphea.*
†May also be observed in patients with congenital erythropoietic porphyria and hepatoerythropoietic porphyria.
§Sclerodermoid changes are typically present at birth.

Table 35.5 Differential diagnosis of sclerodermoid conditions. POEMS, polyneuropathy, organomegaly, endocrinopathy, monoclonal gammopathy, and skin changes.

CLINICAL AND LABORATORY FEATURES OF PRIMARY AND SECONDARY RAYNAUD PHENOMENON		
Feature	**Primary Raynaud**	**Secondary Raynaud**
Sex	F:M 20:1	F:M 4:1
Age at onset	Puberty	>25 years
Frequency of attacks	Usually <5 per day	5–10+ per day
Precipitants	Cold, emotional stress	Cold
Ischemic injury	Absent	Present
Abnormal capillaroscopy	Absent	>95%
Other vasomotor phenomena	Yes	Yes
Antinuclear antibodies	Absent/low titer	90–95%
Anticentromere antibody	Absent	30–40%
Anti-topoisomerase I (Scl-70) antibody	Absent	20–30%
Anti-RNA polymerase III antibody	Absent	10–20%
In vivo platelet activation	Absent	>75%

Table 35.6 Clinical and laboratory features of primary and secondary Raynaud phenomenon. *Adapted from Hochberg MC, Silman AJ, Smolen JS, et al. Rheumatology, 3rd edn. Edinburgh: Mosby, 2003. © Elsevier 2003.*

DIFFERENTIAL DIAGNOSIS OF RAYNAUD PHENOMENON
Structural vasculopathies
Large and medium-sized arteries
• Thoracic outlet syndrome • Brachiocephalic trunk disease (atherosclerosis, Takayasu arteritis) • Buerger disease (thromboangiitis obliterans)* • Crutch pressure
Small arteries and arterioles
• Systemic sclerosis • Systemic lupus erythematosus • Dermatomyositis • Overlap syndromes • Cold injury • Vibration disease (hand–arm vibration syndrome, hypothenar hammer syndrome) • Chemotherapy (bleomycin, vinca alkaloids, cisplatin, carboplatin) • Vinyl chloride disease • Arsenic poisoning
Normal blood vessels – abnormal blood elements
• Cryoglobulinemia (monoclonal or mixed) • Cryofibrinogenemia • Cold agglutinin disease • Myeloproliferative disorders (e.g. essential thrombocythemia)
Normal blood vessels – abnormal vasomotion
• Primary (idiopathic) Raynaud phenomenon • Drug-induced (ergot alkaloids, bromocriptine, interferon, estrogen, cyclosporine, sympathomimetic agents, clonidine, cocaine, nicotine) • Carpal tunnel syndrome • Pheochromocytoma • Carcinoid syndrome • Reflex sympathetic dystrophy • Other vasospastic disorders (migraine, Prinzmetal)
**Can also affect small arteries.*

Table 35.7 Differential diagnosis of Raynaud phenomenon. Paraneoplastic acral vascular syndrome, which can present with Raynaud phenomenon as well as acrocyanosis and gangrene, has been observed in patients with various solid tumors (e.g. lung or ovarian carcinoma). *Adapted from Hochberg MC, Silman AJ, Smolen JS, et al. (Eds.). Rheumatology, 3rd edn. Edinburgh: Mosby, 2003.* *© Elsevier 2003.*

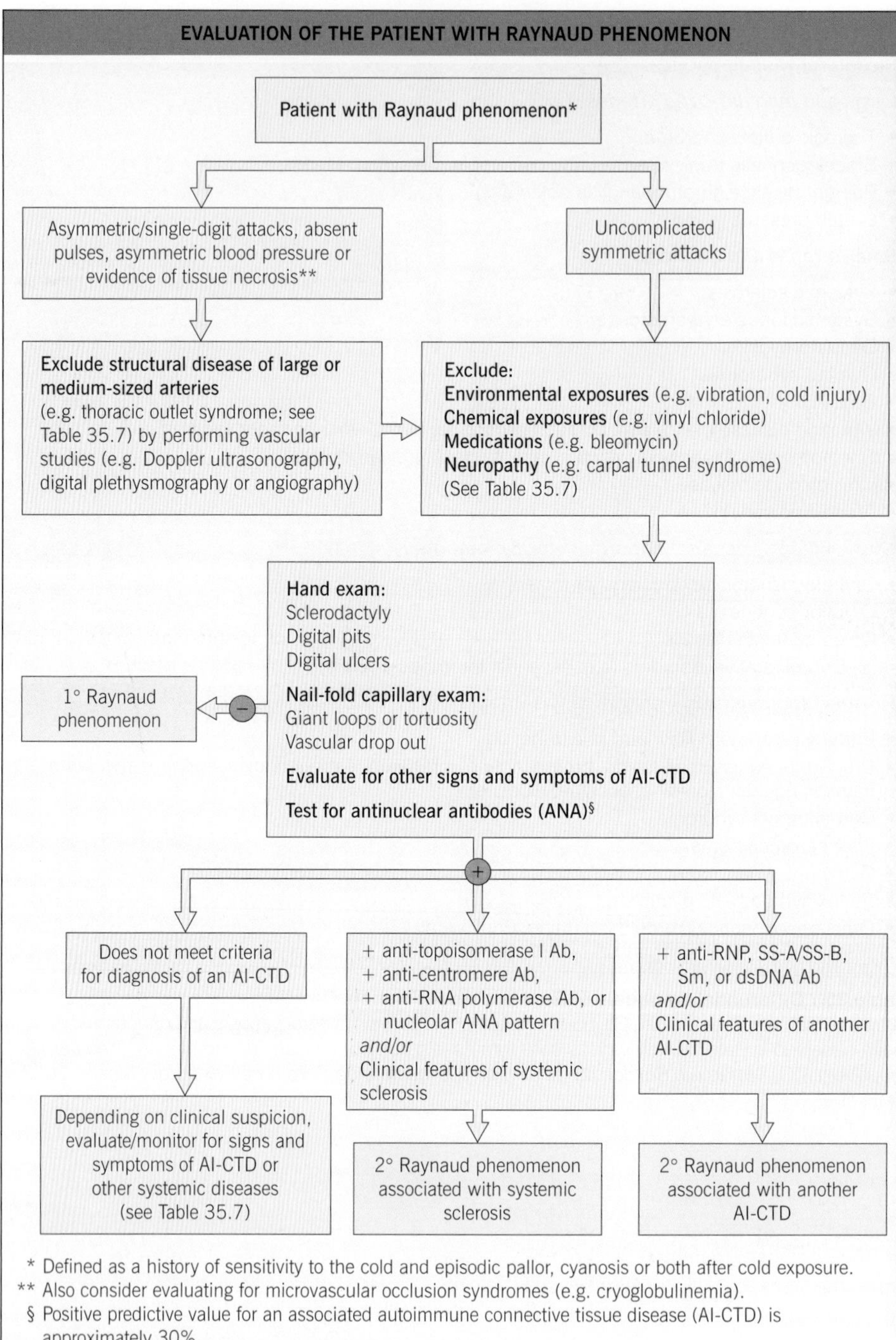

Fig 35.10 Evaluation of the patient with Raynaud phenomenon. RNP, ribonucleoprotein; Sm, Smith; ds, double-stranded.

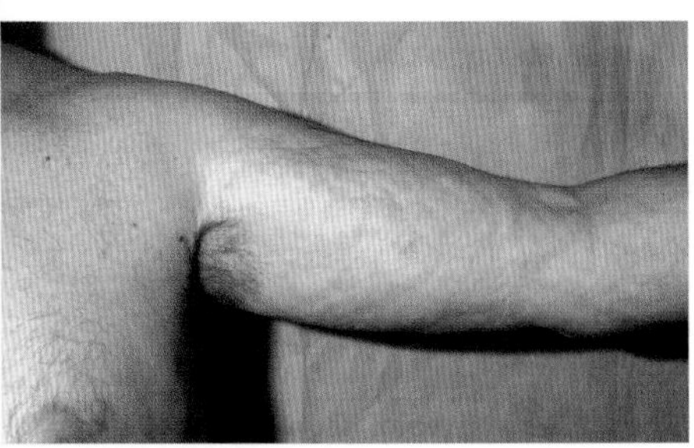

Fig. 35.11 Eosinophilic fasciitis – clinical features. Induration of the arm with a dimpled or "pseudo-cellulite" appearance, also referred to as rippling or puckering. *Courtesy, Edward Cowen, MD.*

Sclerodermoid Disorders

- Disorders with a clinical presentation similar to SSc are referred to as "sclerodermoid disorders" (Table 35.5).

Eosinophilic Fasciitis (Shulman Syndrome)

- Characterized initially by the rapid onset of edema and pain of the extremities, followed by symmetric, woody induration (spares hands, feet, face) (Fig. 35.11), and a dimpled or "pseudo-cellulite" appearance; associated with peripheral eosinophilia; ~30% of cases are preceded by strenuous physical activity.
- May be one of the presentations of chronic GVHD (see Ch. 44)
- Prompt treatment with oral CS is necessary to preserve mobility and function; slow taper over 6–24 months.

Nephrogenic Systemic Fibrosis (NSF)

- Occurs in individuals with impaired renal function, most commonly (~90%) dialysis-dependent chronic kidney disease, in association with exposure to gadolinium-based contrast medium.

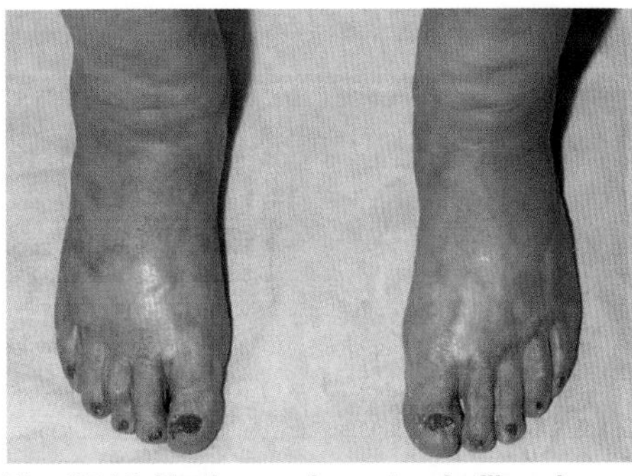

Fig. 35.12 Nephrogenic systemic fibrosis (NSF) – clinical features. Orange-brown indurated plaques. Note the "ameboid" outline of one of the plaques on the left foot. *Courtesy, Edward Cowen, MD.*

- Presents on the extremities with symmetrically distributed, ill-defined, thick, indurated, erythematous to hyperpigmented plaques (Fig. 35.12).
- Confluence of lesions can result in joint contracture, pain, and loss of mobility.
- Systemic fibrosis affecting the heart, lungs, and skeletal muscles can also occur.
- No effective treatment; most helpful intervention is to restore renal function (e.g. via renal transplantation).

Stiff Skin Syndrome

- Congenital or onset in early childhood; pathogenesis unknown, but a subset with fibrillin gene mutations; chronic course with no effective treatment, other than physical therapy to prevent contractures.
- Characterized by "rock hard" induration of the skin and subcutaneous tissues of thighs and buttocks, usually bilateral; noticeable sparing of inguinal folds; associated hypertrichosis of affected areas; joint contractures; typically, no internal organ involvement.

For further information see Ch. 43 from *Dermatology, Fourth Edition*.

For additional online figures and tables visit www.expertconsult.com 

36 Morphea and Lichen Sclerosus

Morphea (Localized Scleroderma)

- An uncommon fibrosing disorder that is limited to the skin, subcutaneous tissues, and occasionally the underlying bone; if present on the face and/or scalp, it can be associated with underlying CNS abnormalities.
- It is distinct from limited systemic sclerosis (SSc; see Ch. 35) in that morphea is not associated with sclerodactyly, Raynaud phenomenon, nail-fold capillary abnormalities, or internal organ involvement.
- Morphea does not transition into SSc, except for a few rare case reports.
- Equal prevalence in adults and children; more common in females and Caucasians.
- Pathogenesis unknown but thought to involve (like SSc) vascular damage, immune activation, and increased connective tissue production by fibroblasts.
- Approximately 2–5% of children and 30% of adults with morphea have a concomitant autoimmune disease (e.g. alopecia areata, vitiligo) as well as a family history of autoimmunity.
- Classified based on clinical presentation, with five major variants recognized (see Fig. 35.1; Table 36.1).
- Early morphea lesions present as erythematous to violaceous patches and plaques (Fig. 36.1); active lesions often have a lilac border with central hypo- or dyspigmentation;

APPROACH TO THE TREATMENT OF MORPHEA	
Morphea variant	**Treatment**
Circumscribed (plaque) morphea	First line* • Topical class I or intralesional CS • Topical tacrolimus Second line • Lesion-limited phototherapy** ***or*** • Topical imiquimod ***or*** • Topical vitamin D analogue under occlusion ± class I topical CS
Generalized morphea	• Phototherapy** (if no joint contractures; see Fig. 36.8) • Weekly methotrexate† ± systemic CS‡ • Mycophenolate mofetil, JAK inhibitors (e.g. tofacitinib)
Linear morphea	***(Involving face or crossing joints)*** First line • Weekly methotrexate† ± systemic CS‡ Second line • CS-sparing agents (e.g. mycophenolate mofetil)
Pansclerotic morphea	See systemic therapies for generalized morphea • Consider tocilizumab for refractory cases

**If not improved after ~8 to 10 weeks, progress to next line of therapy.*
***Phototherapy choice based on local availability (UVA1, PUVA); NB-UVB may be considered for limited plaque disease.*
†Weekly methotrexate doses: adults, 15–25 mg/week; children, 0.3–0.6 mg/kg/week.
‡Especially for early/progressive lesions; pulsed IV or oral daily × 2-3 months, then tapered.

Table 36.1 Approach to the treatment of morphea. Treatment is most effective in active, inflammatory lesions. Topical monotherapy should not be used if any of the following are present: progressing functional impairment, joint contractures or involvement across joints, linear facial involvement.

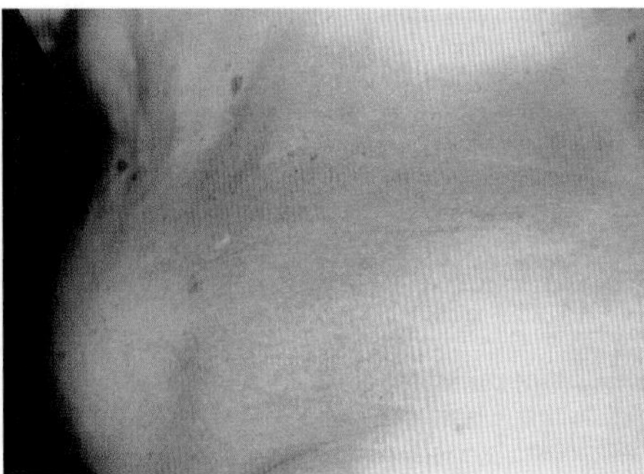

Fig. 36.1 Early inflammatory circumscribed (plaque) morphea of the trunk. Early stage lesion presenting as an erythematous edematous plaque. *Courtesy, Martin Rocken, MD, and Kamran Ghoreschi, MD.*

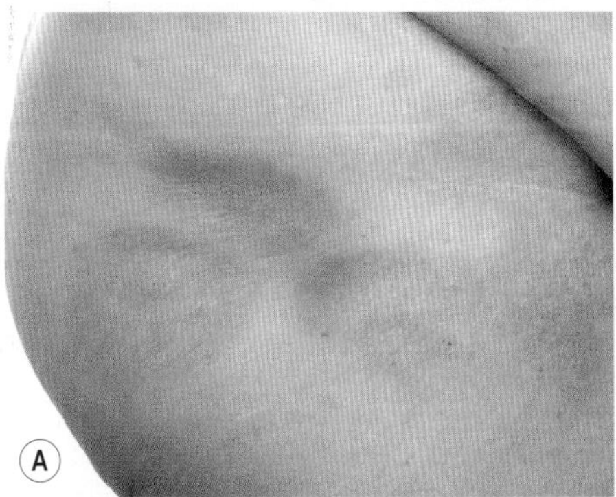

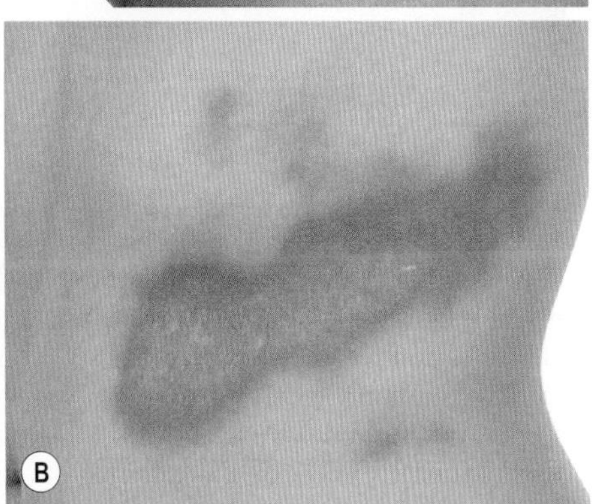

Fig. 36.2 Mid to later stage circumscribed (plaque) morphea. A Sclerotic plaques with the characteristic lilac-colored rim. Histopathologic findings will differ depending upon whether the biopsy specimen is obtained from the inflammatory edge or the central area of the sclerosis. **B** The predominant lesion is a large, well-demarcated, hyperpigmented plaque that is depressed centrally; the trunk is a common location for circumscribed (plaque) morphea. *Courtesy, Martin Rocken, MD.*

inactive lesions are hyperpigmented with variable central sclerosis (Fig. 36.2); usually progresses for several years before regressing; linear variant (below) is more persistent.

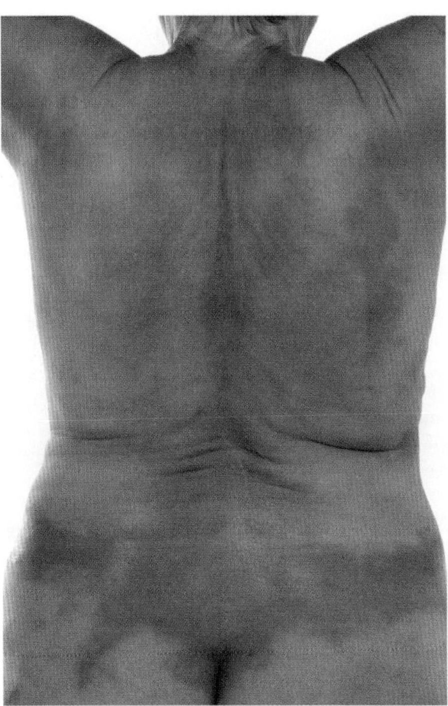

Fig. 36.3 Generalized morphea. Multiple hyperpigmented plaques on the trunk that are becoming confluent. *Courtesy, Martin Rocken, MD.*

- Both ANA and anti-ssDNA Ab can be present.
- *Circumscribed (plaque) morphea* is the most common variant in adults, presenting with ≤3 discrete indurated plaques; the latter favor the trunk and tend to develop in areas of pressure (e.g. hips, waist, and bra line in women); superficial and deep variants (morphea profunda) exist.
- *Generalized morphea* is a rare variant that presents with >3 indurated plaques larger than 3 cm and/or involving ≥2 body sites; spares the face and hands (Figs 36.3, 36.4 and see Fig. 36.8); more likely to have a (+) ANA and systemic symptoms.
- *Linear morphea* is the most common variant in children and may cause a significant degree of morbidity because of either ocular involvement and occasionally CNS involvement in the head variant (Fig. 36.5), or muscle atrophy, discrepancies in limb length, and joint contractures in the limb variant (Fig. 36.6).

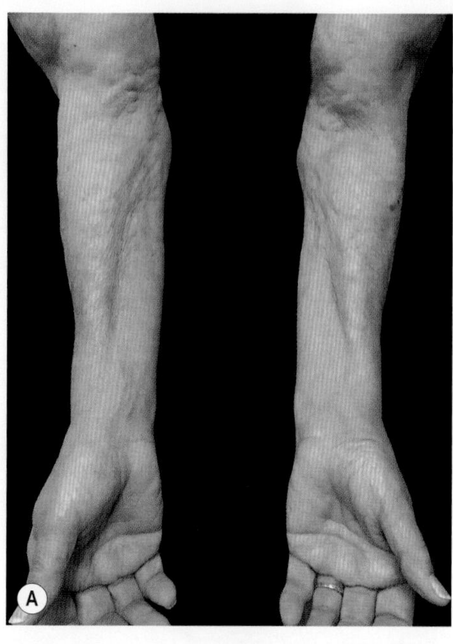

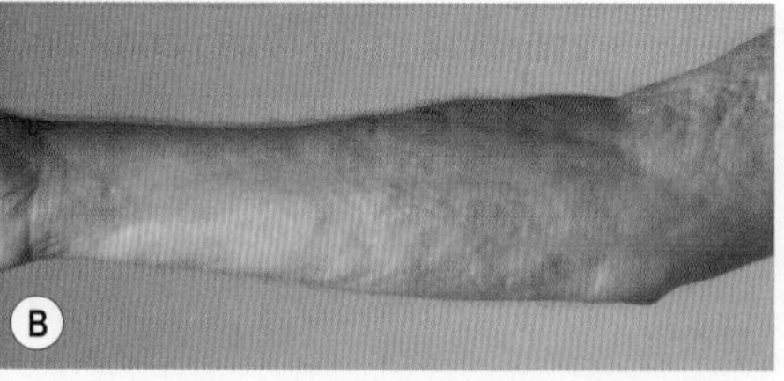

Fig. 36.4 Comparison of deep morphea and eosinophilic fasciitis. It is often difficult to distinguish between deep morphea and eosinophilic fasciitis based upon clinical presentation. **A** Note the "pseudo-cellulite" appearance of the involved skin of the upper arm and the depression or groove in the forearm (due to deep sclerosis) in deep morphea. This patient also had biopsy-proven, generalized morphea on the trunk. The lack of involvement of the hands is a clue that this is not systemic sclerosis (SSc). **B** In eosinophilic fasciitis, the level of fibrosis is also deep, resulting in a similar rippled appearance. This patient had the eosinophilic fasciitis-like form of chronic GVHD, also referred to as chronic GVHD-related fasciitis. *A, Courtesy, Karynne O. Duncan, MD; B, Courtesy, Edward Cowen, MD.*

- *Pansclerotic morphea* is the most debilitating and treatment-resistant variant, but is very rare; it affects the subcutaneous tissues down to and often including the bone; presents as expanding plaques that may eventually coalesce over the entire trunk or extend circumferentially down the extremities; increased risk of cutaneous SCC.
- *Mixed morphea* involves a combination of ≥2 other morphea variants and constitutes ~15% of all morphea cases; overlap with lichen sclerosus can also occur.
- Extracutaneous manifestations are most common in patients with generalized morphea and in children; arthralgia is the most common finding.
- **DDx:** morpheaform disorders (Table 36.2), SSc and sclerodermoid disorders (see Table 35.5), lichen sclerosus, keloids (Fig. 36.7), atrophoderma of Pasini and Perini.
- Morphea and SSc cannot be differentiated by histopathologic examination.
- **Rx:** best utilized during the early, inflammatory stage (see Table 36.1); in general, therapy will not readily reverse established sclerosis; however, the plaques of circumscribed and generalized morphea often soften over a period of years, especially those on the trunk, eventually resembling atrophoderma or completely resolving (Fig. 36.8).

Lichen Sclerosus (LS)

- Formerly called lichen sclerosus et atrophicus.
- A clinically distinct inflammatory disease of the superficial dermis that leads to white, scar-like lesions with surface wrinkling due to epidermal atrophy.
- Most commonly affects female or male genitalia, less often non-genital skin.
- Approximately 80% of LS patients have IgG autoantibodies against extracellular matrix (ECM-1).
- Ultrapotent topical CS are highly effective for treatment of LS; other treatment options are listed in Table 36.3.

Genital LS in Females

- Bimodal presentation: 4–12 years of age and 6th–7th decade.
- Favors vulva and perianal regions; confluent, symmetric involvement of the labial, perineal, and perianal areas has been likened to a "figure 8 configuration".

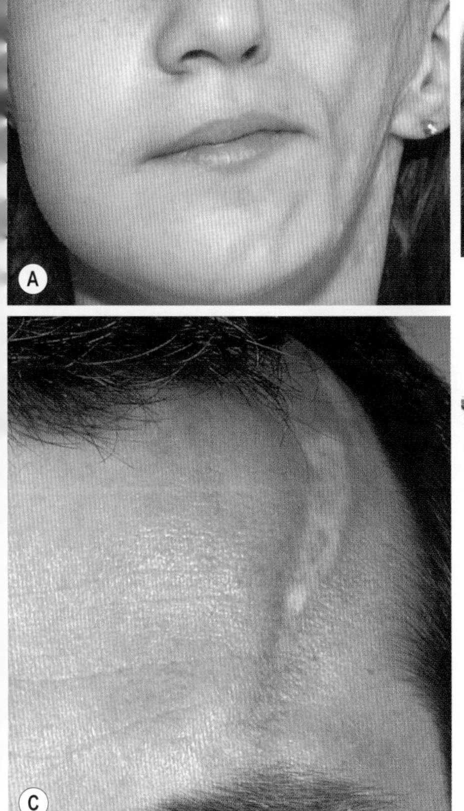

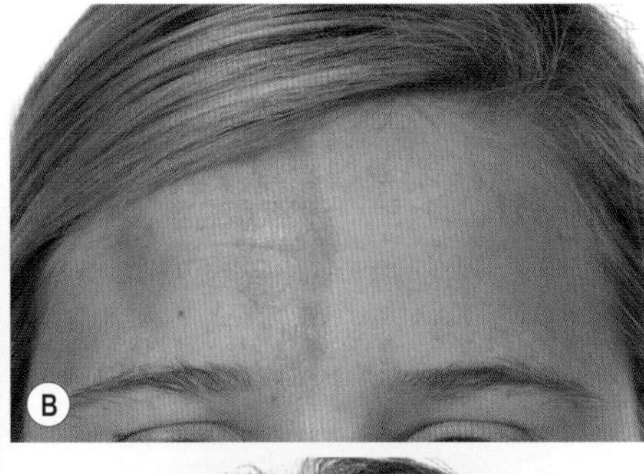

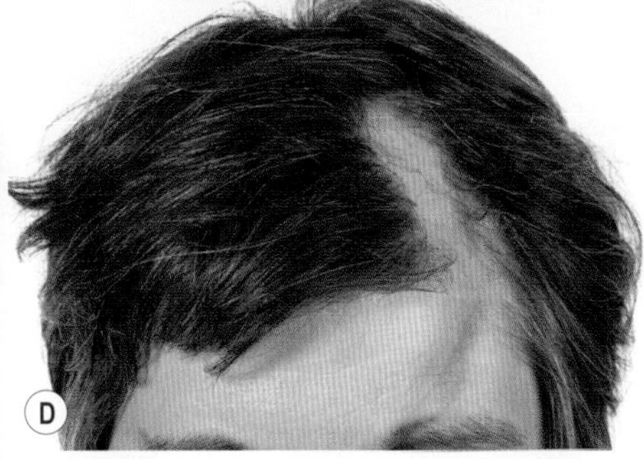

Fig. 36.5 Linear morphea, head variant. **A** Parry–Romberg syndrome, demonstrating unilateral sclerosis and loss of subcutaneous tissue, leading to facial asymmetry. **B–D** *En coup de sabre.* On the forehead, the linear band(s) of sclerosis and atrophy are usually paramedian (rather than midline). **B** Both hyper- and hypopigmentation are present as well as subtle depression. **C** An obviously depressed and sclerotic linear band. **D** When linear morphea extends onto the scalp, it results in scarring alopecia. Note the "lonely hairs" that are seen in various forms of scarring alopecia. *A, Courtesy, Lorenzo Cerroni, MD; B, D, Courtesy, Martin Rocken, MD; C, Courtesy, NYUDSC.*

- **Early:** well-demarcated, erythematous thin plaque(s) ± erosions (Fig. 36.9).
- **Mid:** evolves into dry, hypopigmented sclerotic lesion(s).
- **Late:** obliteration of the labia minora and peri-clitoral structures; narrowing of the vaginal introitus.
- Purpura and perineal fissures are common findings and sometimes mistaken for sexual abuse; lentigines and melanocytic nevi may also be seen within areas of LS.
- Associated symptoms: severe pruritus, soreness, dysuria, dyspareunia, and pain upon defecation.
- May be complicated by possible SCC development, especially if untreated.
- **DDx:** vitiligo, erosive lichen planus, sexual abuse, intraepithelial neoplasia (see Ch. 60), SCC, extramammary Paget disease.

Genital LS in Males

- Also known as balanitis xerotica obliterans.
- Bimodal presentation: prepubertal and older males; more common if uncircumcised.
- Often presents with recurrent balanitis or acquired phimosis; rarely affects perianal region.

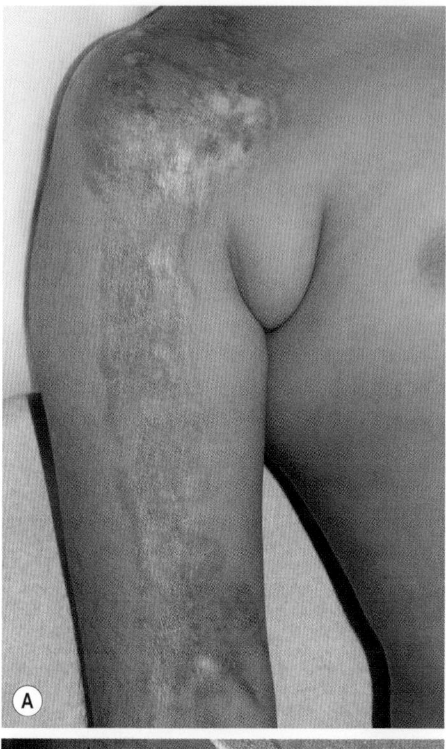

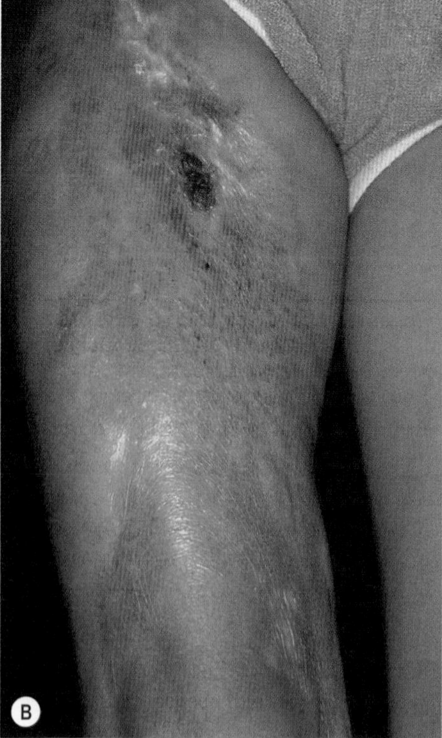

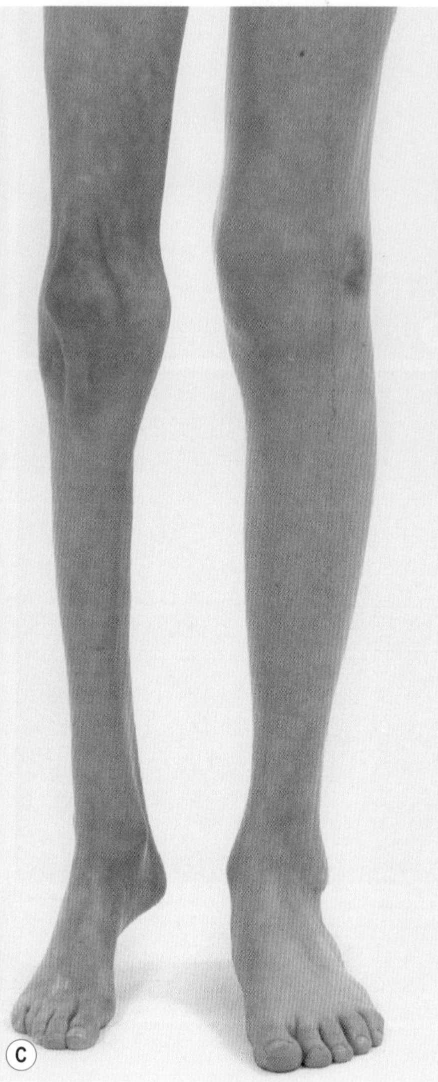

Fig. 36.6 Linear morphea, limb variant. A Linear sclerotic band of the arm with both hyper- and hypopigmentation. The majority of patients with linear morphea have unilateral involvement. **B** More inflammatory phase with ulceration in addition to induration. The differential diagnosis includes linear melorheostosis, which is often associated with underlying candlewax-like linear hyperostosis. **C** Extensive linear morphea of the right leg leading to hypoplasia. In addition to marked hypoplasia, there is induration and a flexion contracture of the knee. *A, Courtesy, Julie V. Schaffer, MD; B, Courtesy, YDRSC; C, Courtesy, Martin Rocken, MD.*

DIFFERENTIAL DIAGNOSIS OF MORPHEAFORM SKIN LESIONS
• Morphea (circumscribed [superficial or deep*], linear, generalized*) • Chronic graft-versus-host disease* • Lichen sclerosus (may coexist with morphea) • Lipodermatosclerosis* • Sclerosis at injection sites** (e.g. vitamin K_1 or B_{12}, silicone or paraffin implants, intralesional bleomycin, interferon-β, glatiramer, enfuvirtide, opioids, vaccinations, antisense oligonucleotides) • Chemical/toxin exposures (e.g. aromatic/chlorinated hydrocarbons*, nephrogenic systemic fibrosis*, toxic oil syndrome [historical]*) • Radiation-induced morphea • Porphyria (e.g. porphyria cutanea tarda) • H syndrome • Stiff skin syndrome*, linear melorheostosis • Reflex sympathetic dystrophy* • Cutaneous metastases (e.g. carcinoma *en cuirasse*)
**Can overlap with sclerodermoid disorders, which are outlined in Table 35.5; in particular, deep morphea and eosinophilic fasciitis may have a similar appearance (see Fig. 36.4).* ***Systemic medications for which there have been reports of an association with morpheaform lesions include bleomycin, taxanes (e.g. paclitaxel, docetaxel), bromocriptine, ethosuximide, valproic acid, appetite suppressants, and penicillamine.*

Table 36.2 Differential diagnosis of morpheaform skin lesions. The location of the morpheaform lesions may offer a clue to the diagnosis, e.g. in lipodermatosclerosis, lesions are located on the lower extremities, and in radiation-induced morphea, lesions are within the radiation port site.

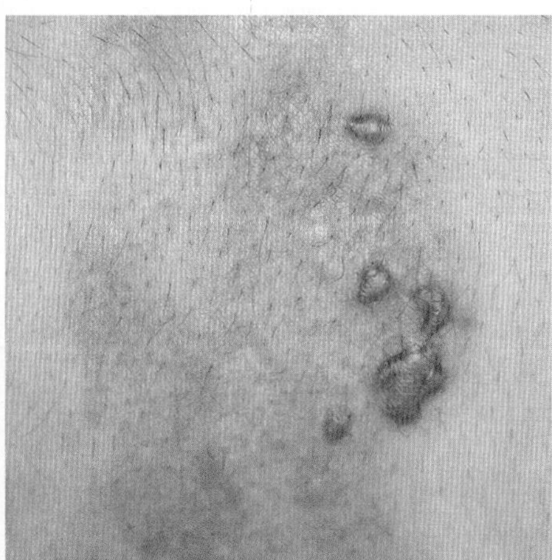

Fig. 36.7 Nodular (keloidal) morphea. Elevated, firm pink papulonodules arising within an area of hyperpigmented induration. *Courtesy, Jean L. Bolognia, MD.*

- **Early:** glans and inner foreskin have well-demarcated, erythematous thin plaques ± erosions.
- **Mid:** evolves into atrophic, white, sclerotic, scar-like lesion(s) (Fig. 36.10).
- **Late:** phimosis or complete occlusion of glans.

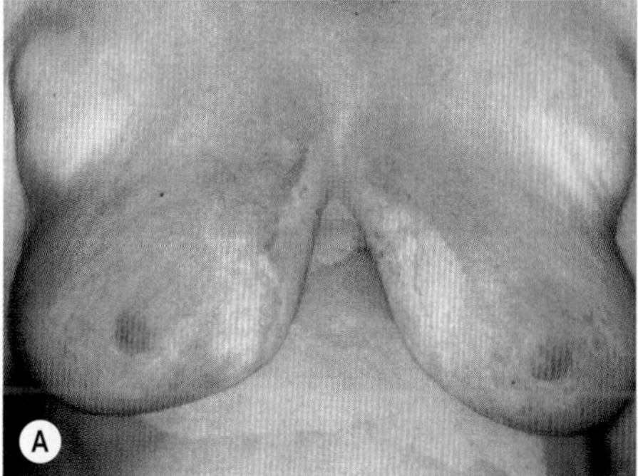

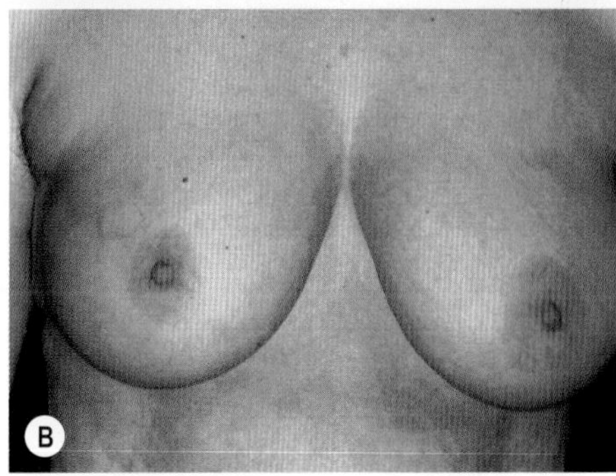

Fig. 36.8 Phototherapy of generalized morphea. Generalized morphea with trunk involvement before **(A)** and after PUVA bath photochemotherapy **(B)**. Note that generalized morphea may involve the breasts but characteristically spares the nipples. *Courtesy, Martin Rocken, MD, and Kamran Ghoreschi, MD.*

TREATMENT OPTIONS FOR LICHEN SCLEROSUS (LS)	
Disease severity	**Treatment**
Mild to moderate	**Clearance**: 6–12 weeks (may need to be repeated yearly if remains clinically active) • Topical class I CS* – daily • Topical calcineurin inhibitors* – daily • Intralesional CS – once to three times during clearance phase, depending upon extent and severity **Maintenance** • Topical petrolatum-based ointments – daily • Topical class VII CS* – daily • Topical class I CS* – occasional, e.g. twice weekly • Topical calcineurin inhibitors* – occasional, e.g. twice weekly
Severe or refractory	• Oral retinoids (acitretin 10–50 mg/day for ≥6 months) • Phototherapy** (e.g. bath PUVA, NB-UVB, UVA1)

**Ointments are preferred over creams for genital LS because they are less irritating.*
***Not recommended for genital LS because increases risk of genital SCC.*

Table 36.3 Treatment options for lichen sclerosus (LS). Some clinicians limit the use of calcineurin inhibitors for genital LS.

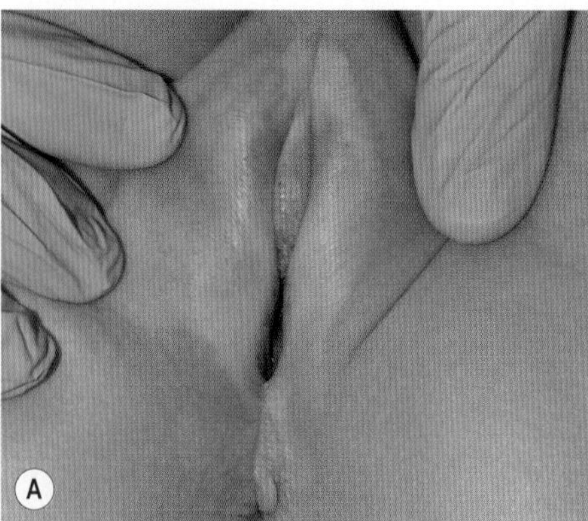

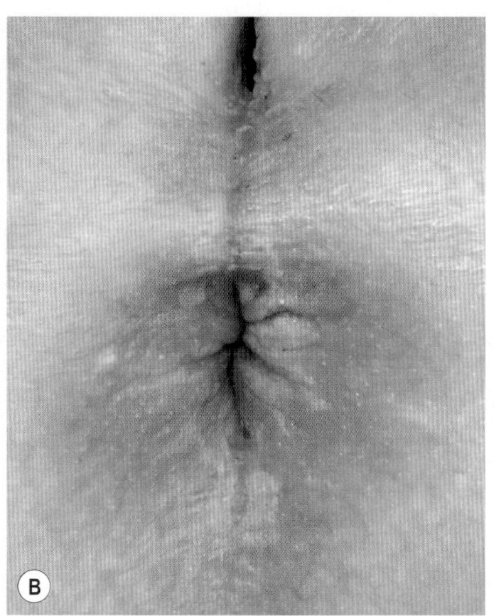

Fig. 36.9 Anogenital lichen sclerosus. **A** Characteristic vulvar, perineal and perianal involvement in a child. Symmetric ivory-colored plaques with a thin pink peripheral rim are seen; a perianal pyramidal protrusion is also present. **B** Perianal lichen sclerosus in which the hypopigmented plaques are accompanied by a linear erosion (skin tear) at 6 o'clock and central fissuring of the perineum. *Courtesy, Martin Rocken, MD.*

• Associated with pruritus and soreness, painful erections, dysuria, urinary obstruction, and possible development of SCC.

• **DDx:** SCC *in situ*, sexual abuse, erosive lichen planus, candidiasis, intraepithelial neoplasia (see Ch. 60), extramammary Paget disease.

Extragenital LS

• Affects all ages with slight female predominance.

• Favors the neck (Fig. 36.11), shoulders, trunk, proximal extremities, flexor wrists, and sites of trauma or pressure; associated xerosis and mild pruritus.

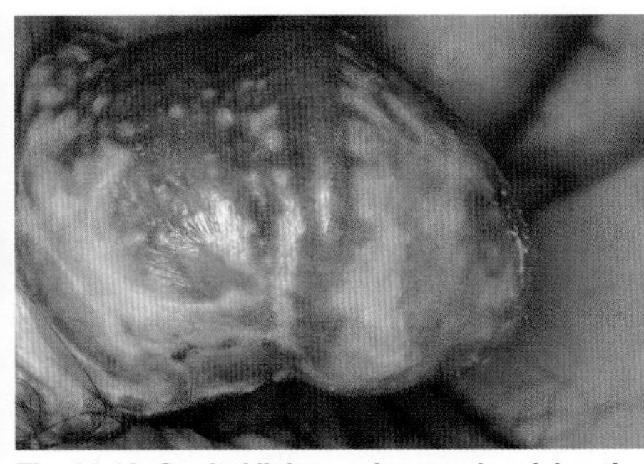

Fig. 36.10 Genital lichen sclerosus involving the penis (balanitis xerotica obliterans). Note the ivory color, erosion, and scarring. *Courtesy, USCDRSC.*

- **Early:** polygonal, white, shiny, papules that often coalesce into plaques.
- **Mid:** evolve into scar-like, atrophic, wrinkled patches and plaques; follicular plugging (Fig. 36.12A).
- **Late:** telangiectasias and occasional hemorrhagic bullae (Fig. 36.12B).
- **DDx:** localized morphea, scar, chronic GVHD; of note, LS (including the genital form) may coexist with morphea and/or vitiligo.

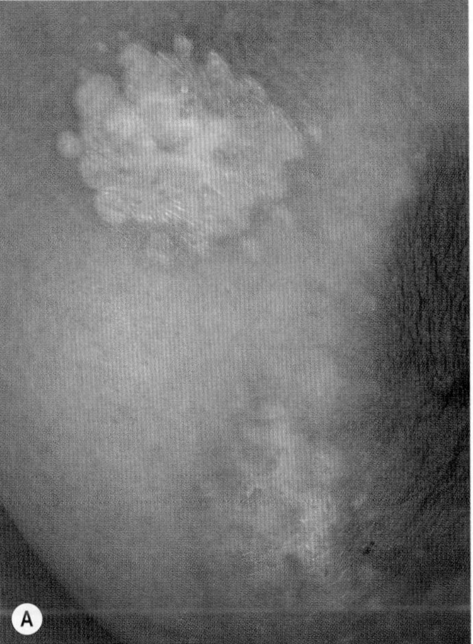

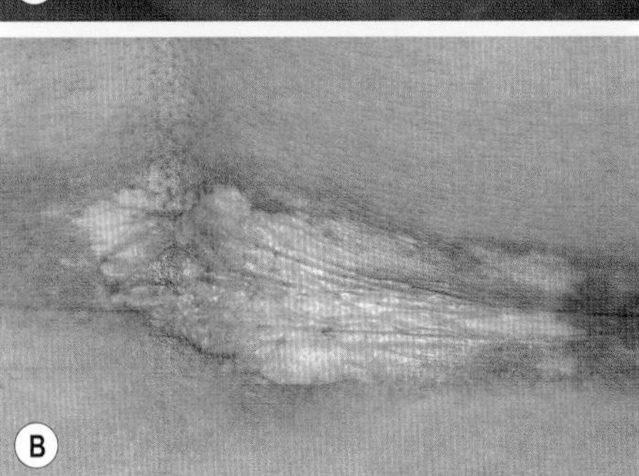

Fig. 36.11 Extragenital lichen sclerosus (LS). Shiny ivory-colored plaques of the breast **(A)** and the lower back **(B)**. Several guttate satellite lesions are present on the breast. *A, Courtesy, Martin Rocken, MD; B, Courtesy, Martin Rocken, MD, and Kamran Ghoreschi, MD.*

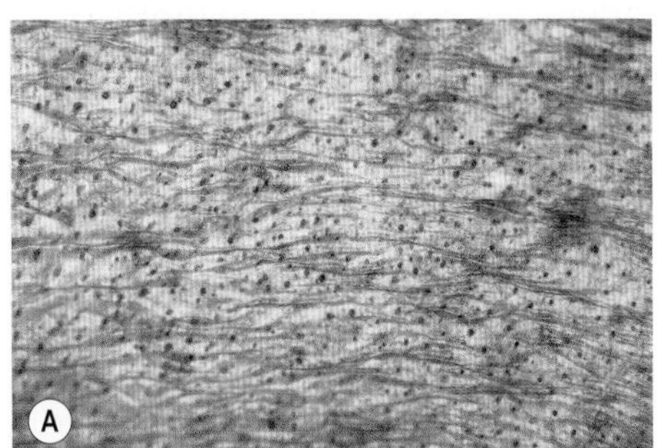

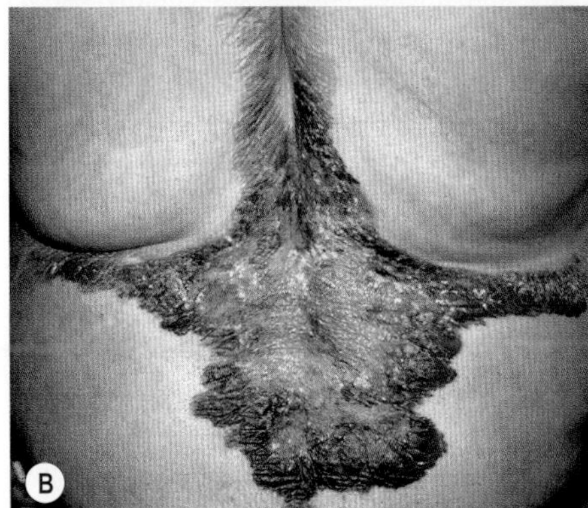

Fig. 36.12 Extragenital lichen sclerosus (LS). A Follicular plugging in a plaque of LS on the back of a patient with chronic GVHD. **B** Hemorrhagic bullae primarily at the periphery of a large plaque on the back. *A, Courtesy, Jean L. Bolognia, MD; B, Courtesy, Luis Requena, MD.*

For further information see Ch. 44 from *Dermatology, Fourth Edition*.

For additional online figures visit www.expertconsult.com 

37 Other Rheumatologic Disorders and Autoinflammatory Diseases

Systemic-Onset Juvenile Idiopathic Arthritis (SoJIA; Still Disease) and Adult-Onset Still Disease (AoSD)

• Among the major types of juvenile idiopathic arthritis (JIA; formerly juvenile rheumatoid arthritis [JRA]), cutaneous manifestations are most common in SoJIA, psoriatic arthritis (see Ch. 6), and rheumatoid factor (RF)-positive polyarthritis (rheumatoid nodules and other findings similar to rheumatoid arthritis [RA]; see below).

• SoJIA can develop at any age prior to 16 years and affects both sexes equally; AoSD has peaks in the second and fourth decades and affects women more often than men.

• Both SoJIA and AoSD are characterized by daily spiking fevers (especially in the late afternoon/early evening) accompanied by an *evanescent* eruption of salmon-pink macules and slightly edematous papules and plaques (Fig. 37.1A; see Table 37.3); these lesions are usually asymptomatic and favor sites of pressure or trauma, often occurring in a linear array.

• Less common skin findings include periorbital edema and persistent pruritic papules and plaques that are scaly, violaceous to reddish brown in color, and linear in configuration (Fig. 37.1B).

• Additional features include a prodromal sore throat and arthralgias/myalgias, arthritis (usually polyarticular; ± carpal ankylosis in AoSD), lymphadenopathy, hepatosplenomegaly, and serositis; occasionally patients may develop macrophage activation syndrome (also characterized by markedly elevated ferritin).

• Leukocytosis with neutrophilia, thrombocytosis, anemia, elevated ESR/CRP, and extremely high serum ferritin levels (e.g. >4000 mg/ml) are common laboratory findings, whereas ANA and RF are usually absent.

• **DDx:** serum sickness-like reactions, urticarial vasculitis, Schnitzler syndrome (in adults; see Ch. 14), other autoimmune connective tissue diseases, rheumatic fever, infections (e.g. parvovirus B19, rat bite fever, malaria), hereditary periodic fever syndromes (see Table 3.2), and malignancies (e.g. leukemia, lymphoma).

• **Rx:** NSAIDs (for mild disease), systemic CS, methotrexate, antagonists of IL-1 (e.g. anakinra, canakinumab) or IL-6 (e.g. tocilizumab), and TNF inhibitors (the latter especially for arthritis).

Rheumatoid Arthritis

• Chronic inflammatory disorder characterized primarily by destructive arthritis.

• Affects 1–3% of adults, with a female:male ratio of 2–3:1 and a peak onset between 35 and 60 years of age.

• RF and anti-cyclic citrullinated peptide (CCP) antibodies represent serologic markers of RA.

• Cutaneous manifestations of RA are presented in Table 37.1 and Fig. 37.2; these findings can serve as diagnostic clues or signs of serious systemic disease.

Sjögren Syndrome

• Autoimmune disorder primarily affecting the lacrimal and salivary glands, resulting in xerophthalmia and xerostomia; may coexist with other AI-CTDs (e.g. LE).

• Affects ~0.5% of the general population, with a female:male ratio of 9:1; peak onset is in the fourth and fifth decades of life, but can occur at any age.

• Cutaneous manifestations include xerosis, palpable purpura due to small vessel

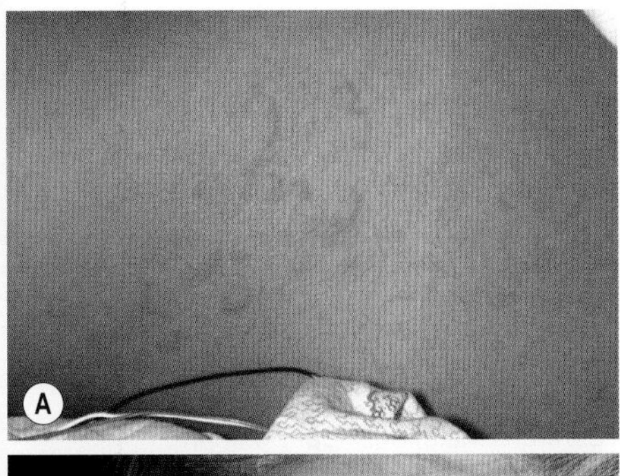

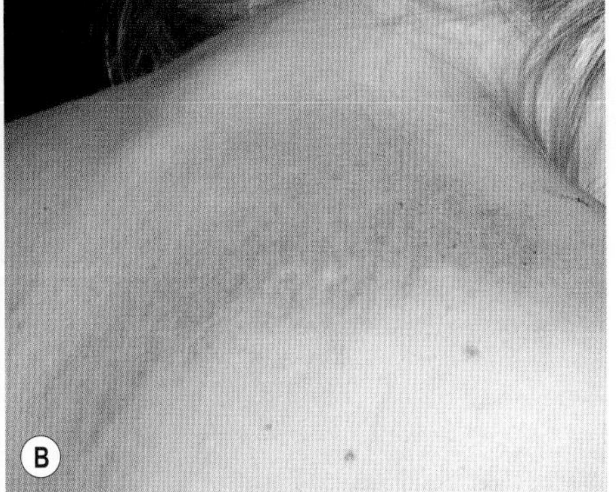

Fig. 37.1 Cutaneous findings in Still disease. **A** Evanescent pink papules and figurate plaques in a child. **B** Flagellate array of pinkish-tan, scaly persistent plaques on the upper back in a teenage girl. *A, Courtesy, YDRSC; B, Courtesy, Julie V. Schaffer, MD.*

vasculitis (including cryoglobulinemic vasculitis), hypergammaglobulinemic purpura of Waldenström, urticarial vasculitis, annular erythema, and Raynaud phenomenon.

- Additional features can include vaginal dryness, arthritis, peripheral neuropathy, internal organ involvement (e.g. kidneys), and development of B-cell lymphoma (often extranodal marginal zone).
- Majority of patients have anti-SSA/Ro and anti-SSB/La antibodies, a positive RF, and an elevated ESR.
- Diagnostic criteria for Sjögren syndrome are presented in Table 37.2.
- **Rx:** mostly symptomatic – use of artificial tears and saliva (e.g. methylcellulose drops), chewing sugar-free gum, meticulous dental hygiene, and treatment of superimposed oral candidiasis; sicca symptoms may improve with cyclosporine eye drops, lifitegrast eye drops, or cholinergic agonists (e.g. pilocarpine, cevimeline); vasculitis or internal involvement often require systemic CS, conventional immunosuppressive agents, or rituximab.

Relapsing Polychondritis

- Uncommon autoimmune condition that affects cartilaginous structures; pathogenesis is thought to involve a reaction against type II collagen.
- Most patients develop erythema, swelling and pain of the cartilaginous portion of the auricle, with sparing of the earlobe (Fig. 37.3A).
- Other manifestations include cutaneous small vessel vasculitis (Fig. 37.3B), aphthae (oral or genital; may overlap with Behçet disease), nasal chondritis (potentially producing a saddle nose deformity), involvement of cartilage of the respiratory tract (e.g. larynx, trachea, bronchi) and costochondral junctions, arthritis, ocular inflammation, audiovestibular damage, and myelodysplastic syndrome.
- **DDx:** *early phase* – erysipelas, cellulitis, infectious chondritis or zoster; *nasal destruction* – granulomatosis with polyangiitis, nasal natural killer/T-cell lymphoma, infections (e.g. mucocutaneous leishmaniasis) (see Table 19.3).
- **Rx:** prednisone (for acute flares), dapsone, immunosuppressive agents, TNF inhibitors; surgical repair of damaged cartilaginous structures.

Mixed Connective Tissue Disease (MCTD)

- Characterized by high-titer anti-U1 ribonucleoprotein (U1-RNP) antibodies plus a constellation of clinical features including arthritis, myositis, and findings of systemic sclerosis; the latter range from swollen hands and Raynaud phenomenon to esophageal dysmotility and pulmonary hypertension (the most serious complication) or fibrosis (often mild).
- Favors women (female:male ratio ~9:1) in the second and third decades of life.
- Edema and erythema of the digits is an early manifestation; digital infarcts, periungual telangiectasias with dropout areas, sclerodactyly, and calcinosis cutis may also develop.
- Poikiloderma on the upper trunk and proximal extremities is common; photosensitivity,

CUTANEOUS MANIFESTATIONS OF RHEUMATOID ARTHRITIS (RA)	
Condition	**Features**
Palisading granulomas	
Rheumatoid nodules	• Affect ~20% of RA patients, often associated with high-titer RF • Firm, semi-mobile papulonodules favoring periarticular locations (e.g. elbows; Fig. 37.2A) and other sites of repetitive trauma or pressure (e.g. the sacral region if bedridden) • **DDx:** subcutaneous granuloma annulare, gouty tophi, synovial hyperplasia/cysts (softer, painful) • Histologically, central zone of eosinophilic fibrin surrounded by palisaded histiocytes
Interstitial granulomatous dermatitis (IGD) and palisaded neutrophilic & granulomatous dermatitis (PNGD)	• See Ch. 78; the PNGD spectrum includes *rheumatoid papules* (Fig. 37.2B) and *superficial ulcerating rheumatoid necrobiosis* (Fig. 37.2C)
Neutrophilic dermatoses	
Rheumatoid neutrophilic dermatitis	• Erythematous papules and plaques that may be vesiculated or crusted; favors extensor extremities • Unlike Sweet syndrome, *not* tender or associated with fevers and malaise
Sweet syndrome and pyoderma gangrenosum (PG)*	• See Ch. 21; Fig. 37.2D
Neutrophilic lobular panniculitis	• Tender red nodules favoring the lower legs; may ulcerate with purulent drainage
Vasculitis and vascular reactions	
Bywaters lesions	• Punctate purpuric papules on the distal digits due to cutaneous small vessel vasculitis (Fig. 37.2E)
Rheumatoid vasculitis	• Associated with long-standing (often "burnt out") joint disease, high-titer RF, and mononeuritis multiplex; may also affect the eyes and internal organs • Cutaneous involvement is usually the first manifestation – *Small vessel vasculitis*: purpuric macules and papules – *Medium-sized vessel vasculitis*: nodules, ulcers, digital gangrene, livedo reticularis, atrophie blanche-like scars • Systemic disease requires aggressive immunosuppressive therapy
Intravascular/intralymphatic histiocytosis	• Erythema, induration and papules in a reticular pattern overlying swollen joints, most often the elbows
Erythema elevatum diutinum	• Firm, red to yellow-brown papulonodules and plaques, usually on extensor surfaces (see Ch. 19)
Complications of therapy for RA	
NSAIDs	• Pseudoporphyria, toxic epidermal necrolysis
Methotrexate >> TNF inhibitors	• Accelerated rheumatoid nodulosis – sudden appearance of multiple papulonodules, especially on the hands (Fig. 37.2F)
TNF inhibitors	• Injection site reactions, urticaria, urticarial eruptions, vasculitis, IGD, cutaneous LE, psoriasiform eruptions, palmoplantar pustulosis, dermatomyositis

"PG-like" leg ulcers are a feature of Felty syndrome, which is characterized by the triad of neutropenia, splenomegaly, and RA; Felty syndrome may be associated with T-cell large granular lymphocyte leukemia.

Table 37.1 Cutaneous manifestations of rheumatoid arthritis (RA).

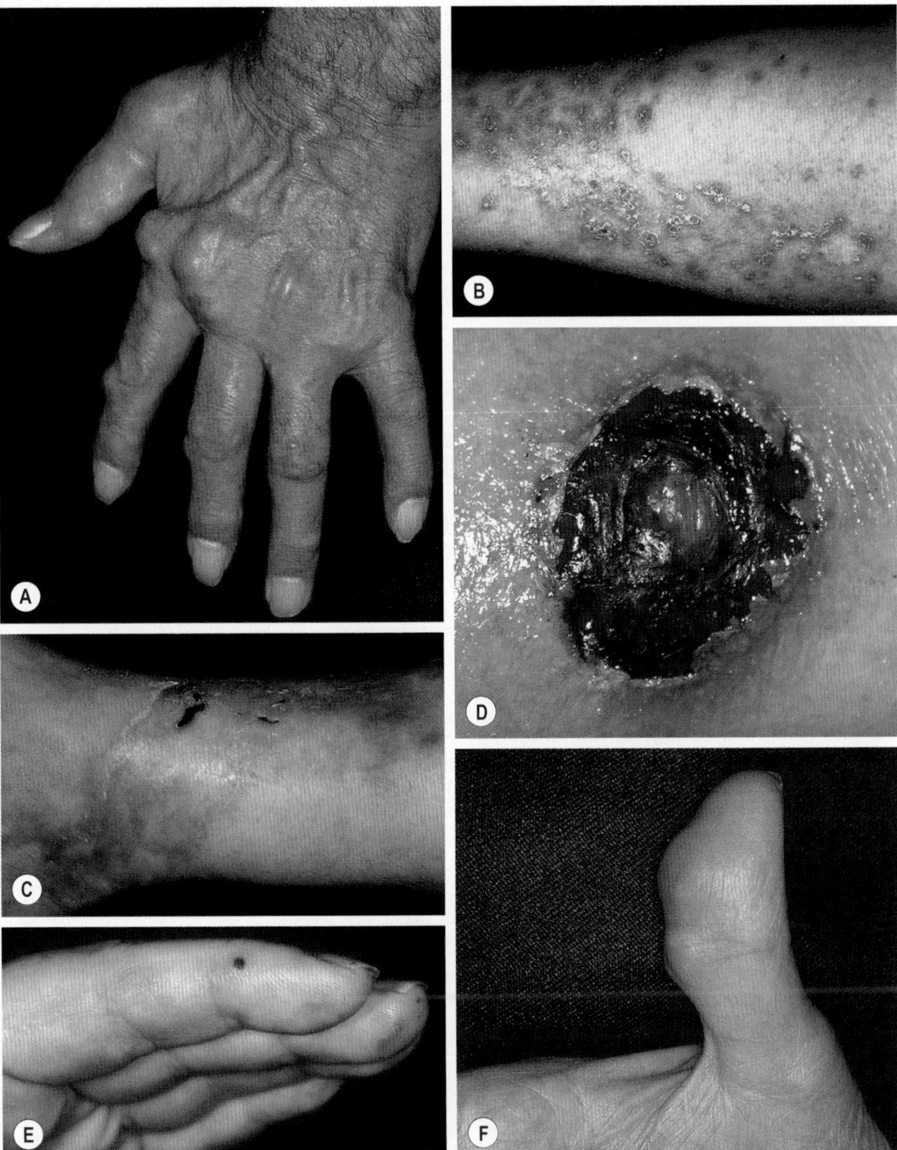

Fig. 37.2 Cutaneous findings in rheumatoid arthritis. **A** Rheumatoid nodules in a periarticular location on the hands. **B** Rheumatoid papules presenting as coalescing red-brown lesions, some with scale-crust, on the lower extremity. **C** Superficial ulcerating rheumatoid necrobiosis manifesting as shiny, yellow-brown plaques with red-brown borders and areas of ulceration; these clinical findings are reminiscent of necrobiosis lipoidica, although both this entity and rheumatoid papules are categorized as forms of palisaded neutrophilic and granulomatous dermatitis (see Ch. 78). **D** Pyoderma gangrenosum resulting in recurrent ulcerations on the lower extremities. **E** Bywaters lesions. These tender purpuric papules on the distal fingers are characterized histologically by leukocytoclastic vasculitis. **F** Methotrexate-induced nodulosis. *A, Courtesy, Kalman Watsky, MD; B, C, E, Courtesy, Jeffrey Callen, MD; D, Courtesy, Carlos Nousari, MD; F, Courtesy, Jean L. Bolognia, MD.*

malar erythema, and subacute cutaneous LE occasionally occur.

- **DDx:** features overlap with those of systemic sclerosis, dermatomyositis/polymyositis, and SLE; for this reason, the debate continues regarding the distinction between MCTD (a specific entity requiring the presence of elevated U1-RNP) and less specific "overlap syndromes" (features of two or more AI-CTDs in a single patient).

AMERICAN COLLEGE OF RHEUMATOLOGY (ACR)/EUROPEAN LEAGUE AGAINST RHEUMATISM (ELAR) 2016 CLASSIFICATION CRITERIA FOR PRIMARY SJÖGREN'S SYNDROME (SjS)	
The classification of primary SjS applies to any individual who meets the inclusion criteria*, does not have any of the conditions listed as exclusion criteria^, and has a score of ≥4 when the weights from the five criteria items below are summed	
Criterion	**Weight/score**
Labial salivary gland with focal lymphocytic sialadenitis and focus score of ≥1 foci/4 mm^2	3
Anti-SSA/Ro-positive	3
Ocular staining score ≥5 (or van Bijsterveld score >4) in at least one eye^^	1
Schirmer's test ≤5 mm/5 min in at least one eye^^	1
Unstimulated whole saliva flow rate ≤0.1 mL/min^^	1

Inclusion criteria apply to any patient with at least one symptom of ocular or oral dryness, defined as a positive response to at least 1 of the following questions: (1) Have you had daily, persistent, troublesome dry eyes for more than 3 months? (2) Do you have a recurrent sensation of sand or gravel in the eyes? (3) Do you use tear substitutes more than 3 times a day? (4) Have you had a daily feeling of dry mouth for more than 3 months? (5) Do you frequently drink liquids to aid in swallowing dry food? or in whom there is suspicion of SjS from the ELAR SjS Disease Activity Questionnaire (at least 1 domain with a positive item).

^Exclusion criteria include prior diagnosis of any of the following conditions: (1) history of head and neck radiation treatment; (2) active hepatitis C infection (with confirmation by PCR); (3) AIDS; (4) sarcoidosis; (5) amyloidosis; (6) GVHD; (7) IgG4-related disease.

^^Patients taking anticholinergic drugs should be evaluated after a sufficient interval without these medications for tests to be valid.

Table 37.2 American College of Rheumatology (ACR)/European League Against Rheumatism (ELAR) 2016 classification criteria for primary Sjögren syndrome. Other possible causes of similar findings include chronic GVHD, primary systemic amyloidosis, sarcoidosis, and radiation therapy of the head and neck. *Adapted from Shiboski et al. Ann Rheum Dis 2017;76:9.*

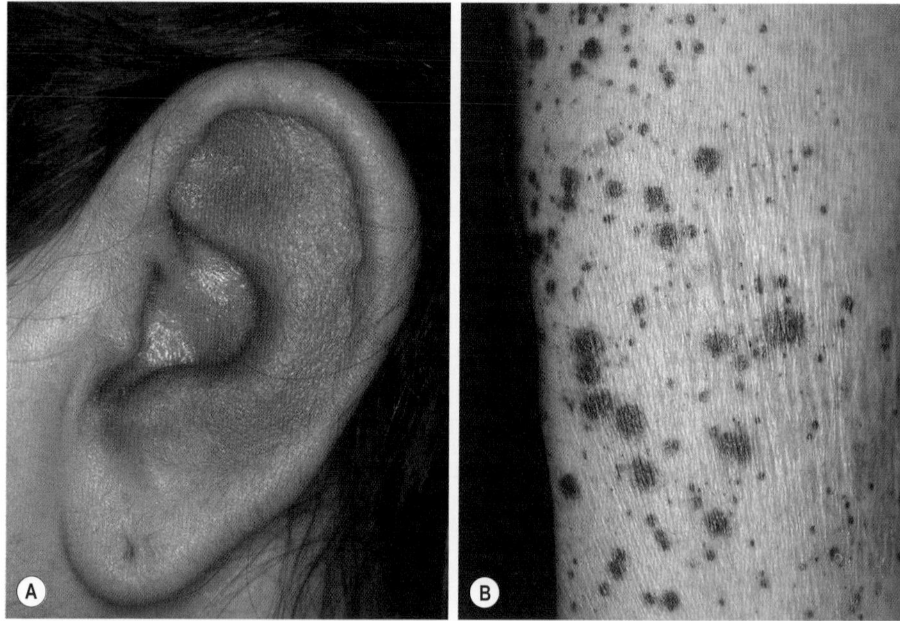

Fig. 37.3 Cutaneous findings in relapsing polychondritis. A Erythema and swelling of the ear with sparing of the earlobe. **B** Small vessel vasculitis presenting as palpable purpura in a patient who also had a myelodysplastic syndrome. *A, Courtesy, Kalman Watsky, MD; B, Courtesy, Jean L. Bolognia, MD.*

- **Rx:** varies depending on the organs involved and disease severity.

Autoinflammatory Diseases

- Monogenic diseases related to aberrant activation of the innate immune system that are characterized by recurrent fevers and/or flares of multi-organ inflammation; the skin is frequently involved as are the musculoskeletal system, eyes, and serosae.
- This group includes the hereditary periodic fever syndromes (see Table 3.2), type I interferonopathies, deficiency of interleukin (IL)-1 receptor (DIRA), and CARD14-mediated pustular psoriasis.
- Cutaneous lesions vary from evanescent urticarial papules and sterile pustules to pyoderma gangrenosum and pernio-like lesions (Table 37.3).
- Increased production of IL-1 via inflammasomes can be seen and several of these entities respond to IL-1 antagonists, e.g. anakinra, rilonacept, canakinumab.
- Complex disorders such as Schnitzler syndrome and systemic-onset juvenile idiopathic arthritis (Still disease) share mechanistic and clinical features.

For further information see Ch. 45 from *Dermatology, Fourth Edition*.

For additional online figures and tables visit www.expertconsult.com 

RANGE OF CUTANEOUS FINDINGS IN INHERITED AUTOINFLAMMATORY DISEASE				
	Cutaneous and histologic features	Inherited autoinflammatory disease(s) – examples		Sporadic or complex disorders with similar findings
		Disorder	Other features†	
	Evanescent maculopapular/urticarial eruption, often cold-induced and (in CAPS) with a dermal neutrophilic infiltrate	CAPS PLAID	• CAPS: conjunctivitis, hearing loss, oral ulcers; LAN, HSM, and aseptic meningitis in NOMID variant • PLAID: recurrent infections, antibody deficiency, autoimmunity; occasionally cutaneous granulomas	• Schnitzler syndrome (Ch. 14) • *Adult-onset Still disease* (pictured) • *Systemic-onset juvenile idiopathic arthritis (SoJIA; Still disease)*
	Ulcerations, with a sterile neutrophilic infiltrate within the dermis* (pyoderma gangrenosum)	PAPA syndrome**	• Arthritis	Pyoderma gangrenosum – idiopathic and in the setting of associated disorders (e.g. ulcerative colitis) (Ch. 21) (pictured)

**Untreated lesion.*
***PASH (pyoderma gangrenosum, acne, and suppurative hidradenitis) and PAPASH (pyogenic arthritis, pyoderma gangrenosum, acne, and suppurative hidradenitis) syndromes are considered variants of PAPA syndrome.*
†Recurrent fevers also occur in many of these disorders.

Table 37.3 *Continued* **Range of cutaneous findings in inherited autoinflammatory diseases.** Disorders discussed in this chapter are in italics. CAPS, cryopyrin-associated periodic syndrome; PAPA, pyogenic arthritis, pyoderma gangrenosum, and acne; PLAID, PLCG2-associated antibody deficiency and immune dysregulation; NOMID, neonatal-onset multisystem inflammatory disease. *Picture courtesies: Diane Davidson, MD (adult-onset Still disease); Gillian Clarke, MD (DIRA); Kalman Watsky, MD (Sweet syndrome); Edward Cowen, MD (ADA2 deficiency); Julie V. Schaffer, MD (AGS, Blau syndrome). Continued*

RANGE OF CUTANEOUS FINDINGS IN INHERITED AUTOINFLAMMATORY DISEASE

	Cutaneous and histologic features	Inherited autoinflammatory disease(s) – examples		Sporadic or complex disorders with similar findings
		Disorder	Other features†	
	Pustules (sterile)	DIRA (pictured) DITRA PAPA syndrome** CAMPS	• DIRA: sterile osteolytic bone lesions, neonatal distress • PAPA: arthritis	Generalized pustular psoriasis Impetigo herpetiformis SAPHO syndrome (Ch. 21) Acne fulminans
	Edematous plaques, with a sterile neutrophilic infiltrate within the dermis or panniculus	Majeed syndrome VEXAS Haploinsufficiency of A20 (Behçet-like) ORAS	• Majeed: sterile multifocal osteomyelitis, dyserythropoietic anemia • VEXAS: periorbital edema, polyarteritis nodosa; myelodysplastic syndrome, arthralgias, polychondritis, pulmonary infiltrates • ORAS: lipodystrophy, joint swelling, diarrhea	Sweet syndrome – idiopathic or occurring in the setting of associated disorders (e.g. acute myelogenous leukemia) (Ch. 21) (pictured) Behçet disease (Ch. 21)

Table 37.3 *Continued* **Range of cutaneous findings in inherited autoinflammatory diseases.** CAMPS, CARD-14-mediated pustular psoriasis; DIRA, deficiency of interleukin-1 receptor antagonist; DITRA, deficiency of interleukin-36 receptor antagonist; ORAS, *OTULIN*-related autoinflammatory syndrome; SAPHO, synovitis, acne, pustulosis, hyperostosis, osteitis; VEXAS, vacuoles, E1 enzyme, X-linked, autoinflammatory, somatic. *Continued*

RANGE OF CUTANEOUS FINDINGS IN INHERITED AUTOINFLAMMATORY DISEASE				
	Cutaneous and histologic features	Inherited autoinflammatory disease(s) – examples		Sporadic or complex disorders with similar findings
		Disorder	Other features†	
	Livedo racemosa with nodules	ADA2 deficiency (pictured)	• Early-onset strokes, HSM, lymphopenia	Sneddon syndrome Sporadic polyarteritis nodosa
	Violaceous plaques that resemble pernio, cutaneous LE, or dermatomyositis; periorbital edema & erythema	PRAAS/CANDLE syndrome‡ Aicardi-Goutières syndrome (AGS) (pictured)/familial chilblain lupus (FCL)‡	• PRAAS: lipomuscular atrophy, joint contractures • AGS: encephalopathy, white matter changes, progressive intellectual disability • FCL: arthritis	Lupus erythematosus Dermatomyositis
	Small papules with dermal granulomatous infiltrate	Blau syndrome (familial juvenile systemic granulomatosis) (pictured)	• Uveitis, polyarticular arthritis	Sarcoidosis

‡*Type I interferonopathies; this group also includes SAVI (STING [stimulator of interferon genes]-associated vasculopathy with onset in infancy), which features acral violaceous plaques/ulcers/gangrene/bone resorption and interstitial lung disease. Of note, the violaceous plaques of PRAAS typically have dermal infiltrates of myeloid cells (immature or mature)*

Table 37.3 *Continued* **Range of cutaneous findings in inherited autoinflammatory diseases.** ADA, adenosine deaminase; CANDLE, chronic atypical neutrophilic

Mucinoses 38

In this group of disorders, there is deposition of glycosaminoglycans, previously referred to as mucopolysaccharides ("mucin"), within the skin, especially the dermis. Most often, the deposit is composed of hyaluronic acid. While several of the entities are idiopathic, underlying disorders include autoimmune thyroid disease, a monoclonal gammopathy, diabetes mellitus, and LE.

Scleredema

- Symmetric diffuse induration of the skin, usually limited to the upper back and posterior neck, that may require palpation to be appreciated; a *peau d'orange* appearance may be present with prominent follicular orifices, and occasionally there is blanching erythema in the sites of involvement (Fig. 38.1).
- While scleredema is often asymptomatic, some patients may complain of tightness or decreased range-of-motion; occasionally there is also involvement of the face and upper extremities and, rarely, the muscles, eyes, or heart.

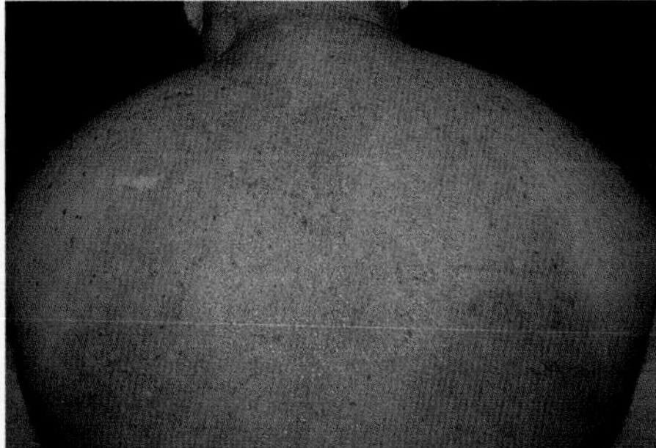

Fig. 38.1 Scleredema in association with diabetes mellitus. Diffuse induration of the upper back and neck with overlying erythema. *Courtesy, USCDRSC.*

- The three major types have different associations: type I – preceding streptococcal infections; type II – monoclonal gammopathy; and type III – diabetes mellitus, with men representing the majority of patients.
- **DDx:** systemic sclerosis (diffuse form), scleromyxedema, and other sclerodermoid disorders (see Table 35.5); occasionally, cellulitis if erythema is present.
- **Rx:** sometimes there is spontaneous resolution, especially with type I disease, but control of underlying diabetes mellitus usually does not lead to improvement; anecdotal therapies include phototherapy (UVA1, PUVA), methotrexate, electron beam therapy, IVIg, and multiple myeloma therapies (e.g. bortezomib) if there is an associated monoclonal gammopathy.

Scleromyxedema/Papular Mucinosis

- A spectrum of clinical findings that varies from multiple linear arrays of firm, 2- to 3-mm, waxy, skin-colored papules (Fig. 38.2) to diffuse induration of the skin with thickened folds, including leonine facies (Fig. 38.3; Table 38.1); involvement is symmetric and often widespread.
- Associated with an underlying monoclonal gammopathy; in addition to skin stiffness, there can be decreased range-of-motion of joints and contractures as well as myositis, peripheral neuropathy, and encephalopathy (dermato-neuro syndrome).
- **DDx:** systemic sclerosis, scleredema; if primarily papules are present, primary systemic amyloidosis, lipoid proteinosis, and especially the various types of skin-limited (localized) mucinoses, e.g. acral persistent papular mucinosis, the discrete papular form of lichen myxedematosus, self-healing cutaneous mucinosis (also has nodules).
- **Rx:** similar to that of multiple myeloma (see primary systemic amyloidosis, Ch. 39),

systemic retinoids, phototherapy (UVA1, PUVA), IVIg.

Pretibial Myxedema

- In the vast majority of patients, associated with hyperthyroidism which is primarily due to Graves disease, an autoimmune disorder with circulating anti-thyroid-stimulating hormone receptor autoantibodies; skin lesions may appear following treatment of the thyroid disease, i.e. when the patient is euthyroid or has developed hypothyroidism.
- Favors the shins but can involve the foot and presents as indurated, waxy nodules or plaques that vary from skin-colored to red-brown (Fig. 38.4); prominent follicular openings may be seen (a *peau d'orange* appearance) and occasionally elephantiasis develops.
- Additional clinical findings include exophthalmos, goiter, and thyroid acropachy.
- **DDx:** obesity-associated lymphedematous mucinosis (no history of hyperthyroidism), lymphedema, lipedema, lichen amyloidosis.

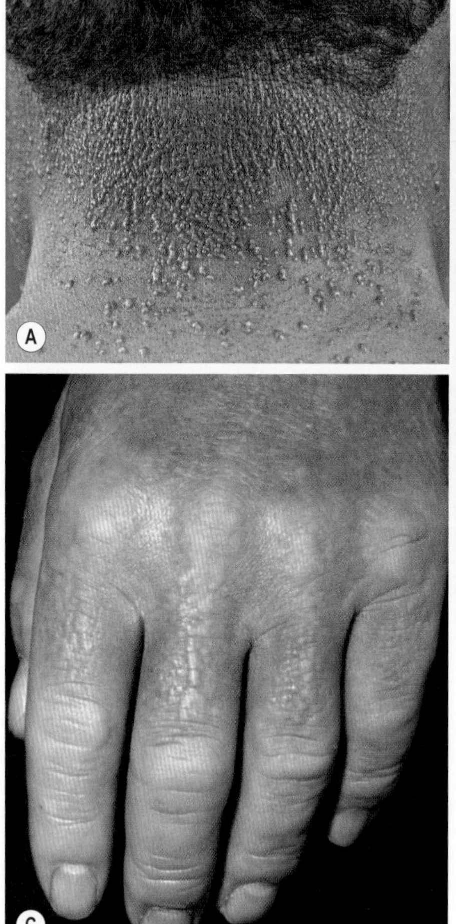

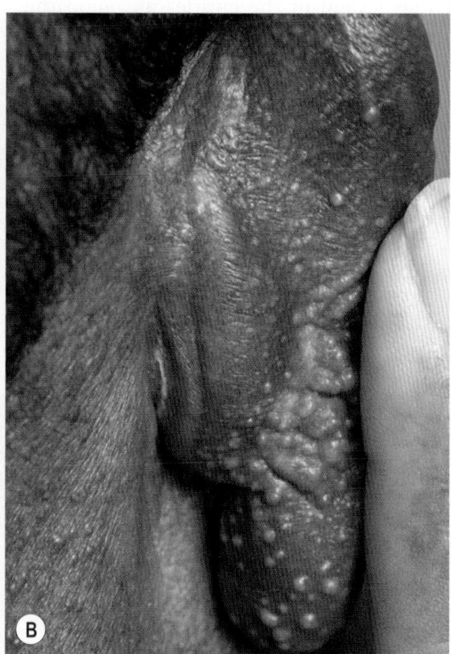

Fig. 38.2 Scleromyxedema/papular mucinosis. A, B Numerous monomorphic, firm, skin-colored to tan papules which can have a striking linear arrangement. This is most obvious on the upper posterior neck. **C** The skin can also become shiny and indurated, leading to a sclerodermoid appearance, but the small firm papules in a linear array are a clue to the diagnosis. *A,B, Courtesy, Edward Cowen, MD; C, Courtesy, Lorenzo Cerroni, MD.*

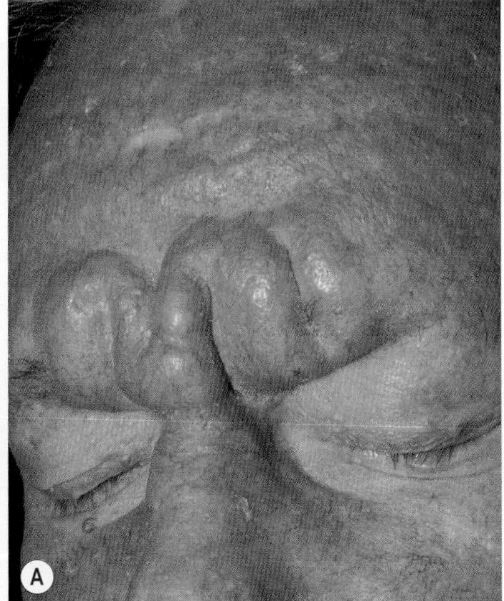

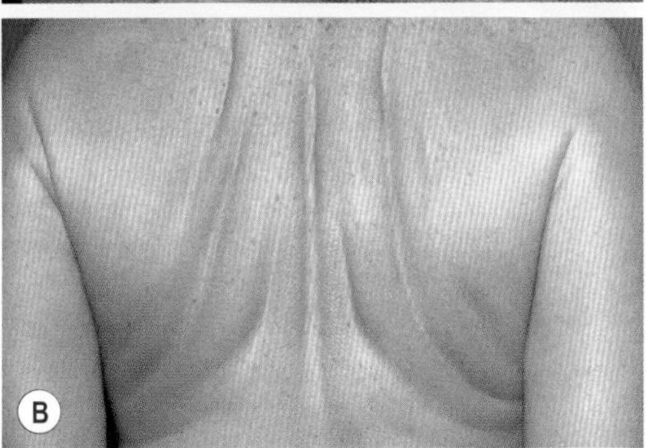

Fig. 38.3 Scleromyxedema. Thickening of the skin of the forehead **(A)** and trunk **(B)**, leading to deep furrows and folds. Scleromyxedema is one of the causes of leonine facies. *A, Courtesy, Joyce Rico, MD; B, Courtesy, Lorenzo Cerroni, MD.*

LEONINE FACIES – ASSOCIATED DERMATOLOGIC DISEASES
• Scleromyxedema/papular mucinosis • Lepromatous leprosy • Leishmaniasis • Cutaneous lymphoma (T-cell, B-cell) • Actinic reticuloid form of chronic actinic dermatitis • Leukemia cutis • Primary systemic amyloidosis • Pachydermoperiostosis • Lipoid proteinosis

Table 38.1 Leonine facies – associated dermatologic diseases. Additional causes include sarcoidosis, mastocytosis, multicentric reticulohistiocytosis, and progressive nodular histiocytosis.

- **Rx:** although lesions may clear spontaneously over a period of several years, treatment of the underlying thyroid disease usually has no effect; anecdotal therapies include topical and intralesional CS, surgical shave removal, and for severe disease, IVIg, rituximab, octreotide, and plasmapheresis. Compression stockings and pneumatic compression can be used for associated lymphedema.

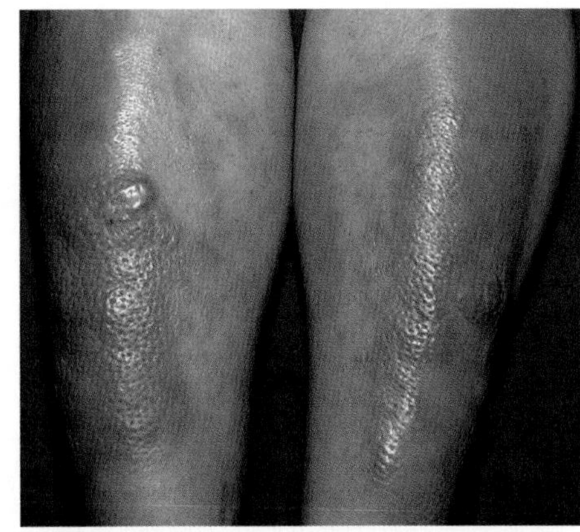

Fig. 38.4 Pretibial myxedema. Purple-brown plaques on the shins of a patient with Graves disease. A *peau d'orange* appearance is present due to prominent follicular openings. *Courtesy, Franco Rongioletti, MD, and Alfredo Rebora, MD.*

Generalized Myxedema

- As a result of profound hypothyroidism, the skin is diffusely dry, cool, and pale, with a waxy appearance; the hair and nails can be brittle, leading to a diffuse non-scarring alopecia of the scalp and alopecia of the lateral eyebrows.
- Additional mucocutaneous findings include eczema craquelé, acquired ichthyosis, carotenoderma, and a puffiness of the hands and the face, including the eyelids; the tongue may be enlarged.
- In the congenital form, developmental delay, stunted growth, poor muscle tone, constipation, somnolence and a large fontanelle are characteristic findings.
- Because the most common underlying disease in adults is Hashimoto thyroiditis, women are more commonly affected; in addition to the skin changes outlined above, patients may gain weight, have cold intolerance and constipation, feel sluggish, and can occasionally develop cutaneous xanthomas.
- **Rx:** thyroid hormone replacement.

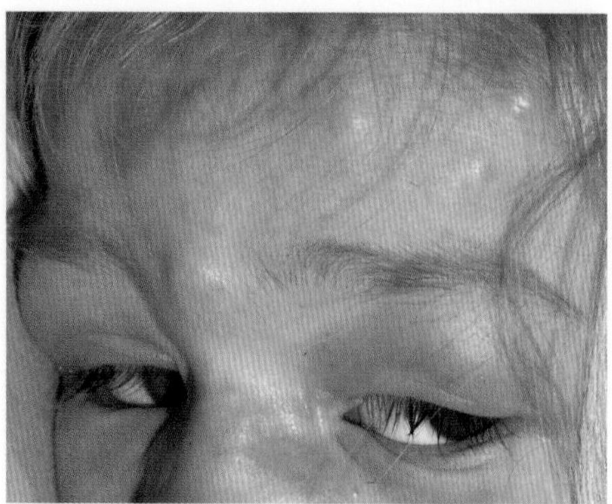

Fig. 38.5 Self-healing cutaneous mucinosis. Pink to skin-colored dermal and subcutaneous nodules as well as periorbital swelling. *Courtesy, Drs. Hansgeorg Müller and Heinz Kofler.*

Self-Healing Cutaneous Mucinosis

- Acute eruption of multiple firm papules and nodules favoring the face (especially the forehead and periorbital region), scalp, and periarticular areas (Fig. 38.5).
- No underlying disorder and characterized by spontaneous resolution over months to years.

Reticular Erythematous Mucinosis (REM)

- Persistent erythematous papules of the central chest and central back that can form a net-like pattern and/or coalesce into plaques (Fig. 38.6); may be photo-aggravated.
- Overlaps with LE tumidus, lymphocytic infiltrate of Jessner (minimal to no dermal mucin), and papulonodular mucinosis (see below).
- **Rx:** topical or intralesional CS, antimalarials (hydroxychloroquine, chloroquine), sunscreens.

Cutaneous Lupus Mucinosis/ Papulonodular Mucinosis (of Gold)

- Occurs in the setting of autoimmune connective tissue diseases, with LE >> dermatomyositis or systemic sclerosis; ~75% of patients with LE who develop these lesions have systemic involvement.
- Skin-colored to erythematous papules and nodules that may require side-lighting to appreciate; favors the back, central chest, and upper extremities (Fig. 38.7).
- Overlaps with LE tumidus, reticular erythematous mucinosis, and lymphocytic infiltrate of Jessner (minimal to no dermal mucin).
- **Rx:** antimalarials (hydroxychloroquine, chloroquine), topical or intralesional CS, sunscreens.

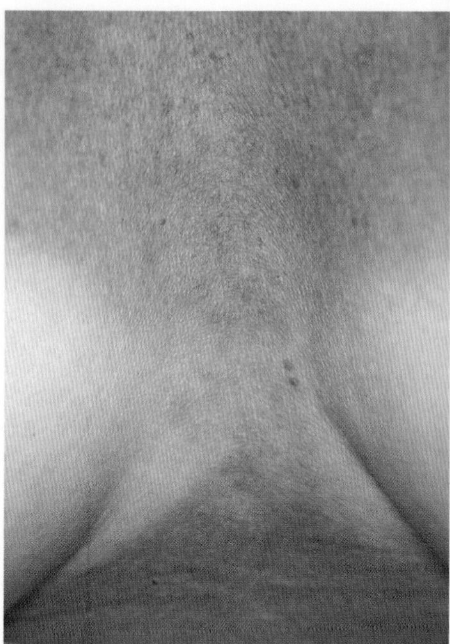

Fig. 38.6 Reticular erythematous mucinosis (REM). Grouped pink papules on the central chest with no surface changes; there is a subtle annular and reticulated configuration. Note the significant tan. *Courtesy, YDRSC.*

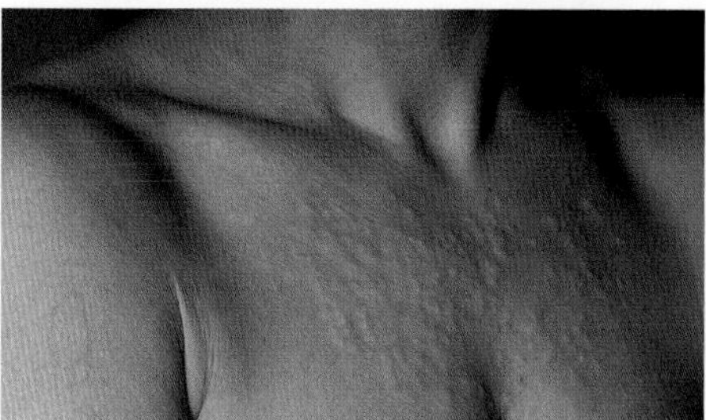

Fig. 38.7 Cutaneous lupus mucinosis/ papulonodular mucinosis. Skin-colored papules and nodules leading to a "lumpy" appearance to the skin that is best appreciated by side-lighting. *Courtesy, Franco Rongioletti, MD, and Alfredo Rebora, MD.*

Follicular Mucinosis (Alopecia Mucinosis)

- In contrast to the other disorders in this chapter, here the mucin is deposited within the epithelium of hair follicles rather than in the dermis.
- In the primary form, there are pink to violet-brown plaques, primarily in the head and neck region, that have associated alopecia and sometimes scale (Fig. 38.8A); in some patients, there are grouped follicular papules (Fig. 38.8B), and in patients with darkly pigmented skin, lesions may be hypopigmented.
- The primary form most commonly occurs in children and young adults and represents a benign, self-limited disease; in older adults, especially when the lesions are more widespread and persistent, the possibility of co-existing mycosis fungoides needs to be considered.
- In addition to the characteristic histopathologic finding of mucin deposition within the follicular epithelium, it is important to comment on the presence or absence of atypical lymphocytes.
- **DDx:** cutaneous LE, tinea faciei or capitis, facial discoid dermatosis, various forms of dermatitis; if diagnosed histologically, consider the possibility it represents an incidental finding (e.g. associated with atopic dermatitis).
- **Rx:** for primary, observation until spontaneous resolution, topical or intralesional CS, antimalarials; if associated with mycosis fungoides, treat the latter (see Ch. 98).

Other Entities

Digital mucous cyst is covered in Chapter 90. Cutaneous mucin deposits can also be seen within tumors (e.g. basal cell carcinomas, cutaneous metastases) and inflammatory disorders (e.g. granuloma annulare, cutaneous LE, dermatomyositis).

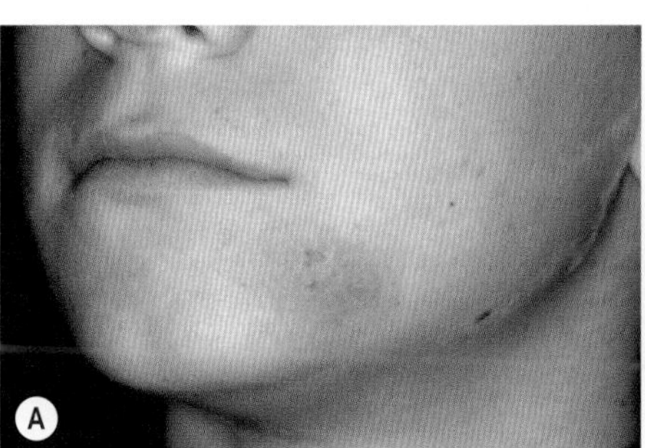

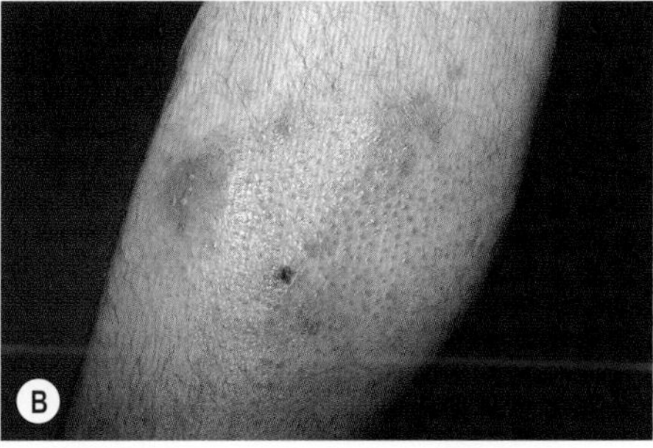

Fig. 38.8 Follicular mucinosis. A Pink plaque containing follicular papules in a young boy. **B** Grouped follicular papules on the leg of an older adult in association with violet-brown plaques; note the associated alopecia. The hemorrhagic crust is the site of a previous biopsy. *A, Courtesy, Lorenzo Cerroni, MD; B, Courtesy, YDRSC.*

For further information see Ch. 46 from *Dermatology, Fourth Edition*.

For additional online figures visit www.expertconsult.com 

39 Amyloidosis

Amyloidosis encompasses a wide range of disorders, several of which have cutaneous manifestations. The common thread is the formation of extracellular deposits that are composed of a β-pleated sheet by X-ray crystallography. In general, amyloid deposits exhibit a red color with Congo red stain and demonstrate birefringence (apple green color) under polarized light. Precursor proteins of amyloid vary from keratin to immunoglobulin (Ig) light chains to transthyretin. If necessary, tandem mass spectrometry can be performed to characterize the specific protein.

In dermatology, the initial distinction is between amyloidosis that is systemic versus skin-limited (Fig. 39.1). The former is less common than the latter.

Systemic Amyloidosis

- *Primary systemic amyloidosis* is due to a plasma cell dyscrasia, but most patients do not fulfill the criteria for symptomatic multiple myeloma (≥10% plasma cells in a bone marrow biopsy *plus* bone lesions, anemia, hypercalcemia, and/or renal disease); the precursor protein is almost always Ig light chains (AL; lambda > kappa) rather than Ig heavy chains (AH).
- Firm, skin-colored to pink to yellow-brown, waxy papules or plaques occur most commonly on the face (Fig. 39.2); infiltration of the tongue can lead to macroglossia (Fig. 39.3), and occasionally there is diffuse waxy induration of the skin (sclerodermoid

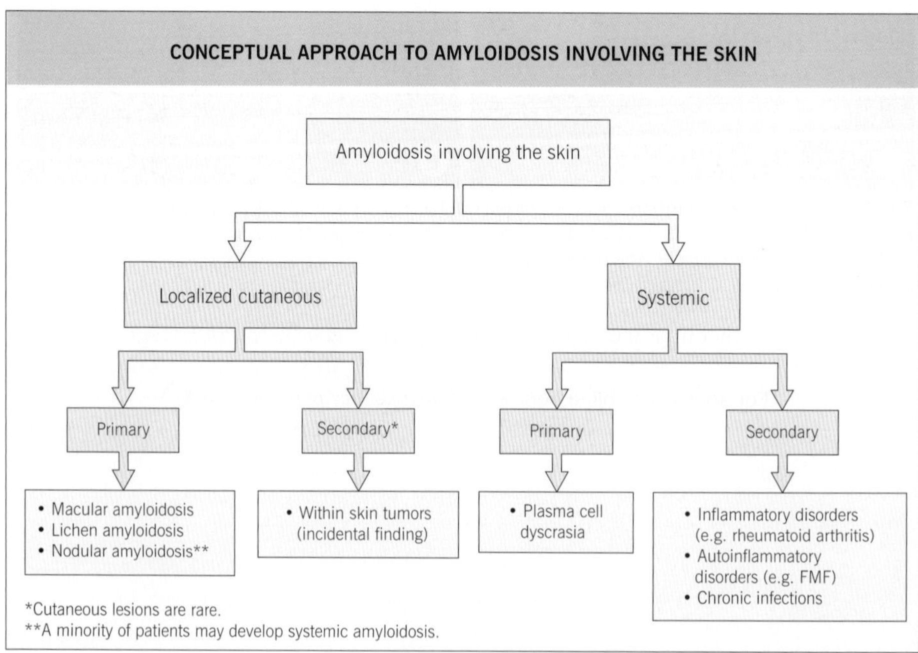

Fig. 39.1 Conceptual approach to amyloidosis involving the skin. FMF, familial Mediterranean fever.

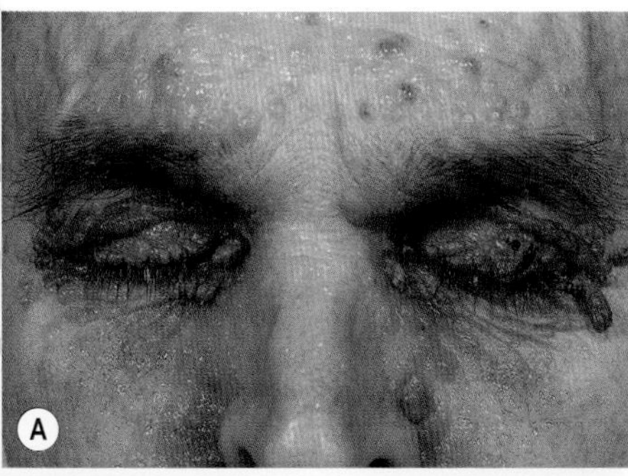

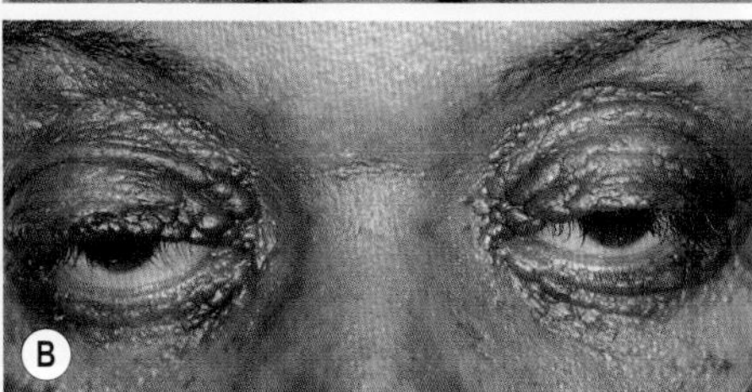

Fig. 39.2 Primary systemic amyloidosis. **A** Numerous waxy translucent facial papules. Some have a yellow to yellow-brown color. **B** Some of the waxy papules have become purpuric, but this may be difficult to appreciate because of the pigmentation of the skin (compare to Fig. 39.4); the periorbital region is a characteristic site of involvement. *A, Courtesy, Jean L. Bolognia, MD; B, Courtesy, Judit Stenn, MD.*

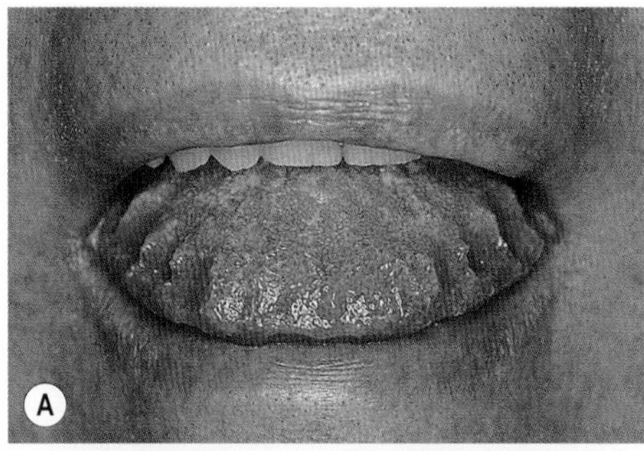

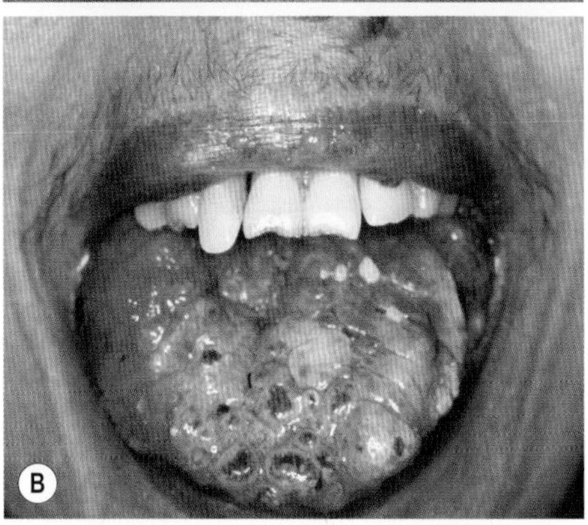

Fig. 39.3 Primary systemic amyloidosis. **A** Macroglossia with dental impressions on the tongue. **B** Papulonodules of the tongue; some are purpuric while others are translucent with a yellowish hue. The combination of macroglossia plus carpal tunnel syndrome is a classic clinical presentation. *A, Courtesy, YDRSC; B, Courtesy, Dennis Cooper, MD.*

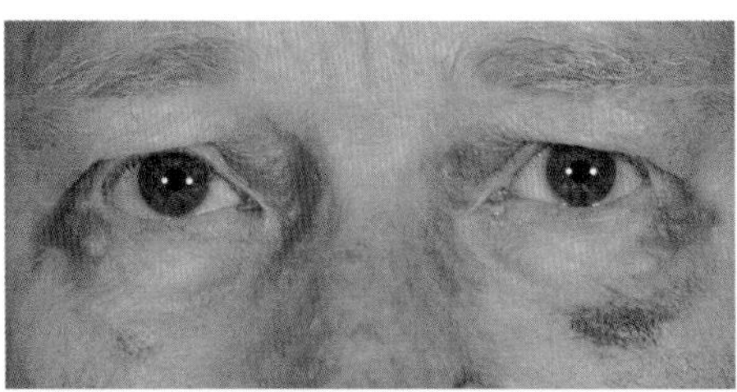

Fig. 39.4 Primary systemic amyloidosis. Purpura and yellow-brown plaques in a periorbital distribution. *Courtesy, Joyce Rico, MD.*

presentation); purpura due to trauma or pinching of the skin can also be seen and is due to the fragility of blood vessels surrounded by amyloid deposits (Fig. 39.4).

- *Secondary systemic amyloidosis* develops in the setting of chronic inflammation, e.g. rheumatoid arthritis, tuberculosis, and in several autoinflammatory disorders (see Ch. 37); the precursor protein is (apo) serum AA, which is produced by the liver; cutaneous lesions rarely occur.
- Amyloid deposits can also lead to a restrictive cardiomyopathy and congestive heart failure as well as renal dysfunction, especially nephrotic syndrome (Fig. 39.5).
- Histologically, cutaneous papules are composed of dermal deposits of amyloid while clinically uninvolved skin (abdominal fat) can show perivascular deposits of amyloid; serum protein electrophoresis (SPEP) and immunofixation electrophoresis (IFE) aid in identifying a gammopathy, but the serum free light-chain assay is the most sensitive test available and the presence of monoclonal free light chains in the blood or urine is required to establish the diagnosis.
- **DDx:** for facial papules, mucinoses, multiple adnexal tumors, colloid milium, lipoid proteinosis (see Fig. 91.16).
- **Rx:** for primary systemic amyloidosis, it is similar to myeloma, e.g. dexamethasone, melphalan, bortezomib or carfilzomib,

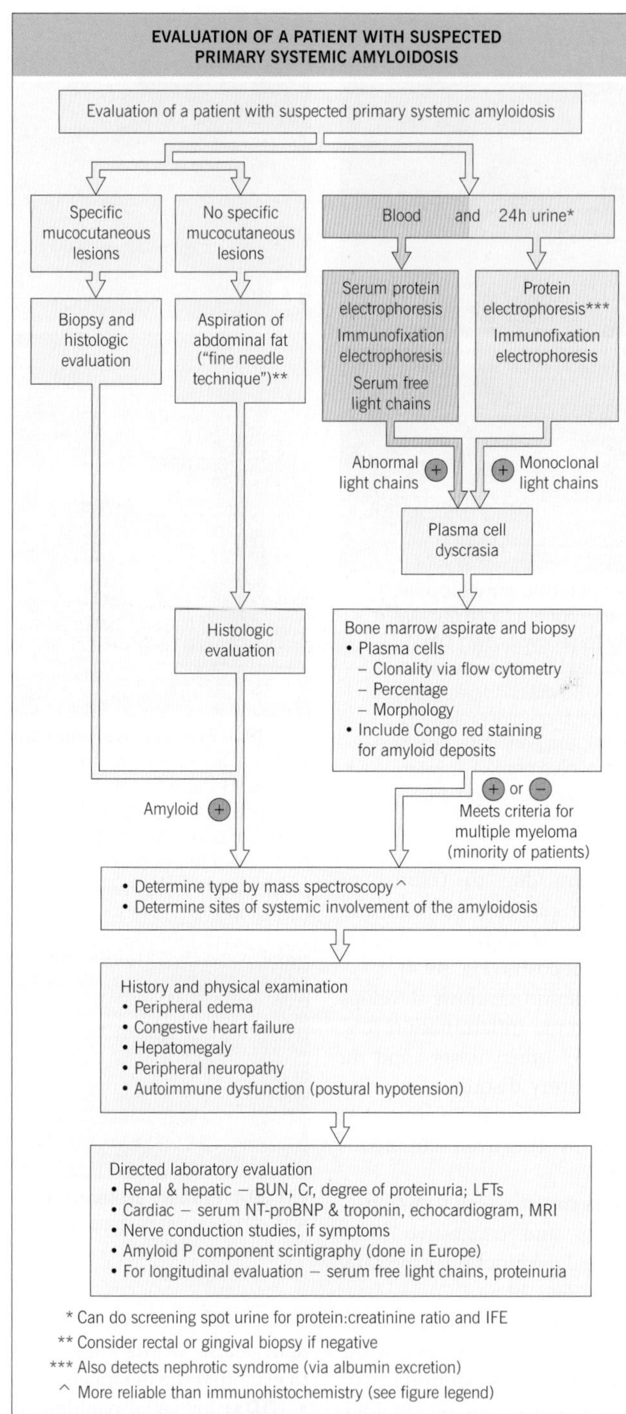

Fig. 39.5 Evaluation of a patient with suspected primary systemic amyloidosis. Because the amyloid is formed from immunoglobulin light chains, an abnormality of light chains in the blood or urine (e.g. increased concentration or abnormal ratio in the blood, positive immunofixation electrophoresis [IFE] of the urine) is required for diagnosis. Mass spectroscopy has become more routine given the potential for misdiagnosis of older patients with wild-type ATTR deposits in the heart or ALect2 deposits in the kidney and liver in the setting of a monoclonal gammopathy of unknown significance. NT-proBNP, N-terminal pro-brain natriuretic peptide.

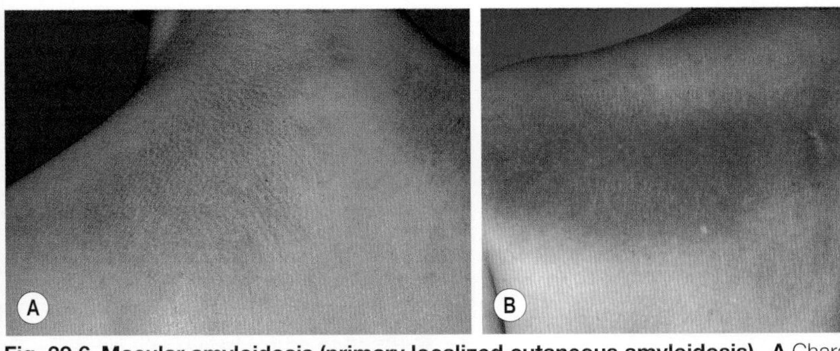

Fig. 39.6 Macular amyloidosis (primary localized cutaneous amyloidosis). A Characteristic rippled hyperpigmentation on the upper back. **B** Occasionally, a linear accentuation is seen. *Courtesy, Richard W. Groves, MD, and Martin M. Black, MD.*

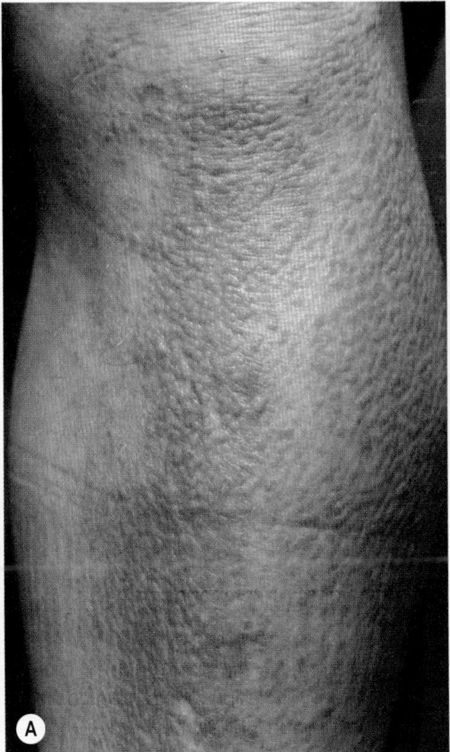

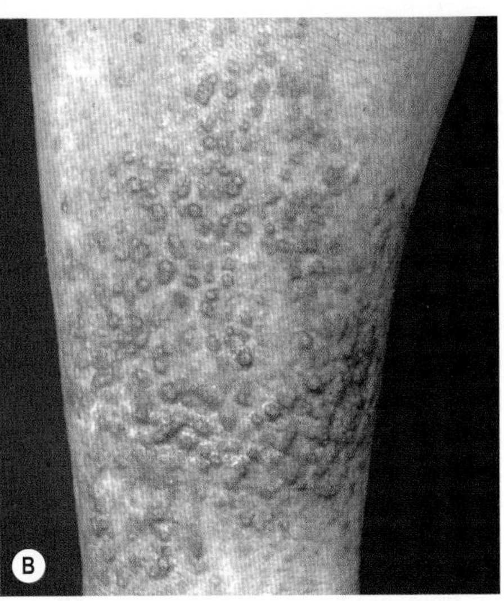

Fig. 39.7 Lichen amyloidosis (primary localized cutaneous amyloidosis). A Numerous monomorphic papules on the shin. The rippled appearance is most obvious laterally. **B** Keratotic, hyperpigmented papules and linear plaques on the shin. *A, Courtesy, YDRSC; B, Courtesy, St. John's Institute of Dermatology.*

lenalidomide or pomalidomide, daratumumab, hematopoietic stem cell transplant (for younger patients).

Localized Cutaneous Amyloidosis

- The three major forms of *primary* localized cutaneous amyloidosis are macular, lichen, and nodular amyloidosis (see Fig. 39.1); an overlap of the first two forms is referred to as biphasic because these two entities exist on a spectrum.
- Both *macular* and *lichen amyloidosis* are due to rubbing, scratching, or friction and have a rippled appearance as well as hyperpigmentation; the macular form favors the upper back of adults while the lichenoid form favors the extensor surfaces of the extremities, primarily the anterolateral shins, and has a palpable component (Figs 39.6 and 39.7).

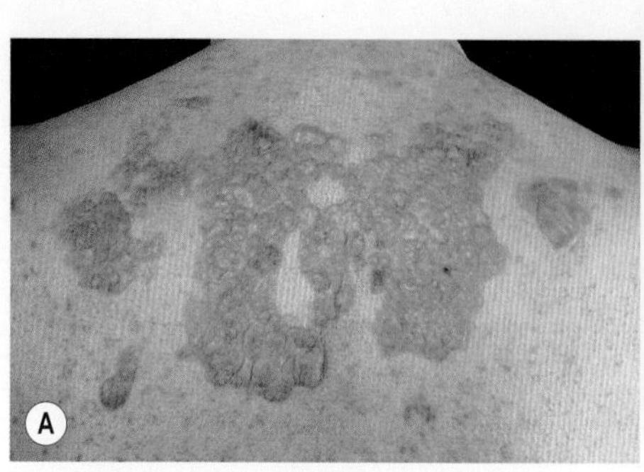

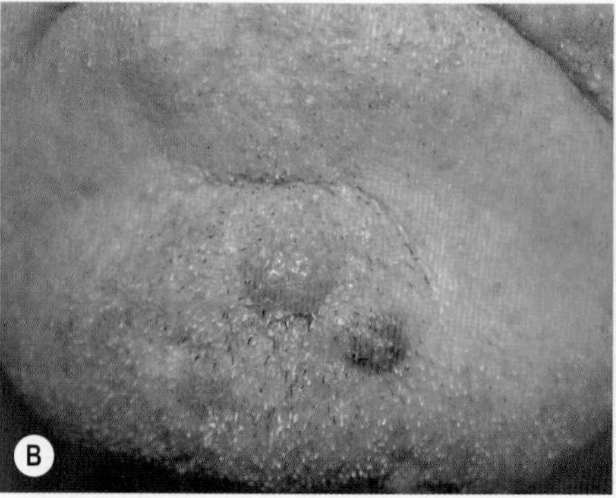

Fig. 39.8 Nodular amyloidosis. A, B Firm waxy plaques and nodules on the back and chin. The color can vary from skin-colored to pink-yellow to violaceous. *A, Courtesy, Richard W. Groves, MD, and Martin M. Black, MD; B, Courtesy, YDRSC.*

- Both forms occur more commonly in individuals with skin phototypes III and IV; cutaneous amyloidosis of the upper back is seen in patients with Sipple syndrome (multiple endocrine neoplasia [MEN] type 2A), but with an onset during childhood.
- In patients with familial primary cutaneous amyloidosis, mutations in three genes have been detected which encode the following proteins: (1) oncostatin M receptor β (a component of the IL-31 receptor); (2) the α subunit of the IL-31 receptor; and (3) GPNMB (dyschromic form in Asians); of note, IL-31 plays a role in pruritus.
- The precursor protein for both macular and lichen amyloidosis is keratin, presumably from nearby keratinocytes; deposits of amyloid in the upper dermis can be subtle, especially in the macular form, and stain positively with anti-keratin antibodies.
- *Nodular amyloidosis* presents as one or more waxy skin-colored to pink-orange plaques or nodules, most commonly on the trunk or extremities (Fig. 39.8); the precursor protein is Ig light chains ± β_2-microglobulin, thought to be produced by cutaneous infiltrates of plasma cells.
- A minority of patients with nodular amyloidosis may develop systemic amyloidosis, so longitudinal evaluation is recommended.
- Occasionally, deposits of amyloid are seen in cutaneous tumors, e.g. basal cell carcinomas, dermatofibromas, intradermal melanocytic nevi, as an inconsequential *secondary* phenomenon.
- **DDx:** back – notalgia paresthetica, lichen simplex chronicus (LSC) with postinflammatory hyperpigmentation; lower extremity – LSC, hypertrophic lichen planus, pretibial myxedema; nodular – cutaneous lesions of systemic amyloidosis, pretibial myxedema, cutaneous lymphoma, BCC.
- **Rx:** difficult; can try topical antipruritics, e.g. pramoxine, topical or intralesional CS; physical coverings, e.g. zinc oxide-impregnated gauze (Unna boot) or hydrocolloid dressings, can lead to improvement but recurrences common when discontinued.

For further information see Ch. 47 from *Dermatology, Fourth Edition*.

For additional online figures visit www.expertconsult.com 

Deposition Disorders 40

A heterogeneous group of disorders in which there are deposits, usually of endogenous materials, within the skin. Entities belonging to this group that are covered in other chapters include mucinoses (Ch. 38), amyloidosis (Ch. 39), porphyrias (Ch. 41), and calcinosis cutis (Ch. 42).

Gout

- Metabolic disorder in which there is hyperuricemia due to increased production and/or decreased excretion of uric acid; often idiopathic but secondary causes include chronic kidney disease and medications such as diuretics or cyclosporine; affects primarily adult men.
- Crystals of monosodium urate can deposit within the skin (tophi) as well as the joints and kidneys; when expressed from the skin or aspirated from the joints, the crystals are needle-like and exhibit negative birefringence under polarized light.
- Tophi present as firm, skin-colored to white or yellow papules and nodules, usually around joints and on the helices of the ears (Figs 40.1 and 40.2); in general, they appear ~10 years after the initial episode of acute arthritis and occur in ~10% of patients with gout.
- Tophi can become inflamed (Fig. 40.3), and they may or may not resolve following normalization of serum uric acid levels.
- **DDx:** rare cutaneous involvement in pseudogout (rhomboid crystals) as well as calcinosis cutis, xanthomas, and rheumatoid nodules. Significant associated inflammation may lead to the misdiagnosis of cellulitis.
- **Rx** for tophi: diet, allopurinol, febuxostat; for refractory disease, pegloticase.

Lipoid Proteinosis

- Autosomal recessive disease due to loss-of-function mutations in *ECM1*, which encodes extracellular matrix protein 1; the result is deposition of hyalin-like material in multiple sites, in particular the brain (seizures) and larynx (hoarseness), as well as the skin and oral mucosa.
- Skin-colored to yellowish waxy papules and nodules favor the face, including the eyelid margin, and the tongue (Fig. 40.4); atrophic scarring, verrucous changes (especially on the elbows and knees), and a diffuse waxy appearance are additional findings; during infancy, fragility, vesicles, and crusting of the face, extremities, and mouth can occur.
- **DDx:** mucinoses, erythropoietic protoporphyria, primary systemic amyloidosis, colloid milium, and in infants, hyaline fibromatosis syndrome (see Ch. 81).

Colloid Milium

- Two major variants – inherited juvenile form and acquired adult form; because the latter is related to cumulative photodamage, it occurs primarily in adults with lightly pigmented skin.

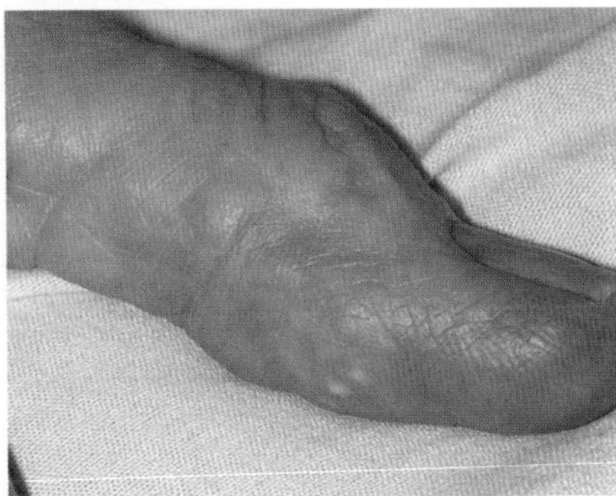

Fig. 40.1 Tophaceous gout of a digit. The deposits create a multilobulated appearance. A small incision over the yellow-white areas followed by microscopic examination of the expressed material would allow a bedside diagnosis. *Courtesy, YDRSC.*

• Dermal deposits lead to dome-shaped, translucent to yellowish papules in chronically sun-exposed sites, in particular the face, ears, posterior neck, and dorsal aspect of the

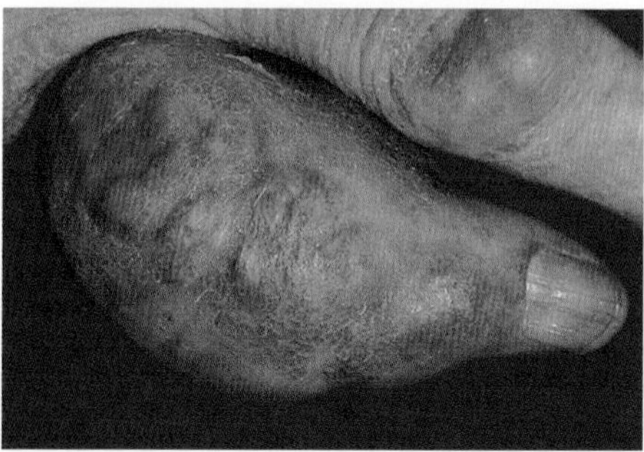

Fig. 40.2 Severe tophaceous gout of a digit leading to a multilobulated appearance. Some of the yellow papules have become erythematous due to associated inflammation. *Courtesy, YDRSC.*

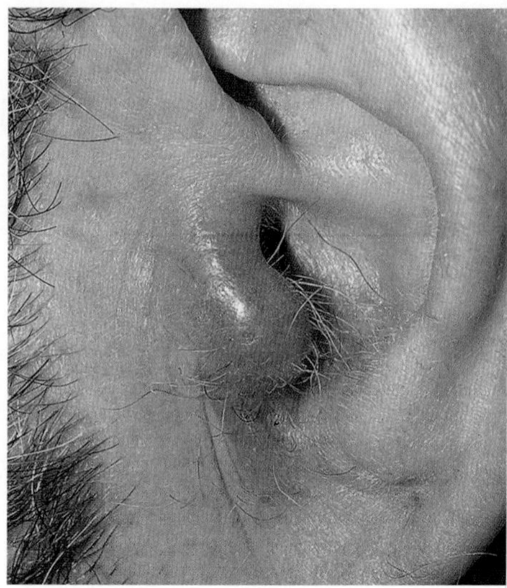

Fig. 40.3 Tophaceous gout of the tragus. The erythema reflects surrounding inflammation. *Courtesy, Harald Gollnick, MD.*

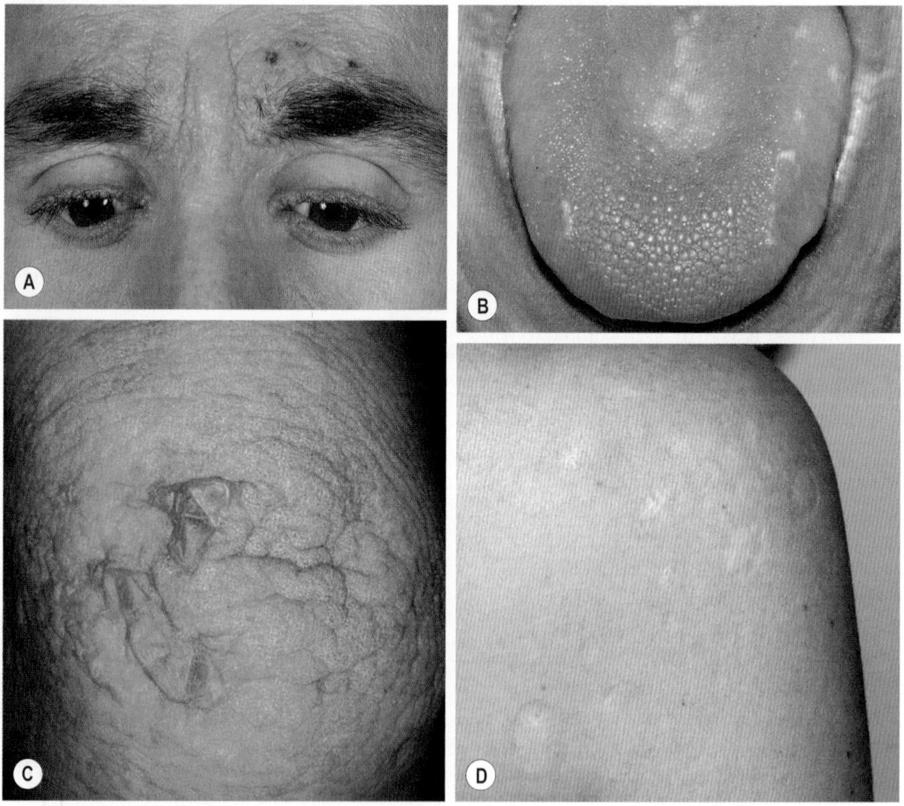

Fig. 40.4 Lipoid proteinosis. A Beaded eyelid papules, hemorrhagic crusts, and confluent waxy papules of the glabella leading to an early leonine facies. **B** A firm tongue with numerous tiny papules on its dorsal surface. **C** Characteristic verrucous changes of the elbow. **D** Multiple, round hypopigmented and depressed scars on the shoulder. *A, Courtesy, NYUDSC; B, D, Courtesy, Julie V. Schaffer, MD; C, Courtesy, Judit Stenn, MD.*

distal extremities; the lesions can become nodular or even pigmented if topical agents such as hydroquinone have been applied.

- **DDx:** similar to that of lipoid proteinosis (see above).
- **Rx:** laser, cryosurgery.

Mucopolysaccharidoses (MPS)

- Group of inherited metabolic disorders in which there is an accumulation of glycosaminoglycans (GAGs; previously referred to as mucopolysaccharides) due to deficiencies in lysosomal enzymes that break down sulfated GAGs (e.g. heparan sulfate, dermatan sulfate).
- The accumulation of GAGs can lead to intellectual disability, hepatosplenomegaly, skeletal and joint disease, corneal clouding, and a coarse facies; in addition to thickening of the skin, some patients have hypertrichosis; in Hunter syndrome (MPS II), grouped skin-colored to white papules can develop in the scapular region ("pebbling"), and in both Hurler syndrome (MPS I) and Hunter syndrome, patients may have extensive dermal melanocytosis.
- Following measurement of urinary GAGs and examination of peripheral leukocytes for vacuoles, genetic analyses can be performed.
- **Rx:** for several of the types (MPS I, II, IVA, VI, VII), enzyme replacement therapy is available; hematopoietic stem cell transplant is another option.

For further information see Ch. 48 from *Dermatology, Fourth Edition*.

For additional online figures visit www.expertconsult.com 

41 Porphyrias

The porphyrias represent a group of metabolic disorders in which there is dysfunction of the enzymes involved in heme synthesis (Fig. 41.1). With the exception of acquired porphyria cutanea tarda (PCT), the underlying etiology is monogenetic mutations. Porphyrins absorb light energy (400–410 nm) and their accumulation within the skin can lead to photosensitization, with water-soluble porphyrins producing blisters and lipophilic porphyrins leading to acute burning and erythema. This chapter focuses on those porphyrias with cutaneous manifestations.

Porphyria Cutanea Tarda (PCT)

- The most common form of cutaneous porphyria; clinical findings typically appear during the 3rd to 4th decade of life.
- Dysfunction of uroporphyrinogen decarboxylase (UD) is usually acquired (type I) but can be inherited in an autosomal dominant manner (type II); the ratio of type I : type II is ~3 : 1.
- In type I PCT, the enzyme is only dysfunctional in the liver, rather than in all tissues; hepatotoxins (e.g. alcohol, iron overload), hepatitis C virus or HIV infection, and estrogens can precipitate or exacerbate PCT.
- In addition to photosensitivity, characteristic skin findings include fragility, erosions, vesiculobullae, milia, and scars in sun-exposed areas, especially on the dorsal aspects of the hands (Fig. 41.2); hypertrichosis (malar region) and hyperpigmentation can develop on the face (Fig. 41.3); a sclerodermoid appearance or morpheaform plaques are seen less often (Fig. 41.4).
- Histologically, if a bulla is biopsied, there is a subepidermal split with minimal inflammation; thickened basement membranes around capillaries in the dermis with festooning of the dermal papillae are also seen.
- Diagnosis is based on the detection of elevated levels of *urinary* uro- and coproporphyrins (water-soluble; Table 41.1) or elevated plasma uroporphyrins or fecal isocoproporphyrins; genetic analysis can be performed for type II PCT.
- Additional evaluation includes serum ferritin and if elevated, analysis of the hemochromatosis gene; screening for hepatitis B or C viral infection; and if risk factors, HIV infection.
- **DDx:** pseudoporphyria due to medications (Table 41.2) or in patients with chronic kidney disease and those undergoing dialysis; phototoxic drug eruption; epidermolysis bullosa acquisita (sites of trauma but not limited to sun-exposed sites); rare forms of porphyria with similar cutaneous findings plus neurologic manifestations similar to acute intermittent porphyria (AIP) – variegate porphyria (see below) and hereditary coproporphyria (elevated coproporphyrins in feces consistently and in urine when symptomatic) – and mild forms of congenital erythropoietic porphyria.
- **Rx:** photoprotection via clothing and sunscreens containing titanium dioxide and zinc oxide (blocks visible light); avoidance of exacerbating factors; phlebotomy, initially 500 ml every 2–3 weeks, depending on the hematocrit; oral antimalarials, but at much lower doses than are used for cutaneous LE, i.e. hydroxychloroquine 200 mg *twice weekly*.
- In the setting of chronic kidney disease or renal dialysis and the associated anemia, the inability to use phlebotomy and/or antimalarials limits therapeutic options.

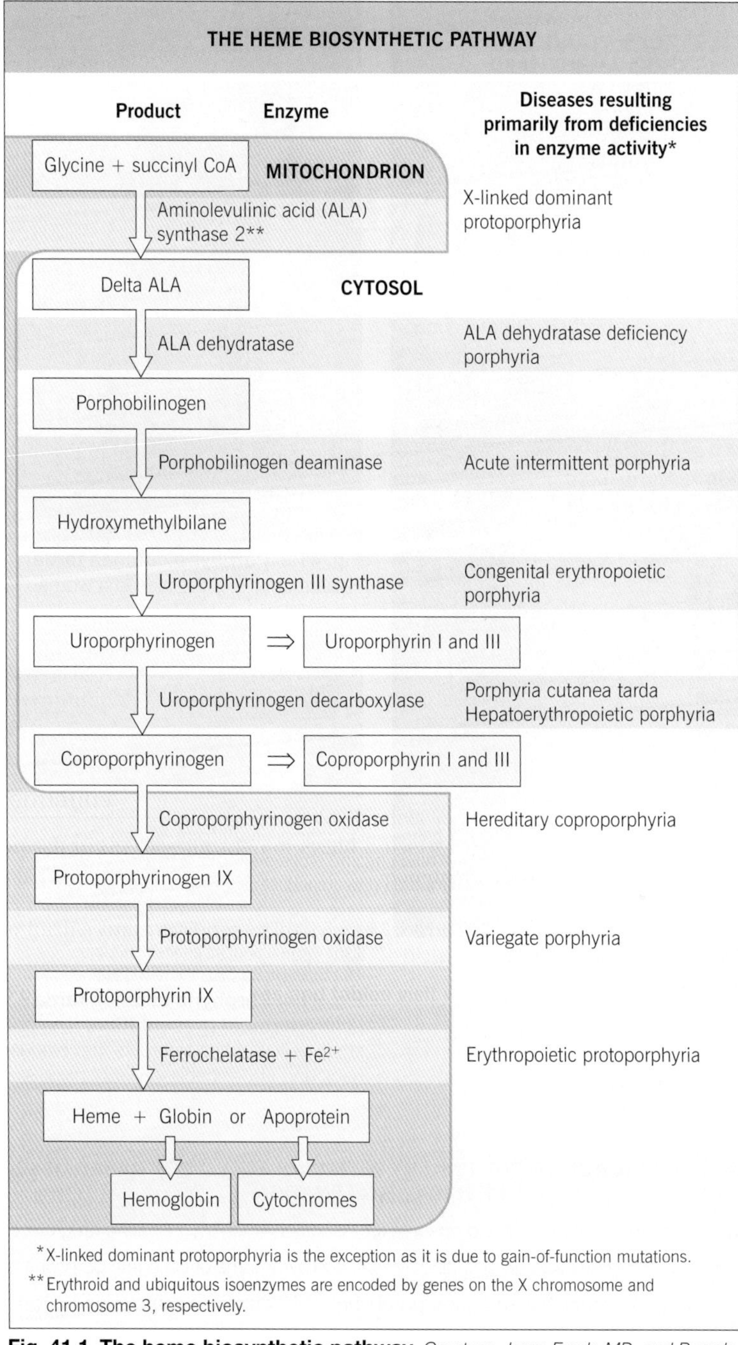

*X-linked dominant protoporphyria is the exception as it is due to gain-of-function mutations.

**Erythroid and ubiquitous isoenzymes are encoded by genes on the X chromosome and chromosome 3, respectively.

Fig. 41.1 The heme biosynthetic pathway. *Courtesy, Jorge Frank, MD, and Pamela Poblete-Gutiérrez, MD.*

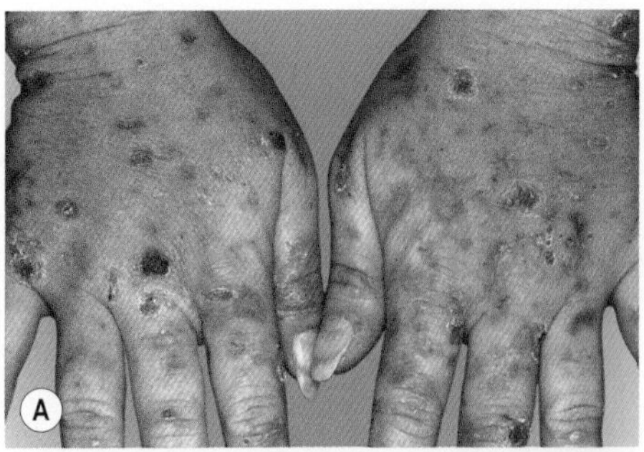

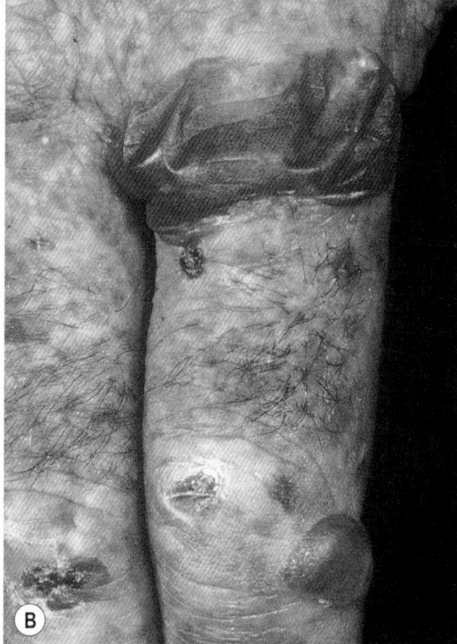

Fig. 41.2 Porphyria cutanea tarda. A Marked fragility with multiple hemorrhagic crusts, erosions, and milia as well as scars. **B** Flaccid bulla and tense vesicle with clear fluid on the forefinger, accompanied by crusts and scars. *A, Courtesy, YDRSC; B, Courtesy, Jorge Frank, MD, and Pamela Poblete-Gutiérrez, MD.*

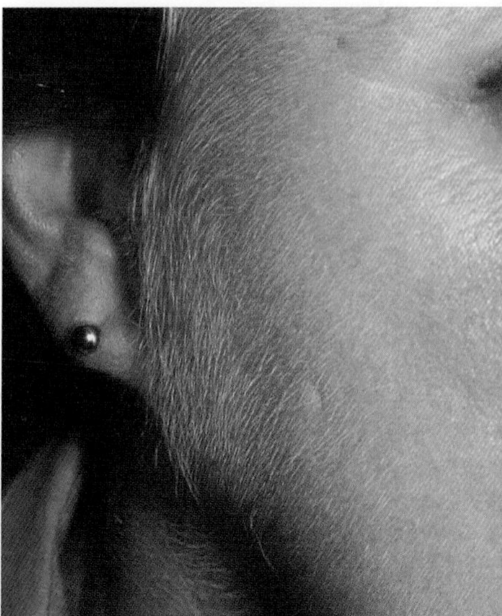

Fig. 41.3 Porphyria cutanea tarda. Hypertrichosis of the face in a woman. *Courtesy, Jeffrey P Callen, MD.*

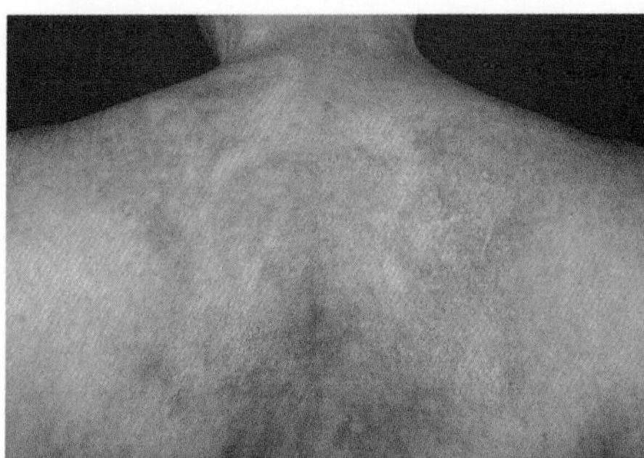

Fig. 41.4 Porphyria cutanea tarda – sclerodermoid presentation. The patient had shiny, yellow-white to brown firm plaques on the neck and upper back. *Courtesy, Jorge Frank, MD.*

BASIC APPROACH TO THE PATIENT WITH SUSPECTED PCT BASED UPON PHYSICAL EXAMINATION
• Review all medications (Table 41.2) and observe for resolution when incriminating drug discontinued
• ROS for chronic kidney disease, precipitating factors, and symptoms of variegate porphyria (see text)
• Measure urinary uroporphyrins and coproporphyrins (24-hour urine sample) and/or plasma uroporphyrins
• If abnormal porphyrin profile for PCT, measure CBC, LFTs, BUN, Cr, and screen for exacerbating factors, in particular HIV, viral hepatitis, and iron overload including hemochromatosis; also consider rare forms of porphyria
• If no elevation of uroporphyrins, consider alternative diagnoses, e.g. EBA, phototoxic drug reaction, pseudo-PCT, rare forms of porphyria

Table 41.1 Basic approach to the patient with suspected PCT based upon physical examination. EBA, epidermolysis bullosa acquisita; ROS, review of systems.

DRUG-INDUCED PSEUDOPORPHYRIA: MOST COMMONLY INCRIMINATED MEDICATIONS	
NSAIDs*	**Diuretics**
Naproxen (proprionic acid derivative)** **Mefenamic acid** Nabumetone Ketoprofen (proprionic acid derivative) Diflunisal Celecoxib	**Furosemide** **Hydrochlorothiazide/triamterene** Chlorthalidone Bumetanide
	Retinoids
	Isotretinoin Acetretin/etretinate
Antibiotics	**Miscellaneous**
Nalidixic acid **Tetracycline, doxycycline** **Ciprofloxacin**	Amiodarone Voriconazole

**When caused by NSAIDs, consider prescribing diclofenac, indomethacin, or sulindac.*
***Most frequently implicated NSAID.*

Table 41.2 Drug-induced pseudoporphyria: most commonly incriminated medications. The most commonly incriminated medications are in **bold**. For a more complete list, see Table 49.5 in *Dermatology, Fourth Edition*. *Courtesy, Misty Sharp, MD.*

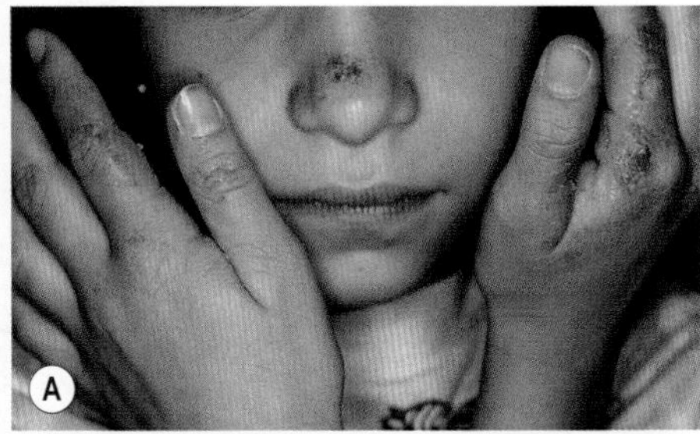

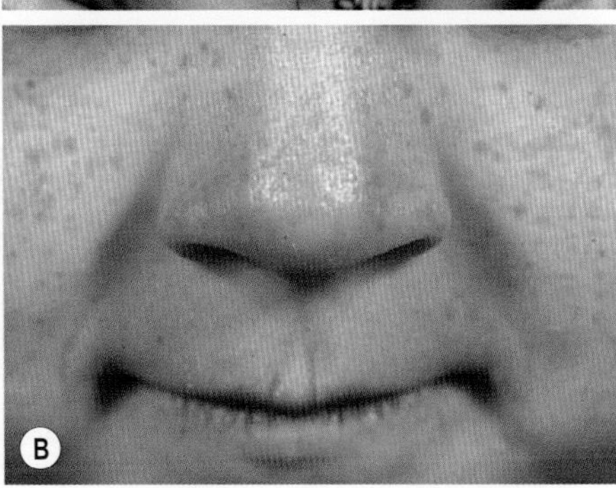

Fig. 41.5 Erythropoietic protoporphyria (EPP). A Erythema, edema, and hemorrhagic crusts on the nose as well as the fingers in a young girl. **B** Subtle scarring on the nose and linear scars on the upper cutaneous lip in a 6-year-old child. *A, Courtesy, YDRSC; B, Courtesy, Gillian Murphy, MD.*

Erythropoietic Protoporphyria (EPP)

- Complaints of erythema, edema, and a painful burning sensation of the skin following sun exposure usually begin during early childhood; purpura and crusts may also be seen and over time, a waxy texture and scarring develop in areas of greatest cumulative UV exposure, i.e. on the nose and dorsal hands (Fig. 41.5).
- Inherited primarily in a semidominant pattern (mutation in one allele and specific polymorphism in second allele); internal manifestations include gallstones and cholestatic liver disease which can lead to liver failure (~5% of patients).
- Diagnosis is based on the detection of elevated levels of *erythrocyte (RBC) free* protoporphyrin (lipophilic); elevated protoporphyrins are also present in the stool and genetic analysis can be performed; of note, zinc protoporphyrins are also elevated but this can be seen in other disorders, e.g. lead poisoning.
- **DDx:** solar urticaria, phototoxic or photoallergic contact dermatitis and drug reactions, hydroa vacciniforme, cutaneous LE, other causes of early onset photosensitivity (e.g. xeroderma pigmentosum, Rothmund–

Thomson syndrome), and a very rare form of porphyria with similar cutaneous and hepatic findings – X-linked dominant protoporphyria.

• **Rx:** photoprotection (see PCT), β-carotene, afamelanotide; cholestyramine or charcoal, if liver disease.

Variegate Porphyria (VP)

• Rare form of porphyria, except in South Africa; autosomal dominant inheritance pattern.

• While the cutaneous findings are similar to PCT, the systemic manifestations are similar to those of AIP, in particular acute attacks of abdominal pain, vomiting, paresthesias, motor and sensory neuropathies, and/or psychosis.

• Diagnosis is based on detection of elevated levels of urinary uro- and coproporphyrins (as in PCT) as well as elevated aminolevulinic acid and porphobilinogen (as in AIP), but these elevations may only be present during periods of symptomatic disease; elevated fecal porphyrins are present consistently and in the plasma, a characteristic peak fluorometric emission at 624–626 nm is observed in symptomatic patients; genetic analysis can also be performed.

• **DDx:** for cutaneous findings, PCT, pseudoporphyria, epidermolysis bullosa acquisita (see PCT **DDx**).

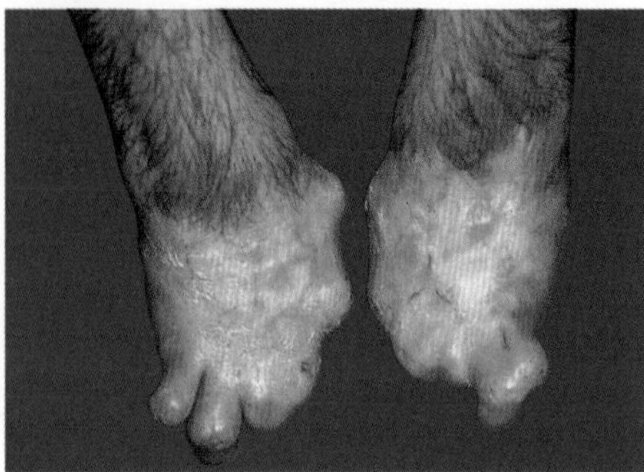

Fig. 41.6 Congenital erythropoietic porphyria. Severe mutilation of the hands due to scarring. *Courtesy, José Mascaro, MD.*

• **Rx:** photoprotection (see PCT); avoidance of exacerbating factors (e.g. alcohol, fasting); for acute attacks, heme preparations.

Congenital Erythropoietic Porphyria (CEP)

• Rare severe form of porphyria in which erythema, edema, blisters, erosions, and scarring, as well as hyperpigmentation and hypertrichosis, develop in sun-exposed areas during infancy; autosomal recessive inheritance.

• Over time, the degree of scarring can become marked, leading to mutilation, e.g. mitten deformities of the hand (Fig. 41.6); additional manifestations include hemolytic anemia, hepatosplenomegaly, and pink-red urine stains and pink-red teeth (erythrodontia).

• Diagnosis is based on detection of elevated levels of uro- and coproporphyrins in the urine, RBCs, and plasma and elevated coproporphyrins in the stool; genetic analysis can also be performed.

• **DDx:** hepatoerythropoietic porphyria, which represents the rare autosomal recessive variant of PCT (Fig. 41.7); other causes of early onset photosensitivity (see EPP above).

• **Rx:** strict photoprotection (see PCT), splenectomy, hematopoietic stem cell transplantation.

Pseudoporphyria (Pseudo-PCT, Bullous Dermatosis of Dialysis)

• Clinical presentation similar to PCT but without abnormal elevation of porphyrins, although patients with renal disease can have borderline elevations in porphyrin levels.

• Seen in patients with chronic kidney disease and those undergoing dialysis, usually hemodialysis (Fig. 41.8); it is also associated with certain medications (Table 41.2).

• Can also occur following tanning bed use.

• **DDx:** see PCT.

• **Rx:** discontinue suspect drug; photoprotection (see PCT).

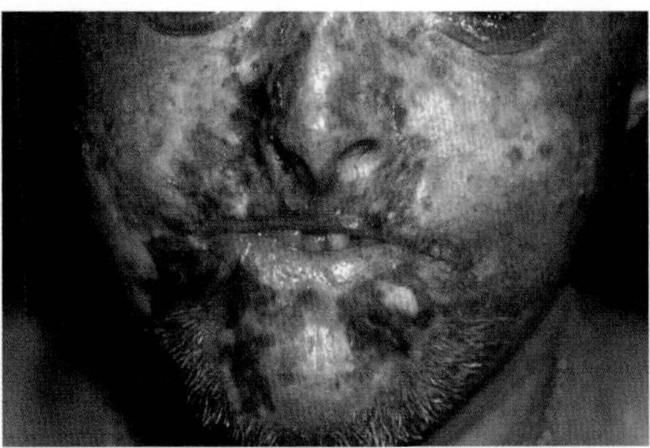

Fig. 41.7 Hepatoerythropoietic porphyria. Hypertrichosis and severe scarring are present, resulting in a clinical appearance similar to congenital erythropoietic porphyria. *Courtesy, José Mascaro, MD.*

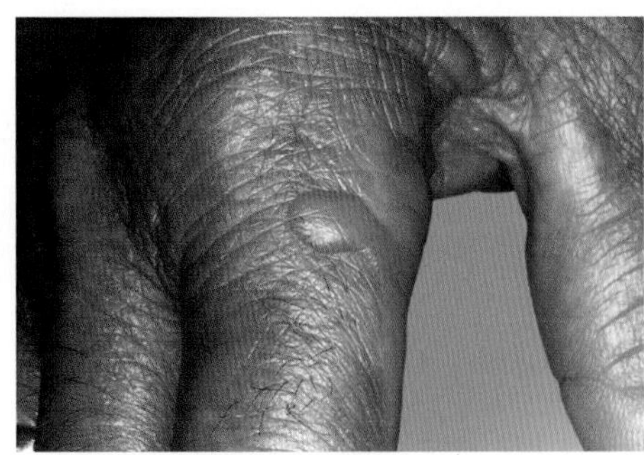

Fig. 41.8 Dialysis-associated pseudo-porphyria. Vesicles filled with clear fluid formed on the dorsal aspects of the hand in this patient with chronic kidney disease. *Courtesy, Kalman Watsky, MD.*

For further information see Ch. 49 from *Dermatology, Fourth Edition*.

For additional online figures visit www.expertconsult.com 

42 Calcinosis Cutis and Osteoma Cutis

There are four major forms of cutaneous calcification (calcinosis cutis): (1) *dystrophic* – locally within sites of pre-existing skin damage; (2) *metastatic* – due to systemic metabolic derangements; (3) *iatrogenic* – secondary to medical treatment or testing; and (4) *idiopathic*. An occasional patient will have a mixed form. Cutaneous ossification (osteoma cutis) occurs in the setting of several genetic disorders, in a miliary form on the face, and within neoplasms and sites of inflammation (secondary).

Calcinosis Cutis

- Deposition of amorphous, insoluble calcium salts within the skin.

Calcinosis Cutis – Dystrophic

- Often seen in autoimmune connective tissue diseases (AI-CTDs), in particular the limited form of systemic sclerosis (previously referred to as CREST syndrome) and childhood dermatomyositis (Figs 42.1 and 42.2); in the former, hard, skin-colored to white papules overlie the bony prominences of the extremities (upper > lower), whereas in the latter the deposits are often larger and sometimes plate-like.
- Extrusion (transepidermal elimination or "perforation"; see Ch. 79) of the calcium deposits appears as a white chalky material and it can be followed by a persistent ulceration.
- Other underlying causes are listed in Table 42.1.
- **Rx:** aggressive treatment of AI-CTDs, when possible, prior to the appearance of calcinosis cutis; excision of symptomatic localized deposits, if feasible; sodium thiosulfate and calcium channel blockers, e.g. diltiazem, may be effective in some patients.

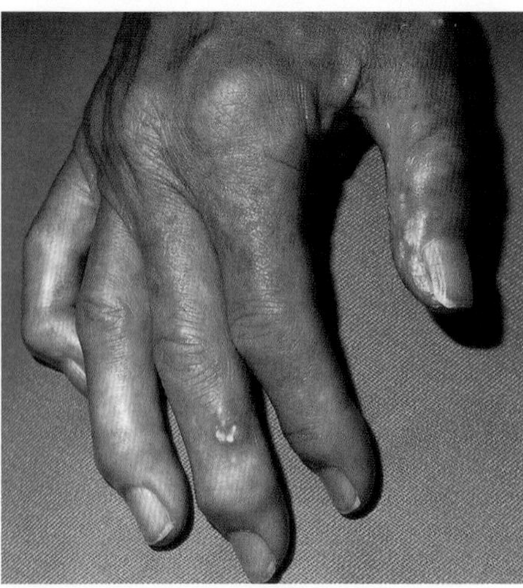

Fig. 42.1 Dystrophic form of calcinosis cutis. Note the cluster of small white papules in this patient with the limited form of systemic sclerosis (previously referred to as CREST syndrome). *Courtesy, Janet Fairley, MD.*

Calcinosis Cutis – Metastatic

- The most common cause is end-stage chronic kidney disease with its associ-

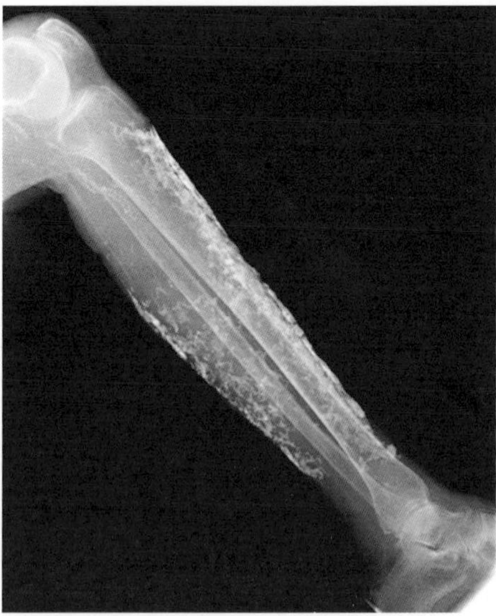

Fig. 42.2 Radiograph of calcinosis cutis in a patient with generalized morphea. Areas that were previously firm became rock-hard, and lesions of perforating calcinosis cutis (transepidermal elimination) developed on both legs. *Courtesy, Jean L. Bolognia, MD.*

DISORDERS OF CUTANEOUS CALCIFICATION
Dystrophic
• Autoimmune connective tissue diseases, especially dermatomyositis and the limited form of systemic sclerosis • Cutaneous tumors or cysts, e.g. pilomatricomas, pilar cysts • Infections, especially when cysts form around larvae or worms • Trauma, including "heel sticks" in neonates (Fig. 42.3), injection sites, surgical scars • Panniculitis, e.g. pancreatic, lupus profundus, subcutaneous fat of the newborn • Genetic disorders, e.g. pseudoxanthoma elasticum, Ehlers–Danlos syndrome (spheroids)
Metastatic
• End-stage chronic kidney disease – Calciphylaxis* – Benign nodular calcification of renal disease • Hypervitaminosis D • Milk–alkali syndrome • Sarcoidosis • Tumoral calcinosis (familial; hyper- or normophosphatemic) • Hyperparathyroidism • Neoplasms (e.g. multiple myeloma, adult T-cell leukemia/lymphoma, SCC of the lung or head and neck)
Idiopathic
• Idiopathic calcified nodules of the scrotum • Subepidermal calcified nodule (favors head and neck of children) • Tumoral calcinosis (sporadic) • Milia-like calcinosis
Iatrogenic
• Extravasation of intravenous solutions containing calcium or phosphate • Application of calcium-containing electrode paste for EMGs and EEGs • Application of calcium alginate dressings to denuded skin • Organ transplantation, especially liver • Gadolinium (nephrogenic systemic fibrosis)

**Can occasionally occur in the setting of severe primary hyperparathyroidism and, less often, in the absence of chronic kidney disease.*

Table 42.1 Disorders of cutaneous calcification.

ated hyperphosphatemia and decreased 1,25-dihydroxyvitamin D levels (Fig. 42.4).

- The two major presentations in patients with chronic kidney disease are: (1) *benign nodular calcification* in which deposits occur within otherwise normal skin, especially around joints; and (2) *calciphylaxis*, which is associated with significant morbidity and mortality.
- Calciphylaxis is characterized by cutaneous ischemia and necrosis which presents as markedly painful retiform purpura and ulcerations (Fig. 42.5); risk factors include obesity and hypercoagulability (e.g. protein C dysfunction, anti-phospholipid Ab); deposits of calcium within blood vessel walls of the subcutis are usually present, but not always, presumably due to sampling error.
- Other etiologies are listed in Table 42.1.

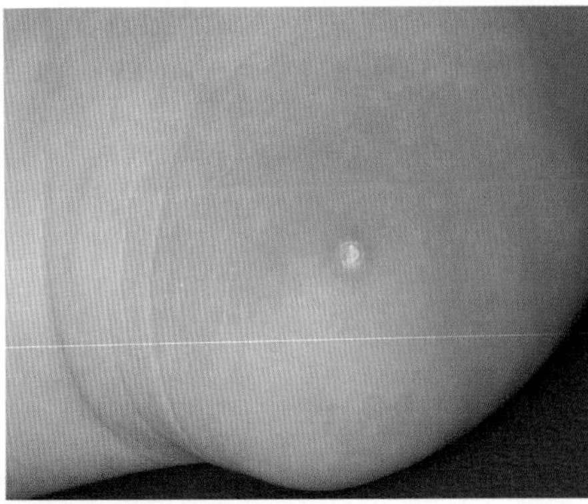

Fig. 42.3 Dystrophic calcification in an infant at the site of a previous "heel stick" for obtaining blood. *Courtesy, Julie V. Schaffer, MD.*

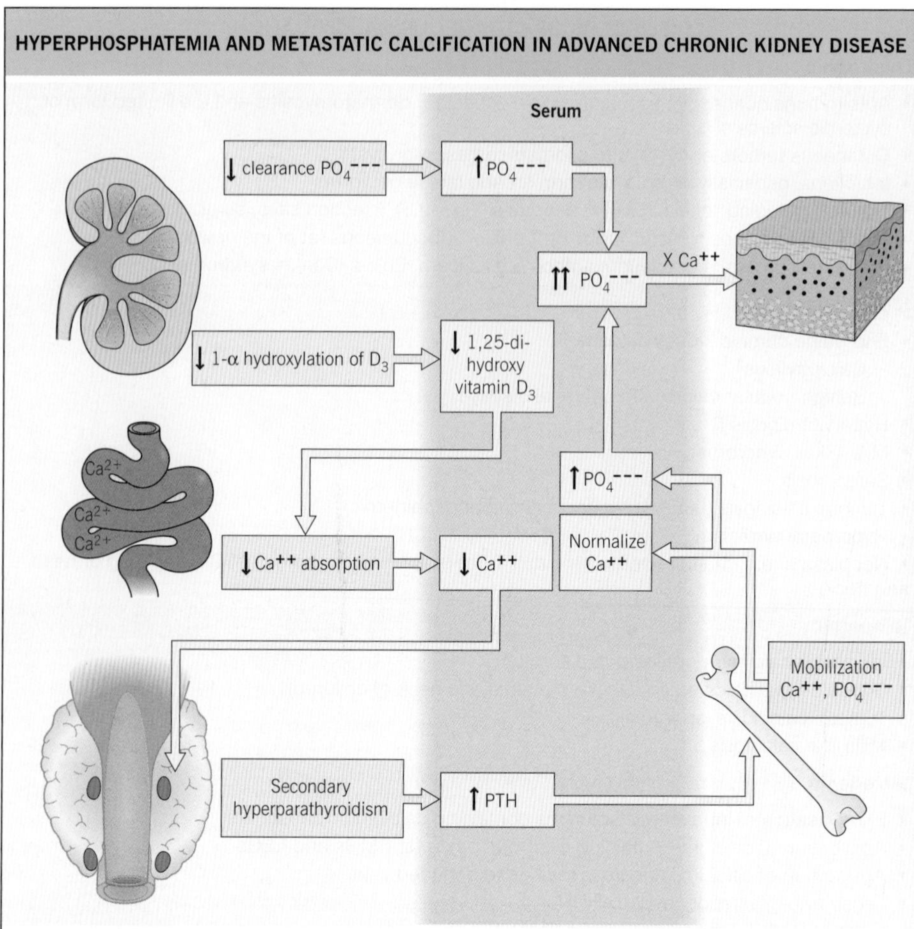

Fig. 42.4 Mechanisms of hyperphosphatemia and metastatic calcification in patients with chronic kidney disease.

- **Rx** of calciphylaxis is difficult but includes aggressive wound care and normalization of the $Ca^{++} \times PO_4^{---}$ product via the use of phosphate binders and sometimes parathyroidectomy; drugs such as sodium thiosulfate and cinacalcet can also be tried as well as local injections of sodium thiosulfate. Anticoagulants such as apixaban can also be prescribed.

Calcinosis Cutis – Iatrogenic and Idiopathic

- Iatrogenic causes and idiopathic forms are listed in Table 42.1.
- Calcification of epidermoid inclusion cysts is the major cause of calcified nodules of the scrotum.
- **Rx:** if symptomatic and feasible, surgical excision.

Osteoma Cutis

- Deposition of a protein matrix plus hydroxyapatite (Ca^{++}, PO_4^{---}) within the skin.
- The four genetic disorders that often have cutaneous or subcutaneous ossification are outlined in Fig. 42.6.
- Miliary osteomas of the face is a rather common entity; small hard papules, whose color can vary from white or skin-colored to blue (Fig. 42.7), gradually appear on the face of adult women > men; the role of preexisting acne vulgaris and its treatment with oral antibiotics is debated.
- Ossification can also occur within cysts and tumors (e.g. pilomatricomas, melanocytic nevi) as well as at sites of inflammation; it is often preceded by cutaneous calcification.

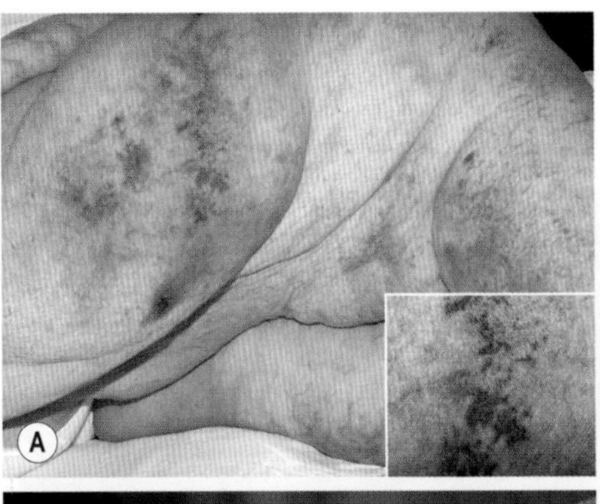

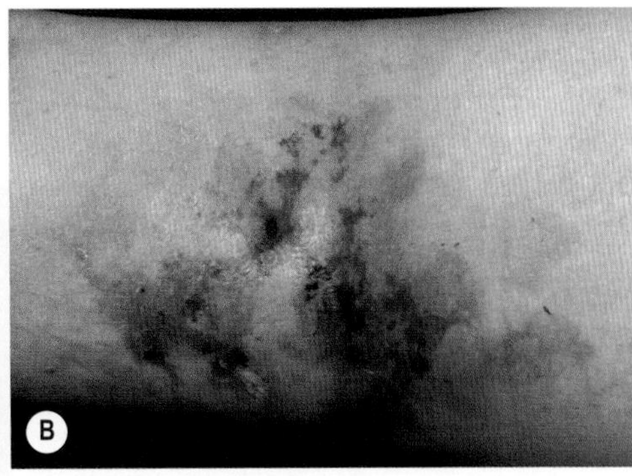

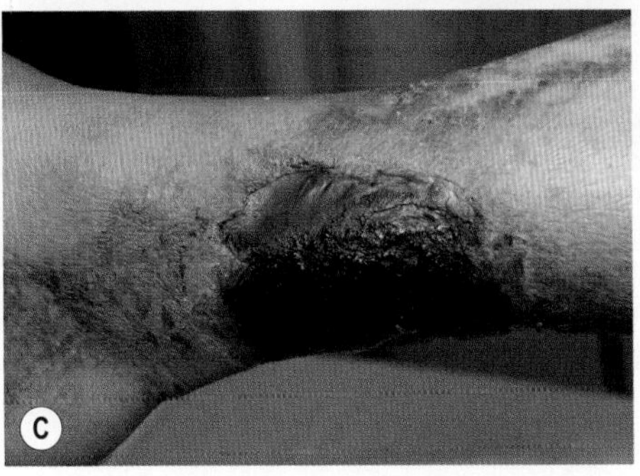

Fig. 42.5 Calciphylaxis. **A** Large reticulated violaceous plaques in an obese woman. Centrally there is retiform purpura (inset) which precedes the ulcerations that are also present. **B** Irregular violaceous plaques on the leg with retiform purpura and hemorrhagic crusts overlying ulcerations. **C** Large ulceration with leathery black eschar. Retiform purpura and scarring are seen in the surrounding skin. *A, B, Courtesy, Lorenzo Cerroni, MD; C, Courtesy, YDRSC.*

ALGORITHM FOR THE EVALUATION OF A PATIENT WITH CUTANEOUS OR SUBCUTANEOUS OSSIFICATION

Cutaneous or subcutaneous ossification

Clinical course
- Progressive
  - Associated features: Malformed great toes → Fibrodysplasia ossificans progressiva
  - Associated features: None → Progressive osseous heteroplasia*
- Limited
  - Associated features: Pseudohypoparathyroidism, Pseudo-pseudohypo-parathyroidism, Obesity, Brachydactyly, Short stature → Albright hereditary osteodystrophy*
  - Associated features: None → Plate-like osteoma cutis*; Miliary osteomas of the face

Fig. 42.6 Algorithm for the evaluation of a patient with cutaneous or subcutaneous ossification. *Associated with mutations in *GNAS1*, which encodes the alpha subunit of the stimulatory G protein that regulates adenyl cyclase activity (thought to be negative regulator of bone formation); clinical phenotype may be a reflection of imprinting.

- **Rx:** if symptomatic and feasible, surgical excision. For removal of miliary lesions of the face, a small incision with a #11 blade can be followed by extraction.
- The evaluation of a patient with calcinosis cutis or osteoma cutis is outlined in Table 42.2.

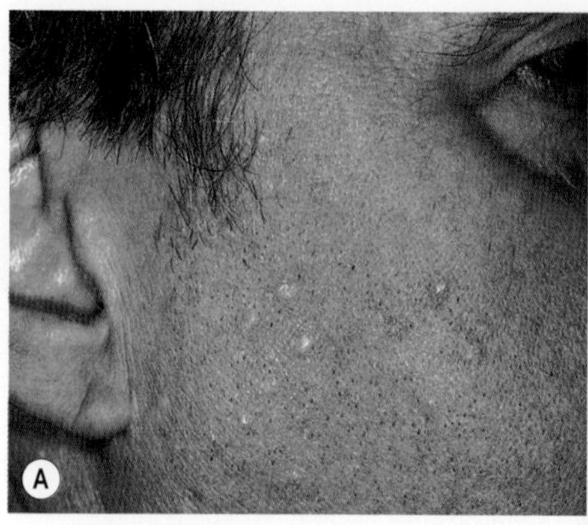

Fig. 42.7 Miliary osteomas of the face. A Small, white, firm papules in a patient without a history of acne. **B** Multiple blue-colored papules in a patient with a history of acne vulgaris. *A, Courtesy, Janet Fairley, MD; B, Courtesy, YDRSC.*

LABORATORY EVALUATION OF PATIENTS WITH CUTANEOUS CALCIFICATION/OSSIFICATION
• Special histopathologic stains for calcium, e.g. von Kossa
• Serum levels of:
– Calcium
– Phosphate
– Parathyroid hormone (PTH)
– 25-OH Vitamin D (routine test); 1,25-di-OH vitamin D (calcitriol; specialized test)
• 24-Hour urinary calcium excretion (in some patients)
• Hypercoagulability evaluation, e.g. protein C activity, anti-phospholipid Ab (if calciphylaxis suspected)
• Genetic analysis (if hereditary disorder suspected; Table 42.1 and Fig. 42.6)

Table 42.2 Laboratory evaluation of patients with cutaneous calcification/ossification. OH, hydroxy.

For further information see Ch. 50 from *Dermatology, Fourth Edition*.

For additional online figures visit www.expertconsult.com 

Nutritional Disorders 43

Malnutrition

- Poor nutrition resulting from an insufficient or poorly balanced diet or from defective digestion or utilization of foods.
- Malnutrition encompasses both deficiencies and excesses (e.g. obesity) (Fig. 43.1; Tables 43.1 and 43.2).
- Primary or exogenous: related to the ingestion of food.
- Secondary or endogenous: inadequate or faulty absorption and/or defective metabolism of food and nutrients.
- In low-income populations, exogenous protein-energy malnutrition (marasmus), due to diminished or inadequate food ingestion, is often observed.
- In high-income populations, obesity due to excessive food consumption and primary or secondary deficiencies due to psychiatric or medical (e.g. cystic fibrosis, Crohn disease) conditions are more commonly seen.

Protein–Energy Malnutrition

- Worldwide is the most prevalent nutritional deficiency; two forms are recognized (see below).
- In developed countries, either form may occur in the setting of "fad" diets or restrictions due to food allergy, e.g. infants given rice milk formula.

Marasmus

- Most commonly seen in young children but can affect all age groups.
- Results from prolonged, inadequate intake of calories and energy.
- Patients present with low body weight (Fig. 43.2) and recurrent infections due to an impaired ability to mount a normal immune response.

Kwashiorkor

- A more acute form of protein–energy malnutrition.
- Patients present with peripheral edema, or even anasarca, in association with hypoalbuminemia (Fig. 43.3).
- Because of edema, body weight is higher than seen with marasmus (~60–80% of expected weight, rather than <40%).
- Most commonly affects weaning children; less often seen in children older than 5 years of age or adults (e.g. in the setting of an acute illness superimposed on a milder state of malnutrition).

Vitamins

- Organic compounds that are biologically active and indispensable for normal physiologic functions.
- Serve as coenzymes of cellular metabolic processes essential for the adequate functioning and growth of tissues.
- Supplied exogenously.
- Both vitamin deficiency (hypovitaminosis) and excess (hypervitaminosis) can cause dermatologic abnormalities (see Tables 43.1 and 43.2; Figs 43.4–43.11).
- Vitamin excess is more common with the fat-soluble vitamins (A, D, K, E).

Vitamin D

- Fat-soluble vitamin that regulates calcium and phosphate homeostasis and bone metabolism; also involved in gene regulation, cell differentiation, and the normal functioning of the innate and adaptive immune system.
- Initial step in synthetic pathway occurs in the skin (Fig. 43.11); many tissues, in addition to the kidney, have been shown to hydroxylate vitamin D precursors to produce the active form.

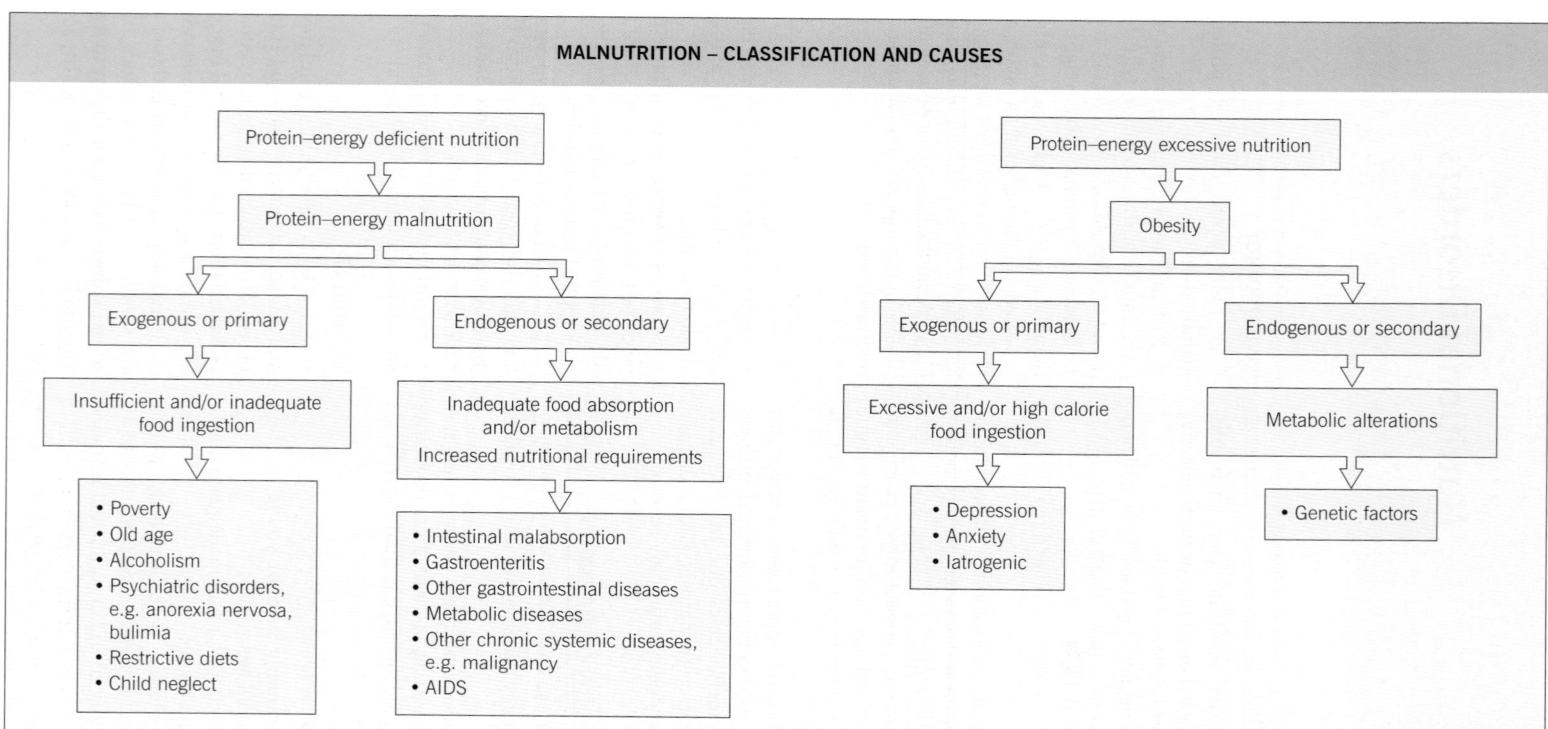

Fig. 43.1 Malnutrition – classification and causes. *Courtesy, Ramón Ruiz-Maldonado, MD.*

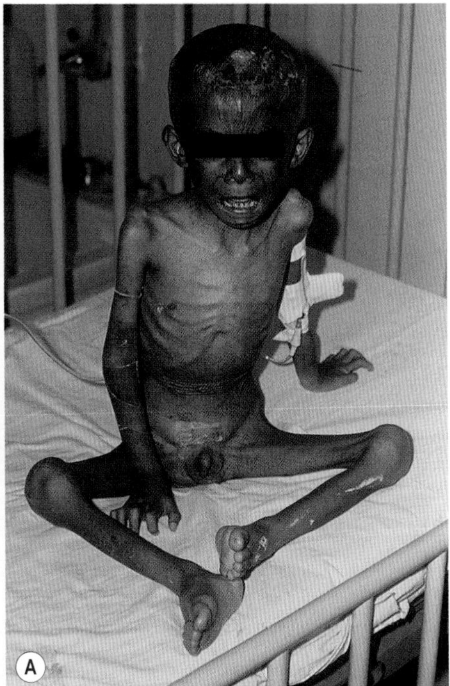

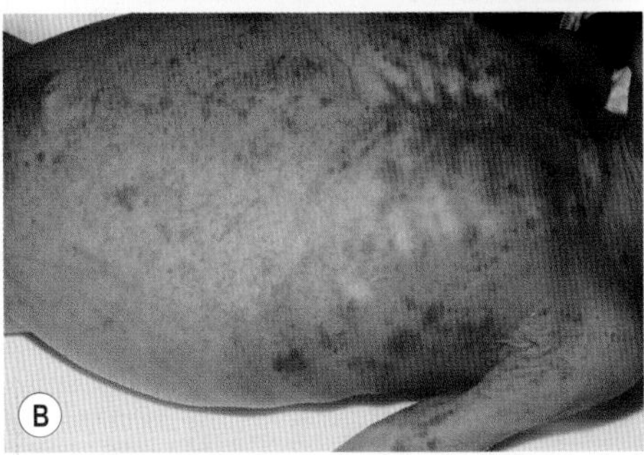

Fig. 43.2 Marasmus. A This child is emaciated and has obvious hyperpigmentation. Both erosions and desquamation are present on the scalp. **B** Multiple sites of purpura are seen. *Courtesy, Ramón Ruiz-Maldonado, MD.*

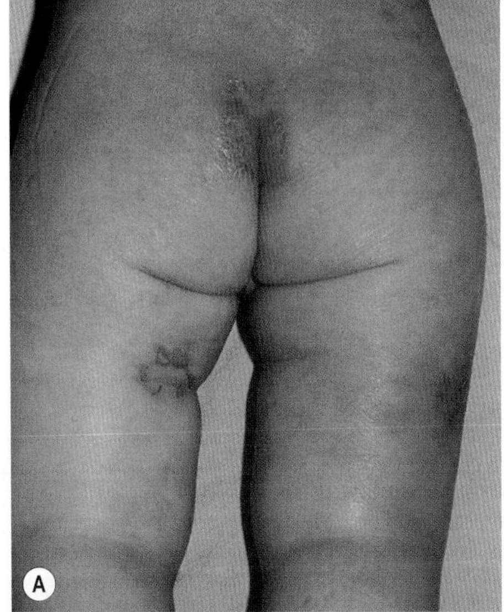

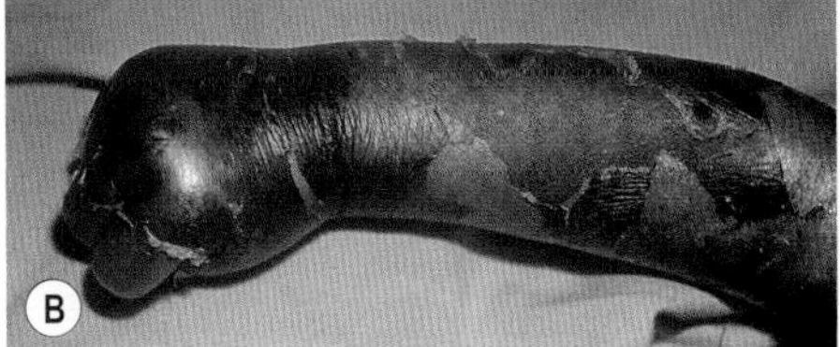

Fig. 43.3 Kwashiorkor. A There is intense edema of the buttocks and lower extremities in addition to areas of erythema with erosions and desquamation. **B** This child's arm has edema and superficial epidermal necrosis with a "flaky paint" appearance. *Courtesy, Ramón Ruiz-Maldonado, MD.*

- Endogenous synthesis and exogenous sources (fortified foods and supplements) represent the major sources.
- Individual vitamin D requirements vary depending on an individual's age, skin pigmentation, underlying diseases, current medications, geographic location, and season of the year; vitamin D receptor polymorphisms may play an important role in disease risk.
- Vitamin D body stores decline with age, during the winter months, and at higher latitudes.
- Phototypes V and VI require about threefold more UVB exposure than phototypes I and II to maintain adequate vitamin D body stores.
- Oral glucocorticoids inhibit the vitamin D-dependent intestinal absorption of calcium.
- Vitamin D *insufficiency* is actually quite common and is thought to contribute to the development of osteoporosis; it has been associated with decreased immune function, bone pain, and possibly cardiovascular disease and certain malignancies.
- True vitamin D *deficiency* is more rare and results in rickets in children and osteomalacia in adults.
- Deficiency of vitamin D can result from inadequate dietary intake, fat malabsorption, lack of adequate UVB exposure, older age with its associated decrease in endogenous

MALNUTRITION-DEFICIENCY SYNDROMES WITH MUCOCUTANEOUS MANIFESTATIONS		
Deficiency syndrome	**Mucocutaneous features**	**Systemic features**
Marasmus (see Fig. 43.2)	Xerotic, thin, pale, lax, wrinkled skin Occasionally fine scaling and hyperpigmentation Follicular hyperkeratosis and folliculitis in adults Ulcerations Lanugo-like hair Slow-growing, thin hair that readily falls out Impaired nail growth and fissured nails Purpura	**Emaciated** appearance <40–60% expected body weight Loss of subcutaneous fat and muscle Suppression of growth "Monkey facies" due to loss of buccal fat Bradycardia, hypotension, and hypothermia
Kwashiorkor (see Fig. 43.3)	Dyschromia Pallor due to distention of skin and loss of pigment **"Enamel"** or **"flaky paint"** areas of superficial desquamation Erythema, petechiae, purpura, and ecchymoses Sparse, dry, lusterless, brittle hair with reddish tinge **"Flag sign"** or alternating light- and dark-colored bands in hair, reflecting intermittent periods of malnutrition Soft and thin nails Cheilitis, xerophthalmia, vulvovaginitis	**Edema** At 60–80% expected body weight Edema or even anasarca Moon facies Anorexia, irritability, apathy Growth retardation and failure to thrive Secondary infections Bilateral parotitis Hepatomegaly Diarrhea Decreased muscle mass
Essential fatty acids	Dry, scaly, leathery skin with underlying erythema Intertriginous erosions (Figs 43.4–43.5) Alopecia and more lightly pigmented hair Increase in transepidermal water loss Petechiae	Growth failure Poor wound healing Impaired fertility Capillary fragility Neurologic damage Increased susceptibility to infections
Vitamin A (Fig. 43.6)	**Phrynoderma** manifests as follicular hyperkeratosis, favoring the extensor surfaces Xerosis Sparse, fragile hair	Ocular abnormalities, including night blindness, xerophthalmia, **Bitot's spots** (gray-white patches on the conjunctiva), keratomalacia, corneal scarring, and blindness Growth and intellectual disability Low serum vitamin A (retinol) levels

Vitamin K	Purpura and ecchymoses	Bleeding diathesis Low plasma vitamin K levels
Vitamin C (ascorbic acid) **Scurvy** (Fig. 43.7)	Follicular hyperkeratosis Corkscrew hairs Perifollicular hemorrhages Petechiae and ecchymoses Gingival hypertrophy with erosions and bleeding gums	Subperiosteal hemorrhage Loose teeth Weakness, fatigue, pseudoparalysis Weight loss, diarrhea, anemia, depression, arthralgias Long-term: edema, hypotension, seizures, increased infections Low plasma vitamin C levels
Thiamine (vitamin B_1) **Beriberi**	Glossitis and glossodynia	**Wernicke encephalopathy*** Korsakoff syndrome** Leigh syndrome†
Riboflavin (vitamin B_2) **Oro-oculo-genital syndrome**	Seborrheic dermatitis-like changes in periorificial sites (see Figs 43.4–43.5) Painless scaly papules Indolent fissures and ulcers Depapillated glossitis Conjunctivitis and photophobia	Anemia Intellectual disability Electroencephalographic changes Low serum and plasma riboflavin levels
Niacin/nicotinic acid (vitamin B_3) **Pellagra** (Fig. 43.8 and see Figs 43.4–43.5) ***Acquired*** Dietary insufficiency, prolonged isoniazid therapy, carcinoid syndrome ***Genetic*** Hartnup disease	Dermatitis begins as a symmetric erythema in sun-exposed areas, that later becomes scarlet or hyperpigmented, with desquamation and crusting **Casal's necklace** is the photosensitive eruption forming a broad band around the neck Shellac-like appearance Perianal inflammation and erosions Painful fissures on palms and soles Mucosal membranes with edema, cheilitis, atrophic glossitis Buccal and vaginal mucosae susceptible to ulceration and secondary infection	**Classic triad** of diarrhea, dementia, and dermatitis Abdominal pain Achlorhydria Low plasma niacin level
Vitamin B_5 (pantothenic acid)	None	Fatigue Headaches Vomiting Paresthesias, dysesthesias "Burning feet syndrome"

Table 43.1 Malnutrition-deficiency syndromes with mucocutaneous manifestations. *Continued*

MALNUTRITION-DEFICIENCY SYNDROMES WITH MUCOCUTANEOUS MANIFESTATIONS

Deficiency syndrome	Mucocutaneous features	Systemic features
Vitamin B_6 (pyridoxine)	Periorificial scaly, seborrheic dermatitis-like eruption (see Figs 43.4–43.5) Glossitis Conjunctivitis Stomatitis	Anorexia, nausea, vomiting Hematologic abnormalities, e.g. sideroblastic anemia, lymphopenia, eosinophilia Neurologic changes, e.g. peripheral neuropathy, weakness, confusion, seizures Low plasma vitamin B_6 levels
Biotin (vitamin H; vitamin B_7) **Multiple carboxylase deficiency** ***Acquired*** – parenteral nutrition deficient in biotin, GI disorders, excessive intake of raw egg whites, chronic anticonvulsant therapy ***Genetic*** 1. **Biotinidase deficiency** (juvenile onset) 2. **Holocarboxylase synthetase deficiency** (neonatal onset)	Alopecia Blepharitis, conjunctivitis Secondary infections Eczematous dermatitis resembling acrodermatitis enteropathica (see Figs 43.4–43.5)	Vomiting Metabolic acidosis Hypotonia, lethargy, seizures Developmental delay Optic atrophy, hearing loss Ataxia Low serum biotin levels
Folic acid (vitamin B_9)	Mucocutaneous features overlap with those seen with B_{12} deficiency Cheilitis, glossitis, and mucosal erosions Gray-brown pigmentation in sun-exposed areas	Megaloblastic anemia, which may present with weakness or congestive heart failure Neuropsychiatric symptoms Low RBC folate levels
Vitamin B_{12} (cyanocobalamin)	Smooth, red, painful tongue Generalized hyperpigmentation with accentuation in flexural areas, palms, soles, nails, and oral cavity Increased incidence of poliosis, vitiligo, and alopecia areata in patients with pernicious anemia	**Pernicious anemia** Megaloblastic anemia Pancytopenia If untreated can lead to degenerative neurologic disease Low serum B_{12} levels[‡]
Zinc (Fig. 43.9) ***Acquired*** – low zinc in maternal milk, deficient parenteral nutrition, GI disorders, high-fiber diets, HIV infection ***Genetic* (acrodermatitis enteropathica)** – onset days–weeks after birth if bottle-fed or onset typically after weaning if breast-fed	Acral and periorificial dermatitis with erythematous patches and plaques, secondary scaling and crust, erosions and possible vesicles and bulla (see Figs 43.4–43.5) Chronic: may see rough, dry skin, seborrheic dermatitis-like eruptions, lichenified psoriasiform plaques, and poor wound healing Necrosis present in severe cases Stomatitis, glossitis, and cheilitis	**Classic triad** of diarrhea, dermatitis, and alopecia Failure to thrive Apathy and irritability Photophobia Low serum zinc and alkaline phosphatase levels

Copper ***Acquired*** – rare; excessive zinc intake, gastrointestinal surgeries, and malabsorptive syndromes ***Genetic* (Menkes disease or kinky hair disease)** (Fig. 43.10) – autosomal recessive; mutation in gene that encodes a copper transporting ATPase	***Acquired*** May rarely see pigmentary dilution of hair and skin Genetic Onset age 2–3 months Diffuse cutaneous pigmentary dilution Characteristic facies with pudgy cheeks, cupid bow of upper lip, and horizontal eyebrows Light-colored, sparse, fragile, **kinky hair** Characteristic structural abnormalities of hair, e.g. pili torti, monilethrix, trichorrhexis nodosa **Obligate female carriers –** as a result of lyonization may see patches of swirled hypopigmentation or pili torti in lines of Blaschko	***Acquired*** Anemia, neutropenia, bone marrow dysplasia Neuropathy Failure to thrive ***Genetic*** Failure to thrive Lethargy, hypotonia Hypothermia Seizures Intellectual disability Osseous alterations Anemia Low serum copper levels
Selenium	Hypopigmentation of skin and hair White nails	Weakness Myalgias and elevated muscle enzymes Cardiomyopathy Low serum selenium levels
Iron	**May see prior to clinically evident anemia** Koilonychia, brittle nails Glossitis, angular cheilitis Pruritus Alopecia; dry, dull, and brittle hair **If significant anemia present** Skin and nail bed pallor	**Anemia and its associated symptoms** Lethargy, fatigue Decreased exercise tolerance Shortness of breath Congestive heart failure Restless legs syndrome Low serum iron and ferritin levels

**Wernicke encephalopathy characterized by ophthalmoplegia, ataxia, confusion.*
***Korsakoff syndrome characterized by peripheral neuropathy, memory loss, confabulation.*
†Leigh syndrome characterized by subacute necrotizing encephalomyopathy; anorexia, weakness, constipation; congestive heart failure; low serum or plasma thiamine levels.
‡Elevated serum homocysteine and methylmalonic acid levels are more reliable indicators of B_{12} deficiency and are useful to obtain if B_{12} deficiency is strongly suspected but serum levels of B_{12} are low–normal.

Table 43.1 *Continued* **Malnutrition-deficiency syndromes with mucocutaneous manifestations.**

MALNUTRITION-EXCESS SYNDROMES WITH MUCOCUTANEOUS MANIFESTATIONS		
Excess syndrome	**Mucocutaneous features**	**Systemic features**
Obesity (Fig. 43.12)	Plantar hyperkeratosis Acanthosis nigricans Acrochordons Striae distensae Intertrigo Frictional hyperpigmentation Hyperhidrosis Stasis dermatitis Leg ulcers, mostly venous > arterial Lipodermatosclerosis, including the pannus Stasis mucinosis	Body mass index >30 Hypertension Diabetes and insulin resistance Gastroesophageal reflux disease Atherosclerotic cardiovascular disease Steatorrhea
Vitamin A	Mucocutaneous findings similar to patients on oral retinoids Xerotic, rough, pruritic, and scaly skin Xerotic cheilitis Diffuse alopecia	Anorexia, weight loss, lethargy Elevated liver enzymes Painful swellings in limbs due to bony changes Radiographic bone changes, e.g. skeletal hyperostosis, extra-spinal tendon and ligament calcification
Beta carotene (the natural pro-vitamin of vitamin A) **Carotenemia**	**Carotenoderma** (Fig. 43.13) – orange-yellow skin pigmentation primarily in sebaceous gland-rich areas (forehead, nasolabial fold) and in areas with a thicker stratum corneum (palms, soles) Differentiated from jaundice, which has prominent yellow discoloration of the sclerae and mucosae	
Copper ***Acquired*** – rare ***Genetic* (Wilson disease)** – autosomal recessive; mutation in gene that encodes a copper-transporting P-type ATPase	***Genetic*** **Kayser–Fleischer** corneal rings	***Genetic*** Liver disease and cirrhosis Dysarthria, dyspraxia, ataxia, and parkinsonian-like extrapyramidal signs
Iron ***Acquired*** – numerous blood transfusions; excess intake ***Genetic* (type I hemochromatosis)** – autosomal recessive; mutation in gene (*HFE*) that regulates absorption of iron; two most common mutations of *HFE* gene are C282Y and H63D	Generalized hyperpigmentation (bronzing)	Chronic fatigue Diabetes Liver disease, cirrhosis Arthritis Cardiac disease Impotence Hypothyroidism

Table 43.2 Malnutrition-excess syndromes with mucocutaneous manifestations.

vitamin D production, impairment in liver and kidney hydroxylation of active vitamin D precursors, and end-organ resistance to vitamin D metabolites.

- Excess vitamin D, typically resulting from prolonged and excessive intake of vitamin D supplements, can present with anorexia, vomiting, diarrhea, headaches, hypercalcemia, hypercalciuria, muscle weakness, and bone demineralization.
- No specific cutaneous features have been described with vitamin D deficiency or excess.
- The best indicator of vitamin D stores is a measurement of the *serum 25-hydroxyvitamin D level*, and this laboratory value is sometimes used to guide individual vitamin D requirements.
- Guidelines for vitamin D supplementation have been in flux, but oral supplementation is generally recommended for exclusively

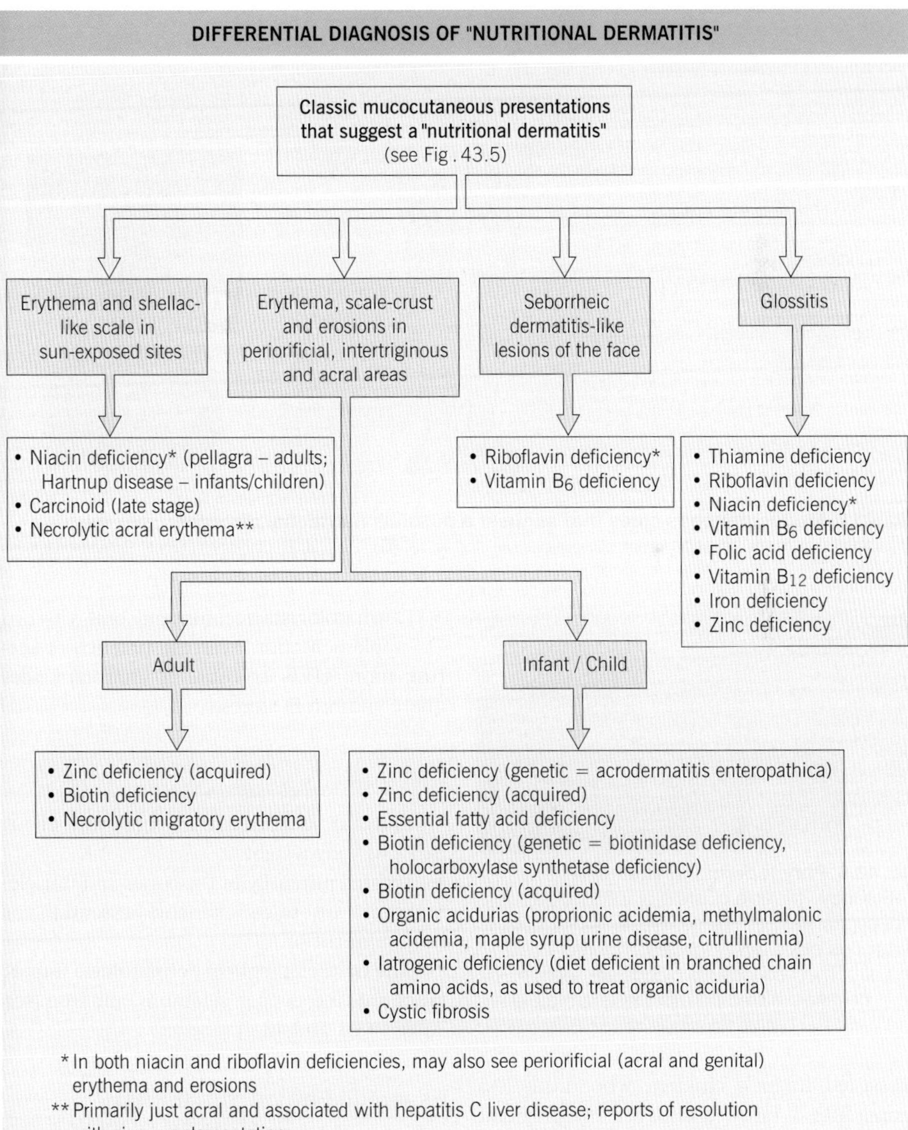

Fig. 43.4 Clinical approach to the patient with a presumed nutritional disorder. Differential diagnosis of "nutritional dermatitis."

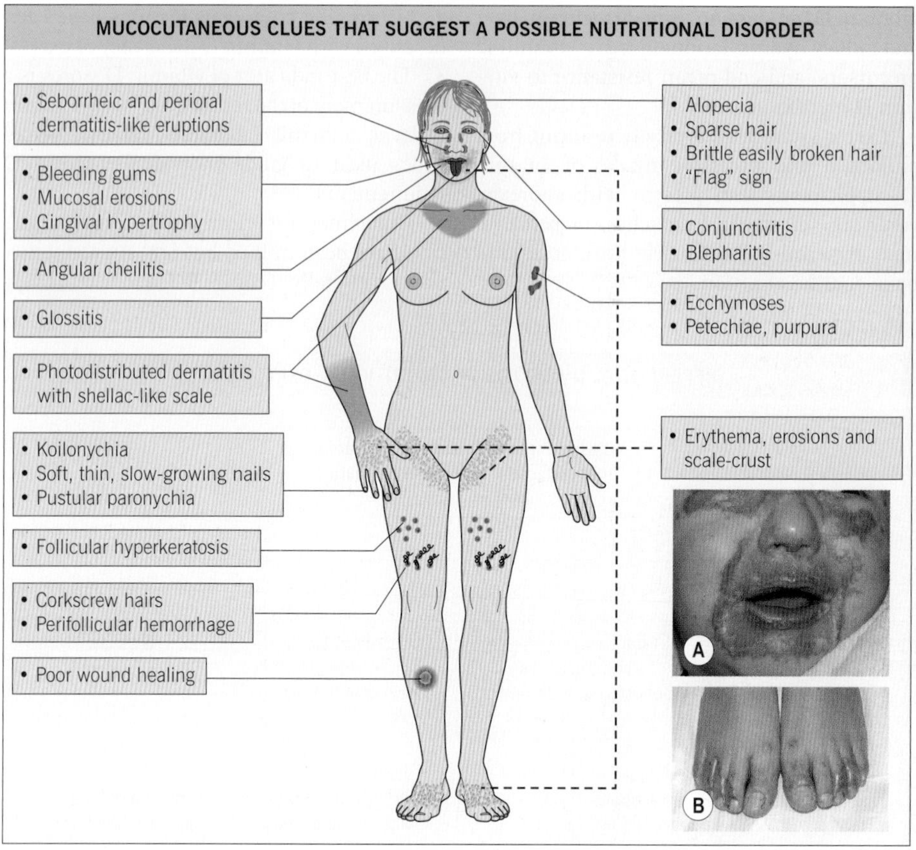

MUCOCUTANEOUS CLUES THAT SUGGEST A POSSIBLE NUTRITIONAL DISORDER

- Seborrheic and perioral dermatitis-like eruptions

- Bleeding gums
- Mucosal erosions
- Gingival hypertrophy

- Angular cheilitis

- Glossitis

- Photodistributed dermatitis with shellac-like scale

- Koilonychia
- Soft, thin, slow-growing nails
- Pustular paronychia

- Follicular hyperkeratosis

- Corkscrew hairs
- Perifollicular hemorrhage

- Poor wound healing

- Alopecia
- Sparse hair
- Brittle easily broken hair
- "Flag" sign

- Conjunctivitis
- Blepharitis

- Ecchymoses
- Petechiae, purpura

- Erythema, erosions and scale-crust

A

B

Fig. 43.5 Mucocutaneous clues that suggest a possible nutritional disorder. Erythema, erosions and desquamation favor periorificial (**A**) and acral (**B**) sites. *A, B, Courtesy, Julie V. Schaffer, MD.*

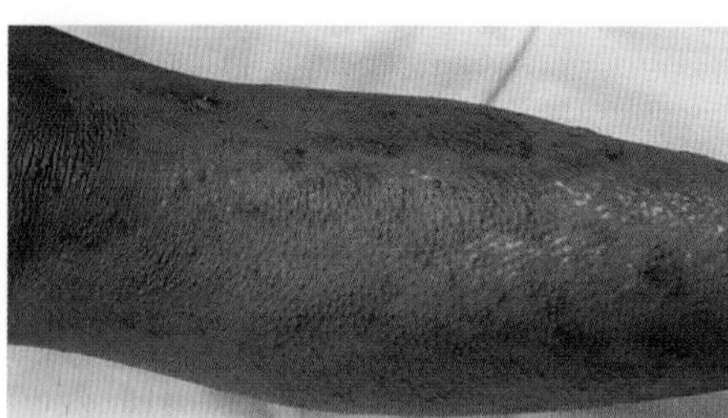

Fig. 43.6 Phrynoderma of vitamin A deficiency. Multiple clusters of follicular papules with central keratotic plugs. Histopathologically, keratinous plugs within follicles, hyperkeratosis and atrophy of sebaceous glands are seen. It must be differentiated from pityriasis rubra pilaris and keratosis pilaris. *Courtesy, Chad M. Hivnor, MD.*

breast-fed infants, children who drink less than a liter of fortified milk per day, pregnant women, the elderly, most adults for the prevention of osteoporosis, and individuals on long-term oral glucocorticoids.

- Dermatologists recommend oral vitamin D supplementation over the practice of getting more UVB exposure to maintain adequate vitamin D stores.

Minerals

- Inorganic elements that constitute about 3–4% of body weight.
- Located primarily in the bones and muscle.
- Some are trace elements essential for human nutrition.
- The trace elements of dermatologic importance are zinc, copper, selenium, and iron (see Tables 43.1 and 43.2).

Essential Fatty Acids (EFAs)

- Unsaturated fatty acids that the body needs but cannot synthesize, and therefore must be obtained from the diet.

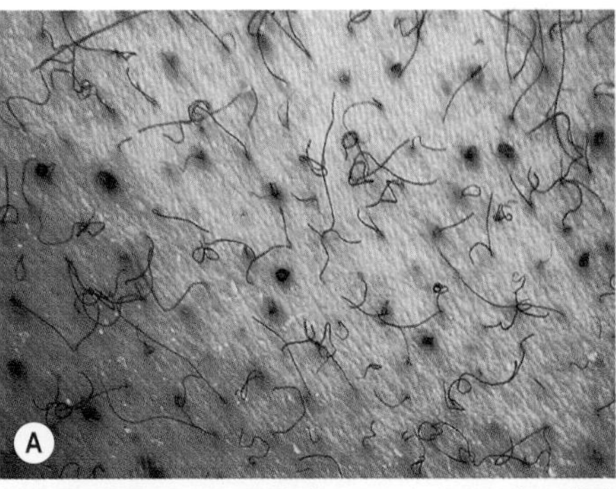

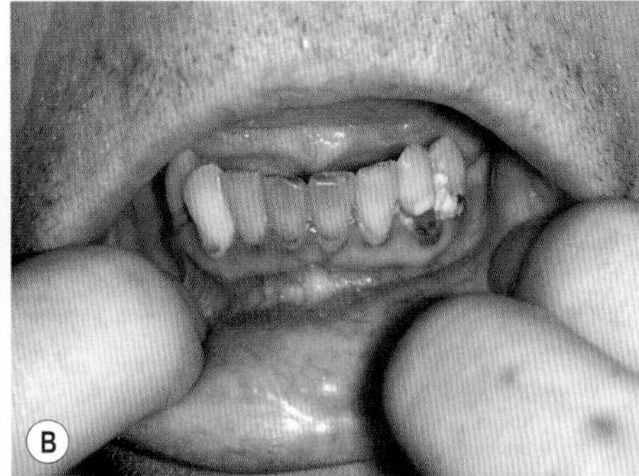

Fig. 43.7 Scurvy. A Corkscrew hairs and perifollicular hemorrhage on the lower extremities. **B** Gingivitis and gingival erosions. *A, Courtesy, YDRSC; B, Courtesy, Jeffrey Callen, MD.*

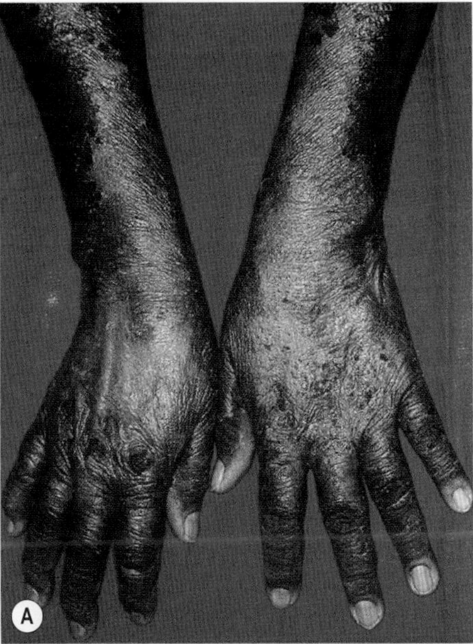

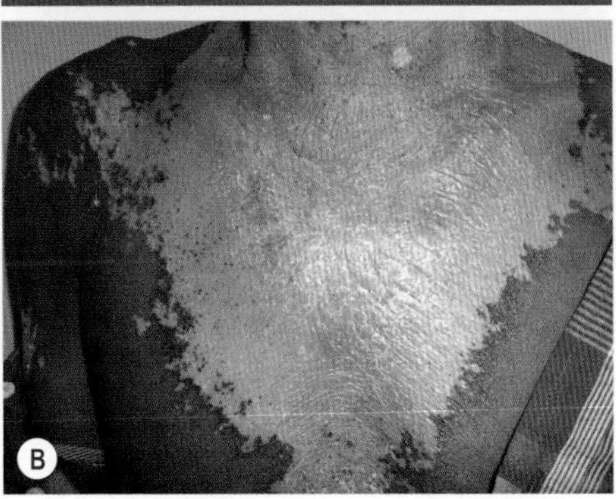

Fig. 43.8 Pellagra. A Hyperpigmentation with desquamation of the dorsal aspects of the hands and forearms. The shellac-like scale is seen best on the forearms. **B** Striking hypopigmentation with peripheral desquamation of the sun-exposed area of the chest in a man from sub-Saharan Africa. *A, Courtesy, YDRSC; B, Courtesy, Rosemarie Moser, MD.*

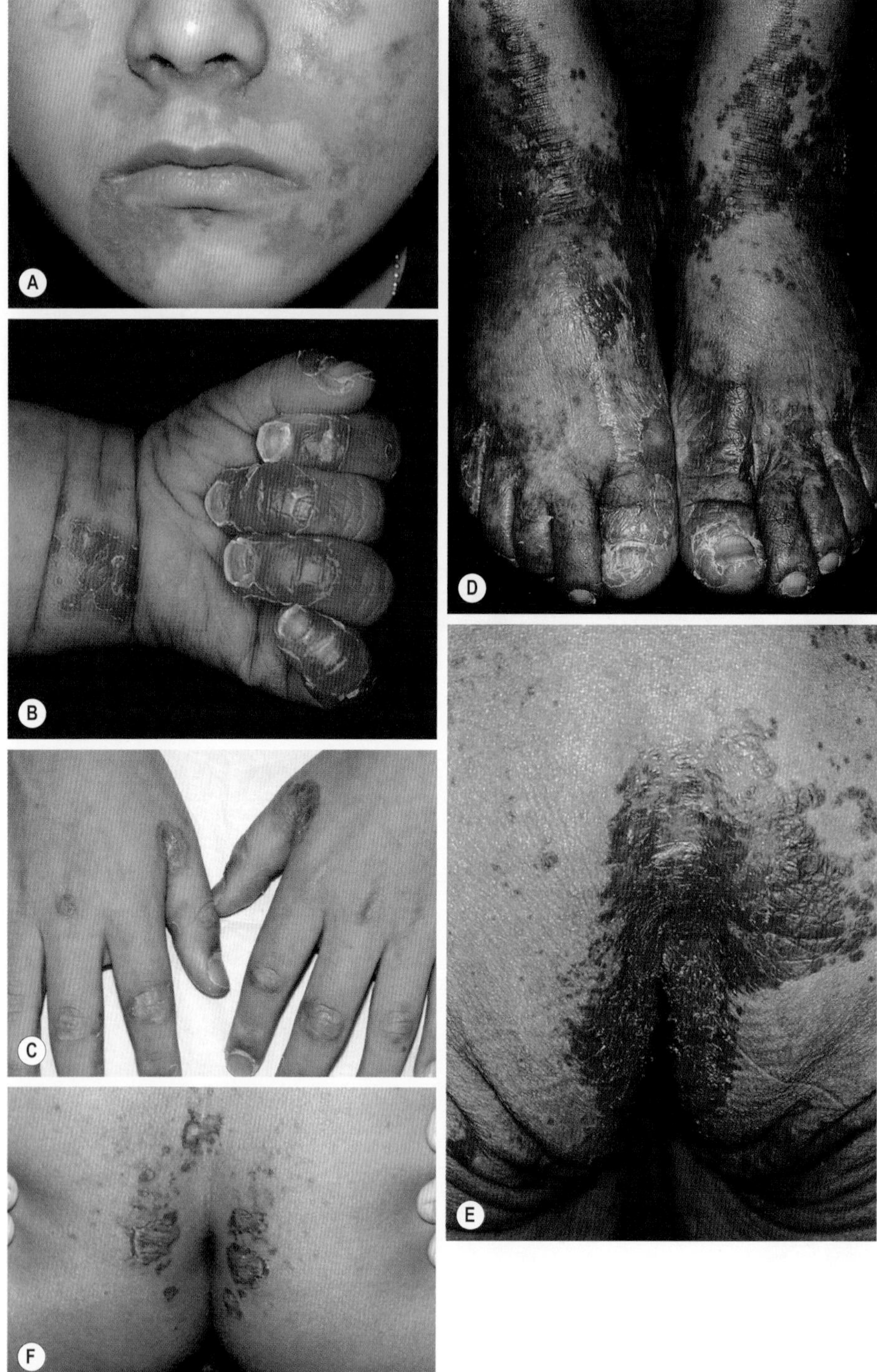

Fig. 43.9 Zinc deficiency. Erythema with erosions and scale-crust that is often shellac-like favors the perioral (**A**), acral (**B–D**), and anogenital (**E, F**) regions. The degree of involvement can vary from subtle to striking and may mimic other types of "nutritional dermatitis" (see Figs 43.4–43.5), necrolytic migratory erythema, and more common disorders such as seborrheic dermatitis and psoriasis.
A, C, F, Courtesy, Julie V. Schaffer, MD; B, D, E, Courtesy, YDRSC.

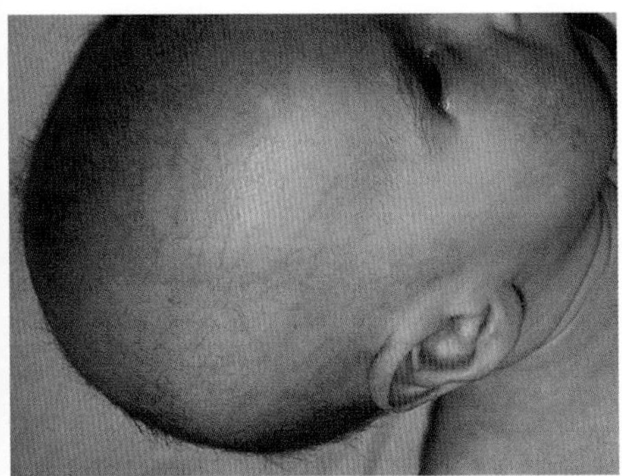

Fig. 43.10 Menkes disease. This child has the characteristic pale skin and sparse kinky hair. *Courtesy, Ramón Ruiz-Maldonado, MD.*

- The three major EFAs are linoleic, linolenic, and arachidonic acids.
- In most patients, EFA deficiency is seen along with other nutritional deficiencies.
- Isolated deficiencies of EFAs are uncommon but can be seen in patients receiving parenteral nutrition without lipid supplementation and with overly aggressive low-fat diets.

Anorexia/Bulimia

- Eating disorders that may lead to nutritional deficiencies.
- Associated cutaneous findings include xerosis, telogen effluvium, lanugo-like hair, brittle nails, carotenoderma, cheilitis, acrocyanosis, and worsening of chilblains (Fig. 43.12).
- In addition, patients with bulimia may develop parotid and salivary gland swelling, erosion of tooth enamel, and abrasions or calluses on the dorsal fingers and knuckles (Russell's sign).

Carotenoderma

- Orange-yellow skin pigmentation (Fig. 43.13) that develops when carotene levels are 3–4 times normal (carotenemia).
- Can result from the high intake of carotenoid-rich foods (carrots) or the inability to convert ingested beta-carotene into vitamin A (some patients with diabetes, hypothyroidism, or anorexia nervosa).
- An excess intake of lycopene-rich foods (tomato, papaya) may induce lycopenemia and skin findings similar to carotenoderma.

Obesity

- Defined as a body mass index (BMI) >30; may be acquired or inherited.
- Predisposing genetic syndromes that result in an earlier, childhood onset include Prader–Willi, Bardet–Biedl, Alström, and Wilson–Turner syndromes.
- Predisposing endocrine conditions include Cushing disease, Cushing syndrome, polycystic ovarian syndrome, and insulin resistance.
- Acquired obesity is at epidemic levels, especially in high-income populations.
- The cutaneous manifestations of obesity are outlined in Table 43.2 and Fig. 43.12.
- May have associated metabolic syndrome (see Ch. 45).
- Post-bariatric surgery patients are at risk for developing nutritional deficiencies due to altered gastrointestinal absorption of micronutrients (e.g. zinc, iron, copper) and vitamins (e.g. A, D, E, folate, B_{12}).

For further information see Ch. 51 from *Dermatology, Fourth Edition*.

For additional online figures visit www.expertconsult.com 

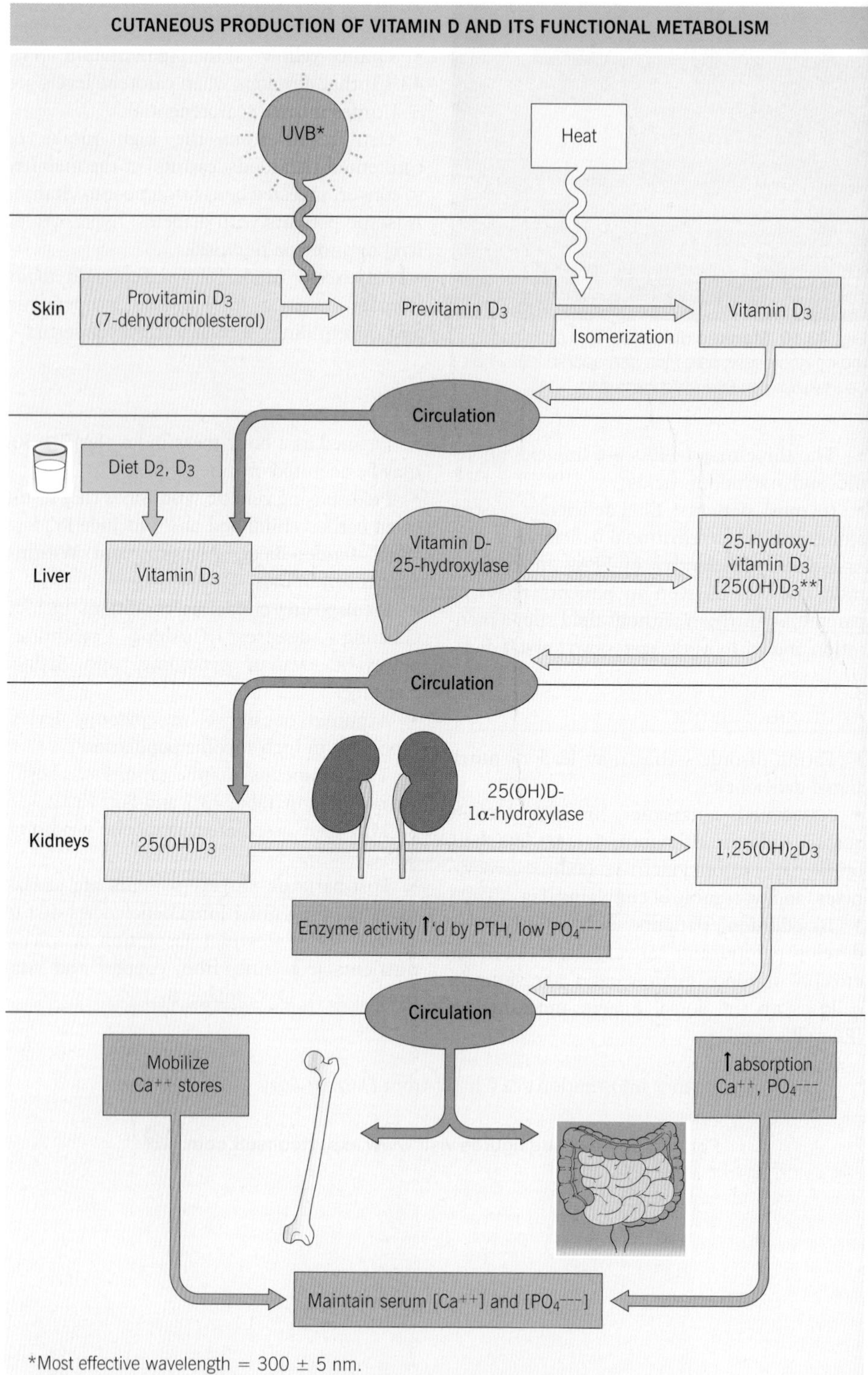

Fig. 43.11 Cutaneous production of vitamin D and its functional metabolism. *See next page for figure legend.*

Fig. 43.11 Cutaneous production of vitamin D and its functional metabolism. During exposure to ultraviolet B radiation, 7-dehydrocholesterol within the skin is converted to previtamin D_3, which is then immediately converted to vitamin D_3 in a heat-dependent process. Of note, the heat from excessive sunlight exposure can degrade previtamin D_3 and vitamin D_3 into inactive photoproducts. Both forms of vitamin D (D_3 and D_2) are biologically inactive and they require activation in the liver and then the kidney. After binding to carrier proteins, vitamin D is transported to the liver, where it is enzymatically hydroxylated to 25-hydroxyvitamin D [25(OH)D], the major circulating form of vitamin D. 25-Hydroxyvitamin D is then converted into its active form, 1,25-dihydroxyvitamin D [1,25$(OH)_2$D], within the kidney by the enzyme 1α-hydroxylase. Of interest, this final hydroxylation step can also occur in keratinocytes when the enzyme CYP27B1 is upregulated in response to wounding or by Toll-like receptor (TLR) activation from microbial-derived ligands. Serum levels of phosphate, calcium, and fibroblast growth factor 23 can either increase or decrease renal production of 1,25$(OH)_2$D. 1,25$(OH)_2$D decreases its own synthesis via feedback inhibition and decreases the synthesis and secretion of parathyroid hormone by the parathyroid glands. 1,25$(OH)_2$D also enhances intestinal calcium absorption in the small intestine by interacting with the vitamin D receptor–retinoic acid X receptor complex (VDR-RXR) to enhance the expression of the epithelial calcium channel and calbindin-D 9K, a calcium-binding protein. In addition, 1,25$(OH)_2$D is recognized by its receptor in osteoblasts, leading to a series of events that maintain calcium and phosphorus levels in the blood which in turn promotes mineralization of the skeleton.

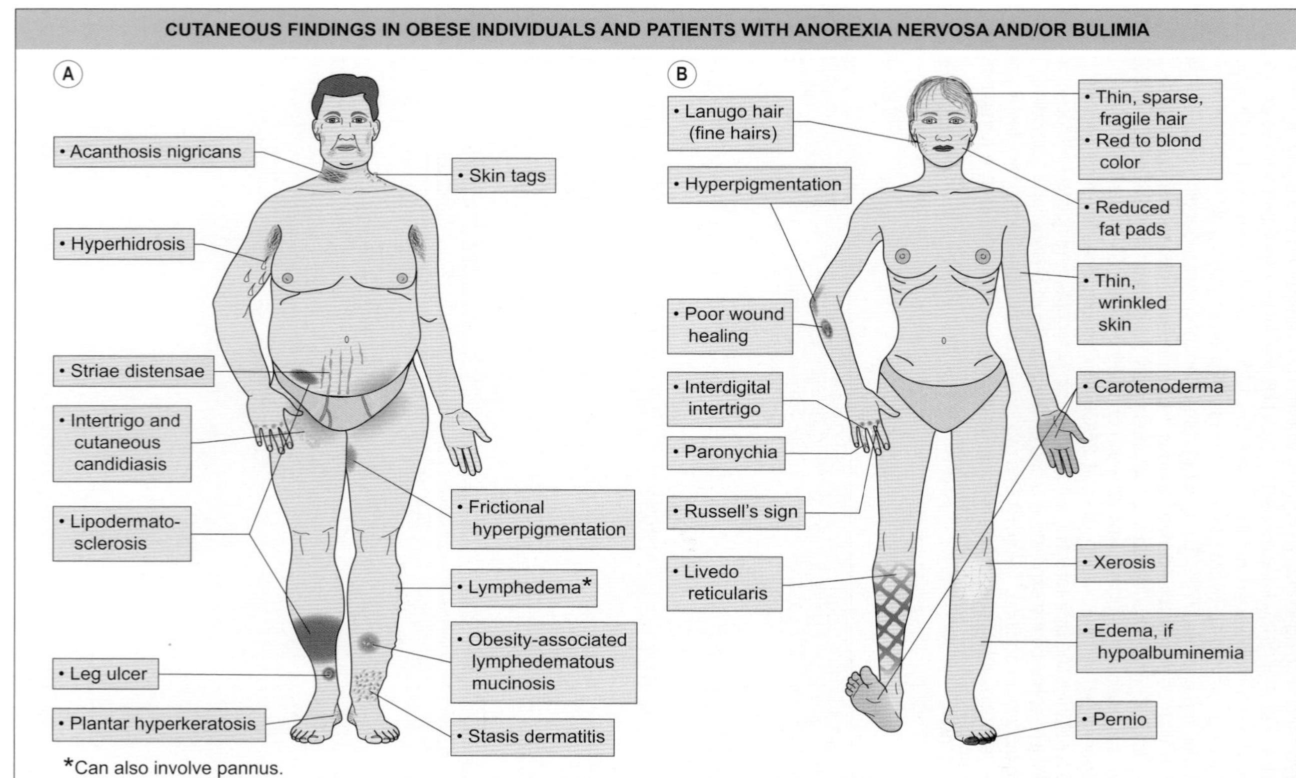

Fig. 43.12 Cutaneous findings in obese individuals (A) and patients with anorexia nervosa and/or bulimia (B). (See Fig. 43.5 for signs of nutritional deficiences).

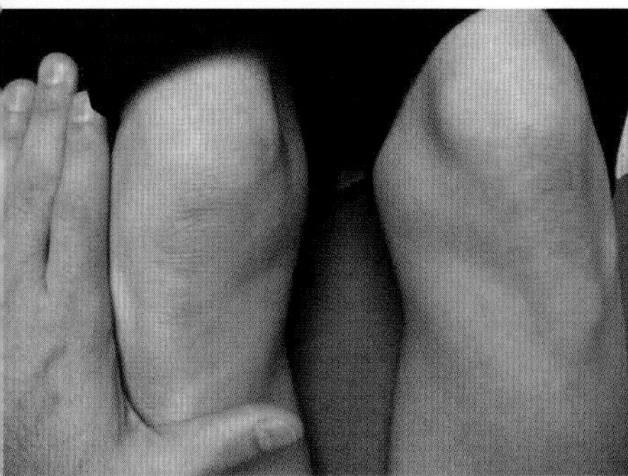

Fig. 43.13 Carotenoderma. The patient's legs are noticeably orange when compared to the photographer's hand. *Courtesy, Chad M. Hivnor, MD.*

44 Graft-Versus-Host Disease

• Multiorgan disorder that most commonly results from the transfer of donor hematopoietic stem cells into a recipient via an allogeneic hematopoietic stem cell transplant (HSCT).
• Despite advances in HSCT procedures and post-transplantation immunosuppressive therapy, more than half of HSCT recipients develop chronic GVHD, which remains a major cause of morbidity and mortality.
• Table 44.1 lists risk factors for GVHD in HSCT recipients.
• Less frequent settings of GVHD include transfusion of non-irradiated blood products to an immunocompromised patient, maternal–fetal transmission to an immunodeficient neonate, and solid organ transplantation.
• Divided into acute and chronic forms based on clinical features.
• Pathogenesis of acute GVHD occurs in three steps: (1) HSCT conditioning regimen leads to epithelial cell injury and activation of *host* antigen presenting cells; (2) activation of *donor* T cells; (3) tissue destruction by cytotoxic T cells, natural killer cells, and soluble factors (e.g. TNF).
• Chronic GVHD shares features (e.g. autoantibody production, cutaneous sclerosis) with autoimmune connective tissue diseases.
• Histopathologically, acute GVHD and epidermal involvement in chronic GVHD are characterized by variable degrees of keratinocyte necrosis (often accentuated in appendages), vacuolar degeneration of the basal layer, and a band-like lymphocytic infiltrate.

Acute GVHD

• Most often arises 4–6 weeks after HSCT with traditional regimens.
• Persistent, recurrent, and delayed variants of acute GVHD can occur during a time period (>100 days post-transplant) traditionally reserved for chronic GVHD, especially following interventions such as tapering of immunosuppression and donor lymphocyte infusions.
• Typically presents as a morbilliform exanthem, often with perifollicular accentuation.
• Initial predilection for acral sites (e.g. dorsal hands and feet, palms, soles, ears), forearms, and upper trunk.
• Clinical staging is based on the proportion of the cutaneous surface involved: Stage 1, <25%; Stage 2, 25–50%; and Stage 3, >50%. Stage 4 represents erythroderma with bullae/epidermal detachment resembling toxic epidermal necrolysis (Fig. 44.1).
• Mucosal surfaces (including the conjunctiva), the gastrointestinal tract (nausea, diarrhea, abdominal pain), and the liver (transaminitis, cholestasis) are frequently affected.
• Histopathologic evaluation is helpful but not necessarily diagnostic, and clinicopathologic correlation is essential.
• **DDx:** drug eruption, viral exanthem, engraftment syndrome (nonspecific erythematous eruption, fever, pulmonary edema; onset day 10–14 post-transplant), toxic erythema of chemotherapy (especially with palmoplantar or intertriginous involvement).
• **Rx:** topical CS if limited cutaneous involvement only; most patients require systemic CS, which are typically added to ongoing prophylactic treatment with a systemic calcineurin inhibitor; second-line treatments include JAK inhibitors (e.g. ruxolitinib) and other immunosuppressive agents (e.g. mycophenolate mofetil [MMF], TNF inhibitors).

Chronic GVHD

• Can occur as a continuation of acute GVHD, as a recurrence following a GVHD-

RISK FACTORS ASSOCIATED WITH THE DEVELOPMENT OF GRAFT-VERSUS-HOST DISEASE (GVHD)
Donor
HLA incompatibility with recipient Unrelated to recipient Female (especially multiparous) with male recipient Older age
Recipient
Age (elderly > middle aged > pediatric)
Stem cell source
Peripheral blood* > bone marrow > cord blood T-cell replete graft
Transplantation protocol**
More intense/myeloablative conditioning regimen (increases risk of acute GVHD) Less aggressive administration of prophylactic immunosuppressive agents
Clinical course
Reduction of immunosuppression ± donor lymphocyte infusions if recurrence of malignancy Reduction of immunosuppression if decrease in donor chimerism

**More rapid engraftment but increased risk of chronic GVHD.*
***Post-transplantation cyclophosphamide administration reduces the risk of GVHD.*

Table 44.1 Risk factors associated with the development of graft-versus-host disease (GVHD). HLA, human leukocyte antigen.

free interval, or without a history of acute GVHD.

- Skin and mucosal involvement are extremely common and highly variable in their presentations (Table 44.2; Fig. 44.2A), and almost any organ system can be affected (Fig. 44.2B).
- Reticulate pink to violet papules with scale (*lichen planus-like*) favoring the dorsal hands and feet, forearms, and trunk represent one characteristic manifestation (Fig. 44.3A).
- The spectrum of sclerotic involvement includes:
  - *Lichen sclerosus-like* shiny, wrinkled, gray-white plaques, ± follicular plugging, favoring the upper trunk (Fig. 44.3B,C)
  - Localized or widespread *morphea-like* indurated, hyperpigmented to skin-colored plaques favoring the trunk (Fig. 44.3D). Longstanding fibrosis may result in skin ulceration, especially of the legs (Fig. 44.3E)
  - *Eosinophilic fasciitis-like* presentations with acute edema and pain evolving into areas of firm skin with subcutaneous rippling ("pseudo-cellulite"; Fig. 44.3F) and linear depressions following a vein or between muscle groups (groove sign); favors the extremities (sparing the hands and feet) and may result in joint contractures
- Often affects the nails and the oral and genital mucosa (Fig. 44.4; see Table 44.2).
- Other frequent sites of involvement include the eyes (keratoconjunctivitis sicca, blepharitis), salivary glands (sicca syndrome), and lungs (bronchiolitis obliterans); may also affect the esophagus (strictures), liver, and pancreas (exocrine insufficiency).
- **DDx:** drug eruption (e.g. lichenoid, photosensitive), AI-CTDs (e.g. lupus erythematosus, morphea), papulosquamous disorders.
- **Rx:** skin-directed with topical CS or calcineurin inhibitors (for superficial disease; tacrolimus under occlusion may increase systemic levels) or phototherapy (narrowband UVB, UVA1, PUVA); for topical treatment of oral disease, see Table 59.2; components of systemic combination therapy may include CS, calcineurin inhibitors, methotrexate, ruxolitinib, ibrutinib, imatinib, rituximab, acitretin, and extracorporeal photopheresis; physical therapy (for joint mobility), sun protection, and regular skin examinations, especially if prolonged immunosuppression.

For further information see Ch. 52 from *Dermatology, Fourth Edition*.

For additional online figures and tables visit www.expertconsult.com 

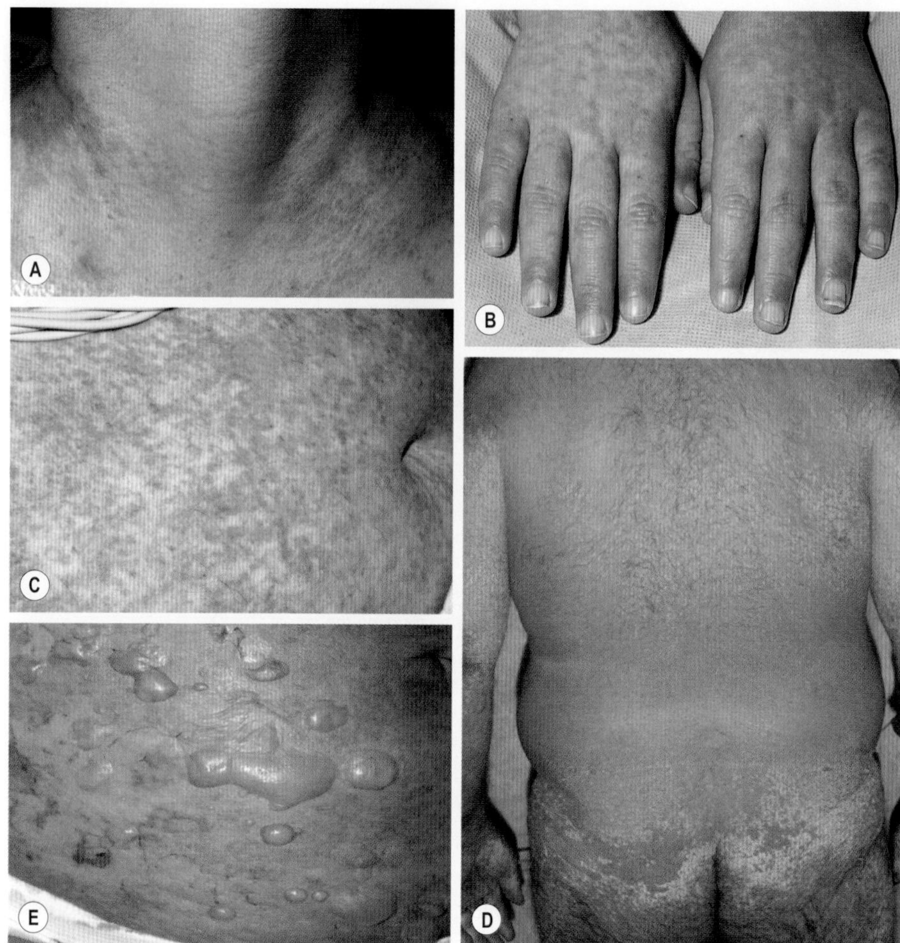

Fig. 44.1 Clinical spectrum of acute cutaneous graft-versus-host disease. A *Stage 1* – discrete and coalescing small pink papules on the upper chest and neck of a woman 6 weeks following allogeneic bone marrow transplant. **B, C** *Stage 2* – pink macules and papules on the dorsal aspect of the hands becoming confluent 4 weeks post allogeneic bone marrow transplant and widespread pink-violet macules and minimally elevated papules on the abdomen in a liver transplant recipient. **D** *Stage 3* – diffuse erythema with desquamation, but without bullae formation. **E** *Stage 4* – widespread bullae and epidermal necrosis in a patient who received a donor lymphocyte infusion following allogeneic bone marrow transplant; note the resemblance to toxic epidermal necrolysis. *A, Courtesy, YDRSC; B, D, E, Courtesy, Edward Cowen, MD; C, Courtesy, Julie V. Schaffer, MD.*

MUCOCUTANEOUS MANIFESTATIONS OF CHRONIC GRAFT-VERSUS-HOST DISEASE (GVHD)
Skin and subcutaneous tissues
Inflammatory manifestations • **Lichen planus-like (lichenoid)** • Psoriasiform, eczematous/dyshidrotic, psoriasiform, pityriasis rosea-like • Photosensitive eruptions resembling subacute cutaneous lupus erythematosus
Sclerotic manifestations • **Lichen sclerosus-like** • **Morphea-like (morpheaform)** • **Scleroderma-like (sclerodermoid)** • **Fasciitis**†
Skin breakdown* • Bullae and ulcerations
Hyperkeratotic and/or adnexal manifestations • Eczema craquelé, keratosis pilaris-like, ichthyosiform • Alopecia (scarring or non-scarring), alopecia areata • Impaired sweating**
Vascular manifestations • **Poikiloderma** • Angiomatous papules/nodules
Pigmentary alterations • Hypo- or depigmentation (e.g. vitiligo-like leukoderma) • Premature graying, leukotrichia • Hyperpigmentation (e.g. leopard-like)
Nail changes • Longitudinal ridging/splitting, brittleness/thinning, onycholysis • Pterygium (dorsal), anonychia
Mucosae
Oral manifestations • **Lichen planus-like** (e.g. lacy white plaques, ulcers) • **Keratotic plaques** • Mucositis, gingivitis, erosions, ulcerations, pseudomembranes • **Restriction of oral opening from sclerosis** • Xerostomia, mucosal atrophy, mucocele
Genital manifestations • **Lichen planus-like** • Erosions/ulcers, fissures (especially of the vulva), balanitis, phimosis • **Vaginal scarring and/or stenosis**

**Often overlying areas of cutaneous sclerosis.*
†Magnetic resonance imaging can help to establish the diagnosis.
***May be related to destruction of eccrine glands.*

Table 44.2 Mucocutaneous manifestations of chronic graft-versus-host disease (GVHD). Diagnostic features are in bold; other signs and symptoms listed are not considered sufficient to establish a diagnosis of chronic GVHD without further testing (e.g. histopathologic assessment) or evidence of other organ system involvement. *Based on Filipovich AH, Weisdorf P, Pavletic S, et al. National Institutes of Health Consensus Development Project on Criteria for Clinical Trials in Chronic Graft-versus-Host Disease: I. Diagnosis and Staging Working Group report. Biol Blood Marrow Transplant. 2005;11:945–956.* For manifestations in other organs (including the eye), see this reference as well as the text.

MANIFESTATIONS OF CHRONIC GRAFT-VERSUS-HOST DISEASE

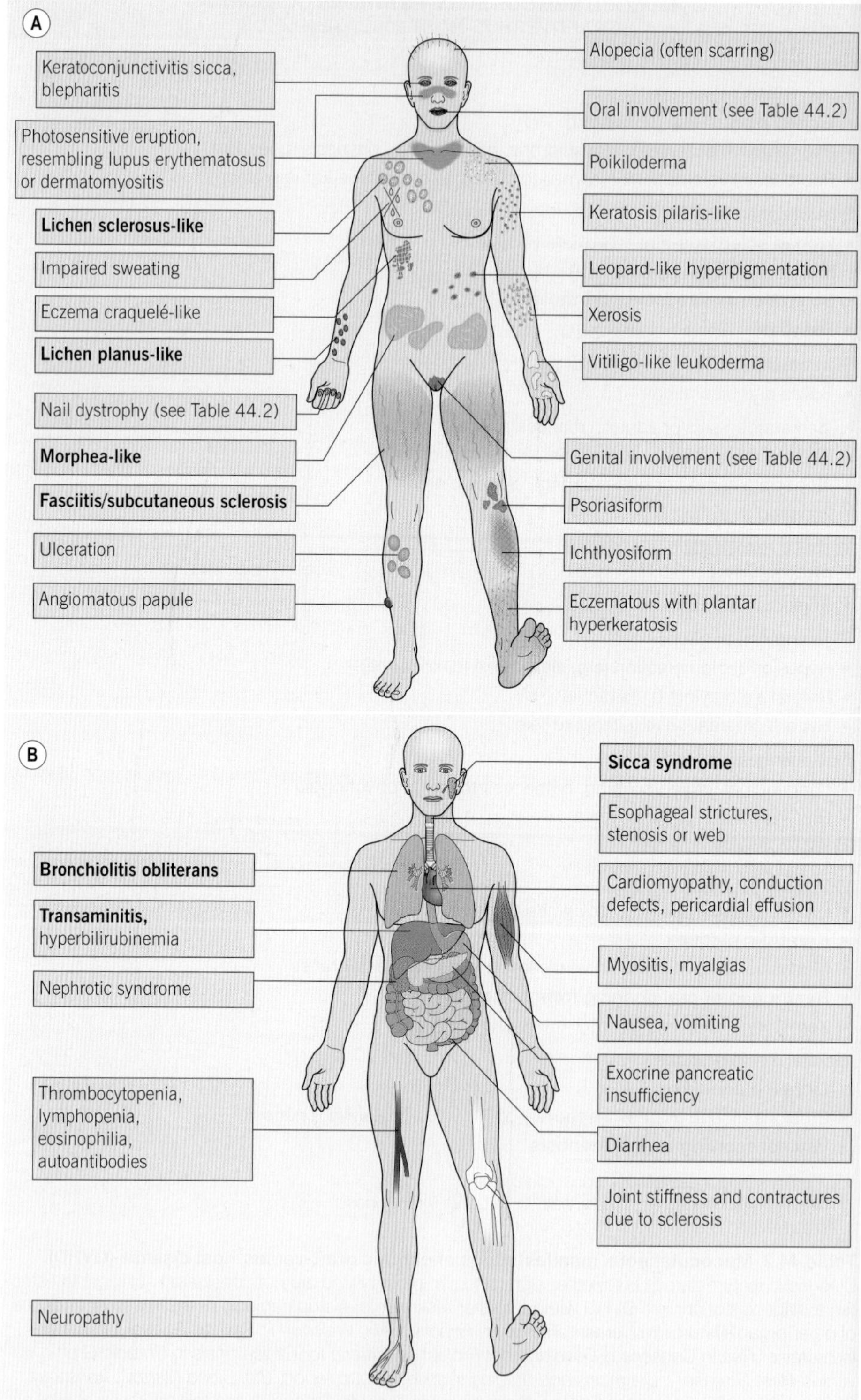

Fig. 44.2 Manifestations of chronic graft-versus-host disease. A Mucocutaneous findings. Lichen sclerosus-like lesions may be prominent on the back. Highly characteristic manifestations are in bold. **B** Internal involvement. The most common manifestations are in bold.

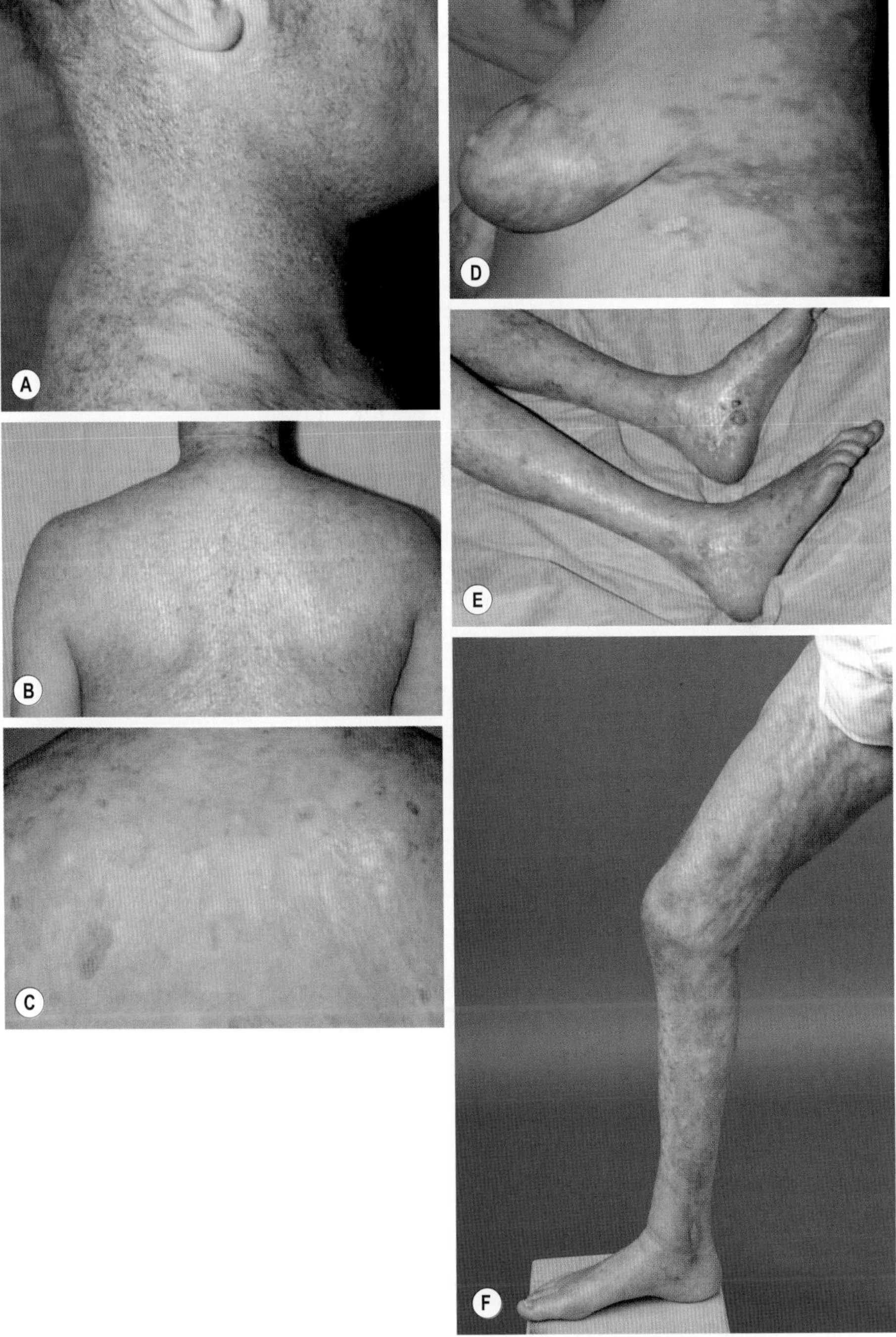

Fig. 44.3 Clinical spectrum of chronic cutaneous graft-versus-host disease. A Lichen planus-like – thin pink-violet papules and plaques with scale, admixed with postinflammatory hyperpigmentation. **B** Lichen sclerosus-like (early) – multiple gray-white thin plaques with obvious wrinkling are present on the mid back. **C** Lichen sclerosus-like (late) – thicker shiny white plaques on the upper back admixed with erosions. **D** Morphea-like (morpheaform) – shiny, hyperpigmented, sclerotic plaques extending from the breast to the lateral trunk. **E** Scleroderma-like (sclerodermoid) – the skin is shiny and bound-down with dyspigmentation, hair loss, angiomatous nodules, multiple erosions and ulceration; range of motion of the ankles is markedly reduced. **F** Eosinophilic fasciitis-like presentation of chronic cutaneous graft-versus-host disease. A rippled appearance and irregular nodular texture to the skin is indicative of involvement of subcutaneous tissues. Especially in the earlier, edematous phase, the presence of hypereosinophilia may be a clue to the diagnosis. *A, B, D–F, Courtesy, Edward Cowen, MD; C, Courtesy, Joyce Rico, MD.*

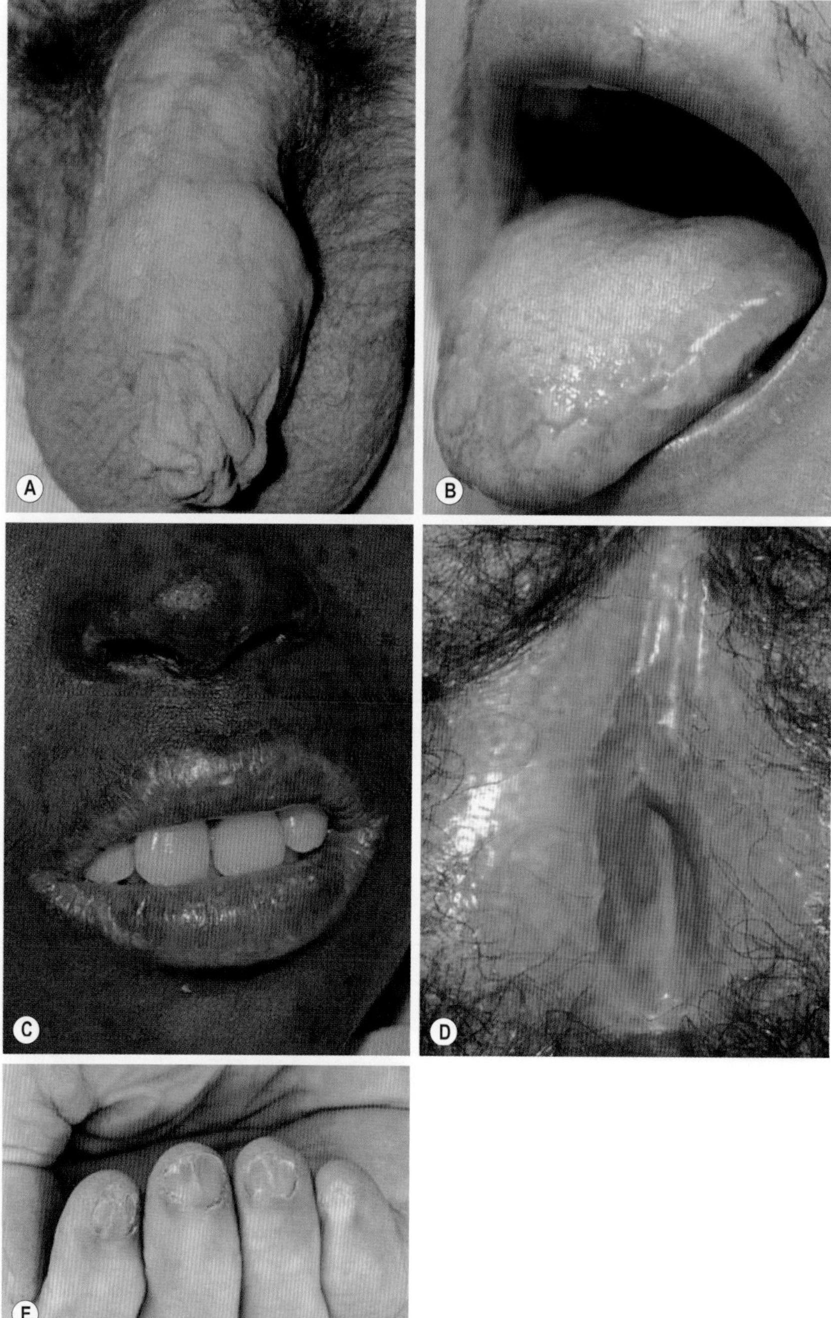

Fig. 44.4 Orogenital and nail involvement in chronic cutaneous graft-versus-host disease. A–C Lichen planus-like – flat-topped violet papules on the penis (**A**), several ulcers on the tongue (**B**), and a lacy white pattern on the lips, distal dorsal tongue, and alar rim (**B, C**). Note the hyperpigmented macules in surrounding skin (**C**). **D** Severe erosive disease of the vulva, with nearly total resorption of the labia minora and agglutination of the lips of the clitoral hood. The vulvar introitus is also markedly narrowed. **E** Nail thinning, splitting and dorsal pterygium formation. *A, D, E, Courtesy, Edward Cowen, MD; B, Courtesy, Jean L. Bolognia, MD; C, Courtesy, Julie V. Schaffer MD.*

Skin Signs of Systemic Disease 45

Introduction

- Recognizing the skin signs of systemic disease is an important aspect of dermatology; however, the vast number of cutaneous manifestations, combined with the infrequency with which each sign is encountered, can be daunting.
- The approach in this chapter is to provide several examples of the most commonly observed or most characteristic cutaneous findings, based on the organ system most often involved – for example, papulonodules of sarcoidosis (lung), diffuse induration of systemic sclerosis (kidney), and melanotic macules of Peutz–Jeghers syndrome (gastrointestinal tract).
- With the exception of endocrinologic disorders and paraneoplastic dermatoses, most of these skin signs have been discussed in other chapters – for example, pyoderma gangrenosum in Chapter 21, telangiectasias of hereditary hemorrhagic telangiectasia (HHT) in Chapter 87, and sebaceous neoplasms of Muir–Torre syndrome in Chapters 52 and 91.

Pulmonary Disease and the Skin

- Table 45.1 and Fig. 45.1.

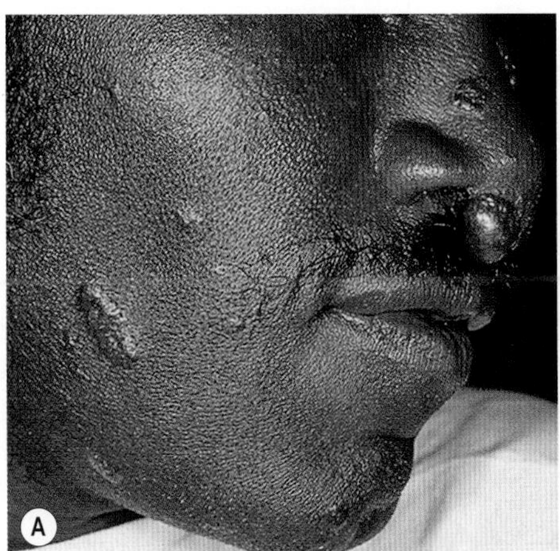

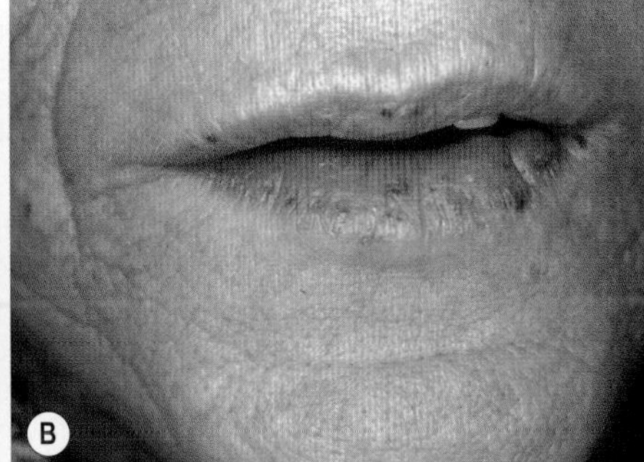

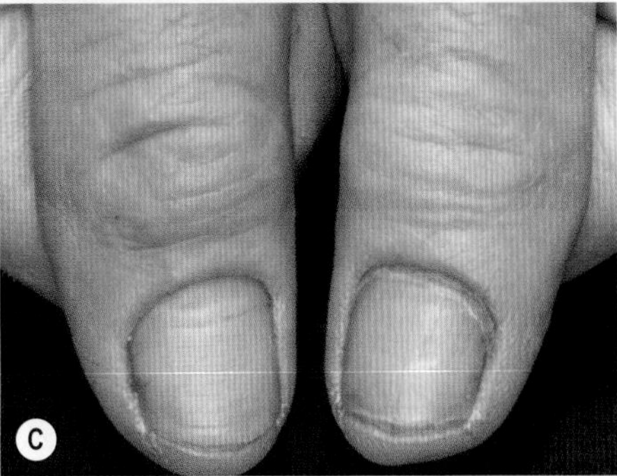

Fig. 45.1 Skin signs of pulmonary disease. **A** Periorificial and facial papules of sarcoidosis. The presence of lesions on the nasal rim is often associated with granulomatous inflammation of the upper respiratory tract. **B** Hereditary hemorrhagic telangiectasia. Several small red macules and papules on the lips. **C** Yellow nail syndrome. *A, Courtesy, Jeffrey P. Callen, MD; B, Courtesy, Irwin Braverman, MD; C, Courtesy, Karynne O. Duncan, MD.*

EXAMPLES OF SKIN SIGNS OF PULMONARY DISEASE		
Disorder	**Cutaneous findings**	**Pulmonary disease**
Genetic		
Birt–Hogg–Dubé syndrome (see Ch. 91)	• Classic triad of fibrofolliculomas, trichodiscomas, and acrochordons	• Lung cysts, spontaneous pneumothoraces
Hereditary hemorrhagic telangiectasia (HHT) (see Ch. 87)	• Mucosal, facial, and acral telangiectatic macules and papules (Fig. 45.1B)	• Pulmonary AVMs
Inflammatory/autoimmune		
Sarcoidosis (see Ch. 78)	• Acute: erythema nodosum • Chronic: papules, nodules (Fig. 45.1A), plaques, lupus pernio, lesions in scars and tattoos; acquired ichthyosis	• Acute: bilateral hilar lymphadenopathy • Chronic: fibrosis due to granulomatous inflammation
Granulomatosis with polyangiitis (Wegener granulomatosis; see Ch. 19)	• Vasculitic lesions (e.g. palpable purpura or nodules), crusted papules due to PNGD, cutaneous granulomas, pyoderma gangrenosum-like ulcers, "strawberry gums" (see Fig. 59.17), oral ulcers (see Fig. 19.10B)	• Dyspnea, cough, hemoptysis, and/or pleuritis • Irregular pulmonary infiltrates or nodules that may cavitate
Eosinophilic granulomatosis with polyangiitis (Churg–Strauss syndrome; see Ch. 19)	• Palpable purpura, urticarial plaques, nodules, crusted papules of the elbows due to PNGD, ulcers	• Asthma • Eosinophilic pneumonia
Yellow nail syndrome (Fig. 45.1C)	• Thickened, slow-growing, excessively curved, yellow-to-green nails with onycholysis, transverse ridging, onychomadesis, and absent cuticles and lunulae	• Bronchopulmonary disease: pleural effusions, bronchiectasis • Lymphedema, sinusitis • Malignancy
Dermatomyositis (see Ch. 34)	• Gottron papules, heliotrope, photodistributed poikiloderma (see Fig. 34.4)	• ILD, aspiration pneumonitis, hypoventilation
Systemic sclerosis (see Ch. 35)	• DcSSc: Raynaud disease (sudden onset); more widespread sclerosis • LcSSc: Raynaud disease (preceding long duration); limited, acrofacial sclerosis	• DcSSc: ILD > PAH • LcSSc: PAH > ILD (see Fig. 35.2)
Neoplastic/paraneoplastic		
Lymphomatoid granulomatosis (see Ch. 99)	• Papulonodules, plaques, ulcers	• Cough, dyspnea and chest pain due to angiocentric, angiodestructive infiltrate of atypical lymphocytes
Paraneoplastic pemphigus (see Ch. 23)	• See Table 45.9 and Fig. 23.8	• Bronchiolitis obliterans

Table 45.1 Examples of skin signs of pulmonary disease. *Continued*

EXAMPLES OF SKIN SIGNS OF PULMONARY DISEASE		
Disorder	**Cutaneous findings**	**Pulmonary disease**
Infectious		
Tuberculosis (see Ch. 62)	• Lupus vulgaris, acute miliary, scrofuloderma, tuberculous gumma, orificial	• Apical infiltrates, cavitating infiltrates; nonproductive or productive cough
Blastomycosis* (see Ch. 64)	• Verrucous, ulcerated plaques or nodules	• Patchy infiltrates or normal chest X-ray
Cryptococcosis (see Ch. 64)	• Variable cutaneous findings, from papulonodules and plaques to molluscum contagiosum-like lesions and cellulitis	• Varies from asymptomatic infection to severe pneumonia and acute respiratory distress syndrome
Aspergillosis (see Ch. 64)	• Plaques with black crusts • Cutaneous emboli: necrotic papules and plaques, often with ulceration and rapidly progressive	• In those with disseminated cutaneous emboli, cavitating infiltrates and nodules
Varicella (see Ch. 67)	• Lesions in various stages of development, including papules, papulovesicles, pustules, and hemorrhagic crusts	• Pulmonary involvement correlates with severity of skin involvement. Interstitial infiltrates or patchy airway disease leads to cough and dyspnea.
Other		
Toxic epidermal necrolysis (TEN) (see Ch. 16)	• Widespread necrosis and detachment	• Acute respiratory distress syndrome

**Primary pulmonary infection also occurs in other systemic mycoses due to dimorphic pathogens, including coccidioidomycosis, histoplasmosis, and paracoccidioidomycosis.*

Table 45.1 *Continued* **Examples of skin signs of pulmonary disease.** Patients with Kaposi sarcoma, urticarial vasculitis, and tuberous sclerosis complex can also have pulmonary disease. AVM, arteriovenous malformation; PNGD, palisaded neutrophilic and granulomatous dermatitis; DcSSc, diffuse cutaneous systemic sclerosis; LcSSc, limited cutaneous systemic sclerosis; ILD, interstitial lung disease; PAH, pulmonary arterial hypertension.

Cardiac Disease and the Skin

- Table 45.2 and Fig. 45.2.

Gastrointestinal Disease and the Skin

- Tables 45.3–45.5 and Figs 45.3 and 45.4.

Liver Disease and the Skin

- Table 45.6 and Fig. 45.5.

Renal Disease and the Skin

- Table 45.7.

Skin Signs of Internal Malignancy

- Tables 45.8 and 45.9 and Figs 45.6 and 45.7.

Skin Signs of Endocrine Disorders and Metabolic Disease

- Tables 45.10–45.13 and Figs 45.8–45.12.

For further information see Ch. 53 from *Dermatology, Fourth Edition*.

For additional online figures visit www.expertconsult.com 

EXAMPLES OF SKIN SIGNS OF CARDIAC DISEASE	
Disorder	**Cardiac disease**
Genetic	
Cardio-facio-cutaneous (CFC) syndrome	• Pulmonic stenosis, atrial septal defects, hypertrophic cardiomyopathy
Heritable connective tissue diseases: cutis laxa, Ehlers–Danlos syndrome (EDS), pseudoxanthoma elasticum, Marfan syndrome (see Ch. 80); cardiac disease varies from mitral valve prolapse to arterial/aortic aneurysms, dissection, and rupture	
Carney complex (NAME and LAMB syndromes) (see Ch. 92)	• Atrial myxomas
Tuberous sclerosis complex (TSC) (see Ch. 50)	• Cardiac rhabdomyomas, arrhythmias
Inflammatory/autoimmune	
Psoriasis (see Ch. 6)	• Increased risk of cardiovascular disease
Systemic lupus erythematosus (see Ch. 33)	• Pericarditis, verrucous endocarditis (Libman–Sacks), coronary artery disease
Neonatal lupus erythematosus (see Ch. 33)	• Congenital heart block
Systemic sclerosis (see Ch. 35)	• PAH, conduction defects, pericarditis, visceral Raynaud phenomenon
Rheumatic fever (see Ch. 15)	• Pancarditis in the acute phase; late manifestations include mitral and/or aortic valve dysfunction
Sarcoidosis (see Ch. 78 and Fig. 45.1A)	• Conduction defects, congestive heart failure
Kawasaki disease (mucocutaneous lymph node syndrome) (see Ch. 3)	• Coronary arteritis, coronary artery aneurysms
DRESS/DIHS (see Ch. 17)	• ECG changes may simulate acute myocardial infarction; acute myocardial dysfunction and hypotension, which may initially appear during taper of CS
Other	
Hyperlipidemia (see Ch. 77)	• Coronary artery disease
Primary systemic amyloidosis (AL) (see Ch. 39)	• Restrictive cardiomyopathy, conduction disturbances
Endocarditis – bacterial or fungal (see Chs 61 and 64)	• Vegetations and dysfunction of the valves
Exfoliative erythroderma (see Ch. 8)	• High-output cardiac failure

Table 45.2 Examples of skin signs of cardiac disease. The cutaneous features of these disorders are discussed in the chapters cited. Cardio-facio-cutaneous syndrome is characterized by generalized ichthyosis-like scaling, keratosis pilaris, café-au-lait macules, sparse curly hair, and developmental delay. Patients with neurofibromatosis 1, hemochromatosis and relapsing polychondritis (see Fig. 45.2) can also have cardiac involvement. PAH, pulmonary arterial hypertension.

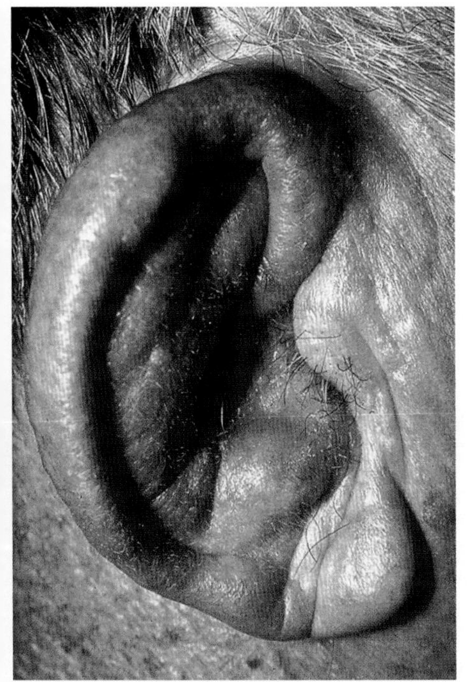

Fig. 45.2 Relapsing polychondritis. The inflammation spares the earlobes, which lack cartilage. Aortic insufficiency and dissecting aortic aneurysm are potential cardiac abnormalities associated with this condition. *Courtesy, Jeffrey P. Callen, MD.*

EXAMPLES OF SKIN SIGNS OF GASTROINTESTINAL (GI) DISEASE	
Disorder	**Gastrointestinal disease/other**
Genetic	
Hereditary hemorrhagic telangiectasia (HHT) (see Ch. 87; Table 45.1; Fig. 45.1B)	• Recurrent hemorrhage in the upper GI tract due to AVMs • Subset of patients have both juvenile GI polyposis due to mutations in *SMAD4*; associated risk of early onset colorectal cancer
Blue rubber bleb nevus syndrome (see Ch. 85; Fig. 45.3A)	• GI vascular malformations
Pseudoxanthoma elasticum (see Ch. 80; Table 45.2)	• Upper or lower GI hemorrhage
Ehlers–Danlos syndrome, vascular type (type IV) (see Ch. 80; Table 45.2)	• GI hemorrhage due to arterial rupture, intestinal perforation
Gardner syndrome (see Chs 90, 91, and 95)	• Hemorrhage from adenomatous colonic polyps. Adenocarcinoma of the colon is universal if the colon is not removed • *C*ongenital *h*ypertrophy of the *r*etinal *p*igment *e*pithelium (CHRPE)
Peutz–Jeghers syndrome (see Ch. 92; Fig. 45.3B)	• Hamartomatous polyps throughout the GI tract. Intussusception or hemorrhage may occur
Cowden disease (multiple hamartoma syndrome; PTEN hamartoma syndrome) (see Chs 52 and 91; Fig. 45.3C)	• Hamartomatous polyps throughout the GI tract. Bleeding is rare
Muir–Torre syndrome (see Ch. 91)	• Colorectal and gastric carcinoma > carcinoma of the small bowel

Table 45.3 Examples of skin signs of gastrointestinal (GI) disease. *Continued*

EXAMPLES OF SKIN SIGNS OF GASTROINTESTINAL (GI) DISEASE	
Disorder	**Gastrointestinal disease/other**
Autoimmune/inflammatory	
Ulcerative colitis (see Ch. 21; Table 45.4)	• Uniform and continuous inflammation of the large bowel. Rectal involvement is present in majority (>95%) of patients. Toxic megacolon may develop
Crohn disease (see Ch. 21; Fig. 45.4; Table 45.4)	• Chronic inflammation, often granulomatous, of the bowel. Skip areas occur
Cronkhite–Canada syndrome	• Adenomatous GI polyps, diarrhea, abdominal pain
Vasculitis (see Ch. 19)	• Ulcerations secondary to vasculitis of the vessels in the bowel. May be more common in IgA-associated vasculitis (Henoch–Schönlein purpura)
Malignant atrophic papulosis (Degos disease) (see Ch. 18)	• Small infarctions in the GI mucosa; hemorrhage and intestinal perforation may result in death
Other	
Scurvy (see Ch. 43)	• Collagen degeneration in the vasculature due to vitamin C deficiency. GI blood loss results in anemia
Kaposi sarcoma (see Ch. 94)	• Similar tumors may occur in the GI tract; possible complications include ulceration, bleeding, perforation and ileus, which are more common in HIV-associated than classic type

Table 45.3 *Continued* **Examples of skin signs of gastrointestinal (GI) disease.** AVMs, arteriovenous malformations.

SKIN FINDINGS IN CROHN DISEASE AND ULCERATIVE COLITIS

- Erythema nodosum – often reflective of active bowel disease
- Urticaria
- Cutaneous small vessel vasculitis
- Cutaneous polyarteritis nodosa
- "Pustular" vasculitis or bowel-associated dermatosis–arthritis syndrome-like lesions
- Pyoderma gangrenosum – primarily the classic (typical) ulcerative form (see Fig. 21.5) or peristomal lesions (Fig. 45.4B); a vegetative pustular variant (pyoderma vegetans; see Fig. 21.9) occasionally occurs. These lesions may or may not reflect activity of the bowel disease
- Other neutrophilic dermatoses, ranging from acneiform lesions to Sweet syndrome and neutrophilic panniculitis
- Oral lesions
  - Granulomatous infiltrates (with Crohn disease only)
  - Aphthosis
  - Angular cheilitis
  - Pyostomatitis vegetans (mucosal variant of pyoderma gangrenosum)
- Contiguous (anogenital) and "metastatic" Crohn disease (Fig. 45.4A)
- Fistulae (perianal and abdominal)
- Genital lymphedema
- Perianal skin tags
- Acquired acrodermatitis enteropathica-like lesions (patients with zinc deficiency and/or essential fatty acid deficiency)
- Epidermolysis bullosa acquisita
- Psoriasis

Table 45.4 Skin findings in Crohn disease and ulcerative colitis.

PERISTOMAL SKIN DISORDERS	
Skin disorder	**Comments**
Irritant contact dermatitis	Most common cause of peristomal dermatitis, especially in patients with an ileostomy. Primarily attributed to exposure to feces or urine
Pre-existing skin disease (e.g. psoriasis, seborrheic dermatitis, atopic dermatitis)	Exclude primary contact dermatitis or infection or superimposed contact dermatitis
Cutaneous infection (*Candida* spp., dermatophyte, herpesvirus [primarily simplex], bacteria [especially *Staphylococcus aureus*])	Colonization with bacteria and/or yeast is common. Recent treatment with antibiotics predisposes to candidiasis. May initially improve and then worsen if treated inappropriately with topical corticosteroids
Allergic contact dermatitis	Relatively uncommon. Potential allergens include adhesive pastes, adhesive ring or wafer of stoma bag, ostomy bag, epoxy resin, rubber, lanolin, and fragrances. Patch test with both standardized allergens and patient's own products
Pyoderma gangrenosum	Infrequent cause of peristomal dermatitis; most common in patients with inflammatory bowel disease (Fig. 45.4B)
Pseudo-verrucous papules and nodules	Seen more commonly in association with urostomies; may be misdiagnosed as verrucae

Table 45.5 Peristomal skin disorders. Peristomal skin disorders are common and may limit use and efficacy of the stoma appliance. When the etiology is uncertain, evaluation can include KOH examination, microbial cultures, patch testing, and histopathologic examination. *Adapted from Lyon CC, Smith AJ, Griffiths CE, et al. The spectrum of skin disorders in abdominal stoma patients. Br J Dermatol. 2000;143:1248–1260.*

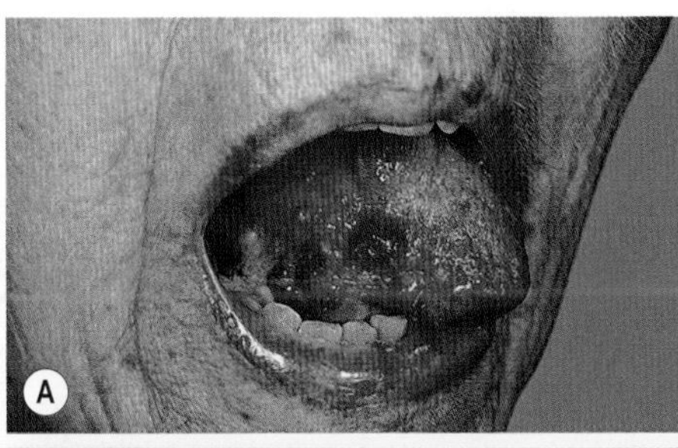

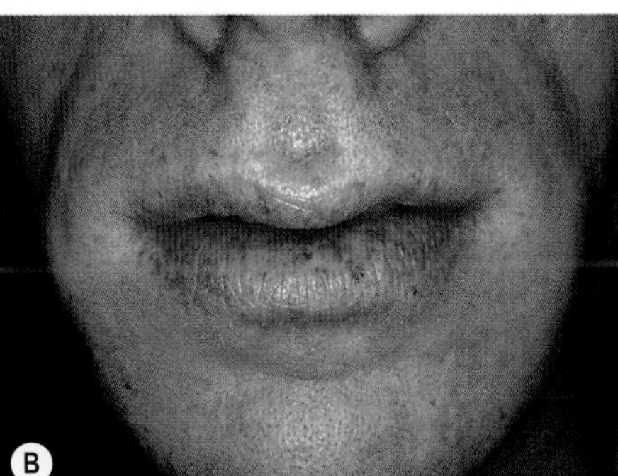

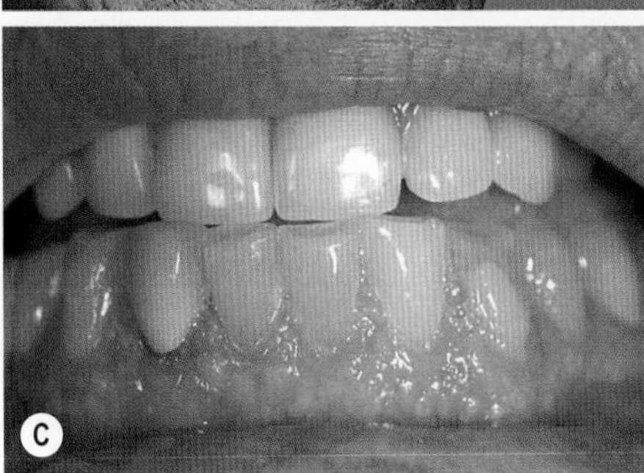

Fig. 45.3 Skin signs of gastrointestinal disease. A Blue rubber bleb nevus syndrome. Several venous malformations are evident on this patient's tongue. **B** Peutz–Jeghers syndrome. Multiple brown macules on the vermilion lips and a few on the lower cutaneous lip. **C** Gingival cobblestoning in Cowden disease. This patient also had tricholemmomas and a "Cowden nodule" or sclerotic fibroma on the neck. *A, C, Courtesy, Jeffrey P. Callen, MD; B, Courtesy, YDRSC.*

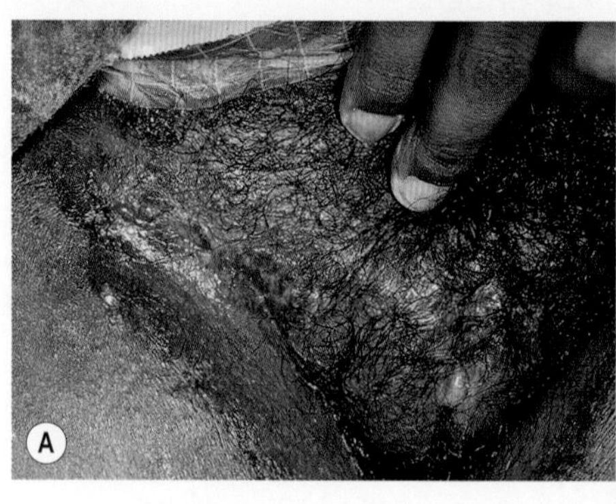

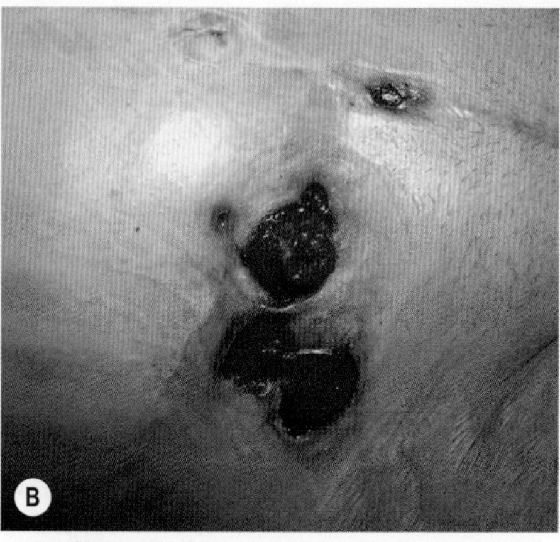

Fig. 45.4 Skin signs of inflammatory bowel disease (IBD). A "Metastatic" Crohn disease. Non-contiguous granulomatous inflammation of the skin is often manifested by deep inflammatory fissures in the inguinal folds. These have been described as "knife-like" fissures. **B** Peristomal pyoderma gangrenosum (PG) in the setting of inflammatory bowel disease. Patients with ostomies, particularly ileostomies, are at risk for peristomal dermatoses, including PG. Patients with IBD can also develop PG elsewhere on the skin (see Ch. 21; Figs 21.5–21.9) *Courtesy, Jeffrey P. Callen, MD.*

EXAMPLES OF SKIN SIGNS OF LIVER DISEASE		
Disorder	**Cutaneous findings**	**Other**
Cirrhosis	• Spider angiomas and other telangiectasias, palmar erythema, Terry and Muehrcke nails (see Ch. 58), pruritus, jaundice	• Gynecomastia • Parotid enlargement
Primary biliary cholangitis (PBC)	• Jaundice, diffuse hyperpigmentation, pruritus, xanthomas (eruptive, planar, sometimes tuberous), may coexist with systemic sclerosis	• Ursodiol, fibrates, cholestyramine, rifampin, sertraline and naloxone may help to relieve the pruritus
Hepatitis B (HBV) and C (HCV) viral infections	• See Table 68.4 • Cutaneous sarcoidosis has been seen with interferon and/ or ribavirin therapy • Necrolytic acral erythema (Fig. 45.5)	• Treatment of chronic HBV and HCV infection depends on the type and severity of disease; includes specific antiviral agents, such as entecavir and tenofovir for HBV infection and direct-acting antiviral agents, often in combination with other agents, for HCV infection
Hemochromatosis ("bronze diabetes")	• Generalized hyperpigmentation	• Due to mutations in *HFE*, most commonly C282Y. Phlebotomy to reduce iron stores or chelation (e.g. deferasirox)
Wilson disease (hepatolenticular degeneration)	• Kayser–Fleischer ring • Blue lunulae • Pretibial hyperpigmentation	• Autosomal recessive; due to mutations in *ATP7B* • Treatment with copper chelating agents (e.g. penicillamine) or metallothionein-inducer drugs (zinc acetate)

Table 45.6 Examples of skin signs of liver disease.

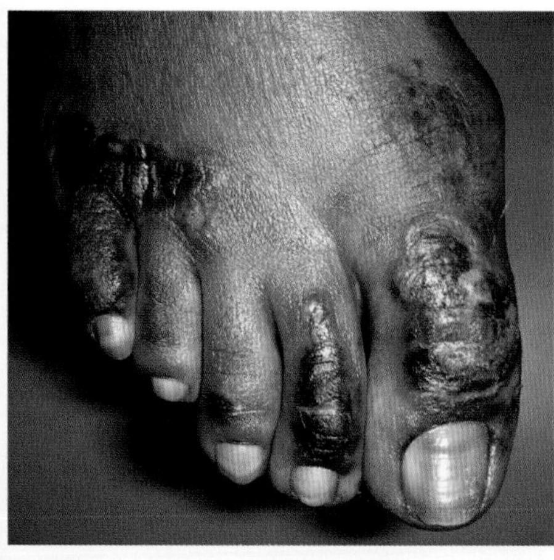

Fig. 45.5 Skin signs of liver disease. Necrolytic acral erythema. This is a manifestation of hepatitis C viral infection. *Courtesy, Jeffrey P. Callen, MD.*

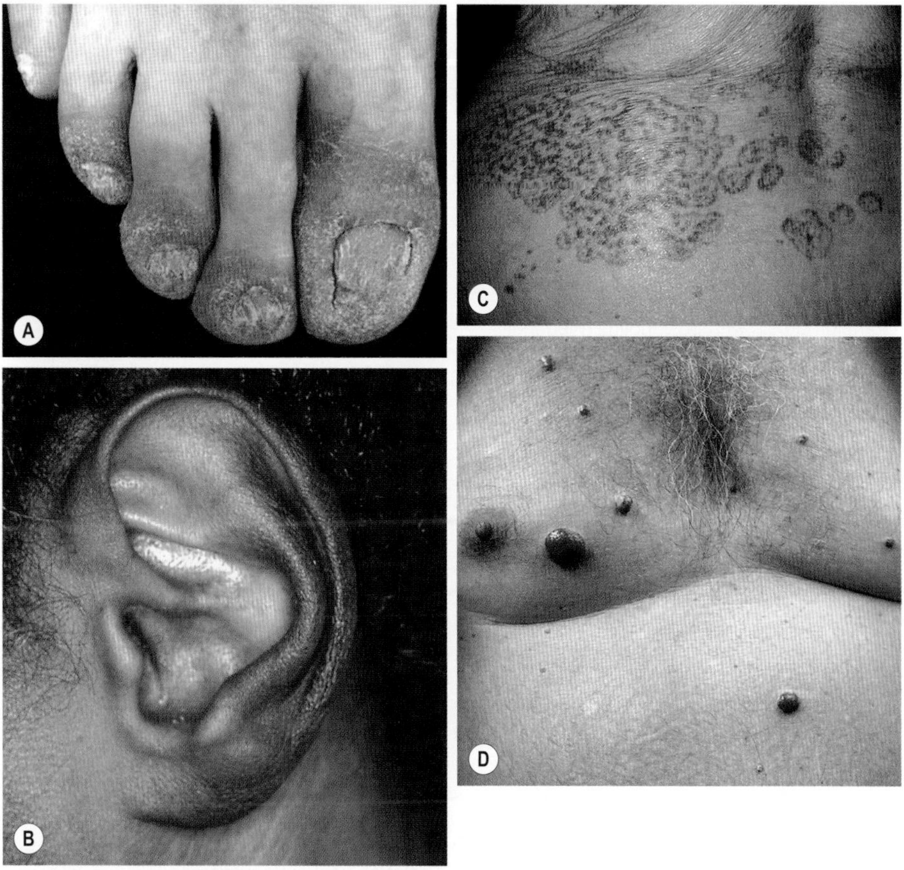

Fig. 45.6 Skin signs that are associated with an internal malignancy in most or all cases. **A, B** Bazex syndrome (acrokeratosis paraneoplastica). Acral psoriasiform lesions that have a violaceous hue, accompanied by nail dystrophy (**A**). This patient had an SCC of the tonsillar pillar. Thin hyperpigmented plaques of the helix and antihelix (**B**) in a patient with SCC of the pharynx. **C** Erythema gyratum repens. This patient had cancer of the breast. **D** POEMS syndrome. This patient had multiple angiomas (glomeruloid hemangiomas histopathologically) on his trunk as well as his face and scalp. In addition, he had peripheral neuropathy, adult-onset diabetes, hypothyroidism, and peripheral edema. His underlying disorder was an osteosclerotic myeloma. *A, C, D, Courtesy, Jeffrey P. Callen, MD; B, Courtesy, Jean L. Bolognia, MD.*

EXAMPLES OF SKIN SIGNS OF RENAL DISEASE	
Disorder	**Renal disease/other**
Genetic	
Tuberous sclerosis complex (TSC) (see Ch. 50; Table 45.2)	• Renal hamartomas (angiomyolipomas). Polycystic kidney disease may occur in a contiguous gene syndrome with *TSC2*
Nail patella syndrome (see Ch. 58)	• Congenital nephrosis, glomerulonephritis
Birt–Hogg–Dubé syndrome (see Ch. 91; Table 45.1)	• Renal tumors, particularly chromophobe, oncocytic, and/or hybrid carcinomas
Hereditary leiomyomatosis and renal cell cancer (HLRCC; Reed syndrome; see Ch. 95)	• Predisposition to develop aggressive renal carcinoma
Inflammatory/autoimmune	
Systemic lupus erythematosus (see Ch. 33; Table 45.2)	• Glomerulonephritis – focal, membranous, or proliferative
Systemic sclerosis (see Ch. 35; Table 45.1)	• Hypertension, renal crisis
Henoch–Schönlein purpura (see Ch. 19)	• IgA-associated glomerulonephritis, which may be chronic
Polyarteritis nodosa (see Ch. 19)	• Renal artery aneurysms, renovascular hypertension, renal failure
Granulomatosis with polyangiitis (Wegener granulomatosis; see Ch. 19; Table 45.1)	• Glomerulonephritis
Cutaneous small vessel vasculitis (CSVV) (see Ch. 19)	• Glomerulonephritis may occur but is less common than in the vasculitides mentioned previously
Other	
Primary systemic amyloidosis (AL) (see Ch. 39; Table 45.2)	• Proteinuria, including nephrotic syndrome, and renal insufficiency
Cutaneous changes of end-stage renal disease	1. Pale color, sallowness 2. Xerosis or acquired ichthyosis (see Fig. 4.3) 3. Pruritus (see Ch. 4) 4. Acquired perforating dermatosis (see Ch. 79 and Figs 4.3, 79.1, and 79.2) 5. Pseudoporphyria (see Ch. 41 and Fig. 41.8) 6. Calciphylaxis (see Ch. 42) 7. Uremic frost
Nephrogenic systemic fibrosis (NSF) (see Ch. 35 and Fig. 35.12)	• Occurs primarily in patients with dialysis-dependent chronic kidney disease in association with exposure to gadolinium-based contrast medium

Table 45.7 Examples of skin signs of renal disease.

PARANEOPLASTIC DERMATOSES		
Disorder	**Cutaneous findings**	**Comments**
Disorders that are associated with cancer in most or all cases		
Bazex syndrome (acrokeratosis paraneoplastica)	Acral psoriasiform plaques, typically with involvement of the nose and helices; often the lesions are violaceous (Fig. 45.6A,B). Longitudinal and horizontal ridging of the nails occurs in 75% of patients	By definition, this condition is linked to malignancy, generally occurring in the upper aero-digestive tract (pharynx, larynx, or esophagus)
Carcinoid syndrome	Flushing and erythema of the head and neck. Pellagra-like dermatitis and sclerodermoid changes may develop in advanced disease	Flushing associated with ~10% of midgut tumors (small intestine, appendix, proximal colon) and liver metastases are required; type III gastric and bronchial carcinoid tumors are also associated with flushing (liver metastases are not required)
Erythema gyratum repens	Concentric erythematous lesions, often giving the appearance of grains of wood (Fig. 45.6C; see Ch. 15)	Variable sites and types of malignancy
Acquired hypertrichosis lanuginosa (malignant down)	Growth of fine lanugo hairs in a generalized distribution or localized to the face. With time, these hairs may become coarser (see Ch. 57)	Associated with a variety of internal malignancies, most often carcinoma of the lung, colon, or breast
AESOP syndrome	Large red to violet-brown patch	Patch overlies a plasmacytoma
Ectopic adrenocorticotropic hormone (ACTH) syndrome	Generalized hyperpigmentation that may be accentuated in sun-exposed sites	Production of ACTH by a tumor (often a small cell carcinoma of the lung) may result in hyperpigmentation and features of Cushing syndrome
Glucagonoma syndrome	Necrolytic migratory erythema, angular cheilitis, glossitis	Due to a glucagon-secreting tumor of the pancreas. Patients are often treated for intertrigo before the syndrome is diagnosed. Weight loss and diabetes mellitus accompany the dermatosis
Paraneoplastic pemphigus	Erosive disease of the mucous membranes (see Fig. 23.8) and erythema multiforme-like, bullous pemphigoid-like, or lichenoid skin lesions (see Ch. 23)	Most often associated with non-Hodgkin lymphoma, chronic lymphocytic leukemia, or Castleman disease (with the latter accounting for the majority of cases in children and Asian populations). Castleman tumors have been shown to produce the autoantibodies responsible for paraneoplastic pemphigus, and their resection can lead to remission of mucocutaneous lesions. Bronchiolitis obliterans is a common complication
Tripe palms	Ridged velvety lesions on the palms	May or may not be accompanied by acanthosis nigricans

Table 45.8 Paraneoplastic dermatoses. *Continued*

PARANEOPLASTIC DERMATOSES		
Disorder	**Cutaneous findings**	**Comments**
Disorders that are strongly associated with cancer in a subset of cases		
Acanthosis nigricans	Rapid onset of hyperpigmented velvety changes of the flexural surfaces (e.g. neck, axillae, and groin). May also involve extensor surfaces (e.g. elbows, knees, and knuckles) and, in malignancy-associated cases, the lips, oral mucosa, and palms (see above, tripe palms). Glossitis is also frequently present in malignancy-associated acanthosis nigricans	Association with adenocarcinoma of the stomach or other sites within the GI or GU tracts; in this setting, acanthosis nigricans is often accompanied by weight loss. Acanthosis nigricans is more commonly associated with endocrinologic abnormalities, particularly insulin resistance (Figs 45.8 and 45.9); such patients are typically overweight, and the onset of the condition is usually insidious
Anti-epiligrin cicatricial pemphigoid*/anti-laminin 332 mucous membrane pemphigoid	Oral ulcerations, conjunctival erosions, and scarring. Tense blisters and erosions of the skin may also develop (see Ch. 24)	Roughly one-third of patients have or develop cancer within the first year following diagnosis. The cancer is usually an adenocarcinoma and is often at an advanced stage at the time of diagnosis, possibly accounting for the high mortality rate
Dermatomyositis (adult)*	Heliotrope, Gottron papules, photodistributed poikiloderma, nailfold overgrowth with dilated capillary loops, pruritus and diffuse scaling of the scalp (see Ch. 34)	Population-based studies demonstrate an overrepresentation of ovarian, lung, colorectal, and pancreatic carcinomas and non-Hodgkin lymphoma in Caucasians
Neutrophilic dermatoses	Sweet syndrome or pyoderma gangrenosum (particularly the atypical bullous form) (see Ch. 21)	Approximately 10–20% of cases are associated with hematologic disorders such as acute myelogenous leukemia or plasma cell dyscrasia (IgA). Underlying solid tumors are rare
Disorders associated with a monoclonal gammopathy**		
Acquired angioedema due to C1 esterase inhibitor dysfunction	Acquired angioedema without associated wheals (see Ch. 14)	Associated with B-cell lymphoproliferative disorders, including lymphomas, as well as monoclonal gammopathy of undetermined significance (MGUS)
Amyloidosis, primary systemic	Waxy, translucent, or purpuric papules; periorbital and pinch purpura; macroglossia (see Ch. 39)	Monoclonal gammopathy due to plasma cell dyscrasia >> multiple myeloma; deposits composed of immunoglobulin light chain (AL)
Cryoglobulinemia, type I	Retiform purpura and necrosis that favors cooler acral sites; acral cyanosis; livedo reticularis (see Ch. 18)	Monoclonal gammopathy due to lymphoplasmocytic disorders
Necrobiotic xanthogranuloma	Indurated xanthomatous plaques with necrosis and ulceration, usually in a periorbital location (see Ch. 76)	Paraproteinemia (>80% of cases, most often IgG with κ light chains); multiple myeloma or a lymphoproliferative disorder develop in a minority of patients

Table 45.8 *Continued* **Paraneoplastic dermatoses.** *Continued*

PARANEOPLASTIC DERMATOSES		
Disorder	**Cutaneous findings**	**Comments**
Normolipemic plane xanthoma	Yellowish patches and thin plaques that favor the skin folds, upper trunk, and periorbital area (see Ch. 77)	Paraproteinemia, due to a plasma cell dyscrasia or lymphoproliferative disorder
POEMS syndrome (*p*olyneuropathy, *o*rganomegaly, *e*ndocrinopathy, *M*-protein, and *s*kin changes)	Although the glomeruloid hemangioma (see Fig. 45.6D) is considered to be pathognomonic, it is present in a minority of patients. Other skin findings include cherry angiomas, hyperpigmentation, hypertrichosis, sclerodermatous thickening, hyperhidrosis, digital clubbing, plethora, acrocyanosis, and leukonychia	Osteosclerotic myeloma, Castleman disease, and plasmacytomas have been reported in patients with POEMS. In addition to the findings designated in the acronym, patients may have peripheral edema, ascites, pulmonary effusions, papilledema, thrombocytosis, polycythemia, and increased serum levels of VEGF
Schnitzler syndrome	Chronic urticarial lesions; histopathologically, a neutrophil-rich dermal infiltrate is often seen (see Ch. 14)	Associated with an IgM usually κ paraproteinemia; lymphoplasmacytic malignancies develop in approximately 15% of patients. Additional manifestations include fevers, arthralgias, and bone pain
Scleromyxedema	Sclerodermoid induration plus firm, waxy papules arranged in linear arrays (see Ch. 38)	Almost always associated with paraproteinemia (usually IgG with λ light chains); multiple myeloma develops in <10% of cases
Disorders that may be associated with cancer in a subset of patients		
Acquired ichthyosis	Resembles ichthyosis vulgaris; most often located on the legs	Lymphoma typically predates the diagnosis of the ichthyosis
Cutaneous small vessel vasculitis	Palpable purpura; may be widespread and/or in unusual locations (see Ch. 19)	Less than 5% of patients with vasculitis have an associated malignancy, most commonly plasma cell dyscrasias, myelodysplasia, myelo- or lymphoproliferative disorders, and hairy cell leukemia
Dermatitis herpetiformis (DH)	Pruritic erosions and blisters on extensor surfaces, scalp, and/or buttocks (see Ch. 25)	Through the association of DH with gluten-sensitive enteropathy, enteropathy-associated T-cell lymphoma occasionally
Exfoliative erythroderma	Diffuse, scaly, erythematous skin (see Ch. 8)	May be associated with cutaneous T-cell lymphoma or, occasionally, with a systemic lymphoma or leukemia
Juvenile xanthogranulomas (JXGs) in the setting of neurofibromatosis 1 (NF1)	Pink-yellow to red-brown, dome-shaped papules and nodules, most often located on the head and neck (see Ch. 76)	A triple association between JXGs, NF1, and JMML has been described
Multicentric reticulohistiocytosis	Nodular lesions, most often on the dorsal aspects of the hands (see Ch. 76)	A variety of associated malignancies have been reported, developing in approximately 25% of adult patients

Table 45.8 *Continued* **Paraneoplastic dermatoses.** *Continued*

PARANEOPLASTIC DERMATOSES		
Disorder	**Cutaneous findings**	**Comments**
Mycosis fungoides	Patch, plaque, or nodular disease (see Ch. 98)	Some studies have demonstrated an increased risk of second malignancies, especially other lymphoid malignancies
Porphyria cutanea tarda (PCT)	Erosions, blisters, and scars on the dorsal aspect of the hands, hyperpigmentation, hypertrichosis, milia (see Ch. 41)	Through its association with hepatitis C virus, PCT may also be associated with primary hepatocellular carcinoma (hepatoma)
Disorders whose association with cancer is controversial		
Sign of Leser–Trélat	Rapid appearance or growth of multiple seborrheic keratoses; keratoses may be inflamed	Often these patients have acanthosis nigricans and generalized pruritus. Controversy continues regarding the existence of this sign in the absence of generalized pruritus and acanthosis nigricans, in part because determining whether seborrheic keratoses are eruptive can be difficult. Eruptive seborrheic keratoses can also develop in erythrodermic patients who do not have an underlying malignancy

**Statistical association.*
***For complete list, see Table 97.4.*

Table 45.8 *Continued* **Paraneoplastic dermatoses.** AESOP syndrome, adenopathy, extensive skin patch overlying (a) plasmacytoma; GU, genitourinary; JMML, juvenile myelomonocytic leukemia; VEGF, vascular endothelial growth factor.

INTERNAL MALIGNANCIES IN FAMILIAL CANCER SYNDROMES WITH CUTANEOUS MANIFESTATIONS

- Cowden disease (breast, thyroid, and GI carcinomas), Muir–Torre syndrome (GI and GU carcinomas), Gardner syndrome (GI carcinoma), Peutz–Jeghers syndrome (various malignancies) – see Table 45.3
- Costello syndrome (rhabdomyosarcoma, bladder carcinoma), Werner syndrome (sarcomas and other malignancies)
- Birt–Hogg–Dubé syndrome, hereditary leiomyomatosis and renal cell cancer – see Tables 45.1 and 45.7
- Howel–Evans syndrome (esophageal carcinoma) – see Ch. 47
- Ataxia–telangiectasia (leukemia, lymphoma, breast cancer) – see Ch. 49 and Fig. 49.1
- Neurofibromatosis (malignant peripheral nerve sheath tumors, JMML, rhabdomyosarcoma, pheochromocytoma, carcinoid, breast cancer), tuberous sclerosis (renal carcinoma) – see Ch. 50
- Multiple endocrine neoplasia syndromes – see Ch. 52, Table 52.2, and Fig. 52.2
- Dyskeratosis congenita (leukemia, Hodgkin lymphoma) – see Table 55.6 and Fig. 55.18
- Basal cell nevus syndrome (medulloblastoma, fibrosarcoma) – see Ch. 88
- Bloom syndrome (lymphoproliferative and GI malignancies), Rothmund–Thomson syndrome (osteosarcoma), xeroderma pigmentosum (brain, especially sarcomas, and oral cavity [not just anterior tongue]) – see Table 73.5
- Familial melanoma (pancreatic carcinoma, neural tumors, renal cell carcinoma, and gliomas, when mutations in *CDKN2A* [p16], *CDKN2A* [p14], *MITF*, and *POT1*, respectively; uveal melanoma, mesothelioma, renal cell carcinoma, and cholangiocarcinoma with *BAP1* mutations)

Table 45.9 Internal malignancies in familial cancer syndromes with cutaneous manifestations. GU, genitourinary; JMML, juvenile myelomonocytic leukemia.

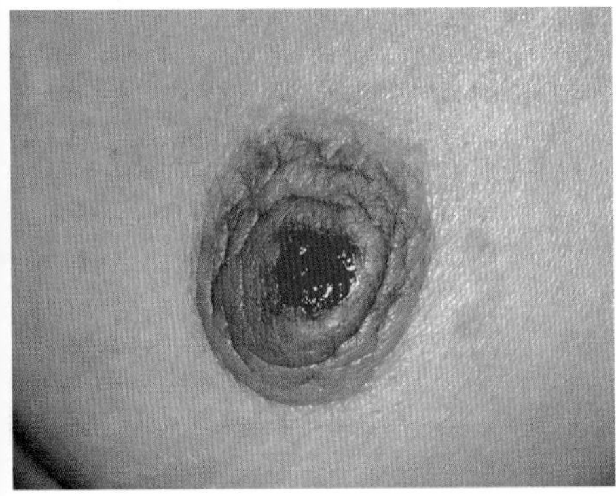

Fig. 45.7 Paget disease of the breast. A chronic, eroded erythematous plaque surrounds the nipple and is due to epidermal extension of an underlying ductal adenocarcinoma of the breast. Paget disease may also occur in extramammary locations (see Ch. 60). *Courtesy, Robert Hartmann, MD.*

SELECTED DERMATOLOGIC ASSOCIATIONS OF DIABETES MELLITUS (DM)		
Dermatosis	**Clinical description**	**Comments**
Acanthosis nigricans (AN)	Velvety hyperpigmentation of the intertriginous/flexural areas (Fig. 45.8A,B) and, less often, extensor surfaces (Fig. 45.8C)	Commonly associated with insulin resistance and most of the patients are obese. More common in Hispanics and individuals of African descent. Recent evidence strongly links AN in children with insulin resistance and diabetes
Acral dry gangrene	Necrosis of the toes > fingertips	Ischemia due to vascular disease in larger vessels
Acral erythema	Erysipelas-like blanching erythema of the hands and/or feet	May be due to small vessel occlusive disease with compensatory hyperemia
Carotenoderma	Diffuse orange-yellow skin color (see Fig. 43.13)	Related to an increase in serum carotene level
Diabetic bullae (bullosis diabeticorum)	Tense non-inflammatory bullae on the lower extremities (Fig. 45.10A)	Unknown pathogenesis
Diabetic cheiroarthropathy	Thickened skin and limited joint mobility of the hands and fingers, leading to flexion contractures (starting with the fifth digit and progressing radially) and an inability to approximate the palmar surfaces of the hands and fingers ("prayer sign"; Fig. 45.10F)	Postulated to result from increased glycosylation of collagen in the skin. Associated with retinopathy, nephropathy, and duration (but not control) of the DM
Diabetic dermopathy	Brown atrophic macules and patches on the legs (Fig. 45.10B)	Possibly precipitated by trauma
Disseminated granuloma annulare	Erythematous, often annular lesions composed of papules	There is controversy about the exact relationship of disseminated granuloma annulare and DM (see Ch. 78)

Table 45.10 Selected dermatologic associations of diabetes mellitus (DM). *Continued*

SELECTED DERMATOLOGIC ASSOCIATIONS OF DIABETES MELLITUS (DM)		
Dermatosis	**Clinical description**	**Comments**
Eruptive xanthomas	Red-yellow papules that appear over a period of weeks to months; favor the extensor surfaces of the extremities and buttocks (Fig. 45.10C and see Ch. 77 and Figs 77.1–77.3)	Associated with elevated serum triglycerides in patients with poorly controlled diabetes. Control of the DM results in a disappearance of the xanthomas (see Ch. 77)
Hemochromatosis	Bronzing of the skin due to an increase in melanin rather than iron	Excess of iron stores associated with cirrhosis and cardiac dysfunction as well as DM. Due to mutations in *HFE*, most commonly C282Y. Also risk factor for porphyria cutanea tarda
Necrobiosis lipoidica	Yellow atrophic patches, most often on the shins. A red-brown rim may indicate activity at the border (Fig. 45.10D). Ulceration can occur and is often slow to heal	Develops in <1% of patients with DM; not always associated with DM (see Ch. 78)
Neuropathic leg ulcers	Non-painful ulcerations at sites of pressure, most commonly on the foot, including the plantar surface (Fig. 45.10E); a keratotic rim is characteristic	Associated with sensory neuropathy (see Ch. 86)
Perforating disorders (e.g. acquired perforating dermatosis)	Keratotic papules, primarily on the extremities	Often occurs in African-American diabetic patients with chronic kidney disease on dialysis (see Ch. 79)
Rubeosis	Chronic, flushed appearance of the face, neck, and upper extremities	Improved by dietary diabetic control. Flares with vasodilator therapies
Scleredema (adultorum of Buschke)	Erythematous induration of the upper back and nape due to glycosaminoglycan deposition; may have overlying erythema	Unknown etiology. No relationship to control of the DM; also referred to as type III scleredema

Table 45.10 *Continued* **Selected dermatologic associations of diabetes mellitus (DM).** Additional cutaneous conditions associated with DM include hirsutism (e.g. related to polycystic ovary syndrome or HAIR-AN – *h*yper*a*ndrogenemia, *i*nsulin *r*esistance, *a*canthosis *n*igricans; see Ch. 57), necrolytic migratory erythema (in the setting of DM due to a glucagon-secreting pancreatic tumor; see Table 45.8), compensatory and gustatory hyperhidrosis, and infections such as mucocutaneous candidiasis, erythrasma (especially the disciform variant), cellulitis, and necrotizing fasciitis. *Adapted from Jorizzo JL, Callen JP. Dermatologic manifestations of internal disease. In: Arndt KA, Robinson JK, LeBoit PE, et al (eds). Cutaneous Medicine and Surgery. Philadelphia: Saunders, 1996:1863–1889.*

CRITERIA FOR THE CLINICAL DIAGNOSIS OF THE METABOLIC SYNDROME
• Elevated waist circumference (population- and country-specific definitions) • Elevated triglycerides (≥150 mg/dl) • Reduced HDL (<40 mg/dl in males; <50 mg/dl in females) • Elevated blood pressure (systolic ≥130 and/or diastolic ≥85 mmHg) • Elevated fasting blood glucose (≥100 mg/dl)

Table 45.11 Criteria for the clinical diagnosis of the metabolic syndrome. Metabolic syndrome is identified by the presence of three or more of these five criteria. Drug treatment for dyslipidemia, hypertension, or hyperglycemia also fulfills the corresponding criterion. Most patients with type 2 diabetes mellitus meet criteria for metabolic syndrome.

DERMATOLOGIC MANIFESTATIONS OF THYROID DISEASE		
	Hyperthyroidism	**Hypothyroidism**
Cutaneous changes	Fine, velvety, smooth skin	Dry, rough, coarse skin
	Warm and moist due to increased sweating	Cold and pale
		Boggy and edematous skin (myxedema)
	Hyperpigmentation – localized or generalized	Yellow discoloration as a result of carotenemia
	Pruritus	Easy bruising (capillary fragility)
Cutaneous diseases	Pretibial myxedema* (see Fig. 38.4), thyroid acropachy (acral soft tissue swelling, periostitis, and clubbing of the digits)	Acquired ichthyosis and palmoplantar keratoderma
		Eruptive and/or tuberous xanthomas
	Urticaria, dermographism	Increased incidence of vitiligo
	Increased incidence of vitiligo	
Hair changes/ diseases	Fine, thin	Dull, coarse, brittle
	Mild, diffuse alopecia	Slow growth (increase in telogen hair phase)
	Increased incidence of alopecia areata	Alopecia of the lateral third of the eyebrows
		Increased incidence of alopecia areata
Nail changes	Onycholysis	Thin, brittle, striated
	Koilonychia	Slow growth
	Clubbing from thyroid acropachy	Onycholysis (rare)

**Can persist when patient is treated and becomes euthyroid or can be associated with euthyroid Graves disease.*

Table 45.12 Dermatologic manifestations of thyroid disease. Serum thyroid-stimulating hormone (TSH) level is the most reliable test of thyroid function; it is usually markedly suppressed in patients with hyperthyroidism. Additional laboratory findings in hyperthyroid patients include elevated free T3 and/or free T4 levels. Patients with primary hypothyroidism have elevated TSH levels and decreased free T4 levels. The detection of anti-thyroid peroxidase and/or anti-thyroglobulin antibodies suggests autoimmune thyroid disease (Hashimoto thyroiditis, Graves disease), while the presence of anti-TSH receptor antibodies points to Graves disease. Ascher syndrome consists of blepharochalasis, double lip, and goiter.

DERMATOLOGIC MANIFESTATIONS OF ADRENAL DISORDERS	
Cushing disease*	**Addison disease**
Altered subcutaneous fat distribution • Rounded "moon" facies • Dorsal cervical fat deposition "buffalo hump" (Fig. 45.11A) • Pelvic girdle fat deposition • Reduced fat in the arms and legs	Hyperpigmentation (MSH-like effect of ACTH) • Diffuse with accentuation in sun-exposed skin (Fig. 45.12) • Prominent at sites of trauma • Axillae, perineum, nipples • Palmar creases • Mucous membranes • Hair • Nails (longitudinal melanonychia) • Melanocytic nevi and lentigines
Skin atrophy • Multiple striae (Fig. 45.11B) • Fragile skin • Prolonged wound healing • Purpura from minor trauma	Loss of androgen-stimulated (axillary, pubic) hair in postpubertal women
Cutaneous infections • Pityriasis (tinea) versicolor • Dermatophytosis and onychomycosis • Candidiasis	Fibrosis and calcification of cartilage, including ear (rare)
Adnexal effects • Acne • Hirsutism	In patients with candidiasis endocrinopathy syndrome, vitiligo and chronic mucocutaneous candidiasis

**Screening tests include late-night salivary cortisol, urine free cortisol (24-hour), 1-mg overnight low-dose dexamethasone suppression test (DST), and longer low-dose DST (2 mg/d for 48 hours).*

Table 45.13 Dermatologic manifestations of adrenal disorders. Both over- and underproduction of adrenal hormones lead to characteristic skin findings. The plasma adrenocorticotropic hormone (ACTH) level is elevated in Cushing disease (pituitary overproduction) and ectopic ACTH syndrome, whereas it is suppressed in patients with adrenal tumors. Plasma ACTH levels are also elevated in patients with primary adrenocortical insufficiency (Addison disease) and suppressed in secondary adrenocortical insufficiency due to exogenous corticosteroid administration. When adrenal insufficiency is suspected, including in patients receiving a prolonged course of corticosteroids, an ACTH stimulation test can provide useful information. MSH, melanocyte-stimulating hormone.

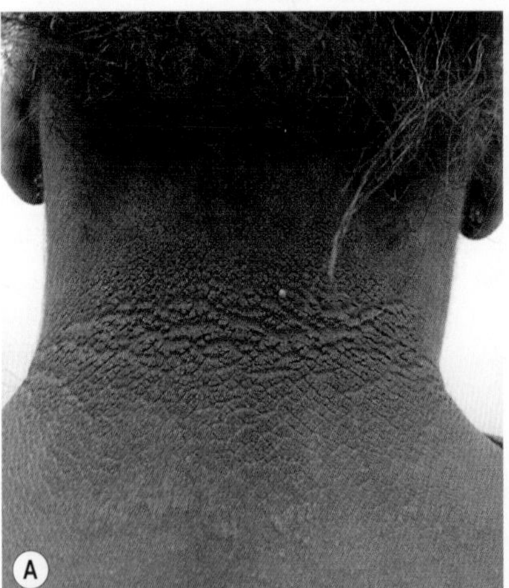

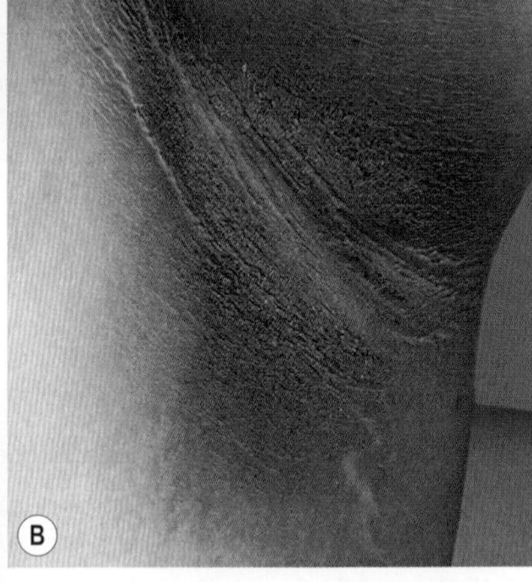

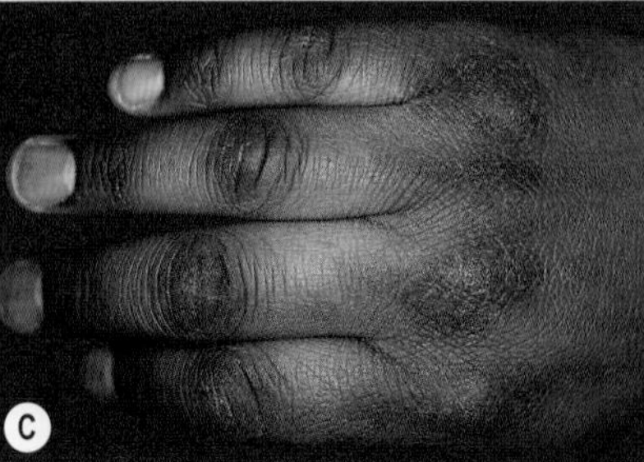

Fig. 45.8 Acanthosis nigricans (AN). **A** Involvement of the posterior neck in a young woman with obesity and insulin resistance. There is also an acrochordon. **B** Axillary involvement in an obese 10-year-old Filipino boy with insulin resistance and a strong family history of type 2 diabetes mellitus. **C** AN over the knuckles. AN can involve extensor surfaces as well as flexural areas. *A, Courtesy, Jeffrey P. Callen, MD; B, Courtesy Julie V. Schaffer, MD; C, Courtesy, Jean L. Bolognia, MD.*

EVALUATION OF THE PATIENT WITH ACANTHOSIS NIGRICANS

Question	Action
Was AN apparent at birth or during early childhood and associated with skeletal abnormalities and/or short stature?	Consider autosomal dominant disorders due to FGFR defects, specially if AN is extensive: • Crouzon syndrome with AN (features craniosynostosis), SADDAN, and thanatophoric dysplasia (*FGFR3* mutations) • Beare–Stevenson cutis gyrata syndrome (features craniosynostosis; *FGFR2* mutations) Consider Costello syndrome • Rabson–Mendenhall syndrome (features dental dysplasia, insulin-resistant diabetes mellitus; compound heterozygote for *INSR* mutation)
Was AN apparent during childhood or adolescence and associated with loss/absence of subcutaneous fat?	Consider generalized lipodystrophy (more extensive AN with congenital variant; see Ch. 84) or partial lipodystrophy (familial > acquired) (see Ch. 84)
Was the onset sudden and accompanied by constitutional symptoms or weight loss?	Consider underlying malignancy, particularly if AN is extensive and involves sites such as the palms and soles. Restaging is required if AN recurs in a patient with a known malignancy
Is the patient overweight or obese?	Evaluate for associated insulin resistance states, especially diabetes mellitus. Consider evaluation for other underlying endocrinopathies, including thyroid disease
Does the patient have striae, hypertension, central obesity and/or a buffalo hump?	Evaluate for Cushing syndrome
If female, does the patient have acne, hirsutism and/or irregular menses?	Evaluate for polycystic ovary syndrome and HAIR-AN syndrome (see Fig. 57.10)
Is the patient on medications such as niacin, human growth hormone, oral contraceptives, corticosteroids or protease inhibitors?	AN may be drug-induced

Fig. 45.9 Evaluation of the patient with acanthosis nigricans (AN). FGFR, fibroblast growth factor receptor; HAIR-AN, *h*yper*a*ndrogenemia, *i*nsulin *r*esistance, *a*canthosis *n*igricans; INSR, insulin receptor; SADDAN, *s*evere *a*chondrodysplasia with *d*evelopmental *d*elay and *AN*.

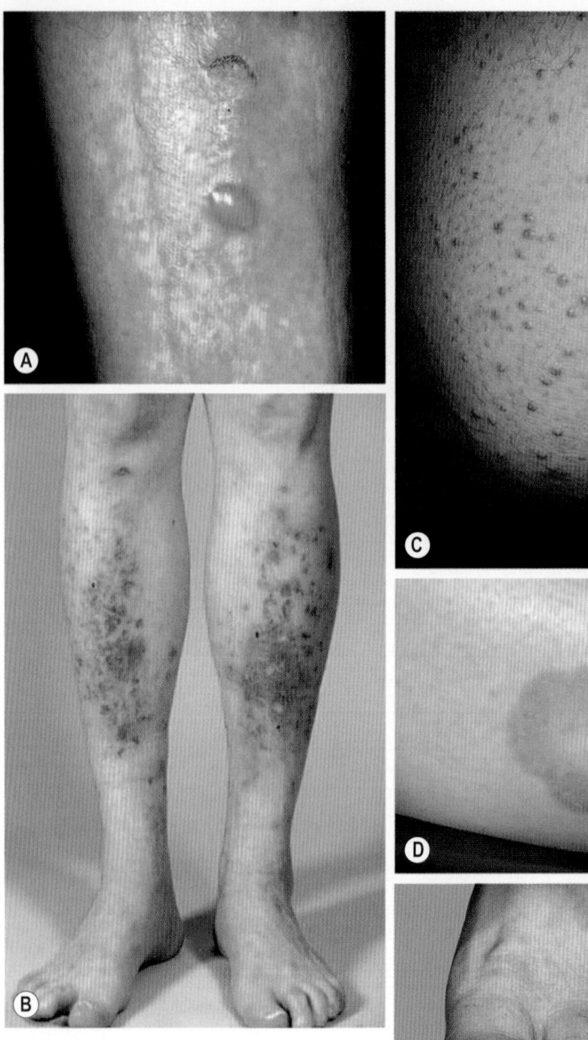

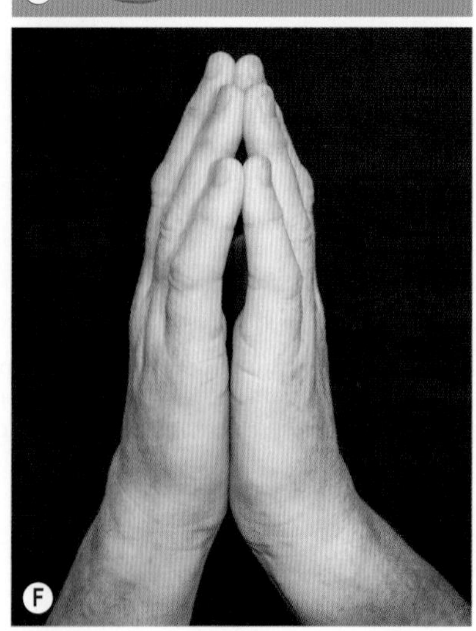

Fig. 45.10 Skin signs of diabetes mellitus. **A** Bullosis diabeticorum (diabetic bullae) with non-inflammatory bullae on the lower extremity. **B** Diabetic dermopathy characterized by brown macules and patches on the shins. **C** Eruptive xanthomas are frequently associated with poorly controlled diabetes mellitus. This patient was first discovered to have diabetes following the appearance of these yellow-red papules. **D** Necrobiosis lipoidica. This plaque on the shin has an inflammatory border and a yellow color with atrophy and telangiectasias centrally. Controversy exists about the exact risk of diabetes mellitus in such patients, but it is more strongly associated with diabetes than is granuloma annulare. **E** Neuropathic ulcers on the toes of a patient with diabetic sensory neuropathy. **F** Diabetic cheiroarthropathy (diabetic stiff hand syndrome). Because of limited joint mobility and thickening of the skin of the hand, the patient is unable to appose the palms ("prayer sign"). *A, C–E, Courtesy, Jeffrey P. Callen, MD; B, F, Courtesy, Jean L. Bolognia, MD.*

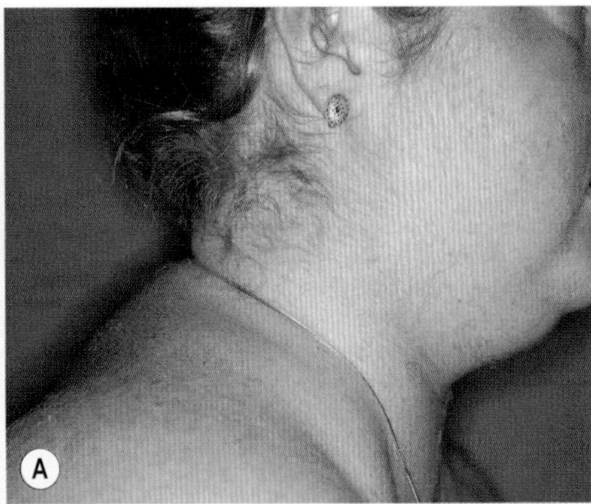

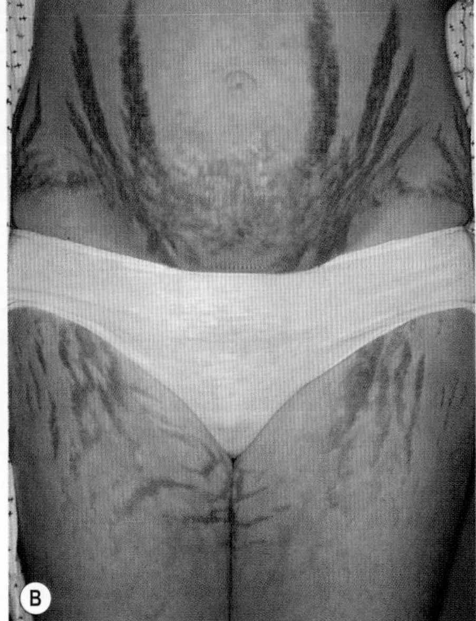

Fig. 45.11 Skin signs of Cushing disease. **A** "Buffalo hump" of Cushing syndrome due to fat redistribution. The patient also has evidence of hirsutism. **B** Cushing syndrome with multiple striae. *Courtesy, Judit Stenn, MD.*

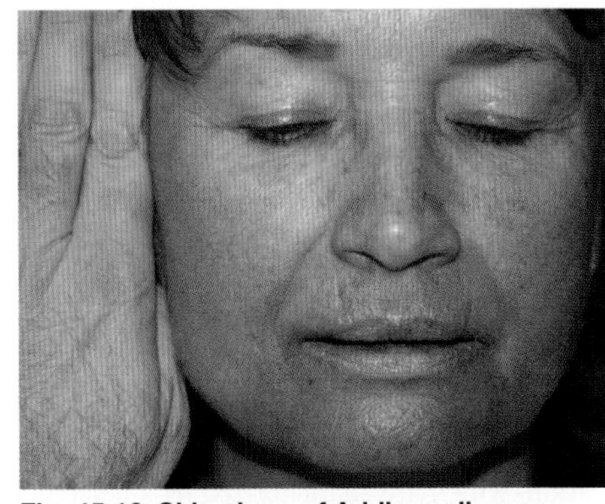

Fig. 45.12 Skin signs of Addison disease. The hyperpigmentation (shown in contrast to the physician's hand) is accentuated in sun-exposed skin and can also involve sites of trauma, skin creases, and mucosae. *Courtesy, Jeffrey P. Callen, MD.*

46 Ichthyoses and Erythrokeratodermas

- Ichthyoses and erythrokeratodermas represent a diverse group of disorders of cornification, which are characterized by a defective epidermal barrier due to abnormal differentiation and/or desquamation of keratinocytes.
- *Ichthyoses* feature diffuse scaling of the skin, often in a widespread distribution, whereas *erythrokeratodermas* present with circumscribed areas of hyperkeratosis without prominent scaling.
- These conditions usually have a genetic basis, with the occasional exception of acquired ichthyosis associated with disorders such as malnutrition, hypothyroidism, sarcoidosis, lymphoma, leprosy, or HIV infection.
- A thorough family history helps in recognizing the inheritance pattern; an affected parent suggests dominant inheritance, whereas inheritance in patients with unaffected parents may be autosomal recessive (especially with affected siblings or parental consanguinity), X-linked recessive (especially for a male patient with affected maternal male relatives), or dominant (e.g. due to a "new" mutation or with incomplete penetrance).
- Clinical features that are useful in determining the type of ichthyosis include the time of presentation (e.g. at birth, ± a collodion membrane, vs later in life), the quality and distribution of the scaling, other cutaneous manifestations (e.g. erythroderma, blistering, abnormal hair), and extracutaneous or laboratory findings (Table 46.1).
- A few ichthyoses such as epidermolytic ichthyosis have characteristic histologic features (see below).
- For conditions with a known molecular etiology, genetic testing can confirm the diagnosis in the patient and affected relatives as well as provide the basis for prenatal/preimplantation testing.

Ichthyosis Vulgaris (IV)

- The most common disorder of cornification, with a prevalence of ~1 in 100 to 1 in 250.
- Autosomal semi-dominant inheritance – mild ichthyosis with a heterozygous filaggrin (*FLG*) mutation and more severe ichthyosis with mutations in both *FLG* alleles.
- Filaggrin deficiency results in impaired cornification, increased transepidermal water loss, enhanced penetration of irritants or allergens, and a propensity for inflammatory responses to the latter; this explains the association of *FLG* mutations with atopic dermatitis and increased risk of contact dermatitis (irritant and allergic) as well as IV.
- IV typically becomes apparent during infancy or early childhood and improves by adulthood; worsens in a cold, dry environment.
- Mild to moderate scaling favors the extensor extremities (Fig. 46.1), ranging from fine white scales to larger adherent scales (especially on the lower legs); the trunk, scalp, and forehead are occasionally affected, and flexural sites are characteristically spared.
- Associated findings include hyperlinear palms (Fig. 46.2), keratosis pilaris, and atopic dermatitis (25–50% of patients).
- **DDx:** xerosis, acquired ichthyosis, X-linked ichthyosis.
- **Rx:** emollients, humectants (e.g. urea), and keratolytic agents (e.g. lactic, salicylic, and glycolic acids); the latter group may be irritating in patients with coexistent atopic dermatitis.

X-Linked Recessive Ichthyosis (XLRI; Steroid Sulfatase Deficiency)

- Incidence of ~1 in 5000 male births; almost exclusively affects boys and men,

CLUES TO THE DIAGNOSIS OF ICHTHYOSES AND ERYTHROKERATODERMAS
Cutaneous findings in neonates
Collodion membrane: lamellar ichthyosis, CIE, "self-healing" form >> SLS, TTD, NLSD, others (e.g. infantile Gaucher disease, ectodermal dysplasias) ***Blisters/erosions/peeling:*** EI, superficial EI, Netherton syndrome, peeling skin syndromes ***Erythroderma:*** EI, CIE, Netherton syndrome, ichthyosis en confetti > SLS, TTD, NLSD, KID, CHH (along lines of Blaschko)
Other findings
Hair shaft abnormalities or hypotrichosis: Netherton, TTD, KID, IFAP ***Ocular findings***: X-linked recessive ichthyosis, SLS, NLSD, TTD, KID§, IFAP§, CHH (unilateral), Refsum ***Sensorineural hearing impairment***: KID, NLSD > Refsum, CHH, CHILD ***Neurologic abnormalities/developmental delay***: SLS, NLSD, TTD, IFAP, Refsum ***Severe pruritus***: ichthyosis vulgaris (with atopic dermatitis), Netherton, SLS, inflammatory peeling skin syndrome Also evaluate for microcephaly, facial dysmorphism, asymmetry, contractures, and hepatosplenomegaly.
Initial evaluation of a neonate/infant with a collodion membrane or other signs of ichthyosis
History • Prenatal diagnoses, prolonged labor (suggestive of steroid sulfatase deficiency), prematurity • Consanguinity makes autosomal recessive ichthyosis more likely • Family history of epidermal nevi, ichthyosis, or erythrokeratoderma Laboratory evaluation and additional assessment • Complete blood count, electrolytes*, hepatic panel**, IgE level†; peripheral blood smear to evaluate for leukocyte vacuoles if suspect NLSD • Trichoscopy and light microscopic evaluation of clipped hairs (scalp and eyebrows) • ± Skin biopsy – e.g. if bullae (to assess for EI), to assess for diminished granular layer if suspect ichthyosis vulgaris, to detect dystrophic calcification if suspect CHH, or after resolution of collodion membrane for TGM-1 immunostaining • Ophthalmologic examination, hearing screen, ± X-rays of epiphyses (if mosaic distribution, for stippling of CHH > CHILD) • ***Consider genetic testing,*** especially a multigene panel if the diagnosis is not evident based on clinical and laboratory findings

§Keratitis has variable onset.
**Hypernatremic dehydration occurs primarily in collodion babies and neonates with Netherton syndrome, EI, or Harlequin ichthyosis.*
***Elevated transaminases are common in NLSD.*
†Increased in Netherton and inflammatory peeling skin syndromes.

Table 46.1 Clues to the diagnosis of ichthyoses and erythrokeratodermas. The disorders in this table are discussed in greater detail in the text or Table 46.2. Other rare ichthyoses and related disorders can also present with these findings. CIE, congenital ichthyosiform erythroderma; CHH, Conradi–Hünermann–Happle syndrome; EI, epidermolytic ichthyosis; CHILD, congenital hemidysplasia with ichthyosiform nevus and limb defects; IFAP, ichthyosis follicularis with atrichia and photophobia; KID, keratitis–ichthyosis–deafness syndrome; NLSD, neutral lipid storage disease; SLS, Sjögren–Larsson syndrome; TGM-1, transglutaminase-1; TTD, trichothiodystrophy.

with transmission by asymptomatic female carriers.

• The underlying steroid sulfatase deficiency is caused by deletion of the entire *STS* gene on chromosome Xp22 in ~90% of patients; ~5% of patients have a larger contiguous gene deletion with manifestations that may also include Kallmann syndrome (hypogonadotropic hypogonadism with anosmia), X-linked recessive chondrodysplasia punctata, ocular albinism, and/or intellectual disability/autism. A higher prevalence of attention deficit hyperactivity disorder has also been reported in children with XLRI.

• Affected neonates may have generalized exfoliation of translucent scales, followed during infancy by the development of characteristic dark brown, polygonal, adherent scales favoring the neck, preauricular area, scalp (especially in young children), extremities,

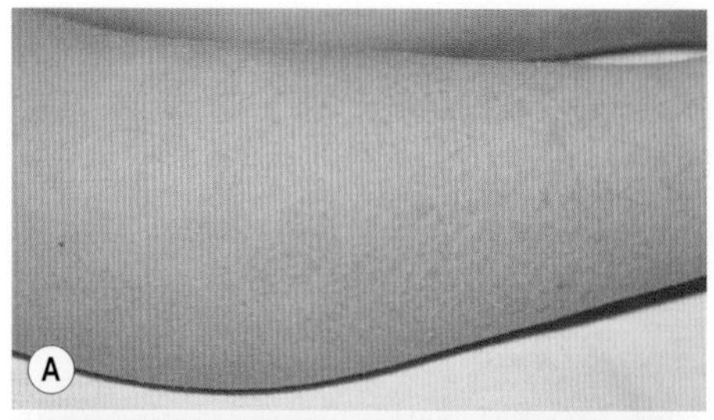

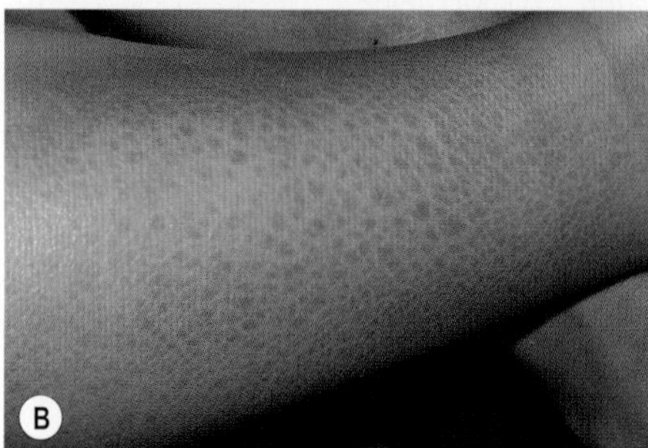

Fig. 46.1 Ichthyosis vulgaris. Fine, whitish, flaky scales (**A**) and larger, darker scales (**B**) on the legs of children with skin phototypes II and IV, respectively. *A, Courtesy, Angela Hernández-Martín, MD; B, Courtesy, Julie V. Schaffer, MD.*

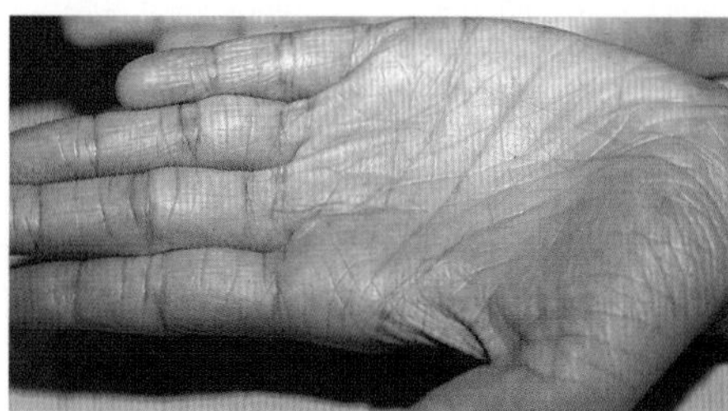

Fig. 46.2 Hyperlinear palms in ichthyosis vulgaris. *Courtesy, S. J. Bale, PhD, and J. J. DiGiovanna, MD.*

and trunk; the palms, soles, and flexural sites tend to be spared (Fig. 46.3).

• Often improves substantially in the summer.

• Associated findings include a perinatal history of prolonged labor due to low placental estrogen production (frequently resulting in birth via cesarean section), cryptorchidism, and asymptomatic corneal opacities.

• **Dx:** fluorescence *in situ* hybridization (FISH) or microarrays (targeted or whole-genome) can detect the underlying deletion in most patients; other methods include genetic testing, detection of increased (hydroxy) cholesterol sulfate (e.g. via increased migration of the β-fraction in serum lipoprotein electrophoresis), and measurement of leukocyte STS activity.

• Prenatal findings include decreased unconjugated estriol levels in maternal serum and the presence of non-hydrolyzed sulfated steroids in maternal urine.

• **Rx:** topical humectants, keratolytics, and retinoids.

Epidermolytic Ichthyosis (EI; Bullous Congenital Ichthyosiform Erythroderma, Epidermolytic Hyperkeratosis [EHK])

• Uncommon autosomal dominant disorder due to mutations in the keratin 1 (*KRT1*) or keratin 10 (*KRT10*) gene; occasionally occurs in the offspring of an individual with an epidermolytic epidermal nevus due to a mosaic *KRT1/10* mutation that involves the gonads as well as the skin.

• Presents at birth with erythroderma, peeling skin, and erosions (Fig. 46.4A); sepsis, dehydration, and electrolyte imbalances may occur.

• Skin fragility decreases over time, with development of widespread hyperkeratosis that forms corrugated ridges in flexures and a cobblestone pattern on extensor surfaces of joints (Fig. 46.4B–D); palmoplantar keratoderma (PPK) is seen in patients with *KRT1* mutations.

• Other manifestations include episodic blistering, secondary skin infections, and a pungent body odor.

• Characteristic histologic changes of epidermolytic hyperkeratosis (e.g. keratinocyte vacuolization and clumped keratin filaments) help to establish the diagnosis.

• **DDx:** *in neonates* – epidermolysis bullosa, staphylococcal scalded skin syndrome, other erosive disorders (see Ch. 28); *in children/adults* – superficial EI, ichthyosis hystrix of Curth–Macklin, other ichthyoses with non-scaling hyperkeratosis (e.g. Sjögren–Larsson and KID syndromes).

• **Rx:** *in neonates* – protective isolation, emollients, and monitoring.

• **Rx:** *in children and adults* – emollients/humectants, mechanical exfoliation of hyperkeratotic areas, antiseptic washes

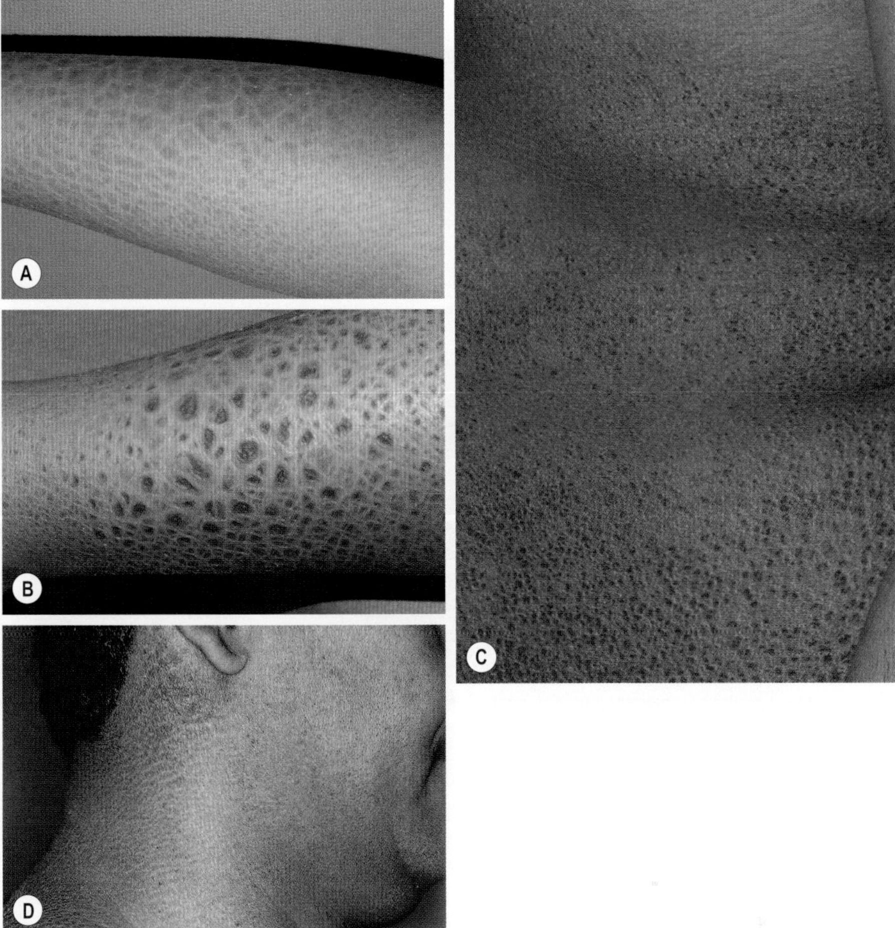

Fig. 46.3 X-linked recessive ichthyosis. Large light brown **(A)** and more prominent dark brown **(B)** scales on the lower leg. **C** Smaller dark brown scales on the trunk, with sparing of the skin folds. **D** Dark scales on the neck, sometimes referred to as a "dirty neck." *A–C, Courtesy, Julie V. Schaffer, MD; D, Courtesy, Gabriele Richard, MD, and Franziska Ringpfeil, MD.*

(e.g. dilute sodium hypochlorite baths), antimicrobial therapy for superinfections; keratolytics and retinoids (topical or oral) can improve hyperkeratosis but may lead to irritation and exacerbate skin fragility; widespread application of concentrated salicylic acid preparations should be avoided due to risk of salicylism.

• ***Superficial epidermolytic ichthyosis (ichthyosis bullosa of Siemens)*** is a related autosomal dominant condition due to mutations in the keratin 2 gene (*KRT2*), which is expressed only in the upper epidermis; affected individuals have milder, more superficial skin shedding ("molting"; Fig. 46.5), minimal erythema, and no PPK.

• ***Ichthyosis hystrix of Curth–Macklin***, which is caused by specific *KRT1* mutations, features hyperkeratosis (sometimes severe and spiky) and PPK similar to epidermolytic ichthyosis, but no skin fragility or histologic evidence of epidermolysis.

• ***Ichthyosis with confetti*** due to heterozygous frameshift mutations in *KRT10* > *KRT1* presents with ichthyosiform erythroderma at birth, with subsequent development of numerous small, confetti-like "islands" of normal skin that reflect revertant clones.

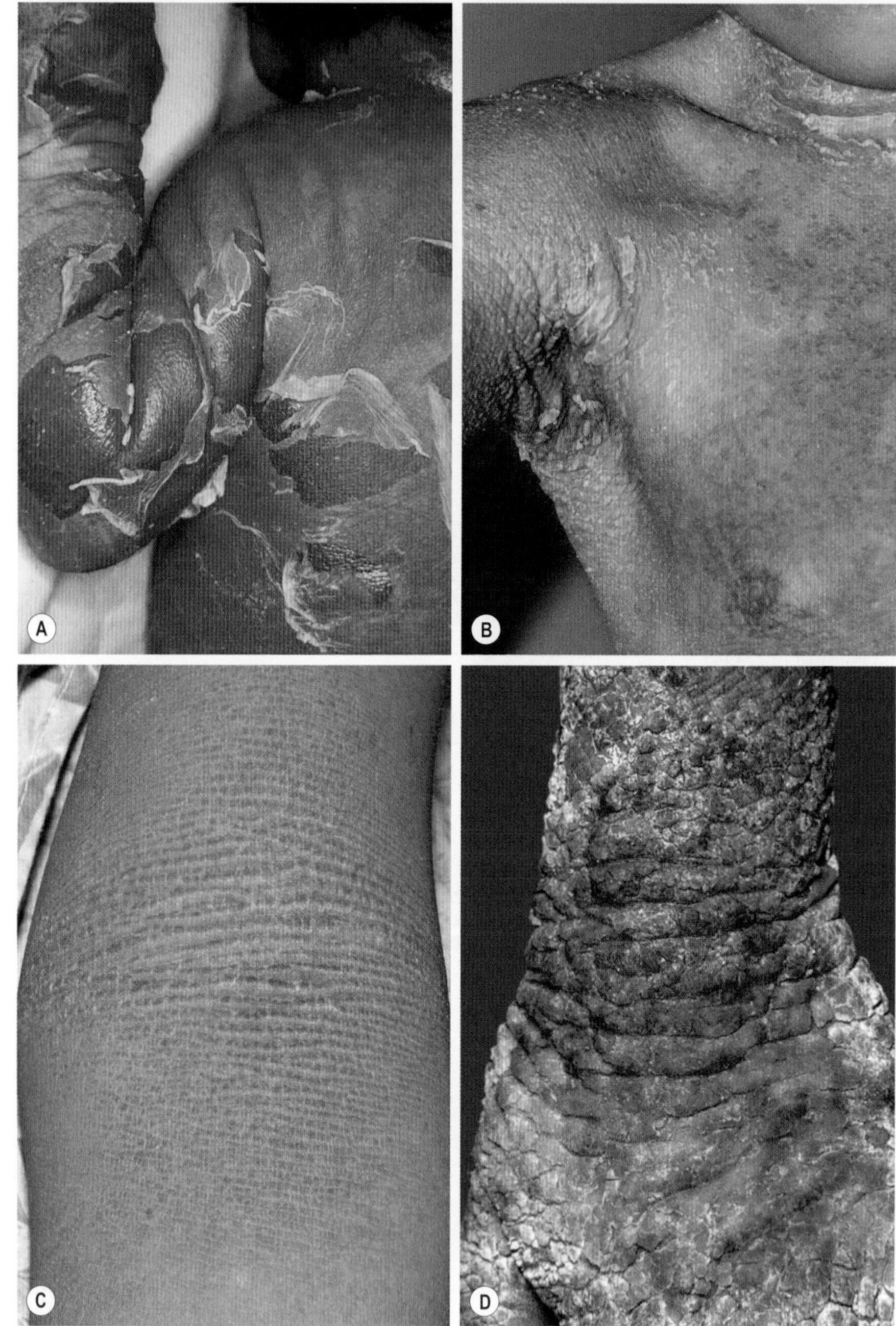

Fig. 46.4 Epidermolytic ichthyosis. A Erythroderma with widespread peeling and erosions during the neonatal period. **B** Later development of marked hyperkeratosis with focal erosions. **C** Corrugated hyperkeratosis in the antecubital fossa. **D** Hyperkeratosis with a cobblestone pattern on the dorsal hand. *A, Courtesy, Eugene Mirrer, MD; B, C; D, Courtesy, S. J. Bale, PhD, and J. J. DiGiovanna, MD.*

Continued

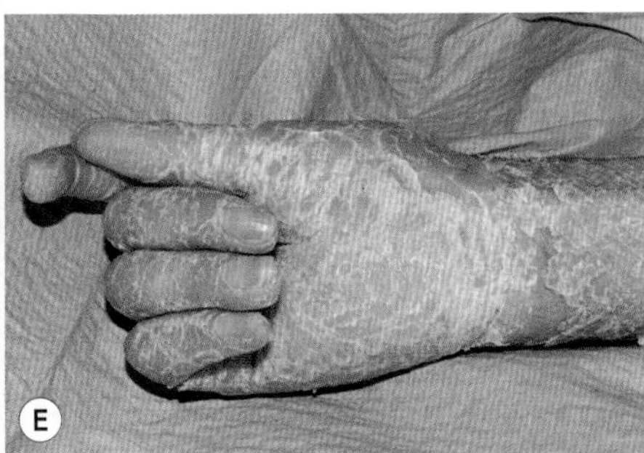

Fig. 46.4 *Continued* **Epidermolytic ichthyosis. E** Severe palmoplantar keratoderma with digital contractures in a patient with a *KRT1* mutation. *E, Courtesy, Julie V. Schaffer, MD.*

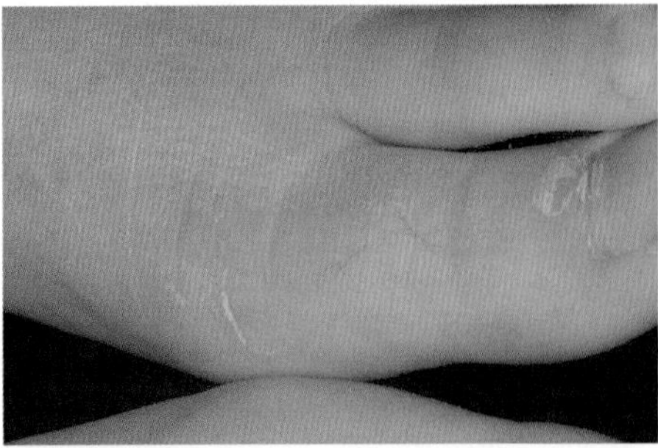

Fig. 46.5 Superficial epidermolytic ichthyosis. Increased skin markings and "collarettes" where the skin has been superficially shed ("Mauserung"). *Courtesy, Anthony Mancini, MD.*

Nonsyndromic Autosomal Recessive Congenital Ichthyosis (ARCI): Lamellar Ichthyosis and Congenital Ichthyosiform Erythroderma (CIE)

- Lamellar ichthyosis and CIE exist on a phenotypic spectrum, and nonsyndromic ARCI with these clinical findings can be caused by mutations in at least 11 different genes, including those encoding transglutaminase 1 (*TGM1*; most common), two lipoxygenases (*ALOX12B*, *ALOXE3*), and an ABC lipid transporter (*ABCA12*).

Collodion Baby

- Infants with ARCI (and occasionally other ichthyoses; see Table 46.1) are often born covered by a taut, shiny, transparent membrane resembling plastic wrap, which leads to ectropion, eclabium, and distortion of the nose and ears (Fig. 46.6).
- Neonatal complications can include impaired sucking, restricted ventilation, fluid and electrolyte imbalances, skin infections, and sepsis.
- **Rx:** humidified incubator, emollients, and monitoring for complications; keratolytic agents and manual debridement of the membrane are *not* advised due to risk of systemic absorption and infection, respectively.
- Within 2 weeks, the membrane peels off in sheets and a transition to the underlying disease phenotype takes place; a subset of collodion babies with underlying mutations in *TGM1*, *ALOX12B*, *ALOXE3*, or other genes have a *self-improving collodion ichthyosis* phenotype where the skin is fairly normal in appearance when the membrane resolves.

Lamellar Ichthyosis

- Characterized by large, brown, plate-like scales with little or no associated erythema (Fig. 46.7).
- Usually generalized, although involvement is limited to the trunk and scalp in the South African "bathing suit ichthyosis" variant (due to a particular *TGM1* mutation).
- Associated findings can include ectropion (which may result in conjunctivitis or keratitis), eclabium, scarring alopecia (especially of the peripheral scalp), PPK, nail dystrophy, and heat intolerance due to disruption of sweat ducts.
- **Rx:** oral retinoids (e.g. acitretin) for severe disease; use of topical retinoids (e.g. tazarotene) and keratolytics is limited by irritation and (for the latter agents) potential systemic absorption if applied to an extensive area; longitudinal ophthalmologic care can help to prevent complications of ectropion.

Congenital Ichthyosiform Erythroderma

- Characterized by erythroderma and small white scales, often with a powdery consistency, in a generalized distribution (Fig. 46.8).
- The degree of erythema and type of scale varies, and phenotypic overlap with lamellar ichthyosis is often observed; for example, larger, darker scales may be evident, especially on the lower extremities, and some patients have relatively small scales but little associated erythema.
- PPK and nail dystrophy are frequently present, but ectropion and scarring alopecia are less common than in lamellar

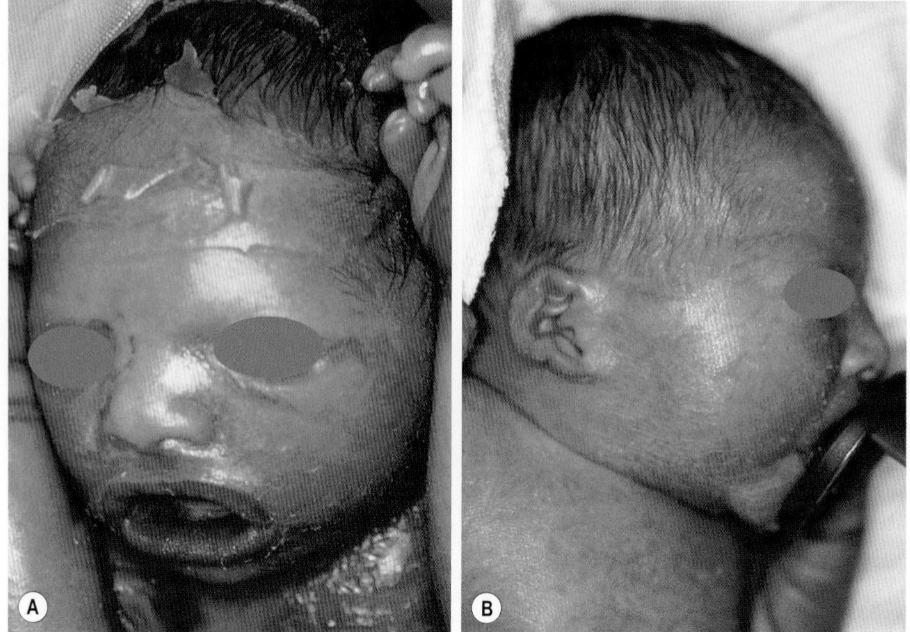

Fig. 46.6 Collodion baby. A Day 1 with ectropion and eclabium. **B** Day 8 with erythema and diffuse mild scaling and misshapen ears. *Courtesy, YDRSC.*

ichthyosis; severe exfoliative erythroderma represents a substantial metabolic stress that can result in poor growth and failure to thrive in children.

• **Rx:** similar to lamellar ichthyosis, although oral retinoids are more beneficial for scaling than the associated erythema; increased intake of fluids, calories, and protein is required for erythrodermic patients. Considering that Th17-associated inflammation plays a role in this and other forms of ichthyosiform erythroderma, drugs that block this pathway may have potential therapeutic benefit.

Other Ichthyoses and Erythrokeratodermas

• Major features of several additional ichthyoses and erythrokeratodermas are summarized in Table 46.2 (Figs 46.9–46.15); many other rare disorders of cornification with diverse cutaneous and extracutaneous manifestations also exist.

For further information see Ch. 57 from *Dermatology, Fourth Edition*.

For additional online figures visit www.expertconsult.com 

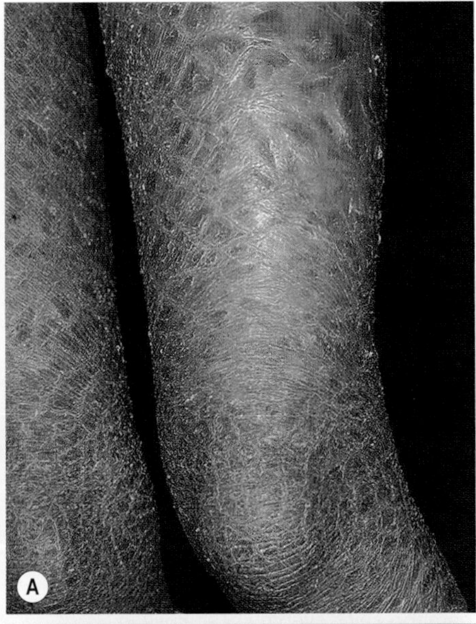

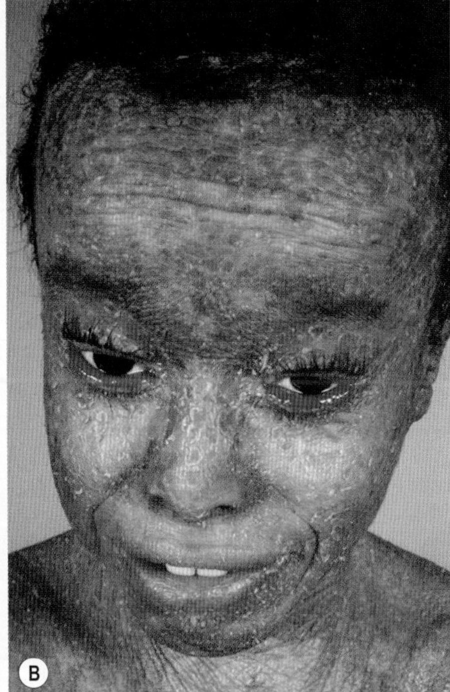

Fig. 46.7 Lamellar ichthyosis. A Large, plate-like scales on the lower extremities forming a mosaic pattern. **B** Obvious ectropion as well as plate-like scales. *A, Courtesy, Gabriele Richard, MD, and Franziska Ringpfeil, MD; B, Courtesy, NYUDSC.*

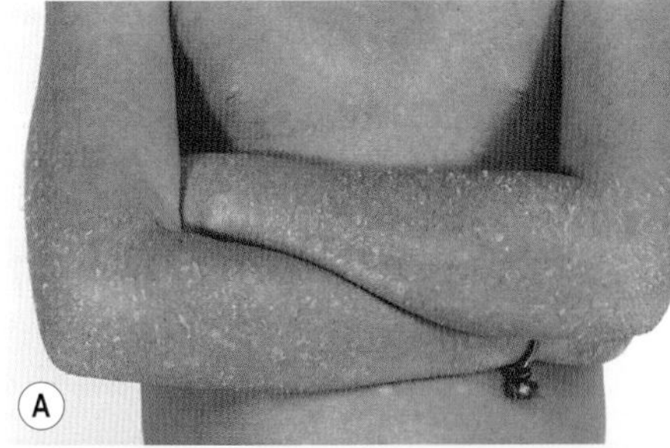

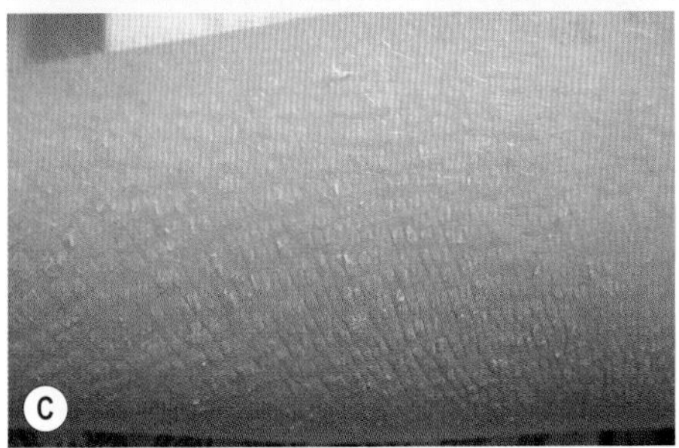

Fig. 46.8 Congenital ichthyosiform erythroderma. The differential diagnosis may include other causes of erythroderma (see Ch. 8). **A** Intense redness and fine, flaky, white scale on the trunk and arms. Close-up of fine white **(B)** and coarser yellowish **(C)** scale in a background of prominent erythema. *A, B, Courtesy, S. J. Bale, PhD, and J. J. DiGiovanna, MD; C, Courtesy, YDRSC.*

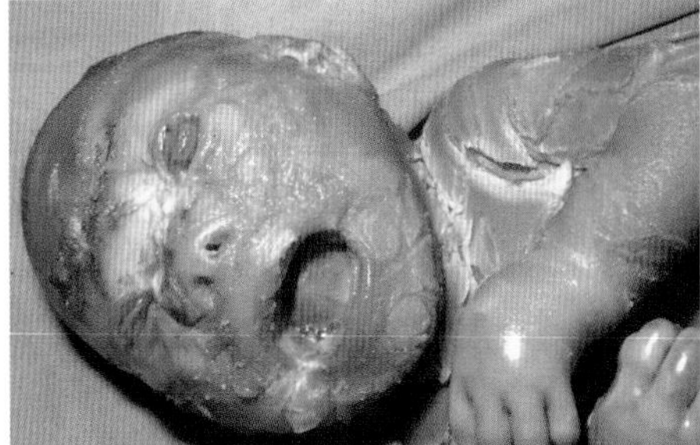

Fig. 46.9 Harlequin ichthyosis. Severe hyperkeratosis with fissuring as well as eclabium and ectropion. *Reproduced from Morillo M, Novo R, Torrelo A, et al. Feto arlequin. Actas Dermosifiliogr 1999;90:185–7.*

MAJOR FEATURES OF OTHER SELECTED ICHTHYOSES AND ERYTHROKERATODERMAS		
Diagnosis	**Gene, inheritance pattern**	**Major features**
Other nonsyndromic ichthyoses		
Harlequin ichthyosis	*ABCA12* (or rarely *KDSR*), AR	• Extremely thick, armor-like plates of scale with deep fissures encase the neonate (Fig. 46.9) • Extreme ectropion, eclabium, and deformities of the ear, nose, and hands/feet • Often premature birth and neonatal death due to sepsis or respiratory insufficiency • Acitretin therapy may allow survival with a severe CIE-like phenotype
Syndromic ichthyoses presenting in the neonatal period		
Netherton syndrome	*SPINK5*, AR	• Erythroderma and peeling in neonates, with risk of hypernatremic dehydration and FTT • Later ichthyosis linearis circumflexa (circinate erythematous plaques bordered with double-edged scale) or a CIE-like phenotype (Fig. 46.10A–C) • Fragile hair with trichorrhexis invaginata ("bamboo hair"; eyebrow > scalp) (Fig. 46.10D) • Pruritus, eczematous dermatitis, food allergies, elevated serum IgE, recurrent infections • **DDx:** generalized inflammatory peeling skin syndrome (corneodesmosin mutations)
Sjögren–Larsson syndrome (SLS)	*ALDH3A2*, AR	• Pruritic non-scaling hyperkeratosis (Fig. 46.11) > scaling (fine to plate-like); favors abdomen, neck, flexures • Spastic di- and tetraplegia, intellectual disability, perifoveal glistening white dots
Neutral lipid storage disease with ichthyosis (NLSD)	*ABHD5*, AR	• Generalized scaling (fine, plate-like on legs) with variable erythema • Hepatomegaly, myopathy, developmental delay, hearing impairment, cataracts • Lipid-containing vacuoles in leukocytes
Trichothiodystrophy with ichthyosis (TTD; Tay syndrome, [P]IBIDS)	*ERCC2* > *ERCC3* > *GTF2H5*, AR	• *P*hotosensitivity; *I*chthyosis: generalized scaling with minimal erythema beyond infancy • *B*rittle hair (tiger-tail banding, trichoschisis) and nails • *I*ntellectual impairment, *D*ecreased fertility, *S*hort stature, cataracts (occasionally)

Table 46.2 Major features of other selected ichthyoses and erythrokeratodermas. *ABCA12*, ATP-binding cassette, subfamily A, member 12; *ABHD5*, abhydrolase domain-containing 5; *ALDH3A2*, aldehyde dehydrogenase 3A2; AR, autosomal recessive; CIE, congenital ichthyosiform erythroderma; *ERCC2/3*, excision repair cross-complementing 2/3; FTT, failure to thrive; *GTF2H5*, general transcription factor IIH, polypeptide 5; *KDSR*, 3-ketodihydrosphingosine reductase; *SPINK5*, serine protease inhibitor Kazal type 5. *Continued*

MAJOR FEATURES OF OTHER SELECTED ICHTHYOSES AND ERYTHROKERATODERMAS		
Diagnosis	**Gene, inheritance pattern**	**Major features**
Syndromic X-linked dominant ichthyosiform conditions		
CHILD (congenital hemidysplasia with ichthyosiform nevus & limb defects) syndrome	*NSDHL*, X-D	• Unilateral erythematous, thickened skin with striking midline demarcation and a waxy surface or adherent scale in neonates (Fig. 46.12) • Later less erythematous and more verrucous, with affinity for skin folds • Ipsilateral skeletal abnormalities and organ hypoplasia
Conradi–Hünermann–Happle syndrome (CHH)	*EBP*, X-D	• Ichthyosiform erythroderma with feathery, adherent scale along the lines of Blaschko in neonates (Fig. 46.13) • Later follicular atrophoderma along lines of Blaschko and patchy scarring alopecia • Unilateral cataracts, asymmetric skeletal abnormalities, chondrodysplasia punctata (infants)
Erythrokeratodermas		
Keratitis–ichthyosis–deafness (KID) syndrome	*GJB2*, AD	• Transient neonatal erythroderma; later well-demarcated, erythematous, furrowed hyperkeratotic plaques favoring the face and extremities (Fig. 46.14A) > diffusely thickened, grainy skin • Cheilitis, stippled PPK (Fig. 46.14B), follicular keratoses, follicular occlusion triad, cysts • Congenital sensorineural hearing impairment; progressive keratitis and conjunctivitis • Recurrent mucocutaneous infections (especially candidiasis); risk of SCC (oral and cutaneous) • **DDx:** *I*chthyosis *F*ollicularis, *A*trichia and *P*hotophobia (IFAP) syndrome (*MBTPS2*)
Erythrokeratodermia variabilis (EKV)	*GJB3* or *GJB4* > *GJA1*, AD	• Transient erythematous patches (Fig. 46.15A), especially in childhood (occasionally circinate) • Fixed, geographic hyperkeratotic plaques on extremities and trunk (Fig. 46.15B); ± PPK • **DDx:** progressive symmetric erythrokeratoderma (no transient lesions, often affects face), including *KDSR*-related erythrokeratoderma (thrombocytopenia)

Table 46.2 *Continued* **Major features of other selected ichthyoses and erythrokeratodermas.** Additional rare conditions include ichthyosis prematurity syndrome, Refsum disease, and erythrokeratodermia–cardiomyopathy syndrome. AD, autosomal dominant; *EBP*, emopamil binding protein (sterol isomerase); *GJB2/3/4* and *GJA1*, gap junction β2/3/4 and α1 (encoding connexins 26/31/30.3 and 43); *KDSR*, 3-ketodihydrosphingosine reductase; MBTPS2, membrane bound transcription factor peptidase, site 2; PPK, palmoplantar keratoderma; SCC, squamous cell carcinoma; X-D, X-linked dominant.

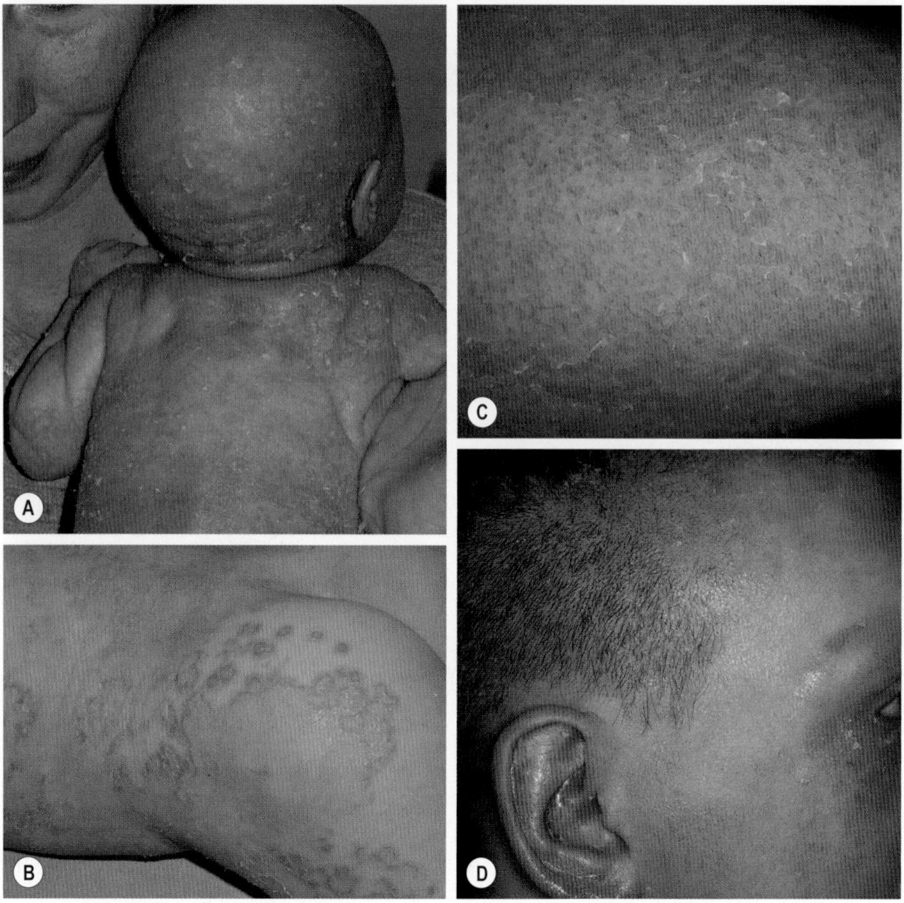

Fig. 46.10 Netherton syndrome. A Erythroderma in a neonate who also presented with hypernatremic dehydration. **B** Ichthyosis linearis circumflexa. Note the double-edged scale. **C** Close-up showing "peeling" quality of the scale. **D** Short, thin hair on the scalp, sparse eyebrows, and a lack of eyelashes. *A, Courtesy, Julie V. Schaffer, MD; B, Courtesy, Antonio Torrelo, MD; C, D, Courtesy, YDRSC.*

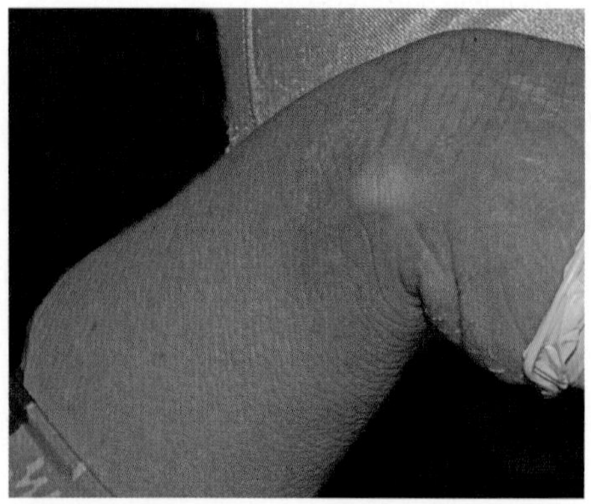

Fig. 46.11 Sjögren–Larsson syndrome. Yellowish-brown hyperkeratosis with accentuated skin markings. *Courtesy, Julie V. Schaffer, MD.*

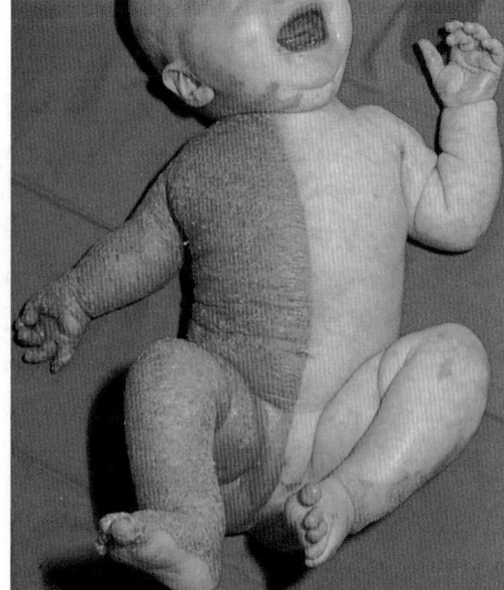

Fig. 46.12 CHILD syndrome. Note the sharp midline demarcation on the trunk. *From Happle R, Mittag H, Kuster W. Dermatology 1995;191:210–6, with permission. Courtesy, Rudolph Happle, MD.*

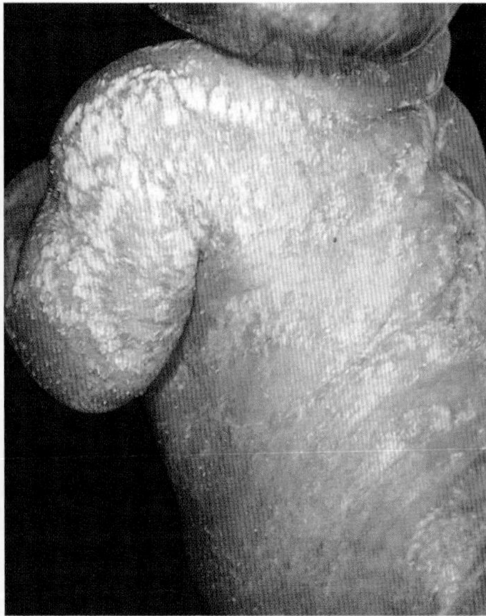

Fig. 46.13 Conradi–Hünermann–Happle syndrome. Erythroderma and linear streaks and whorls of hyperkeratosis. *Courtesy, Rudolph Happle, MD.*

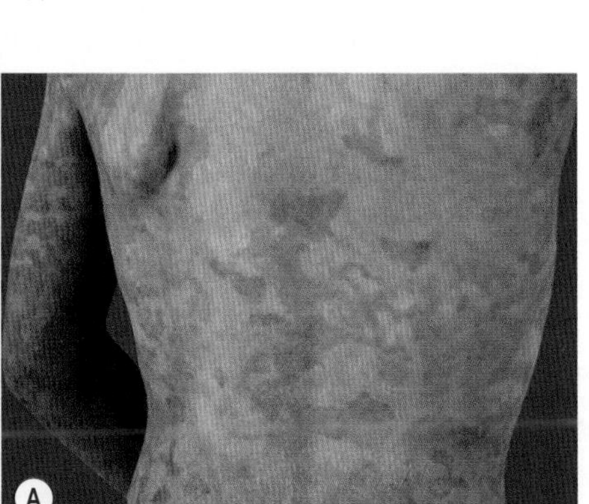

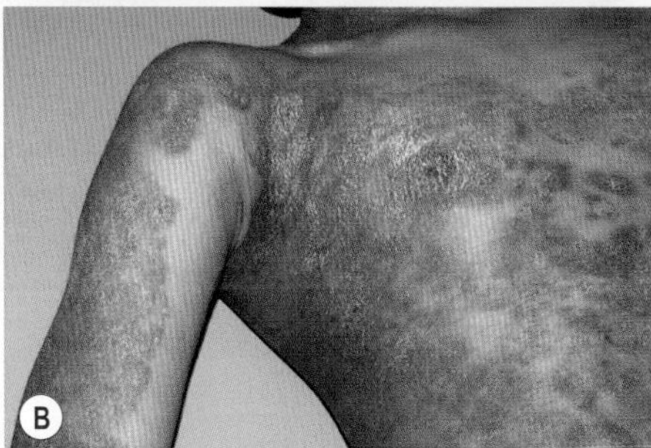

Fig. 46.15 Erythrokeratodermia variabilis. **A** Transient erythematous patches and generalized brownish hyperkeratosis. **B** Symmetrically distributed hyperkeratotic plaques with hypertrichosis. *A, Courtesy, Gabriele Richard, MD, and Franziska Ringpfeil, MD; B, Courtesy, Julie V. Schaffer, MD.*

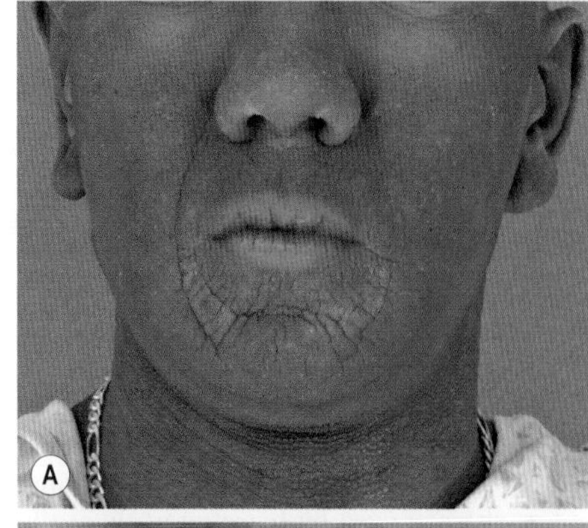

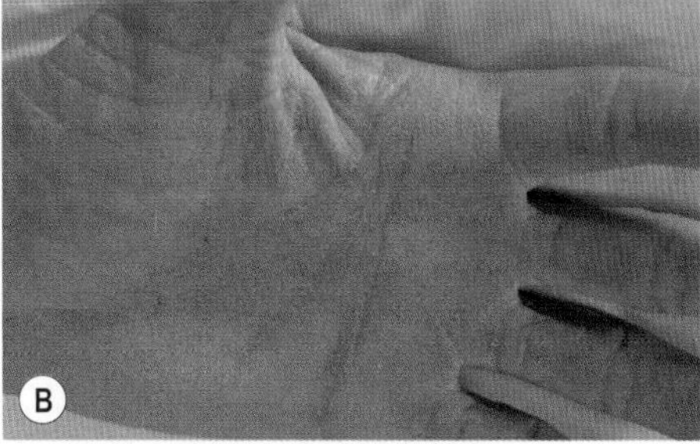

Fig. 46.14 KID syndrome. **A** Diffusely thickened, hyperkeratotic skin with a coarse-grained texture and an erythematous component; note the characteristic radial furrows around the mouth. **B** Bright pink, keratotic periorificial plaques with crusting. *Courtesy, Julie V. Schaffer, MD.*

47 Keratodermas

- Palmoplantar keratodermas (PPKs) represent a group of hereditary and acquired disorders characterized by hyperkeratosis of the skin on the palms and soles.
- Three major types of involvement:
  - *Diffuse PPK*: confluent over the entire palmoplantar surface; onset by early childhood in hereditary forms, with initial erythema evolving into thick, yellow hyperkeratosis that may be waxy or verrucous (Fig. 47.1)
  - *Focal PPK*: primarily in areas of friction or pressure; the *areata/nummular* (oval) pattern affects the soles (Fig. 47.2A) > palms; the *striate* (linear) pattern extends from the palms to the volar fingers (Fig. 47.2B)
  - *Punctate PPK*: small (≤1 cm) keratotic papules on the palms and soles; onset is usually in adolescence or early adulthood, with initial pinhead-sized translucent papules that may become larger and callus-like (Fig. 47.3)
- Other possible features include hyperhidrosis, an erythematous border (see Fig. 47.1C), extension beyond the palmoplantar

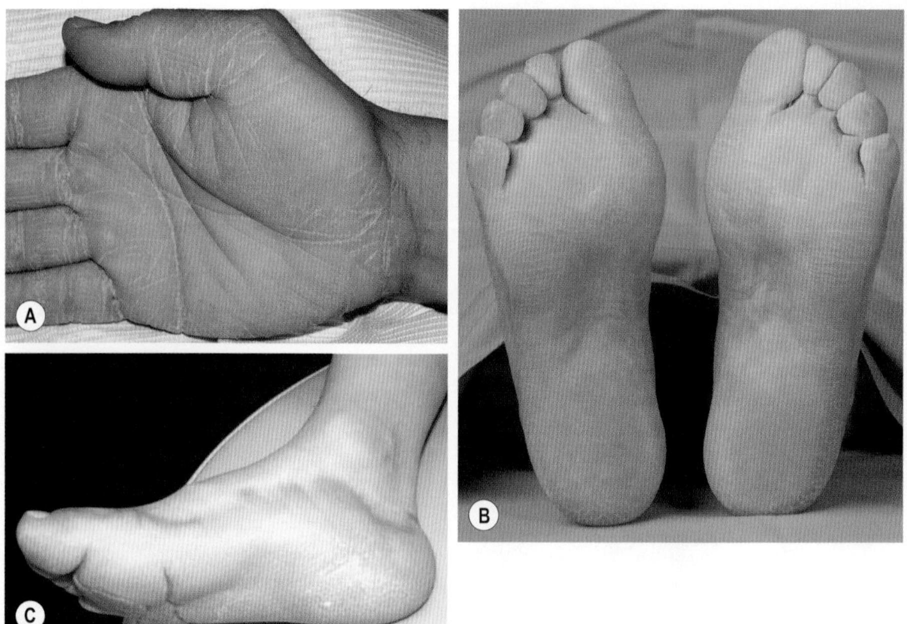

Fig. 47.1 Diffuse palmoplantar keratoderma. A Non-epidermolytic keratoderma with sharp demarcation at the wrist and side of the thumb. **B** Epidermolytic keratoderma with greater thickness in sites of pressure. **C** Epidermolytic keratoderma with prominent erythema at the border. In general, epidermolytic and non-epidermolytic forms cannot be distinguished clinically. *A, Courtesy, Julie V. Schaffer, MD; B, Courtesy, Dieter Metze, MD, and Vinzenz Oji, MD; C, Courtesy, Alfons L. Krol, MD, and Dawn Siegel, MD.*

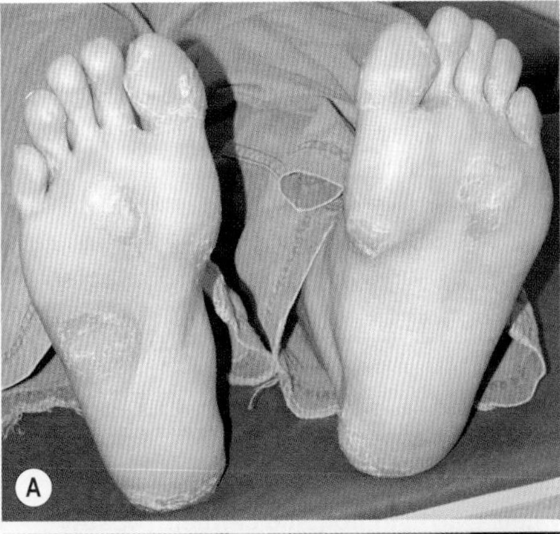

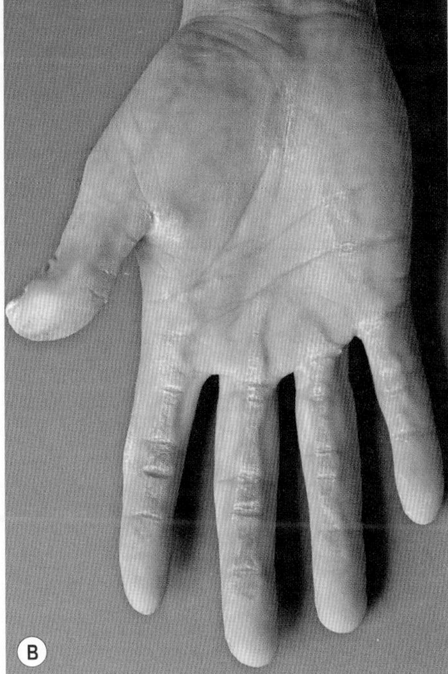

Fig. 47.2 Focal palmoplantar keratoderma. **A** Areata type on the soles. **B** Striate type on the palm. *A, Courtesy, Alfons L. Krol, MD, and Dawn Siegel, MD; B, Courtesy, Dieter Metze, MD, and Vinzenz Oji, MD.*

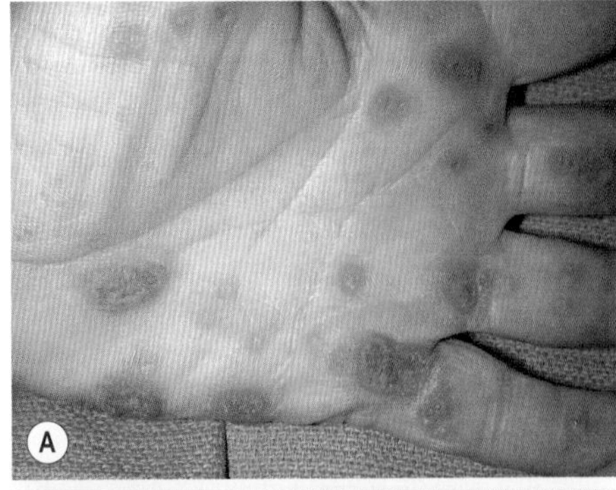

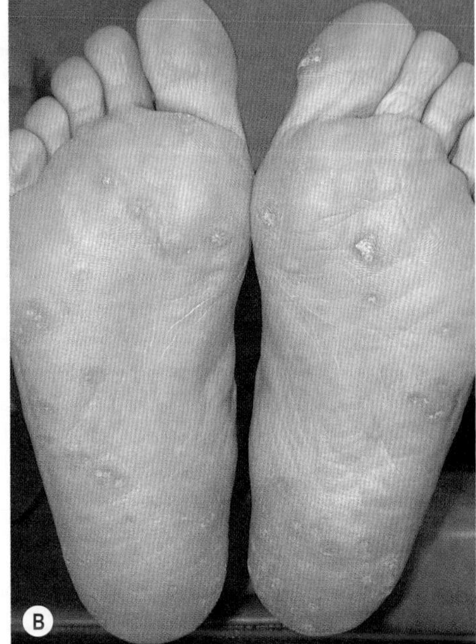

Fig. 47.3 Punctate palmoplantar keratoderma. Keratotic papules, some coalescing to form plaques, on the palm **(A)** and soles **(B).** *A, Courtesy, Kalman Watsky, MD; B, Courtesy, YDRSC.*

skin (e.g. onto dorsal hands/feet, flexor wrists; "transgrediens"), digital constriction bands (pseudoainhum; Fig. 47.4B), and the histopathologic finding of epidermolytic hyperkeratosis ("epidermolytic PPK").

- Table 47.1 outlines major forms of PPK, either isolated or associated with additional cutaneous and extracutaneous manifestations (Figs 47.4–47.11).
- **Rx:** keratolytics (e.g. salicylic acid 4–6% in petrolatum, urea 40%), mechanical debridement, topical or oral retinoids; treatment of secondary fungal and bacterial infections.

For further information see Ch. 58 from *Dermatology, Fourth Edition*.

For additional online figures and a table on palmoplantar pits, visit www.expertconsult.com 

MAJOR FORMS OF PALMOPLANTAR KERATODERMA (PPK)	
Forms with primarily cutaneous manifestations	**Forms with adnexal and/or extracutaneous manifestations**
Hereditary diffuse PPK	
• **Isolated epidermolytic PPK**, *Vörner(–Unna–Thost) type* (AD, keratin 9 > 1) • **Isolated non-epidermolytic PPK** (AD) • Other: e.g. ichthyoses & erythrokeratodermas (see Ch. 46), epidermolysis bullosa simplex (see Fig. 26.4B), Mal de Meleda (malodorous transgredient PPK)	• **Deafness**[*] + **"honeycombed" PPK** (AD, connexin 26) (Fig. 47.4) • *Hidrotic ectodermal dysplasia* (*Clouston syndrome*): **hypotrichosis + nail dystrophy + grid-like acral papules** (Fig. 47.5, see Ch. 52) • *Olmsted syndrome:* **mutilating PPK + periorificial plaques** • *Papillion–Lefèvre syndrome:* **periodontitis + psoriasiform plaques + pyogenic infections**
Hereditary diffuse *or* focal PPK (with infantile onset)	• **Woolly hair + arrhythmogenic cardiomyopathy**[†]: *Naxos disease* (**diffuse PPK**; AR, plakoglobin), *Carvajal syndrome* (**striate PPK**; AR>>AD, desmoplakin)
Hereditary focal PPK	
• **Isolated striate/areata PPK**: onset usually in childhood, increased severity with repetitive friction (AD; desmoglein 1, desmoplakin, keratin 1 or 6c)	• *Pachyonychia congenita:* **painful areata PPK** (soles > palms; often hyperhidrosis, blisters) + **hypertrophic nail dystrophy** with wedge-shaped subungual hyperkeratosis (Fig. 47.7) ± follicular keratoses, oral leukokeratosis, steatocystomas/other cysts (esp. PC-17) > natal teeth (PC-17), pili torti (AD, keratin 6a > 16 or 17 > 6b or 6c) • *Howel–Evans syndrome:* **esophageal carcinoma** (in adulthood) **+ areata PPK** (Fig. 47.6) **+ oral leukokeratosis + follicular keratoses** (AD) • *Richner–Hanhart syndrome:* **dendritic keratitis** (in infancy) **+ areata PPK** (Fig. 47.8) **+ intellectual disability**
Hereditary punctate PPK	
• **Isolated punctate PPK**[§] (AD) • **Punctate keratoses of the palmar creases**[§] (Fig. 47.9) • *Acrokeratoelastoidosis/focal acral hyperkeratosis:* **small papules at margins of hands/feet** (Fig. 47.10) (AD) • **Spiny keratoderma** (AD)	• Other: e.g. Darier disease[§] (see Ch. 48), PTEN hamartoma tumor syndrome[§] (see Ch. 52) • DDx: warts, punctate porokeratosis[§] (see Ch. 89), arsenical keratoses (see Ch. 74)
Acquired PPK	
• *Keratoderma climactericum:* **focal PPK on heels/weight-bearing areas of soles, esp. in women >45 y of age**; associated with obesity, cold climate, backless shoes • DDx: see Table 13.1 and Fig. 13.1	• Associations: **hypothyroidism**, **cancer** (e.g. lung, GI), **drugs** (e.g. sorafenib) • *Aquagenic PPK:* **thickening + white/translucent "pebbling" of palms > soles upon water immersion** (Fig. 47.11); usually isolated, but affects >50% of cystic fibrosis patients

[*]*Deafness + PPK may also occur in mitochondrial disorders.*

[†]*Cardiac disease usually becomes evident after puberty and can present with sudden death; desmocollin 2 mutations have also been described.*

[§]*May leave a pit upon removal of the keratotic plug; DDx of palmoplantar pits also includes pitted keratolysis (see Ch. 61) and basal cell nevus syndrome (see Ch. 88).*

Table 47.1 Major forms of palmoplantar keratoderma (PPK). The most common types in children and adults are shaded pink and yellow, respectively. Selected genetic etiologies are in parentheses. AD, autosomal dominant; AR, autosomal recessive.

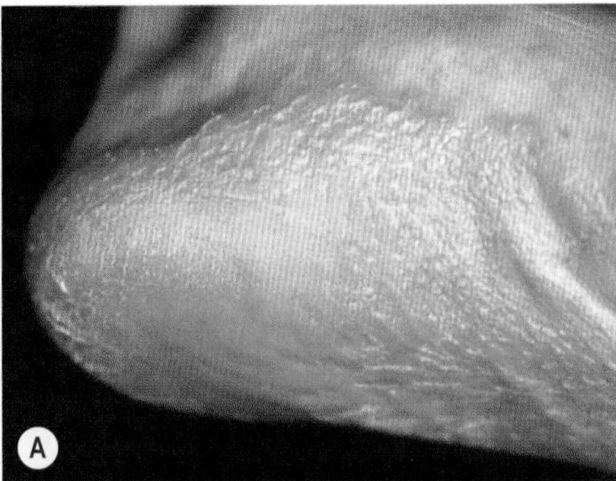

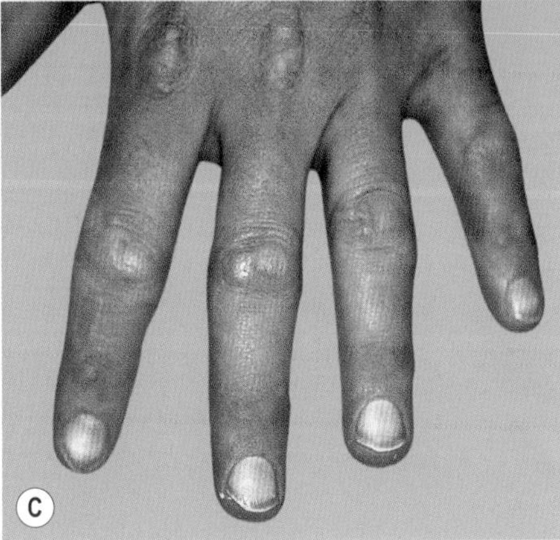

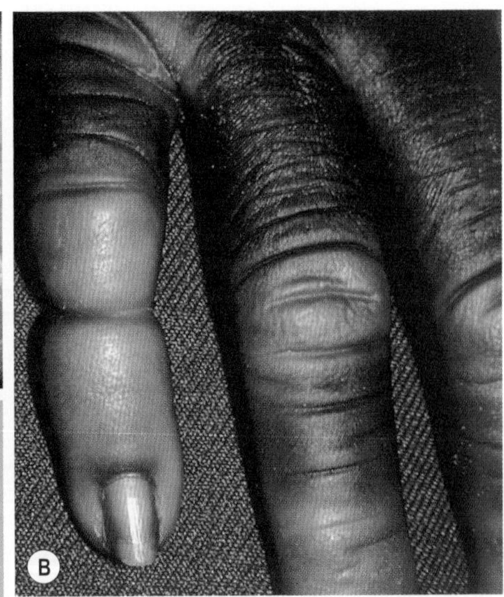

Fig. 47.4 Palmoplantar keratoderma associated with deafness due to connexin 26 mutations. A Diffuse "honeycombed" keratoderma on the sole. **B** Pseudoainhum formation in Vohwinkel syndrome, which can also feature "starfish" keratoses on the knuckles. **C** Leukonychia and knuckle pads in Bart–Pumphrey syndrome. *A, C, Courtesy, Alfons L. Krol, MD, and Dawn Siegel, MD; B, Courtesy, YDRSC.*

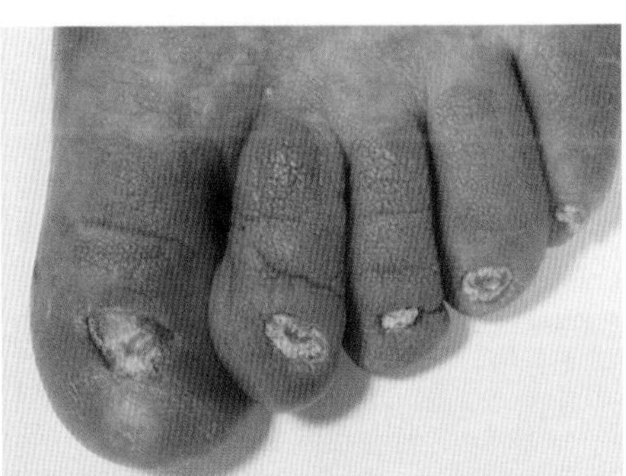

Fig. 47.5 Hidrotic ectodermal dysplasia (Clouston syndrome). Note the "pebbled" skin on the dorsal aspect of the toes as well as the dystrophic nail plates. *Courtesy, D. Sasseville, MD, and R. Wilkinson, MD.*

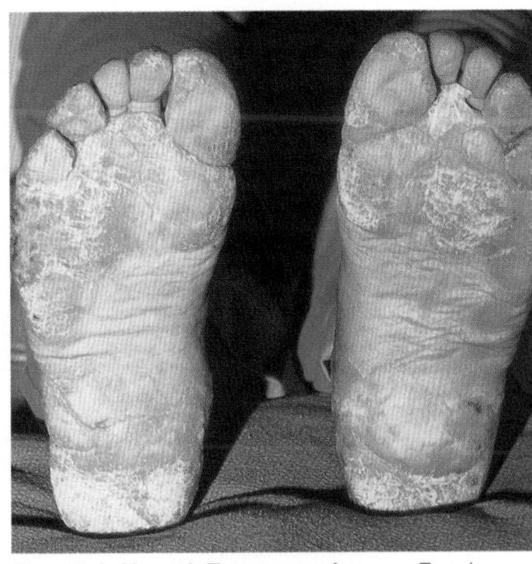

Fig. 47.6 Howel–Evans syndrome. Focal palmoplantar keratoderma, usually with onset at 5–15 years of age, associated with development of carcinoma of the esophagus in adulthood. *Courtesy, Alfons L. Krol, MD, and Dawn Siegel, MD.*

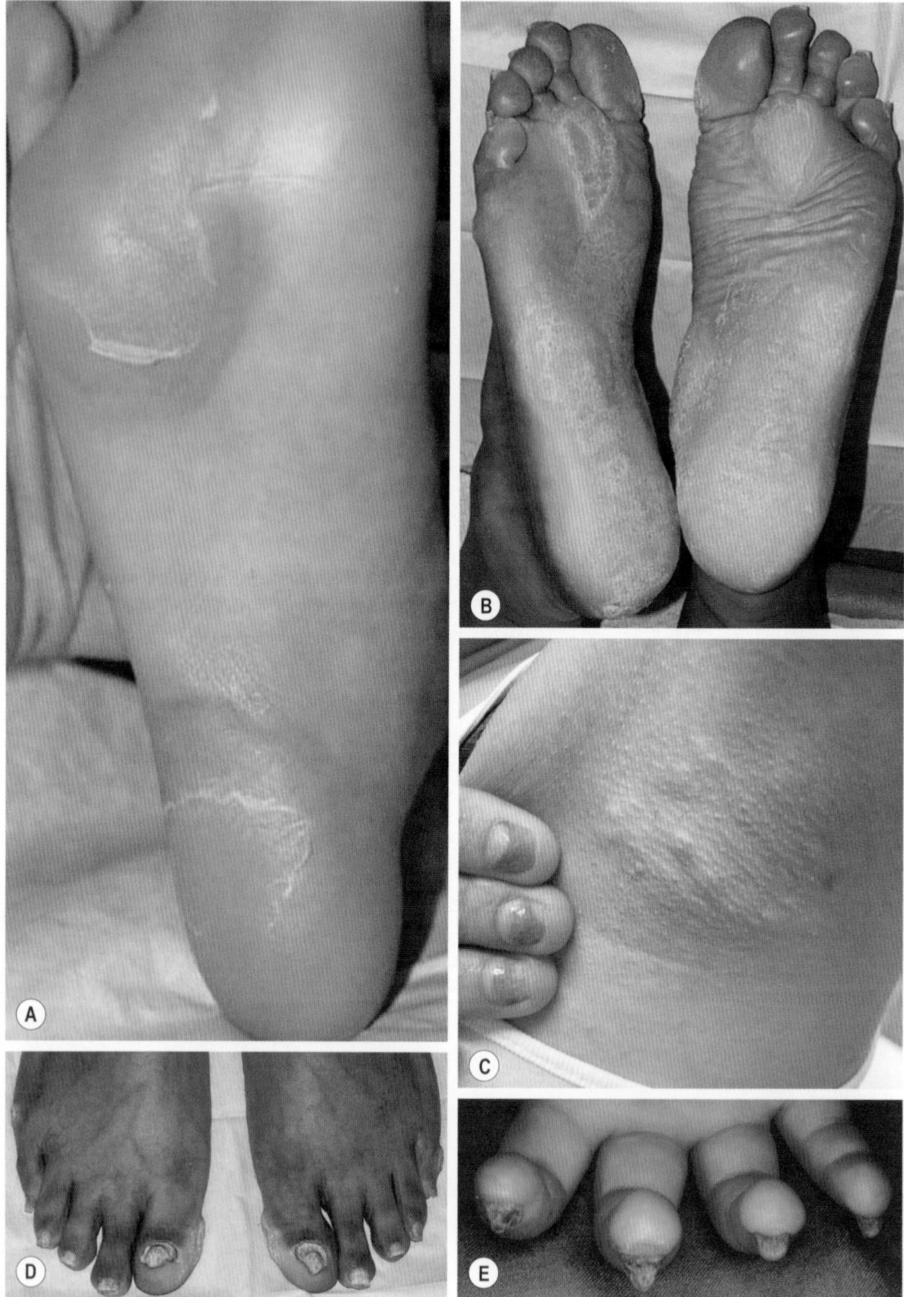

Fig. 47.7 Pachyonychia congenita. **A** Painful focal plantar keratoderma with associated erythema and blistering. **B** Plantar hyperkeratosis accentuated over pressure points. **C** Steatocystomas in the axilla. **D, E** Hypertrophic nail dystrophy with wedge-shaped subungual hyperkeratosis. *A, Courtesy, Alfons L. Krol, MD, and Dawn Siegel, MD; B, D, Courtesy, Julie V. Schaffer, MD; C, Courtesy, J. Valverde, MD; E, Courtesy, YDRSC.*

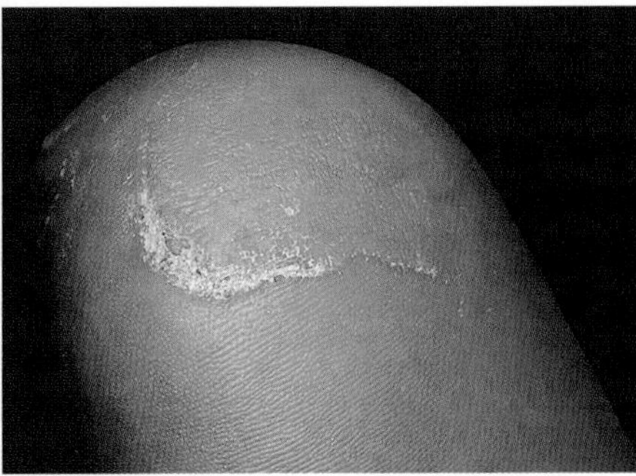

Fig. 47.8 Richner–Hanhart syndrome (tyrosinemia II). Focal painful keratoses on the plantar surface in a patient with corneal ulcers and intellectual disability. In this disorder, the onset of keratoderma ranges from early childhood to adolescence. *Courtesy, Jean L. Bolognia, MD.*

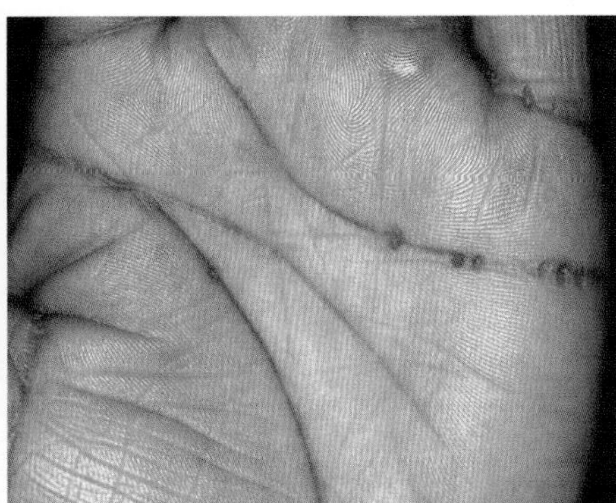

Fig. 47.9 Punctate keratoses of the palmar creases in an African American. *Courtesy, YDRSC.*

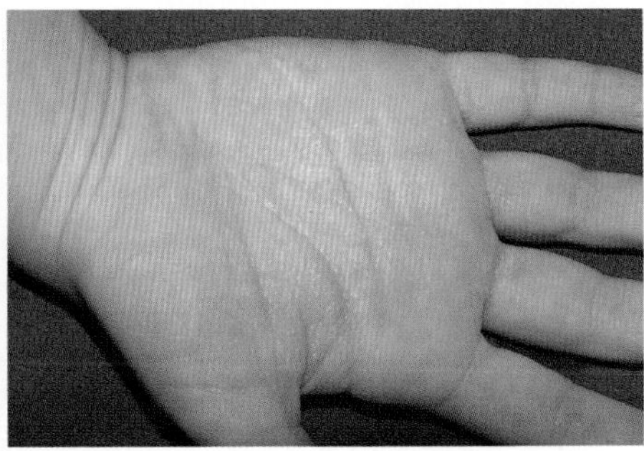

Fig. 47.11 Aquagenic keratoderma. White "pebbly" changes on the palm following immersion in water for a few minutes in a healthy teenage girl. *Courtesy, Julie V. Schaffer, MD.*

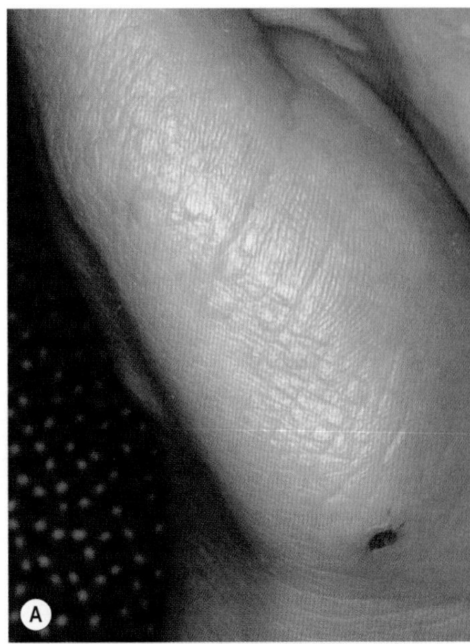

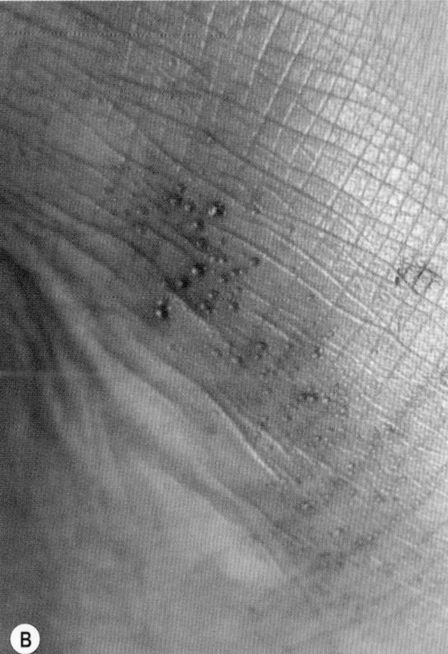

Fig. 47.10 Marginal papular keratoderma. **A** Acrokeratoelastoidosis presenting with multiple skin-colored to yellowish papules at the margin of the palmar skin. **B** Focal acral hyperkeratosis presenting with umbilicated keratotic papules at the margin of volar skin in an African-American woman. *A, Courtesy, YDRSC; B, Courtesy, Boni Elewski, MD.*

48 Darier Disease and Hailey–Hailey Disease

Darier Disease (Keratosis Follicularis)

- Autosomal dominant.
- Mutation in *ATP2A2* leads to dysfunction of SERCA2 protein, interfering with cellular calcium signaling.
- Clinical features:
  - Onset usually between ages 6 and 20 years, with peak during adolescence
  - Chronic course, often worse in summer
  - Crusted, pink-red to brown papules that may coalesce into plaques (Fig. 48.1) in a "seborrheic" and sometimes intertriginous distribution (Figs 48.2–48.3)
  - Hypopigmented macules may be the predominant feature, especially in darker skin types (Fig. 48.4)
  - Itching and malodor can be prominent
  - Flat-topped, skin-colored to brown papules (resembling flat warts) on the dorsal hands and feet (Fig. 48.5)
  - Palmoplantar keratotic papules (Fig. 48.6)
  - Nail changes, e.g. distal notching with longitudinal erythronychia (Fig. 48.7; see Ch. 58)
  - Whitish papules of the oral mucosa (Fig. 48.8)
- Rare subtypes – acral hemorrhagic, segmental (see Ch. 51).
- Exacerbating factors include sunlight, heat, occlusion, sweat, bacterial colonization.
- There may be an association with neuropsychiatric disease (e.g. major depression).
- Complications include bacterial (e.g. *Staphylococcus aureus*), fungal (e.g. tinea corporis), viral (e.g. HSV) infections; consider Kaposi varicelliform eruption due to HSV in a patient with a sudden onset of uniform hemorrhagic crusts, fever, and malaise (Fig. 48.9).
- Histopathologic features – acantholytic dyskeratosis above suprabasilar clefting.
- **DDx:** mild forms – severe seborrheic dermatitis, Grover disease; predominantly intertriginous – Hailey–Hailey disease, pemphigus vegetans, blastomycosis-like pyoderma, papular acantholytic dyskeratosis (vulvar); acral lesions – acrokeratosis verruciformis of Hopf (may be an allelic disorder or forme fruste; Fig. 48.10), flat warts, stucco keratoses, Flegel disease.
- **Rx:**
  - General measures: lightweight clothing, sunscreen, antimicrobial cleansers, keratolytic emollients
  - For symptomatic disease: topical retinoids ± topical CS (to decrease irritation from the former), oral retinoids (e.g. isotretinoin)
  - As-needed basis: topical and oral antibiotics and antifungals, systemic antivirals (e.g. acyclovir) for Kaposi varicelliform eruption, destructive modalities (e.g. laser treatment) for refractory lesions

Hailey–Hailey Disease (Familial Benign Chronic Pemphigus)

- Autosomal dominant.
- Mutation in *ATP2C1* gene causing dysfunction of a Golgi-associated protein and interference with cellular calcium signaling.
- Clinical features:
  - Onset during the second or third decade but sometimes delayed into the fourth or fifth decade
  - Variable course with remissions and flares
  - Mainly affects the major body folds (see Fig. 48.2), including inframammary in women (Fig. 48.11); sometimes other sites affected, e.g. trunk (Fig. 48.12)
  - Moist, malodorous plaques, with erosions, fissures, and flaccid blisters (see Fig. 48.11); circinate plaques with eroded/crusted borders (see Fig. 48.12)
- Rare subtype – segmental (see Ch. 51).

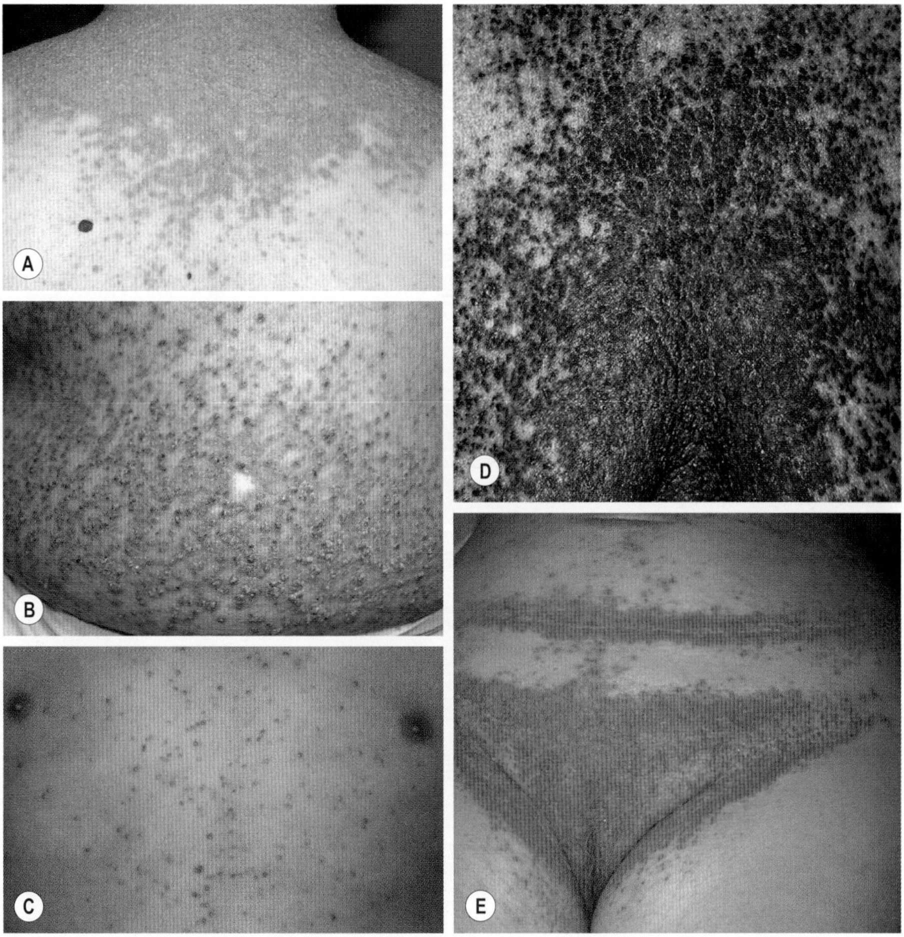

Fig. 48.1 Darier disease. Truncal involvement with a predilection for seborrheic areas **(A–D)**. Keratotic papules can vary from red **(A, B)** to brown **(C, D)** in color and may become confluent. **E** Severe intertriginous involvement. *A, C, Courtesy, Julie V. Schaffer, MD; B, D, Courtesy, YDRSC; E, Courtesy, Daniel Hohl, MD.*

- Exacerbating factors include friction, heat, sweat, bacterial colonization, application of adhesive tape; complications the same as for Darier disease (see above).
- Histopathologic features – acantholysis of the majority of the epidermis.
- **DDx:** intertrigo, irritant contact dermatitis, cutaneous candidiasis, pemphigus vegetans, Darier disease.
- **Rx:**
  - General measures: lightweight clothing, antimicrobial cleansers
  - For symptomatic disease: intermittent topical/intralesional CS, other topicals including calcineurin inhibitors, botulinum toxin type A to decrease sweat production, oral low-dose naltrexone
  - As-needed basis: topical and oral antibiotics and antifungals, destructive modalities (e.g. surgical excision, laser treatment) for refractory lesions

For further information see Ch. 59 from *Dermatology, Fourth Edition*.

For additional online figures visit www.expertconsult.com 

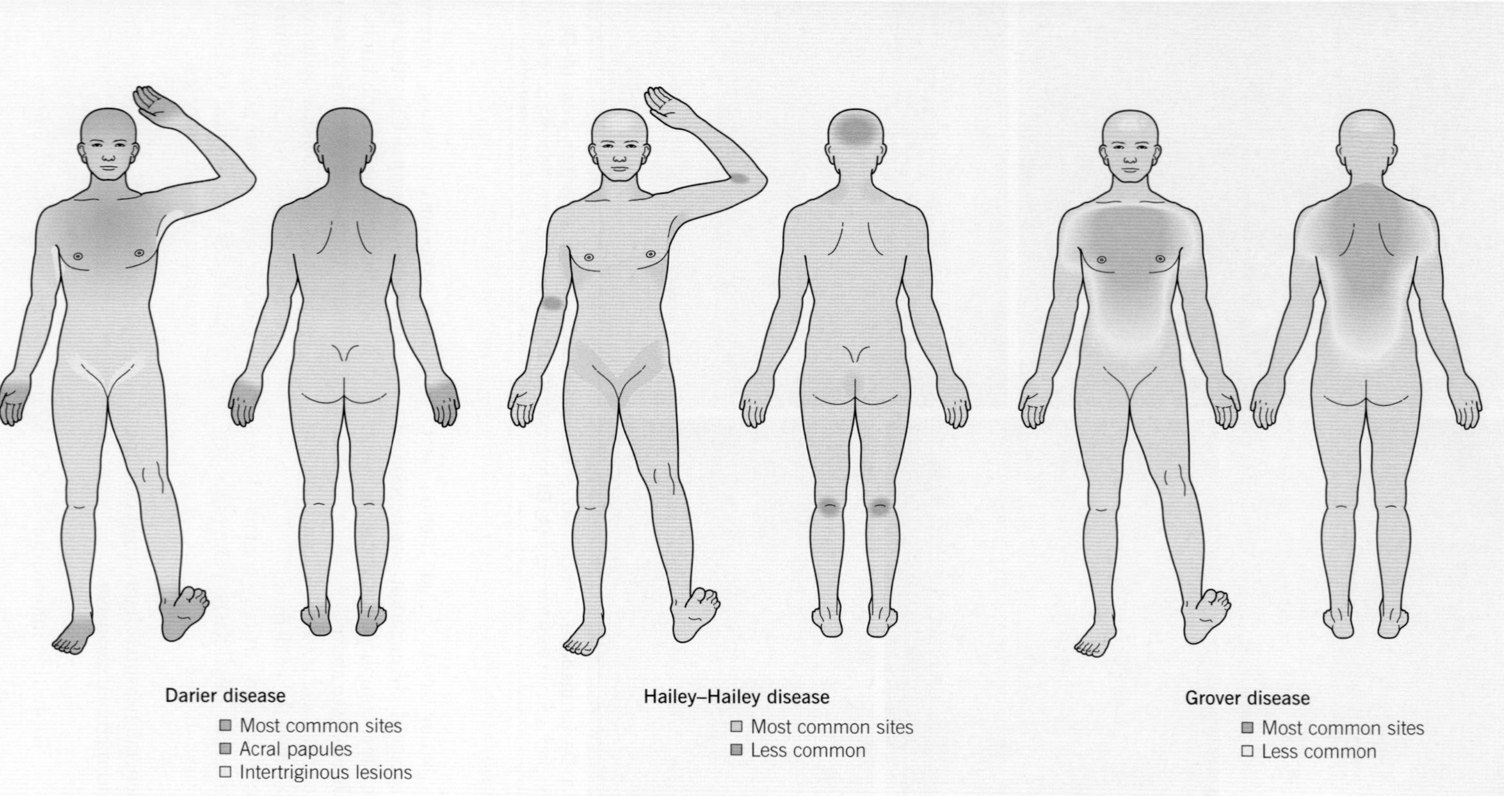

Fig. 48.2 Distribution patterns for Darier, Hailey–Hailey, and Grover disease.

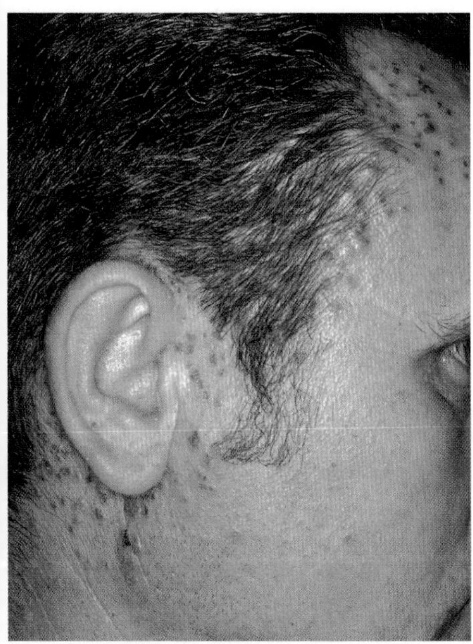

Fig. 48.3 **Darier disease.** Crusted papules at the hairline on the face and in the posterior auricular area. *Courtesy, Daniel Hohl, MD.*

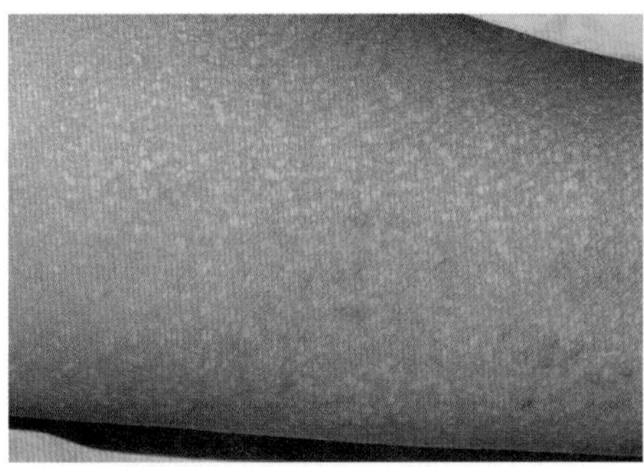

Fig. 48.4 Darier disease. Observed most commonly in individuals with darkly pigmented skin, a guttate leukoderma may be seen in patients with Darier disease, including the segmental form. *Courtesy, Julie V. Schaffer, MD.*

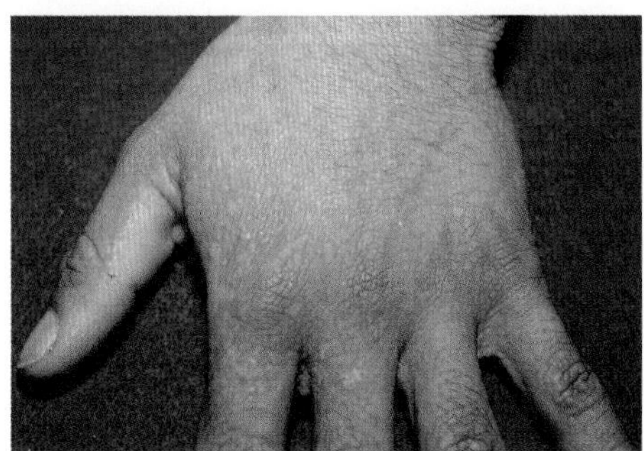

Fig. 48.5 Darier disease. Multiple flat-topped papules on the dorsal aspect of the hand. *Courtesy, Daniel Hohl, MD.*

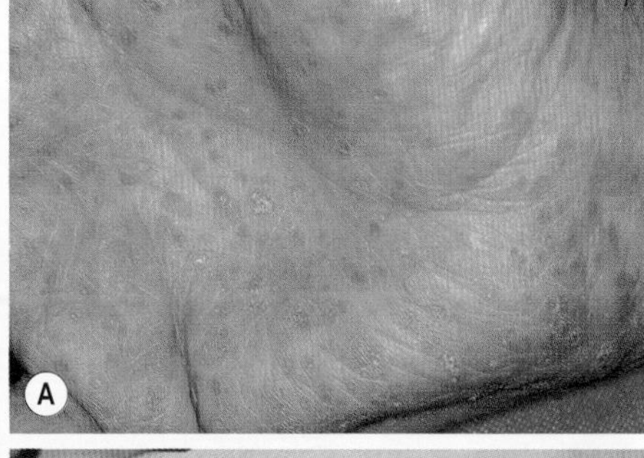

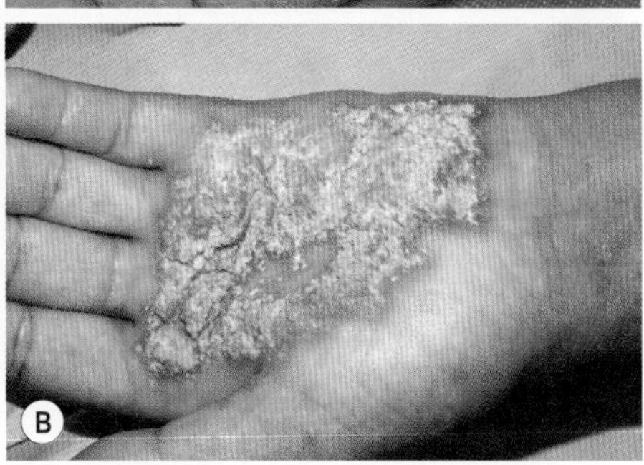

Fig. 48.6 Palmar involvement in Darier disease. A Both keratotic papules and keratin-filled depressions are seen. **B** Less commonly, a thick, spiked focal keratoderma is observed. *A, Courtesy, Kalman Watsky, MD; B, Courtesy, Julie V. Schaffer, MD.*

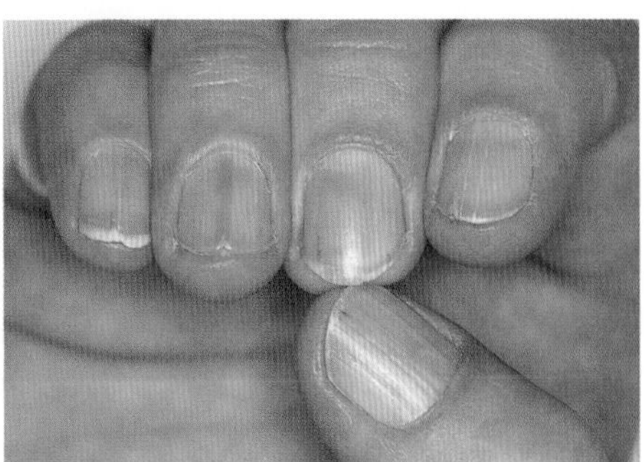

Fig. 48.7 Darier disease. Alternating longitudinal red and white streaks as well as notching of the free edge of the nail plate. *Courtesy, Antonella Tosti, MD.*

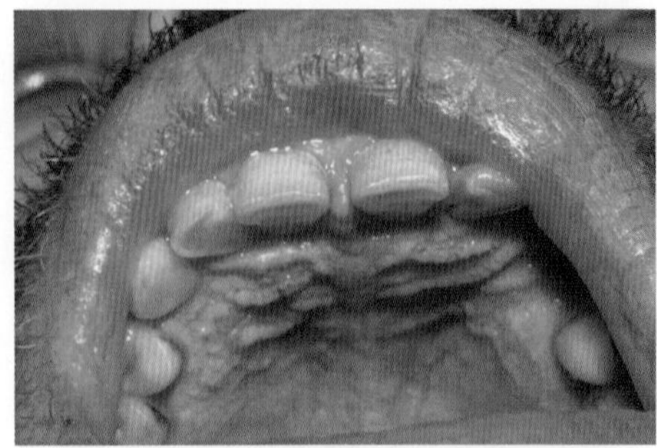

Fig. 48.8 Oral mucosal Darier disease. Whitish papules on the palate. *Courtesy, Daniel Hohl, MD.*

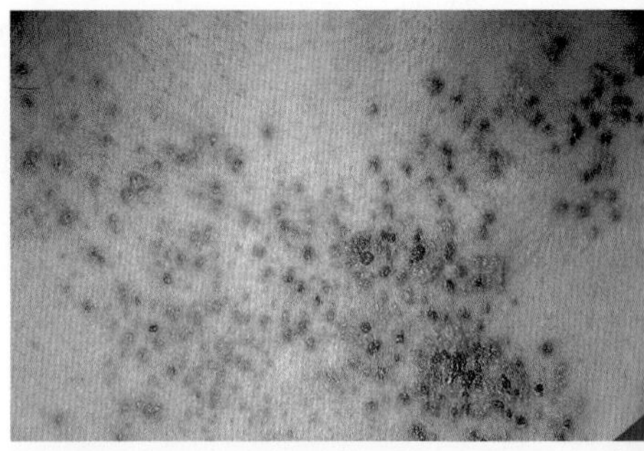

Fig. 48.9 Darier disease with superimposed HSV infection (Kaposi varicelliform eruption). Multiple hemorrhagic crusts of a similar size are seen. *Courtesy, YDRSC.*

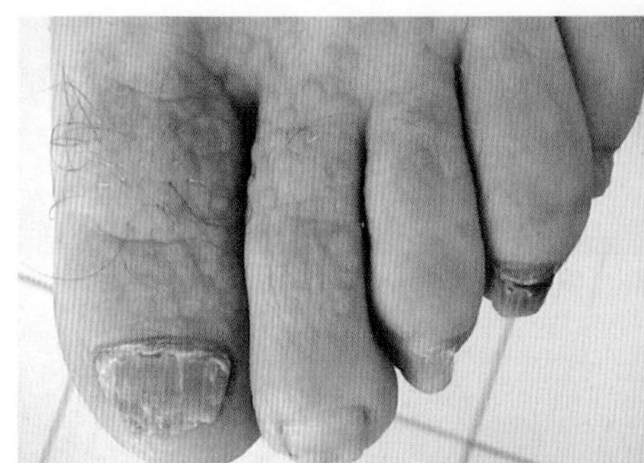

Fig. 48.10 Acrokeratosis verruciformis of Hopf. Involvement of the dorsal aspect of the foot with flat-topped papules. *Courtesy, YDRSC.*

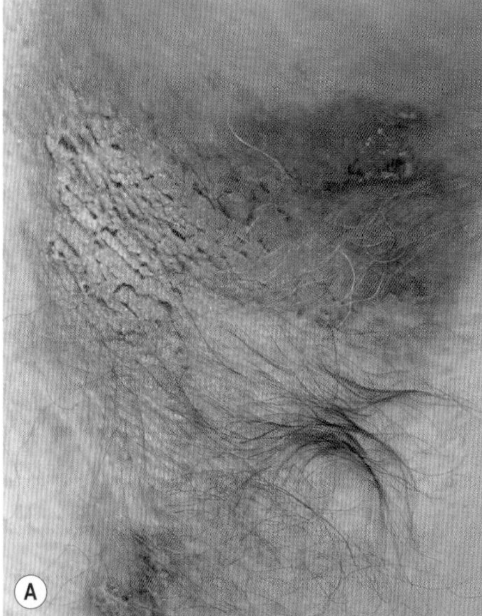

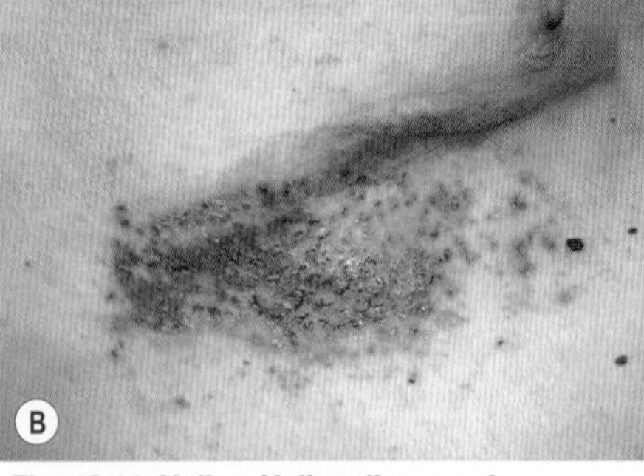

Fig. 48.11 Hailey–Hailey disease. A Erythematous, eroded plaque in the axilla. Note the intact flaccid vesicles at 2 and 7 o'clock. **B** Chronic submammary lesion with erosions in a worm-eaten pattern. *Courtesy, YDRSC.*

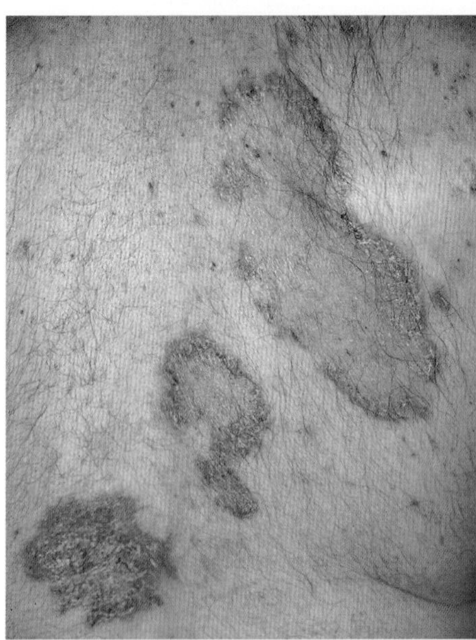

Fig. 48.12 Hailey–Hailey disease. Circinate plaques on the back with erosions and crusting in the active borders. *Courtesy, Louis A. Fragola, Jr., MD.*

Primary Immunodeficiencies 49

- Heterogeneous group of disorders characterized by immune system defects that result in increased susceptibility to various infections, often with additional manifestations such as autoimmunity, allergy, and risk of malignancy.
- The genetic basis has been determined for >200 primary immunodeficiencies.
- Many immunodeficiency syndromes present with dermatologic findings that can facilitate early diagnosis (Table 49.1; Figs 49.1–49.9); these features may be divided into three categories:
  - Recurrent, severe, atypical or recalcitrant mucocutaneous infections, most often with *Staphylococcus aureus*, *Candida* spp., and human papillomaviruses
  - Patterns of cutaneous inflammation that are shared by several immunodeficiencies, e.g. eczematous dermatitis, non-infectious granulomas, lupus erythematosus-like lesions, small vessel vasculitis, and ulcers
  - More specific skin findings suggestive of particular disorders, e.g. oculocutaneous telangiectasias in ataxia–telangiectasia and maternofetal GVHD in severe combined immunodeficiencies (SCID)
- In addition to extracutaneous infections with unusual organisms and increased frequency (e.g. pneumonia ≥2 times or otitis media ≥4 times yearly) or severity, signs of immunodeficiency in children may include failure to thrive, chronic diarrhea, lymphadenopathy (or lack of expected lymph nodes), and hepatosplenomegaly.

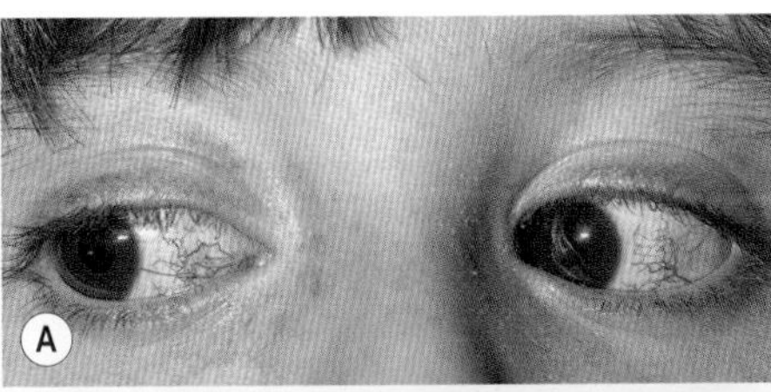

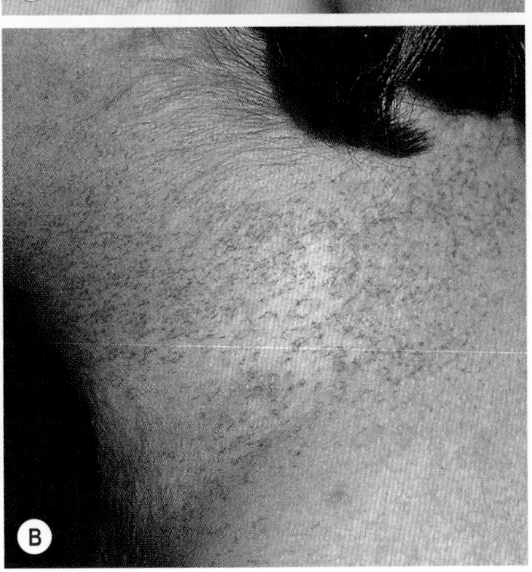

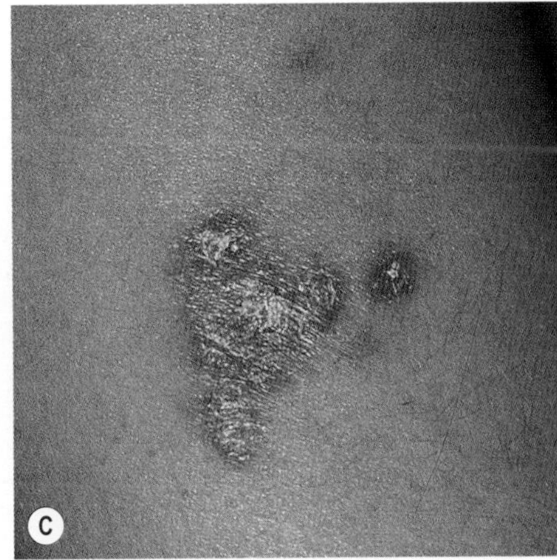

Fig. 49.1 Ataxia–telangiectasia.
A Characteristic linear telangiectasias on the medial and lateral bulbar conjunctivae. Punctate and smaller linear telangiectasias are also present on this girl's eyelids. **B** Extensive telangiectasias on the neck of a young woman. **C** Persistent granulomatous plaques on the leg of a child. These lesions often ulcerate and are difficult to manage. *A, Courtesy, Edward Cowen, MD; B, C, Courtesy, Amy Paller, MD.*

CUTANEOUS FINDINGS IN PRIMARY IMMUNODEFICIENCY (ID) DISORDERS

Disorder	*S. aureus* infections*	CMC	Warts**	Eczematous dermatitis	Granulomas***	LE	SVV	Ulcers (PG-like)	Additional mucocutaneous findings	Other major clinical features
Ataxia–telangiectasia (Fig. 49.1)	+			+ (facial)	+ (often ulcerates)				Oculocutaneous telangiectasias (onset age 3–6 y; favor ears, cheeks), CALMs, progeric changes	Cerebellar ataxia (onset age 1–2 y), sinopulmonary infections, leukemia/lymphoma, sensitivity to IR
Chédiak–Higashi syndrome (DDx includes Griscelli syndrome type 2; see Ch. 54)	+							+	Pigmentary dilution, hyper- or dyspigmentation in sun-exposed sites, silvery hair, gingivitis	Bleeding diathesis, lymphoproliferative "accelerated phase", neurologic degeneration
Chronic granulomatous disease (XR>AR) (Fig. 49.2)	++	+		+	++ (nodular, necrotic)	+		+	Sweet syndrome, oral ulcers; DLE in female carriers	LAN (often suppurative), HSM, internal granulomas, pneumonias
CMC syndromes (Figs 49.3 & 49.4)		++			(++) (candidal)				See text	See text
Complement deficiencies	+	+				++	+	+	See Table 49.3	See Table 49.3
DiGeorge (22q11.2 deletion) syndrome		+		+	+				Erythroderma	Thymic hypoplasia, ↓ Ca^{+2} due to hypoparathyroidism, congenital heart defects, craniofacial anomalies
Hyper-IgE syndromes (Figs 49.5 & 49.6)	++	+	+ (AR)	++					See text	See text

Immunoglobulin deficiencies										
• Agammaglobulinemia (XR>AR)	+			+	+				Dermatomyositis-like (due to echovirus); ecthyma gangrenosum	Bacterial and viral infections (e.g. lungs, GI)
• Hyper-IgM syndromes	+		+		+	+		+	Oral & anogenital ulcers	Infections (e.g. lungs, GI), autoimmunity
• Common variable ID (CVID) (Fig. 49.7)	+	+	+	+	++	+	+	+	Dermatophyte infections, vitiligo, alopecia areata	Variable infections (e.g. lungs, GI), autoimmunity (e.g. cytopenias), granulomas
• IgA deficiency†	+	+		+		+	+	+	Vitiligo, lipodystrophy	Similar to CVID but milder
Idiopathic CD4+ lymphocytopenia (<300/mm³ or <20%)		+	++			+			HSV infections, non-tuberculous mycobacterioses	Cryptococcal meningitis, lymphoma; *HIV infection excluded*
Leukocyte adhesion deficiency (Fig. 49.8)	++ (necrotic, little pus)							++	Poor wound healing, delayed umbilical stump separation, gingivitis	Pneumonias > severe bacterial or fungal infections
Severe combined ID (SCID)	+	+	+	+	+***				GVHD, erythroderma, Omenn syndrome‡	Severe infections, diarrhea, failure to thrive
Wiskott–Aldrich syndrome (XR) (Fig. 49.9)	++			++	+		+		Petechiae, ecchymoses	Platelet dysfunction, sinopulmonary infections, autoimmunity, atopy, lymphoma

**Including abscesses and superficial pyoderma.*

***Extensive warts are also a characteristic finding in warts, hypergammaglobulinemia, infections and myelokathexis (WHIM) syndrome.*

****Non-infectious unless otherwise noted; extensive granulomas (including destructive mid facial lesions) are associated with hypomorphic RAG1 or RAG2 mutations.*

†Prevalence of ~1:500, with clinical manifestations in only ~15% of affected individuals; profound IgA deficiency is occasionally associated with reactions to blood products containing IgA.

‡Neonatal onset of erythrodermic eczematous dermatitis, alopecia, lymphadenopathy, hepatosplenomegaly, and peripheral eosinophilia.

+, occasional finding.

++, common finding.

Table 49.1 Cutaneous findings in primary immunodeficiency (ID) disorders. Infectious conditions are in darker blue shading and non-infectious conditions in lighter blue shading. AR, autosomal recessive; CALMs, café-au-lait macules; CMC, chronic mucocutaneous candidiasis; DLE, discoid lupus erythematosus; HSM, hepatosplenomegaly; IR, ionizing radiation; LAN, lymphadenopathy; PG, pyoderma gangrenosum; SVV, small vessel vasculitis; XR, X-linked recessive (affects primarily boys/men).

• The primary feature of some immunodeficiency disorders is lymphoproliferation due to immune dysregulation (e.g. familial hemophagocytic lymphohistiocytosis, X-linked and autoimmune lymphoproliferative syndromes), whereas others involve predisposition to a specific type of infection, such as severe mycobacterial infections with defects in the IL-12/interferon-γ axis.

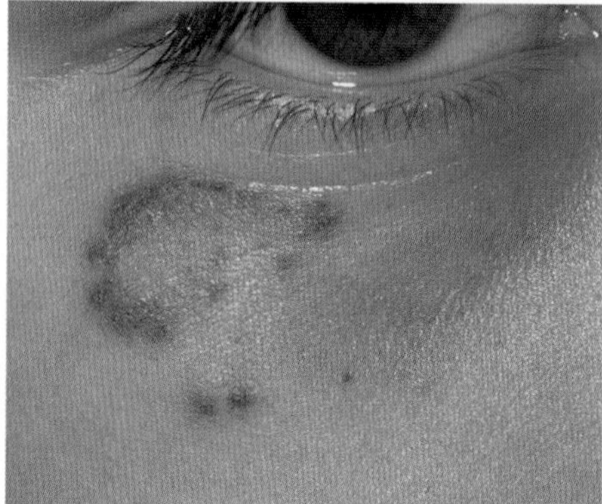

Fig. 49.2 Chronic granulomatous disease. Lupus erythematosus-like annular plaques and papules on the infraorbital cheek. *Courtesy, Edward Cowen, MD.*

• Initial laboratory evaluation for patients suspected to have an immunodeficiency is outlined in Table 49.2.

Chronic Mucocutaneous Candidiasis (CMC)

• Heterogeneous group of conditions characterized by recurrent and severe infections of the skin, nails, and mucous membranes with *Candida albicans*, together with variable autoimmunity and susceptibility to other infections (see Table 49.1).

• These disorders share an underlying impairment in Th17 responses, e.g. due to autoantibodies neutralizing Th17 cytokines in APECED (see below) and mutations in the genes encoding IL-17F, the IL-17 receptor A or C, or STAT1 (*s*ignal *t*ransducer and *a*ctivator of *t*ranscription *1*) in other forms of CMC.

• Clinical manifestations include recalcitrant oral thrush, dystrophic nails, and granulomatous plaques with scale-crust favoring the scalp, face, and skin folds (see Figs 49.3 and 49.4).

• The *a*utoimmune *p*oly*e*ndocrinopathy–*c*andidiasis–*e*ctodermal *d*ystrophy syndrome (APECED) is caused by mutations (usually

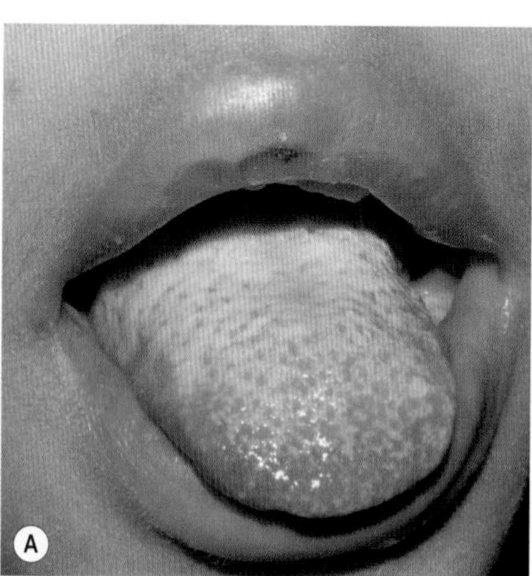

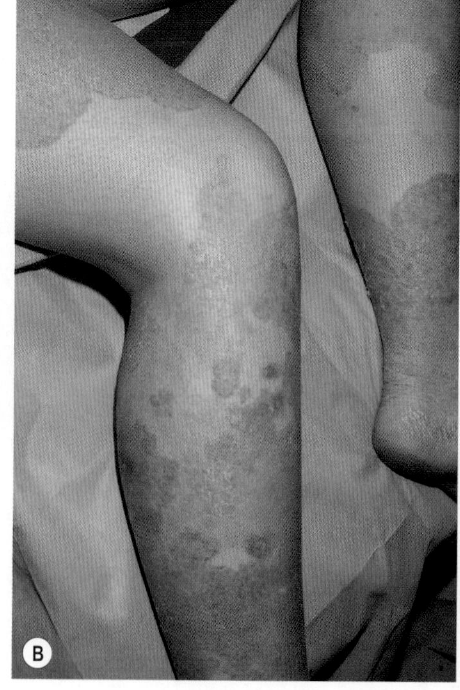

Fig. 49.3 Chronic mucocutaneous candidiasis due to increased STAT1 signaling. A Recalcitrant thrush on the tongue of a 6-year-old child. **B** Extensive tinea corporis with coalescing annular and polycyclic plaques on the legs. *A, Courtesy, Julie V. Schaffer, MD; B, Courtesy, Edward Cowen, MD.*

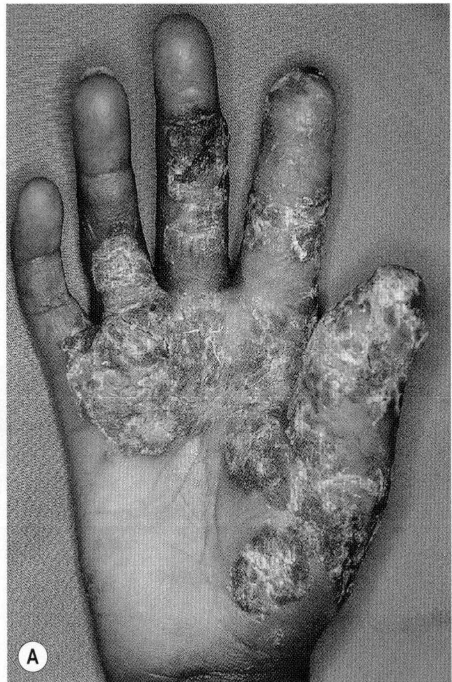

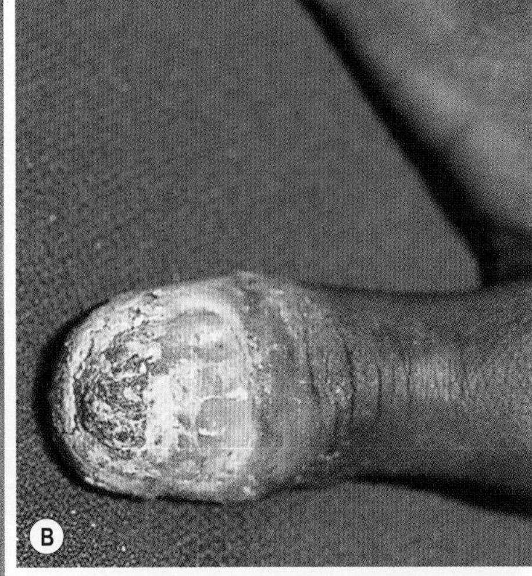

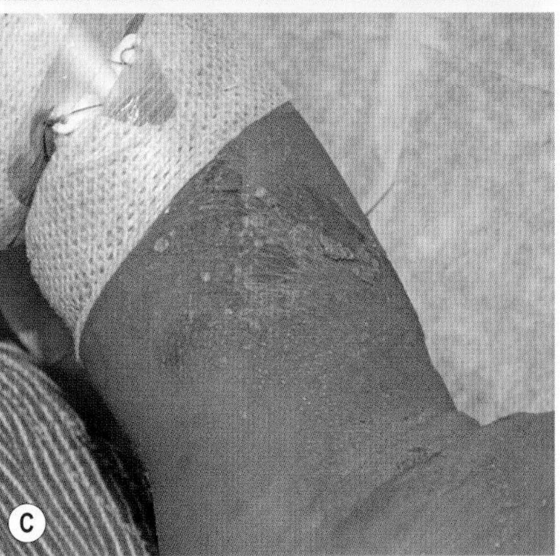

Fig. 49.4 Chronic mucocutaneous candidiasis (CMC). A Non-syndromic CMC presenting as crusted granulomatous plaques on the palm. **B** Non-syndromic CMC presenting as marked onychodystrophy with significant paronychial swelling and erythema. **C** Recurrent cutaneous candidiasis in an infant with DiGeorge syndrome. Note the erythema, pustules, and scale-crust near the site of an intravenous line on the arm. *A, Courtesy, YDRSC; B, Courtesy, Amy Paller, MD; C, Courtesy, Julie V. Schaffer, MD.*

with autosomal recessive inheritance) in the *a*uto*i*mmune *re*gulator gene (*AIRE*), which result in failure to delete autoreactive T cells in the thymus; patients present with a variety of autoimmune disorders (e.g. hypoparathyroidism, hypoadrenocorticism, alopecia areata) in addition to CMC.

- The most common form of CMC is autosomal dominant due to an activating *STAT1* mutation; additional manifestations can include autoimmunity, predisposition to other infections (e.g. viral, invasive fungal), and aneurysms (see Fig. 49.3).

Complement Disorders

- Clinical manifestations of various complement deficiencies are presented in Table 49.3.

Hyperimmunoglobulin E Syndromes (HIESs)

- HIESs feature eczematous dermatitis, recurrent staphylococcal skin (including "cold" abscesses and impetigo) and respiratory tract infections, mucocutaneous candidiasis, and markedly elevated serum IgE levels (usually > 2000 IU/ml) (see Fig. 49.6A).
- *Classic HIES* has autosomal dominant inheritance and is caused by mutations in the *STAT3* gene, which encodes a signaling protein that promotes production of cytokines (e.g. IL-6, IL-10, IL-17, IL-22) important to fighting infections at epithelial surfaces and controlling inflammation.
  - Usually presents in the first month of life with a non-infectious papulopustular eruption on the face, scalp, and diaper area

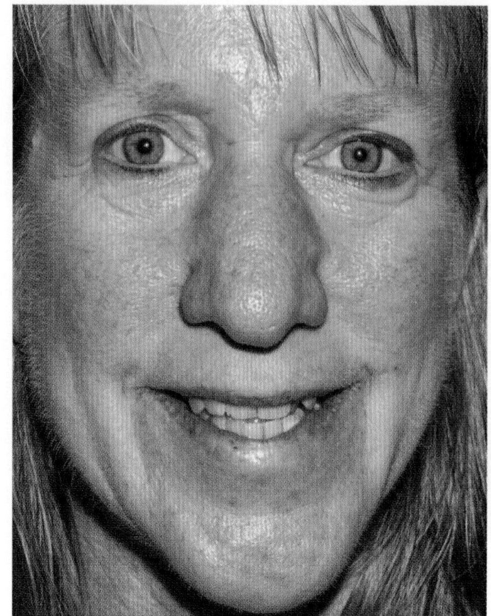

Fig. 49.5 Autosomal dominant hyper-immunoglobulin E syndrome (AD-HIES). Coarse facial features that developed progressively over time in an affected woman. Note the prominent follicular ostia, doughy skin, and broad nasal bridge. *Courtesy, Edward Cowen, MD.*

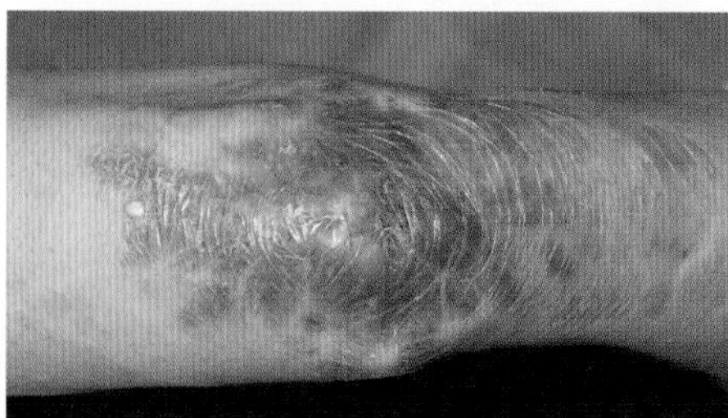

Fig. 49.7 Persistent granulomatous plaques in a patient with common variable immunodeficiency (CVID). *Courtesy, Edward Cowen, MD.*

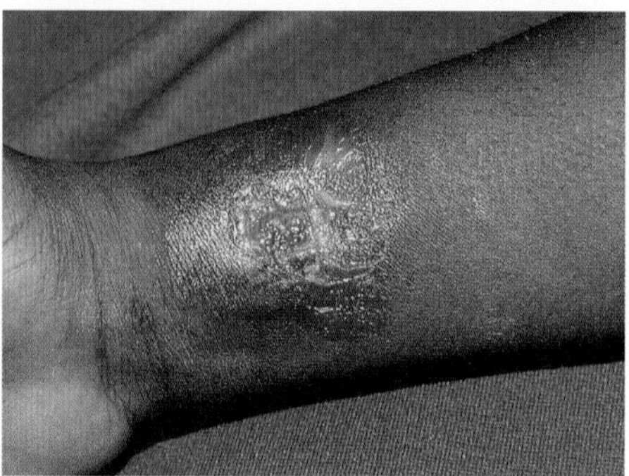

Fig. 49.8 Leukocyte adhesion deficiency type I. This 7-year-old boy was scratched by his sister, resulting in a large gaping wound that healed poorly. *Reprinted with permission from Schachner L, Hansen R (Eds.). Pediatric Dermatology, 4th edn. London: Mosby, 2011.*

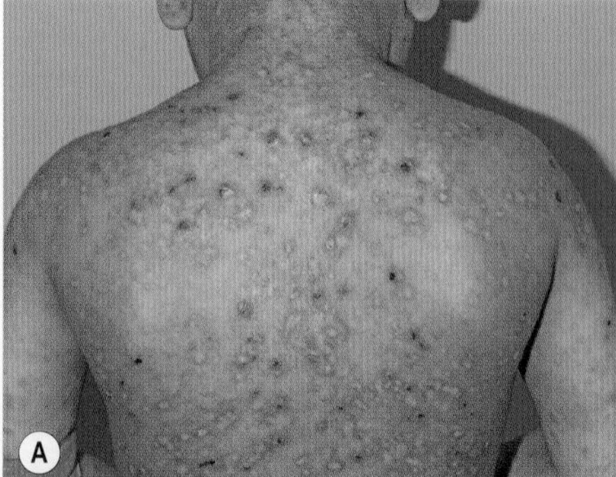

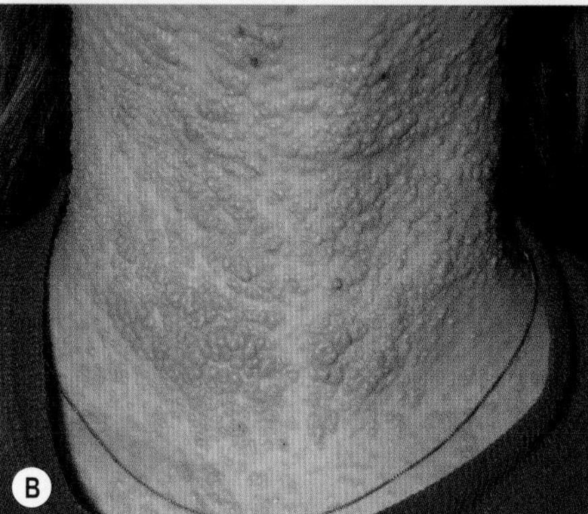

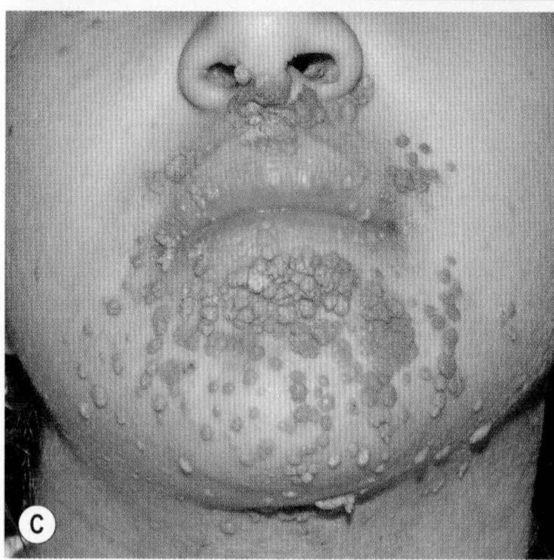

Fig. 49.6 Autosomal recessive hyper-immunoglobulin E syndrome (AR-HIES) due to *DOCK8* deficiency. A Eczematous dermatitis with prurigo nodularis lesions. **B** Extensive molluscum contagiosum. **C** Numerous coalescing facial warts. *A, B, Courtesy, Edward Cowen, MD; C, Julie V. Schaffer, MD.*

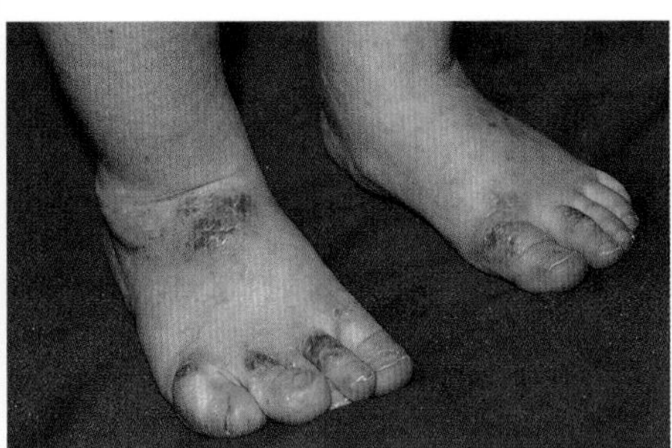

Fig. 49.9 Wiskott–Aldrich syndrome. This young boy presented with widespread, severe atopic dermatitis. Following successful treatment with hematopoietic stem cell transplantation, his dermatitis virtually cleared. *Reprinted with permission from Schachner L, Hansen R (Eds.). Pediatric Dermatology, 4th edn. London: Mosby, 2011.*

- Other findings include progressive facial coarsening with pitted scarring (see Fig. 49.5), retention of primary teeth, a high-arched palate, osteopenia with minimal-trauma fractures, scoliosis, pneumatocele formation, and increased risk of B-cell lymphomas
- Absent Th17 cells

• An *autosomal recessive form of HIES (AR-HIES)* can be caused by mutations in the *d*edi*c*ator *o*f *c*yto*k*inesis 8 (*DOCK8*) gene.

- Characterized by severe viral (e.g. warts, molluscum contagiosum, HSV, VZV; see Fig. 49.6B, C) and opportunistic infections, other atopic manifestations, CNS vasculitis, and increased

INITIAL LABORATORY EVALUATION FOR A PATIENT SUSPECTED TO HAVE A PRIMARY IMMUNODEFICIENCY (ID)		
Test	**Potential finding**	**Examples of disorders identified**
Complete blood count with differential, platelet count, and examination of smear	• Giant granules within neutrophils, ± neutropenia	• Chédiak–Higashi syndrome
	• Neutrophilia	• Leukocyte adhesion deficiency
	• Small platelets, thrombocytopenia, eosinophilia	• Wiskott–Aldrich syndrome
	• Marked eosinophilia	• Hyper-IgE syndromes • Omenn syndrome
Quantitative immunoglobulins	• All Ig ↓	• Agammaglobulinemia
	• IgA ↓, IgG ↓, ± IgM ↓	• Common variable ID
	• IgA ↓ or IgM ↓	• IgA or IgM deficiency
	• IgM ↑, other Ig ↓	• Hyper-IgM syndrome
	• IgA ↓, IgE ↓, $IgG_{2,4}$ ↓	• Ataxia telangiectasia
	• IgE ↑↑	• Hyper-IgE syndromes
	• IgM ↓, ± IgG ↓, IgA ↑, IgE ↑	• Wiskott–Aldrich syndrome
Total hemolytic complement (CH50)	• Marked ↓	• Various complement deficiencies
Nitroblue tetrazolium (NBT) reduction assay	• <10% of normal NBT reduction	• Chronic granulomatous disease
T- and B-cell analysis by flow cytometry	• Lack of T cells ± B cells	• Severe combined ID
Hair shaft examination (if silvery hair color)	• Small, regular melanin clumps	• Chédiak–Higashi syndrome
	• Large, irregular melanin clumps	• Griscelli syndrome

Table 49.2 Initial laboratory evaluation for a patient suspected to have a primary immunodeficiency (ID). Antibody titers to previously administered vaccines can also be assessed.

COMPLEMENT DISORDERS		
Complement component(s)	**Susceptibility to infectious agents**	**Autoimmune/inflammatory disorders**
Classical pathway		
C1q/r/s, C4, C2*	**Encapsulated bacteria** (especially *Streptococcus pneumoniae*) > *Candida* (C1q)	• **SLE**: risk with deficiency of C1q (~90%) > C4 > C1r/s > C2 (~20%) – C1q/r/s or C4 deficiency: often childhood onset (F = M); photosensitivity, renal disease – C2 deficiency: usually adult onset (median age ~30 years; ~8 F:1 M); photosensitivity, SCLE > DLE, oral ulcers – ANA may be – or low-titer; anti-Ro/SSA usually + • Uncommon associations include dermatomyositis, Henoch–Schönlein purpura, urticaria, and atrophoderma
C1 inhibitor		Hereditary angioedema (see Ch. 14)
Lectin pathway		
Mannose-binding lectin (MBL)§	Encapsulated bacteria, especially *N. meningitides*	• SLE, dermatomyositis
C3 and alternative pathway		
C3, factor H, factor I	**Encapsulated bacteria** (severe infections for C3)	• SLE, vasculitis, partial lipodystrophy (C3), glomerulonephritis, atypical HUS • "Leiner phenotype" (C3): erythroderma, failure to thrive, chronic diarrhea, recurrent infections
Properdin¶, factor D	***Neisseria* spp.** (fulminant infections)	
Membrane attack complex		
C5, C6, C7, C8, C9†	***Neisseria* spp.** (recurrent infections)	• SLE (rarely); "Leiner phenotype" (C5)

**C2 deficiency is the most common homozygous complement disorder.*
§Very low penetrance, usually in young children and immunocompromised individuals.
¶X-linked recessive, so occurs primarily in male patients.
†Prevalence of ~1:1000 in Japan; milder than other etiologies.

Table 49.3 Complement disorders. Unless otherwise specified, refers to homozygous/biallelic deficiencies. DLE, discoid lupus erythematosus; F, female; HUS, hemolytic–uremic syndrome; M, male; SCLE, subacute cutaneous lupus erythematosus.

risk of mucocutaneous SCC as well as lymphoma
- Decreased $CD4^+$ T cells and low IgM levels

- **DDx:** atopic dermatitis; Wiskott–Aldrich, Netherton, Omenn, and IPEX (*i*mmune dysregulation, *p*olyendocrinopathy, *e*nteropathy, *X*-linked) syndromes.

For further information see Ch. 60 from *Dermatology, Fourth Edition*.

For additional online figures and tables visit www.expertconsult.com 

Neurofibromatosis and Tuberous Sclerosis Complex 50

• Neurofibromatosis (NF) and tuberous sclerosis complex (TSC) are neurocutaneous disorders (phacomatoses) characterized by skin lesions as well as neoplasms of the central and peripheral nervous systems.
• Cutaneous manifestations (especially pigmentary findings) are often the first clinical signs of NF type 1 (NF1) and TSC.
• Both disorders have autosomal dominant inheritance, although ~30–50% of patients have unaffected parents and harbor new, spontaneous mutations.
• Education of patients/parents about the condition, attention to psychosocial concerns, and genetic counseling represent important components of care.

Neurofibromatosis Type 1

• Incidence of approximately 1 in 3000 births.
• The *NF1* tumor suppressor gene encodes the neurofibromin protein, which negatively regulates the RAS-mitogen-activated protein kinase (MAPK) pathway that promotes cell survival and proliferation.
• Patients with NF1 have a constitutive (germline) *NF1* mutation plus a somatic "second hit" mutation inactivating the other copy of the gene in affected tissues, e.g. Schwann cells in neurofibromas and melanocytes in café-au-lait macules (CALMs).
• The major clinical features of NF1 are outlined in Table 50.1 and depicted in Figs 50.1–50.5; Fig. 50.6 shows the time course of their development.
• Revised diagnostic criteria for NF1 (Table 50.2) developed by an international consensus group were published in 2021.
• An approach to infants or young children with ≥6 CALMs is presented in Fig. 50.7.
• Comprehensive *NF1* gene analysis with ≥95% sensitivity is available; this can help to establish the diagnosis in atypical presentations or young children not yet meeting criteria.
• **DDx:** other disorders that can manifest with multiple CALMs are summarized in Table 50.3.
• Management of NF1 requires a multidisciplinary approach (Table 50.4). Selumetinib, a MEK inhibitor, is FDA-approved for the treatment of symptomatic plexiform neurofibromas.

Tuberous Sclerosis Complex (TSC)

• Incidence of approximately 1 in 10,000 births.
• Hamartomatous disorder caused by mutations in either the *TSC1* or *TSC2* gene; both encode proteins (hamartin and tuberin, respectively) that negatively regulate the *m*ammalian *t*arget *o*f *r*apamycin (mTOR) pathway that promotes cell growth.
• *TSC2* mutations are associated with more severe disease and are threefold more common than *TSC1* mutations in TSC patients overall.
• Fig. 50.9 shows the time course for the development of cutaneous findings in TS.
• Hypomelanotic macules may be very subtle or inapparent in individuals with lightly pigmented skin, and a Wood's light can help to identify them.
• The hypomelanotic macules in TS patients vary in number (few to >100) and size (<1 to >10 cm); their shapes are polygonal more often than resembling an "ash leaf" – rounded at one end, tapered at the other (Fig. 50.10A).
  – **DDx:** nevus depigmentosus is a common (1–5% of healthy children) cause of one or two hypopigmented macule(s) or patch(es); Fig. 50.11 presents an approach to infants/young children with ≥3 hypomelanotic macules

MAJOR CLINICAL FEATURES OF NEUROFIBROMATOSIS TYPE 1 (NF1)

Cutaneous findings

- Café-au-lait macules (CALMs) (>90%; often evident within first year of life)
  - Tan to dark brown, uniformly pigmented macules/patches with regular borders (Fig. 50.1A–C)
  - Most patients have ≥6 by early childhood
- Axillary and/or inguinal freckling (Crowe sign) (~80%; usually present by 4–6 years of age)
  - 1- to 3-mm brown macules, more akin to lentigines than ephelides
  - Favor intertriginous sites (Fig. 50.1B) and the neck, but may be widespread (Fig. 50.1C,D)
- *Cutaneous* neurofibromas (70–90%; typically begin to appear around puberty)
  - Skin-colored to pink-tan, soft papulonodules that invaginate with gentle pressure ("button-hole" sign); dome-shaped, pedunculated, or barely elevated (early lesions) (Figs 50.2 and 50.3)
  - Range from a few millimeters to several centimeters in diameter and <10 to >1000 in number
- *Plexiform* neurofibromas (PNF) (25%; congenital origin, enlarge during first 4–5 years of life)
  - Deeper nodules or masses resembling a "bag of worms" upon palpation (Fig. 50.4)
  - May have overlying hyperpigmentation (Fig. 50.4A) ± hypertrichosis and associated soft tissue overgrowth
- Nevus anemicus (30–50%; congenital), a pale area with irregular outline favoring the chest and more apparent after rubbing the skin
- Juvenile xanthogranuloma (JXG) (~15–30%; typically develops in first 2–3 years of life)
  - Pink (early) to yellow-brown papule/nodule (see Ch. 76); may be associated with additional increased risk of JML in NF1 patients (who already have a higher risk of JML)
- Glomus tumors of the fingers and toes (see Ch. 94)

Ocular lesions

- Lisch nodules (iris hamartomas) (>90% by 20 years of age; begin to appear at ~3 years of age)
  - 1- to 2-mm yellow-brown papules, best seen on slit-lamp examination (Fig. 50.5)
- Choroidal abnormalities (~80% of adults, 60-70% of children)
  - Nodules detected by optical coherence tomography/near infrared reflectance imaging

Skeletal anomalies

- *Cranial*: macrocephaly (20–50%), hypertelorism (25%), sphenoid wing dysplasia (<5%)
- *Spinal*: scoliosis (5–10%)
- *Limbs*: cortical thinning ± pseudoarthrosis (2%; e.g. tibial bowing)

Extracutaneous tumors

- Optic glioma (10–15%; childhood) (± precocious puberty), other CNS tumors (~5%)
- Malignant peripheral nerve sheath tumor (3–15%, peak in young adults), usually arising from a PNF
  - Rapid growth, increased firmness, or persistent pain in established PNF; new neurologic deficit
- Other, e.g. pheochromocytoma (1%), JML, GIST, rhabdomyosarcoma (especially GU), breast cancer

Neurologic manifestations

- Unidentified bright objects (UBO) on MRI (50–75%)
- Learning difficulties (30–50%), ADD, intellectual impairment (severe in <5%), seizures (~5%)

Cardiovascular manifestations

- Hypertension (~30%): essential > from renal artery stenosis (~2%) or pheochromocytoma (1%)
- Pulmonic stenosis (~1%), cerebrovascular anomalies (2–5%)

Table 50.1 Major clinical features of neurofibromatosis type 1 (NF1). ADD, attention deficit disorder; GIST, gastrointestinal stromal tumors; GU, genitourinary; JML, juvenile myelomonocytic leukemia.

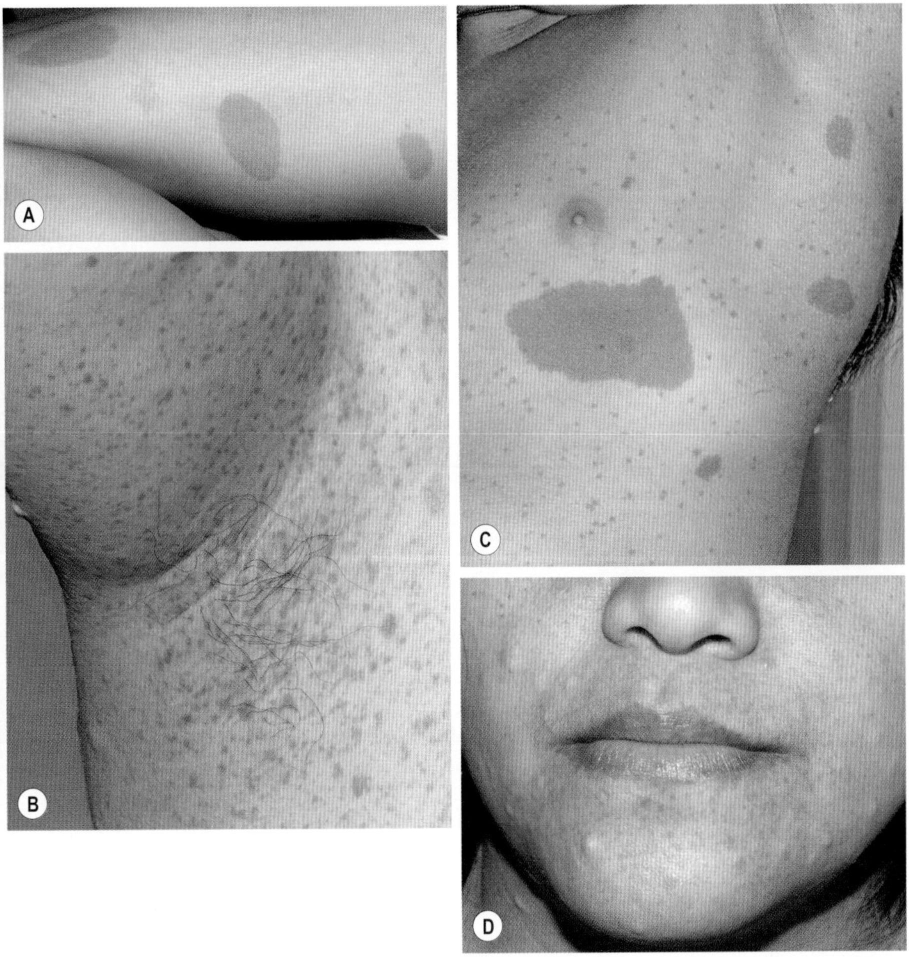

Fig. 50.1 Café-au-lait macules and "freckling". Oval-shaped, light- to medium-brown patches with regular borders and uniform pigmentation **(A–C).** Numerous 1- to 3-mm lentigines are most commonly found in the axilla (Crowe sign) **(B)** but can also develop in other sites such as the chest (**C**) and perioral region **(D)**. *Courtesy, Julie V. Schaffer, MD.*

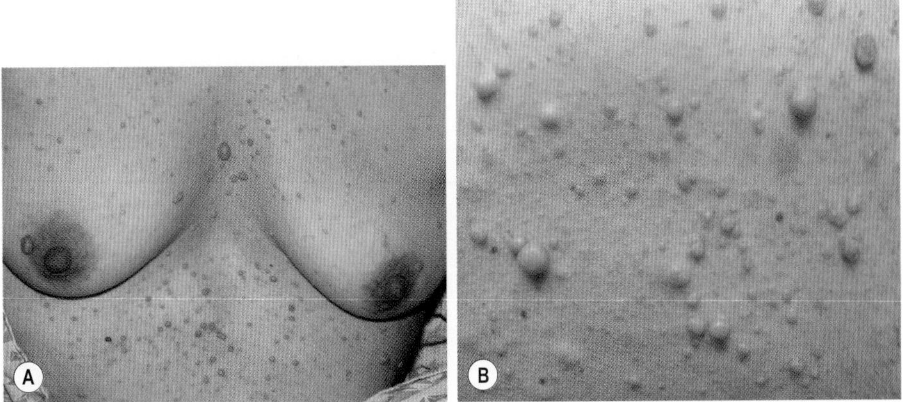

Fig. 50.2 Multiple cutaneous neurofibromas. Soft, skin-colored to pinkish tan, dome-shaped or polypoid, well-demarcated papules and nodules of various sizes **(A, B)** in patients with NF1. Neurofibromas may be superimposed on café-au-lait macules and lentigines **(B)**. *A, Courtesy, Julie V. Schaffer, MD; B, Courtesy, Hensin Tsao, MD, and Su Luo, MD.*

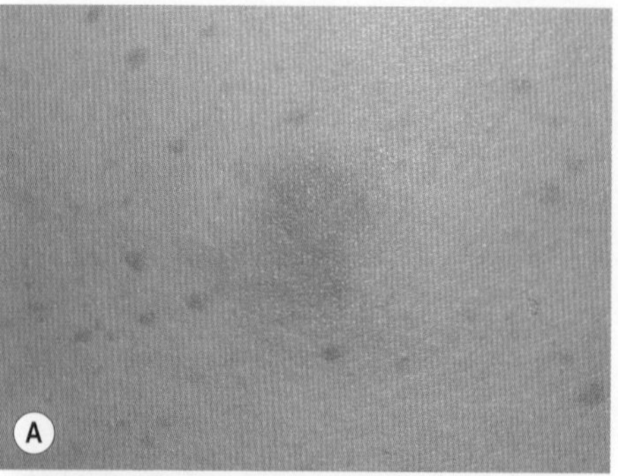

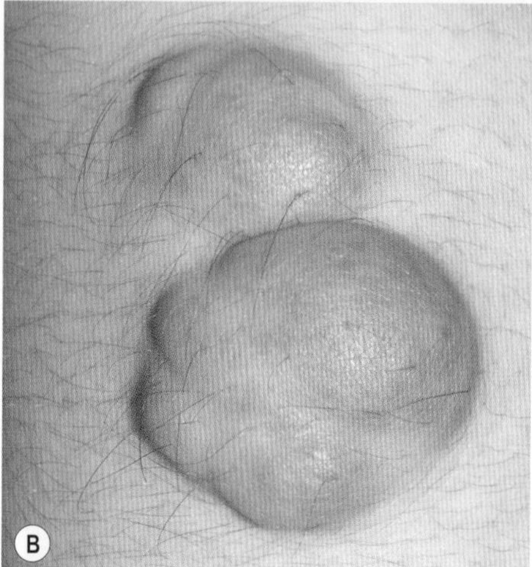

Fig. 50.3 Spectrum of cutaneous neurofibromas. Lesions range from subtle blue-red macules **(A)** to exophytic nodules with associated hypertrichosis **(B)**. *Courtesy, Julie V. Schaffer, MD.*

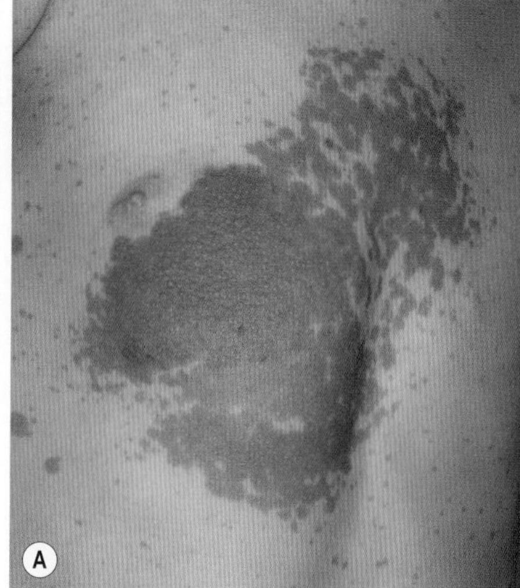

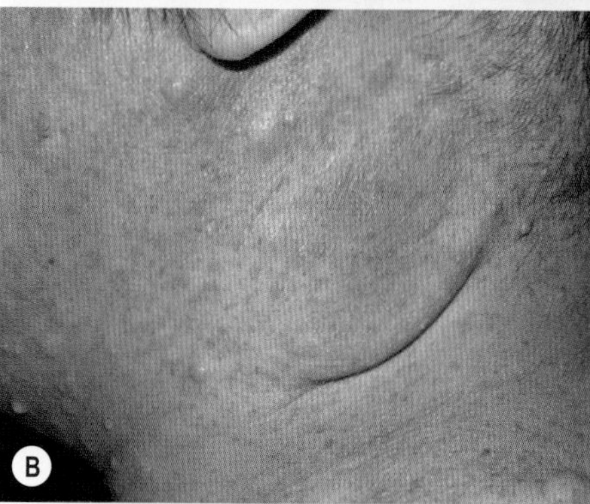

Fig. 50.4 Plexiform neurofibromas. A A hyperpigmented plaque that may be misdiagnosed as a congenital melanocytic nevus or (if not palpated) a café-au-lait macule. Note the widespread "freckling" on the trunk. **B** A poorly circumscribed, sagging pink mass. *Courtesy, Julie V. Schaffer, MD.*

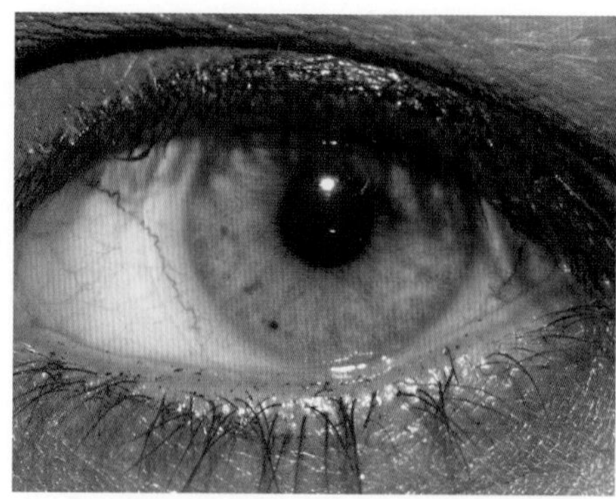

Fig. 50.5 Lisch nodules. Multiple yellow-brown papules of the iris. Although best seen using a slit lamp, Lisch nodules may also be evident on clinical examination in patients with lightly pigmented eyes. *Courtesy, Julie V. Schaffer, MD.*

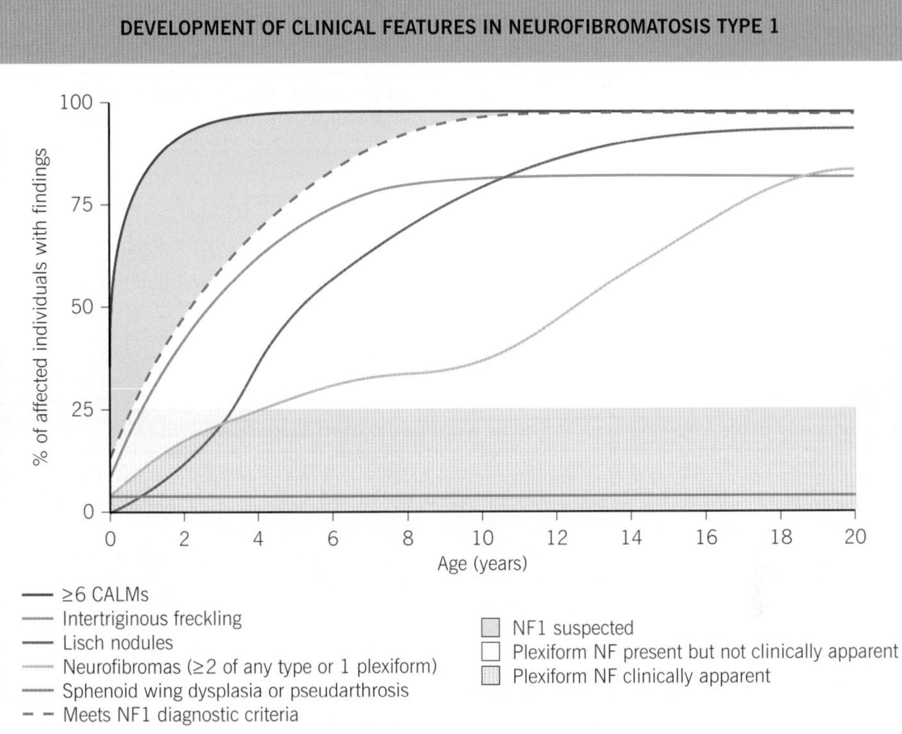

Fig. 50.6 Development of clinical features in neurofibromatosis type 1. The time course of major diagnostic lesions that develop in NF1. During the first few years of life, a child may have only café-au-lait macules. *Adapted from DeBella K, Szudek J, Friedman JM. Use of the National Institutes of Health criteria for diagnosis of neurofibromatosis 1 in children. Pediatrics 2000;105:608–614.*

- Numerous small, confetti-like hypopigmented macules (especially on the extremities) represent a relatively specific finding for TS (Fig. 50.10B).
- Angiofibromas (formerly known as "adenoma sebaceum") are smooth, dome-shaped, pink to red-brown papules (Fig. 50.12); they favor the central face and sometimes coalesce to form plaques.
  - **DDx:** one or two angiofibromas (fibrous papules) can occur in the general population, and multiple facial angiofibromas can develop in multiple endocrine neoplasia type 1 (MEN1) and Birt–Hogg–Dubé syndrome (see Ch. 91)
- Variants of angiofibromas include cephalic fibrous plaques (e.g. on forehead or other facial sites) (see Fig. 50.12), ungual fibromas (Koenen tumors; toes > fingers) (Fig. 50.13), and molluscum pendulum (resembling large skin tags) in flexural sites.
- Shagreen patches are collagenomas with a predilection for the lower back; they present as skin-colored, hyperpigmented or (less often) hypopigmented plaques with an uneven, pigskin-like surface (Fig. 50.14).
- Infantile spasms affect ~70% of TS patients, typically beginning at 3–6 months of age; the spectrum of *T*SC-*a*ssociated *n*europsychiatric *d*isorders (TAND) can also include intellectual impairment, autism, attention deficit disorder, and psychiatric conditions.
- Additional extracutaneous manifestations and diagnostic criteria are listed in Table 50.5.

REVISED DIAGNOSTIC CRITERIA FOR NEUROFIBROMATOSIS TYPE 1 (NF1) AND MOSAIC NF1
Diagnostic criteria for NF1
Requires **two or more** of the following in an individual ***without a parent diagnosed with NF1*** and **one or more** of the following in an individual ***with a parent diagnosed with NF1***: • Six or more café-au-lait macules >5 mm in prepubertal individuals and >15 mm in postpubertal individuals* • "Freckling" in the axillary or inguinal region* • Two or more neurofibromas of any type *or* one plexiform neurofibroma • Optic pathway glioma • Two or more Lisch nodules (iris hamartomas) or two or more choroidal abnormalities • A distinctive osseous lesion such as sphenoid dysplasia, anterolateral bowing of the tibia, or pseudoarthrosis of a long bone • A heterozygous pathogenic *NF1* variant with a variant allele fraction of 50% in apparently normal tissue (e.g. white blood cells)
Diagnostic criteria for mosaic NF1
Requires any of the following in an individual ***without a parent diagnosed with NF1***: • A heterozygous pathogenic *NF1* variant with a variant allele fraction of significantly <50% in apparently normal tissue (e.g. white blood cells) **AND** one of the other NF1 criteria above • An identical heterozygous pathogenic *NF1* variant in two anatomically independent affected tissues, in the absence of a pathogenic *NF1* variant in unaffected tissue • A clearly segmental distribution of café-au-lait macules or cutaneous neurofibromas **AND** *either* another NF1 criterion** *or* offspring diagnosed with NF1 • One of the *clinical* NF1 criteria above *other than* café-au-lait macules **AND** offspring diagnosed with NF1
**If only café-au-lait macules and freckling are present, at least one should be bilateral; the diagnosis is most likely NF1 but may rarely be another condition such as Legius syndrome.* ***If only café-au-lait macules and freckling are present, the diagnosis is most likely mosaic NF1 but may rarely be mosaic Legius syndrome or constitutional mismatch repair deficiency syndrome (see Table 50.3).*

Table 50.2 2021 revised diagnostic criteria for neurofibromatosis type 1 (NF1) and mosaic NF1. *Adapted from Legius E, Messiaen L, Wolkenstein P, et al. Revised diagnostic criteria for neurofibromatosis type 1 and Legius syndrome: an international consensus recommendation. Genet Med 2021;23:1506-13.*

- Recommendations for evaluation and management are presented in Table 50.6.
- **Rx:** systemic administration of mTOR inhibitors (rapamycin [sirolimus], everolimus) for astrocytomas, renal angiomyolipomas, and pulmonary lymphangioleiomyomas; topical rapamycin (0.1–1%), lasers (pulsed dye or ablative), and electrosurgery to treat angiofibromas; sun protection to potentially prevent development of angiofibromas.

For further information see Ch. 61 From *Dermatology, Fourth Edition*.

For additional online figures visit www.expertconsult.com 

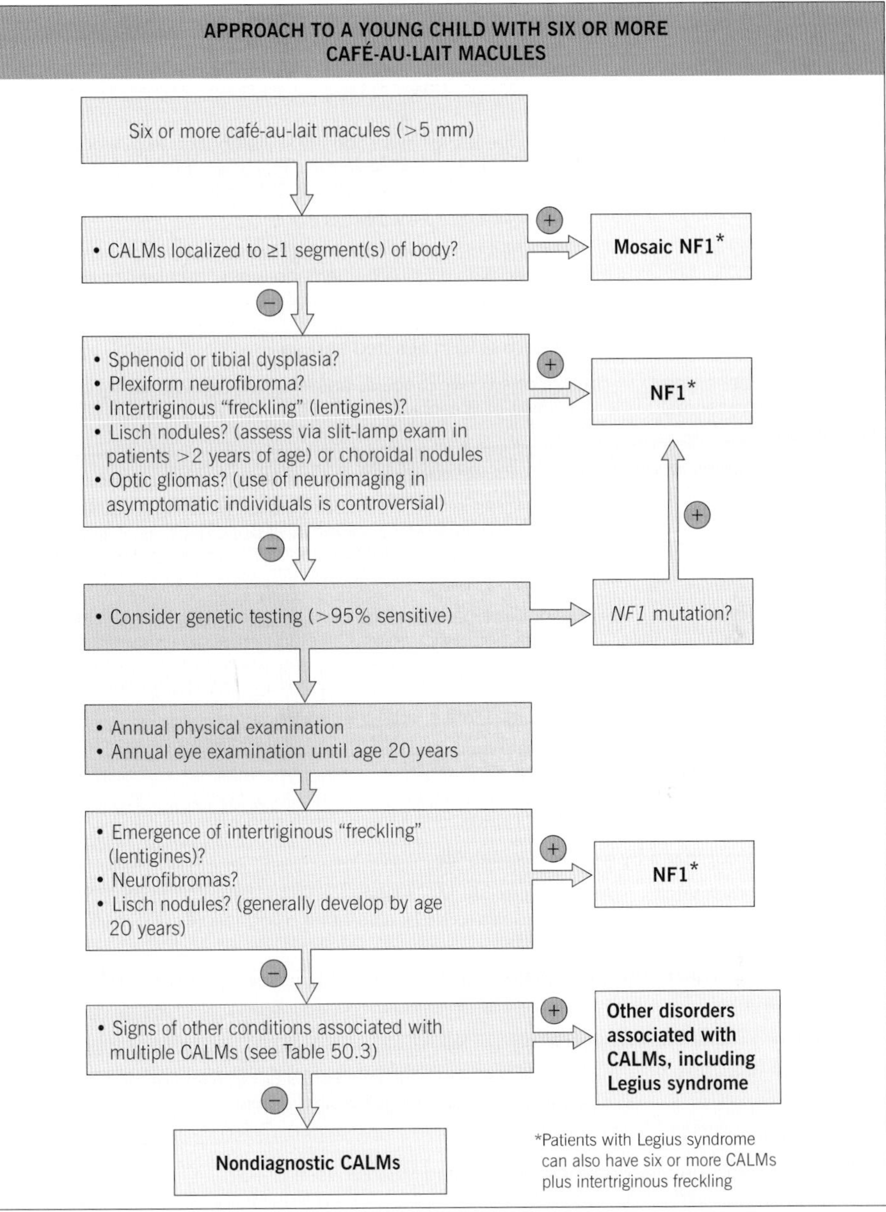

Fig. 50.7 Approach to a young child with six or more café-au-lait macules (CALMs). More than half of these patients will eventually be diagnosed with NF1 or, less often, another CALM-associated syndrome (see Table 50.3). The latter should be considered if other signs of NF1 do not develop.

OTHER DISORDERS ASSOCIATED WITH MULTIPLE CAFÉ-AU-LAIT MACULES (CALMs)	
Disorder	**Additional features**
Mosaic conditions	
Mosaic (segmental) NF1 (see Table 50.2)†	CALMs ± "freckling" in a segmental distribution (e.g. block-like) (Fig. 50.8A); can also have neurofibromas (Fig. 50.8B); post-zygotic *NF1* mutations – if in gonads, could potentially pass on generalized NF1 to offspring
McCune–Albright syndrome	CALMs often block-like or in broad bands along the lines of Blaschko with midline demarcation and irregular ("coast of Maine") borders; polyostotic fibrous dysplasia; endocrine hyper-function (e.g. precocious puberty); activating *GNAS1* mutations (encodes $G_s\alpha$) in affected tissues
"Pigmentary mosaicism" due to chromosomal anomalies	CALMs often have irregular borders; may be segmental or follow the lines of Blaschko (see Ch. 51)
Other RASopathies (characterized by increased MAPK signaling)	
Legius syndrome	AD; ≥6 CALMs in >80% ± intertriginous "freckling" (~50%); *lacks* neurofibromas, Lisch nodules, and optic gliomas; often macro-cephaly, learning disabilities; loss-of-function *SPRED1* muta-tions
Noonan syndrome*	AD; lymphedema, webbed neck; KP (atrophicans); nevi; short stat-ure, characteristic facies, developmental delay; cardiac defects, especially pulmonic stenosis; activating mutations in *PTPN11* > *SOS1*, *RAF1*, *RIT1* > *KRAS*, *NRAS*, *MAP2K1*; Noonan-like: *SHOC12* (loose anagen hair), *CBL* (JML)
Noonan syndrome with multiple lentigines (LEOPARD syndrome)	Called "café noir" macules due to dark color; *l*entigines, *e*lectrocar-diogram abnormalities, *o*cular hypertelorism, *p*ulmonary steno-sis, *a*bnormalities of genitalia, *r*etardation of growth, *d*eafness; *PTPN11* mutations
Disorders characterized by genomic instability	
Constitutional mismatch repair deficiency syndrome	AR; multiple CALMs, axillary freckling, neurofibromas, CNS glio-mas (similar to NF1); also other malignancies (e.g. hematologic, colorectal)
Fanconi anemia* (see Ch. 55), Bloom syndrome* (see Ch. 73), ataxia–telangiectasia* (see Ch. 49)	
Other tumor predisposition syndromes	
Neurofibromatosis type 2*	AD; cutaneous and bilateral vestibular schwannomas; meningiomas, spinal tumors; *NF2* gene
Tuberous sclerosis*	See text
PTEN hamartoma tumor syndrome*, MEN1*, and MEN2B* (see Ch. 52)	
Disorders of pigmentation	
Piebaldism (CALMs in leukodermic and uninvolved skin; see Ch. 54), familial progressive hyper- and hypopigmentation (see Ch. 55)	

†DDx may include a large speckled lentiginous nevus (nevus spilus) or partial unilateral lentiginosis (see Ch. 92).
**Multiple CALMs in small minority of affected individuals.*

Table 50.3 Other disorders associated with multiple café-au-lait macules (CALMs). Of note, approximately 30% of the general population has at least one CALM. AD, autosomal dominant; AR, autosomal recessive; JML, juvenile myelomonocytic leukemia; KP, keratosis pilaris; MAPK, mitogen-activated protein kinase; NF1, neurofibromatosis type 1.

EVALUATION AND MANAGEMENT OF NEUROFIBROMATOSIS 1 (NF1) PATIENTS
At time of diagnosis and annually
Dermatologic examination (especially if a plexiform neurofibroma [PNF] is present) • Surgical consultation if painful or disfiguring neurofibromas • PET/CT if rapid growth, increased firmness, or persistent pain in an established PNF
Neurologic examination • MRI and/or other studies (e.g. PET/CT if related to a PNF) if neurologic signs/symptoms*
Cardiac assessment (*at initial diagnosis*) and measurement of blood pressure • Renal arteriography and 24-hour urine collection for catecholamines and metanephrines if hypertension
At the time of diagnosis and annually, depending on the age of the patient
Evaluation for scoliosis and other bony defects (e.g. tibial bowing) (*annually only in children/adolescents*) Neurodevelopmental/behavioral evaluation (*annually only in children/adolescents*)
Ophthalmologic examination with visual assessment (*prior to 8 years of age*) • Orbital/brain MRI if signs/symptoms of optic glioma (e.g. visual compromise, proptosis) Assessment for precocious pubertal development (*prior to ~8 years of age*) Measurement of head circumference (*in young children*)
Screening for breast cancer with clinical examination + mammography ± MRI (*in women, beginning by age 30 years*)

**The role of neuroimaging in asymptomatic patients is controversial.*

Table 50.4 Evaluation and management of neurofibromatosis 1 (NF1) patients. PET/CT, positron emission tomography/computed tomography.

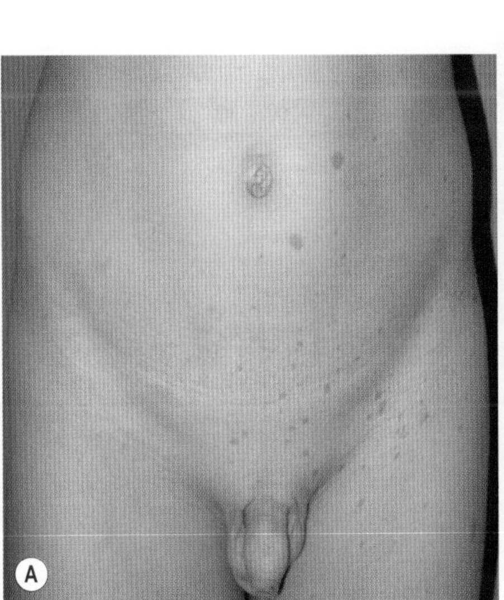

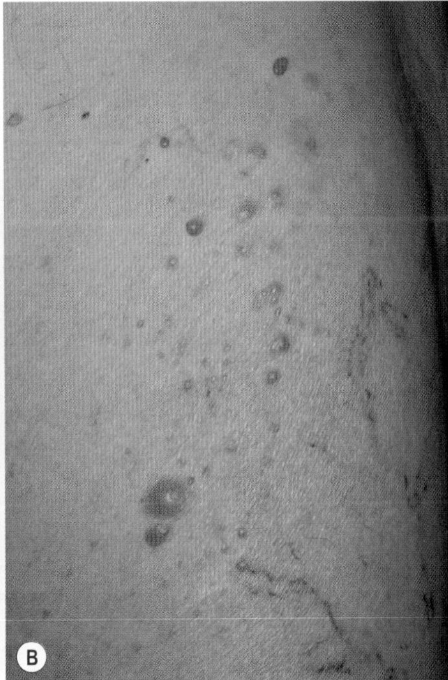

Fig. 50.8 Mosaic neurofibromatosis. A Multiple small café-au-lait macules and "freckling" limited to the left side of the trunk and groin, with slight extension past the midline. **B** A cluster of soft, pink to pink-brown papules limited to the thigh. There were no associated café-au-lait macules. *A, Courtesy, Antonio Torrelo, MD; B, Courtesy, Jean L. Bolognia, MD.*

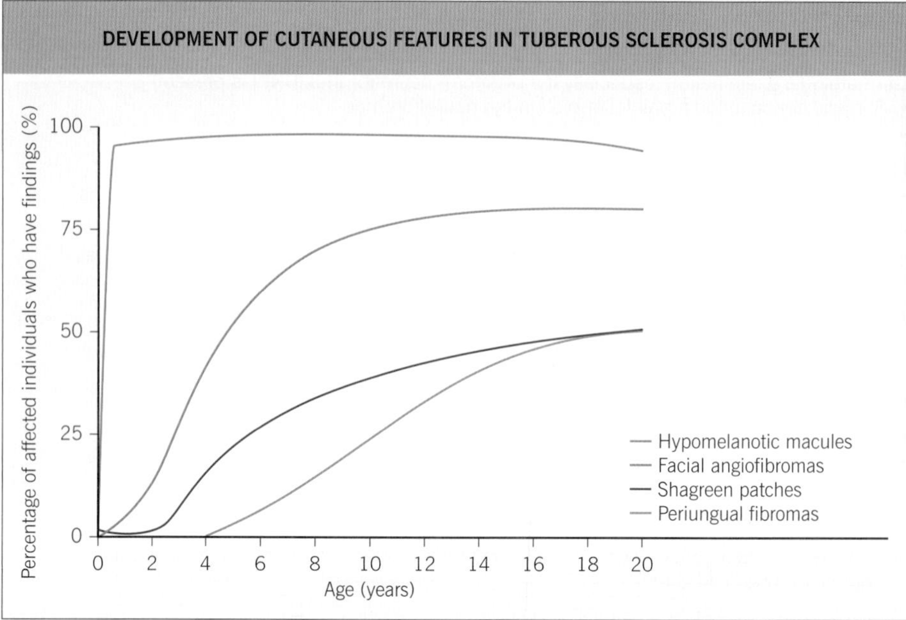

Fig. 50.9 Development of cutaneous features in tuberous sclerosis complex. Hypomelanotic macules are usually the only cutaneous finding at birth.

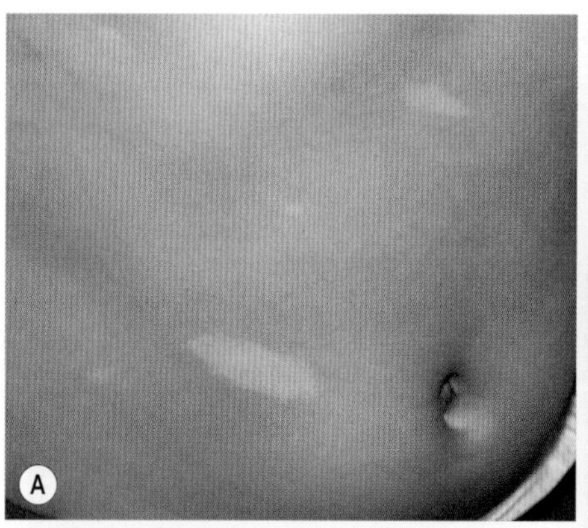

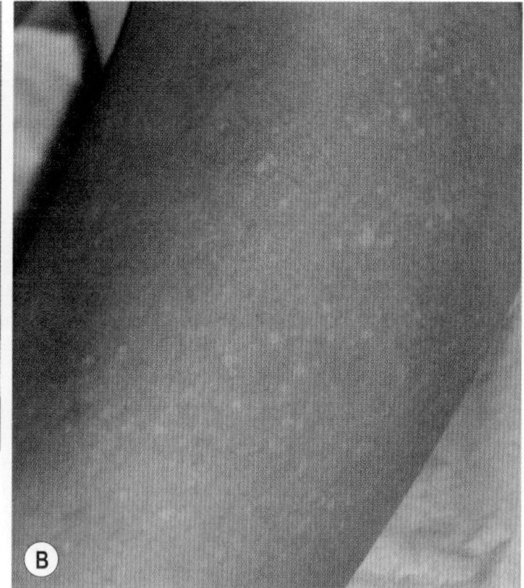

Fig. 50.10 Hypopigmentation in tuberous sclerosis complex. A Ash leaf macules. **B** "Confetti" macules of guttate leukoderma. *A, Courtesy, Julie V. Schaffer, MD; B, Courtesy, Jean L. Bolognia, MD.*

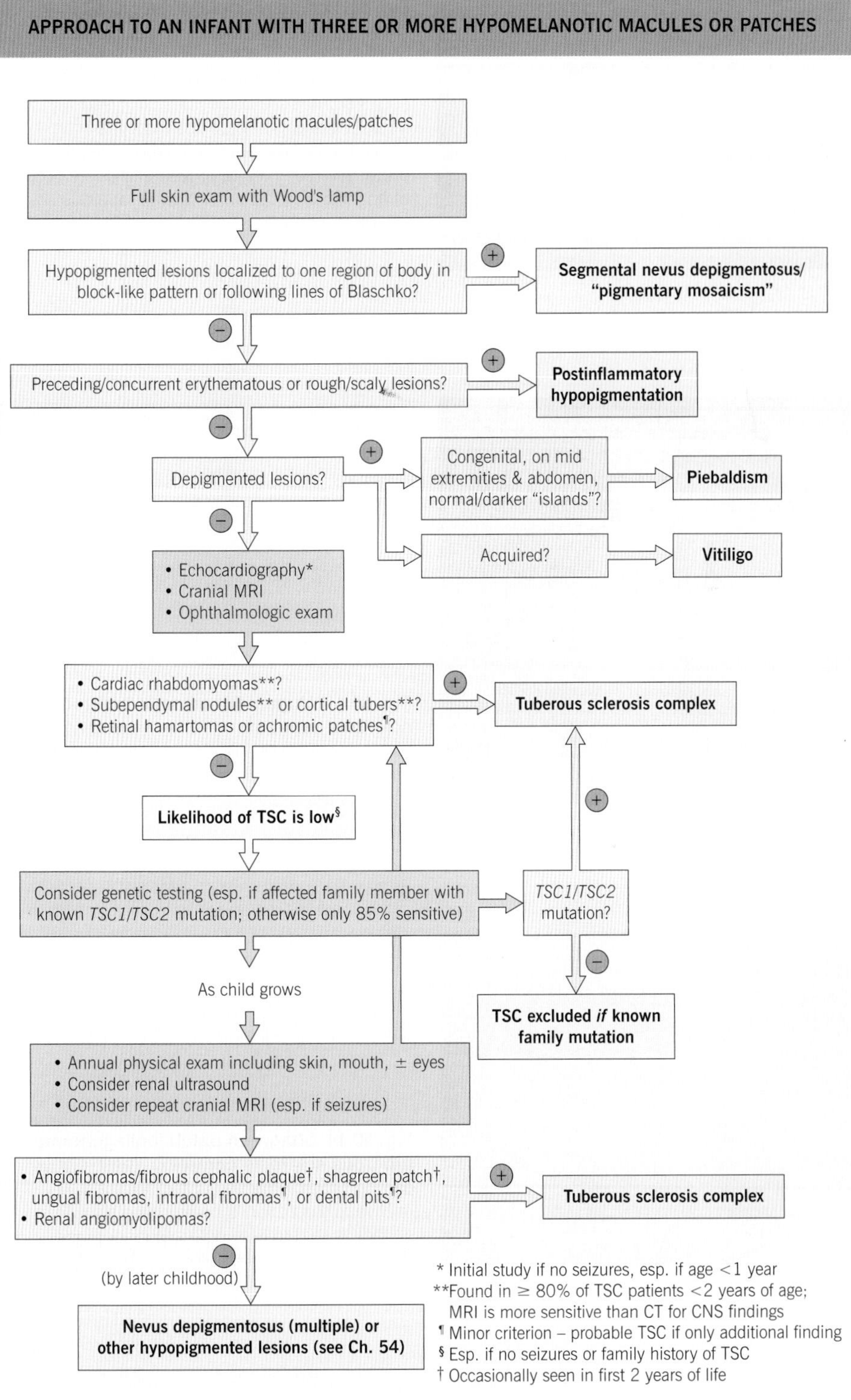

Fig. 50.11 Approach to an infant with three or more hypomelanotic macules or patches. A child with fewer than three macules and no family history of tuberous sclerosis complex (TSC) has an extremely low likelihood of having this disease.

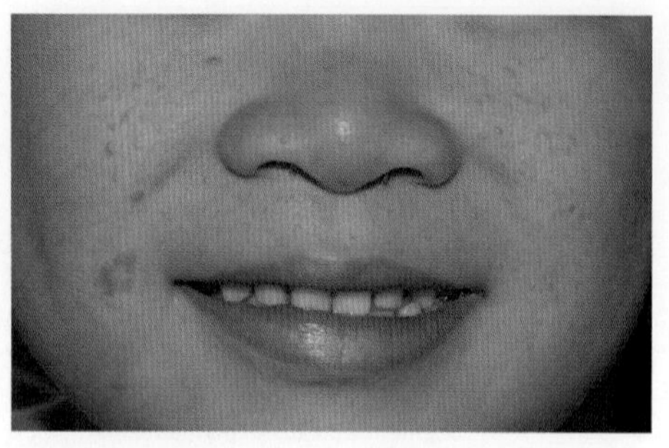

Fig. 50.12 Facial angiofibromas. Multiple small, pink-tan, dome-shaped papules on the cheeks and nose of a young boy. Note the brown fibrous plaque on the lower right cheek. Early angiofibromas are sometimes confused with acne, but taking photos at two points in time will show that individual lesions are persistent. Sun protection may help to prevent the development of angiofibromas in patients with tuberous sclerosis complex, as UV-induced DNA damage has been implicated in the development of these lesions. *Courtesy, Julie V. Schaffer, MD.*

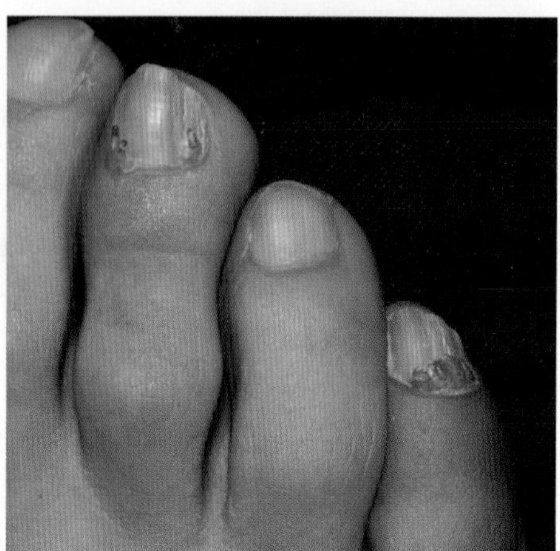

Fig. 50.13 Ungual fibromas of tuberous sclerosis complex. Multiple fibromas of the toes arising in a periungual location. Note the associated longitudinal grooves. *Courtesy, Julie V. Schaffer, MD.*

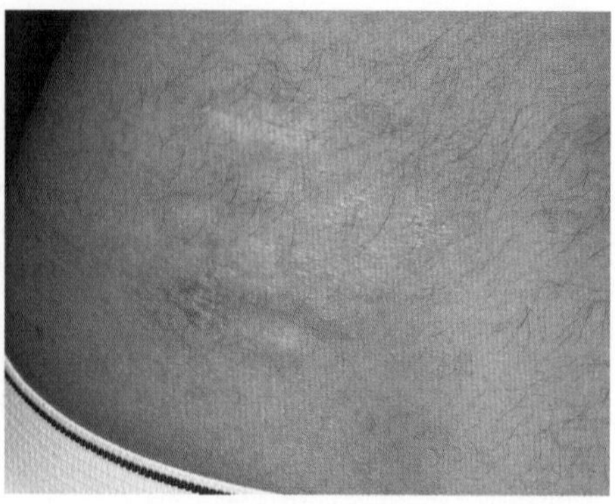

Fig. 50.14 Shagreen patch (collagenoma) in tuberous sclerosis complex. These plaques can be hyperpigmented or hypopigmented relative to the patient's background skin. The surface is said to resemble leather or pigskin. *Courtesy, Julie V. Schaffer, MD.*

2012 REVISED DIAGNOSTIC CRITERIA FOR TUBEROUS SCLEROSIS COMPLEX (TSC)	
Major features	
Hypomelanotic macules (≥3, diameter ≥5 mm) Facial angiofibromas (≥3) or fibrous cephalic plaque Ungual fibromas (≥2) Shagreen patch	
Multiple retinal hamartomas Cortical dysplasias (including tubers and cerebral white matter radial migration lines) Subependymal nodules Subependymal giant cell astrocytoma Cardiac rhabdomyoma Lymphangioleiomyomatosis Angiomyolipomas (≥2; renal >> other organs, e.g. liver)	
Minor features	
"Confetti" skin lesions	
Dental enamel pits (≥3) Intraoral fibromas (≥2) Retinal achromic patch Multiple renal cysts Non-renal hamartomas	
Definite *clinical* diagnosis • Either two major features* *or* one major feature plus ≥2 minor features **Possible *clinical* diagnosis** • Either one major feature or ≥2 minor features **Definite *genetic* diagnosis**† • Identification of a pathogenic mutation in either *TSC1* or *TSC2* in DNA from the blood or normal tissue	
Key: *Cutaneous*	*Extracutaneous*

With the exception of lymphangioleiomyomatosis + angiomyolipomas.
†Genetic testing is recommended when the diagnosis of TSC is suspected but cannot be clinically confirmed, as well as to assist in genetic counseling and family planning; 10–15% of patients who meet clinical diagnostic criteria for TSC have no pathogenic mutation identified by conventional genetic testing.

Table 50.5 2012 revised diagnostic criteria for tuberous sclerosis complex.

EVALUATION AND MANAGEMENT OF TUBEROUS SCLEROSIS COMPLEX (TSC) PATIENTS
Evaluation for TSC-associated neuropsychiatric disorder (TAND): at diagnosis and then annual screening, with comprehensive evaluation at ages 0–3, 3–6, 6–9, 12–16, and 18–25 years
Ophthalmologic examination: at diagnosis
Brain MRI with and without gadolinium*: at diagnosis and every 1–3 years until age 25
Electroencephalogram (EEG): at diagnosis
Electrocardiogram (ECG)†: at diagnosis and every 3–5 years; **echocardiography**: at diagnosis if <3 years of age
Abdominal MRI (favored over CT or ultrasound) to detect angiomyolipomas and renal cysts: at diagnosis and every 1–3 years
Assess blood pressure and determine GFR: at diagnosis and at least annually
High-resolution chest CT and PFTs to assess for lymphangioleiomyomatosis: in adult women at diagnosis and then CT every 5–10 years
Dental examination: at diagnosis and every 6 months, with panoramic radiographs by age 7 years
Dermatologic examination: at diagnosis and annually
Genetic testing/counseling: offer to patients of reproductive age

Findings may correlate with seizure activity and cognitive deficits; assess for enlarging lesions suggestive of giant cell astrocytomas (most common during childhood).
†Arrhythmias are more common in patients with TSC than the general population.

Table 50.6 Evaluation and management of tuberous sclerosis complex (TSC) patients. More frequent evaluation may be required for patients with symptoms and/or abnormal findings. GFR, glomerular filtration rate; PFTs, pulmonary function tests.

51 Mosaic Skin Conditions

- A mosaic organism is composed of ≥2 genetically distinct cell populations derived from a homogeneous zygote.
  - *Genomic mosaicism* results from alteration in the DNA sequence, affecting genes or chromosomes
  - *Functional (epigenetic) mosaicism* results from changes in gene expression (but not the DNA sequence) that are passed on during cellular replication; an important example is *lyonization* in female embryos, where random inactivation of one of the two X chromosomes occurs in each cell during early development
- Clinical findings in mosaic skin conditions depend not only on the underlying genetic alteration but also on: (1) the timing of its origin, with earlier onset generally leading to more widespread involvement; and (2) the types of cells or tissues affected (cutaneous ± extracutaneous).
  - For example, mosaicism for an activating *HRAS* mutation can produce the combination of a nevus sebaceus (keratinocytes affected), speckled lentiginous nevus (melanocytes affected), and occasionally CNS abnormalities (nerve cells affected) in patients with phakomatosis pigmentokeratotica
- The accessibility of the skin allows visualization of mosaic patterns.
  - The *lines of Blaschko* are streaks and swirls that represent pathways of epidermal cell (e.g. keratinocyte) migration during embryonic development (Fig. 51.1)
  - Segmental (e.g. block-like) patterns can also reflect cutaneous mosaicism involving melanocytes, mesodermal cells, or nerve cells
- Types of cutaneous lesions that can follow the lines of Blaschko or have a block-like/segmental pattern are outlined in Tables 51.1 and 51.2, respectively (Fig. 51.2).
- In *chimerism*, different cell populations reflect a genetically heterogeneous zygote, e.g. from fusion of two zygotes or fertilization of one egg by two sperm; this may manifest with a checkerboard, linear, or irregular pattern of pigmentary variation.

Epidermal Nevi and "Epidermal Nevus Syndromes"

- Epidermal nevi (see Ch. 89) present as streaks and swirls of thickened (e.g. verrucous, hyperkeratotic, or velvety) skin along the lines of Blaschko, usually with hyperpigmentation and sometimes with adnexal involvement (e.g. in a nevus sebaceus or nevus comedonicus) (Fig. 51.3).
- The heterogeneous genetic etiologies and potential systemic associations ("epidermal nevus syndromes") of various types of epidermal nevi are presented in Table 51.3 (Fig. 51.4).

Mosaicism in Autosomal Dominant Skin Conditions

- When evaluating a patient with skin lesions in a mosaic pattern, it can be helpful to consider whether the findings would resemble an autosomal dominant genodermatosis if present in a more generalized distribution.
- Type 1, type 2, and revertant forms of mosaicism occurring in autosomal dominant skin disorders are summarized in Fig. 51.5.
- Some dominant mutations in autosomal genes are only observed in a mosaic state, as they would not be compatible with life if present in all the cells of the body; examples

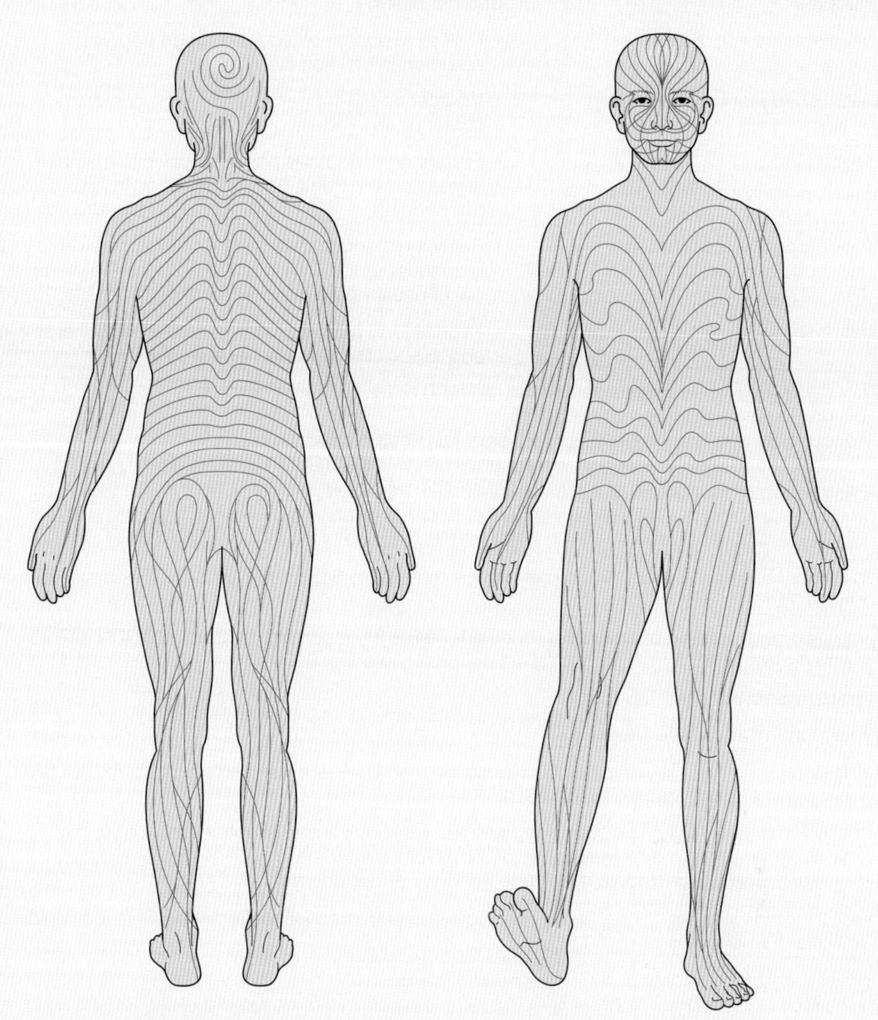

Fig. 51.1 Lines of Blaschko. Note the S-shape of lines on the abdomen, the V-shape on the central back, perpendicular lines on the face, and swirls on the posterior scalp.

include Proteus, Schimmelpenning (nevus sebaceus), and McCune–Albright syndromes (see Tables 50.3 and 51.3).

Mosaicism in X-Linked Conditions

- In X-linked disorders, functional mosaicism due to lyonization occurs in female patients and carriers.
- *X-linked dominant* conditions are typically lethal in male embryos and are therefore seen almost exclusively in a mosaic pattern in female patients with a heterozygous mutation; male patients occasionally survive due to underlying mosaicism, e.g. in the setting of Klinefelter syndrome (47,XXY karyotype) or a postzygotic mutation.
- In conditions traditionally referred to as *X-linked recessive*, male patients have generalized disease and female patients or "carriers" are affected to a variable (usually lesser) degree, often in a mosaic pattern; an example is hypohidrosis and hyperpigmentation following the lines of Blaschko in female "carriers" of X-linked hypohidrotic ectodermal dysplasia (Fig. 51.6A).

SKIN FINDINGS THAT CAN OCCUR ALONG THE LINES OF BLASCHKO	
Inflammation	
Examples	**Clinical clues**
Lichen striatus (Fig. 51.2A)	• Pink to hypopigmented flat-topped papules; common in children (see Ch. 9)
Linear lichen planus (Fig. 51.2B)	• Violaceous flat-topped papules with Wickham striae; often in adults
"Blaschkitis"	• Pruritic erythematous papulovesicles in multiple streaks on the trunk; usually develops in adults and often recurs
Inflammatory linear verrucous epidermal nevus (ILVEN) (Fig. 51.2C)	• Scaly, erythematous psoriasiform plaques with prominent pruritus and lack of response to therapy; onset usually by childhood
Linear psoriasis (Fig. 51.2D)	• Psoriasiform plaques, often responding to therapy and associated with psoriasis elsewhere
Other conditions resembling lichen planus: linear GVHD, lupus erythematosus > dermatomyositis, drug eruptions *Other conditions with a keratotic and/or vesiculobullous component*: • Variable onset: linear Darier (Fig. 51.2E) and Hailey–Hailey (Fig. 51.2F) diseases • Early onset: linear porokeratosis (see Fig. 89.8D), PEODDN, IP* stages 1–2 (see Figs 28.10 and 51.7A), epidermolytic epidermal nevus*, Conradi–Hünermann–Happle syndrome* (see Fig. 46.13)	
Verrucous lesions – e.g. epidermal/sebaceous nevi (Table 51.3; see Fig. 51.3), IP stage 2 (see Fig. 51.7B)	
Spines/comedones – e.g. nevus comedonicus (Table 51.3; see Fig. 51.3G), PEODDN (favors palms/soles), linear lichen planopilaris (later onset; see Fig. 9.5H)	
Hypopigmentation (see Table 54.3)	
Hyperpigmentation (see Table 55.4)	
Hairlessness – e.g. X-linked hypohidrotic ectodermal dysplasia (female "carriers"; Fig. 51.6A), Goltz syndrome, IP stage 4 (Fig. 51.7C)	
Atrophy – e.g. linear lichen sclerosus (epidermal wrinkling), linear atrophoderma of Moulin (hyperpigmented and depressed; Fig. 51.6B), Goltz syndrome (Fig. 51.8A,B), IP stage 4, Conradi–Hünermann–Happle syndrome (follicular atrophoderma)	
Papulonodular lesions** – e.g. adnexal neoplasms (e.g. trichoepitheliomas), BCCs, basaloid follicular hamartomas	

**Inflammatory manifestations occur primarily during infancy.*
***In addition to conditions with inflammatory or verrucous papulonodules noted above.*

Table 51.1 Skin findings that can occur along the lines of Blaschko. IP, incontinentia pigmenti; PEODDN, porokeratotic eccrine ostial and dermal duct nevus.

SKIN FINDINGS THAT CAN HAVE A SEGMENTAL PATTERN THAT REFLECTS MOSAICISM
Hypopigmentation – e.g. nevus depigmentosus, segmental vitiligo (see Ch. 54) **Hyperpigmention** ± **hypertrichosis** – e.g. CALM, Becker melanosis (nevus)/smooth muscle hamartoma (see Table 50.3 and Ch. 55) **Hypertrichosis** – e.g. X-linked congenital generalized hypertrichosis (female "carriers") **Vascular lesions** – e.g. port wine stain,† CMTC, unilateral nevoid telangiectasia, venous malformation,* plaque-type glomuvenous malformation,** segmental infantile hemangioma (see Ch. 85) **Papulonodular lesions** – e.g. segmental leiomyomas** or neurofibromas**

†Associated with mosaic activating mutations in the GNAQ gene encoding the Q-class G protein α-subunit; mutations in this gene have also been associated with dermal melanocytosis, which occurs as "twin spots" with port wine stains in phakomatosis pigmentovascularis.
**Type 1 segmental manifestation of an autosomal dominant disorder (Fig. 51.5).*
***Type 2 segmental manifestation of an autosomal dominant disorder (Fig. 51.5).*

Table 51.2 Skin findings that can have a segmental pattern that reflects mosaicism. CALM, café-au-lait macule; CMTC, cutis marmorata telangiectatica congenita.

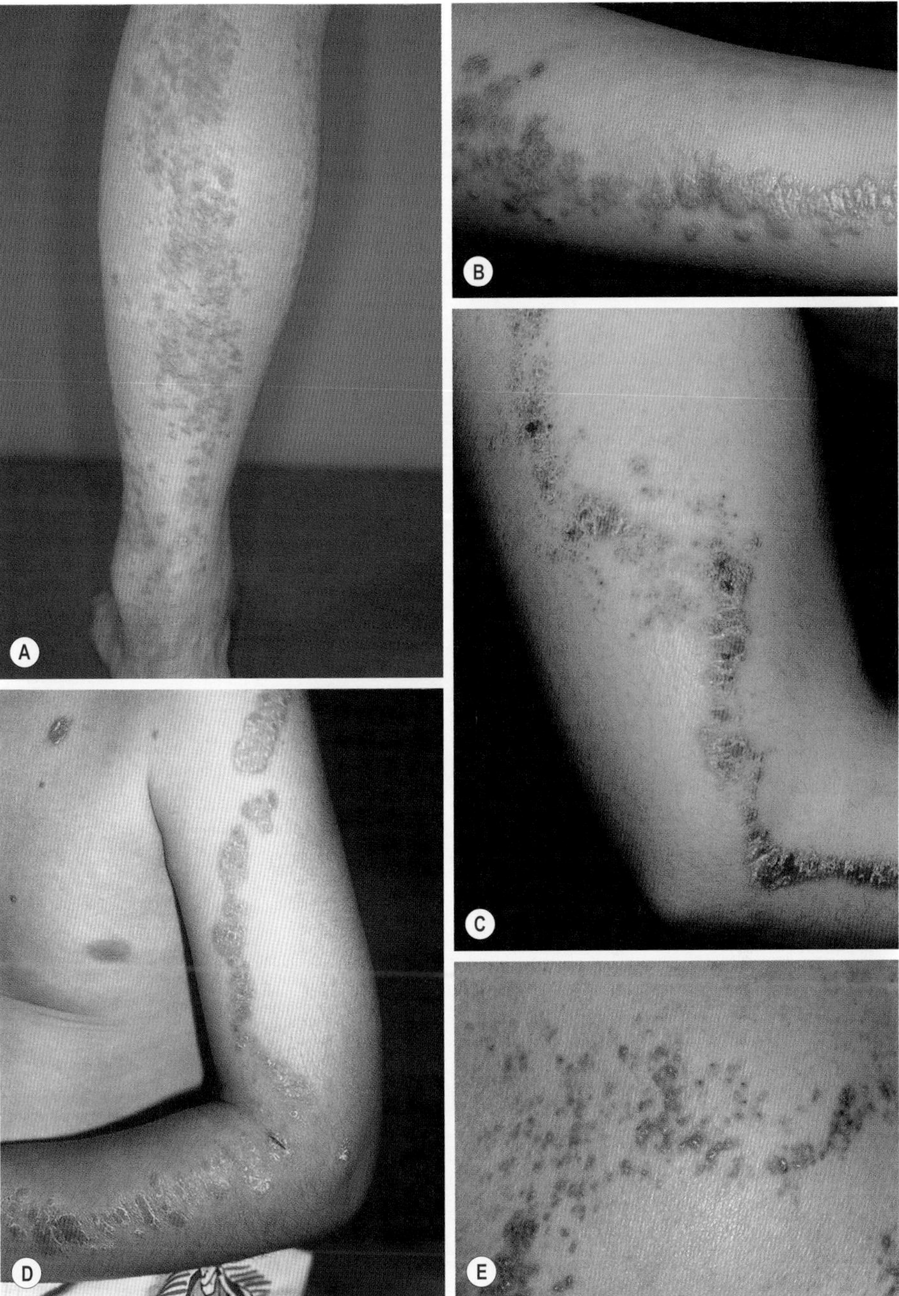

Fig. 51.2 Inflammatory lesions along the lines of Blaschko. **A** Lichen striatus on the leg presenting as linear streaks composed of multiple pink papules with variable scale. **B** Linear lichen planus presenting as a band of coalescing violaceous papules and plaques with Wickham striae on an extremity. Note the postinflammatory hyperpigmentation proximally. **C** Inflammatory linear verrucous epidermal nevus (ILVEN) featuring persistent, extremely pruritic, scaly psoriasiform plaques. **D** Linear psoriasis with erythema and scale that responded to treatment with a high-potency topical CS. Small scattered psoriasiform lesions are also present. **E** Linear Darier disease presenting with keratotic papules in an adult, representing type 1 mosaicism (see Fig. 51.5A). *A, Courtesy, Tetsuo Shiohara, MD, and Yoshiko Mizukawa, MD; B, Courtesy, Joyce Rico, MD; C, E, Courtesy, YDRSC; D, Courtesy, Celia Moss, MD.* Continued

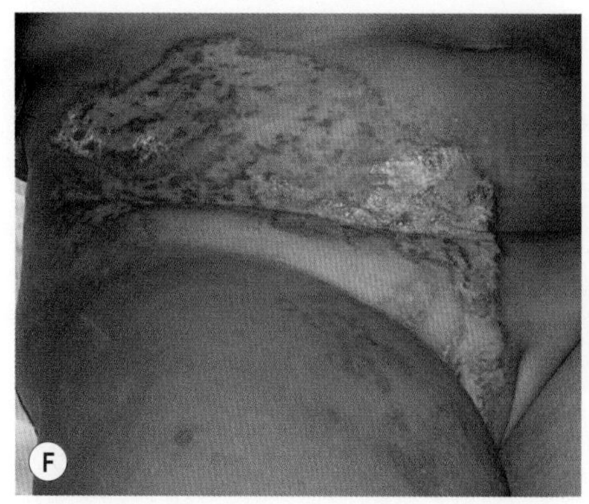

Fig. 51.2 *Continued* **Inflammatory lesions along the lines of Blaschko. F** Linear Hailey–Hailey disease presenting with recurrent blistering and erosions in a young girl, representing type 2 mosaicism with earlier and more severe involvement in the affected region due to a "second hit" mutation (see Fig. 51.5B). *F, Courtesy, Julie V. Schaffer, MD.*

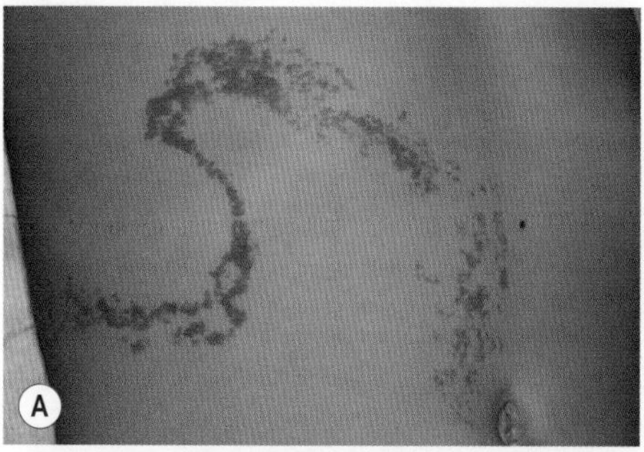

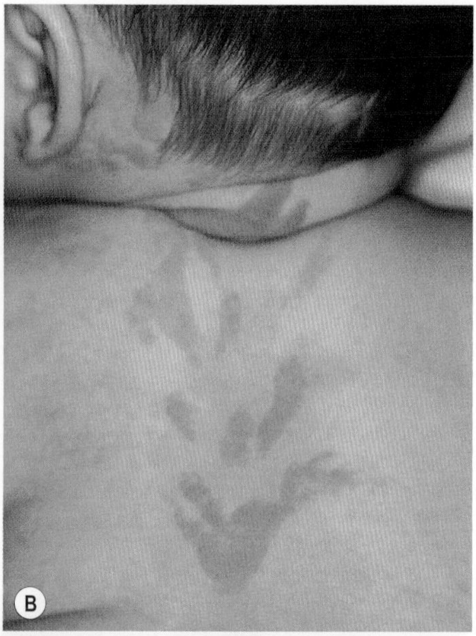

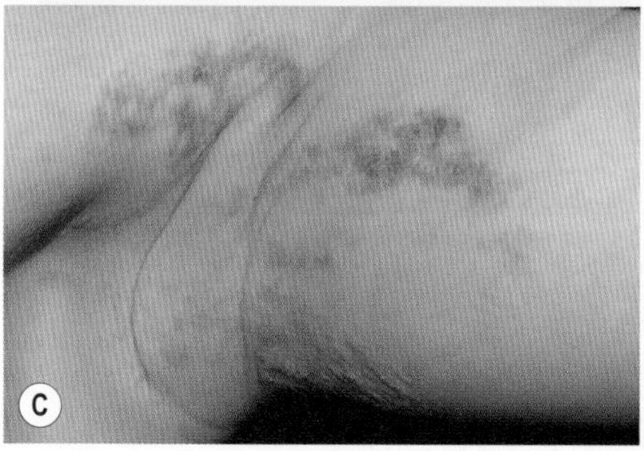

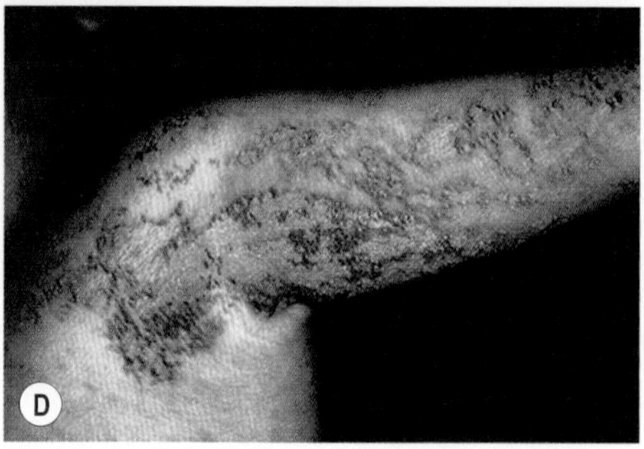

Fig. 51.3 Epidermal nevi (EN). A Non-epidermolytic EN presenting as S-shaped hyperpigmented papillomatous streaks on the abdomen with sharp midline dermarcation. **B** Non-epidermolytic EN in a V-shaped pattern on the mid back. **C** Non-epidermolytic EN with hyperpigmented keratotic streaks accentuated in skin folds. **D** Epidermolytic EN with shedding of scale and associated hypopigmentation. *A, C, Courtesy, Julie V. Schaffer, MD; B, D, Courtesy, YDRSC. Continued*

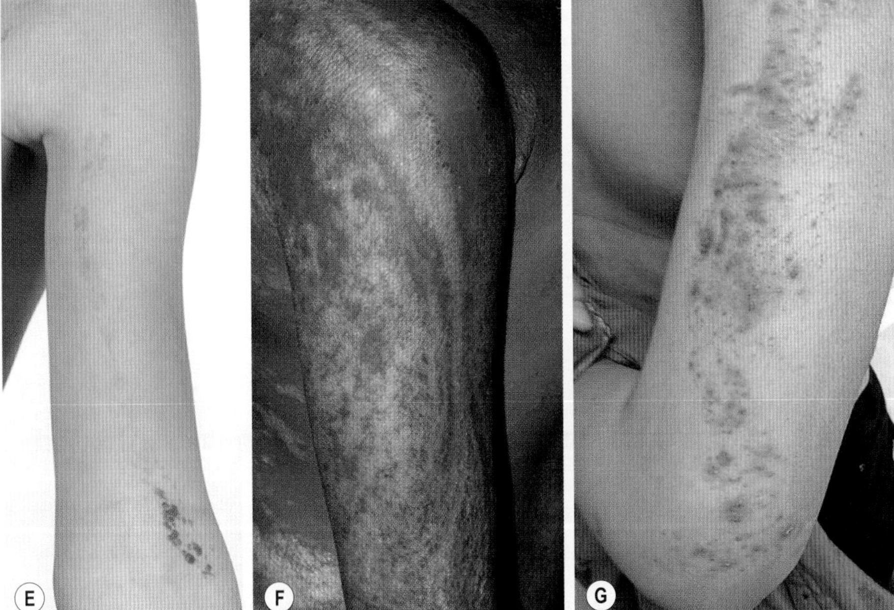

Fig. 51.3 *Continued* **Epidermal nevi (EN). E** Non-epidermolytic EN due to a *FGFR3* mutation, representing a mosaic counterpart of the acanthosis nigricans in thanatophoric dysplasia, an autosomal dominant neuroskeletal syndrome. This explains the flexural accentuation of the epidermal nevus. **F** Extensive non-epidermal EN presenting as hypopigmented streaks with variable adherent scale. **G** Nevus comedonicus with inflammatory papulonodules as well as comedones in an adolescent. The lesion initially presented as a congenital hypopigmented streak. *E, Courtesy, Celia Moss, MD; F, G, Courtesy, Julie V. Schaffer, MD.*

Incontinentia Pigmenti (IP)

- X-linked dominant disorder caused by mutations in the *N*F-κB *e*ssential *mo*dulator (*NEMO; IKBKG*) gene, which encodes a protein that protects against TNF-α-induced apoptosis; male patients with milder *NEMO* mutations may present with hypohidrotic ectodermal dysplasia with immune deficiency (see Table 52.5).
- IP has four stages, which may be absent or overlapping, of cutaneous findings that follow the lines of Blaschko (with the exception of stage 4) (Fig. 51.7; see Fig. 28.10):
  - *Vesicular* streaks favoring the extremities and scalp in neonates, often associated with peripheral blood leukocytosis and eosinophilia; may recur during childhood febrile illnesses
  - *Verrucous* linear plaques favoring the extremities in infants; acral keratotic nodules sometimes develop after puberty
  - *Hyperpigmented* grayish-brown streaks and swirls favoring the trunk and intertriginous areas from infancy through adolescence
  - *Hypopigmented/atrophic* "Chinese character"-like bands lacking hair and sweat glands, favoring the calves in adolescents and adults
- Other manifestations can include alopecia (often at the vertex in a swirled pattern), missing or conical teeth, CNS abnormalities (e.g. seizures, developmental delay), and retinal vascular anomalies that require monitoring with ophthalmologic examinations during infancy.

Goltz Syndrome (Focal Dermal Hypoplasia)

- X-linked dominant condition caused by mutations in the *PORCN* gene, which encodes a protein that regulates Wnt signaling.
- Skin lesions following the lines of Blaschko are characterized by vermiculate dermal atro-

EPIDERMAL NEVI: SELECTED VARIANTS AND POTENTIAL SYNDROMIC ASSOCIATIONS			
Type of epidermal nevus (EN)	**Gene**	**Generalized conditions caused by constitutional mutations***	**Potential syndromic associations with the EN**
Epidermolytic verrucous EN	*KRT1, KRT10*	Epidermolytic ichthyosis, PPK *(KRT1)*	None
Non-epidermolytic verrucous EN	Mosaic RASopathies (also nevus sebaceus [see below] and woolly hair nevi)		
	HRAS > *NRAS* > *KRAS*, *BRAF*	Costello, Noonan, and cardio-facio-cutaneous syndromes (see Table 50.3)	Cutaneous skeletal hypophosphatemic syndrome (CSHS); phakomatosis pigmentokeratotica with speckled lentiginous nevus
	Mosaic FiGRopathies (also nevus sebaceous and acneiform nevi; see below)		
	FGFR3§ > *FGFR2*	Thanatophoric dysplasia, SADDAN, Beare–Stevenson cutis gyrata	Asymmetric craniofacial malformations, intellectual disability
	Mosaic AKTopathies (see Ch. 85)		
	PIK3CA§	Cowden syndrome variant (rare)	Asymmetric overgrowth, lipomatosis, vascular anomalies, digital anomalies, macrocephaly; cerebriform connective tissue nevi of palms/soles (Proteus)
	AKT1	Not reported	
	PTEN	PTEN hamartoma (e.g. Cowden) syndrome	
Nevus sebaceus	*HRAS* > *KRAS*; rarely *FGFR2*	See above	Schimmelpenning syndrome (CNS, ocular, skeletal); CSHS (see above)
Munro acne nevus (hypopigmented background skin)	*FGFR2*	Apert syndrome	Digital anomalies, intellectual disability
Nevus comedonicus	*NEK9*	Skeletal dysplasia (with biallelic mutations)	Digital anomalies, scoliosis
Porokeratotic adnexal ostial nevus¶	*GJB2*	Keratitis–ichthyosis–deafness (KID) syndrome	
Inflammatory linear verrucous epidermal nevus (ILVEN)	*GJA1* ?*NSHDL*	Erythrokeratodermia variabilis et progressiva ? CHILD syndrome (mosaic)	Distal limb reductions

**Could potentially occur in the offspring of an epidermal nevus patient who has gonadal as well as cutaneous mosaicism.*
§Somatic activating mutations are also found in seborrheic keratoses, dermatosis papulosa nigra, stucco keratoses, and solar lentigines; the PIK3CA-related overgrowth spectrum includes Klippel–Trenaunay syndrome, megalencephaly–capillary malformation, and CLOVES (see Ch. 85).
¶Includes porokeratotic eccrine ostial and dermal duct nevus (PEODDN) and other spiny hyperkeratotic EN.
Mosaic RAS mutations found in epidermal nevi are often (but not always) different from those in generalized conditions, suggesting that the former represent more severe, lethal mutations rescued by mosaicism.

Table 51.3 Epidermal nevi: selected variants and potential syndromic associations. CHILD, congenital hemidysplasia with ichthyosiform erythroderma/nevus and limb defects; FGF, fibroblast growth factor; GJA1/B2, gap junction α1/β2; KRT, keratin; PPK, palmoplantar keratoderma; SADDAN, severe achondroplasia with developmental delay and acanthosis nigricans.

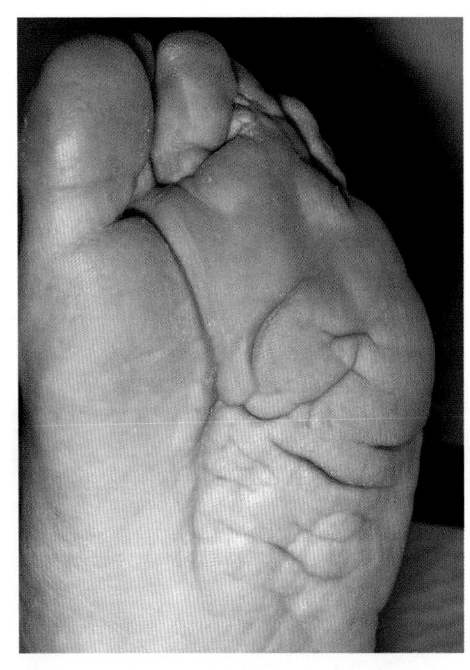

Fig. 51.4 Plantar cerebriform connective tissue nevus in a man with Proteus syndrome. *Courtesy, Odie Enjolras, MD.*

MOSAICISM FOR AUTOSOMAL DOMINANT (AD) TRAITS

	A	B	C
	Type 1 in AD	Type 2 in AD	Revertant in AD
Background genotype	Normal	Heterozygous	Heterozygous
Background phenotype	Normal	Abnormal	Abnormal
"Line" genotype	Heterozygous	Homozygous abnormal	Homozygous normal
"Line" phenotype	Abnormal	Very abnormal	Normal
Mosaic event	Somatic mutation ("gain of heterozygosity")	Loss of heterozygosity	Reversion to normal
Examples	Type 1 linear Darier (see Fig. 51.2E) or Hailey–Hailey disease	Type 2 linear Darier or Hailey–Hailey (see Fig. 51.2F) disease	Ichthyosis en confetti

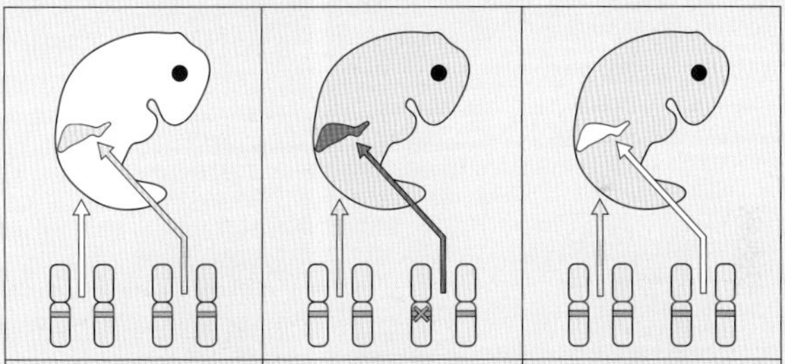

Normal gene
Dominant mutation
Loss of heterozygosity
Normal phenotype
Abnormal phenotype
Very abnormal phenotype

Fig. 51.5 Mosaicism for autosomal dominant (AD) traits. A *See next page for figure legend.*

Fig. 51.5 Mosaicism for autosomal dominant (AD) traits. A *Type 1 mosaicism* features a linear distribution of the skin lesions that characterize an AD genodermatosis in the absence of involvement elsewhere on the body. This results from a postzygotic heterozygous mutation in the underlying gene that is only present in the affected region. **B** *Type 2 mosaicism* presents with a more severe linear lesion superimposed on the background of a generalized AD genodermatosis. This reflects a constitutional (in all the cells of the body) heterozygous mutation plus a "second hit" in the other allele of the gene within the more severely affected region. **C** In *revertant mosaicism*, an area of normal-appearing skin occurs in the background of a generalized AD genodermatosis due to a reversion ("back" mutation) to normal or another correction of the underlying heterozygous mutation in that region. Of note, mosaicism can also occur in autosomal recessive conditions, with revertant mosaicism potentially leading to a spared area (e.g. in epidermolysis bullosa).

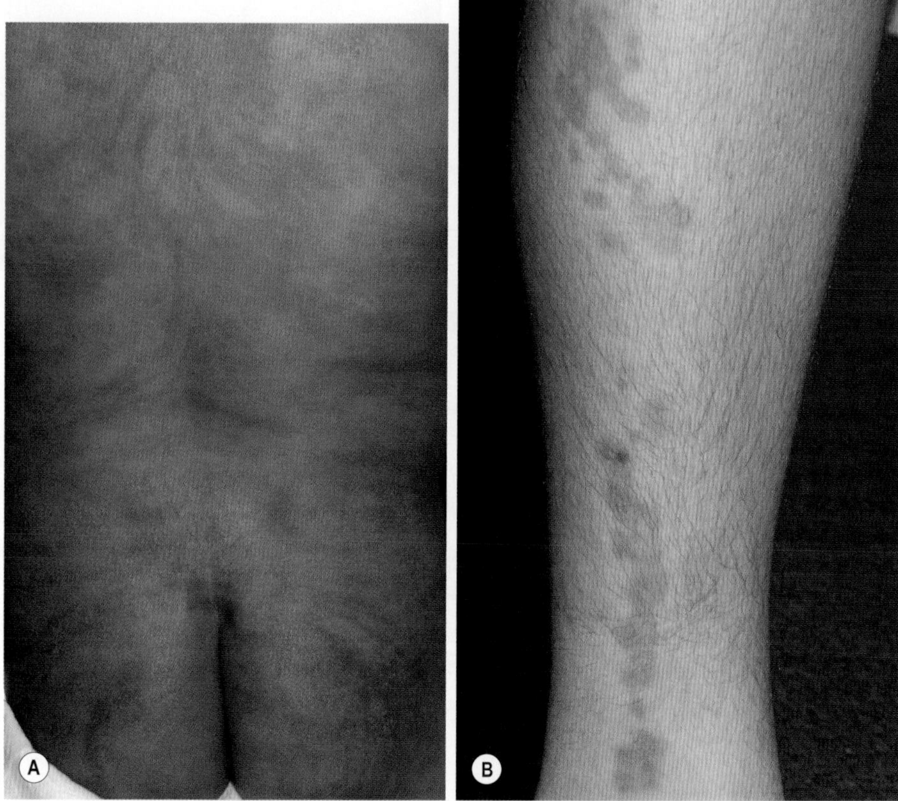

Fig. 51.6 Hyperpigmentation along the lines of Blaschko. A In this 2-year-old female "carrier" of X-linked hypohidrotic ectodermal dysplasia, the skin within the hyperpigmented streaks and swirls is extremely smooth. Starch-iodine testing on the back disclosed a patchy distribution of active sweat glands. The patient also had whorled areas of sparse hair on the posterior scalp and several cone-shaped teeth. **B** Linear atrophoderma of Moulin presenting as streaks of hyperpigmented depressions with "cliff-drop" borders. The morphology resembles atrophoderma of Pasini and Pierini. *A, B, Courtesy, Julie V. Schaffer, MD.*

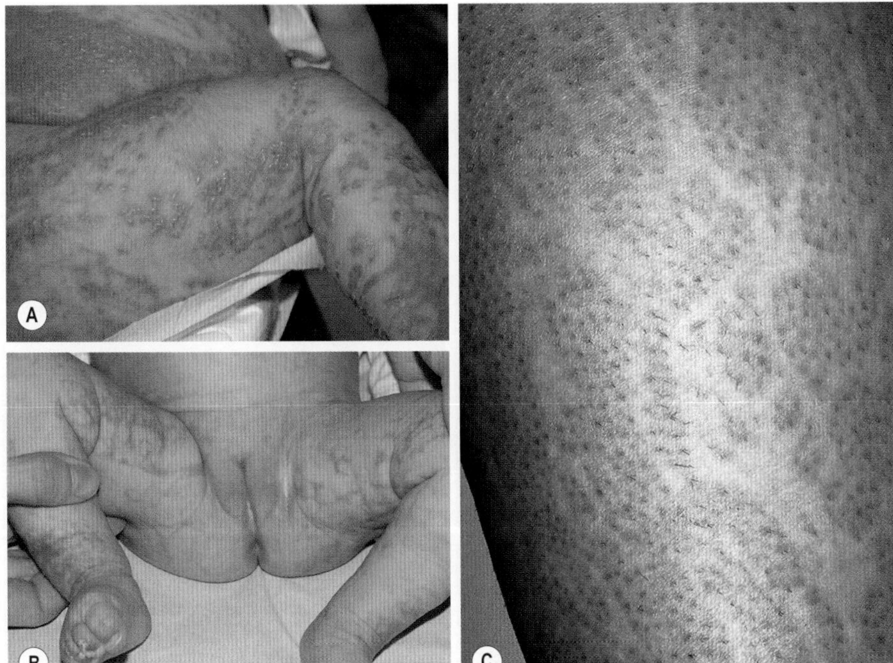

Fig. 51.7 Incontinentia pigmenti. A Stage 1 with streaks of erythema and vesicles in a neonate. **B** Stages 2 (verrucous) and 3 (hyperpigmented). Note the keratotic lesions on the toes. The scalloped edges of the hyperpigmented streaks reflect growth of normal keratinocytes into areas of apoptosis. **C** Stage 4 (atrophic and hypopigmented). Note the absence of hairs within the streaks on the calf. *A, Courtesy, Robert Silverman, MD; B, Courtesy, Julie V. Schaffer, MD; C, Courtesy, USCDRSC.*

phy, outpouchings of fat, telangiectasias, and hypo- > hyperpigmentation (Fig. 51.8).

• Additional features include periorificial raspberry-like papillomas, dystrophic nails, sparse hair, abnormal teeth, split hand/foot ("lobster claw") malformations, ocular abnormalities (e.g. microphthalmia), and the radiographic finding of osteopathia striata in long bones.

X-Linked Dominant Ichthyosiform Conditions

• Examples include *c*ongenital *h*emidysplasia with *i*chthyosiform nevus and *l*imb *d*efects (CHILD) and Conradi–Hünermann–Happle syndromes (see Table 46.2).

Mosaic Manifestations of Acquired Skin Conditions

• Multifactorial skin disorders with environmental as well as genetic components occasionally occur along the lines of Blaschko or in a segmental distribution, presumably reflecting mosaicism for a "susceptibility" mutation; as a result, such conditions often develop in older children or adults following an environmental trigger, and they are sometimes superimposed on a pre-existing mosaic lesion (e.g. psoriasis within an epidermal nevus).

• Other examples include linear lichen planus, linear GVHD, and segmental vitiligo (see Fig. 51.2B, D).

For further information see Ch. 62 from *Dermatology, Fourth Edition*.

For additional online figures visit www.expertconsult.com 

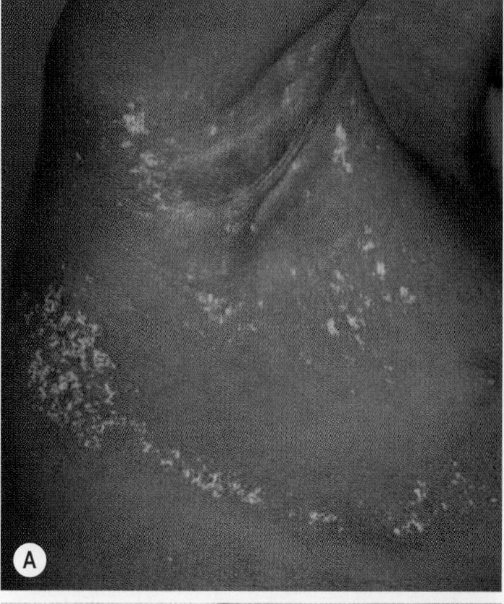

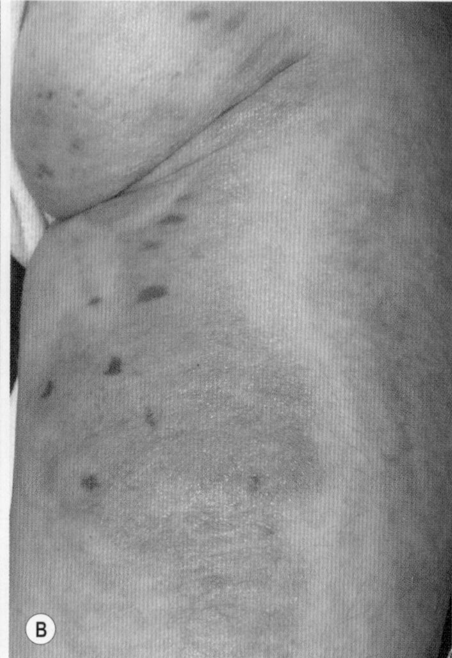

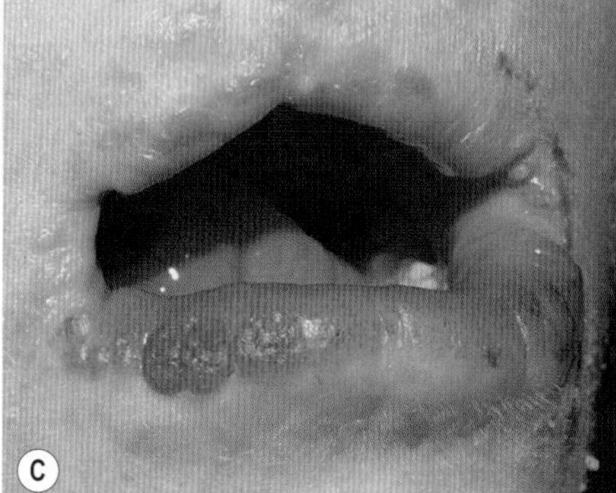

Fig. 51.8 Goltz syndrome. A Hypopigmented streaks of vermiculate atrophy. **B** Bands of telangiectatic erythema, dermal atrophy with fat "herniation," and hyperpigmented macules on the posterior thigh. **C** Raspberry-like papules on the lower lip. Similar lesions can occur in the anogenital region and may be confused with warts. *A–C, Courtesy, Julie V. Schaffer, MD.*

Other Genodermatoses 52

This chapter discusses genetic skin diseases that are not covered in other chapters, including conditions featuring extracutaneous tumorigenesis, enzyme deficiencies, premature aging, and ectodermal dysplasia.

Disorders Featuring Extracutaneous Tumorigenesis

Cowden Syndrome and Other Forms of PTEN Hamartoma Tumor Syndrome

- Spectrum of autosomal dominant multisystem disorders that feature characteristic skin findings (Fig. 52.1), macrocephaly, hamartomatous overgrowth of a variety of tissues, and a predisposition to certain cancers (Table 52.1).
- Due to mutations in the phosphatase and tensin homolog tumor suppressor gene (*PTEN*), which negatively regulates the AKT/mammalian target of rapamycin (mTOR) pathway of increased cellular growth and survival.

Multiple Endocrine Neoplasia Syndromes

- Group of autosomal dominant disorders associated with neoplasia or hyperplasia in two or more endocrine organs, often presenting with mucocutaneous findings that serve as clues to the diagnosis (Table 52.2; Fig. 52.2).

Muir–Torre Syndrome (MTS)

- Subtype of hereditary nonpolyposis colorectal cancer (Lynch) syndrome characterized by sebaceous neoplasms (e.g. sebaceous adenoma, sebaceoma, sebaceous carcinoma; Fig. 52.3, see Table 91.2) and keratoacanthomas (± sebaceous differentiation) as well as internal malignancies (Table 52.3).
- Caused by heterozygous constitutional mutations in a DNA mismatch repair gene, e.g. *MSH2* (70–90% of patients), *MLH1*, and *MSH6*.

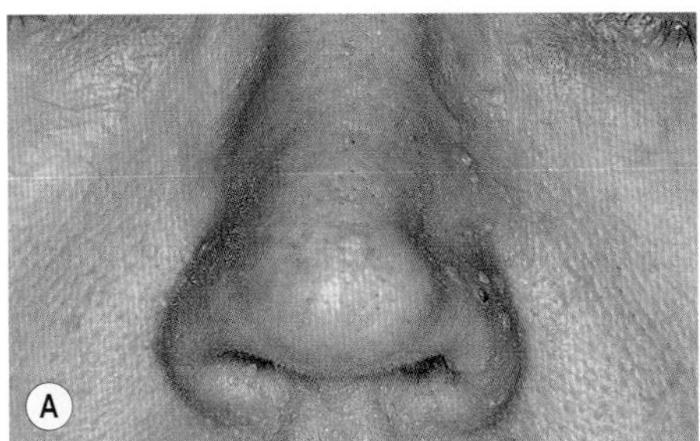

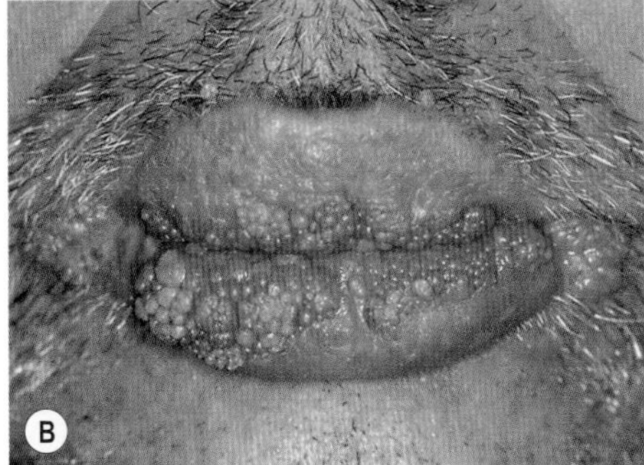

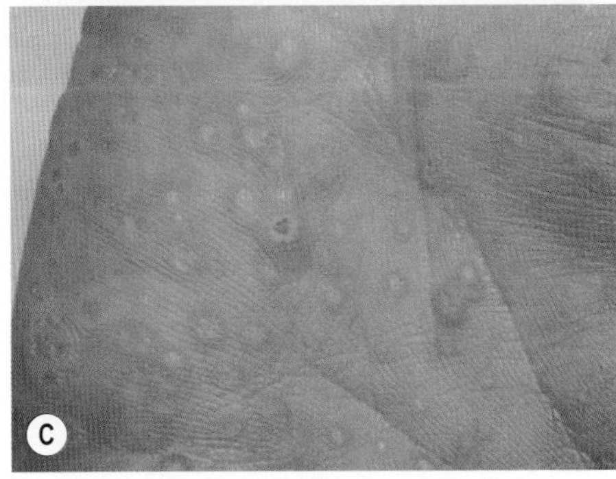

Fig. 52.1 Cowden syndrome. A Multiple skin-colored papules on the face, especially the nose, some of which are verrucous. **B** Coalescing papules with a cobblestone-like appearance on the vermilion lips. **C** Multiple palmar keratoses, many with a glassy appearance or depression centrally. *A, Courtesy, Kalman Watsky, MD; B, Courtesy, Jean L. Bolognia, MD; C, Courtesy, Joyce Rico, MD.*

MAJOR CLINICAL MANIFESTATIONS OF PTEN HAMARTOMA TUMOR SYNDROME		
	Onset at birth or in childhood – *classic features of BRR*	**Onset in adolescence or adulthood – *classic features of Cowden syndrome***
Mucocutaneous	• Pigmented genital macules (penis > vulva) • Lipomas • Vascular anomalies* • Epidermal nevi • Café-au-lait macules • Neuromas (acrofacial, mucosal)	• Multiple facial tricholemmomas (Fig. 52.1A; see Ch. 91) and other verrucous papules (especially periorificial and on ears) • Multiple oral papillomas (lips, tongue) (Fig. 52.1B) • Acral/palmoplantar keratoses (Fig. 52.1C) • Sclerotic fibromas • Multiple acrochordons, acanthosis nigricans
Extracutaneous	• Macrocephaly, intracranial developmental venous anomalies • High-arched palate, adenoid facies • Scoliosis/kyphosis, pectus excavatum • GI: ganglioneuromas, hamartomatous polyps • CNS: developmental delay, autism	• Breast: fibrocystic disease, fibroadenomas, carcinoma (25–50% of women, mean age = 40 years; occasionally in men) • Thyroid: goiter, adenomas, carcinoma (10–15% of patients; often follicular) • GU: testicular lipomatosis, ovarian cysts, uterine leiomyomas, endometrial carcinoma (5–10% of women), renal cell carcinoma • GI: colon carcinoma • CNS: Lhermitte–Duclos disease†

**Typically with fast-flow channels, intramuscular involvement, and ectopic fat; may have capillary, venous, and/or lymphatic components and associated soft tissue/bony overgrowth.*
†Hamartomatous dysplastic gangliocytoma of the cerebellum.

Table 52.1 Major clinical manifestations of PTEN hamartoma tumor syndrome. This categorization reflects general tendencies, as the age of onset or recognition of these findings can vary. Criteria for PTEN gene testing and guidelines for surveillance in patients suspected to have Cowden syndrome are available at http://www.nccn.org/professionals/physician_gls/PDF/genetics_screening.pdf. BRR, Bannayan–Riley–Ruvalcaba syndrome.

• Cutaneous findings develop at a mean age of ~55 years, presenting as yellow to pink papulonodules on the face (the usual site of sebaceous neoplasms outside of MTS) or trunk > extremities.

Gardner Syndrome

• Variant of familial adenomatous polyposis syndrome with prominent extraintestinal involvement as well as premalignant GI polyps (typically by age 20 years) and colorectal carcinoma (usually by age 40 years); caused by heterozygous mutations in the adenomatous polyposis coli gene (*APC*).

• Epidermoid cysts often develop during childhood; pilomatricomas, fibromas, desmoid tumors (e.g. within abdominal scars), lipomas, and jaw osteomas are additional manifestations.

• *C*ongenital *h*ypertrophy of the *r*etinal *p*igment *e*pithelium (CHRPE) is an early sign.

Birt–Hogg–Dubé Syndrome

• Autosomal dominant genodermatosis caused by mutations in the folliculin gene (*FLCN*).

• Onset during early adulthood of multiple fibrofolliculomas > trichodiscomas, presenting as small whitish papules on the face, ears, and neck (see Figs 91.4 and 91.16); also flexural acrochordons.

CLASSIC MULTIPLE ENDOCRINE NEOPLASIA (MEN) SYNDROMES			
MEN type	**Gene**	**Major extracutaneous features**	**Cutaneous features**
1 (Wermer)	*MEN1* (*MENIN*)	• **Pituitary** neoplasia (e.g. prolactinoma) • **Parathyroid** hyperplasia/adenoma • **Pancreatic** islet cell hyperplasia/adenoma/carcinoma	• Multiple facial angiofibromas • Collagenomas (Fig. 52.2A), lipomas • Multiple gingival papules • Guttate hypopigmented macules
2A (Sipple)	*RET* (especially codon 634)	• **Parathyroid** hyperplasia/adenoma • **Thyroid** medullary carcinoma • **Adrenal** pheochromocytomas	• Pruritus/notalgia paresthetica → macular or lichen amyloidosis on the upper back (often with childhood onset)
2B (multiple mucosal neuroma syndrome)	*RET* (especially codon 918)	• **Thyroid** medullary carcinoma • **Adrenal** pheochromocytoma • **GI ganglioneuromatosis** • Marfanoid habitus	• Multiple mucosal neuromas (especially on eyelid margins/conjunctiva, lips, tongue; Fig. 52.2B); rarely neuromas of perinasal skin

Table 52.2 Classic multiple endocrine neoplasia (MEN) syndromes.

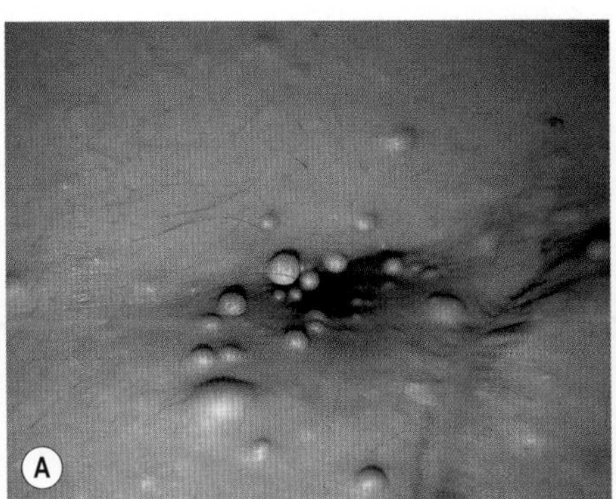

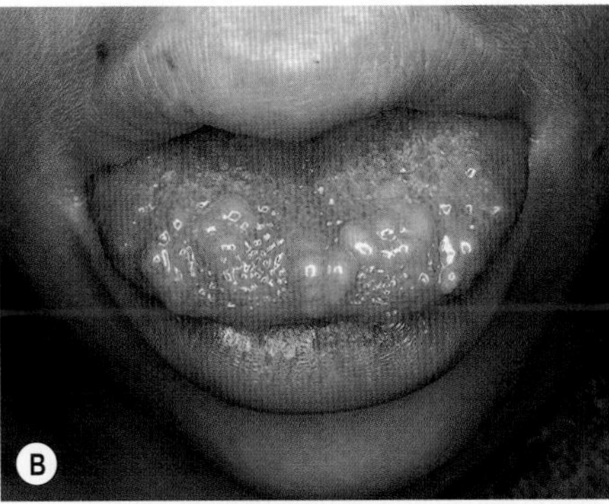

Fig. 52.2 Mucocutaneous findings in multiple endocrine neoplasia (MEN). A Multiple collagenomas in a patient with MEN type 1. **B** Enlarged nodular lips and multiple mucosal neuromas on the lateral and distal tongue in a patient with MEN type 2B. *A, Courtesy, Susan Bayliss, MD; B, Courtesy, YDRSC.*

- Increased risk of spontaneous pneumothoraces and renal cell carcinoma (especially oncocytic and chromophobe subtypes).

Reed Syndrome (Hereditary Leiomyomatosis and Renal Cell Cancer Syndrome)

- Discussed in Chapter 95.

Enzyme Deficiency Disorders

Alkaptonuria

- Rare autosomal recessive disorder due to homogentisic acid oxidase deficiency.
- Urine that darkens on standing and brown-black cerumen represent early findings.
- Blue-gray discoloration of the axillary skin, ear (Fig. 52.4), and sclera typically ap-

pears during early adulthood, when arthritis and valvular heart disease often develop.

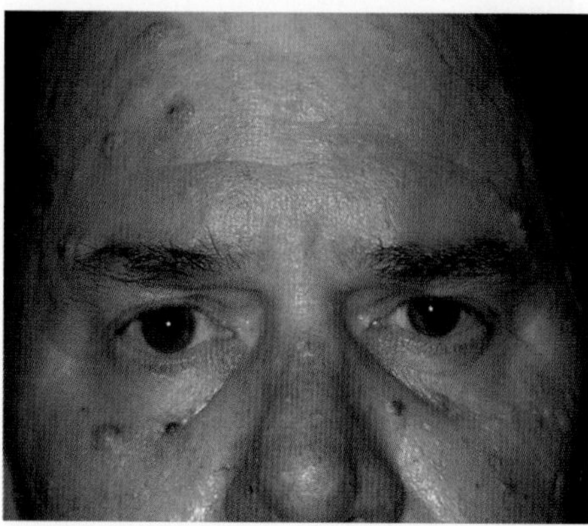

Fig. 52.3 Muir–Torre syndrome with multiple sebaceous neoplasms. *Courtesy, Dan Ring, MD.*

Fabry Disease

- X-linked lysosomal storage disorder due to α-galactosidase A deficiency, which leads to glycosphingolipid accumulation within endothelial cells and results in progressive renal, coronary, and cerebrovascular insufficiency.
- Female heterozygotes have variable clinical manifestations, often with later onset than those in affected men.
- *Angiokeratoma corporis diffusum* presents as punctate dark red macules and papules clustered between the umbilicus and knees ("bathing trunk" distribution) (Fig. 52.5); serves as an early sign of Fabry disease, typically developing in childhood or adolescence along with paresthesias of the extremities, hypohidrosis, and whorled corneal opacities.

RISK ASSESSMENT FOR MUIR–TORRE SYNDROME (MTS)	
Higher likelihood of MTS	**Lower likelihood of MTS**
Clinicopathologic characteristics of skin lesions	
• ≥2 sebaceous neoplasms **[2]** • Located outside of the head and neck region • Sebaceous neoplasm with high specificity for MTS, e.g. a cystic lesion or seboacanthoma	• Single sebaceous neoplasm • Located in photodamaged facial skin • Sebaceous hyperplasia
Characteristics of patient and family history	
• Age <60 years **[1]** • Personal history of colorectal cancer* and/or other Lynch syndrome-related malignancies (e.g. small bowel, gastric, endometrial, bladder, ureteral, renal, biliary, pancreatic, glioblastoma) **[1]**, especially if more than one • Colorectal cancer and/or other Lynch syndrome-related malignancies in family member(s) **[1]**, especially if before 50 years of age and in first-degree relative(s)	• Elderly patient with no history of a Lynch syndrome-related malignancy • No family members with colorectal cancer/other Lynch syndrome-related malignancies
Additional analysis of sebaceous neoplasms	
• Loss of MSH2, MLH1, MLH6, and/or PMS2 expression shown by immunohistochemical staining‡ • Evidence of MSI in lesional tissue (more specific)§	• Expression of MLH1, MSH2, MSH6, and PMS2 shown by immunohistochemical staining • No evidence of MSI in lesional tissue§

**Especially if MSI-high histology – presence of tumor-infiltrating lymphocytes, Crohn disease-like lymphocytic reaction, medullary growth pattern, or signet ring/mucinous differentiation.*

‡MSH2 and MSH6 proteins form a heterodimer, so lack of one can lead to the absence of the other; likewise, PMS2 is unstable without a functional MLH1 protein.

§Testing can be performed on paraffin-embedded tissue; diagnostic yield may be higher for colonic neoplasms.

Table 52.3 Risk assessment for Muir–Torre syndrome (MTS). A clinical score of ≥2 based on the sum of the applicable numbers in [ ] has a sensitivity of nearly 100% and a specificity of ~80% for predicting a germline mutation in a mismatch repair gene. MSI, microsatellite instability.

• Fig. 52.6 compares the clinical features of Fabry disease and *fucosidosis*, one of several other lysosomal storage disorders associated with angiokeratomas.
• **Rx:** intravenous α-galactosidase A replacement therapy; migalastat, an oral pharmacologic chaperone that stabilizes mutant forms of α-galactosidase, is an alternative in patients with suitable mutations.

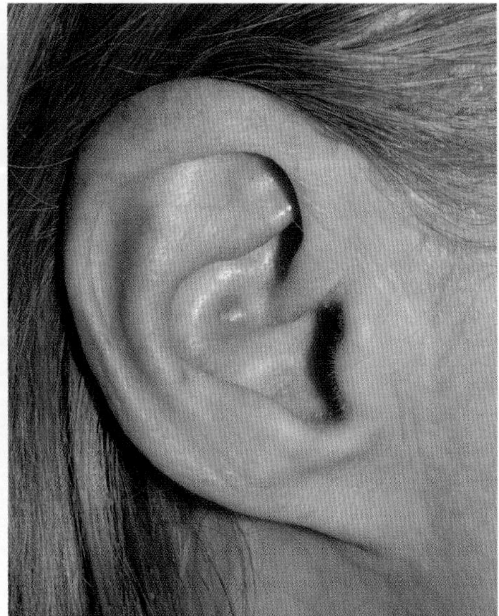

Fig. 52.4 Blue-gray discoloration of the pinna in a woman with alkaptonuria. *Courtesy, Julie V. Schaffer, MD.*

Phenylketonuria

• Autosomal recessive disorder due to phenylalanine hydroxylase deficiency.
• Cutaneous findings can include diffuse pigmentary dilution (skin, hair, eyes), eczematous dermatitis, sclerodermatous skin changes favoring the proximal extremities (Fig. 52.7), and sweat with a musty odor; pigmentary banding of the hair can occur as a reflection of nonadherence to the diet.
• Newborn screening allows prevention of intellectual disability and skin changes through early nutritional intervention (e.g. a phenylalanine-restricted diet).

Mitochondrial Disorders

• This heterogeneous group of conditions can present with a wide variety of cutaneous manifestations (Table 52.4) as well as neuromuscular and visceral dysfunction.

Premature Aging Disorders

Inherited photosensitivity disorders (see Ch. 73) and Kindler syndrome (see Ch. 26) may also have features of premature aging.

Hutchinson–Gilford Progeria Syndrome

• Accelerated aging due to heterozygous mutations in the *LMNA* gene; the mutant lamin A protein ("progerin") remains farnesylated and disrupts nuclear scaffolding.
• Onset during infancy of growth failure, facial findings (e.g. frontal bossing, protruding

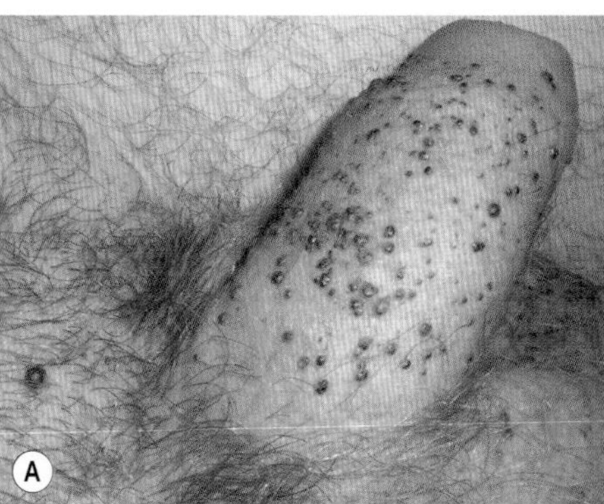

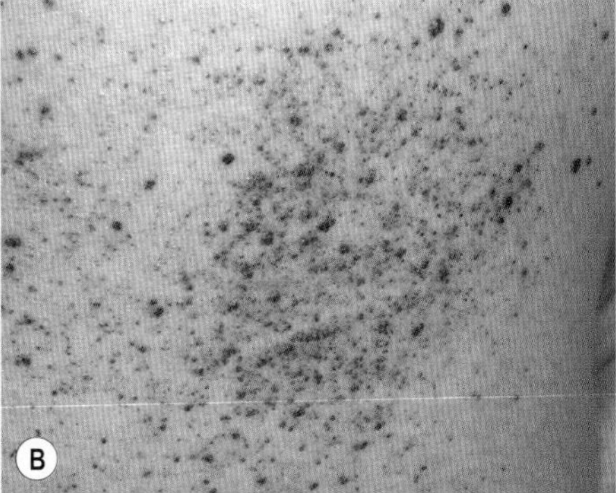

Fig. 52.5 Angiokeratomas of Fabry disease. Multiple dark red to red-brown macules and papules located: (**A**) on the penis, an uncommon site for angiokeratomas in the general population, as well as on the scrotum; and (**B**) on the lower trunk within a "bathing trunk" distribution. *Courtesy, Paula Luna, MD.*

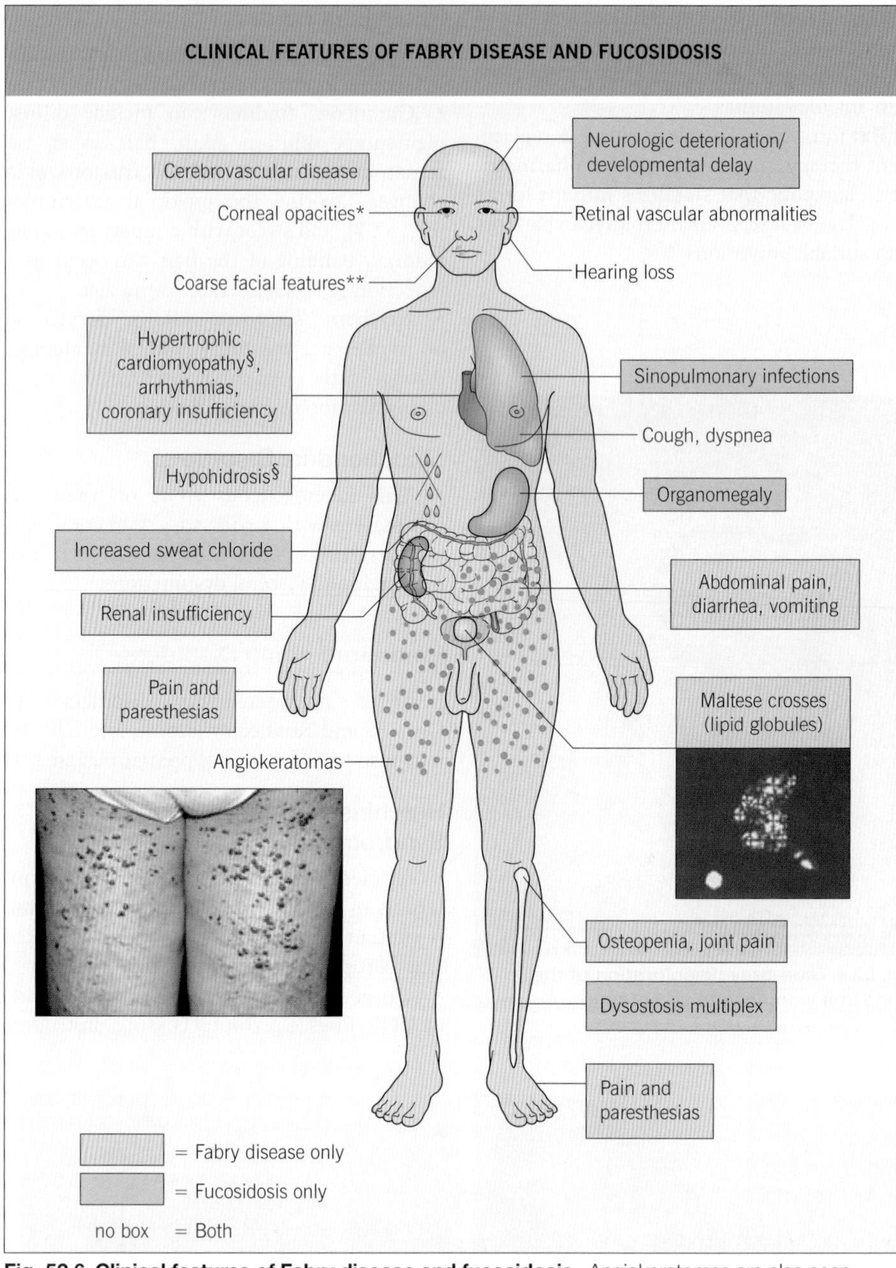

Fig. 52.6 Clinical features of Fabry disease and fucosidosis. Angiokeratomas are also seen in other metabolic disorders, including galactosialidosis, GM1 gangliosidosis, Kanzaki disease, β-mannosidosis, sialidosis, and aspartylglucosaminuria. *Also lenticular in Fabry disease. **Milder in Fabry disease. §Occasionally observed in fucosidosis. *Angiokeratomas of Fabry disease, courtesy, Luis Requena, MD; photomicrograph of urinary sediment demonstrating Maltese crosses (via polarization), courtesy, Robert J. Desnick, MD, PhD.*

eyes, prominent veins), decreased subcutaneous fat, and cutaneous manifestations such as thin dry skin, acral wrinkling, mottled hyperpigmentation, sclerodermoid changes (especially on the lower trunk and thighs), and alopecia.

- Progressive atherosclerosis results in a median life span of 14 years.

CUTANEOUS MANIFESTATIONS OF MITOCHONDRIAL RESPIRATORY CHAIN DISORDERS
• Alopecia • Hair shaft abnormalities – trichoschisis, pili torti, longitudinal grooving, trichorrhexis nodosa • Hypertrichosis • Absent or excessive sweating • Pigmentary abnormalities – mottled or reticulated pigmentation • Palmoplantar keratoderma (linked with deafness) • Hypoplastic nails • Lipomas • Acrocyanosis

Table 52.4 Cutaneous manifestations of mitochondrial respiratory chain disorders.

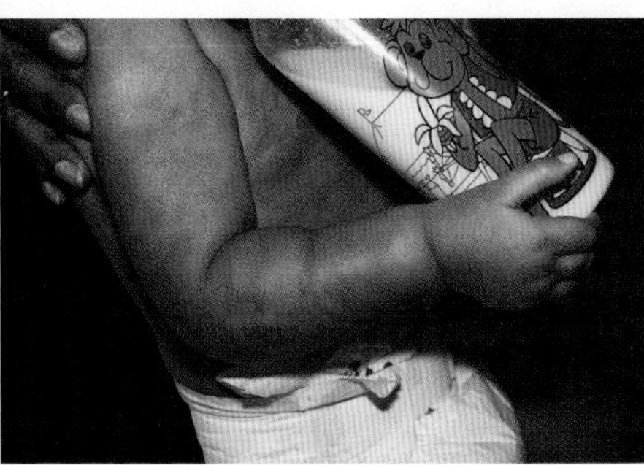

Fig. 52.7 Phenylketonuria (PKU). Infant with PKU and sclerodermoid skin changes. *Courtesy, New York Medical College.*

• **Rx:** inhibitors of farnesylation (e.g. lonafarnib) may be of benefit.

Werner Syndrome

• Autosomal recessive disorder characterized by premature aging beginning in the second decade of life; caused by mutations in the *RECQL2* gene, which encodes a DNA helicase.

• Cutaneous findings include atrophy, mottled hyperpigmentation, sclerodermoid changes, keratoses and ulcers over pressure points (especially acrally), and premature graying of hair.

• Short stature, characteristic facies (e.g. thin with beaked nose), atherosclerosis, osteoporosis, diabetes mellitus, and an increased risk of sarcomas are additional features; median survival ~50 years.

Ectodermal Dysplasias

• Large, heterogeneous group of genetic disorders characterized by abnormalities in ≥2 major ectodermal structures: the hair, sweat glands, nails, and teeth. Other ectodermal structures, e.g. sebaceous or mucous glands, may also be affected.

• Major features of several classic forms of ectodermal dysplasia are presented in Table 52.5 and Figs 52.8–52.11.

For further information see Ch. 63 from *Dermatology, Fourth Edition*.

For additional online figures and tables visit www.expertconsult.com 

SELECTED ECTODERMAL DYSPLASIA (ED) SYNDROMES						
Syndrome	**Inheritance (gene)**	**Scalp hair**	**Sweating**	**Nails**	**Teeth**	**Other features**
Hypohidrotic ED (Figs 52.8 and 52.9)	XLR (*EDA*)* > AD, AR (*EDAR* > *EDARADD*)	Sparse–absent; often lightly pigmented in childhood	↓↓, often leads to hyperpyrexia	Normal	Hypodontia, conical	• Frontal bossing, saddle nose, everted lips, periorbital wrinkling/hyperpigmentation, sebaceous hyperplasia • ± Collodion-like membrane at birth; eczema later • Frequent respiratory tract infections, thick cerumen
Hypohidrotic ED-immune deficiency	XLR (*NEMO*)** > AD (*NFKBIA*)	Sparse	↓	Normal	Hypodontia, conical	• Intertrigo, seborrheic-like dermatitis, erythroderma • Colitis; recurrent infections (pyogenic, opportunistic); ↑ IgM, IgA; ↓ IgG • Rare osteopetrosis, lymphedema
Hidrotic ED (Clouston syndrome) (Fig. 52.10)	AD (*GJB6*), most common in French Canadians	Wiry/brittle, variable alopecia	Normal	White in infants→ thickened with distal separation	Normal	• Diffuse PPK, "pebbled" skin on dorsal digits with EFSA • Blepharitis, conjunctivitis
WNT10A-associated ED†	AR > AD (*WNT10A*)	Thin, sparse	± ↓	Dystrophic or absent	Hypodontia	• Facial telangiectasias, reticulated erythema, atrophy • PPK with ESFA, xerosis
AEC (Hay–Wells) syndrome‡ (Fig. 52.11)	AD (*p63*, SAM domain)	Wiry/coarse, lightly pigmented, patchy alopecia	± ↓	Thickened > absent	Hypodontia, often conical	• Neonatal erythroderma with peeling skin/ erosions • Erosive scalp dermatitis • Ankyloblepharon • Cleft palate ± lip; GER • ± Syndactyly
EEC syndrome	AD (*p63*, DNA-binding domain)	Coarse, lightly pigmented, ± sparse	Usually normal	Transverse ridges, pitting	Hypodontia, premature loss	• PPK, xerosis • Cleft palate + lip • Ectrodactyly > syndactyly

**Variable phenotype with mosaic pattern (e.g. hypohidrosis and hyperpigmentation along the lines of Blaschko lines) in female "carriers" of XLR form.*
***Female carriers may have mild features of incontinentia pigmenti (see Ch. 51).*
†Includes odonto-onycho-dermal dysplasia and Schöpf–Schulz–Passarge syndrome, which also features eyelid hidrocystomas.
‡Rapp–Hodgkin syndrome is now included in the AEC spectrum.

Table 52.5 Selected ectodermal dysplasia (ED) syndromes. AD, autosomal dominant; AEC, ankyloblepharon–ED–clefting; AR, autosomal recessive; EDA, ectodysplasin A; EDAR, EDA receptor; EDARADD, EDAR-associated death domain; EEC, ED–ectrodactyly–clefting; ESFA, eccrine syringofibroadenomatosis; GER, gastroesophageal reflux;

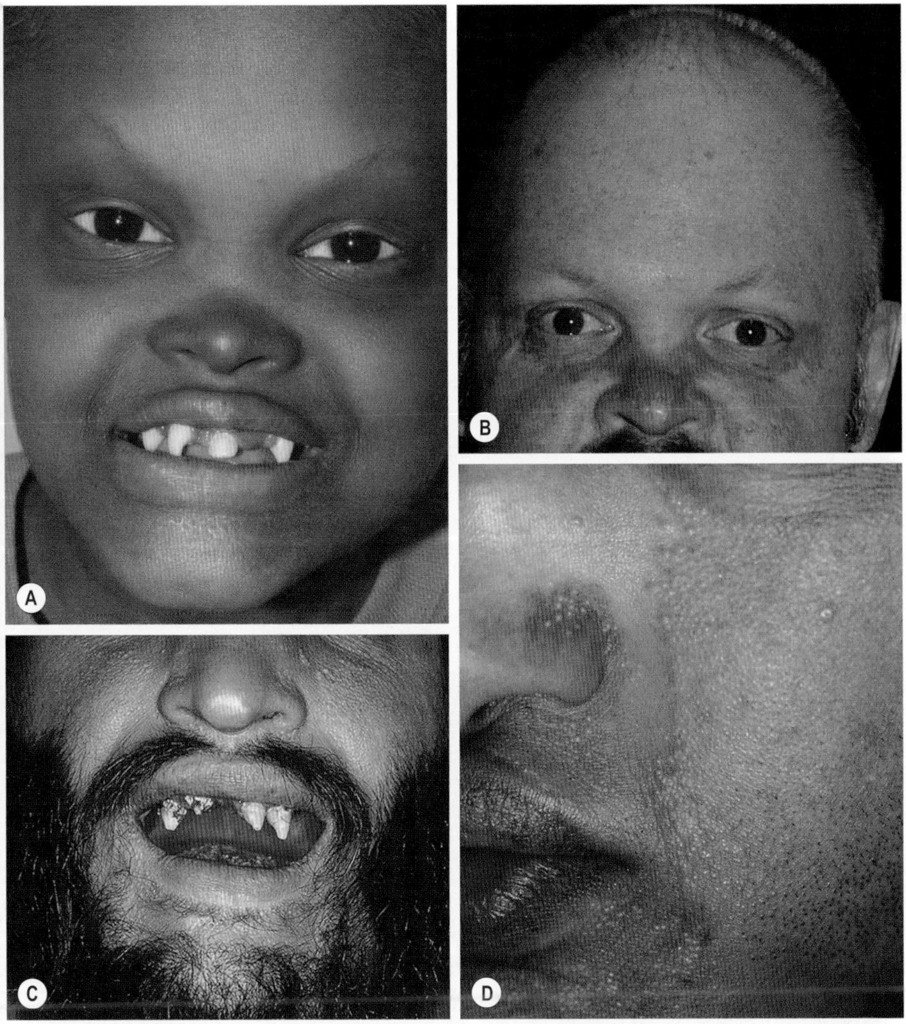

Fig. 52.8 Male patients with hypohidrotic ectodermal dysplasia. Note the flat nasal bridge, depressed nasal tip, sparse hair (scalp, eyebrows, eyelashes), peg-shaped teeth, full lips, and sebaceous hyperplasia. Also note the normal secondary hair in adults. *A, Courtesy, Julie V. Schaffer, MD; B, D, Courtesy, Mary Williams, MD; C, Courtesy, YDRSC.*

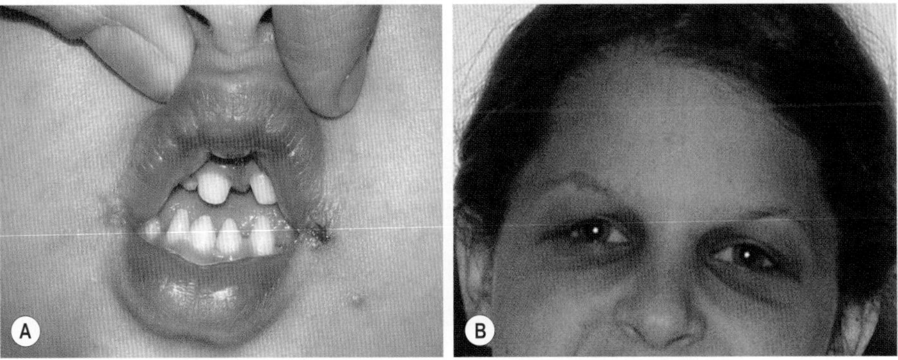

Fig. 52.9 Female patients with X-linked hypohidrotic ectodermal dysplasia. A Full lips, peg-shaped teeth, and hypodontia. **B** Periorbital hyperpigmentation. *A, Courtesy, Julie V. Schaffer, MD. Continued*

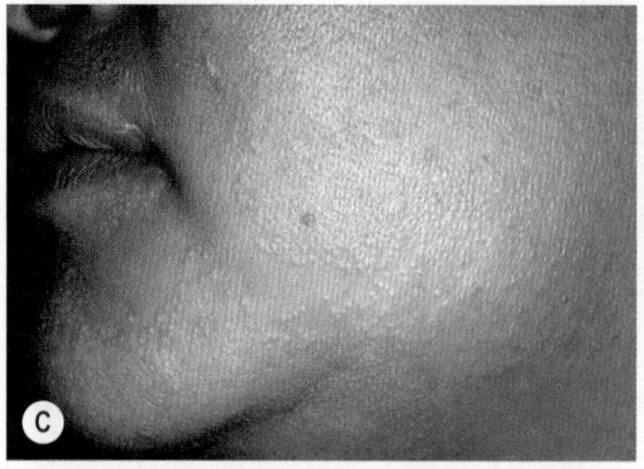

Fig. 52.9 *Continued* **Female patients with X-linked hypohidrotic ectodermal dysplasia.** **C** Sebaceous hyperplasia.

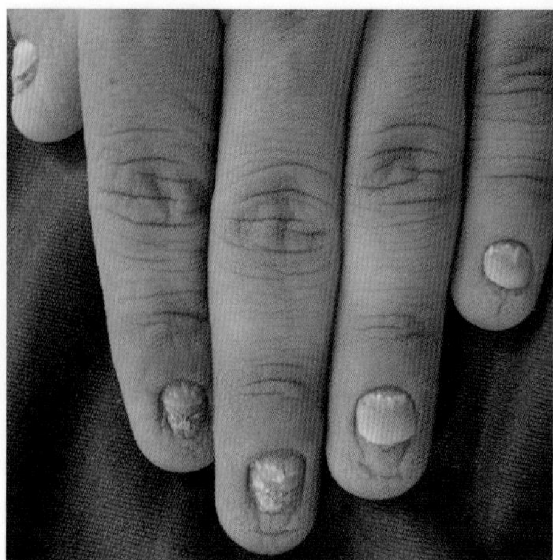

Fig. 52.10 Hidrotic ectodermal dysplasia (Clouston syndrome). Note the thickened, shortened nails with distal separation and the tiny papules in a regular distribution on the dorsal fingertips. *Courtesy, Virginia Sybert, MD, and Alanna Bree, MD.*

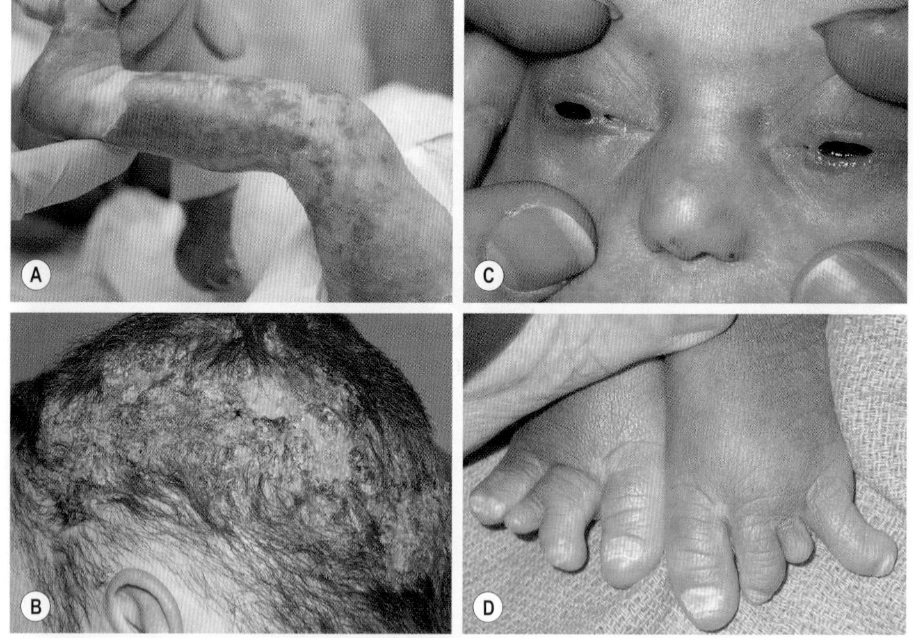

Fig. 52.11 Ankyloblepharon–ectodermal dysplasia–clefting syndrome. A Extensive erosions in an infant who succumbed to sepsis. **B** Chronic erosive scalp dermatitis with thick scale-crust and alopecia. **C** Strands of tissue between the eyelids (ankyloblepharon filiforme adnatum). **D** Digital abnormalities (including syndactyly) and nail dystrophy. *A, C, D, Courtesy, Virginia Sybert, MD, and Alanna Bree, MD; B, Courtesy, Julie V. Schaffer, MD.*

Developmental Anomalies 53

Developmental anomalies are a diverse group of congenital disorders that result from faulty *in utero* morphogenesis. When they affect the skin, developmental anomalies can range in severity from isolated minor physical findings to potentially life-threatening conditions or cutaneous signs of significant extracutaneous defects.

Midline Lesions of the Nose or Scalp

- A midline mass or pit on the nose or scalp due to a dermoid cyst, cephalocele, nasal glioma, or other heterotopic brain/meningeal tissue (Fig. 53.1) may have a deeper component with intracranial extension.
- These lesions are typically apparent at birth or during early childhood.
- *Hair collar sign*: a peripheral ring of long, dark hair often surrounds ectopic neural tissue or membranous aplasia cutis congenita (ACC) on the scalp (Figs 53.2 and 53.3); the latter is thought to represent a forme fruste of a neural tube defect.
- **DDx:** outlined in Table 53.1 for nasal masses; epidermoid cysts, tricholemmal cysts, and granuloma annulare for scalp lesions (especially in older children).
- **Rx:** avoid biopsy or aspiration, which could lead to a CNS infection (e.g. meningitis); MRI and/or CT is required to assess extent prior to surgical intervention, which should include exploration to exclude intracranial extension and repair of any bony/dural defects.

Dermoid Cysts

- Result from sequestration of ectodermal tissue along embryonic fusion planes.
- Recognized at birth or when they enlarge or become inflamed during infancy or childhood.
- Firm, noncompressible, skin-colored to pink subcutaneous nodules that often reach a size of 1–4 cm in diameter; some have a sinus ostium, which may be heralded by protruding hairs.
- Most often located around the eyes, especially the lateral eyebrow region (Fig. 53.4); midline lesions on the nose, scalp, or back may have intracranial extension.
- **Rx:** surgical excision, following imaging if midline.

Cephaloceles

- Neural tube defect characterized by congenital herniation of brain + meninges (*encephalocele*) or meninges (*cranial meningocele*) through a skull defect (see Fig. 53.3).
- Midline or paramedian location at the occiput or vertex > nasal region.
- Soft, compressible, pulsatile mass, often with a bluish color; covered with normal skin or a glistening membrane.
- Clues to the diagnosis include transillumination and transient expansion with crying or the Valsalva maneuver; nasal lesions may present with cerebrospinal fluid (CSF) rhinorrhea or a broad nasal bridge.
- **Rx:** MRI followed by neurosurgical repair.

Nasal Gliomas, Other Heterotopic Brain Tissue, and Rudimentary Meningoceles

- A *nasal glioma* is a congenital mass of heterotopic brain tissue (HBT) at the nasal root/glabella > intranasally; the skin overlying this firm, noncompressible nodule tends to be red with prominent telangiectasias (mimicking an infantile hemangioma) (Fig. 53.5).

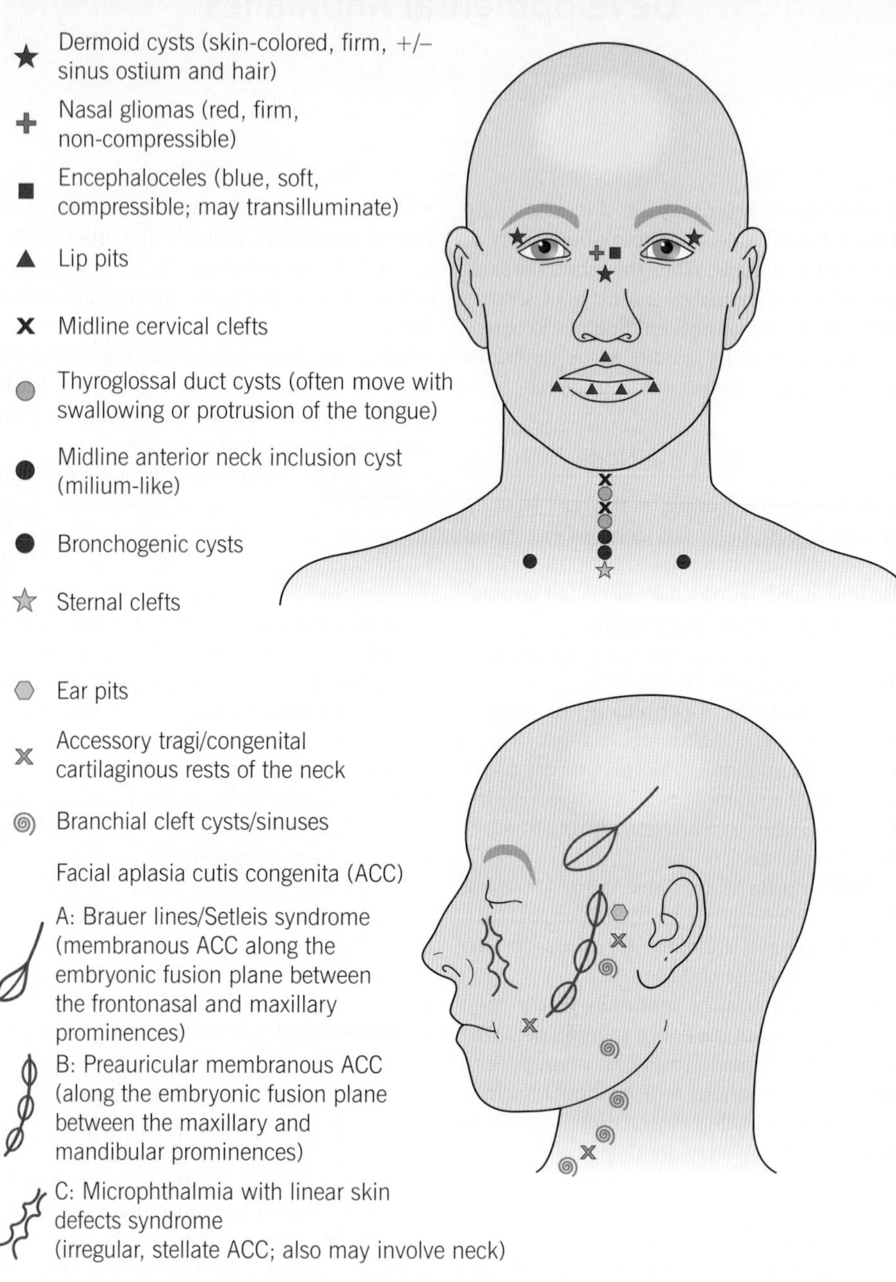

Fig. 53.1 Common sites of developmental anomalies of the face and neck. *Courtesy, Julie V. Schaffer, MD.*

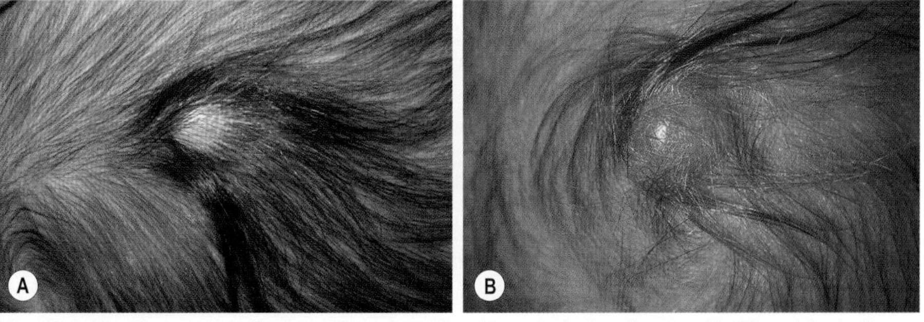

Fig. 53.2 Membranous aplasia cutis congenita. Note the hair collar sign **(A, B)** and the bullous appearance **(B)**. *A, Courtesy, Julie V. Schaffer, MD; B, Courtesy, YDRSC.*

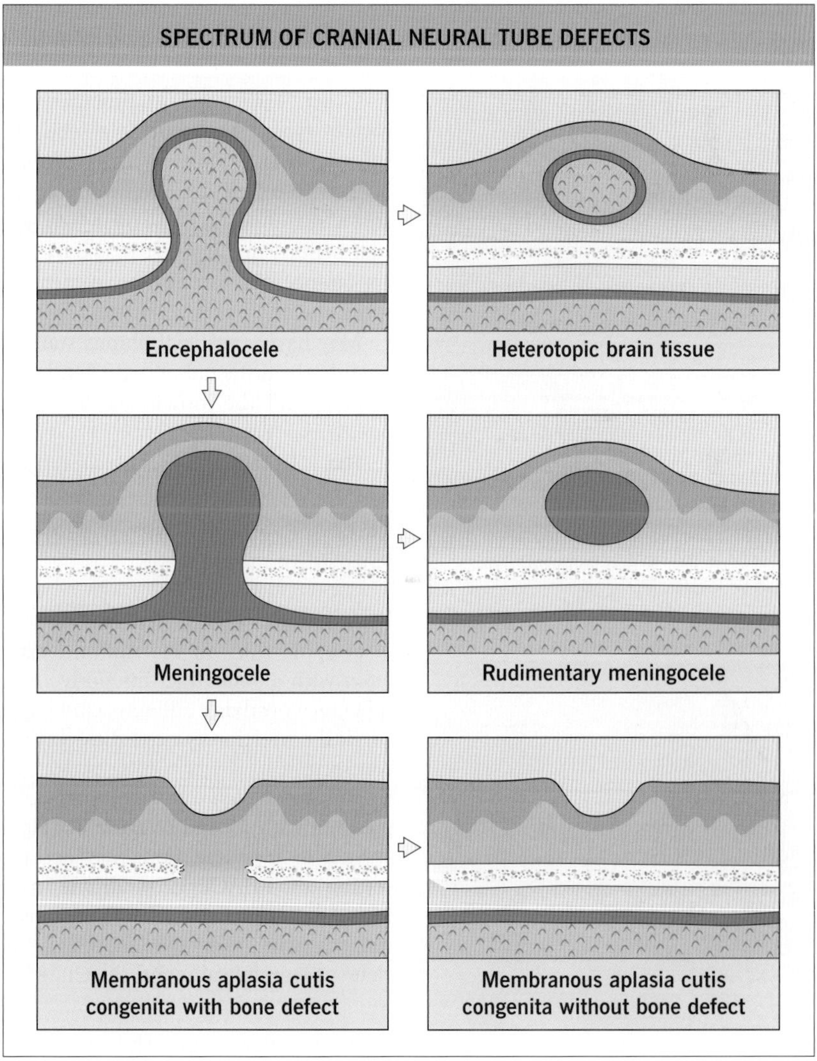

SPECTRUM OF CRANIAL NEURAL TUBE DEFECTS

Encephalocele

Heterotopic brain tissue

Meningocele

Rudimentary meningocele

Membranous aplasia cutis congenita with bone defect

Membranous aplasia cutis congenita without bone defect

Fig. 53.3 Spectrum of cranial neural tube defects.

DIFFERENTIAL DIAGNOSIS OF NASAL MASSES PRESENTING AT BIRTH OR DURING INFANCY
Cysts and developmental defects
Midline lesions (see Fig. 53.1)
• Dermoid cyst, nasal glioma, cephalocele
Other lesions
• Vascular malformation (e.g. lymphatic, venous; see Ch. 85) • Epidermoid cyst (see Ch. 90), pilomatricoma (see Ch. 91), nasolacrimal duct cyst
Benign neoplasms and hamartomas
• Infantile hemangioma (see Ch. 85), neurofibroma (see Ch. 95) • Hamartomas (e.g. chondromesenchymal, lipomatous), teratoma*
Malignant neoplasms
• Rhabdomyosarcoma > fibrosarcoma, neuroblastoma

*May also be malignant.

Table 53.1 Differential diagnosis of nasal masses presenting at birth or during infancy.

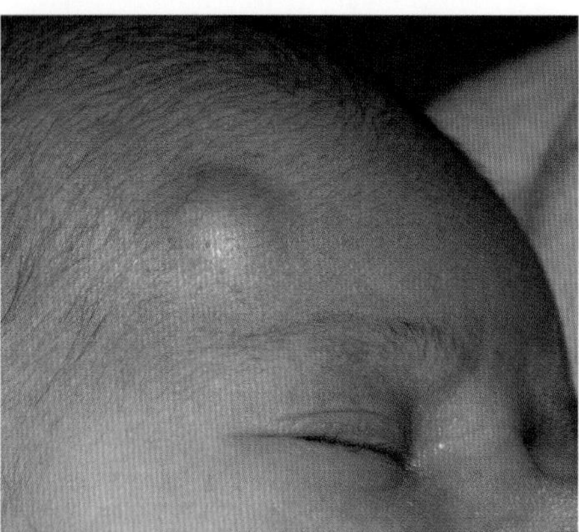

Fig. 53.4 Dermoid cyst. This dermoid cyst presented in an infant as a firm subcutaneous nodule superior to the right lateral eyebrow. *Courtesy, Julie V. Schaffer, MD.*

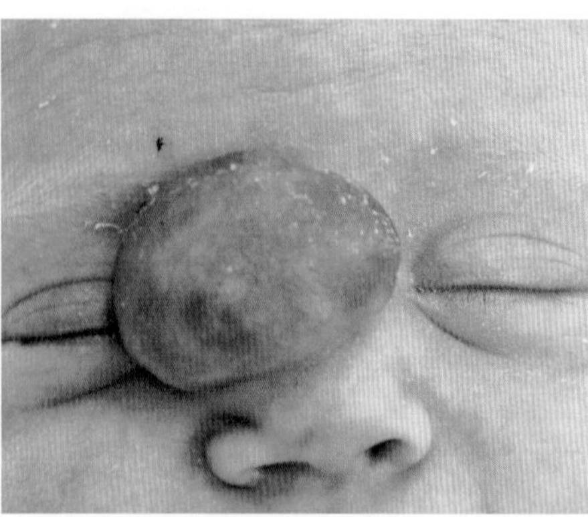

Fig. 53.5 Nasal glioma. A mass was noted on prenatal ultrasound, and this reddish, slightly pedunculated, rubbery nodule was evident at birth. *Courtesy, Mary Chang, MD.*

- Other HBT and rudimentary meningoceles typically present as a solid or cystic subcutaneous nodule on the midline scalp, often with a blue-red hue, overlying alopecia and a surrounding hair collar (see above); a rudimentary meningocele may have a bullous appearance and can also be located over the spine.
- May have a vestigial fibrous stalk extending into the intracranial space, but lack a connection with the intracranial leptomeninges or CSF (see Fig. 53.3).
- **Rx:** MRI followed by surgical excision.

Midline Cervical, Sternal, and Supraumbilical Clefts

- A *midline cervical cleft* is a vertical band of atrophic skin on the mid anterior neck, often with a sinus tract inferiorly and a protuberance overlying a fibrous cord superiorly; surgical correction is needed to prevent neck contracture.
- A *sternal cleft* or *supraumbilical raphe* presents with a band of atrophic (Fig. 53.6), scarred or ulcerated skin; may occur in the setting of PHACE(S) syndrome (*p*osterior fossa malformations; *h*emangiomas; *a*rterial, *c*ardiac, and *e*ye anomalies; *s*ternal cleft/*s*upraumbilical raphe; see Ch. 85).

Midline Lesions Overlying the Spine

- Midline cutaneous lesions serve as a valuable marker for "occult" spinal dysraphism

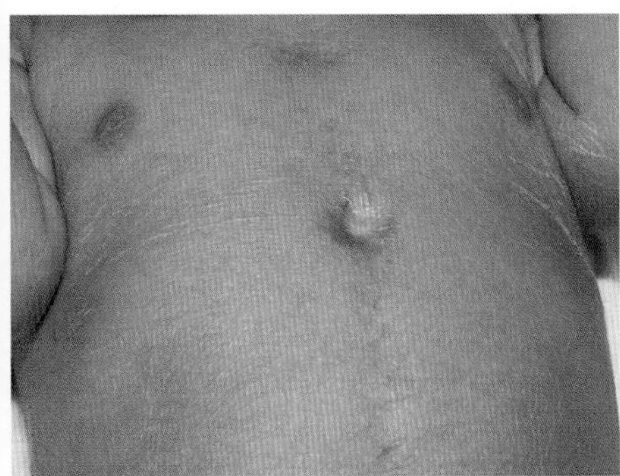

Fig. 53.6 Sternal cleft. Note the atrophic skin overlying the defect and prominent veins in the midline chest. Generalized desquamation is also evident in this 1-day-old post-term neonate. She did not develop an infantile hemangioma and had no cardiac defects or other features of PHACE(S) syndrome. *Courtesy, Julie V. Schaffer, MD.*

and are present in ~80% of affected individuals (most of whom have >1 type of skin lesion), compared to <3% of the general population; shallow coccygeal dimples and deep gluteal clefts, which are considered as normal variants, occur in an additional 4% of infants.

- Skin lesions associated with spinal dysraphism are presented in Table 53.2 and Fig. 53.7.
- **Rx:** Fig. 53.8 outlines an approach to patients with skin signs of spinal dysraphism.

Aplasia Cutis Congenita (Congenital Absence of Skin)

- ACC is a physical finding: areas of skin (localized or widespread) that are absent or scarred at birth.
- Possible causes of ACC include genetic factors, vascular compromise, trauma, teratogens, and intrauterine infections.
- The morphology and distribution of the skin defects (Figs 53.9 and 53.10) and the presence or absence of associated abnormalities represent clues to the etiology of ACC (Table 53.3).
- The most common form is *membranous ACC*, which favors the scalp (especially the vertex) and presents as a sharply marginated, round to oval defect that is covered by a thin translucent membrane and often surrounded by a hair collar (see Fig. 53.2 and above); may have a bullous appearance in neonates, evolving into an atrophic scar.
- An autosomal dominant form of scalp ACC presents with hypertrophic scarring. Another ACC morphology is stellate or angulated ulcerations, which may result from vascular abnormalities and/or intrauterine ischemic events (see Table 53.3).
- **DDx:** obstetric trauma, rudimentary meningocele (especially if bullous).
- Imaging is recommended for irregular and membranous lesions on the scalp, in particular those that are large and/or deep, to assess for underlying skull defects and vascular anomalies.
- **Rx:** topical antibiotic ointment until re-epithelialization occurs; early surgical repair of large, deep stellate scalp lesions to prevent life-threatening hemorrhage, thrombosis, or meningitis.

Congenital Lip and Ear Pits

- *Commissural lip pits*: most common form of lip pits (1–2% of newborns), found bilaterally at angles of mouth (Fig. 53.11A); usually isolated, occasionally associated with branchio-otic syndrome (preauricular pits, deafness).
- *Lower lip pits*: typically bilateral at apex of conical elevation (Fig. 53.11C); isolated > associated with Van der Woude (cleft lip/palate, hypodontia) or popliteal pterygium syndrome.
- *Upper lip pits*: along philtrum or paramedian (Fig. 53.11B); isolated > associated findings (e.g. hypertelorism) or branchio-oculo-facial syndrome (see below).
- *Ear pits*: affect 0.5–1% of newborns, presenting as an invagination (Fig. 53.11D) > cystic nodule in the upper preauricular area (unilateral > bilateral); usually isolated (± autosomal dominant inheritance), occasionally associated with hearing impairment or malformation syndromes (e.g. branchio-oto-(±)renal syndrome, hemifacial microsomia).

Accessory Tragi (Preauricular Tags)

- Congenital anomalies of the first branchial arch that are found in ~5 per 1000 newborns.
- Soft or firm (due to a cartilaginous core) skin-colored papules or nodules covered by vellus hairs.

SKIN LESIONS OF THE SPINAL AXIS ASSOCIATED WITH DYSRAPHISM	
Lesion	**Features**
Hypertrichosis	A V-shaped patch of long, coarse or silky hair (see Fig. 53.7B,C); "faun tail"
Lipomas	Soft subcutaneous mass, asymmetric buttocks, curved gluteal cleft (see Fig. 53.7A); most common sign of spinal dysraphism
Dimples	Above the gluteal cleft or >2.5 cm from the anal verge in neonates (see Fig. 53.7A,D); >0.5 cm in size or deep*
Dermal sinuses	Hair may be present at the ostium*
Acrochordons	May be associated with a dimple or dermal sinus
Pseudotails	Caudal protrusion due to prolonged vertebrae or hamartomatous elements, e.g. adipose tissue or cartilage (see Fig. 53.7A,D)
True tails	Persistent vestigial appendage with a central core of mature adipose tissue, muscle, blood vessels, and nerves May be capable of spontaneous or reflex motion
Infantile hemangiomas	Usually superficial with a segmental pattern (see Fig. 53.7D) and often ulcerated; represents a component of LUMBAR syndrome
Telangiectasias	May represent an early, minimal/arrested growth or regressed infantile hemangioma
Vascular malformations**	Capillary malformations are typically found together with other skin lesions Cobb syndrome: spinal arteriovenous malformation associated with segmental skin lesions mimicking a CM or angiokeratomas
Aplasia cutis congenita (ACC)	Ulcer, scar, or atrophic skin
Connective tissue nevus	Typically found together with other skin lesions
Hypo/depigmentation	May represent a nevus depigmentosus (typically found together with other skin lesions) or the residua of ACC
Hyperpigmentation	Typically found together with other skin lesions
Congenital melanocytic nevi	Spinal dysraphism has been reported in patients with neurocutaneous melanosis
Subcutaneous masses	May represent (lipomyelo)meningoceles or teratomas

**Due to a potential risk of meningitis, these lesions should not be probed.*
***The common occipital nevus simplex ("stork bite") and lumbosacral capillary stains in the setting of additional nevus simplex lesions on the head/neck (but no other lumbosacral skin lesions) are generally not considered to be signs of spinal dysraphism.*

Table 53.2 Skin lesions of the spinal axis associated with dysraphism. The presence of two or more types of lesions increases the risk of a spinal anomaly. LUMBAR, lumbosacral hemangiomas and lipomas, urogenital anomalies and ulceration, myelopathy, bony deformities, anorectal and arterial malformations, renal anomalies.

- Located in preauricular area > mandibular cheek or anterolateral neck (*congenital cartilaginous rests of the neck* or *"wattles"*) (Fig. 53.12).
- Usually an isolated finding; occasionally associated with hearing impairment or malformation syndromes (e.g. hemifacial microsomia).
- **Rx:** assessment of hearing; excision, with care to remove any cartilaginous component.

Branchial Cleft Cysts, Sinuses, and Fistulae

- Located on the neck along the anterior border of the sternocleidomastoid muscle or in the mandibular or preauricular region (see Fig. 53.1).
- *Branchial cleft cysts* lack a primary cutaneous opening and typically present in older children and adults when they become infected or inflamed.

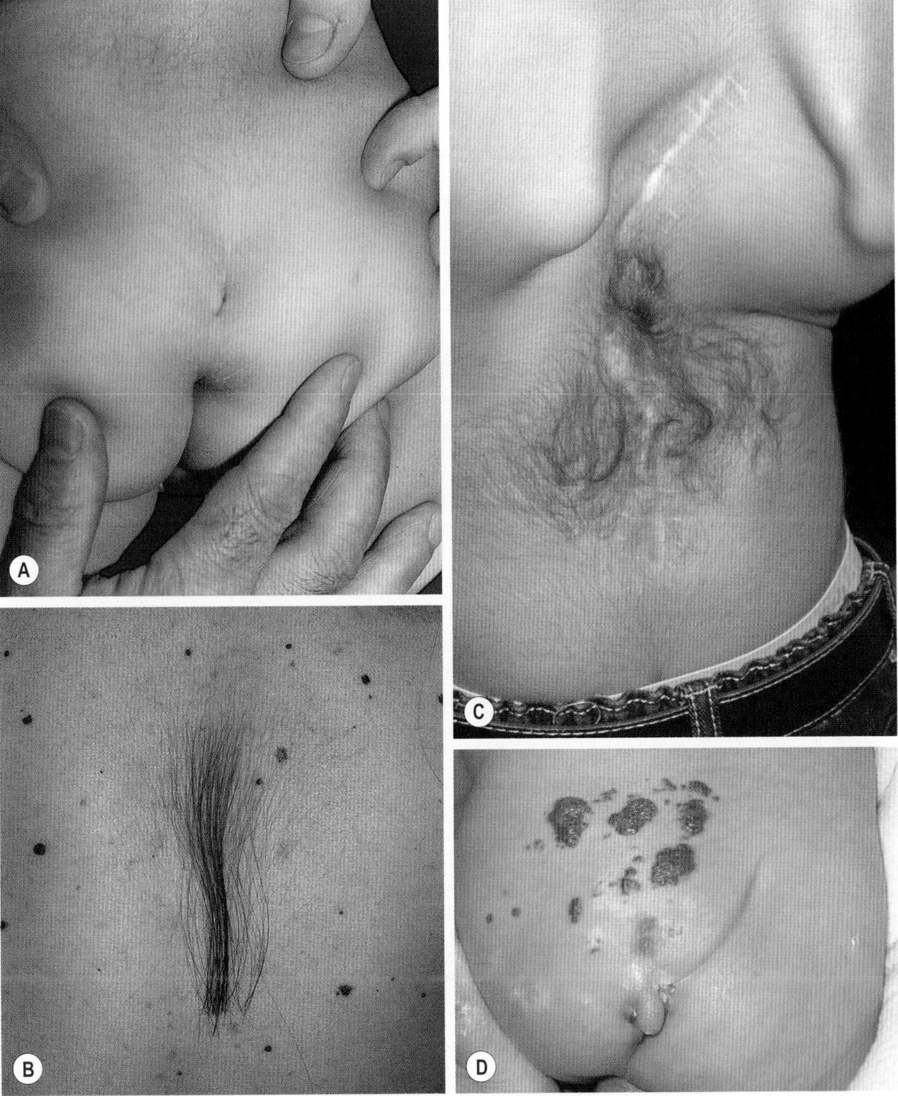

Fig. 53.7 Skin findings associated with spinal dysraphism. **A** Midline deep sacral dimple located above the gluteal cleft in association with a small pseudotail. In contrast, a shallow dimple within the gluteal cleft is a common finding and not a sign of spinal dysraphism. **B** Circumscribed midline hypertrichosis overlying the lower thoracic spine in a patient with occult dysraphism. The patient periodically clips the distal ends. **C** V-shaped patch of long, coarse hair on the mid back in a boy born with a large thoracic myelomeningocele. Severe scoliosis remains after multiple surgeries. **D** This infant with segmental infantile hemangiomas, a dimple, a pseudotail, and a deviated gluteal cleft had an underlying lipomyelomeningocele. *A, Courtesy, Seth Orlow, MD; B, Courtesy, Jean L. Bolognia, MD; C, Courtesy, Julie V. Schaffer, MD; D, Courtesy, Richard Antaya, MD.*

- *Branchial cleft sinuses/fistulae* usually have a sinus ostium with mucus discharge that is evident at birth or during the first few years of life.
- Usually an isolated anomaly, but occasionally associated with branchio-oto-(±) renal and branchio-oculo-facial (with eroded/"hemangiomatous" overlying skin) syndromes.
- **Rx:** surgical excision after delineation of extent with MRI or fistulography (via CT or intraoperatively).

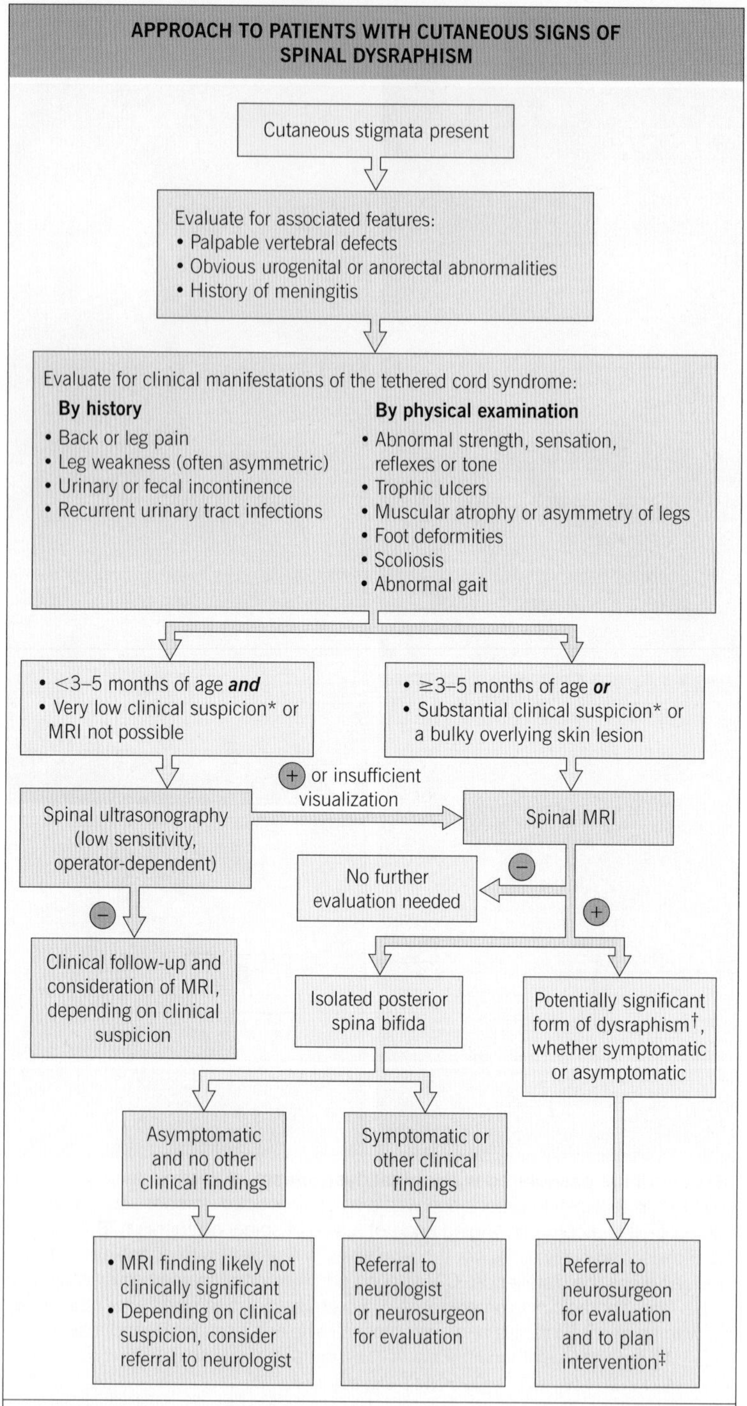

APPROACH TO PATIENTS WITH CUTANEOUS SIGNS OF SPINAL DYSRAPHISM

Cutaneous stigmata present

↓

Evaluate for associated features:
- Palpable vertebral defects
- Obvious urogenital or anorectal abnormalities
- History of meningitis

↓

Evaluate for clinical manifestations of the tethered cord syndrome:

By history
- Back or leg pain
- Leg weakness (often asymmetric)
- Urinary or fecal incontinence
- Recurrent urinary tract infections

By physical examination
- Abnormal strength, sensation, reflexes or tone
- Trophic ulcers
- Muscular atrophy or asymmetry of legs
- Foot deformities
- Scoliosis
- Abnormal gait

↓

Left branch:
- <3–5 months of age ***and***
- Very low clinical suspicion* or MRI not possible

→ Spinal ultrasonography (low sensitivity, operator-dependent)
- (+) or insufficient visualization → Spinal MRI
- (−) → Clinical follow-up and consideration of MRI, depending on clinical suspicion

Right branch:
- ≥3–5 months of age ***or***
- Substantial clinical suspicion* or a bulky overlying skin lesion

→ Spinal MRI
- (−) → No further evaluation needed
- (+) →
  - Isolated posterior spina bifida
    - Asymptomatic and no other clinical findings → • MRI finding likely not clinically significant • Depending on clinical suspicion, consider referral to neurologist
    - Symptomatic or other clinical findings → Referral to neurologist or neurosurgeon for evaluation
  - Potentially significant form of dysraphism†, whether symptomatic or asymptomatic → Referral to neurosurgeon for evaluation and to plan intervention‡

* See Table 53.2; the presence of ≥2 types of skin lesions increases the risk of dysraphism

† E.g., meningocele, intraspinal lipoma, lipomyelomeningocele, diastematomyelia (split cord), syringomyelia (fluid within the cord), tight filum terminale, dermoid cyst/dermal sinus

‡ If indicated, surgery should be performed prior to the development of symptoms and potentially irreversible neurologic damage

Fig. 53.8 Approach to patients with cutaneous signs of spinal dysraphism.
Courtesy, Julie V. Schaffer, MD.

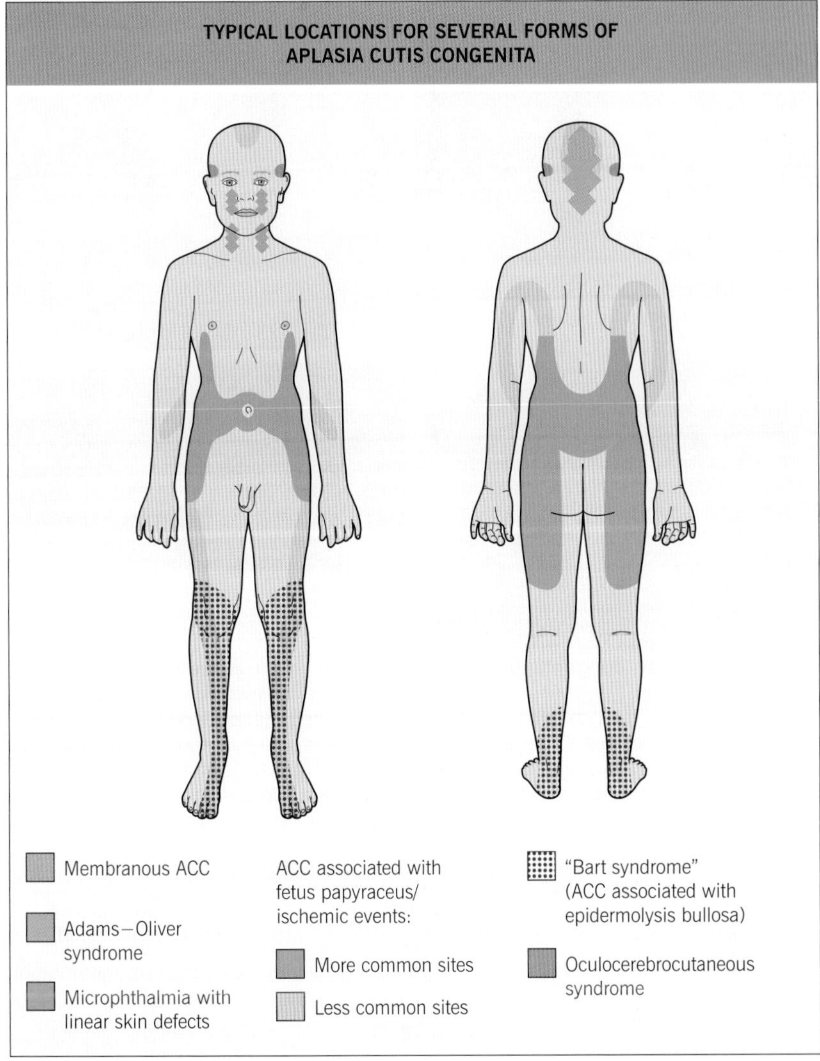

Fig. 53.9 Typical locations for several forms of aplasia cutis congenita (ACC). See Fig. 53.1 for Brauer lines/Setleis syndrome and preauricular membranous ACC. *Courtesy, Julie V. Schaffer, MD.*

Thyroglossal Duct Cysts and Bronchogenic Cysts (See Fig. 53.1)

- *Thyroglossal duct cysts* present in children and young adults as a nodule on the mid anterior neck that moves with swallowing.
- *Cutaneous bronchogenic cysts* typically appear as a congenital papule or nodule, most often in the suprasternal notch or surrounding areas; mucus discharge is sometimes noted.
- **Rx:** surgical excision.

Omphalomesenteric Duct Cysts and Urachal Cysts

- Defective closure of the omphalomesenteric duct, the embryonic connection between the midgut and yolk sac, can result in an umbilical-enteric fistula, umbilical sinus or *omphalomesenteric duct cyst*, which typically presents as an umbilical polyp (Fig. 53.13).
- A patent urachus, which connects the fetal bladder to the umbilicus, results in leakage of urine from the umbilicus; in contrast, a *urachal*

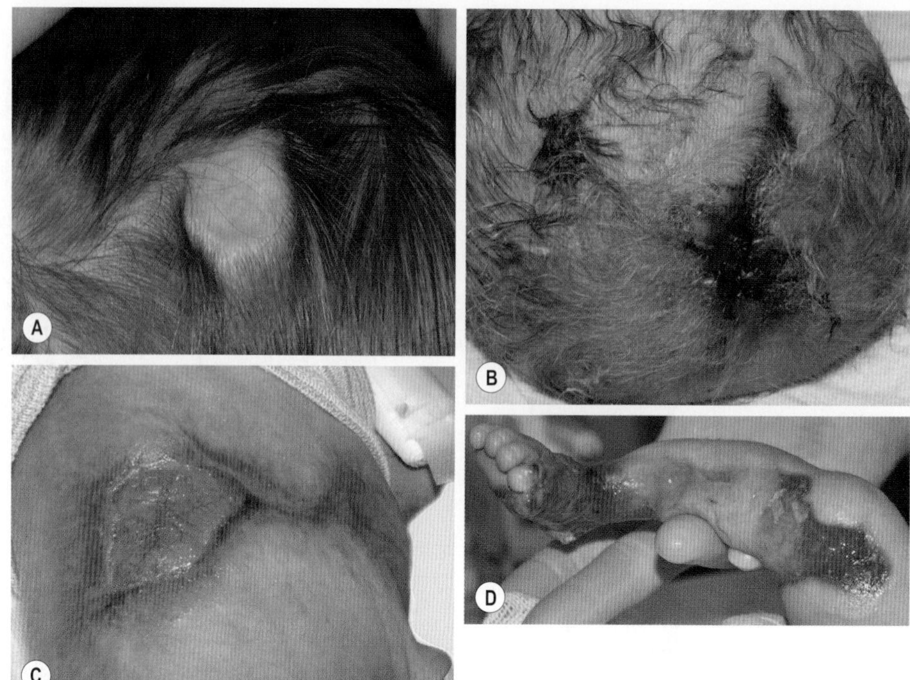

Fig. 53.10 **Aplasia cutis congenita (ACC). A** This hairless, round, scarred plaque on the scalp of a 6-month-old was present at birth. **B** Stellate ACC on the midline scalp of a neonate with mosaic trisomy 13. This hemorrhagic lesion was associated with an underlying skull defect and cerebrovascular anomalies. **C** Stellate ACC on the lateral trunk of a neonate born of an initial sextuplet gestation for which fetal reduction was performed. The lesions had a bilateral, symmetric distribution. **D** ACC on the leg in a neonate with epidermolysis bullosa. *A, Courtesy, Anthony J. Mancini, MD; B, C, Courtesy, Julie V. Schaffer, MD; D, Courtesy, Emily Berger MD.*

CLASSIFICATION SCHEME FOR APLASIA CUTIS CONGENITA (ACC)		
Group	**Inheritance**	**Location, features, and associated abnormalities**
1. Isolated scalp ACC (see Figs 53.2 and 53.10A)	Sporadic > AD	• Favors vertex: membranous with hair collar
	Often AD	• Favors vertex: irregular hypertrophic scars
2. Scalp ACC associated with Adams–Oliver syndrome (limb reductions, CMTC)	AD > AR	• Large, irregular lesions on midline scalp • Frequent skull defect and dilated scalp veins
3. Scalp ACC associated with epidermal, sebaceous, and/or large congenital melanocytic nevi	Sporadic	• Scalp, often unilateral and membranous • ± Ipsilateral ophthalmologic or CNS abnormalities
4. ACC overlying embryologic malformations	Variable	• Scalp with hair collar (heterotopic brain/meningeal tissue) • Lumbosacral (spinal dysraphism) • Anterior trunk (sternal defect, omphalocele)
5. ACC associated with fetus papyraceus* (see Fig. 53.10C), placental infarct, or other ischemic events	Sporadic	• Scalp, chest, flanks, axillae, extremities • Multiple, symmetric • Stellate/angulated morphology

Table 53.3 Classification scheme for aplasia cutis congenita (ACC). *Continued*

CLASSIFICATION SCHEME FOR APLASIA CUTIS CONGENITA (ACC)		
Group	**Inheritance**	**Location, features, and associated abnormalities**
6. ACC associated with epidermolysis bullosa (simplex, junctional, or dystrophic; see Ch. 26 and Fig. 53.10D)	AD or AR	• Lower extremities ("Bart syndrome") or widespread
7. ACC localized to extremities without blistering	Variable	• Pretibial areas, extensor forearms (± radial dysplasia), dorsal hands/feet
8. ACC caused by teratogens (e.g. methimazole), maternal conditions (e.g. antiphospholipid syndrome), or intrauterine infections (e.g. varicella, HSV)	Not inherited	• Scalp with drugs • Any site with congenital infections
9. ACC associated with malformation syndromes	Variable	• Favors scalp, e.g. in trisomy 13 (see Fig. 53.10B), 4p- syndrome, and Goltz syndrome

Due to second trimester death of a co-twin/triplet.

Table 53.3 *Continued* **Classification scheme for aplasia cutis congenita (ACC).** CMTC, cutis marmorata telangiectatica congenita.

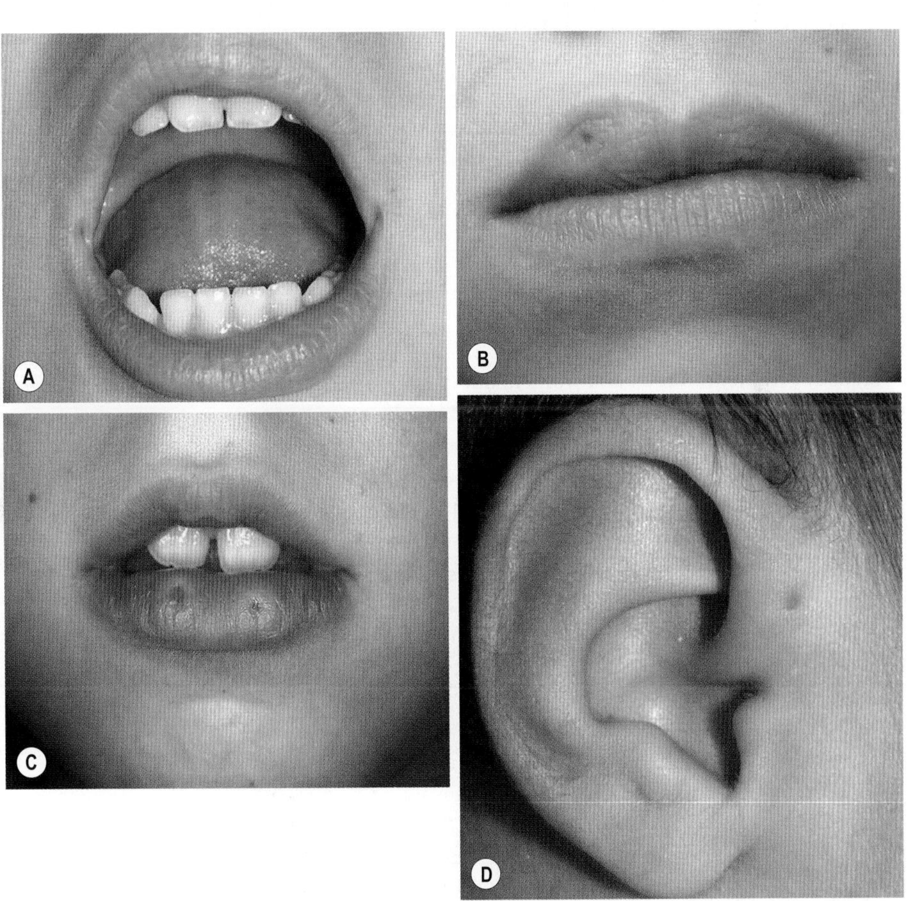

Fig. 53.11 Lip and ear pits. A Bilateral commissural lip pits. **B** Unilateral right-sided upper lip pit. **C** Bilateral paramedian lower lip pits, each located on the apex of a conical elevation. **D** Ear pit. In all of these patients, the pits represented an isolated finding. *A, B, Courtesy, Richard Antaya, MD; C, Courtesy, NYUDSC; D, Courtesy, Julie V. Schaffer, MD.*

cyst typically presents with an umbilical mass, often in the setting of a secondary infection.

- **DDx:** umbilical granuloma (persistent granulation tissue after cord separation).
- **Rx:** excision after radiographic studies to determine extent.

Rudimentary Supernumerary Digits (Rudimentary Polydactyly)

- Found in 0.5–1:1000 white newborns and 5–10:1000 black newborns.
- Soft-tissue duplications without a skeletal component, usually arising from the ulnar side of the fifth finger (postaxial location) (Fig. 53.14).
- Range from small, fleshy or wart-like papules to pedunculated nodules that may contain cartilage or a vestigial nail; frequently bilateral.
- Typically an isolated finding, often with an autosomal dominant inheritance pattern.
- **Rx:** surgical excision; removal via ligation with suture material increases risk of infection and often leaves a residual papule that becomes a painful neuroma.

Supernumerary Nipples and Other Accessory Mammary Tissue

- Present in 2–5% of the population, representing remnants of the embryonic "milk lines" (Fig. 53.15A).
- Equally prevalent in men and women, but often become more prominent at puberty or during pregnancy in female patients.
- Found on the inframammary chest > axilla, vulva, or upper medial thigh.
- Small, soft, pink or brown papules, with or without a surrounding areola (Fig. 53.15B, C); ectopic glandular breast tissue is occasionally present (± a nipple/areola), especially in the axilla or vulva.
- Usually an isolated finding; controversial potential association with malformations of the kidneys or urinary tract, and occasionally seen together with a Becker's nevus or malformation syndrome.
- **Rx:** excision if symptomatic or cosmetically undesirable; accessory mammary tissue can develop the same disorders as normal breasts and requires periodic breast cancer screening.

Amniotic Band Sequence and Disorganization Syndrome

- Various congenital anomalies of the limbs, head, body wall, and viscera with asymmetric, seemingly haphazard distribution patterns.
- Characterized by fibrous bands that form constriction rings and lead to amputations of limbs/digits.
- Extrinsic (entanglement in torn amnion) and intrinsic (endogenous "disorganization syndrome") hypotheses for its pathogenesis; latter is favored by the presence of duplicated structures and internal malformations.
- **Rx:** surgical release of constriction bands.

For further information see Ch. 64 from *Dermatology, Fourth Edition*.

For additional online figures visit www.expertconsult.com 

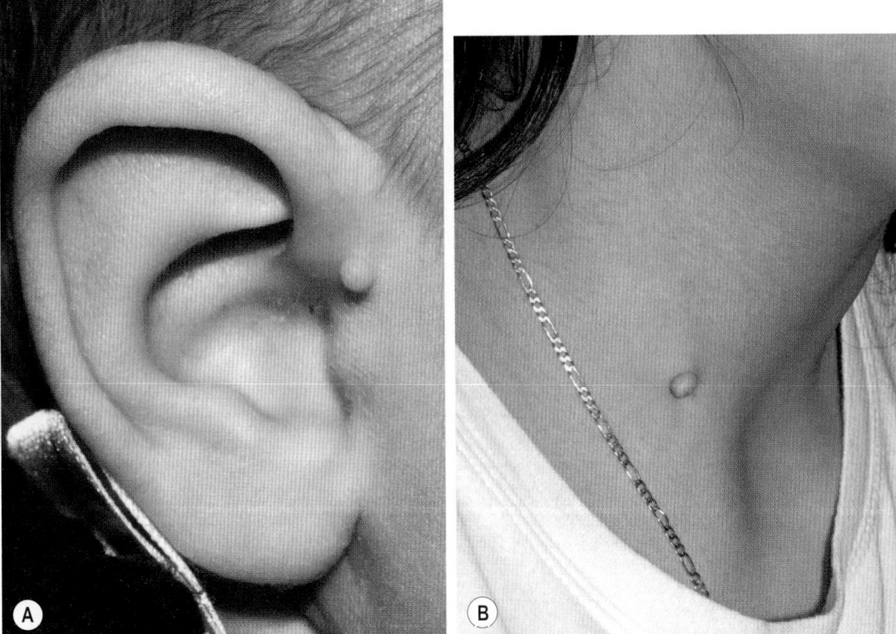

Fig. 53.12 Accessory tragi. **A** Typical small preauricular papule. **B** Congenital cartilaginous rest on the neck, which is considered to represent a cervical subtype of accessory tragus. *Courtesy, Julie V. Schaffer, MD.*

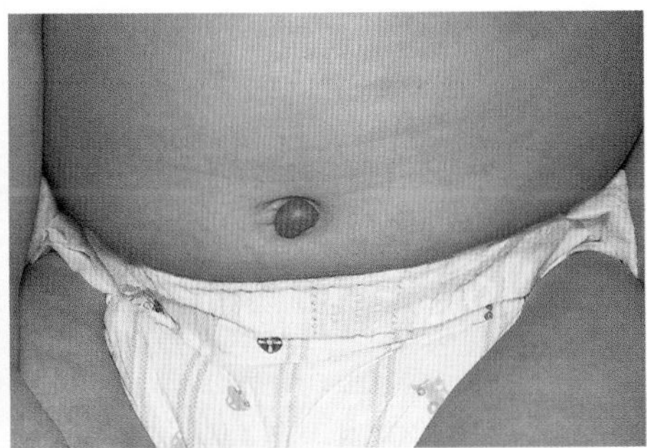

Fig. 53.13 Omphalomesenteric duct cyst. The pink papule in the umbilicus of this infant showed gastrointestinal epithelium histologically. *Courtesy, Mary S. Stone, MD.*

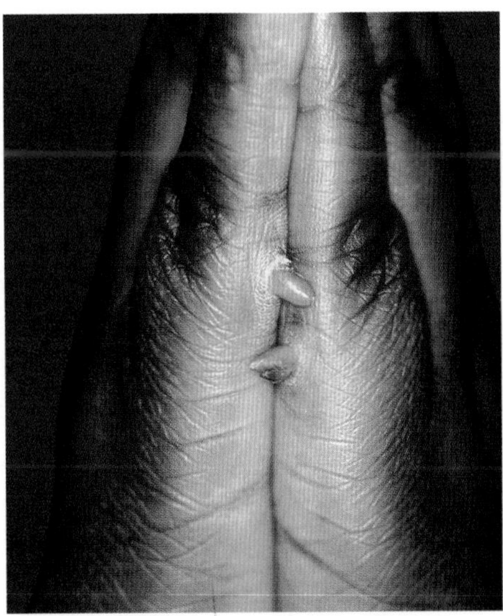

Fig. 53.14 Bilateral rudimentary supernumerary digits. The ulnar side of the fifth digit is the most common location (referred to as postaxial). *Courtesy, YDRSC.*

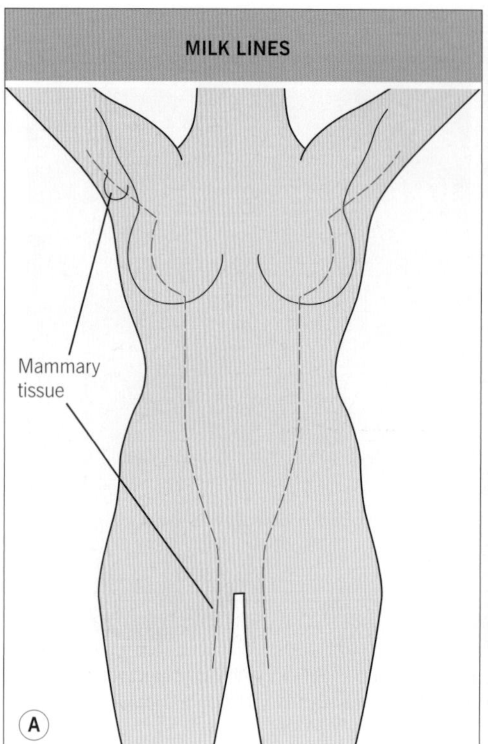

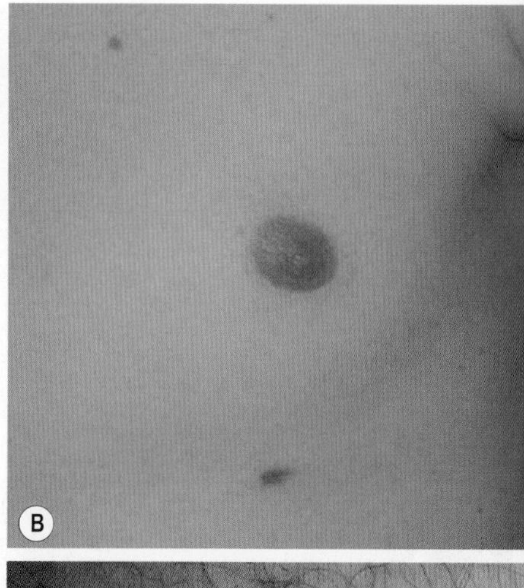

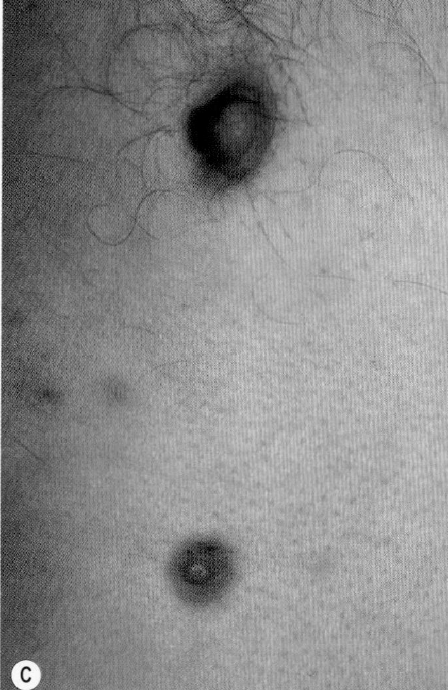

Fig. 53.15 Supernumerary nipples. A Supernumerary nipples and other forms of accessory mammary tissue represent focal remnants of the embryologic mammary ridges ("milk lines") that extend from the anterior axillary fold to the upper medial thigh bilaterally. **B** Brown papule that might be mistaken for a melanocytic nevus. **C** Nipple with a surrounding areola. *A, B, Courtesy, Julie V. Schaffer, MD; C, Courtesy, Jean L. Bolognia, MD.*

Vitiligo and Other Disorders of Hypopigmentation

54

Introduction/Definitions

• **Leukoderma** and **hypopigmentation**: areas of skin are lighter in color than uninvolved skin, due primarily to a decrease in melanin; decreased blood supply to the skin (e.g. nevus anemicus) can be another cause of leukoderma.

• **Hypomelanosis**: an absence or reduction of melanin in the skin that may be due to any one or a combination of the following:

1. A decrease in the number of melanocytes (e.g. vitiligo).
2. A decrease in melanin synthesis by a normal number of melanocytes (e.g. albinism).
3. A decrease in the transfer of melanin to keratinocytes (e.g. postinflammatory hypopigmentation).

• **Amelanosis**: total absence of melanin in the skin.

• **Depigmentation**: usually implies a total loss of skin color (e.g. as in vitiligo).

• **Pigmentary dilution**: a generalized lightening of the skin, hair, and eyes (e.g. oculocutaneous albinism); sites of melanin production include the epidermis, hair follicles, pigmented retinal epithelium, and uveal tract.

• **Poliosis**: a lock of scalp hair, eyebrows, or eyelashes that is white in color.

• **Canities**: generalized depigmentation of scalp hair.

• **Wood's lamp examination**: the greater the loss of epidermal pigmentation, the more marked the contrast with uninvolved skin on Wood's lamp examination (see Table 2.1 and Fig. 61.10B).

• All disorders of hypopigmentation are more easily observed in darkly pigmented individuals or after a suntan.

Approach to Disorders of Hypopigmentation

• Assess the following parameters:

1. Age of onset (e.g. birth/infancy vs. childhood vs. adulthood).
2. Presence or absence of preceding inflammation.
3. Distribution pattern (see below) and anatomic location.
4. Degree of pigment loss.

• The distribution patterns can be divided into *circumscribed* (e.g. vitiligo), *diffuse* (e.g. albinism), *linear*, or *guttate* (e.g. idiopathic guttate hypomelanosis).

• An approach to leukoderma is outlined in Fig. 54.1.

Vitiligo

• An acquired disease, due to autoimmune destruction of melanocytes, that is characterized by circumscribed, amelanotic macules or patches of the skin and mucous membranes (Fig. 54.2); hairs within involved areas may be depigmented or pigmented; the uveal tract and retinal pigmented epithelium can also be affected.

• Two major subtypes of vitiligo: *generalized* (most common) and *localized* (Fig. 54.3).

• A polygenic disorder, i.e. involving multiple susceptibility genes, plus environmental factors (mostly unknown).

• There is an increased incidence of other autoimmune disorders (e.g. thyroid disease > Addison disease, pernicious anemia, SLE, rheumatoid arthritis, type I diabetes mellitus) in individuals with vitiligo as well as in family members; associated autoimmune skin disorders include halo melanocytic nevi, alopecia areata, and lichen sclerosus.

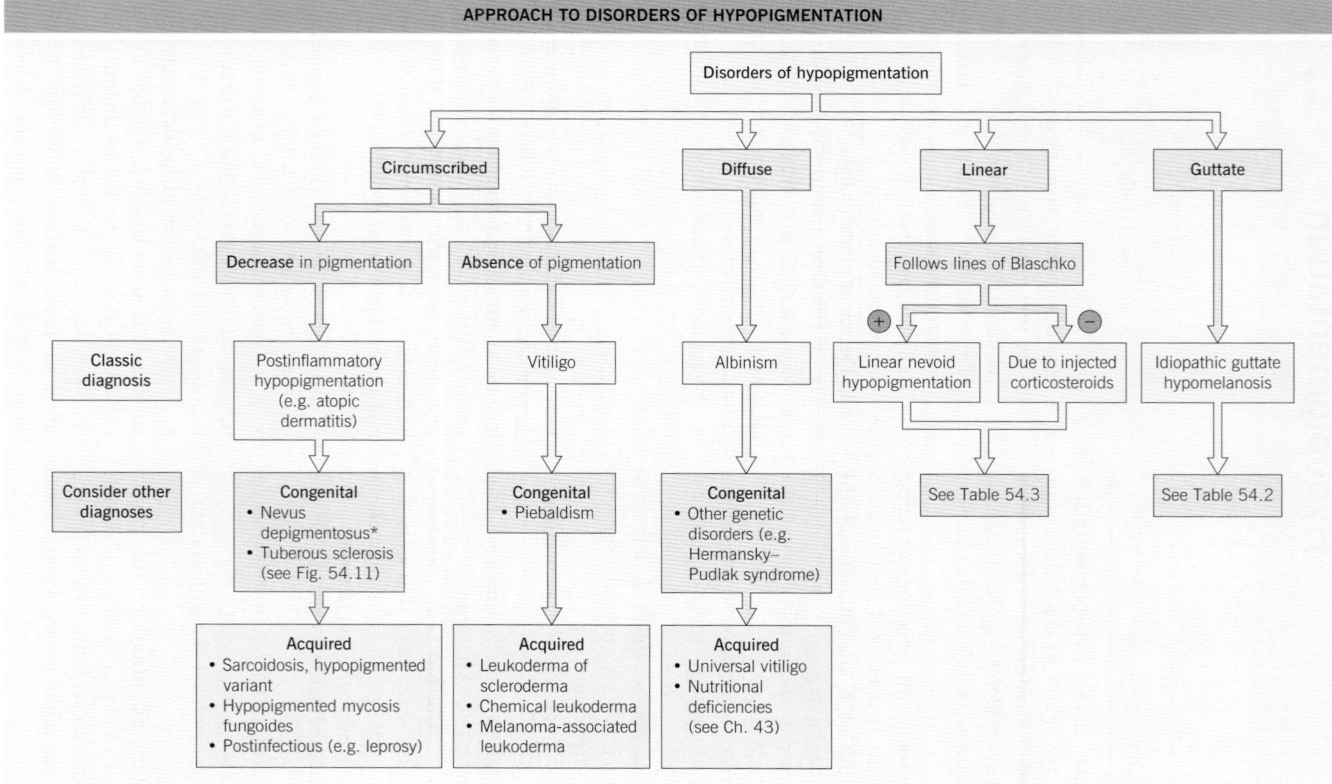

Fig. 54.1 Approach to disorders of hypopigmentation.

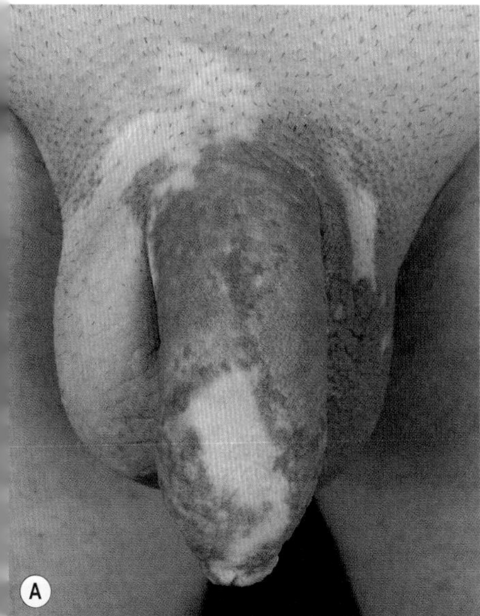

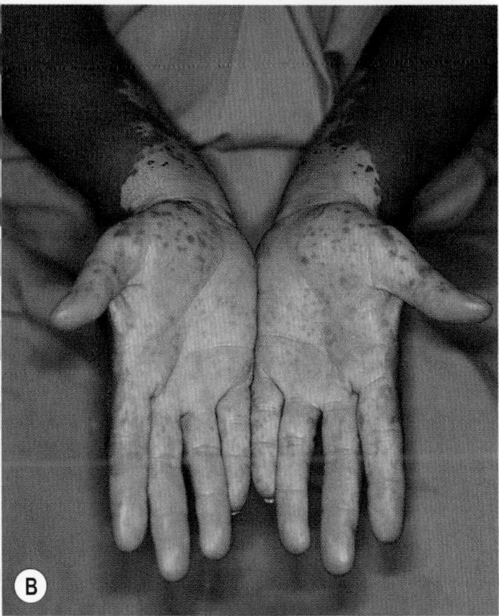

Fig. 54.2 Vitiligo. A Complete loss of pigment on the penis and scrotum. Note the lack of any secondary changes. **B** Depigmentation of the volar wrists as well as the palmar surfaces; easily recognizable in darkly pigmented individuals. *A, Courtesy, Lorenzo Cerroni, MD; B, Courtesy, Jean L. Bolognia, MD.*

- ***Generalized vitiligo.***
  - Includes acrofacial, vulgaris, and universal variants (see Fig. 54.3); occasionally an inflammatory edge is seen (Fig. 54.4)
  - Affects ~1% of the population worldwide; males = females; onset in ~50% before age 20 years; onset after age 50 years is unusual and prompts widening of the **DDx** (see below)
  - The typical lesion is an asymptomatic, amelanotic macule or patch that is milk or chalk-white in color; early on the pigment loss may not be complete; margins are fairly discrete and convex
  - Course is unpredictable, but often progressive
- ***Segmental vitiligo.***
  - Usually begins in childhood; typically presents in a unilateral, segmental pattern that respects the midline, most often with an initial rapidly progressive phase followed by stabilization within ~1–2 years (Fig. 54.5)
  - **DDx:** nevus depigmentosus (decreased but not total absence of pigment)
- **DDx** of depigmented lesion(s).
  - **In a child:** if 1–2 isolated circular or oval macules, stage 3 halo nevus; piebaldism, Waardenburg syndrome (see below)
  - **In an adult:** chemical leukoderma, melanoma-associated leukoderma, leukoderma of scleroderma, Vogt–Koyanagi–Harada syndrome, onchocerciasis, and postinflammatory *de*pigmentation (see below)
  - With the exception of onchocerciasis, or in areas of sclerosis or inflammation, a biopsy is not particularly helpful
- **Vitiligo and ocular disease.**
  - Uveitis is the most significant ocular abnormality; asymptomatic depigmented areas of the ocular fundus can also be seen
  - Uveitis is a major component of the *Vogt–Koyanagi–Harada syndrome*, in which patients also develop aseptic meningitis, otic involvement (e.g. dysacousia), poliosis, and vitiligo, especially of the head and neck region
  - *Alezzandrini syndrome* is a rare disorder characterized by unilateral facial vitiligo, poliosis, and ipsilateral ocular involvement
- **Rx:** primarily directed at halting the progression of disease and at repigmentation (Fig. 54.6); there is some evidence that earlier initiation of treatment is more effective.

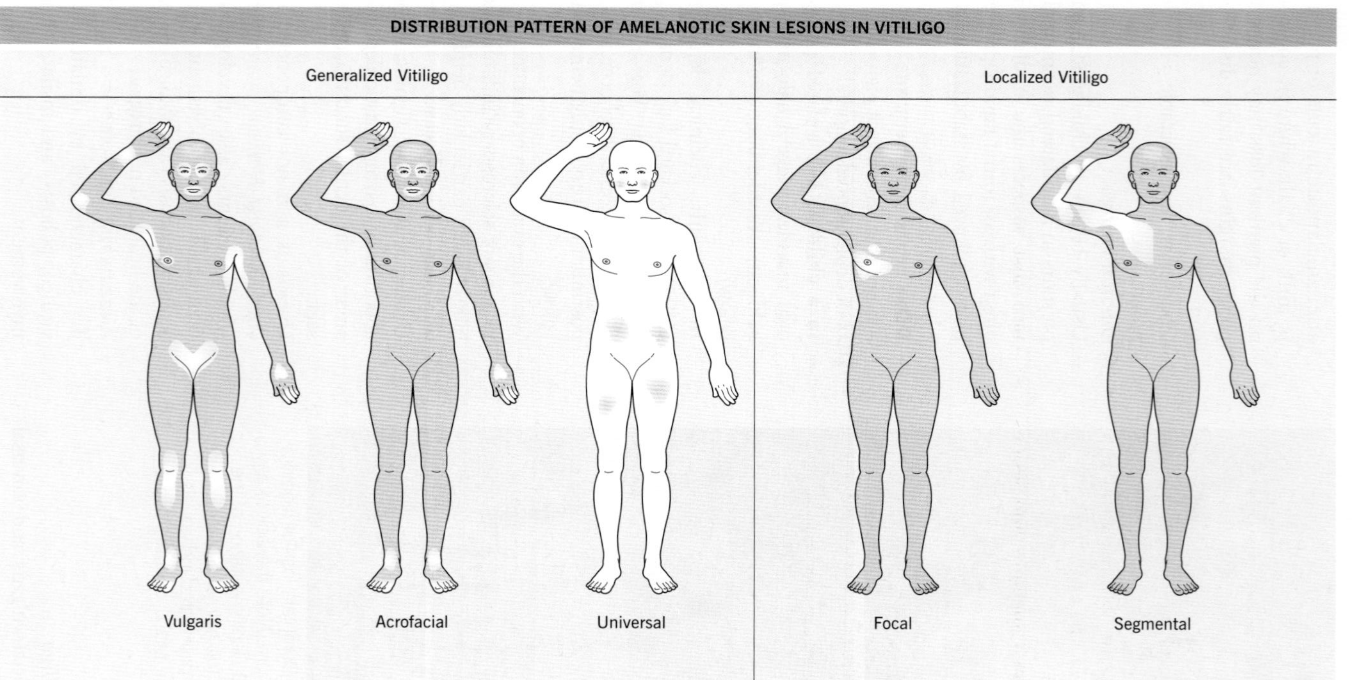

Fig. 54.3 Distribution of amelanotic skin lesions in vitiligo. Vitiligo is clinically divided into two broad categories: *generalized* and *localized*. The three distribution patterns in *generalized* vitiligo include *vulgaris*, *acrofacial*, and *universal*. In *focal* vitiligo, the amelanotic macules or patches are limited to one or only a few areas, but not necessarily in a segmental pattern, as in *segmental* vitiligo, which is also unilateral and respects the midline. *Adapted with permission from Le Poole C, Boissy RE. Vitiligo. Semin Cutan Med Surg 1997;16:3–14.*

- The choice of treatment depends upon the extent, location and activity of the vitiligo, as well as the patient's age, skin type, and motivation for treatment
- Treatment of progressive disease more difficult than stable disease
- Repigmentation usually appears in a perifollicular pattern (Fig. 54.7) and/or from the periphery of lesions; vitiligo in areas with hair (e.g. face, neck, mid extremities) is typically more responsive to treatment compared to distal digits and lips, which lack hair
- 10–20% monobenzyl ether of hydroquinone (MBEH) is sometimes used as depigmentation therapy for widespread or treatment-resistant vitiligo, but it can be permanent and lead to loss of pigment in areas distant to the sites of application

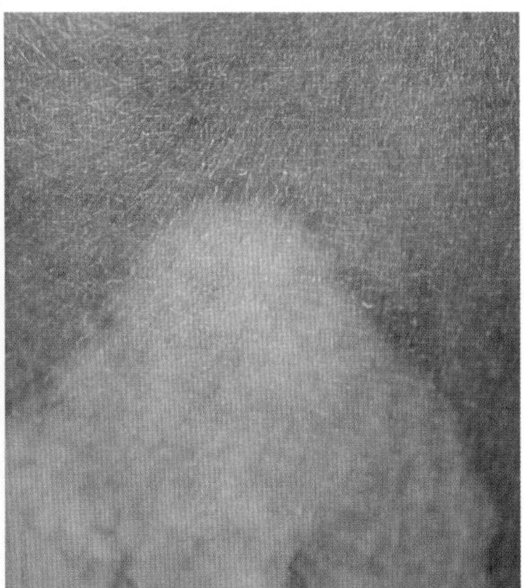

Fig. 54.4 Inflammatory vitiligo. An erythematous inflammatory border is evident. Such lesions are sometimes misdiagnosed as tinea corporis. *Courtesy, Thierry Passeron, MD.*

Hereditary Hypomelanosis

Oculocutaneous Albinism (OCA)

- A group of genetic disorders characterized by pigmentary dilution due to a partial or total absence of melanin within the skin, hair follicles, and eyes; the number of melanocytes is normal.
- Estimated frequency is 1:20,000, but may be 1:1500 in areas of Africa.
- Multiple types of OCA (Table 54.1) exist; nearly always inherited in an autosomal recessive manner; OCA1 and OCA2 constitute ~90% of all cases of OCA.
- The ocular manifestations are due to a decrease of melanin within eye structures (e.g. photophobia, reduced visual acuity) or the misrouting of optic nerve fibers during development (e.g. strabismus, nystagmus, lack of stereoscopic vision).
- Early ophthalmologic consultation and strict photoprotection are mandatory; the development of aggressive SCCs (Fig. 54.8A) is a significant cause of morbidity and mortality.

Disorders of Melanocyte Development

PIEBALDISM

- A rare autosomal dominant congenital disorder resulting primarily from mutations

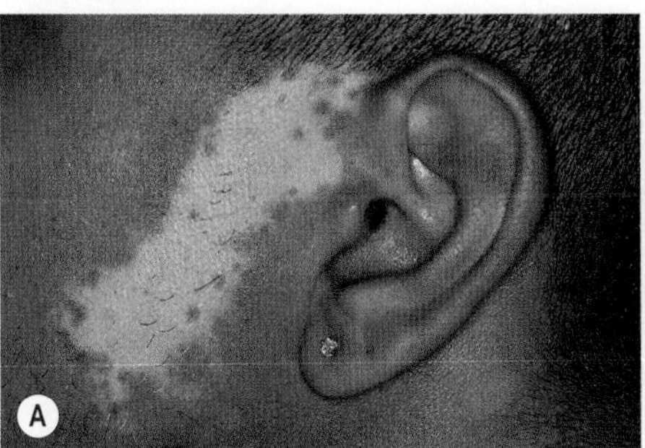

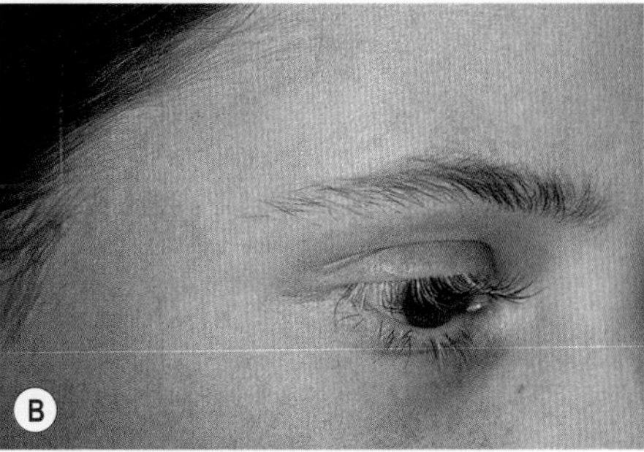

Fig. 54.5 Segmental vitiligo. A Unilateral band of depigmentation on the face, the most common location for segmental vitiligo. Note the pigmented and depigmented hairs within the affected area. **B** Under normal light, vitiligo can be subtle in lightly pigmented individuals. The clue to the diagnosis is the poliosis of the eyelashes. *A, Courtesy, Kalman Watsky MD; B, Courtesy, Jean L. Bolognia, MD.*

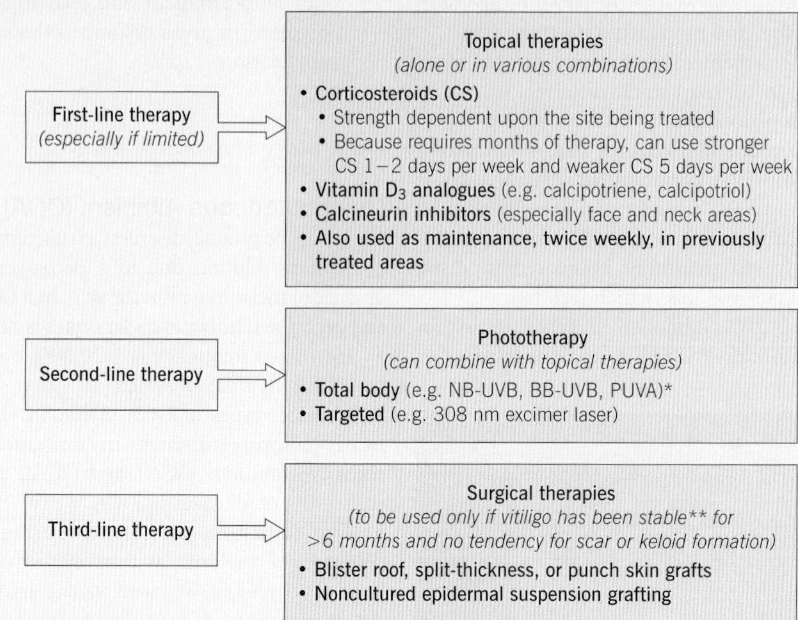

Fig. 54.6 Treatment options for vitiligo. Treatment of vitiligo is directed at halting the progression of disease and at repigmentation of patient-desired areas. Some clinicians may use oral or IM CS in the short term to help stabilize aggressive or rapidly progressive disease, in conjunction with other modalities. Camouflage can be offered to all patients for temporary (e.g. makeup, self-tanners) or more permanent (e.g. tattoos) cosmetic relief. Referral to a support group (e.g. Vitiligo Support International [vitiligosupport.org]) may also be helpful. 10–20% monobenzyl ether of hydroquinone (MBEH) is sometimes used (see text). Non-FDA-approved systemic therapies include an alpha-melanocyte-stimulating hormone analogue (afamelanotide) and JAK inhibitors, in combination with NB-UVB.

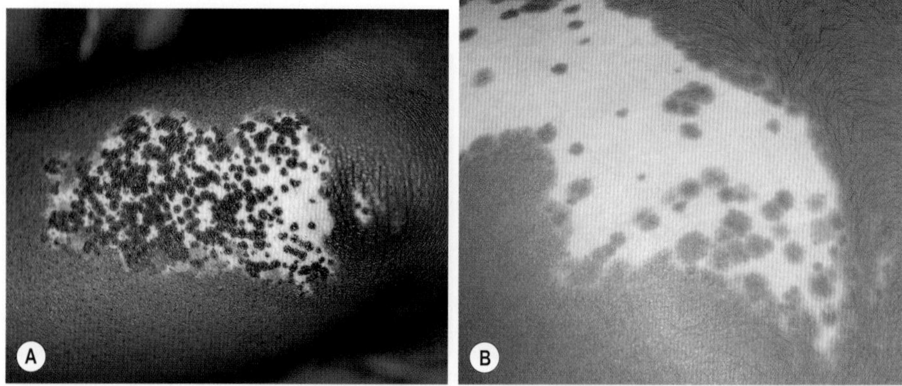

Fig. 54.7 Perifollicular repigmentation. Vitiligo on the elbow **(A)** and segmental vitiligo on the back **(B)** responding to PUVA and narrowband UVB therapy, respectively, with repigmentation in a prominent perifollicular pattern as well as from the periphery. The areas of repigmentation are darker in color than the uninvolved skin in **(A)**. *A, Courtesy, Jean L. Bolognia, MD; B, Courtesy, Julie V. Schaffer, MD.*

CLASSIFICATION OF OCULOCUTANEOUS ALBINISM (OCA)	
Type (gene mutation)	**Clinical features**
OCA1A (*TYR*) *absent* tyrosinase activity	• **At birth:** white hair, milk-white skin, blue-gray eyes, pink nevi • No increase in pigmentation over time, except for the denaturing (yellow color) of hair • Most severe ocular abnormalities (see text)
OCA1B (*TYR*) *reduced* tyrosinase activity	• **At birth:** similar to OCA1A • Majority acquire some pigmentation of hair and skin during first two decades of life • Ocular abnormalities less severe than in OCA1A
OCA2 *(OCA2)*	• **At birth:** more pigmentation compared to OCA1A • Over time, pigmented nevi may develop and large, stellate lentigines appear in photodistributed sites (Fig. 54.8B)
OCA3 *(TYRP1)*	• Red-bronze skin, ginger-red hair, blue or brown irides
OCA4 *(SLC45A2)*	• Similar clinical presentation as OCA2, with variability in pigmentation

Table 54.1 Classification of oculocutaneous albinism (OCA). Three additional, less common OCA subtypes include OCA5, OCA6, OCA7. SLC45A2, solute carrier family 45 member 2; TYR, tyrosinase; TYRP1, tyrosinase-related protein-1.

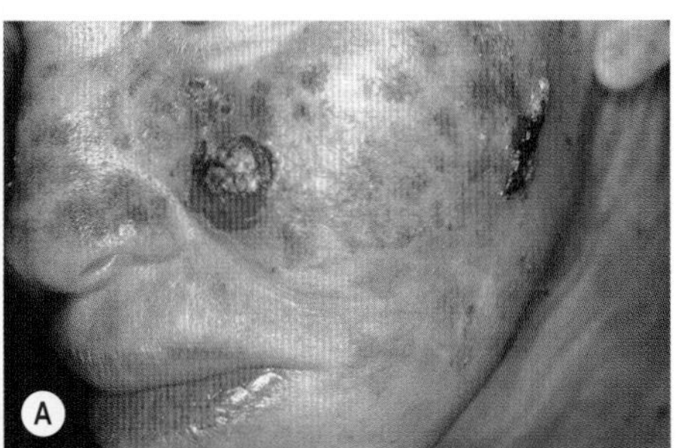

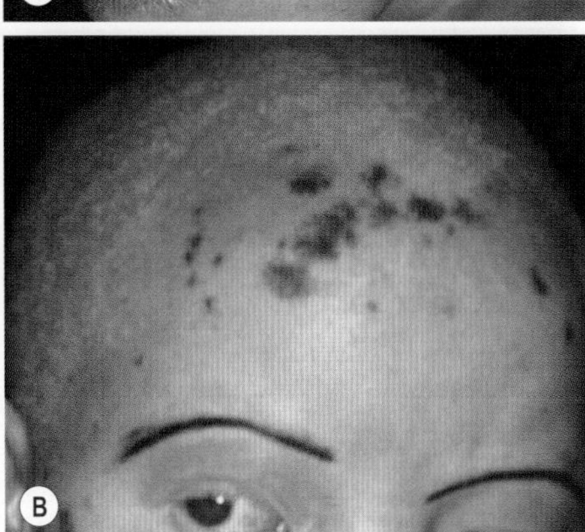

Fig. 54.8 Oculocutaneous albinism type 2 (OCA2). A African patient with obvious squamous cell carcinomas on the cheek as well as multiple pigmented lentigines. **B** African patient with hypopigmented hair and large pigmented lentigines. *Courtesy, James Nordlund, MD.*

in the *KIT* proto-oncogene, causing abnormal melanocyte development.

- Presents at birth with poliosis of the mid frontal scalp and stable circumscribed areas of amelanosis in a characteristic distribution pattern, favoring the anterior trunk, mid extremities, and central forehead (Fig. 54.9).
- Areas of amelanosis contain normally pigmented and hyperpigmented macules and patches within them (see Fig. 54.9); the latter can be seen in uninvolved skin.
- **Rx:** amenable to autologous skin grafting given its stability.

WAARDENBURG SYNDROME (WS)

- A rare autosomal dominant or recessive disorder characterized by:
  - Skin lesions resembling piebaldism, including the white forelock
  - Congenital deafness (10–40%)
  - Partial or total heterochromia iridis
  - Medial eyebrow hyperplasia (synophrys)
  - Broad nasal root
  - Dystopia canthorum (increase in the distance between the inner canthi with normal interpupillary distance)
- Four clinical subtypes have been described:
  - WS1: classic form
  - WS2: lacks dystopia canthorum (Fig. 54.10)

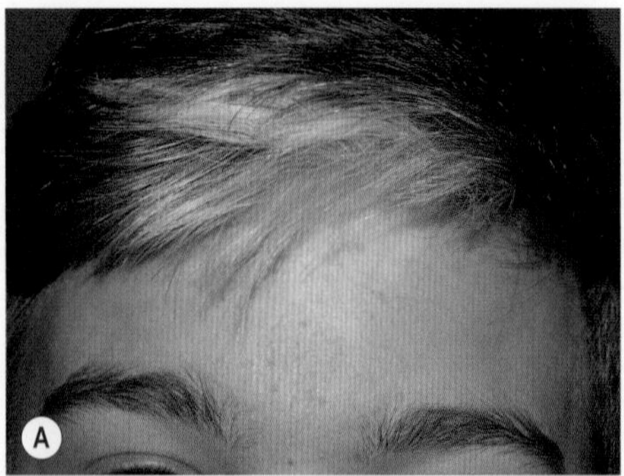

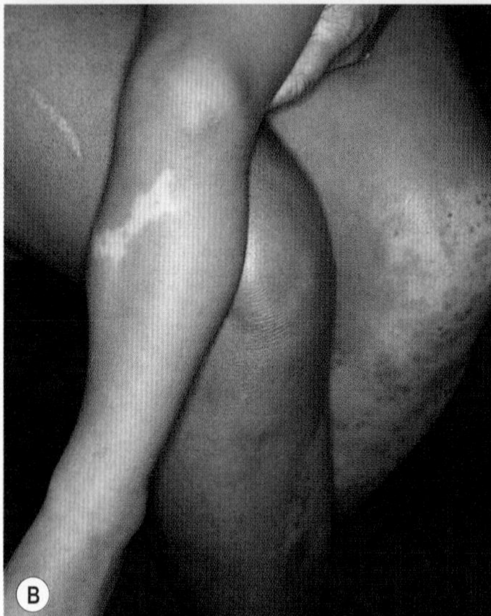

Fig. 54.9 Piebaldism. A White forelock (poliosis) and characteristic triangular amelanotic patch on the mid-forehead. **B** Mother and son with the characteristic involvement of the mid-extremities. Note the normally pigmented macules within the leukoderma. *A, Courtesy, Julie V. Schaffer, MD; B, Courtesy, Jean L. Bolognia, MD.*

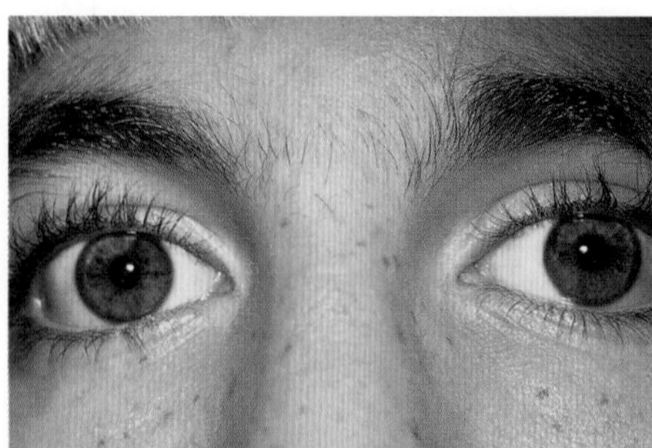

Fig. 54.10 Waardenburg syndrome type 2. Heterochromia irides in the absence of dystopia canthorum. The white forelock is seen in the upper left corner. *Courtesy, Daniel Albert, MD.*

 - WS3: associated limb abnormalities
 - WS4: associated with Hirschsprung disease

Disorders of Melanosome Biogenesis

- Because biosynthesis of lysosome-related organelles, e.g. platelet-dense granules and lytic granules of cytotoxic lymphocytes and natural killer cells, are also affected, patients can have a bleeding diathesis and immunodeficiency.

HERMANSKY–PUDLAK SYNDROME (HPS)

- Autosomal recessive inheritance; eight subtypes; HPS1 and HPS3 are the most common subtypes seen in Puerto Ricans.
- Characterized by variable pigmentary dilution of skin, hair, and eyes, depending on ethnicity; ocular manifestations of OCA; bleeding tendency; normal platelet count with a prolonged bleeding time.
- Depending on HPS subtype, may develop fatal pulmonary fibrosis and/or granulomatous colitis; average life span is 30–50 years.
- No specific treatment other than platelet transfusions prior to surgery.

CHÉDIAK–HIGASHI SYNDROME (CHS)

- Characterized by silvery hair, OCA skin and ocular findings, bleeding diathesis, progressive neurologic dysfunction, and infections due to severe immunodeficiency.
- Giant lysosomes within neutrophils seen on peripheral blood smear.
- Death is often in childhood secondary to infection, bleeding, or an accelerated lymphoma-like phase.
- **Rx:** hematopoietic stem cell transplant.

Disorders of Melanosome Transport and/or Transfer to Keratinocytes

- Consequences of this disrupted transport are pigmentary dilution and silvery hair (which contains melanin clumps in the hair shafts).

GRISCELLI SYNDROME (GS)

- Autosomal recessive; three subtypes, based on sites of expression of three mutated genes; all characterized by silvery hair and pigmentary dilution; patients can also have neurologic impairment (GS1) or immune abnormalities and hemophagocytic syndrome (GS2).

Other

TUBEROUS SCLEROSIS COMPLEX (TSC) (See Ch. 50)

- Hypomelanotic macules are often the first sign of TSC.
- These hypomelanotic macules are typically multiple in number; polygonal is the most common shape, followed by lance-ovate or "ash leaf" (Fig. 54.11); less often, the macules are "thumbprint"-like, guttate/confetti, or segmental (see Fig. 54.11; Table 54.2); lesions favor the trunk or extremities.

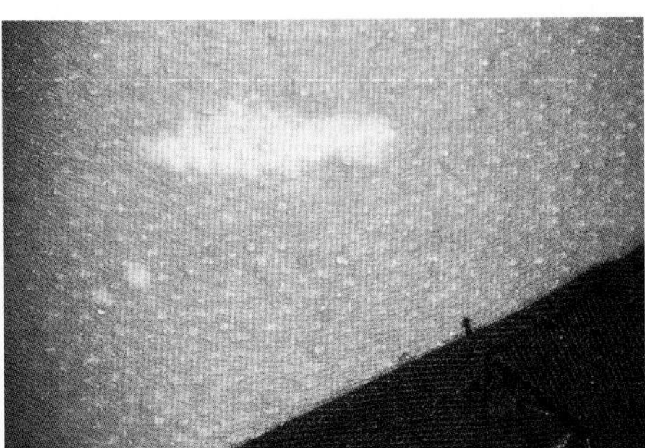

Fig. 54.11 Tuberous sclerosis complex (TSC). Two types of hypomelanotic macules, lance-ovate (ash leaf) and confetti (idiopathic guttate hypomelanosis-like). *Courtesy, David Strobel, MD.*

Hypopigmentation in Mosaic Patterns

- Several patterns of hypopigmentation can result from a mosaic "clone" of skin cells with decreased potential for pigment production ("pigmentary mosaicism").
- Hypopigmented areas may be apparent at birth or become evident during childhood, especially in patients with fair skin.

LINEAR NEVOID HYPOPIGMENTATION

- Localized or widespread streaks and swirls of hypopigmentation that follow the lines of Blaschko, which represent pathways of epidermal cell migration during embryogenesis (Fig. 54.12; see Fig. 51.1).
- ~10–20% of affected individuals have associated extracutaneous abnormalities, most often affecting the CNS (e.g. seizures, developmental delay), eyes, or musculoskeletal system; more severe involvement is usually

DIFFERENTIAL DIAGNOSIS OF GUTTATE LEUKODERMA
Idiopathic guttate hypomelanosis (see Fig. 54.23)
Pityriasis lichenoides chronica (see Fig. 7.3E)
Lichen sclerosus (see Fig. 54.17)
Confetti-like lesions of tuberous sclerosis (see Fig. 50.10B)
Tinea versicolor (especially on the face of children; see Fig. 54.18B)
Pityriasis alba (favors the cheeks of children)
Achromic verrucae planae*
Frictional lichenoid dermatosis*
Clear cell papulosis*
Vitiligo ponctué
Darier disease (usually admixed with keratotic lesions; see Fig. 48.4)
Xeroderma pigmentosum
In association with chromosomal abnormalities
Following PUVA therapy (leukoderma punctata, disseminated hypopigmented keratoses*)

**Minimally elevated flat-topped papules.*

Table 54.2 Differential diagnosis of guttate leukoderma. Guttate hypopigmentation may also be seen in the setting of dyschromatoses (see Ch. 55). *Adapted from Bolognia JL, Shapiro PE. Albinism and other disorders of hypopigmentation. In Arndt KA, et al. (Eds.). Cutaneous Medicine and Surgery. Philadelphia: Saunders, 1995.*

apparent in infancy and evaluation is directed by clinical findings.

- The term *hypomelanosis of Ito* has been used in studies focusing on linear nevoid hypopigmentation associated with systemic manifestations, and it should be reserved for this subset of patients.
- **DDx:** outlined in Table 54.3 (Fig. 54.13).

NEVUS DEPIGMENTOSUS

- Present in ~1:50 children, generally as an isolated finding.

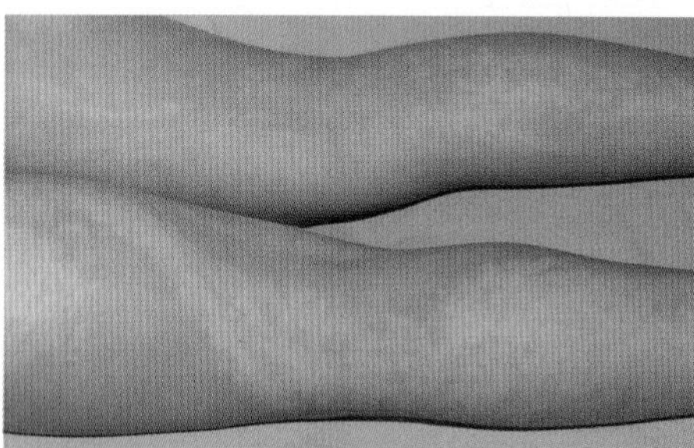

Fig. 54.12 Linear nevoid hypopigmentation. Hypopigmented streaks with various widths along the lines of Blaschko on the posterior lower extremities. *Courtesy, Antonio Torrelo, MD.*

- Lesions are typically hypopigmented, not depigmented as implied by the name.
- *Classic form*: ovoid or irregular hypopigmented patch, often breaking up into smaller macules at its periphery (Fig. 54.14).
- *Segmental form* (hypopigmented variant of *"segmental pigmentation disorder"*): block-like hypopigmented patch with midline demarcation and less distinct lateral borders.

PHYLLOID HYPOMELANOSIS

- Leaf-shaped and oblong hypopigmented macules and patches in an arrangement resembling a floral ornament, usually in the setting of mosaic trisomy 13 and associated with CNS abnormalities.

Postinflammatory Hypomelanoses

- Inflammatory skin conditions can potentially result in postinflammatory *hypo*pigmentation or *hyper*pigmentation or both (see Ch. 55).
- Postinflammatory hypopigmentation is a very common skin disorder that follows a wide variety of dermatoses, most commonly atopic dermatitis, seborrheic dermatitis, and psoriasis,

DISORDERS WITH LINEAR HYPOPIGMENTATION
Lesions usually follow lines of Blaschko
Linear nevoid hypopigmentation*/hypomelanosis of Ito (see Fig. 54.12) Lichen striatus (see Ch. 9 and Fig. 54.15D) Focal dermal hypoplasia (Goltz syndrome; see Fig. 51.8A) Menkes kinky hair disease (female carrier; see Ch. 43) Conradi–Hünermann–Happle syndrome (see Ch. 46) Epidermal nevus In association with Munro acne nevus (see Fig. 51.3G) Linear lichen sclerosus (see Ch. 36) Guttate macules in linear keratosis follicularis and linear basaloid follicular hamartoma
Lesions may follow lines of Blaschko
Segmental vitiligo (see Fig. 54.5) Segmental ash leaf spot Fourth stage of incontinentia pigmenti (see Fig. 54.13)
Lesions do not follow lines of Blaschko
Linear hypopigmentation secondary to intralesional corticosteroids (see Fig. 54.22A) Pigmentary demarcation lines, type C (see Ch. 55)

**Block-like hypopigmentation (segmental pigmentation disorder) represents another pattern of "pigmentary mosaicism" and may coexist with linear lesions; previous terms include "systematized" nevus depigmentosus with a linear configuration.*

Table 54.3 Disorders with linear hypopigmentation. *Adapted from Bolognia JL, Shapiro PE. Albinism and other disorders of hypopigmentation. In Arndt KA, et al. (Eds.). Cutaneous Medicine and Surgery. Philadelphia: Saunders, 1995.*

as well as pityriasis lichenoides chronica, lichen striatus, and lichen sclerosus (Fig. 54.15).

- It typically coexists or co-localizes with the inflammatory lesions, but occasionally only hypopigmented lesions are seen; the size, shape, and distribution pattern often provide clues to the underlying inflammatory dermatosis and the clinician can imagine the lesions being pink, red or red-brown.
- Most commonly there is a decrease in pigmentation; rarely there is an absence (e.g. severe atopic dermatitis).
- Histopathologic examination is often nonspecific, but in certain diseases (e.g. sarcoidosis and hypopigmented mycosis fungoides) can be diagnostic.
- **Rx** of underlying dermatosis is followed by gradual resolution.

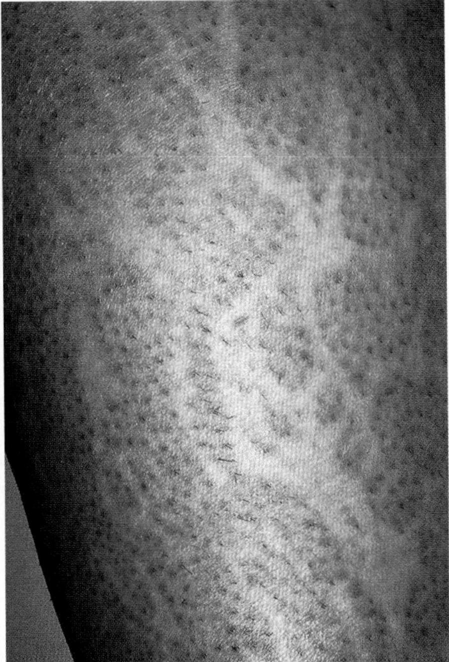

Fig. 54.13 Stage 4 of incontinentia pigmenti. Note the absence of hairs within the irregular streaks on the calf. *Courtesy, USCDRSC.*

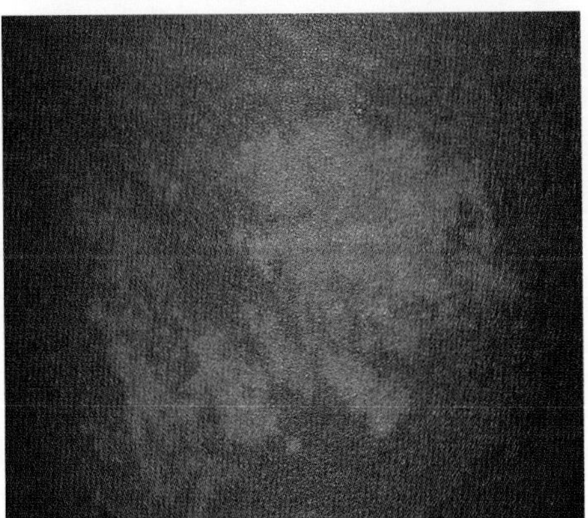

Fig. 54.14 Nevus depigmentosus. Hypomelanotic patch with a decrease, but not absence, of pigmentation. *Courtesy, YDRSC.*

Pityriasis Alba (See Ch. 10)

- A very common, asymptomatic disorder seen primarily during childhood and adolescence.
- One to several slightly scaly, hypopigmented macules and patches are seen, typically on the cheeks; the lesions are usually ill-defined and occasionally there is associated mild erythema.
- The hypomelanosis often becomes more apparent during the summer months; emollients, sunscreens, or low-strength topical CS (e.g. hydrocortisone 2.5%) may be helpful.
- **DDx:** tinea versicolor, early vitiligo, and postinflammatory hypopigmentation from seborrheic dermatitis or atopic dermatitis.

Sarcoidosis

- Sarcoidosis occurs more commonly in African-Americans, and the hypopigmented variant of cutaneous sarcoidosis may go undiagnosed; this form has no associated prognostic significance and may spontaneously repigment.
- Hypopigmented papules, plaques, or sometimes nodules are seen; range in size from 1 to several cm.
- Histopathology reveals noncaseating granulomas.

Hypopigmented Mycosis Fungoides (MF) (See Ch. 98)

- A variant of early stage MF that is most commonly observed in darkly pigmented individuals (see Fig. 54.15E); seen in adults, as well as children and adolescents.
- Atrophy can be observed within the hypopigmented patches.
- Histopathology reveals typical features of MF.
- **DDx:** hypopigmented parapsoriasis, pityriasis lichenoides chronica (PLC).

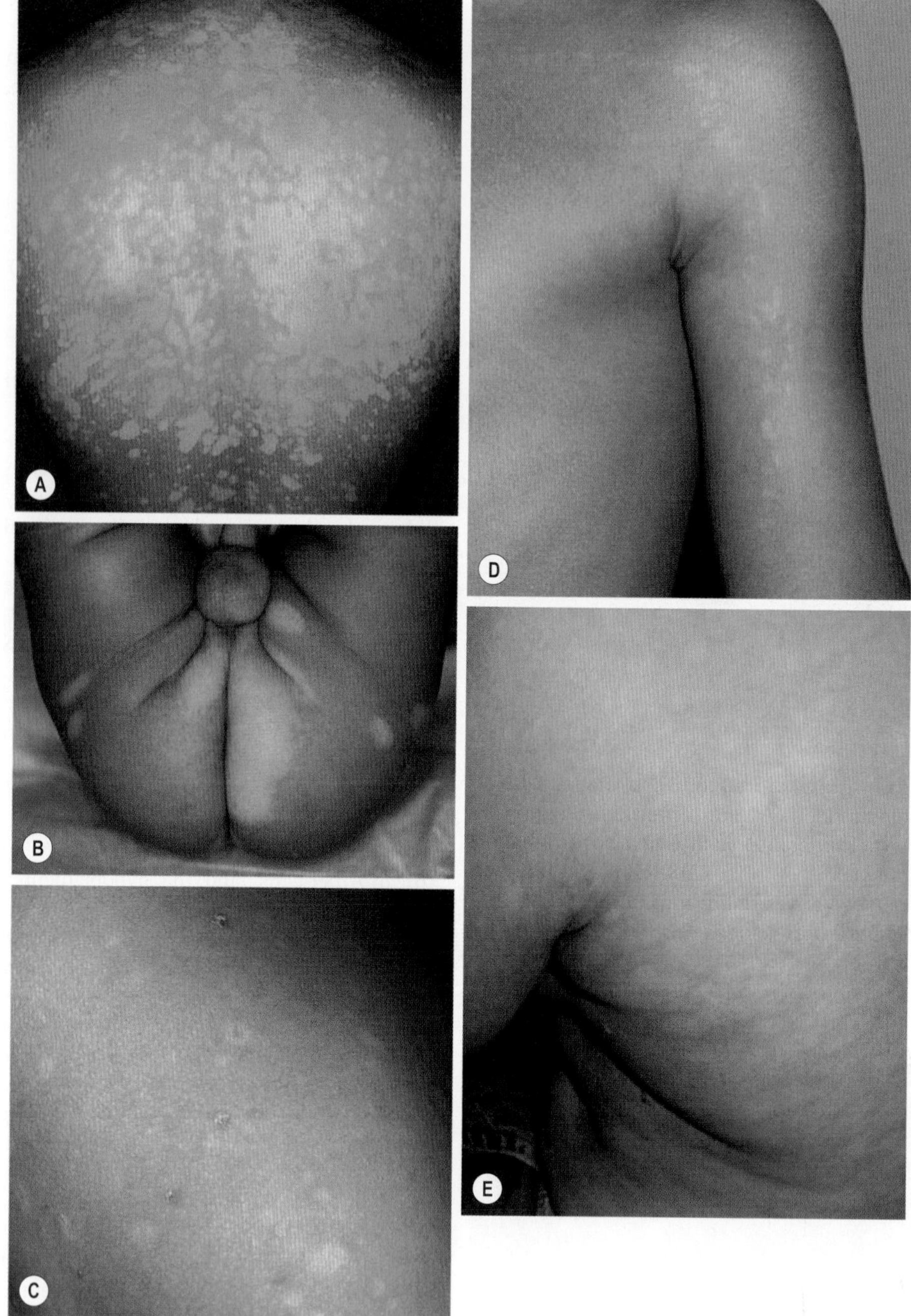

Fig. 54.15 Postinflammatory hypomelanosis. Hypopigmentation secondary to psoriasis **(A),** seborrheic dermatitis in an infant **(B),** pityriasis lichenoides chronica **(C)**, lichen striatus (note the flat-topped papules) **(D),** and hypopigmented mycosis fungoides **(E)**. *Continued*

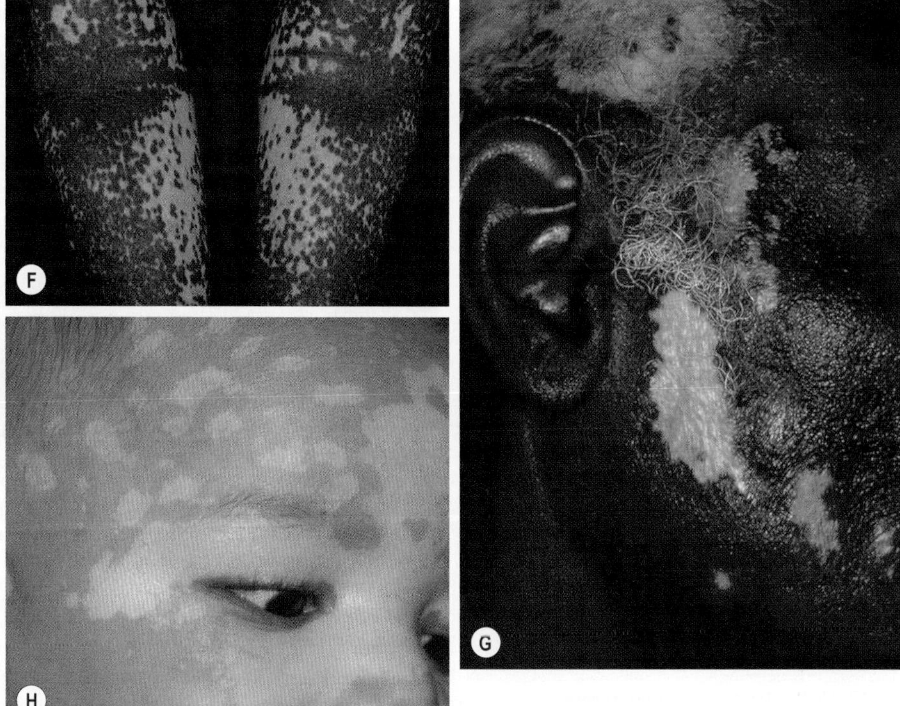

Fig. 54.15 *Continued* **Postinflammatory hypomelanosis.** Complete pigment loss in patients with severe atopic dermatitis **(F)**, discoid lupus erythematosus **(G)**, and neonatal lupus erythematosus **(H)**. *A, E–G, Courtesy, YDRSC; B, Courtesy, Jean L. Bolognia, MD; C, Courtesy, SUNYSBDRSC; D, H, Courtesy, Julie V. Schaffer, MD.*

Cutaneous Lupus Erythematosus (LE) (See Ch. 33)

- In discoid LE (DLE), hypomelanosis is often seen centrally within well-developed lesions and the lesions also have cutaneous atrophy, scarring, erythema (if active) and a hyperpigmented rim; pigmentary changes tend to be persistent (see Fig. 54.15G).
- In subacute cutaneous LE (SCLE), hypomelanosis typically occurs within the center of annular lesions and is usually reversible.

Systemic Sclerosis (SSc) (See Ch. 35)

- Patients with SSc can develop several pigmentary abnormalities, including diffuse hypermelanosis with photoaccentuation, mixed hyper- and hypopigmentation in areas of chronic sclerosis, and a characteristic leukoderma in both sclerotic and nonsclerotic skin (Fig. 54.16).
- This leukoderma of systemic sclerosis presents as circumscribed areas of depigmentation but with perifollicular and supravenous retention of pigment (see Fig. 54.16).
- This peculiar leukoderma is rather specific for SSc as it occasionally occurs in two other clinical settings, an overlap syndrome (that includes SSc) and scleromyxedema.
- Although clinically similar to the perifollicular repigmentation seen in treatment-responsive vitiligo, it is different in that in vitiligo the perifollicular macules represent *new* pigmentation, whereas in SSc the macules represent *old* or retained pigmentation.

Lichen Sclerosus (LS) (See Ch. 36)

- Genital and extragenital lesions of LS are often hypopigmented, but in addition display cutaneous atrophy, follicular plugging (extragenital), and purpura (genital).
- Occasionally extragenital LS presents as guttate leukoderma (Fig. 54.17; see Table 54.2).

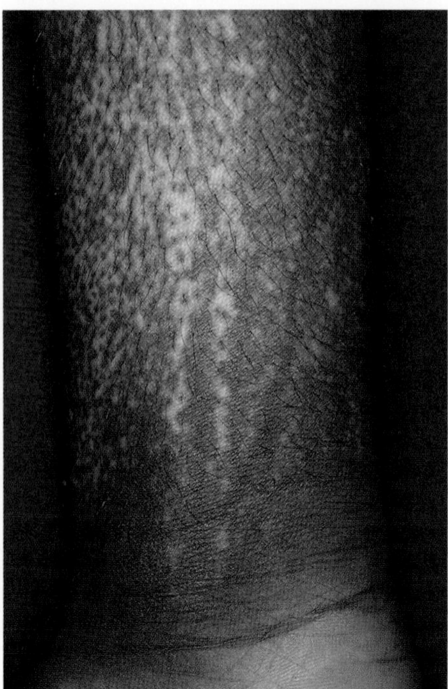

Fig. 54.16 Leukoderma of systemic sclerosis (scleroderma). Uniform retention of perifollicular pigment within areas of leukoderma. Hyperpigmentation is also seen overlying a superficial vein. *Courtesy, YDRSC.*

Infectious and Parasitic Hypomelanosis

Tinea (Pityriasis) Versicolor (See Ch. 64)

- A very common superficial cutaneous mycosis caused by *Malassezia* spp.; although there is usually minimal inflammation, this infection can lead to either hyper- or hypopigmentation.
- Typically presents symmetrically on the upper trunk and shoulders or flexural areas (e.g. groin and inframammary) as round to oval macules or thin papules that coalesce into patches or thin plaques; the lesions vary in color from pink to light tan to brown, hence the term *versicolor* (Fig. 54.18).
- Lesions often coalesce and when untreated, there is usually a subtle overlying fine scale that is more readily apparent upon scratching or stretching the skin.
- Diagnosis is easily confirmed by KOH examination of the associated scale.

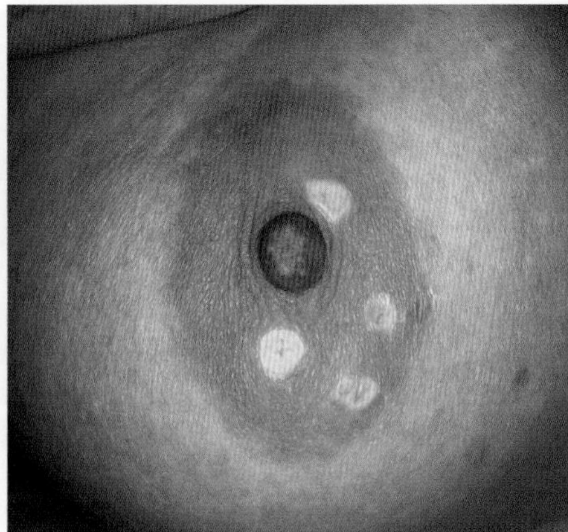

Fig. 54.17 Guttate lichen sclerosus involving the areolae. *Courtesy, YDRSC.*

- Hypomelanosis without any scaling may remain for months after treatment.

Leprosy (See Ch. 62)

- *Tuberculoid leprosy* (Fig. 54.19): fewer larger hypopigmented patches with discrete, often raised, borders; favor posterolateral aspects of extremities, back, buttocks, face; associated anhidrosis, alopecia, and loss of sensation.
- *Borderline leprosy*: occasionally, ill-defined hypomelanotic macules are seen.
- *Indeterminate leprosy*: erythematous to hypomelanotic macules asymmetrically distributed on exposed sites; normal hair.
- *Lepromatous leprosy*: hypomelanotic macules may be the earliest manifestation; often small, multiple, subtle, and ill-defined; favor the face, extremities, and buttocks; minimal or no anhidrosis or loss of sensation.

Treponematoses (See Chs 61 and 69)

- Non-venereal treponematoses (e.g. pinta, yaws, bejel) and venereal syphilis may be associated with hypomelanosis, especially during their untreated phase.

Onchocerciasis (River Blindness) (See Ch. 70)

- A filarial infestation that predominantly affects cutaneous and ocular tissues and is caused by the transmission of *Onchocerca volvulus* from the bite of a black fly in tropical areas of Africa > Central and South America.

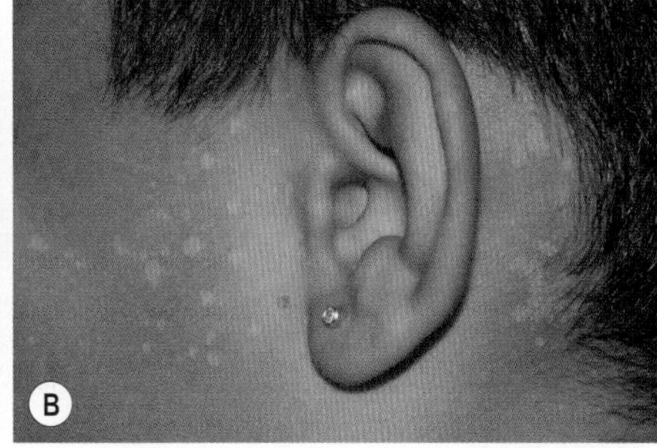

Fig. 54.18 Tinea (pityriasis) versicolor. **A** Hypopigmented variant with obvious scale. **B** Guttate hypopigmented lesions on the cheek; note the classic scaly lesions in the posterior auricular area. *A, Courtesy, YDRSC; B, Courtesy, Julie V. Schaffer, MD.*

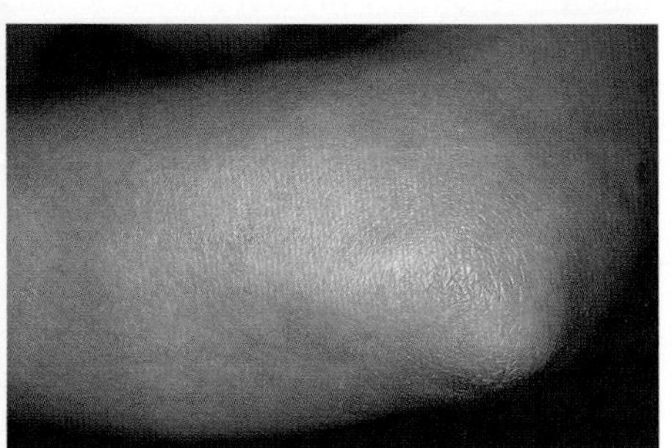

Fig. 54.19 Tuberculoid leprosy. Large thin hypopigmented plaque on the elbow with a raised light pink border. *Courtesy, YDRSC.*

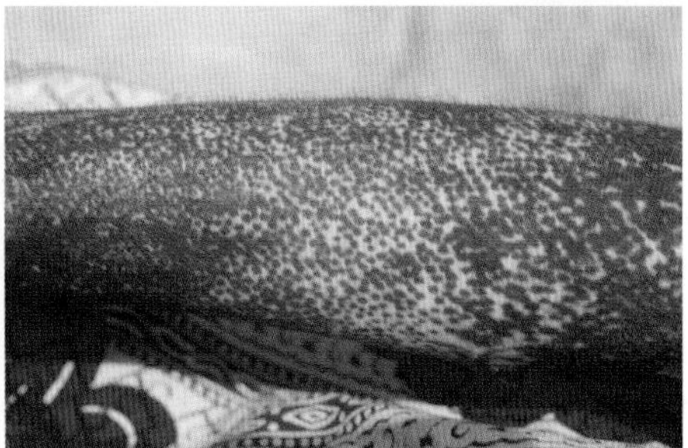

Fig. 54.20 Onchocerciasis (leopard skin). Depigmentation of the shin with follicular repigmentation or retention of perifollicular pigment, a common site for the associated leukoderma. Clinically resembles repigmenting vitiligo or the leukoderma of scleroderma. *Courtesy, Jean-Paul Ortonne, MD.*

- A later cutaneous finding is leukoderma of the shins with follicular pigmentation, resembling leopard skin (Fig. 54.20).
- **DDx:** atopic dermatitis with postinflammatory depigmentation, or atopic dermatitis plus vitiligo with Koebner phenomenon.

Other

- Hypopigmentation may also result from cutaneous bacterial or viral infections, e.g. herpes zoster.

Melanoma-Associated Leukoderma (See Ch. 93)

- Vitiligo-like depigmentation can occur in patients with cutaneous or ocular melanoma, either spontaneously or in the setting of immunotherapy (e.g. ipilimumab, pembrolizumab, nivolumab).
- Thought to result from an immune reaction directed against shared antigens on normal and malignant melanocytes (Fig. 54.21).
- Whereas the spontaneous form points to the need for re-staging, the treatment-associated form can portend a better prognosis.

Chemical Leukoderma

- Contact with a number of chemical agents can lead to hypomelanosis of the skin and hair (Fig. 54.22).
- Depigmenting compounds have chemical structures that are similar to melanin precursors; they include catechols, phenols, or quinones (e.g. hydroquinone [HQ] or monobenzyl ether of HQ [MBEH]).
- HQ induces a reversible hypopigmentation, whereas MBEH depigmentation is often permanent and occurs not only at the site of application but also at distant sites.
- Topical and injected CS can also lead to hypopigmentation (see Fig. 54.22).

Miscellaneous

Idiopathic Guttate Hypomelanosis (IGH)

- A very common disorder that increases in incidence with age; occurs in all races and skin types (Fig. 54.23).

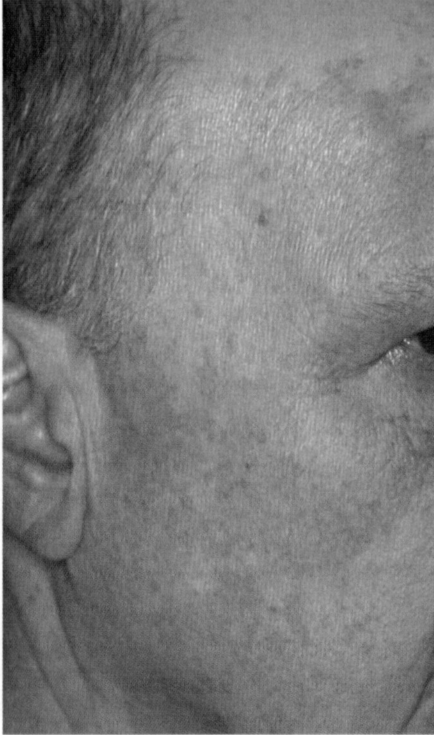

Fig. 54.21 Melanoma-associated leukoderma. Vitiligo-like leukoderma associated with ipilimumab, an anti-cytotoxic T-lymphocyte-associated antigen-4 (CTLA-4) antibody, administered for metastatic melanoma. *Courtesy, Jean L. Bolognia, MD.*

- Typically presents as multiple, asymptomatic, small (guttate), well-circumscribed white macules on the extensor forearms and shins; the surface is smooth, often with accentuation of the skin markings.
- **DDx:** other guttate leukodermas (see Table 54.2).

Progressive Macular Hypomelanosis of the Trunk (PMH)

- Characterized by asymptomatic, poorly defined, small, round to oval, non-scaly, hypopigmented macules and patches, primarily on the trunk and proximal upper extremities, often with confluence of lesions (Fig. 54.24).
- A less common variant is seen in Afro-Caribbean females as larger patches.
- **DDx:** previously treated tinea versicolor.

Hair Hypomelanosis

- Circumscribed (poliosis) versus generalized (canities).
- Graying of hair, either localized or generalized, is characterized by an admixture of normally pigmented, hypomelanotic and amelanotic hairs.
- Whitening of hair is the endpoint of graying of hair, and both are due to defective maintenance of melanocyte stem cells.
- Premature graying of the hair has been associated with a number of genetic disorders (e.g. Werner syndrome, piebaldism) as well as vitiligo.
- Diffuse hypomelanosis of hair has been associated with both hereditary (e.g. Fanconi syndrome) and acquired causes (e.g. tyrosine kinase inhibitors, antimalarials).

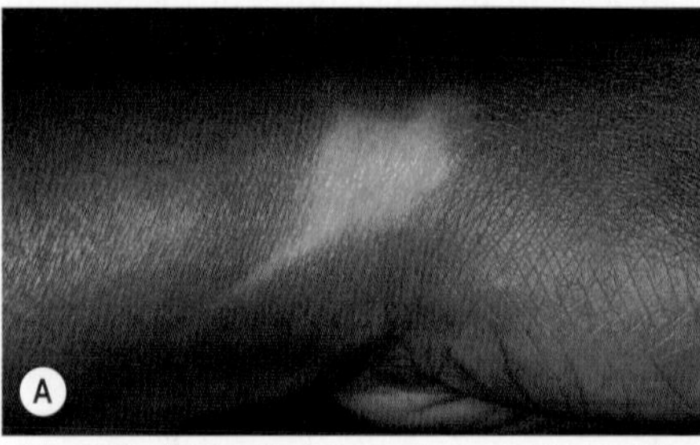

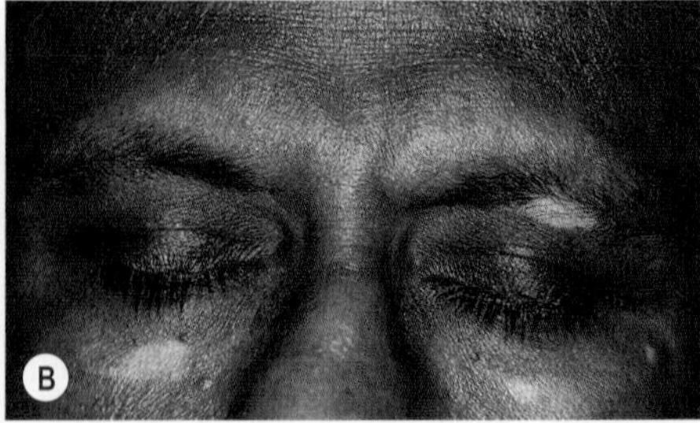

Fig. 54.22 Chemical leukoderma. A Hypopigmentation due to injection of corticosteroids into the anatomic snuff box. The outline is both stellate and linear. Typically appears several weeks to months after the injection. In most cases repigmentation occurs within one year after stopping the injections. **B** Depigmentation developed at sites of contact with rubber swimming goggles. *A, Courtesy, YDRSC; B, Courtesy, Kalman Watsky, MD.*

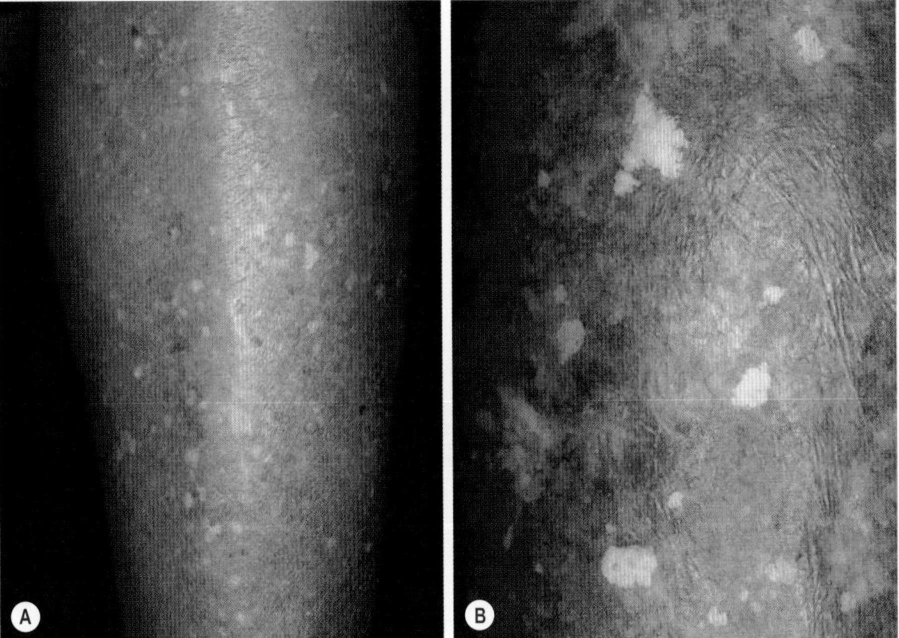

Fig. 54.23 Idiopathic guttate hypomelanosis. **A** Typical 1- to 5-mm macules on the shin. **B** Occasionally there is an admixture of larger lesions. *Courtesy, YDRSC.*

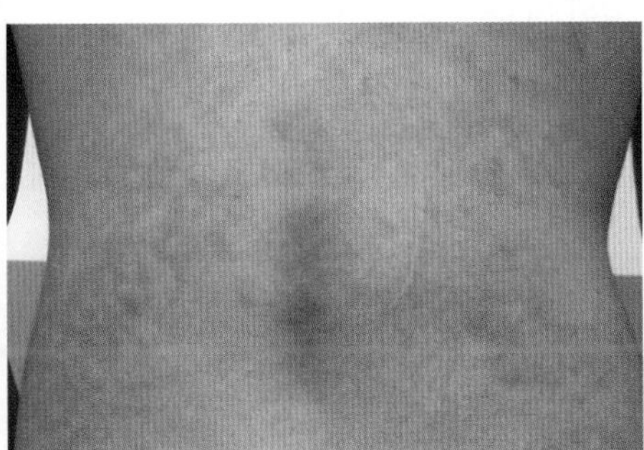

Fig. 54.24 Progressive macular hypomelanosis. Note the coalescence of the non-scaly hypopigmented macules on the center of the back. *Courtesy, Jean-Paul Ortonne, MD.*

For further information see Chs 65 and 66 from *Dermatology, Fourth Edition*.

For additional online figures and tables visit www.expertconsult.com 

55 Disorders of Hyperpigmentation

Definitions

- **Hyperpigmentation**: a term used to describe disorders characterized by darkening of the skin; encompasses hypermelanosis.
- **Hypermelanosis**: a more specific term that denotes an increase in the melanin content of the skin; typically due to an increase in melanin production but occasionally from an increase in the density of active melanocytes.
- **Discoloration**: a term used to describe an abnormal color of the skin; may be due to deposition of substances such as drugs, drug complexes (e.g. with melanin or iron), or heavy metals within the dermis.
- **Dyschromatosis**: a disorder characterized by the presence of both hypo- and hyperpigmentation.
- **Pigment incontinence**: the presence of melanin within dermal macrophages (melanophages); the source of the melanin is the epidermis, and this typically results from inflammation at the dermal–epidermal junction.
- **Epidermal pigmentation**: denotes increased melanin within the epidermis, which typically leads to a light brown to dark brown color.
- **Dermal pigmentation**: denotes increased melanin in the dermis, primarily within melanophages; characteristically presents as a gray-blue to gray-brown color.

Approach to Disorders of Hyperpigmentation

- Disorders of hyperpigmentation usually result from an increase in melanin production and occasionally from an increase in the density of active melanocytes.
- The clinical approach to these disorders is simplified by dividing them into four patterns, namely *circumscribed*, *diffuse*, *linear*, and *reticulated* (Fig. 55.1).
- The most common clinical pattern is *circumscribed*; observation of the sites of involvement, shape, configuration, and size can provide clues to the diagnosis.
- The dyschromatoses are discussed separately.

Circumscribed Hyperpigmentation

- The three major entities in this category are postinflammatory hyperpigmentation, melasma, and drug-induced hyperpigmentation.

POSTINFLAMMATORY HYPERPIGMENTATION

- Represents an acquired excess of melanin pigment following cutaneous inflammation (e.g. acne, psoriasis) or injury (e.g. burns or friction).
- Depending on the disorder, postinflammatory hypopigmentation may also occur and is discussed in Chapter 54.
- Can occur anywhere on the body, including the mucosae or nail unit; increased pigmentation is localized to areas of inflammation and becomes more apparent once the associated erythema resolves (likened to "a shadow left behind").
- The preceding inflammation may be obvious, transient, or subclinical (Table 55.1; Fig. 55.2).
- The hyperpigmented macules and patches can range in color from light brown to dark brown (epidermal melanin) or gray-blue to gray-brown (dermal melanin).
- In general, postinflammatory epidermal pigmentation eventually resolves as long as the underlying disorder is treated effectively, but this may take months or even years; postinflammatory dermal pigmentation can be persistent.

APPROACH TO DISORDERS OF HYPERPIGMENTATION

Disorders of hyperpigmentation
- Circumscribed
  - Postinflammatory hyperpigmentation → See Table 55.1
  - Melasma
  - Drug-induced → See Table 55.3
- Diffuse → See Fig. 55.9
- Linear → See Table 55.4
- Reticulated → Exclude reticulated erythema (e.g. livedo reticularis, early stage erythema ab igne) → Exclude poikiloderma (e.g. poikiloderma of Civatte, dermatomyositis, lupus erythematosus) → See Table 55.6
- Exclude dyschromatosis → See text; See Figs 55.21, 55.22

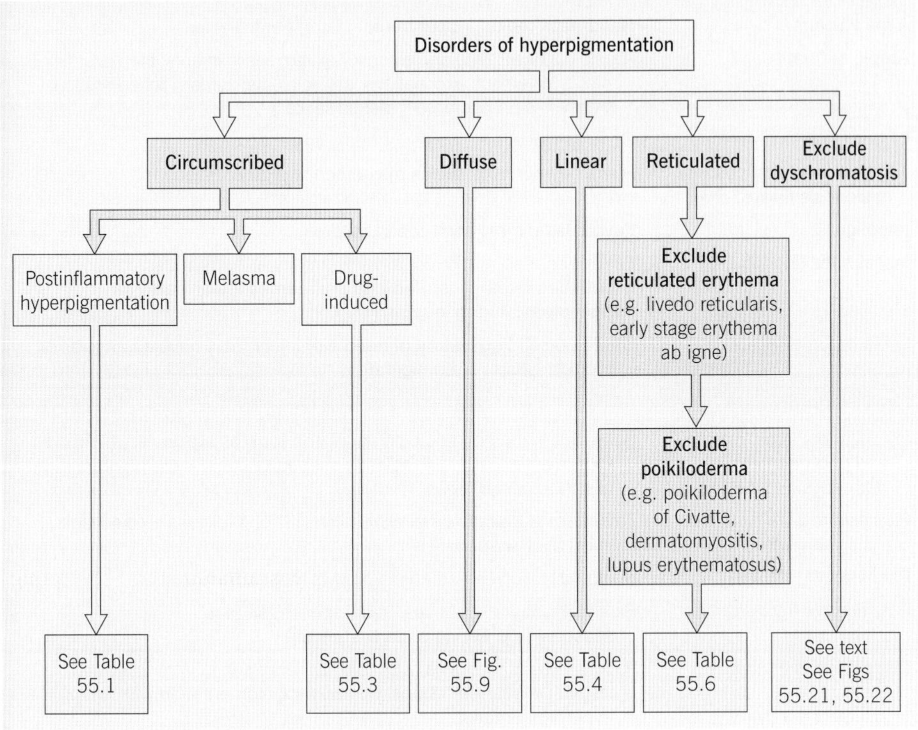

Fig. 55.1 Approach to disorders of hyperpigmentation.

• May also be exacerbated by UVR exposure, and photoprotection is an important part of treatment.

• **DDx:** see Table 55.1; occasionally a skin biopsy will assist in establishing the diagnosis.

• Causes of postinflammatory hyperpigmentation that often present without obvious prior inflammation include the following:
- Primary (localized) cutaneous amyloidosis (see Ch. 39 and Figs 39.6 and 39.7)
- Erythema dyschromicum perstans (EDP or ashy dermatosis) (see Ch. 9 and Figs 9.10 and 55.3A)
- Lichen planus pigmentosus (LPP) (see Ch. 9, Table 9.1, and Figs 9.5G and 55.3B)
- ***Mastocytosis*** (see Ch. 96 and Fig. 96.4)
- ***Tinea (pityriasis) versicolor*** (see Chs 54 and 64 and Fig. 64.1)
- ***Atrophoderma of Pasini and Pierini*** (see Ch. 82)
  - There is some debate as to whether this represents a distinct entity or is an end-stage (i.e. "burned-out" stage) of morphea
  - Typically seen in young healthy adults as several 3- to 6-cm, oval, hyperpigmented, minimally depressed patches on the posterior trunk
  - Lacks an inflammatory phase
  - **Rx:** In addition to treating the underlying inflammatory disorder and photoprotection, the following topical agents may be used: hydroquinone 2–4%; a combination of hydroquinone, tretinoin, and a low-strength CS; azelaic acid 15%; α-hydroxy acids (e.g. glycolic acid)

MELASMA

• A very common, acquired disorder characterized by symmetric, hyperpigmented patches with irregular borders, resulting from an increase in epidermal and/or dermal melanin; favors the face (see below) > mid-upper chest and extensor forearms.

DISORDERS ASSOCIATED WITH POSTINFLAMMATORY HYPERPIGMENTATION	
Inflammatory disease	**Clinical clues**
Common	
Acne vulgaris	Head/neck region, upper trunk; <1 cm; perifollicular
Atopic dermatitis	Atopic diathesis; face and extensor extremities in infants, then later flexural involvement; excoriations; atopic pleats; xerosis; lichenification; transverse nasal crease ("allergic salute")
Lichen simplex chronicus	Common locations: posterior neck, ankle, scrotum
Transient neonatal pustular melanosis (Fig. 55.2D)	Black newborns; pustules may precede pigmentation
Impetigo	Favors face; most common in children
Insect bites (Fig. 55.2A)	Favor exposed areas; usually <1 cm; lower extremities common with flea bites; clustered and sometimes linear patterns ("breakfast–lunch–dinner")
Linear trauma	Often a preceding history of trauma or injury; may have an angular or irregular shape or configuration
Less common	
Irritant and allergic contact and photocontact dermatitis (Fig. 55.2E)	Sites determined by etiologic agent and form of exposure; phytophotodermatitis leads to irregularly shaped or linear hyperpigmentation in sun-exposed areas
Pityriasis rosea	Favors trunk and proximal extremities; lesions follow skin cleavage lines; oval-shaped
Psoriasis (Fig. 55.2B)	Scalp/nail involvement; knees/elbows most common sites
Polymorphic light eruption	Extensor upper extremities, mid upper chest, face; seasonal (e.g. spring or early summer)
Discoid lupus erythematosus	Face and conchal bowls, with follicular plugging in latter site; oral lesions; in scarred lesions, central hypopigmentation with rim of hyperpigmentation
Lichen planus (LP) (Fig. 55.3B)	Wrists, shins, and presacral area in classic LP; face, neck and intertriginous sites in LP pigmentosus; nail/oral involvement
Erythema dyschromicum perstans* (EDP; ashy dermatosis) (Fig. 55.3A)	Neck, proximal upper extremities, trunk; round or oval in shape with gray-brown to blue-gray color; long axis can follow skin cleavage lines (similar to pityriasis rosea); less commonly observed in fair-skinned individuals
Idiopathic eruptive macular pigmentation*	Trunk, proximal extremities, neck, face; round or oval in shape with gray-brown to blue-gray color; barely elevated plaques with a subtle velvety texture; affects primarily children and adolescents; lasting months to years
Fixed drug eruption (Fig. 55.2C)	Circular; favors perioral, acral, and genital sites; recurrence at same site(s) with repeated exposure
Morbilliform drug eruption	Widespread; usually discrete lesions; history of drug exposure
Viral exanthem	Widespread; usually discrete lesions; history of associated symptoms
Morphea	Trunk or extremities; large-sized except in guttate variant; may be linear; induration and later dermal atrophy
Atrophoderma of Pasini and Pierini	Trunk; large-sized; depressed with "cliff sign" at periphery; no induration
Neurotic (psychogenic) excoriation, acne excoriée	Favors face, scalp, extensor surface of arms, upper back (reachable areas); linear or angular shapes; multiple stages of evolution, from erosions/ulcerations to scars

**Typically no preceding inflammatory phase evident clinically or histopathologically.*

Table 55.1 Disorders associated with postinflammatory hyperpigmentation. Disorders in the blue rows are characterized by inflammation at the dermal-epidermal junction. Such inflammation can lead to dermal melanin within melanophages (pigment incontinence), which can be resistant to treatment and take longer to resolve. Most disorders result in epidermal hyperpigmentation and eventually resolve if the underlying disorder is treated effectively. *Adapted from Bolognia JL. Disorders of hypopigmentation and hyperpigmentation. In: Harper J, Oranje A, Prose N (Eds.), Textbook of Pediatric Dermatology, 2nd edn. Oxford: Blackwell Science, 2006;997–1040.*

- Seen primarily in women; increased prevalence in individuals with skin phototypes III–IV.
- Pathogenesis is thought to be related to hyperfunctional melanocytes that are stimulated by exacerbating factors, such as sun exposure and hormones (e.g. pregnancy, oral contraceptives).
- Three classic clinical patterns based on distribution: centrofacial (most common), malar, and mandibular (Fig. 55.4).
- Classically, melasma was also classified based on findings from Wood's lamp examination: lesions that enhance imply an increase in epidermal melanin and lesions that do not enhance imply an increase in dermal melanin; however, mixed epidermal and dermal melasma patterns are common.
- In northern latitudes, lesions tend to fade during the winter months; melasma tends to be more persistent in darkly pigmented individuals.
- **DDx:** postinflammatory hyperpigmentation, drug-induced (e.g. minocycline, amiodarone), acquired bilateral nevus of Ota-like macules (especially in Asian women), actinic lichen planus, pigmented contact dermatitis, exogenous ochronosis due to the application of hydroquinone-containing bleaching agents (Fig. 55.5), erythromelanosis faciei.
- These other disorders are distinguished from melasma based on historical aspects (e.g. drug ingestion, application of topical medications or cosmetics, previous inflammation), color (e.g. clusters of nevus of Ota-like macules are typically blue-gray in color), distribution pattern, histopathologic features, and primary lesions, if present.
- Treatment options are outlined in Table 55.2; typically, epidermal hyperpigmentation responds best to treatment.

DRUG-INDUCED CIRCUMSCRIBED HYPERPIGMENTATION AND DISCOLORATION

- A wide range of medications and chemicals can cause hyperpigmentation or discoloration in circumscribed, diffuse, and even linear patterns; longitudinal or horizontal melanonychia may also be present.
- The most common culprits of drug-induced circumscribed hyperpigmentation and discoloration are minocycline and the antimalarials (Table 55.3; Figs 55.5–55.8).
- The pathogenesis involves varying mechanisms, from increased melanin production to deposition of drug complexes or heavy metals within the dermis.
- The hyperpigmentation or discoloration typically resolves upon discontinuation of the offending drug, but the course may be prolonged.

Diffuse Hyperpigmentation

- Diffuse hyperpigmentation has multiple causes, including drug-induced, metabolic and endocrine abnormalities, nutritional deficiencies, exposure to heavy metals, and inherited syndromes.
- May be accentuated in sun-exposed sites.
- An approach to the patient with diffuse hyperpigmentation is presented in Fig. 55.9.

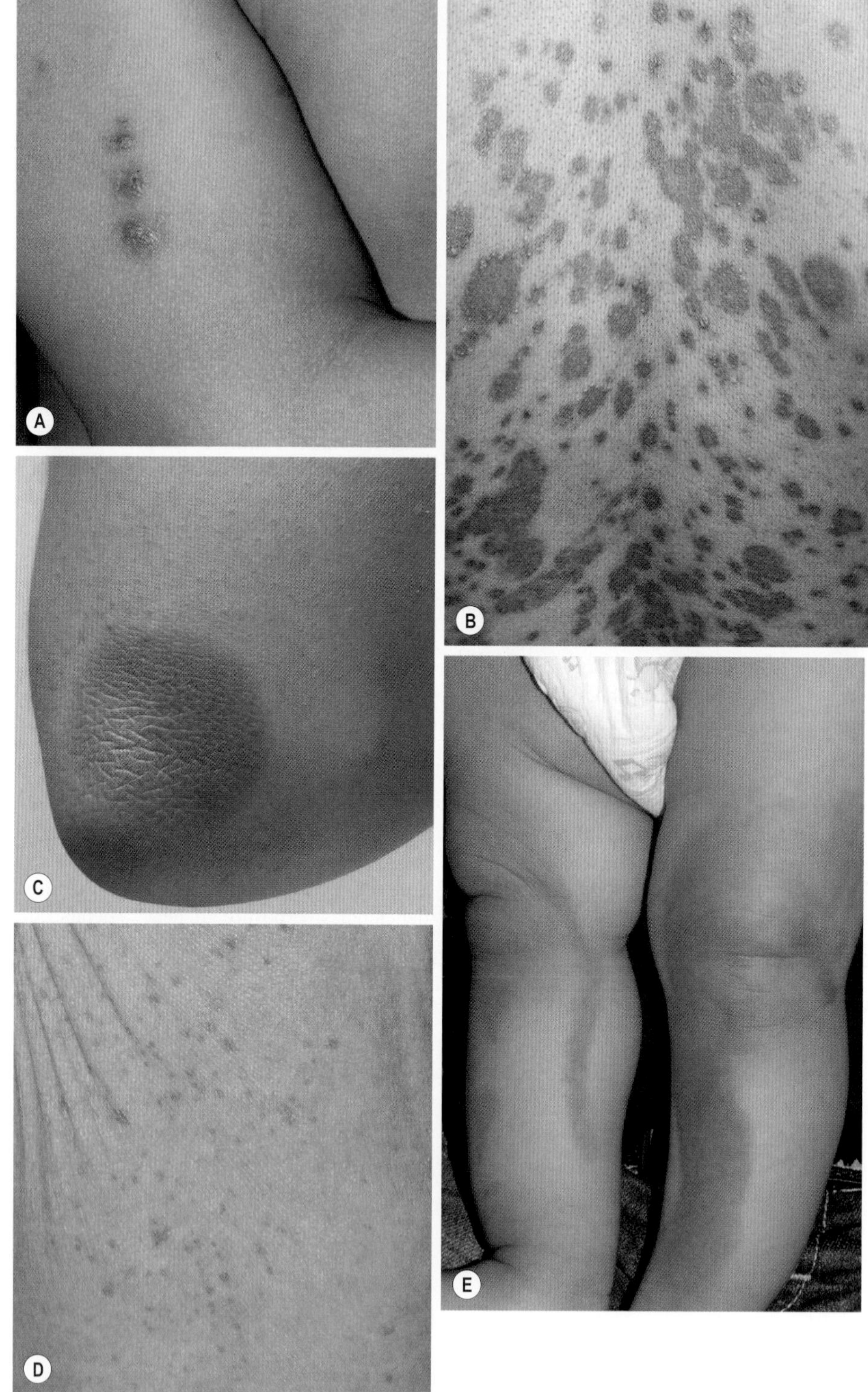

Fig. 55.2 Epidermal postinflammatory hyperpigmentation. The lesions were caused by insect bite reactions **(A)**, psoriasis **(B)**, a fixed drug eruption induced by trimethoprim–sulfamethoxazole **(C)**, and transient neonatal pustular melanosis **(D)**. Note the residual inflammation and "breakfast–lunch–dinner" configuration in **(A)**. **E** Linear epidermal postinflammatory hyperpigmentation due to phytophotodermatitis, which requires contact with a plant (e.g. lime) containing a photosensitizing chemical followed by UVR exposure. *A, D, E, Courtesy, Julie V. Schaffer, MD; B, C, Courtesy, Justin Finch, MD.*

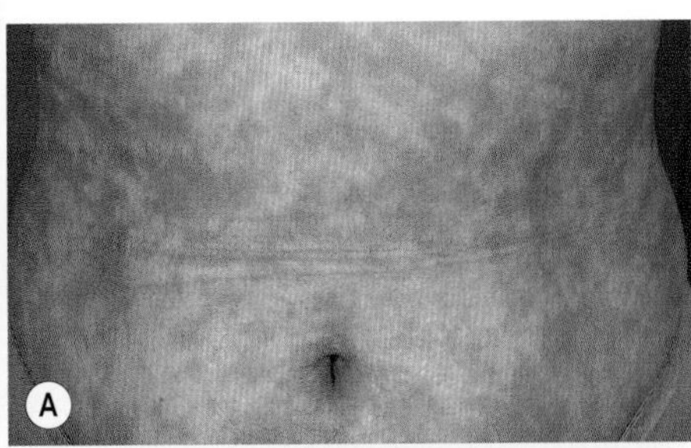

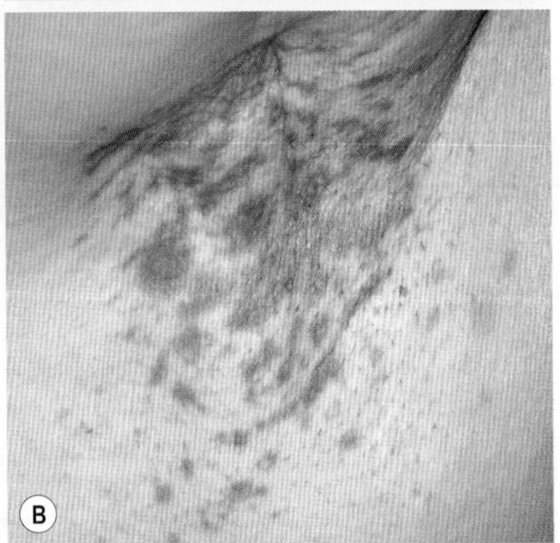

Fig. 55.3 Dermal postinflammatory hyperpigmentation. A Erythema dyschromicum perstans (EDP or ashy dermatosis). Multiple gray-brown macules and patches on the abdomen. The "ashy" color is characteristic. **B** Lichen planus pigmentosus. Multiple coalescing brown to gray-brown macules in the axilla of a middle-aged woman. *A, Courtesy, NYUDSC; B, Courtesy, YDRSC.*

Linear Hyperpigmentation

- Linear hyperpigmentation, like linear hypopigmentation (see Ch. 54), can result from multiple etiologies; one of the initial steps is determining if the lesions do or do not follow the lines of Blaschko (see Ch. 51).
- The differential diagnosis of linear hyperpigmentation is presented in Table 55.4 (Figs 55.10–55.16).

HYPERPIGMENTATION ALONG THE LINES OF BLASCHKO AND IN OTHER MOSAIC PATTERNS

- Hyperpigmentation can follow the lines of Blaschko or have other mosaic patterns (e.g. block-like [see Ch. 51]).
- Hyperpigmented streaks along the lines of Blaschko has been termed ***"linear and whorled nevoid hypermelanosis" (LWNH)*** or linear nevoid hyperpigmentation, and they reflect pigmentary mosaicism (see Fig. 55.10).
- In a minority of patients, LWNH is associated with systemic abnormalities (e.g. CNS, musculoskeletal, or ocular); hyperpigmented streaks usually appear in infancy.
- Patients presenting with hypo- or hyperpigmented streaks along the lines of Blaschko can be approached in a similar fashion, with a physical examination and further evaluation (e.g. genetic) directed by clinical findings.
- Hyperpigmentation can also occur in a block-like configuration, also referred to as ***segmental pigmentation disorder*** (see Fig. 55.11); the **DDx** includes Becker melanosis (nevus) and segmental CALM, either isolated or syndromic (e.g. McCune–Albright syndrome [see Table 50.3]); in the latter, the CALM may be more geographic in configuration.

LINEAR HYPERPIGMENTATION THAT IS NOT ALONG THE LINES OF BLASCHKO

- ***Pigmentary demarcation lines*** (see Fig. 55.14)
  - In humans, the dorsal skin surfaces are relatively hyperpigmented, compared to the ventral surfaces
  - In patients with darker pigmentation, visible lines of demarcation between dorsal and ventral surfaces are more apparent
  - These demarcation lines are present from infancy and persist throughout life; they are most prevalent on the anterolateral upper arm and posteromedial thigh (see Fig. 55.15)
  - Several forms of pigmentary demarcation lines exist and are presented in Table 55.5 and Fig. 55.14
- ***Flagellate pigmentation from bleomycin***
  - Occurs in ~10–20% of patients treated with systemic bleomycin
  - The pigmentation appears to be dose dependent but the pathogenesis is not well understood
  - Presents as linear hyperpigmented streaks on the chest, back, and occasionally extremities (see Fig. 55.16); typically in a configuration that suggests a relationship to scratching, but attempts to reproduce lesions by scratching have in general been unsuccessful; an erythematous phase, which is typically pink in light-skinned individuals, can precede the hyperpigmentation

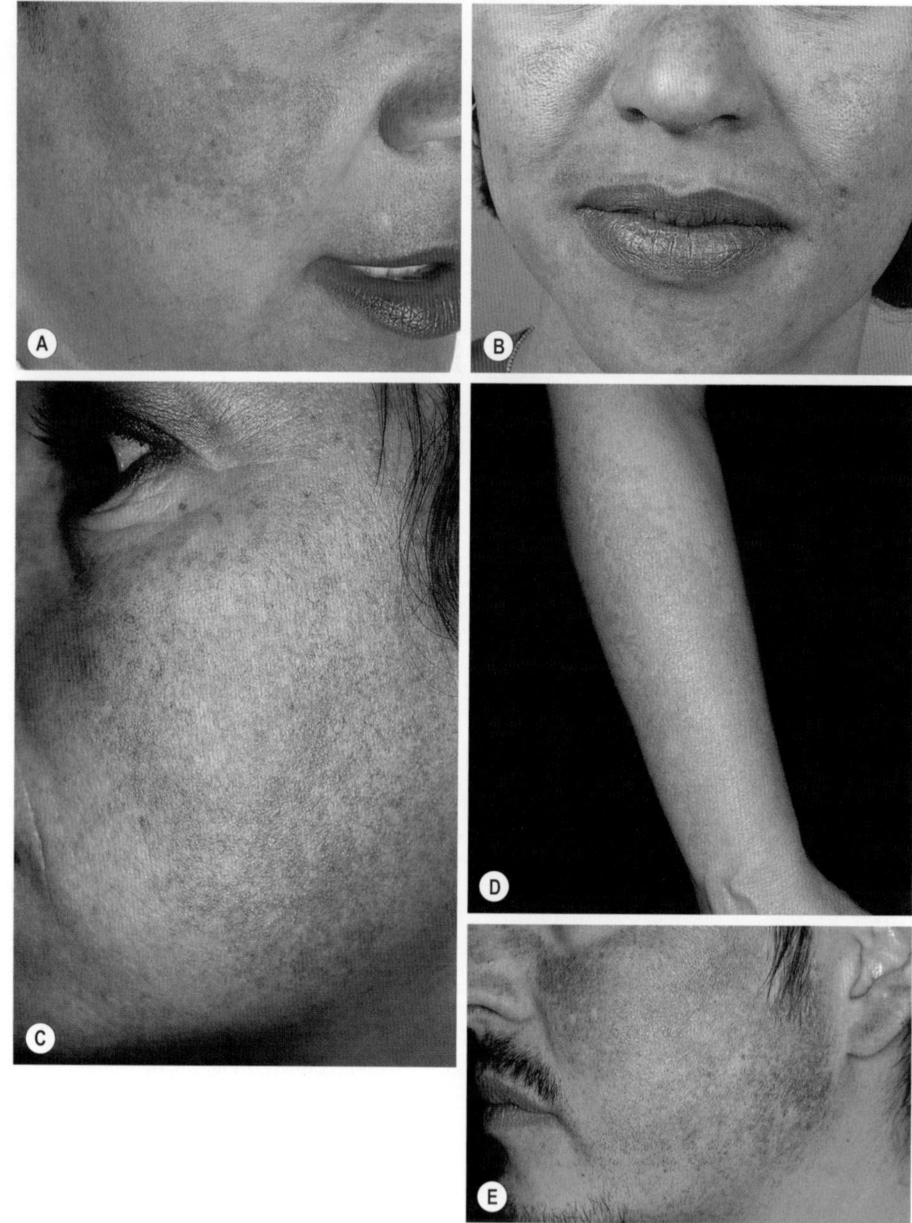

Fig. 55.4 Various forms of melasma and melasma-like hyperpigmentation. **A** Malar variant. **B** Mild centrofacial type with sparing of the philtrum. **C** Extension of the hyperpigmentation onto the mandible. **D** Involvement of the extensor forearm; note the same irregular outline as seen on the face. **E** Melasma-like appearance in a patient with previous acute cutaneous lupus erythematosus.
A, B, Courtesy, NYUDSC; C–E, Courtesy, Jean L. Bolognia, MD.

SELECTED TREATMENT OPTIONS FOR MELASMA
Recommendations for all patients
• Avoidance of sun exposure and tanning beds • Daily use of broad-spectrum sunscreen (ideally SPF ≥30 with physical blocker such as zinc oxide or titanium dioxide) • Sun-protective hats and clothing • Camouflage makeup • Discontinue oral contraceptives, if possible
Active/intense treatment options*,**
First-line topical therapies
• Triple combination of HQ + retinoid + CS† at bedtime • 4% HQ daily, typically at bedtime • Azelaic acid (15–20%)
Adjunctive topical therapy
• L-ascorbic acid (10–15%) • Kojic acid (1–4%) • Tranexamic acid (2–5%)
Second-line therapies
• Glycolic (typically start at 30% and increase as tolerated) or salicyclic acid (20–30%) peels every 4–6 weeks
Third-line therapies‡
• Laser (e.g. fractional) and intense pulsed light therapy (IPL)
Long-term maintenance recommendations
• Daily sunscreen and sun protective measures (see above) • Topical retinoid • Topical α-hydroxy acid (e.g. glycolic acid cream) • Other topicals (e.g. L-ascorbic acid [10–15%], azelaic acid [15–20%], kojic acid [1–4%], tranexamic acid [2–5%])

**Results from topical treatments may take up to 6 months to appreciate; depending on the patient, HQ and combination HQ + retinoid + CS are typically used daily for 2–4 months and then decreased in frequency to 1–2 times per week; prolonged daily use can result in side effects such as perioral dermatitis, telangiectasias, atrophy (CS) and ochronosis (HQ; see Fig. 55.5).*
***While topical HQ can cause an allergic contact dermatitis, all topical agents may cause an irritant contact dermatitis, which can result in worsening of the dyspigmentation; if this is a concern, a small, non-facial site test can be performed prior to widespread facial application.*
†Typically a Class 5–7 topical CS is used (see Appendix).
‡Potential risk of post-procedural dyspigmentation; a site test should be performed prior to widespread facial laser or light therapy.

Table 55.2 Selected treatment options for melasma. HQ, hydroquinone.

- The hyperpigmentation is usually reversible once the bleomycin is discontinued, but it may take 3–4 months to fade
- Other skin findings can include circumscribed hyperpigmentation overlying the small joints of the hands as well as sclerodermoid changes

• ***Flagellate mushroom dermatitis***
- Occurs after eating large amounts of raw or partially cooked shiitake mushrooms
- A second form occurs in persons who cultivate shiitake mushrooms
- Presents initially with pruritic papules and vesicles that develop on the face, scalp, trunk, and proximal extremities; scratching of these lesions then leads to long, flagellate streaks composed of petechiae or papules, followed finally by linear patterns of discoloration (due to hemosiderin) or postinflammatory hyperpigmentation

LINEAR HYPERPIGMENTATION THAT MAY OR MAY NOT BE ALONG THE LINES OF BLASCHKO

• ***Linear postinflammatory hyperpigmentation***
- More common in individuals with darkly pigmented skin
- Occurs after linear trauma (e.g. burn, abrasion, dermatitis artefacta) and along

DRUGS AND CHEMICALS ASSOCIATED WITH CIRCUMSCRIBED HYPERPIGMENTATION OR DISCOLORATION	
Drug or chemical	**Clinical features**
Chemotherapeutic agents	
Mechlorethamine (nitrogen mustard)	• Hyperpigmentation at sites of topical application
Bleomycin (intravenous or intralesional)	See text
Anthracyclines (e.g. daunorubicin, doxorubicin)	• Hyperpigmentation of sun-exposed areas • Hyperpigmentation overlying the small joints of the hand and involving the palms (especially the creases), soles, and oral mucosa (buccal, tongue) • Transverse brown-black melanonychia
5-Fluorouracil	• Hyperpigmentation in sun-exposed areas (~5% of patients treated systemically; often follows an erythematous photosensitivity reaction) • Hyperpigmentation of skin overlying veins in which the drug was infused • Other sites include the dorsal aspects of the hands, palms/soles, and radiation ports • Transverse or diffuse melanonychia; lunular pigmentation
Antimalarials	
Chloroquine, hydroxychloroquine, quinacrine	• Gray to blue-black discoloration, usually pretibial, with (hydroxy) chloroquine; face, hard palate, sclerae, and subungual areas may be involved • Diffuse yellow to yellow-brown discoloration with quinacrine • Discoloration affects up to 25% of patients
Heavy metals	
Arsenic (see Ch. 74)	• Areas of bronze hyperpigmentation ± superimposed "raindrops" of lightly pigmented skin; favors axillae, groin, palms, soles, nipples, and pressure points (see Fig. 74.7A)
Bismuth	• Generalized blue-gray discoloration of the face, neck, and dorsal hands • Oral mucosa and gingivae may be involved
Gold (chrysiasis)	• Permanent blue-gray discoloration in sun-exposed areas, mostly around the eyes
Iron	• Permanent brown discoloration at injection sites or in areas of application of ferric subsulfate (Monsel's) solution as a hemostatic agent • Dermal hemosiderin deposits (due to lysis of extravasated red blood cells and release of their iron stores) are commonly observed in the setting of venous hypertension, in pigmented purpuric dermatoses, at sites of previous solar purpura, and as a side effect of sclerotherapy of superficial veins
Lead	• "Lead line" in gingival margin • Nail discoloration
Mercury	• Slate-gray discoloration, particularly in skin folds

Table 55.3 Drugs and chemicals associated with circumscribed hyperpigmentation or discoloration. *Continued*

DRUGS AND CHEMICALS ASSOCIATED WITH CIRCUMSCRIBED HYPERPIGMENTATION OR DISCOLORATION	
Drug or chemical	**Clinical features**
Silver (argyria)	• Sites of topical application (e.g. of silver sulfadiazine to burns or ulcers) • Diffuse slate-gray discoloration, increased in sun-exposed areas; occurs in settings of occupational exposure, alternative medications, or systemic absorption from use of silver sulfadiazine on extensive burns/wounds • The nail unit (diffuse or localized to the lunulae) and sclerae may also be affected
Hormones	
Oral contraceptives, hormone replacement therapy	• Melasma; increased pigmentation of nipples and nevi
Miscellaneous compounds	
Amiodarone	• Slate-gray to violaceous discoloration of sun-exposed skin, especially the face (less common than erythema from photosensitivity) • Fair-skinned patients after long-term, continuous therapy; usually fades over months to years after discontinuation of the drug, but may persist
Azidothymidine (zidovudine, AZT)	• Longitudinal > transverse and diffuse melanonychia (up to 10% of patients); blue lunulae • Mucocutaneous hyperpigmentation (e.g. widespread diffuse, acral, oral macules); most common in patients with darkly pigmented skin, and may be accentuated in areas of friction or sun exposure
Clofazimine	• Violet-brown to blue-gray discoloration, especially lesional skin (Fig. 55.7) • Diffuse red to red-brown discoloration of skin, conjunctivae
Diltiazem	• Slate-gray to gray-brown discoloration of sun-exposed skin in patients with skin phototypes IV–VI (see Fig. 73.12); perifollicular accentuation and a reticular pattern may be observed
Hydroquinone	See text and Fig. 55.5
Minocycline	• *Type I:* blue-black discoloration in sites of inflammation and scars, including those due to acne (Fig. 55.8C) • *Type II:* blue-gray macules/patches (1 mm–10 cm in size) within previously normal skin, most often on the shins (Fig. 55.8A,B); sometimes misdiagnosed as ecchymoses • *Type III:* diffuse "muddy brown" pigmentation that is most prominent in sun-exposed areas • Blue-black discoloration may also involve nails, sclerae, oral mucosa, bones, thyroid, and teeth
Psychotropic drugs (e.g. chlorpromazine, amitriptyline)	• Slate-gray discoloration in sun-exposed areas

Table 55.3 *Continued* **Drugs and chemicals associated with circumscribed hyperpigmentation or discoloration.** Additional drugs include busulfan (causes more diffuse hyperpigmentation), hydroxyurea (hyperpigmentation over pressure points and mucosal [see Fig. 55.6], melanonychia), methotrexate (sun-exposed sites), imatinib (localized or diffuse, may involve nails and mucosa). Diffuse hyperpigmentation and discoloration is discussed in Fig. 55.9.

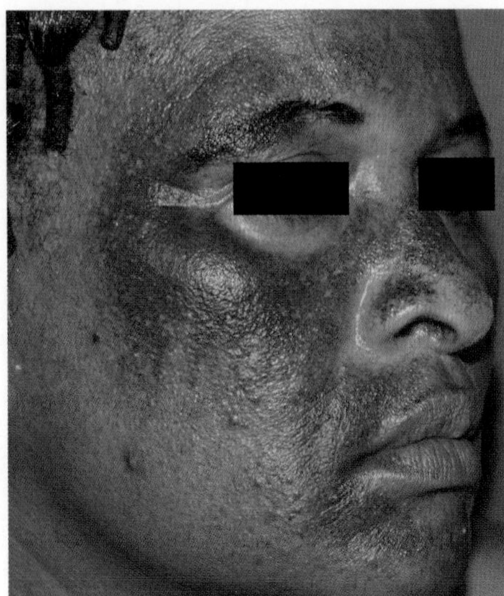

Fig. 55.5 Exogenous ochronosis secondary to topical hydroquinone. This cause of progressive darkening is seen more commonly in Africa. *Courtesy, Regional Dermatology Training Centre, Moshi, Tanzania.*

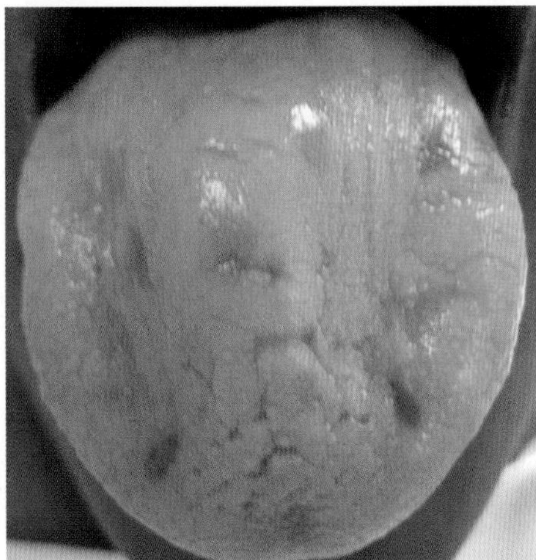

Fig. 55.6 Hydroxyurea-induced hyperpigmentation of the oral mucosa. Circumscribed hyperpigmented macules on the dorsal tongue. *Courtesy, Brian Horvath, MD.*

veins (e.g. phlebitis, intravenous drug abuse, systemic sclerosis); also follows linear inflammatory dermatoses, most often allergic contact dermatitis due to plants (e.g. poison ivy/oak dermatitis) or phytophotodermatitis, which requires both plant exposure and UVR (see Fig. 55.2E)

- Occasionally, postinflammatory hyperpigmentation may follow the lines of Blaschko due to the configuration of the antecedent inflammatory dermatosis (e.g. linear lichen planus, Blaschkitis)

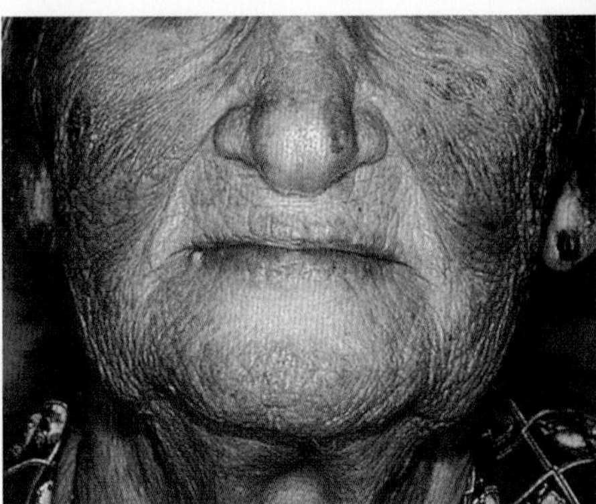

Fig. 55.7 Blue-violet discoloration of previous leprosy lesions in a patient treated with clofazimine. *Courtesy, Anne Burdick, MD.*

Reticulated Hyperpigmentation

- Disorders characterized by true reticulated macular hyperpigmentation are unusual and are primarily rare genodermatoses (Table 55.6; Figs 55.17–55.20).
- It is more common to encounter disorders where the reticulated hyperpigmentation represents just one of several components; as an example, confluent and reticulated papillomatosis (CARP) of Gougerot and Carteaud also has papillomatosis and slight hyperkeratosis (see Fig. 55.17).
- In addition, it is necessary to exclude cutaneous disorders characterized by reticulated erythema (e.g. livedo reticularis) or poikiloderma (e.g. poikiloderma of Civatte).
- Reticulated hyperpigmentation can also correspond to the pattern of the venous plexus (e.g. later stage of erythema ab igne); the clinical clue is a wider spacing than in genodermatoses.

Dyschromatoses

- The dyschromatoses are characterized by the presence of both hypo- and hyperpigmentation; often at least one component of the dyspigmentation is guttate in configuration.
- These disorders can be divided into three groups:
  - *Genetic* (e.g. dyschromatosis symmetrica hereditaria [Fig. 55.21] and dyschromatosis universalis hereditaria [Fig. 55.22])

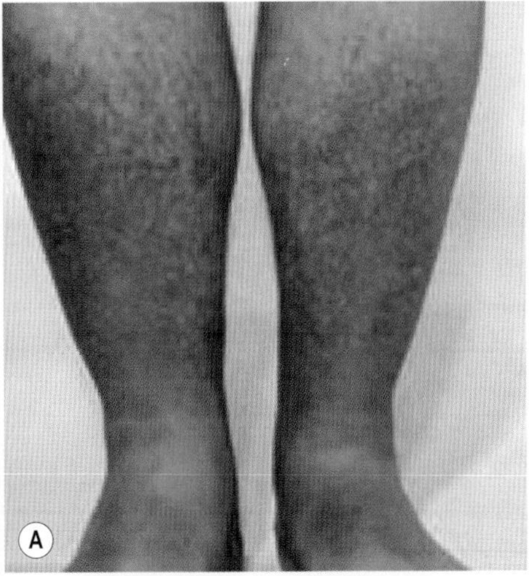

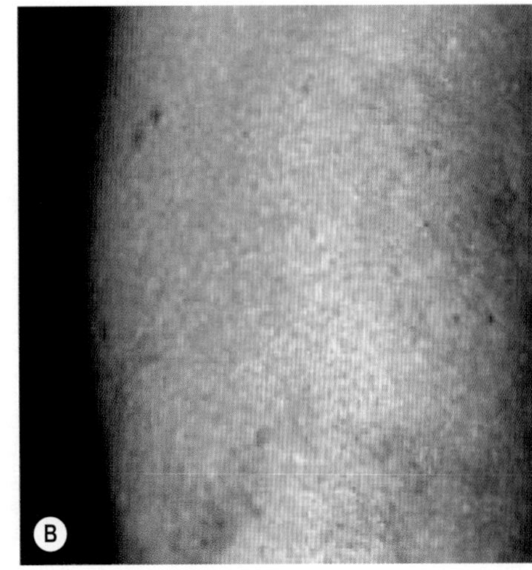

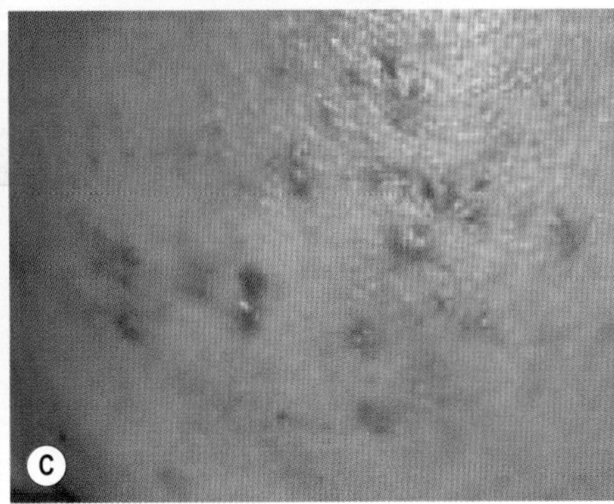

Fig. 55.8 Minocycline-induced discoloration. **A** The distribution on the shins and the gray-blue color can be similar to that seen with antimalarials. **B** Sometimes the discoloration is misdiagnosed as ecchymoses, but the subsequent color changes of green and yellow do not occur. **C** Blue-black pigmentation within acne scars and inflammatory papules.
A, Courtesy, Mary Wu Chang, MD; B, Courtesy, YDRSC; C, Courtesy, Richard Antaya, MD.

- *Exposure-induced* (e.g. arsenic [see Fig. 74.7A], monobenzyl ether of hydroquinone [MBEH], diphenylcyclopropenone [DPCP], betel leaf)
- *Infection-related* (e.g. secondary syphilis, pinta [see Ch. 61])

• There is also a variant of cutaneous amyloidosis that is dyschromic.

For further information see Ch. 67 from *Dermatology, Fourth Edition*.

For additional online figures and tables visit www.expertconsult.com 

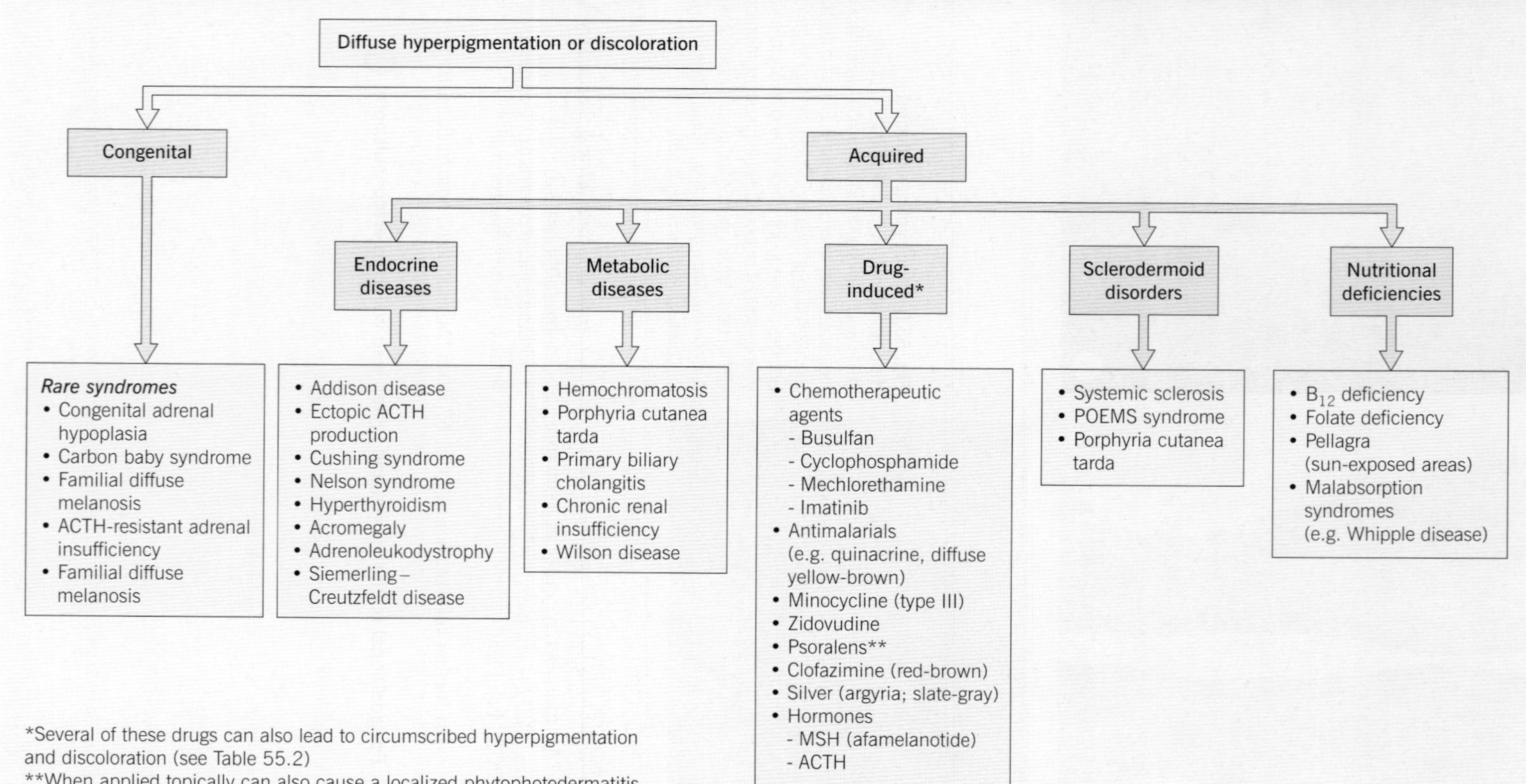

Fig. 55.9 Differential diagnosis and clinical

DISORDERS WITH LINEAR HYPERPIGMENTATION
Follows the lines of Blaschko
Inherited/early onset
Linear and whorled nevoid hypermelanosis ("pigmentary mosaicism"*; see Fig. 55.10) Early or subtle epidermal nevus Third stage of incontinentia pigmenti** (see Fig. 55.12) X-linked reticulate pigmentary disorder** Focal dermal hypoplasia** (Goltz syndrome; hyperpigmented macules within linear streaks, along with cribriform dermal atrophy, fat "herniation", hypopigmentation, and/or telangiectasias) X-linked hypohidrotic ectodermal dysplasia** Conradi–Hünermann–Happle syndrome** Café-au-lait macules of McCune–Albright syndrome (more often broad bands or block-like) Chimerism (more often block-like or ill-defined pattern)
Acquired/often later onset
Linear lichen planus, lichen planus pigmentosus, erythema dyschromicum perstans, or fixed drug eruption Linear atrophoderma of Moulin (see Fig. 55.13), possibly linear morphea Postinflammatory hyperpigmentation due to Blaschkitis Linear biphasic cutaneous amyloidosis‡
Does *not* follow the lines of Blaschko
Pigmentary dermarcation lines (see Figs 55.14 and 55.15, Table 55.5) Linea nigra (Fig. 22.7B) Phytophotodermatitis (see Fig. 55.2E) Sock- or mitten-line hyperpigmentation Flagellate hyperpigmentation – e.g. from bleomycin (see Fig. 55.16), shiitake mushroom dermatitis, dermatomyositis, persistent plaques of Still disease Serpentine supravenous hyperpigmentation, e.g. from phlebitis, intravenous drug use, systemic sclerosis Additional causes of linear postinflammatory hyperpigmentation – excoriations, trauma/abuse, burns, allergic contact dermatitis (especially to plants), koebnerized lesions (e.g. psoriasis, lichen planus), coining

**Pigmentary mosaicism can also present with hyperpigmentation in a block-like pattern, referred to as segmental pigmentation disorder (see Fig. 55.11).*
***Primarily in female patients, due to functional mosaicism (via lyonization) in these X-linked disorders; occasionally in male patients with somatic mosaicism or Klinefelter syndrome.*
‡Single case.

Table 55.4 Disorders with linear hyperpigmentation.

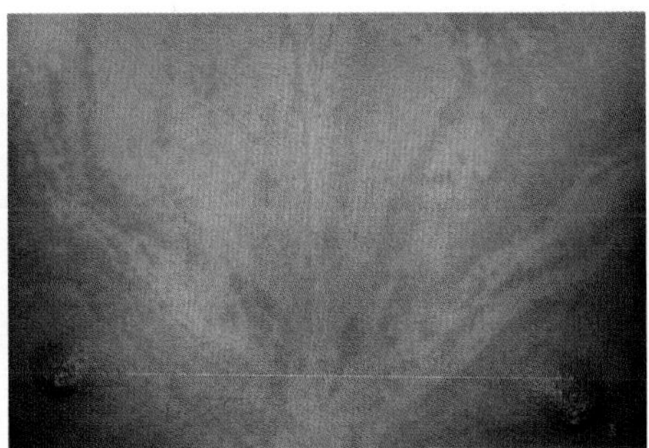

Fig. 55.10 Linear and whorled nevoid hypermelanosis (LWNH) on the trunk. This young African-American girl had developmental delay. Note the distribution along the lines of Blaschko. *Courtesy, Julie V. Schaffer, MD.*

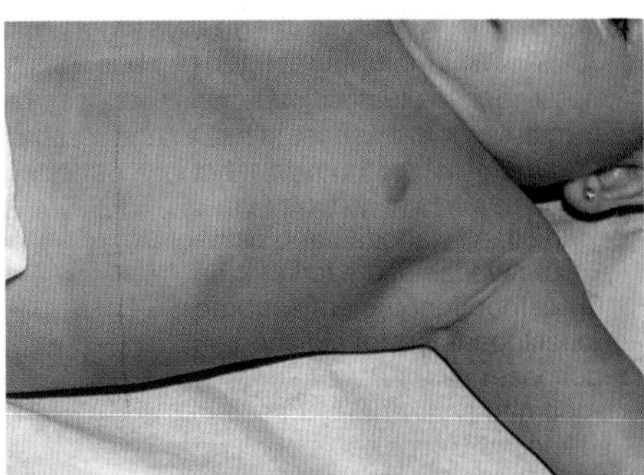

Fig. 55.11 Segmental pigmentation disorder. Unilateral block-like hyperpigmentation on the chest, abdomen and upper arm of an infant. Note the midline demarcation inferiorly. *Courtesy, Julie V. Schaffer, MD.*

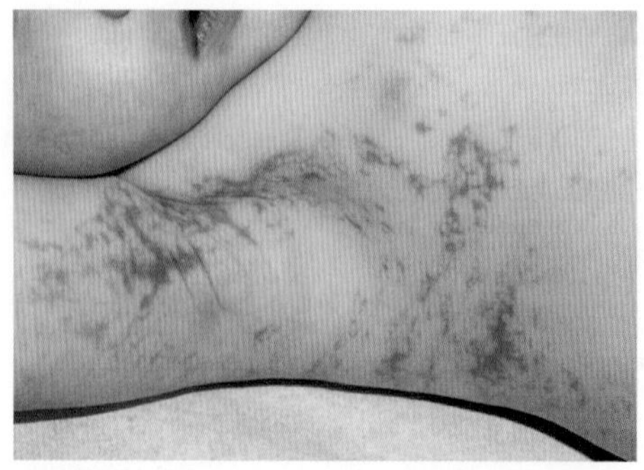

Fig. 55.12 Stage 3 incontinentia pigmenti in a 2-year-old child. Note the characteristic gray-brown color, and the distribution along the lines of Blaschko. *Courtesy, Julie V. Schaffer, MD.*

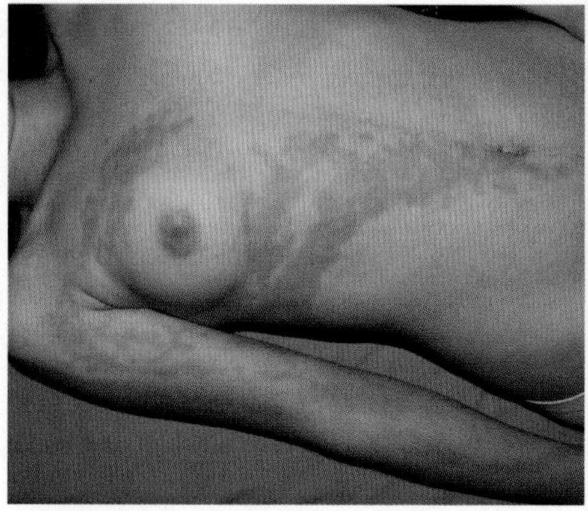

Fig. 55.13 Linear hyperpigmentation due to atrophoderma of Moulin. Note the subtle depression of the lesions. *Courtesy, Antonio Torrelo, MD.*

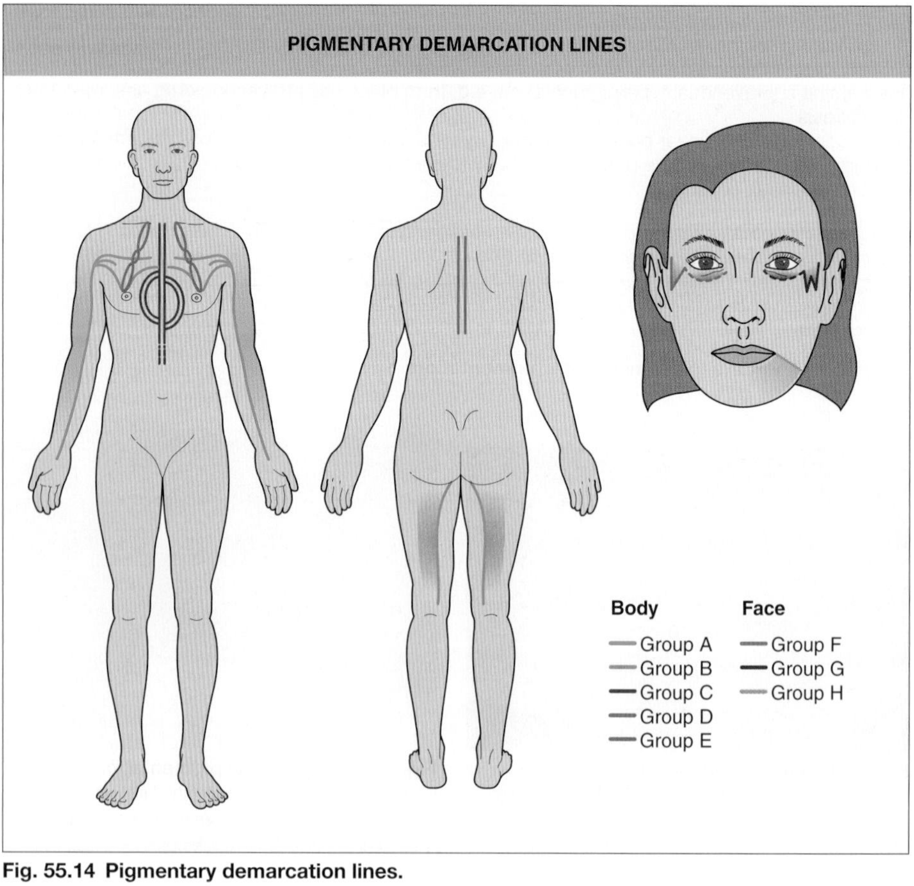

PIGMENTARY DEMARCATION LINES

Body
Group A
Group B
Group C
Group D
Group E

Face
Group F
Group G
Group H

Fig. 55.14 Pigmentary demarcation lines.

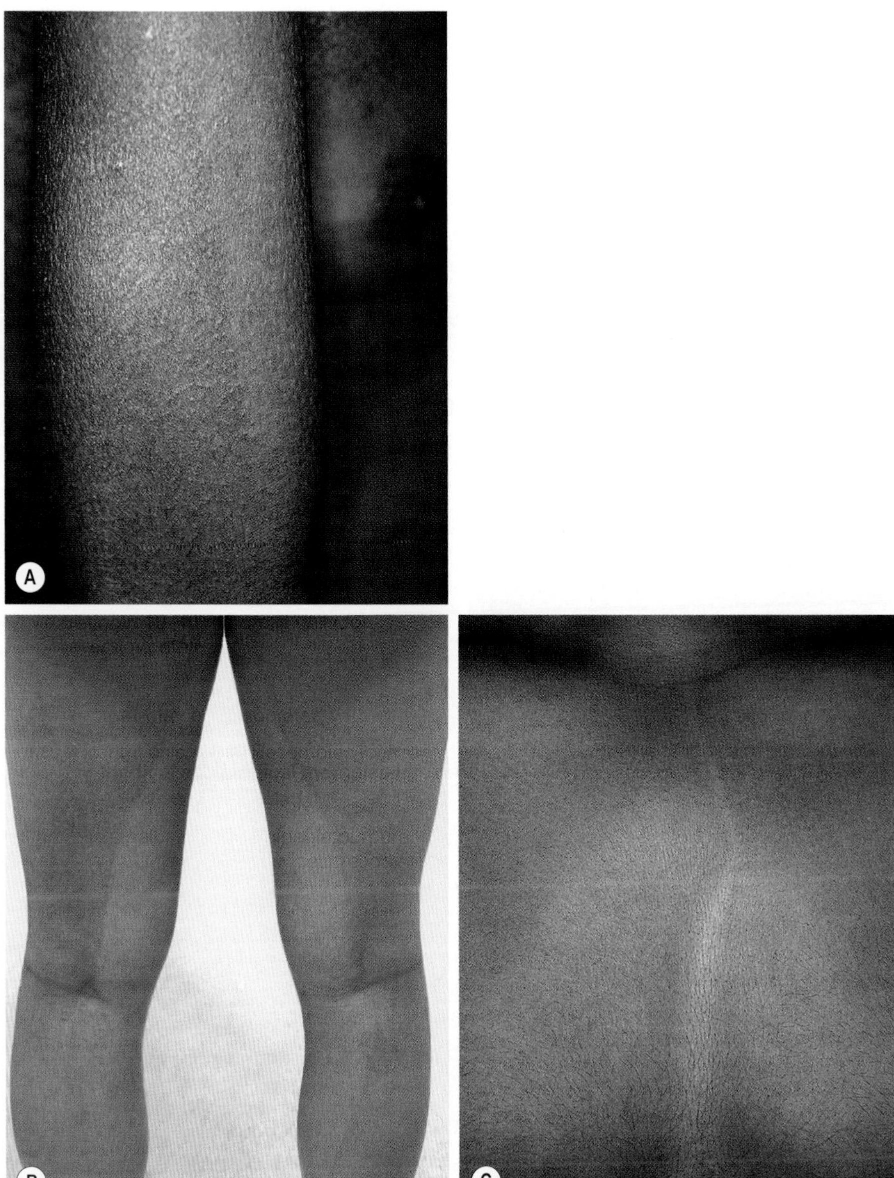

Fig. 55.15 Pigmentary demarcation lines (PDLs). A The most common PDL (Type A) is on the upper arm, with relative hypopigmentation on the ventral surface. **B** Type B PDLs on the posterior thighs, with relative hypopigmentation medially. **C** Type C PDL (composed of parallel lines) may be confused with linear nevoid hypopigmentation. *A, C, Courtesy, Jean L. Bolognia, MD; B, Courtesy, Justin Finch, MD.*

PIGMENTARY DEMARCATION LINES: FIVE MAJOR TYPES (A-E) AND PROPOSED FACIAL TYPES (F-H)	
Type	**Description**
A	A vertical line along the anterolateral portion of the upper arm that may extend into the pectoral region (most commonly observed type; see Fig. 55.15A)
B	A curved line on the posteromedial thigh that extends from the perineum to the popliteal fossa and occasionally to the ankle (see Fig. 55.15B)
C	A vertical or curved hypopigmented band on the mid chest that results from two parallel pigmentary demarcation lines (see Fig. 55.15C)
D	A vertical line in a pre- or paraspinal location
E	Bilateral chest markings (hypopigmented macules and patches) in a zone that runs from the mid third of the clavicle to the periareolar skin
F&G	“V”- or “W”-shaped lines between the lateral temple and malar prominence; a curved line may extend medially in the infraorbital area
H	A diagonal line from the angle of the mouth to the lateral aspect of the chin

Table 55.5 Pigmentary demarcation lines: five major types (A–E) and proposed facial types (F–H). Also see Fig. 55.14.

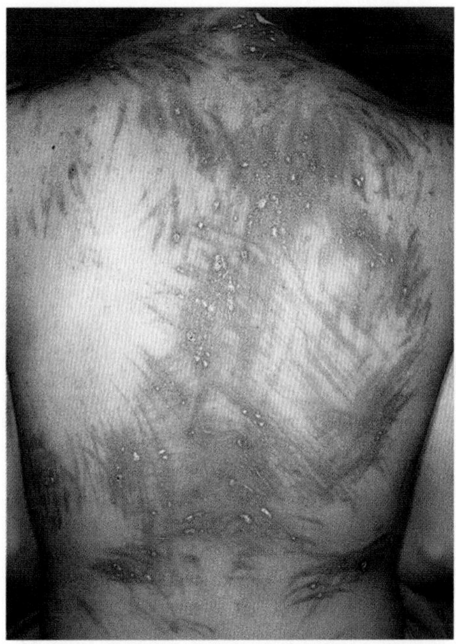

Fig. 55.16 Flagellate pigmentation. This young man had received bleomycin as a treatment for his lymphoma. Note the linear excoriations. *Courtesy, David E. Cohen, MD, MPH.*

DISORDERS CHARACTERIZED BY RETICULATED HYPERPIGMENTATION	
Disorder	**Key features**
Reticulated hyperpigmentation with additional cutaneous features	
Confluent and reticulated papillomatosis (CARP) of Gougerot and Carteaud (Fig. 55.17)	• Elevated, favors neck and upper trunk; treated with minocycline • Often appears during adolescence
Erythema ab igne (later stage) (Fig. 74.3)	• Widely spaced net that corresponds to vascular pattern • Due to heat injury, including from heating pads (back) or laptop computer batteries (anterior thighs)
Atopic dirty neck	• Anterolateral neck • Favors children
Epidermolysis bullosa simplex (EBS) herpetiformis (Dowling–Meara) and EBS with mottled pigmentation*	• "Mottled" appearance; AD, due to *KRT 5/14* mutations • Onset during early childhood
Prurigo pigmentosa	• Typically young Asian (primarily Japanese) women • Favors the back, neck, and chest • Recurrent crops of pruritic papulovesicles that resolve with a reticulated pattern of hyperpigmentation
True reticulated macular hyperpigmentation – onset in infancy or early childhood	
X-linked reticulate pigmentary disorder	• XLR, due to *POLA1* mutations • *Males* present with generalized reticulated pigmentation, neonatal colitis, recurrent pneumonia, hypohidrosis, photophobia, ± amyloid deposits in adults • *Female carriers* present with hyperpigmented streaks along lines of Blaschko
Dyskeratosis congenita* (Fig. 55.18)	• XLR form more common than AD and AR forms • ~50% due to mutations in the *TERT*, *TERC*, *DKC1*, or *TINF2* genes • Pterygium, leukoplakia, pancytopenia, mucosal squamous cell carcinoma, leukemia
Fanconi anemia*	• AR, with at least 11 complementation groups; rarely XLR • More diffuse hyperpigmentation, radial ray bony defects, pancytopenia, leukemia
Dermatopathia pigmentosa reticularis (Fig. 55.19)	• AD; due to *KRT14* mutations • Persistent hyperpigmentation, alopecia, nail dystrophy; absent dermatoglyphics in some patients
Naegeli–Franceschetti–Jadassohn syndrome	• AD; due to *KRT14* mutations • Fading hyperpigmentation, hypohidrosis, dental anomalies, palmoplantar hyperkeratosis, reduced/missing dermatoglyphics, nail dystrophy
True reticulated macular hyperpigmentation – onset in adolescence or adulthood	
Dowling–Degos disease (DDD) (Fig. 55.20)	• AD; due to mutations in *KRT5, POFUT1,* and *POGLUT1* • Reticulated hyperpigmentation of major flexures, comedones on the back and neck, pitted facial scars
Galli–Galli disease	• Acantholytic variant of DDD
Haber syndrome	• Rosacea-like facial eruption plus the clinical features of DDD
Pigmentatio reticularis faciei et colli	• Possible variant of DDD • Hyperpigmentation of the face and neck plus multiple epidermoid cysts
Reticulate acropigmentation of Kitamura	• AD; due to *ADAM10* mutations • Atrophic, acral lentigo-like lesions, palmoplantar and dorsal phalangeal pitting

*Also dyschromatosis.

Table 55.6 Disorders characterized by reticulated hyperpigmentation. The two most common disorders are in bold. Additional disorders include Mendes da Costa disease*, Cantu syndrome, reticulate genital hyperpigmentation associated with localized vitiligo*, and mitochondrial disorders. AD, autosomal dominant; *ADAM10, a disintegrin and metalloproteinase 10*; AR, autosomal recessive; *KRT5/14,* keratin 5 or 14; *POFUT1,* protein O-fucosyltransferase 1; *POGLUT1,* protein O-glucosyltransferase 1; *POLA1,* DNA polymerase-α 1, catalytic subunit; XLR, X-linked recessive.

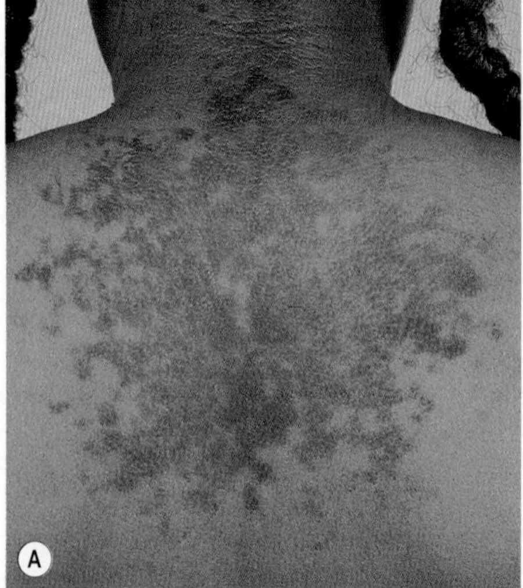

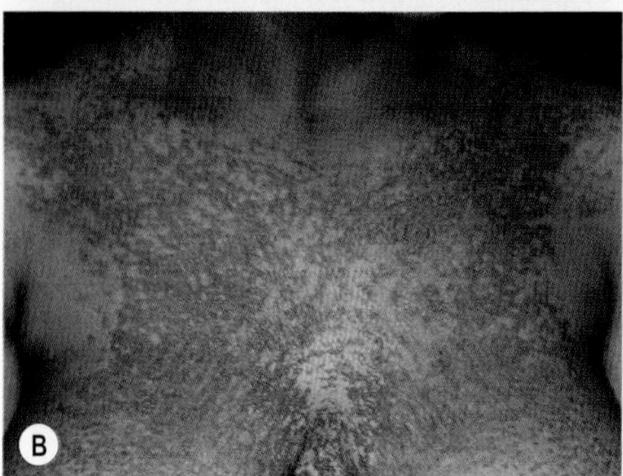

Fig. 55.17 Confluent and reticulated papillomatosis of Gougerot and Carteaud. A On the neck and back of a teenage girl. **B** On the chest of an older woman. *A, Courtesy, Seth Orlow, MD, PhD; B, Courtesy, YDRSC.*

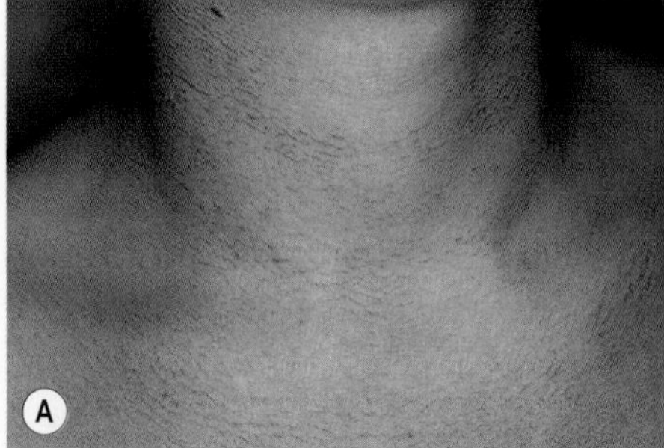

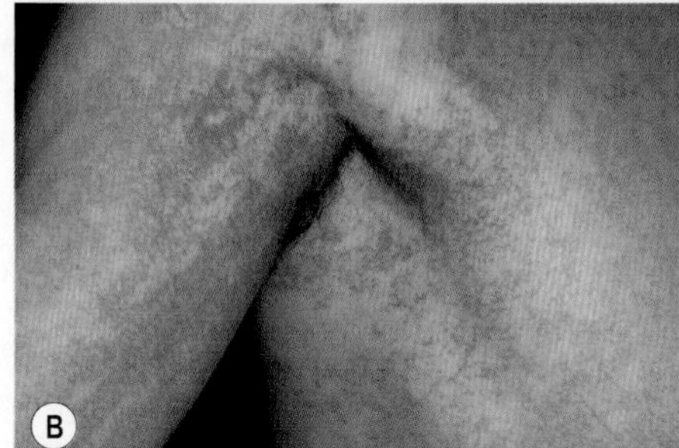

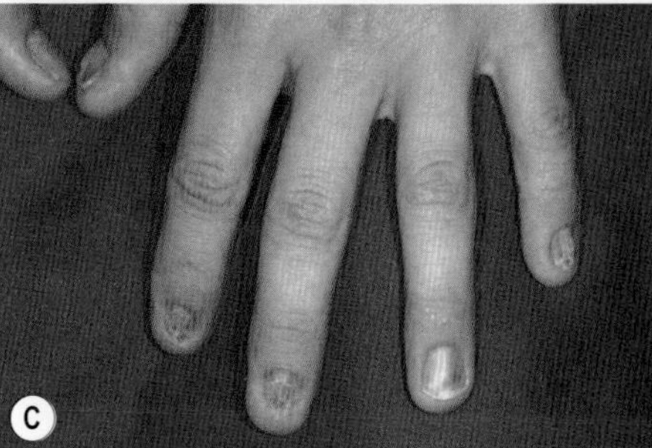

Fig. 55.18 Dyskeratosis congenita. A Reticulated hyperpigmentation on the chest and neck of a teenage boy. **B** More pronounced reticulated and confluent hyperpigmentation on the shoulder and axilla. **C** Longitudinal ridging, splitting, and early pterygium formation in another teenage boy. *A, Courtesy, Seth Orlow, MD, PhD; B, Courtesy, Eugene Mirrer, MD; C, Courtesy, Anthony Mancini, MD.*

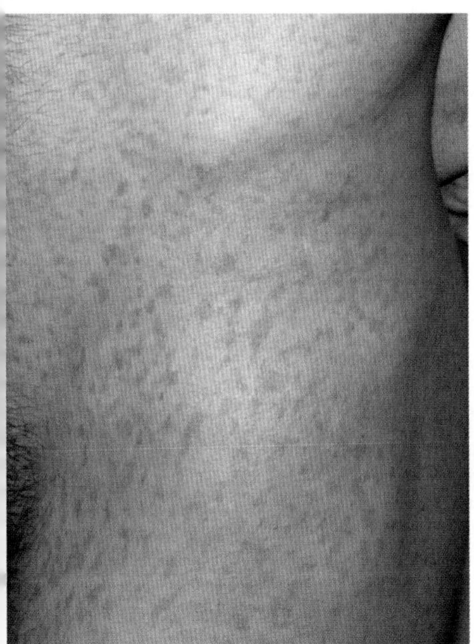

Fig. 55.19 Dermatopathia pigmentosa reticularis. Persistent hyperpigmentation in a reticulated pattern extending from the lower abdomen to the thigh in a young man. *Courtesy, Julie V. Schaffer, MD.*

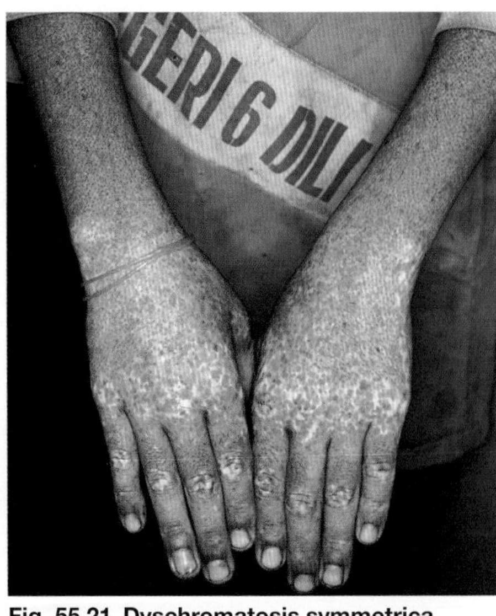

Fig. 55.21 Dyschromatosis symmetrica hereditaria. An autosomal dominant disorder characterized by mutations in *ADAR* (*DSRAD*) (encodes an adenosine deaminase) and mixed hypo- and hyperpigmentation on the distal hands and feet. Note that the hands are more involved than the forearms. *Courtesy, Peter Ehrnstrom, MD.*

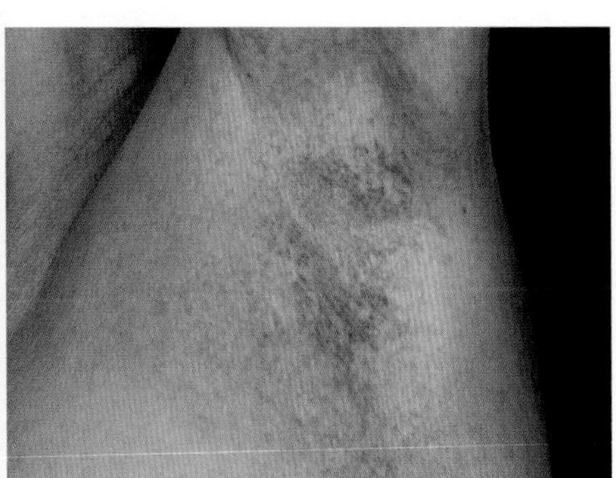

Fig. 55.20 Dowling–Degos disease. Hyperpigmented macules forming a reticulated pattern in the axilla. *Courtesy, Thomas Schwarz, MD.*

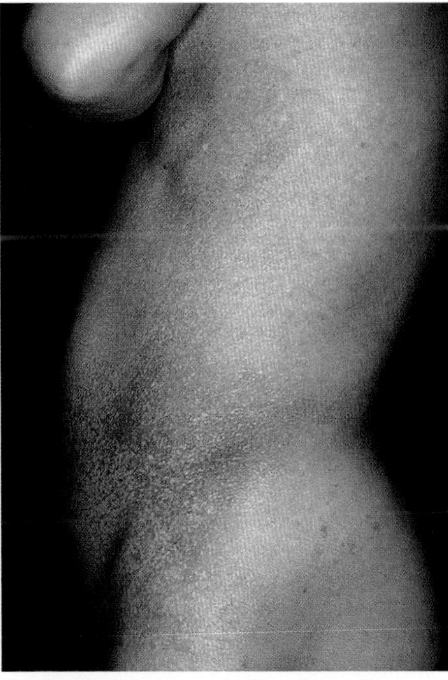

Fig. 55.22 Dyschromatosis universalis hereditaria. Widespread distribution of both hypo- and hyperpigmented macules. *With permission from Urabe K, Hori Y. Dyschromatosis. Semin Cutan Med Surg 1997;16:81–5.*

56 Alopecias

- In a normal scalp, 90–95% of hairs are in anagen phase, 5–10% in telogen phase (Fig. 56.1).
- About 50–100 hairs normally shed daily.
- Alopecias can be categorized as diffuse vs circumscribed, patterned vs non-patterned, and non-scarring vs scarring loss (Fig. 56.2).

Non-Scarring Alopecias

Male and Female Pattern Hair Loss (Androgenetic Alopecia)

- 80% of Caucasian men are affected by age 70 years.
- Women are less likely than men to have a family history of the disorder.
- Related to hormonal effects of dihydrotestosterone (DHT), converted from testosterone by 5-alpha reductase.
- Sensitivity of scalp hair to androgen hormones causes gradual miniaturization of hairs on the frontal/midline/vertex regions of men and the midline and crown of women (Fig. 56.3).
- In women, the frontal hairline is spared (except in the setting of virilization) and a Christmas tree pattern of widening of the hair part may be seen.
- May first become clinically apparent with superimposed telogen effluvium >> alopecia areata, especially in women.
- Should exclude hyperandrogenism (e.g. ovarian or adrenal source) in younger women or in women with signs of virilization (see Ch. 57).
- **Rx:** topical minoxidil 2% or 5% solution (BID) or foam (daily) for both genders; finasteride or dutasteride (inhibits 5-alpha reductase) in men; spironolactone in women; hair transplantation (using occipital hair as the source).

Telogen Effluvium

- Sometimes a definable precipitating event ~3 months prior precedes diffuse shedding, leading to a reduced density of hair on the entire scalp and occasionally other areas of body hair (Table 56.1).

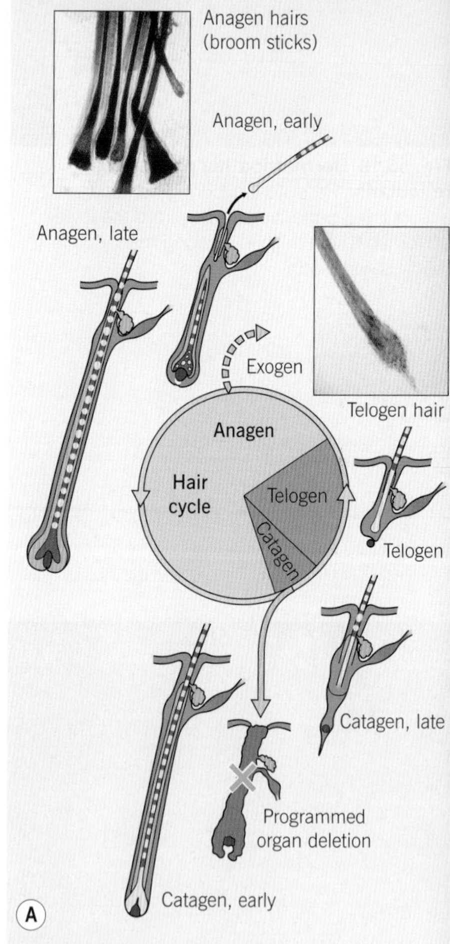

Fig. 56.1 General concepts. A Hair follicle development and cycling. *Courtesy, Ralf Paus, MD; Anagen hairs, Courtesy, Maria K. Hordinsky, MD; Telogen hair, Courtesy, Leonard C. Sperling, MD.* *Continued*

SCHEMATIC OF THE SCALP, SHOWING FRONTAL, TEMPORAL, AND CROWN/VERTEX REGIONS

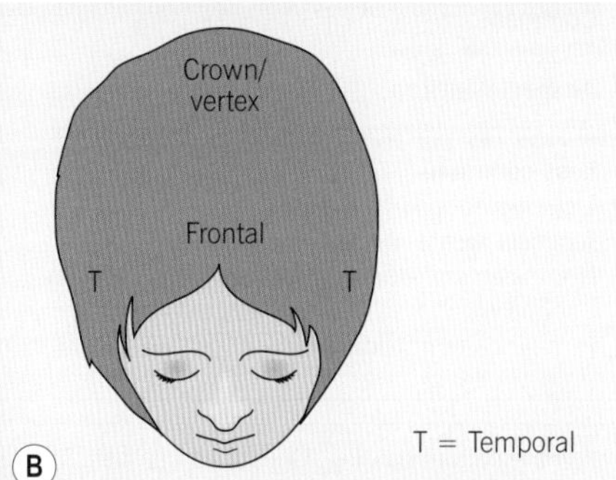

Fig. 56.1 *Continued* **General concepts. B** Schematic of the scalp, showing frontal, temporal, and crown/vertex regions.

- Shed hairs are predominantly telogen hairs (Fig. 56.1).
- Generally complete hair regrowth occurs after months to years.
- Some women have chronic telogen effluvium without a definable cause.
- **Rx:** discontinue any potentially offending drugs, exclude thyroid abnormality and etiologies listed in Table 56.1.

Alopecia Areata

- Autoimmune disease with increased T-cells present in the hair matrix.
- Associated with atopy and other autoimmune diseases (e.g. autoimmune thyroid disease, vitiligo, inflammatory bowel disease, autoimmune polyendocrinopathy syndrome type 1).
- Average lifetime risk for developing this disease is 1–2%.
- Circular to oval areas of alopecia that may progress to total scalp hair loss (alopecia totalis) or total body hair loss (alopecia universalis) (Fig. 56.4).
- May see exclamation point hairs at borders (Fig. 56.4).
- Positive pull test (easily extractable telogen hairs at periphery of oval areas of loss) correlates with active disease.
- Ophiasis pattern is a band-like pattern of loss along the temporal/occipital scalp (Fig. 56.4) that may be less responsive to therapy.
- When there is a single, long-standing lesion in the temporal region, the possibility of temporal triangular alopecia should be considered.
- Associated nail findings = nail pitting, trachyonychia >> brittle nails, onycholysis, koilonychia, onychomadesis (see Ch. 58).
- **Rx:** *for regrowth of hair* – high-potency topical or intralesional CS (e.g. 5 mg/ml); topical irritants (e.g. anthralin or tazarotene), topical immunotherapy (e.g. squaric acid dibutyl ester), topical minoxidil 5%; in rapidly progressive disease, occasionally oral CS are given for a limited trial period (e.g. pulsed therapy over 2–3 months); for severe disease, JAK/STAT pathway inhibitors.

Trichotillomania

- Self-induced twirling, pulling, and/or breaking of hair.
- May be related to a psychologic disorder or stress.
- Plucking of scalp hair results in patchy >> diffuse alopecia, sometimes in a wave-like pattern or centrifugally; hairs tend to be of different lengths (see Fig. 5.5).
- Occiput often spared.
- In difficult cases, can distinguish from alopecia areata by shaving a defined area of involvement and observing for regrowth.
- **Rx:** counseling and treat any underlying psychiatric illness (see Ch. 5).

Postoperative (Pressure-Induced Alopecia)

- Most commonly secondary to a long surgical procedure.
- Generally alopecia seen on occiput as a solitary, oval patch.
- Usually hair regrows completely.

Drug-Induced Alopecia

- Chemotherapeutic agents (e.g. cyclophosphamide, doxorubicin, paclitaxel, etoposide) are common causes of anagen effluvium (see Table 17.8).
- Anagen effluvium can also be secondary to exposure to metals, e.g. arsenic, gold.
- Telogen effluvium can be drug-induced (see Table 56.1).

Secondary Syphilis

- Patchy, "moth-eaten" alopecia in 7% of patients with secondary syphilis.
- Telogen effluvium has also been described.

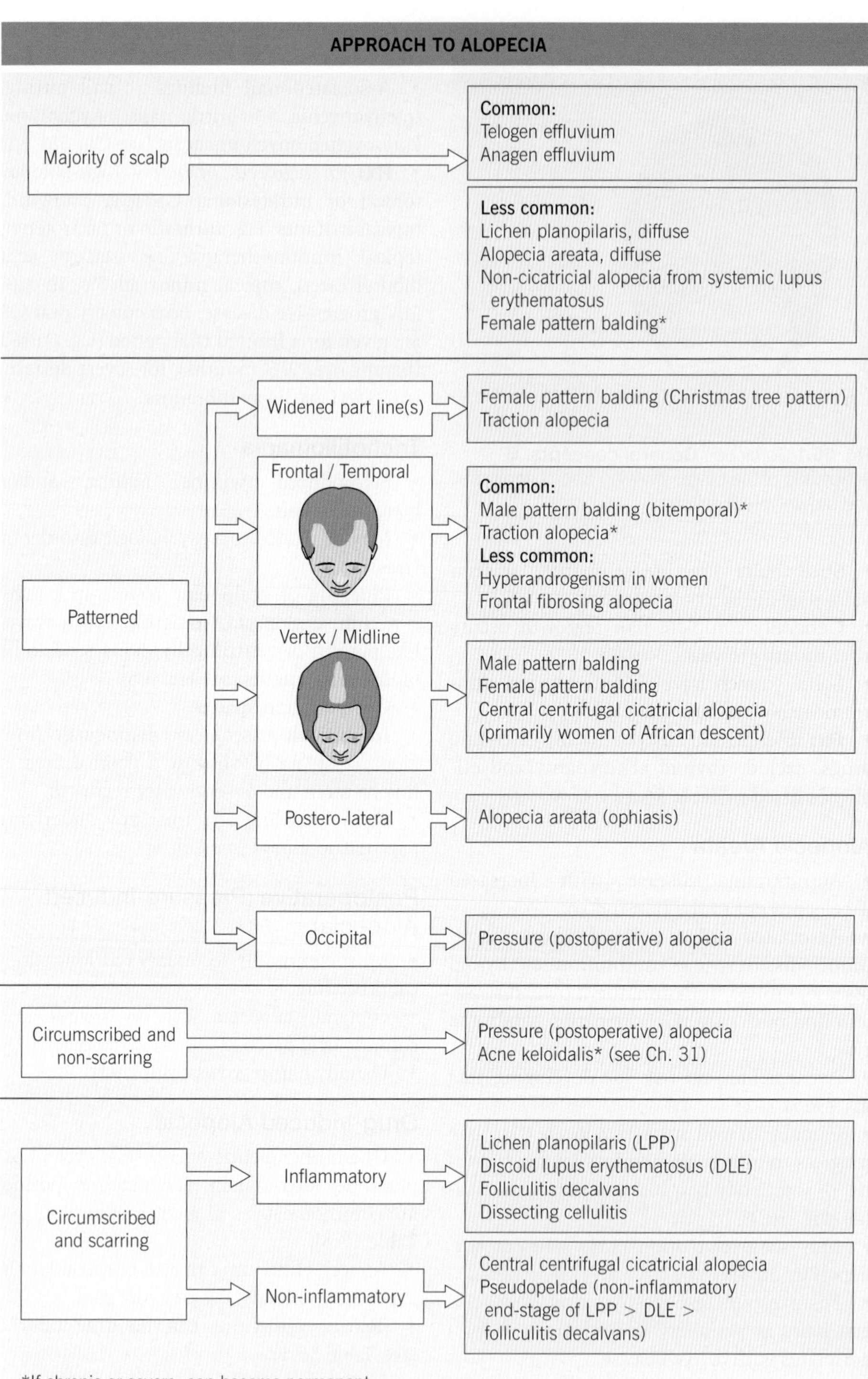

Fig. 56.2 Approach to alopecia.

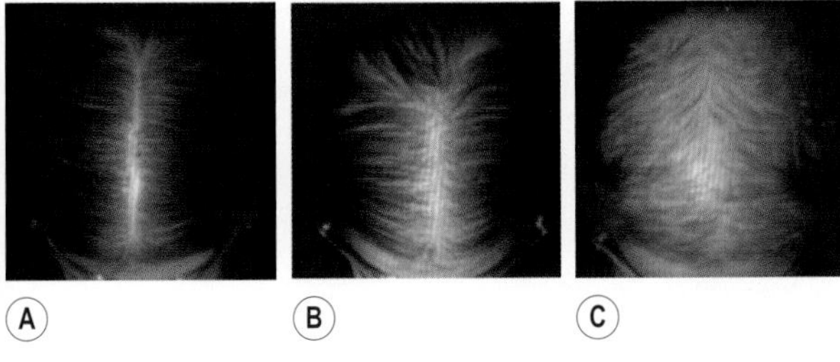

Fig. 56.3 Androgenetic alopecia. Widening of the central part line in early disease (**A**) with further widening and translucency of hairs along the border in more severe disease (**B**). Rarely, hair loss is extensive in advanced disease (**C**). *Courtesy, Rodney D. Sinclair, MD.*

CAUSES OF TELOGEN EFFLUVIUM
• Shedding of the newborn (physiologic)
• Postpartum (physiologic)
• Chronic telogen effluvium (no attributable cause or illness)
• Postfebrile (extremely high fevers, e.g. malaria)
• Severe infection
• Severe chronic illness (e.g. HIV disease, systemic lupus erythematosus)
• Severe, prolonged psychological stress
• Postsurgical (implies major surgical procedure)
• Hypothyroidism and other endocrinopathies (e.g. hyperparathyroidism)
• Crash or liquid protein diets; starvation/malnutrition
• Drugs
– Retinoids (acitretin, isotretinoin)
– Discontinuation of birth control pills
– Anticoagulants (especially heparin)
– Antidepressants
– Lithium
– Antithyroid (propylthiouracil, methimazole)
– Anticonvulsants (e.g. phenytoin, valproic acid, carbamazepine)
– Interferon-α-2b
– Heavy metals
– β-blockers (e.g. propranolol)

Table 56.1 Causes of telogen effluvium. Some authors also propose vitamin B_{12} or iron deficiency as causes.

Psoriatic Alopecia

- Areas of hair loss that in some patients are associated with shedding of thick psoriatic plaques.
- Most commonly non-scarring.

Scarring (Cicatricial) Alopecias

- Classically defined as loss of hair follicles with scarring (e.g. lupus erythematosus, lichen planopilaris) *or* an alopecia in which hair does not grow back (e.g. chronic, long-standing traction alopecia).
- Non-scarring alopecias that may eventually result in permanent hair loss include male and female pattern hair loss > alopecia areata.
- In *secondary* scarring alopecia, the hair is destroyed nonspecifically, i.e. secondary to burns, radiation dermatitis, cutaneous malignancy (see Ch. 100), sarcoidosis, morphea, necrobiosis lipoidica, infections (e.g. severe kerion), mucous membrane (cicatricial) pemphigoid.

Central Centrifugal Cicatricial Alopecia (CCCA)

- Most commonly observed in black women.
- May be related to the use of chemical hair relaxers or thermal relaxers (e.g. flat iron).
- Slowly progressive; centered on the crown/vertex and midline (Fig. 56.5).
- Symptoms may be mild or absent.

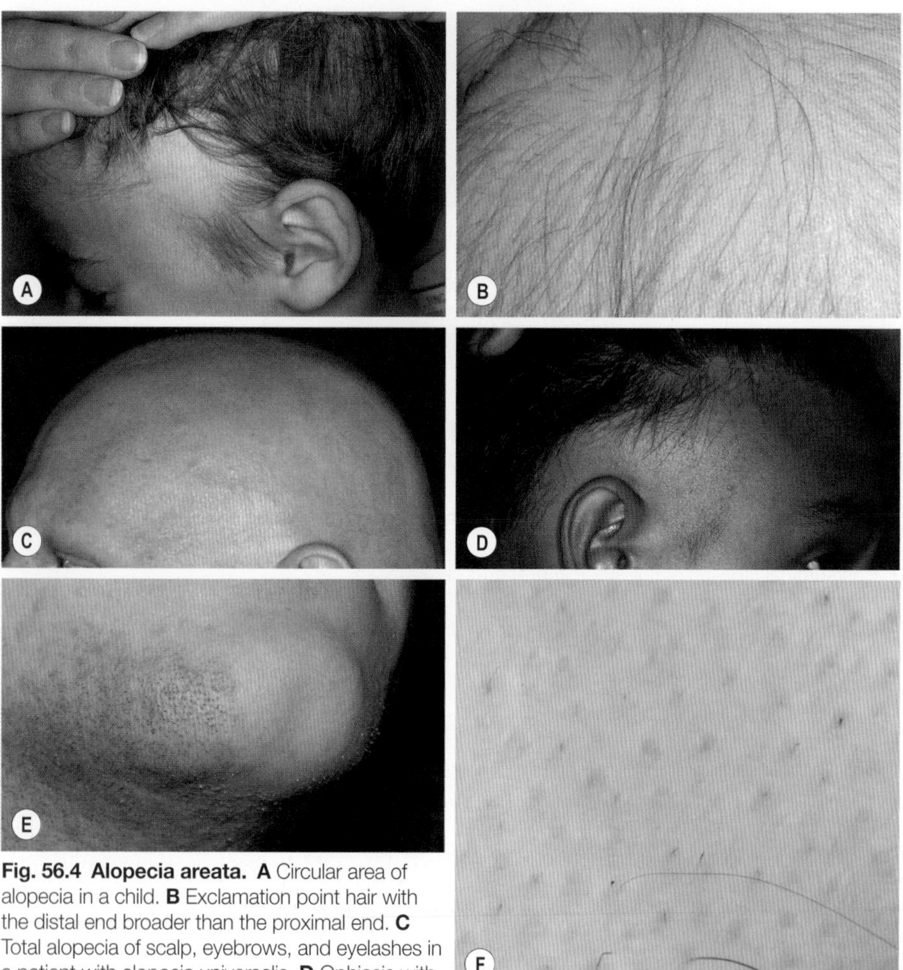

Fig. 56.4 Alopecia areata. **A** Circular area of alopecia in a child. **B** Exclamation point hair with the distal end broader than the proximal end. **C** Total alopecia of scalp, eyebrows, and eyelashes in a patient with alopecia universalis. **D** Ophiasis with a band-like pattern of hair loss along the periphery of the temporal and occipital scalp. **E** Alopecia areata with just beard involvement. **F** Typical yellow dots seen dermoscopically in alopecia areata. *A, D, Courtesy, YDRSC; B, Courtesy, Julie V. Shaffer, MD; C, Courtesy, Leonard C. Sperling, MD; E, Courtesy, Maria K. Hordinsky, MD; F, Courtesy, Iris Zalaudek, MD.*

- Occasionally patients have secondary changes, especially crusting or pustules.
- **Rx:** mild disease – oral tetracycline plus potent topical CS; severe disease – oral rifampin plus oral clindamycin; occasionally intralesional CS if an inflammatory component is present.

Lichen Planopilaris

- Women > men, more common in Caucasians.
- 30% may have associated lichen planus involving the skin (see Table 9.1), mucous membranes, or nails (see Chs 9 and 58).
- Usually several foci of alopecia with loss of follicles and scarring centrally (may be clinically subtle); peripheral follicles having a central, keratotic plug and a rim of inflammation (pink to violet in color) (Fig. 56.6).
- Centered on the crown/vertex or midline.

Frontal Fibrosing Alopecia

• Predominantly affecting the frontal hairline and eyebrows ("frontal fibrosing alopecia") (Fig. 56.7), or rarely a diffuse pattern. Lonely hairs and absence of solar lentigines may be present.

Graham Little Syndrome

• Scalp alopecia, alopecia of axillary/pubic areas, and grouped spinous follicular papules on trunk/extremities.
• **Rx:** topical or intralesional CS, oral doxycycline, oral antimalarials (e.g. hydroxychloroquine), oral retinoids, oral mycophenolate mofetil (if severe).

Discoid Lupus Erythematosus (DLE)

• A type of chronic cutaneous lupus erythematosus.
• More common in adult women, especially black women.
• Minority of patients fulfill the criteria for systemic lupus erythematosus (see Ch. 33), but patients need to be evaluated at the time of diagnosis of DLE and followed longitudinally.
• Circular lesions of erythema, atrophy, dilated/plugged follicles, and scale as well as alopecia.
• As lesions age, central hypopigmentation and peripheral hyperpigmentation may appear, along with scarring (Fig. 56.8).
• May see similar-appearing lesions elsewhere (especially face and ears).
• **Rx:** discussed in Chapter 33.

Acne Keloidalis

• Favors young black men (see Ch. 31).
• Occipital scalp most common site, but sometimes involves the crown/vertex.
• Smooth, firm papules > pustules.
• Initial lesions resolve with alopecia and/or protuberant papules.
• Coalescence of lesions leads to alopecia.
• **Rx:** intralesional CS, oral antibiotics, excision (see Table 31.6).

Dissecting Cellulitis

• May be associated with "follicular occlusion tetrad," which includes this entity,

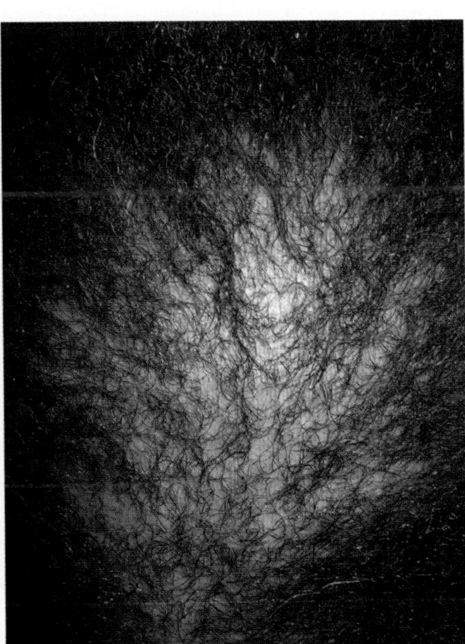

Fig. 56.5 Central centrifugal cicatricial alopecia in an African-American woman. Alopecia is most prominent on the crown/vertex and the midline. *Courtesy, Leonard C. Sperling, MD.*

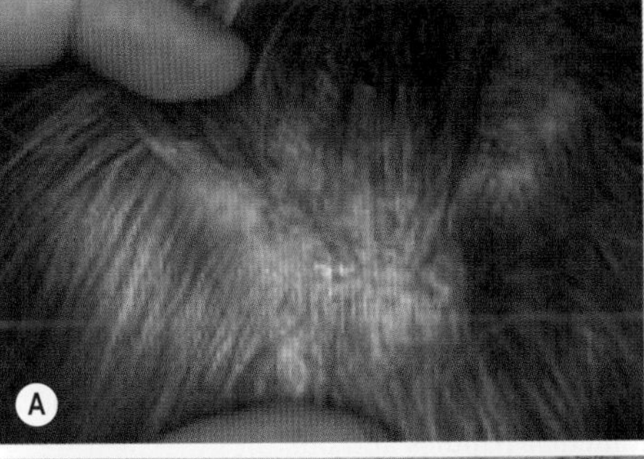

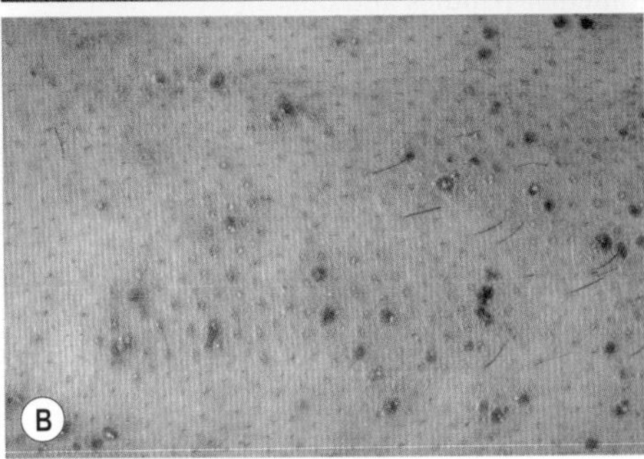

Fig. 56.6 Lichen planopilaris. A Perifollicular erythema in association with scale. **B** Multiple clusters of follicular keratotic plugs on the leg admixed with small violaceous papules, some of which are folliculocentric. *A, Courtesy, Jean L. Bolognia, MD; B, Courtesy, NYUDSC.*

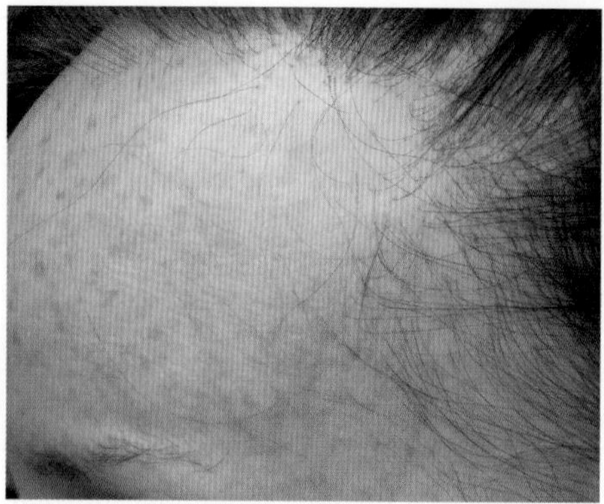

Fig. 56.7 Frontal fibrosing alopecia. Progressive hair loss along the frontotemporal hairline. Note eyebrow hair loss as well as the presence of isolated "lonely" hairs on the upper forehead. *Courtesy, Leonard C. Sperling, MD, and Rodney D. Sinclair, MD.*

hidradenitis suppurativa, acne conglobata, and pilonidal cyst/sinus.

- Affects young adult men, especially black men.
- Multiple, firm scalp nodules over crown/vertex/occiput that become boggy and fluctuant with purulent discharge; often interconnecting.
- Sometimes little pain.
- **Rx:** intralesional CS, antibiotics based on cultures, incision and drainage, excision.

Folliculitis Decalvans

- Inflammatory scarring alopecia with perifollicular papules and pustules.
- **Rx:** dapsone, oral antibiotics (e.g. tetracycline or doxycycline for anti-inflammatory effects; combination of rifampin and clindamycin).

Pseudopelade (of Brocq)

- Considered by most to be the end-stage, burned-out phase of different scarring alopecias (Fig. 56.9), especially lichen planopilaris.

Traction Alopecia (Late-Stage)

- Occurs after years of hair styling that causes traction.
- Generally seen in black women on the bitemporal/frontal scalp line (Fig. 56.10).

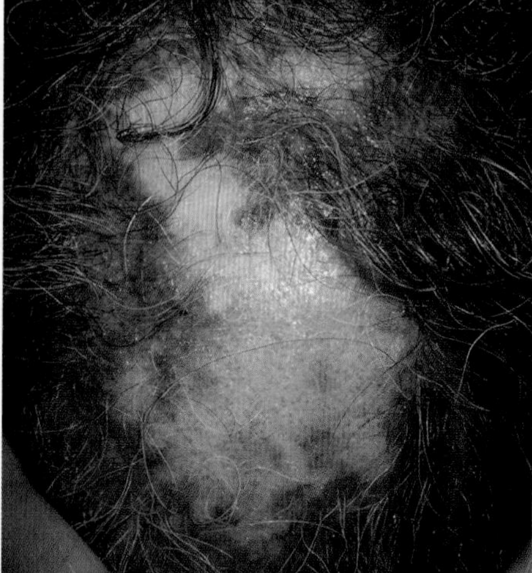

Fig. 56.8 Discoid lupus erythematosus. Coalescing areas of alopecia in which there is obvious erythema. Central hypopigmentation is accompanied by peripheral hyperpigmentation. *Courtesy, Leonard C. Sperling, MD, and Rodney D. Sinclair, MD.*

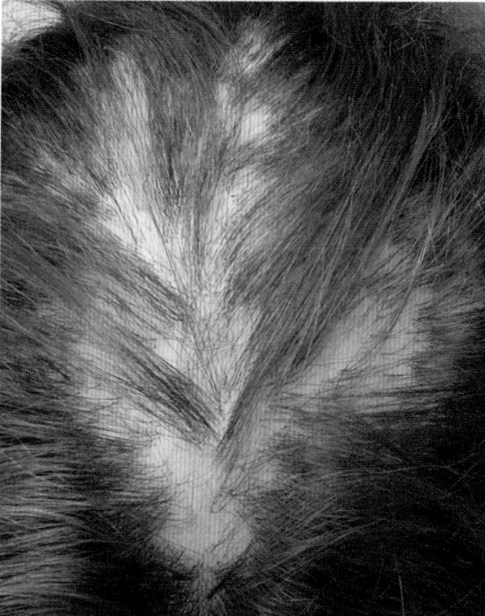

Fig. 56.9 Pseudopelade (end-stage scarring alopecia). Irregularly shaped areas of scarring alopecia along the midline. *Courtesy, Kalman Watsky, MD.*

Hair Shaft Abnormalities

- Four main categories: (1) *fractures* (trichorrhexis nodosa and invaginata, trichoschisis); (2) *irregularities* (monilethrix); (3) *twisting* (pili torti, woolly hair, trichonodosis); and (4) *extraneous matter* (Fig. 56.11).

• Can also divide into *increased breakage* (bubble hair, monilethrix, pili torti, trichorrhexis invaginata and nodosa, trichothiodystrophy) and *no increased breakage* (loose anagen, pili annulati, spun-glass hair, woolly hair).

• Trichorrhexis nodosa – common hair shaft abnormality that leads to increased breakage; hair shaft fractured with the appearance of two brushes pushing against each other; seen with hair straightening.

• Loose anagen hair syndrome – common cause of sparse, short hair especially in young children, with improvement over time; anagen hairs are poorly anchored and therefore easily shed or pulled, but breakage is not increased.

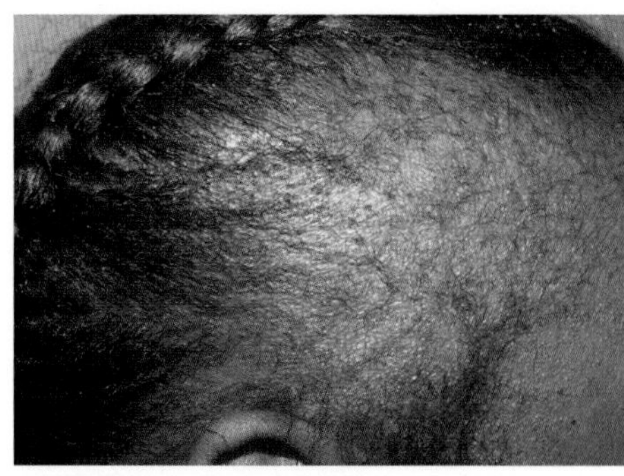

Fig. 56.10 Traction alopecia. Favors frontotemporal area in African-American women and is due to traumatic types of hair styling. *Courtesy, Leonard C. Sperling, MD.*

Trichoscopy (Fig. 56.12)

For further information see Ch. 69 from *Dermatology, Fourth Edition*.

For additional online figures visit www.expertconsult.com 

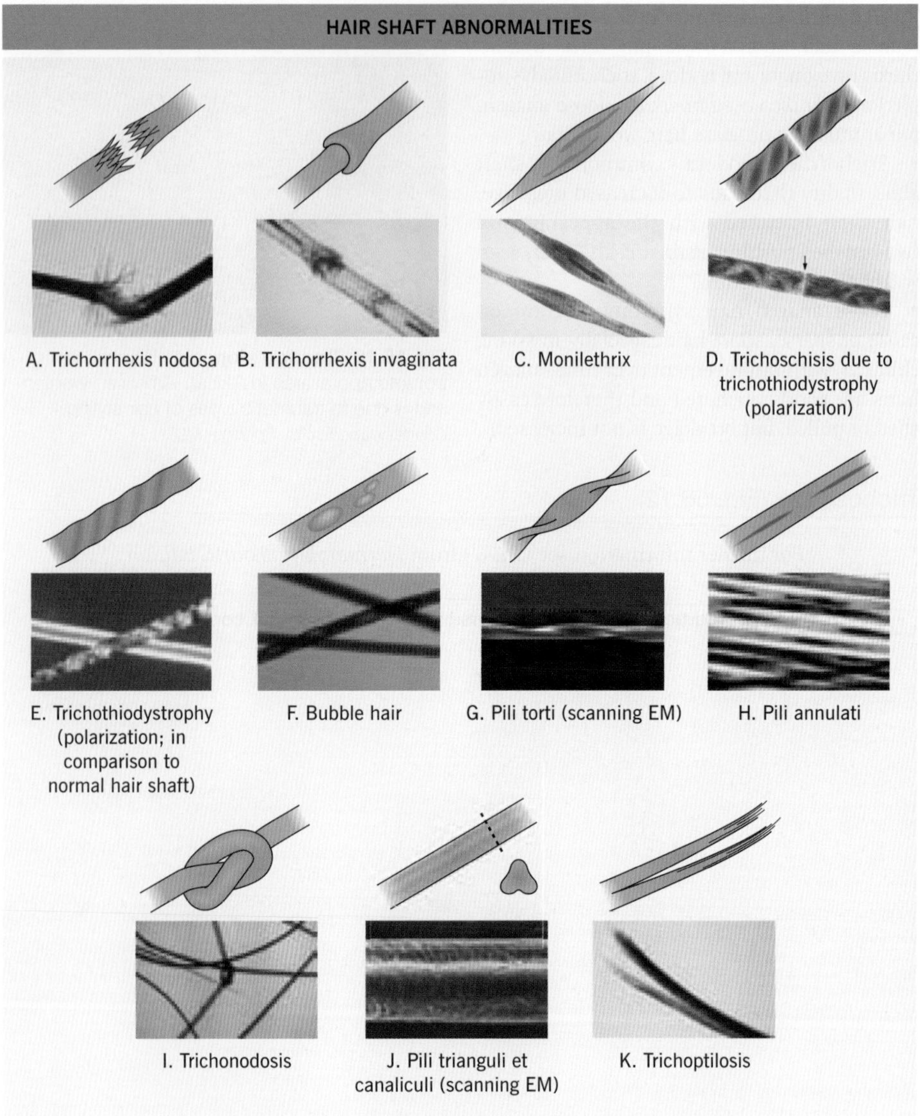

HAIR SHAFT ABNORMALITIES

A. Trichorrhexis nodosa

B. Trichorrhexis invaginata

C. Monilethrix

D. Trichoschisis due to trichothiodystrophy (polarization)

E. Trichothiodystrophy (polarization; in comparison to normal hair shaft)

F. Bubble hair

G. Pili torti (scanning EM)

H. Pili annulati

I. Trichonodosis

J. Pili trianguli et canaliculi (scanning EM)

K. Trichoptilosis

Fig. 56.11 Schematic drawings and microscopic appearance of hair shaft abnormalities. **A** Trichorrhexis nodosa. **B** Trichorrhexis invaginata. **C** Monilethrix. **D** Trichoschisis (due to trichothiodystrophy). **E** Trichothiodystrophy (polarization; in comparison to normal hair shaft). **F** Bubble hair. **G** Pili torti (scanning electron microscopy [EM]). **H** Pili annulati. **I** Trichonodosis. **J** Pili trianguli et canaliculi ("spun glass hair"). **K** Trichoptilosis. Some of the hair shaft abnormalities are seen in genetic syndromes (e.g. trichorrhexis invaginata in Netherton syndrome, trichoschisis in trichothiodystrophy). *A, B, Courtesy, Maria K. Hordinsky, MD; C–E, G, H, J, K, Courtesy, YDRSC; F, Courtesy, Jean L. Bolognia, MD.*

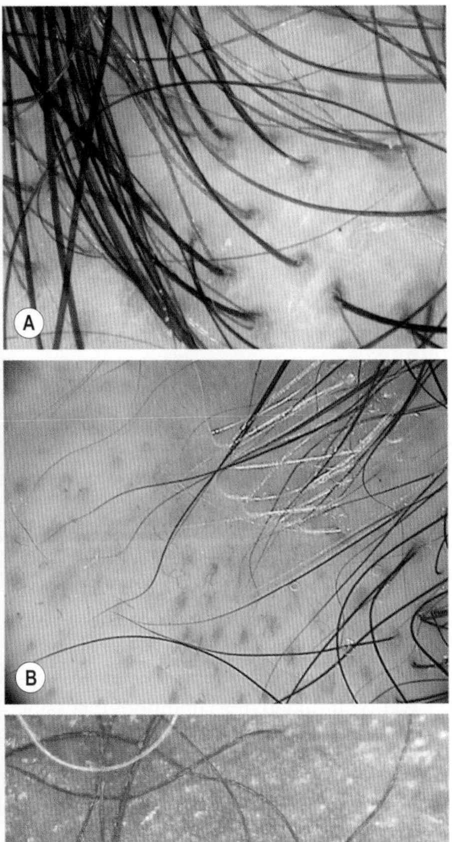

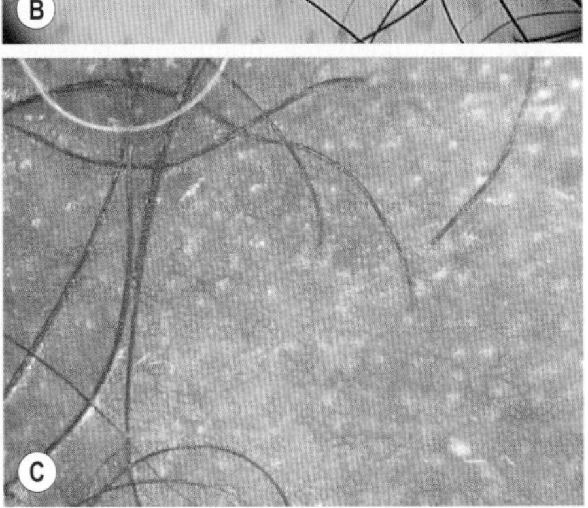

Fig. 56.12 Trichoscopy. A Androgenetic alopecia: a diversity of hair shaft diameters affects >20% of the hairs. Brown halos around hair shafts (peripilar sign) is a subtle clue. **B** Discoid lupus erythematosus (DLE): follicular red dots are a characteristic sign and they correspond histopathologically to dilated vessels, extravasated erythrocytes, and keratin plugs. **C** Lichen planopilaris: discrete white dots due to loss of melanin over scarred fibrotic tracts and perifollicular fibrosis. The fibrosis in DLE is more diffuse. Trichoscopic findings in alopecia areata are shown in Fig. 56.4F. *A, Courtesy, Leonard C. Sperling, MD, and Rodney D. Sinclair, MD; B, C, Courtesy, Antonella Tosti, MD.*

57 Hypertrichosis and Hirsutism

Definitions

- **Hypertrichosis**: excessive hair growth on any area of the body, beyond what is normally expected for a patient's demographic group.
- **Hirsutism**: excessive terminal hair growth in women or children in a pattern typically seen in adult men.
- **Lanugo hair**: long fine hair that is grown *in utero*, covers the fetus, and is normally shed either *in utero* or during the first few weeks of life.
- **Vellus hair**: short, non- or lightly pigmented hair that covers most areas of the body; occasionally so fine as to not be appreciated clinically.
- **Terminal hair**: thick pigmented hair that is typical of the scalp and androgen-dependent areas, such as the axillae and pubic region in both sexes, as well as the beard, trunk, and limbs in adult males.
- **Hyperandrogenism**: elevated serum levels of testosterone, DHEAS, and/or androstenedione; cutaneous findings include hirsutism, severe or treatment-resistant acne, androgenetic alopecia, and seborrhea.
- **Virilization**: in women, clinical features of hyperandrogenism plus clitoromegaly, deepened voice, increased muscle mass, breast atrophy, and increased libido.
- **Depilation**: removal of a portion of the hair at some point along its shaft.
- **Epilation**: removal of the entire hair shaft.

Hypertrichosis

- Can be classified based on the **distribution** (generalized vs. localized), **age of onset** (congenital or early onset vs. acquired), and **type of hair** (lanugo vs. vellus vs. terminal).
- Three mechanisms of hypertrichosis are generally recognized:
    1. Conversion of vellus to terminal hair (e.g. localized hypertrichosis in an area of chronic rubbing or scratching).
    2. Changes in the hair growth cycle (e.g. intranasal and ear hairs in older males due to prolongation of anagen phase).
    3. Increase in hair follicle density beyond what is normal for a given site (e.g. congenital melanocytic nevus).
- **Rx:** treat underlying condition, if possible, otherwise see Table 57.2.
- Shaving of hairs does not increase the thickness or pigmentation of the hairs, contrary to common belief.

Generalized Hypertrichosis

- The presence of lanugo hair, excess vellus hair, or terminal hair on most of the body.
- An approach to a patient with *generalized hypertrichosis* is presented in Fig. 57.1.
- In young girls, constitutional prepubertal hypertrichosis is the most common form of generalized hypertrichosis.

Localized Hypertrichosis

- Most often involves a switch from vellus to terminal hair in sites that normally do not have terminal hairs.
- ***Congenital localized hypertrichosis*** is usually related to an underlying hamartoma or occurs at a specific anatomic site (Table 57.1; Figs 57.2–57.5).
- ***Acquired localized hypertrichosis*** most often develops after repeated trauma, friction, irritation, or inflammation (see Table 57.1; Figs 57.6–57.7).

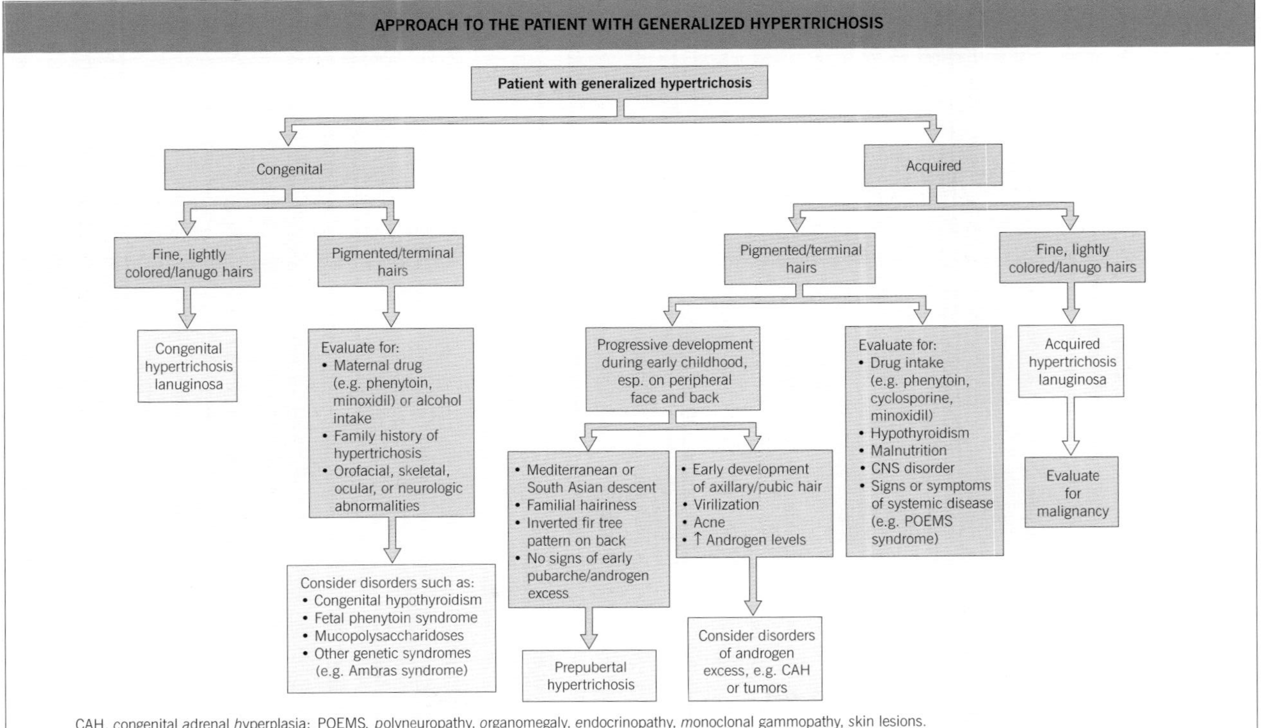

Fig. 57.1 Approach to the patient with generalized hypertrichosis. Acquired hypertrichosis lanuginosa occasionally may involve only the face.

CLASSIFICATION AND KEY FEATURES OF SELECTED DISORDERS OF LOCALIZED HYPERTRICHOSIS	
Condition	**Key features**
Congenital localized hypertrichosis	
Congenital melanocytic nevus	• Hyperpigmented and usually elevated (see Ch. 92)
Plexiform neurofibroma	• Palpable component and often hyperpigmented (see Ch. 50)
Nevoid hypertrichosis (Fig. 57.2)	• Circumscribed area of terminal hair growth • *Primary*: skin normally pigmented; no underlying hamartoma • *Secondary*: can be associated with lipodystrophy, hemihypertrophy, scoliosis, and abnormalities of underlying vasculature
Smooth muscle hamartoma	• Exists on a clinical spectrum with Becker melanosis (nevus) (see Ch. 95)
Becker melanosis (nevus) (Fig. 57.3)	• Hamartoma characterized by macular hyperpigmentation with irregular borders; often on the upper lateral trunk; onset in first decade of life • Hypertrichosis (variable) usually appears in second decade, correlating with puberty • Males > females • Occasionally associated with asymmetry of the extremities and hyper- or hypoplasia of the affected areas
Spinal hypertrichosis (see Ch. 53)	• Tufts of terminal hairs along the dorsal midline • May signify underlying *spinal dysraphism*
Hair collar sign (see Ch. 53)	• Peripheral ring of hypertrichosis surrounding membranous aplasia cutis or ectopic neural tissue in the scalp • MRI can detect underlying skull defect; do *not* biopsy
Anterior cervical hypertrichosis (see Fig. 57.5)	• Tuft of terminal hair above laryngeal prominence • Isolated > associated with a neuropathy or intellectual disability
Hypertrichosis cubiti (hairy elbow syndrome) (Fig. 57.4)	• Symmetric excessive hair growth on the elbow region • Occasionally associated with short stature
Facial hypertrichosis	• Genetic syndromes (e.g. Cornelia de Lange syndrome)
Acquired localized hypertrichosis	
Due to repeated trauma, friction, inflammation, or irritation (Fig. 57.6)	• Hair within the affected area becomes longer and thicker • Typical scenarios: repeated scratching or LSC; fractured limb or orthopedic casts and splints; sack carriers
Chemical-induced	• Exposure to iodine or topical agents (e.g. minoxidil, tacrolimus, CS)
Facial hypertrichosis	• May be due to familial predisposition, PCT (see Fig. 41.3), systemic medications (e.g. CSA) or topical medications (e.g. minoxidil), malnutrition
Hypertrichosis singularis	• One long "wild" hair
Trichomegaly of eyelashes (Fig. 57.7)	• May be due to topical ophthalmic medications (e.g. bimatoprost), systemic medications (e.g. EGFR inhibitors, tacrolimus, CSA, topiramate), HIV infection, malnutrition
Systemic disease	• Complex regional pain syndrome (hypertrichosis in affected area) • Juvenile dermatomyositis (hypertrichosis in infrapatellar region) • Pretibial myxedema (anterior shins) • In association with cutaneous sclerosis (e.g. H syndrome, linear melorheostosis)

Table 57.1 Classification and key features of selected disorders of localized hypertrichosis. CSA, cyclosporine; LSC, lichen simplex chronicus; PCT, porphyria cutanea tarda.

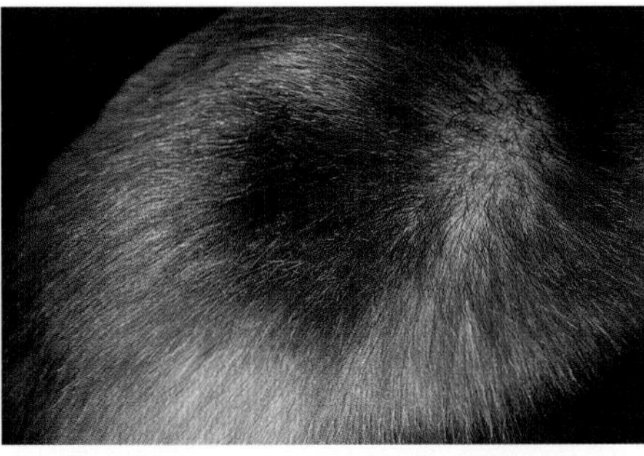

Fig. 57.2 Nevoid hypertrichosis in the scalp of a young boy. There was no underlying melanocytic nevus or hyperpigmentation. *Courtesy, Jean L. Bolognia, MD.*

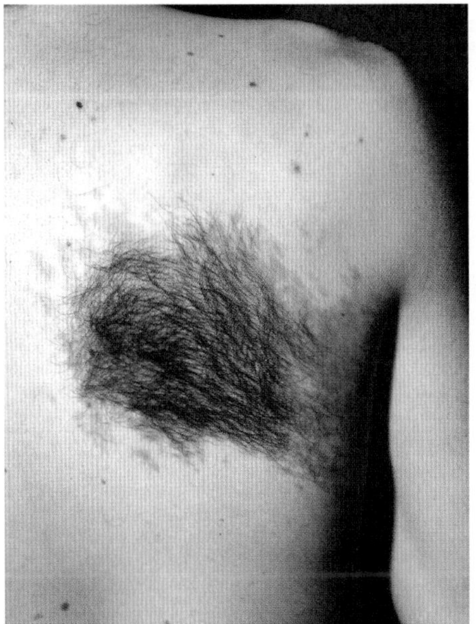

Fig. 57.3 Becker melanosis (nevus) on the mid back in a young man. In addition to hyperpigmentation, there is marked hypertrichosis. The degree of hypertrichosis can vary. When it is marked, as in this patient, the clinical differential diagnosis includes congenital melanocytic nevus, especially when there is an underlying smooth muscle hamartoma. *Courtesy, Francisco M. Camacho Martinez, MD.*

Hirsutism

- Affects ~5–10% of females of reproductive age; can also affect postmenopausal women.
- Due to hyperandrogenism (exogenous or endogenous) or increased sensitivity of the hair follicle to normal androgen levels and is the most commonly used clinical criterion of androgen excess.

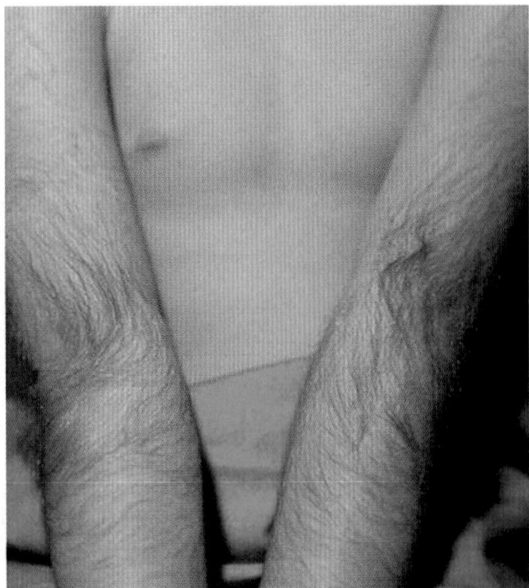

Fig. 57.4 Hypertrichosis cubiti. Multiple terminal hairs on both elbows in a child. *Courtesy, Francisco M. Camacho Martinez, MD.*

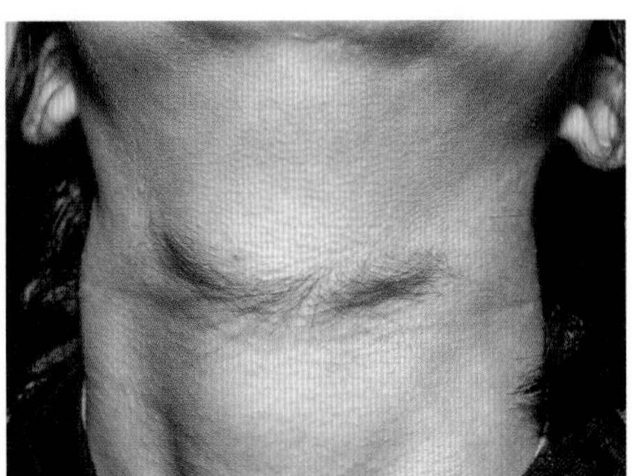

Fig. 57.5 Anterior cervical hypertrichosis. *Courtesy, Harvey Lui, MD.*

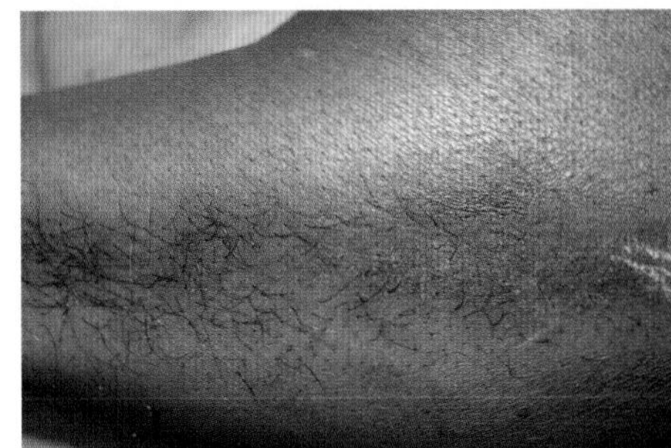

Fig. 57.6 Acquired localized hypertrichosis. Hypertrichosis, hyperpigmentation, and epidermal hyperplasia at the site of friction. Some authors refer to this as "frictional asymmetric darkening of the extensor surfaces", when there is primarily hyperpigmentation. *Courtesy, YDRSC.*

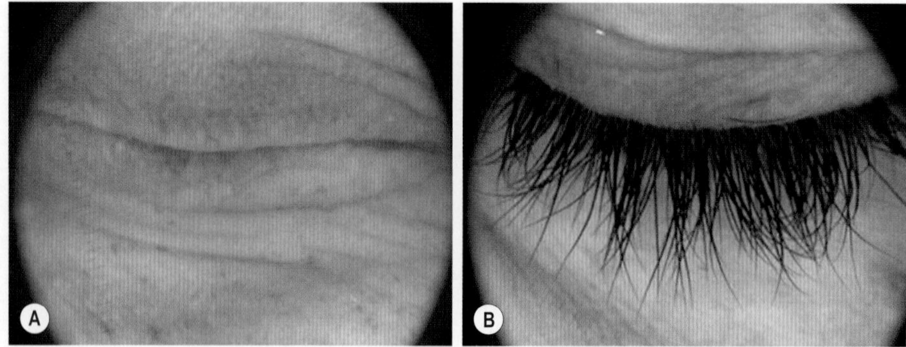

Fig. 57.7 Treatment of eyelash alopecia in a patient with alopecia universalis. A Prior to treatment. **B** Following daily application of topical latanoprost ophthalmic 0.005% solution for 6 months, there was regrowth of eyelashes. *Courtesy, Francisco M. Camacho Martinez, MD.*

THE MODIFIED FERRIMAN–GALLWEY (mFG) HIRSUTISM SCORING SYSTEM – NINE SITES OF ASSESSMENT

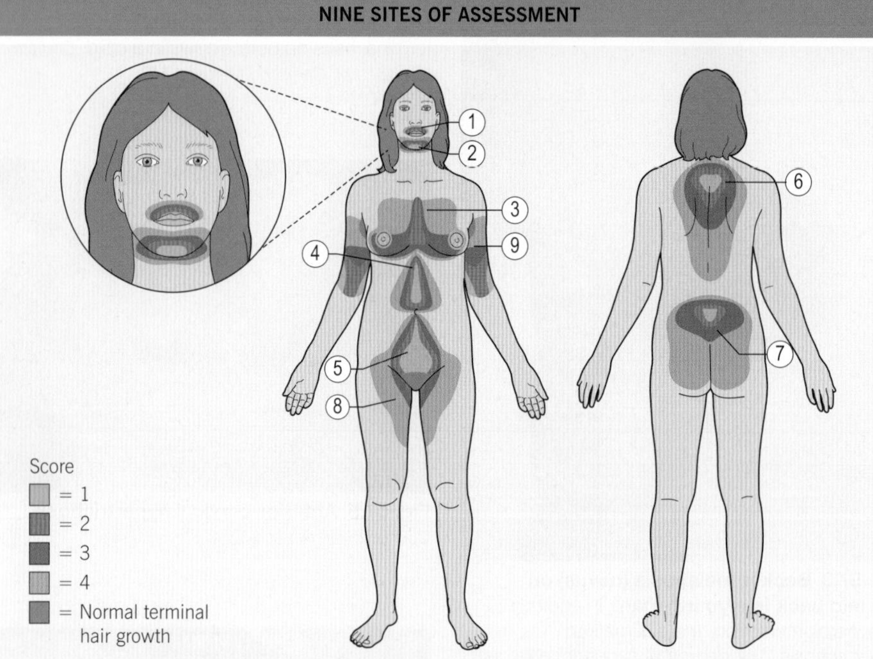

Fig. 57.8 The modified Ferriman–Gallwey (mFG) hirsutism scoring system. In this system, nine body areas are evaluated for the amount of terminal hair growth. A score of "0" (no hair) up to "4" (frankly virile) is given to each of the nine areas and these are added together to compute a hormonal hirsutism score (mFG score). Total scores that define hirsutism in women of reproductive age are as follows: US and UK black or white women, ≥8; Mediterranean, Hispanic and Middle Eastern women, ≥9 to 10; South American women, ≥6; and Asian women, a range of ≥2 for Han Chinese women to ≥7 for Southern Chinese women.

- Quantified using the modified Ferriman–Gallwey (mFG) method (Fig. 57.8).
- Etiologies of hyperandrogenism and hirsutism in *premenopausal* females include:
  - *Most common*: polycystic ovary syndrome (PCOS), idiopathic (end-organ sensitivity; Fig. 57.9)
  - *Less common*: nonclassic congenital adrenal hyperplasia (NC-CAH), ovarian hyperthecosis, tumoral
  - *Must exclude*: pregnancy; drugs (e.g. androgens, anabolic steroids, valproic acid, supplements)

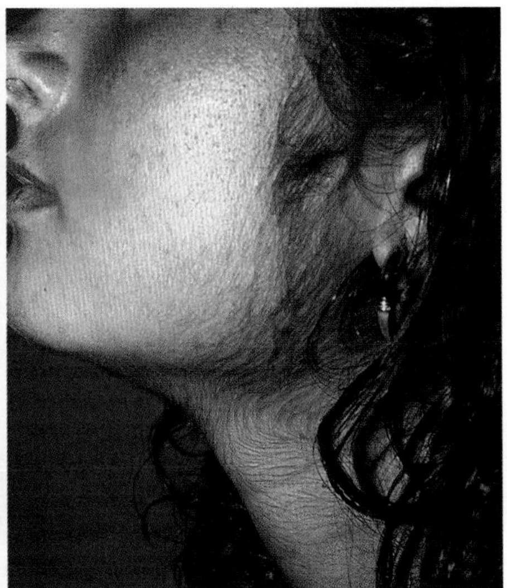

Fig. 57.9 Facial hirsutism in a young female. This can be due to hyperandrogenism or end-organ sensitivity. *Courtesy, Francisco M. Camacho Martinez, MD.*

- Etiology in *postmenopausal* women (new onset) is most likely ovarian hyperthecosis or tumoral hirsutism.
- Suggested algorithms for the evaluation of hirsutism and for hyperandrogenism are shown in Figs 57.10 and 57.11, respectively.

Polycystic Ovary Syndrome (PCOS)

- Diagnosed by the presence of ≥2 of the following criteria *and* the exclusion of other possible etiologies (see Fig. 57.11):
  1. Oligo- or anovulation (<8 menses/year or cycles >35 days).
  2. Clinical and/or biochemical signs of hyperandrogenism (Fig. 57.12).
  3. Polycystic ovaries (pelvic [preferably trans-vaginal] ultrasound).
- Luteinizing hormone (LH): follicle-stimulating hormone (FSH) ratio is >3 in ~95% of cases
- Occurs only during the reproductive years, and although the majority of patients are obese, some are of normal weight.
- Other associated findings may include acanthosis nigricans and insulin resistance; patients are at increased risk for the metabolic syndrome (see Table 45.11), infertility, obstructive sleep apnea, endometrial carcinoma, depression and anxiety.
- **Rx** of hirsutism: hormonal agents (Table 57.3) as well as general hair removal methods (see Table 57.2).

Idiopathic Hirsutism

- Usually characterized by mild hirsutism, regular ovulation, and normal testosterone levels.
- Diagnosis of exclusion.

Nonclassic Congenital Adrenal Hyperplasia (NC-CAH)

- Autosomal recessive disorder due to partial deficiency in 21-hydroxylase activity (mutations in *CYP21A2*), leading to increased 17-hydroxyprogesterone (17-OHP) levels.
- More prevalent in Ashkenazi Jews, Hispanics, and Slavics.
- Usually presents in the peripubertal and young adult years with hirsutism, menstrual irregularities, infertility, androgenetic alopecia, and acne.
- Initial testing includes measuring an early morning 17-OHP level during the follicular phase of menstrual cycle; if equivocal, a high-dose ACTH stimulation test and/or genotyping for *CYP21A2* can be performed.
- **Rx** of hirsutism: overlaps with that of PCOS, but may also include systemic CS (see Tables 57.2 and 57.3).

Ovarian Hyperthecosis

- Occurs in both premenopausal and postmenopausal females.
- Due to the differentiation of ovarian interstitial cells into steroidogenically active luteinized stromal cells, resulting in greater production of androgens.
- Clinical features are similar to those of PCOS but with more pronounced and long-standing hirsutism, an increased likelihood of virilization (Fig. 57.13), and the occurrence postmenopausally.
- Testosterone levels are often quite elevated (>200 ng/dl); DHEAS can be normal or increased (see Fig. 57.11).
- Compared to tumoral hirsutism, a slower onset of symptoms and more gradual worsening over years.
- Increased risk of insulin resistance, type 2 diabetes, and endometrial carcinoma.

Tumoral Hirsutism

- Can be caused by a variety of benign or malignant ovarian or adrenal androgen-secreting tumors.
- Typically presents with either sudden onset or rapid progression of hirsutism and other clinical features of hyperandrogenism; virilization more likely.

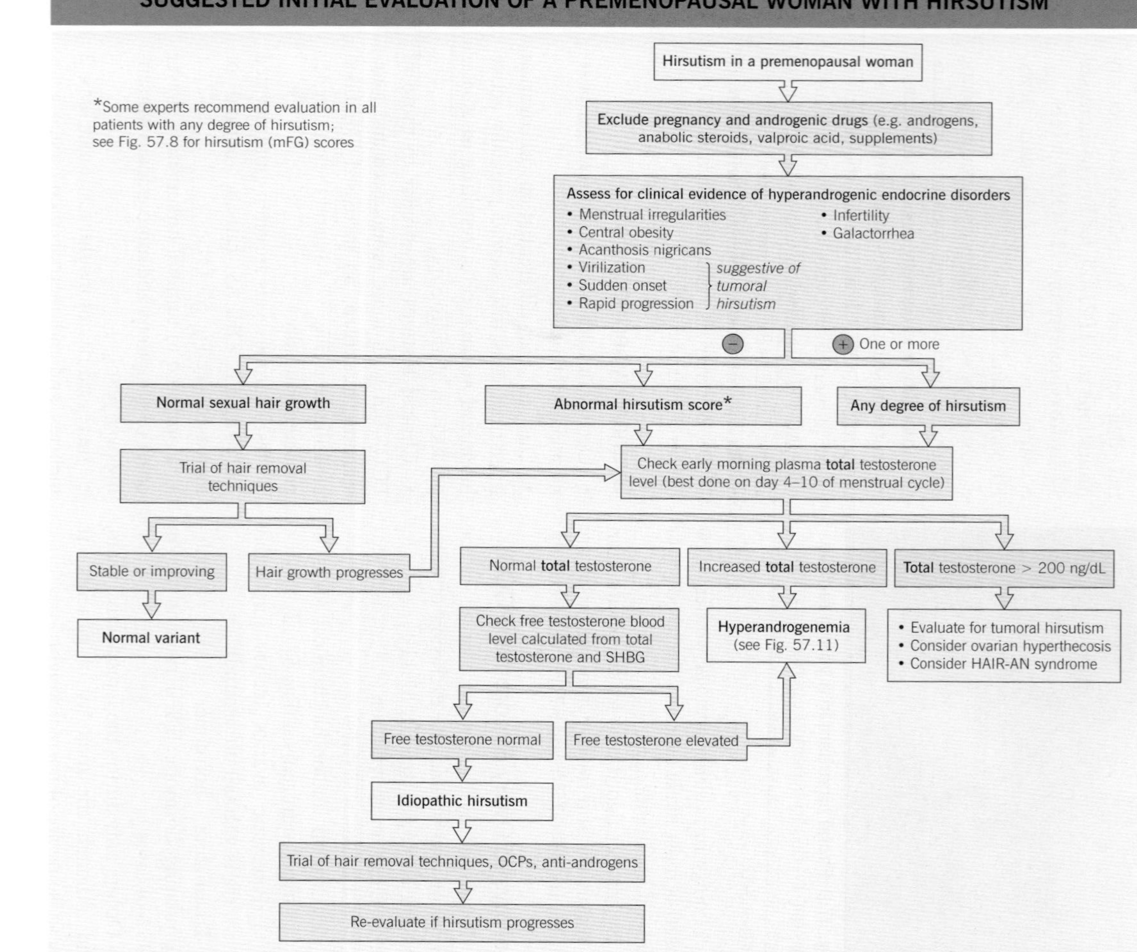

Fig. 57.10 Suggested initial evaluation of a premenopausal female with hirsutism. HAIR-AN

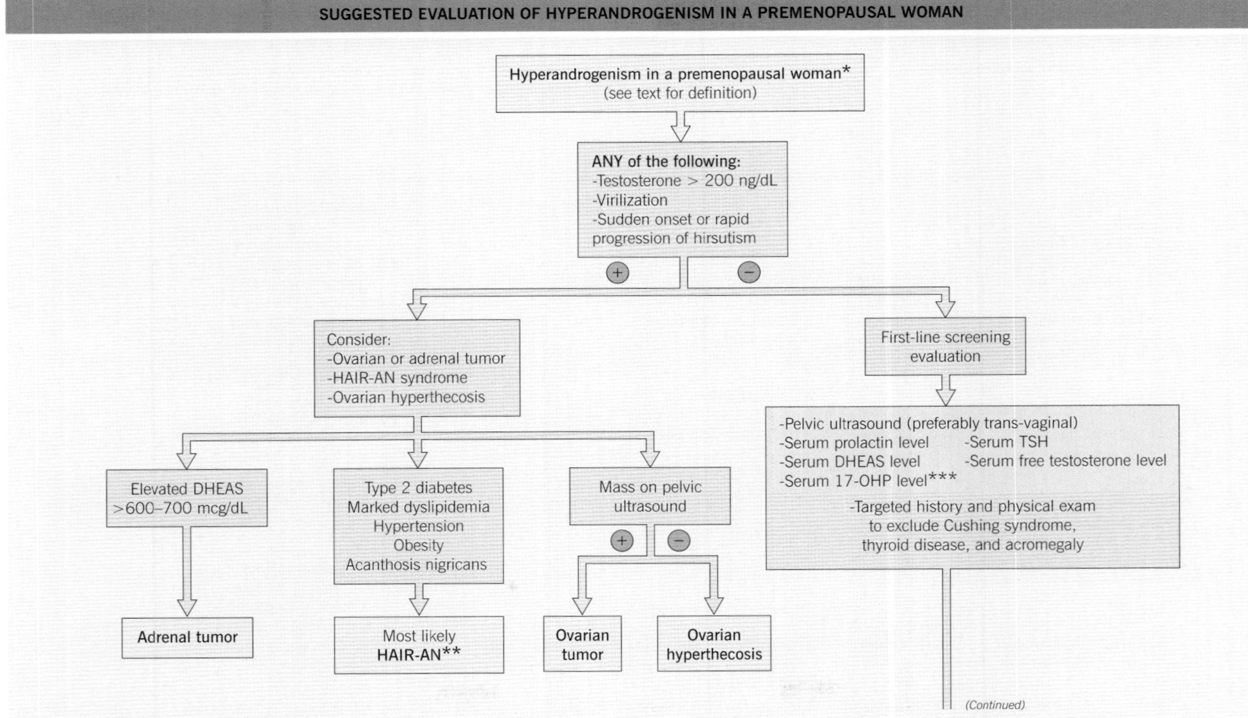

Fig. 57.11 Suggested evaluation of hyperandrogenism in a premenopausal woman. *Continued*

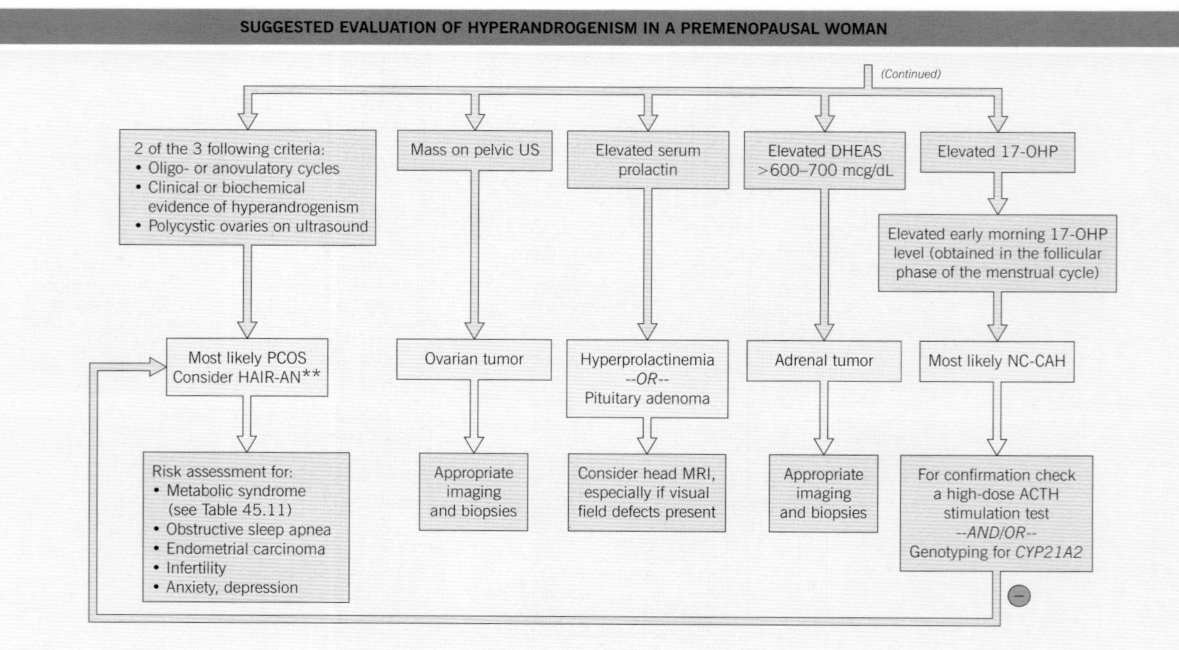

Fig. 57.11 *Continued* **Suggested evaluation of hyperandrogenism in a premenopausal woman.** 17-OHP, 17-hydroxyprogesterone; ACTH, adrenocorticotropic hormone; HAIR-AN, *h*yper*a*ndrogenism, *i*nsulin *r*esistance, and *a*canthosis *n*igricans; NC-CAH, nonclassic congenital adrenal hyperplasia; PCOS, polycystic ovarian syndrome.

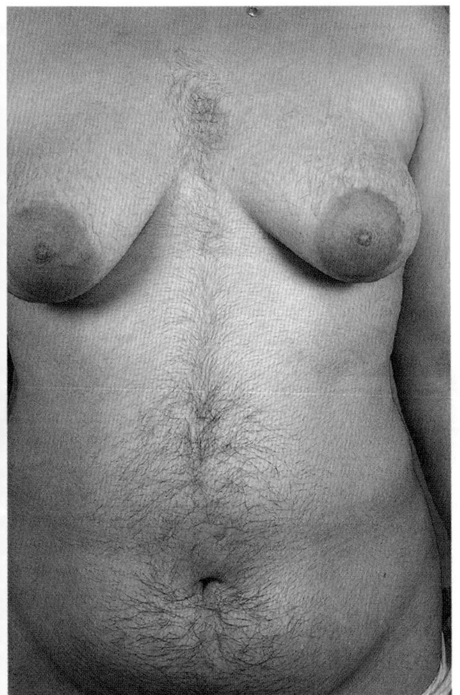

Fig. 57.12 Hirsutism in a young woman with polycystic ovarian syndrome (PCOS). Modified Ferriman–Gallwey (mFG) score of 9 based on three sites: chest, upper abdomen, and lower abdomen. *Courtesy, NYUDSC.*

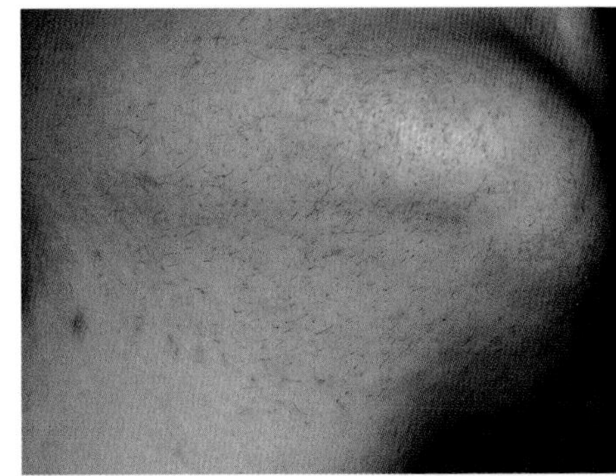

Fig. 57.13 Facial hirsutism (mFG score 4) due to ovarian hyperthecosis. *Courtesy, Robert Hartman, MD.*

- Diagnostic clues are extremely elevated levels of testosterone (>200 ng/dl, seen in ovarian and adrenal tumors) or DHEAS (>600–700 mcg/dl, seen in adrenal tumors).
- If suspected, an appropriate imaging study is recommended (e.g. CT scan, MRI, and/or ultrasound).

HAIR-AN Syndrome

- *H*yper*a*ndrogenism, *i*nsulin *r*esistance, and *a*canthosis *n*igricans syndrome.

TREATMENT OPTIONS FOR HYPERTRICHOSIS AND UNWANTED HAIR		
Camouflage	**Hair removal techniques**	**Retardation of hair growth**
• Make-up • Lightening of hair color with commercial bleach or 6–12% hydrogen peroxide	Depilation ***Chemical*** 1. Barium sulfate creams* 2. Calcium thioglycolate creams ***Mechanical*** 1. Hair trimming 2. Shaving Epilation • Tweezing • Waxing • Threading • Sugaring • Electrolysis** • Thermolysis** • Lasers or other light sources** (e.g. Nd:YAG, diode, alexandrite, IPL)	• Eflornithine hydrochloride cream (best used in conjunction with other hair removal techniques)

**More effective than calcium thioglycolate but more irritating and odiferous.*
***These epilatory methods are operator-dependent and have the potential for permanent hair removal results.*

Table 57.2 Treatment options for hypertrichosis and unwanted hair. Epilation technique results typically last longer than those of depilation. Chemical depilatories work by dissolving hair shafts, specifically by breaking disulfide bonds. IPL, intense pulsed light.

• Marked insulin resistance leads to secondary increased insulin levels and resultant increased ovarian androgen production.
• More likely than PCOS to have overt type 2 diabetes, hypertension, and cardiovascular disease.
• Marked hyperandrogenism and often frank virilization; total testosterone levels are often markedly increased.
• Evaluation involves excluding an androgen-secreting tumor and PCOS.

Hirsutism Associated with Other Endocrine Abnormalities

• Cushing syndrome, hyperprolactinemia, pituitary adenoma, acromegaly, and thyroid dysfunction may present with hirsutism and other signs of hyperandrogenism, but typically manifest with other distinguishing and diagnostic features specific to the underlying disease (see Ch. 45).

TREATMENT OF HIRSUTISM AND HYPERANDROGENISM – SYSTEMIC AGENTS AND CLINICAL SCENARIOS		
Systemic agents		
Oral contraceptives (OCPs)* • All OCPs appear to be equally effective for treating hirsutism • If relatively higher risk for venous thromboembolism (e.g. obesity or age > 39 years), then choose an OCP with the lowest effective dose of ethinyl estradiol (usually 20 mcg) and a low-risk progestin (e.g. norethindrone, levonorgestrel, norgestimate) **Antiandrogens***** • Spironolactone 100–200 mg/day (usually given in divided doses, twice daily) • CPA (cyproterone acetate); given on days 5–15 of menstrual cycle)** • Finasteride > flutamide (not recommended because of potential hepatotoxicity) **GnRH agonists** (risk of severe estrogen deficiency) **Insulin-lowering agents** (e.g. metformin > thiazolidinediones; improves metabolic syndrome and reproductive function but not hirsutism as a single agent) **Glucocorticoids** (e.g. low-dose hydrocortisone [children], prednisone or dexamethasone [adolescents and adults]; *restricted to second-line treatment of women with NC-CAH or for those seeking ovulation induction*)		
Clinical scenarios and recommended treatment†		
Premenopausal female	**First-line**: OCP **Second-line**: OCP + spironolactone or CPA**	**Severe or refractory:** Finasteride or GnRH agonist; plus an OCP if premenopausal
Postmenopausal female	**First-line**: Spironolactone or CPA**	
NC-CAH	**First-line:** OCP ± spironolactone or CPA** **Second-line or if seeking ovulation induction:** Glucocorticoids	

**Should avoid in females who smoke or who have risk factors for hypercoagulability and thrombosis.*
***CPA is not available in the United States.*
****Requires concomitant reliable contraceptive method because of the risk of feminization of the male fetus.*
†A waiting period of 6 months is recommended after initiating a treatment and before adding or changing medications.

Table 57.3 Treatment of hirsutism and hyperandrogenism – systemic agents and clinical scenarios. For hirsute women with obesity, including those with polycystic ovary syndrome, lifestyle changes are also recommended. GnRH, gonadotropin releasing hormone; NC-CAH, nonclassic congenital adrenal hyperplasia.

For further information see Ch. 70 from *Dermatology, Fourth Edition*.

For additional online figures and tables visit www.expertconsult.com 

Nail Disorders 58

- The nail matrix, which is the growth area, has proximal and distal components (Fig. 58.1).
  - The proximal nail matrix forms the top (surface) of the nail plate
  - The distal nail matrix forms the underside of the nail plate; therefore, biopsies of the distal matrix are less likely to produce a deformity of the surface of the nail plate
- Fingernails grow ~1–3 mm per month and are replaced every 6 months.
- Toenails grow ~0.5–1 mm per month and are replaced every 12 months.
- Therefore, nail plate abnormalities such as Beau's lines that are due to insults to the nail matrix can be dated by their distance from the cuticle.
- **Rx** of common nail disorders is given in Table 58.1.

TREATMENT OF COMMON NAIL DISORDERS	
Disorder	**Treatment**
Psoriasis	Systemic treatment of psoriasis may be helpful Topical vitamin D analogues or tazarotene Injection of CS into nail matrix or nail bed Topical CS under occlusion
Lichen planus	Injection of CS into nail matrix
Beau's lines Onychomadesis	Await spontaneous resolution
Paronychia, acute	Incision and drainage (may have occurred spontaneously) If mild, topical mupirocin or retapamulin Oral antibiotics (directed against *Staphylococcus aureus*)
Paronychia, chronic	Avoid trauma to cuticle Strict avoidance of irritants Topical CS for 2–3 weeks
Onycholysis*	Keep nails short, reduce trauma and friction to nail Strict avoidance of irritants Can consider topical antifungal solution If due to psoriasis, see above
Green nails*	1% acetic acid solution soaks Topical antibiotic (e.g. gentamycin, tobramycin, or ciprofloxacin ophthalmic solution)
Onychorrhexis	Topical 20% urea, 12% lactic acid, or retinoids; nail hardener; and/or biotin (2.5 mg PO daily)
Ingrown toenails	Correct predisposing factors (e.g. change to a larger toebox) Trim nail properly (straight across) Elevate lateral border of nail with piece of gauze, cotton, or dental floss Warm soaks If severe, matrixectomy (partial or total)

**Cut back portions of detached nail plate.*

Table 58.1 Treatment of common nail disorders.

NAIL UNIT ANATOMY

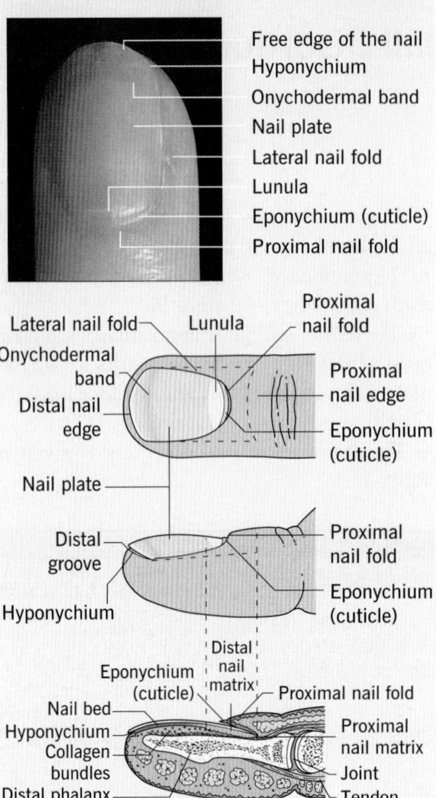

Fig. 58.1 Nail unit anatomy.

Common Nail Findings

Ingrown Toenails (Onychocryptosis)

- Painful inflammation of lateral fold with growth of granulation tissue.
- Usually due to horizontal overcurvature of the nail plate with aging; most commonly involves the great toes.
- Overgrowth of granulation tissue from systemic medications, e.g. systemic retinoids, can embed the lateral nail plate.
- **Rx:** see Table 58.1.

Longitudinal Melanonychia

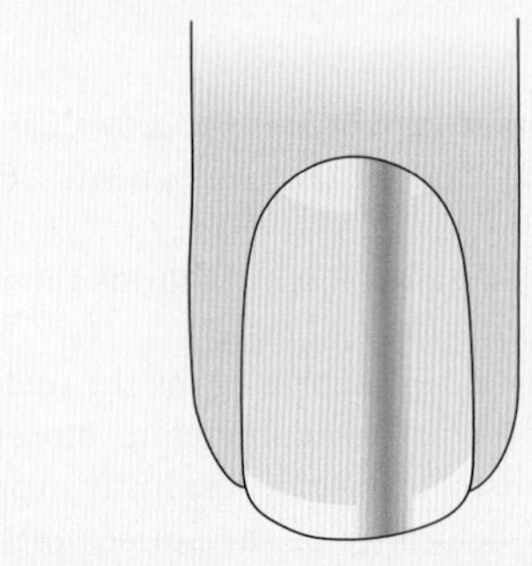

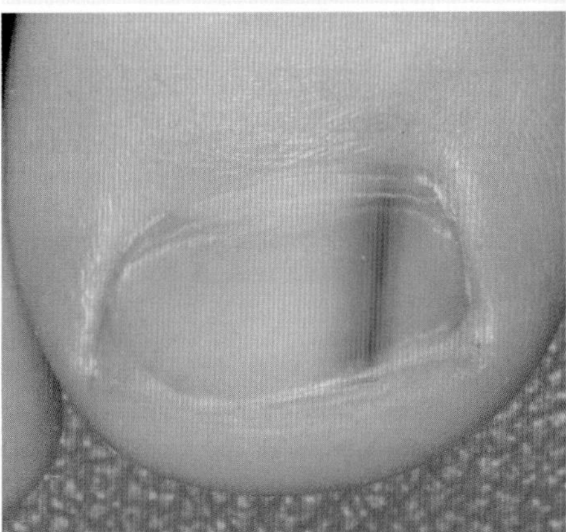

- Longitudinal brown-to-black band.
- Multiple bands common in darker skin types (physiologic); also can be due to trauma (Table 58.2).
- Single band may be a sign of nail melanoma (Table 58.3; Fig. 58.2).
- When melanoma is suspected, the nail matrix must be biopsied (see Fig. 58.1).

CAUSES OF LONGITUDINAL MELANONYCHIA	
Melanocyte activation	Racial
	Trauma • Manicures • Nail biting/onychotillomania • Frictional, primarily in toenails
	Drugs • Cancer chemotherapeutic agents, e.g. doxorubicin, 5-fluorouracil • Zidovudine (AZT) • Psoralens
	Pregnancy
	Laugier–Hunziker syndrome/Peutz–Jegher syndrome
	Addison disease
	HIV infection
	Postinflammatory • Lichen planus • Pustular psoriasis • Onychomycosis (*T. rubrum* and *Scytalidium* spp.) • Chronic radiodermatitis
Non-melanocytic tumors and proliferations	Bowen disease Verrucae Basal cell carcinoma Subungual keratosis Myxoid cyst
Melanocyte hyperplasia	
Nail matrix nevus	
Nail matrix melanoma	

Table 58.2 Causes of longitudinal melanonychia.

ABCDEF RULE FOR CLINICAL SUSPICION OF NAIL MELANOMA	
A	• Age (peak incidence – 5th to 7th decades of life) • African-Americans, Asians, and Native Americans (of all nail melanoma cases) • Asymmetry
B	• Brown to black • Breadth (3 mm or wider) • Borders (variegated, blurred)
C	• Change in the nail band (color/size) • Lack of change in the nail morphology despite presumed adequate treatment
D	• Digit most commonly involved (thumb and big toe)
E	• Extension of the pigment into the proximal and/or lateral nail fold (Hutchinson's sign)
F	• Family or personal history of melanoma

Table 58.3 ABCDEF rule for clinical suspicion of nail melanoma. *Adapted from Levit EK, et al. The ABC rule for clinical detection of subungual melanoma. J Am Acad Dermatol 2000;42:269–74; Benati E, et al. Clinical and dermoscopic clues to differentiate pigmented nail bands: an International Dermoscopy Society study. J Eur Acad Dermatol Venereol 2017;31:732–6; Ohn J, et al. Assessment of a predictive scoring model for dermoscopy of subungual melanoma in situ. JAMA Dermatol 2018;154:890–6.*

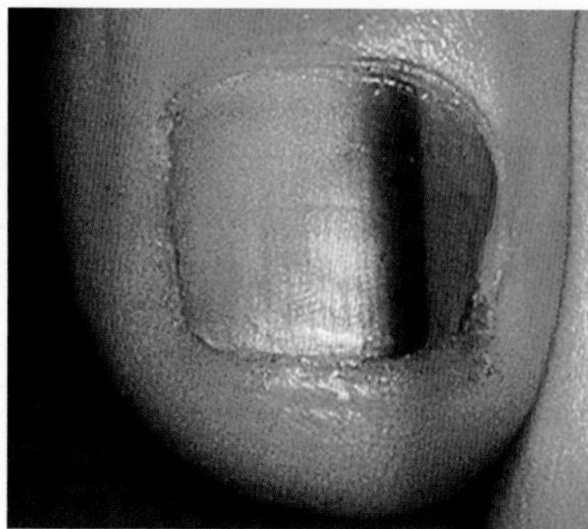

Fig. 58.2 Melanoma *in situ* of the nail. Darkly pigmented band in the nail bed and matrix.
Courtesy, Frank O. Nestle, MD.

Onycholysis

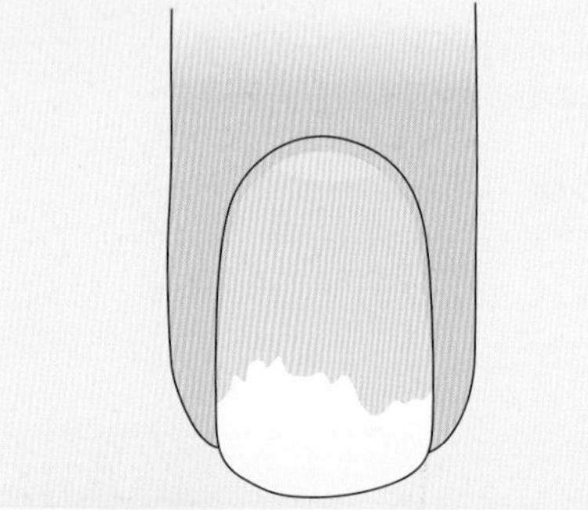

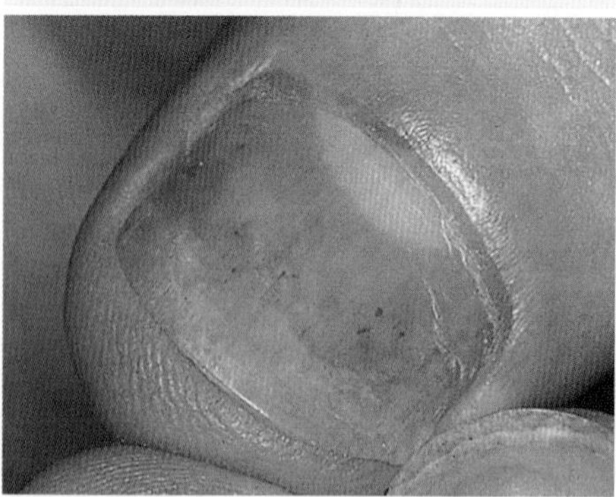

- Distal nail plate detachment, causing nail to look white to yellow-white (Fig. 58.3).
- Additional exogenous pigments beneath the nail plate (e.g. pyocyanin from *Pseudomonas*) may cause yellow to green-black coloration.
- Chronic exposure to water and irritants (e.g. soaps) is a common cause of fingernail onycholysis whereas onycholysis of the great toe is often due to biomechanical forces.
- Associated with psoriasis (see Fig. 6.14), onychomycosis, hyperthyroidism, and medications (Table 58.4).

Onychomycosis

- See Chapter 64.

Onychorrhexis

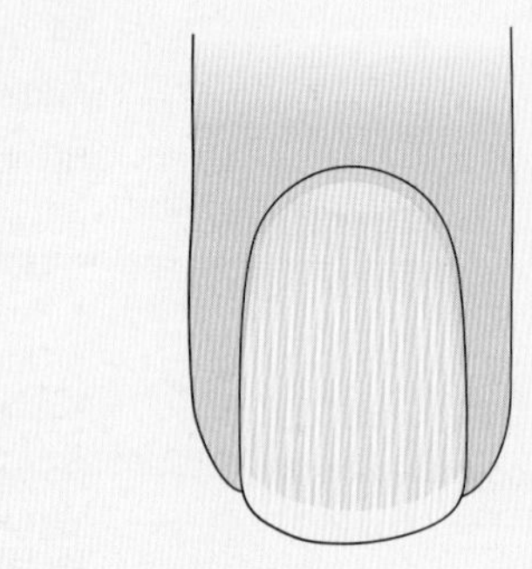

- Thinning and longitudinal ridging.
- May develop fissuring or notching.
- Less pronounced than trachyonychia.
- Sometimes secondary to trauma but more commonly an age-related phenomenon.

Onychoschizia

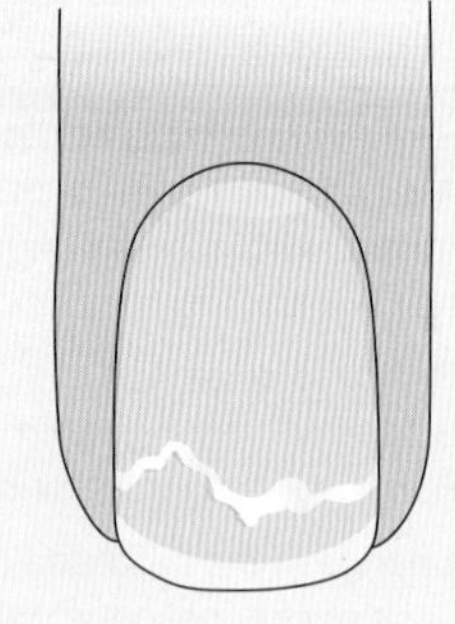

- Lamellar splitting of distal nail into multiple layers.
- Associated with the use of soap and irritants.
- Normal finding with aging.

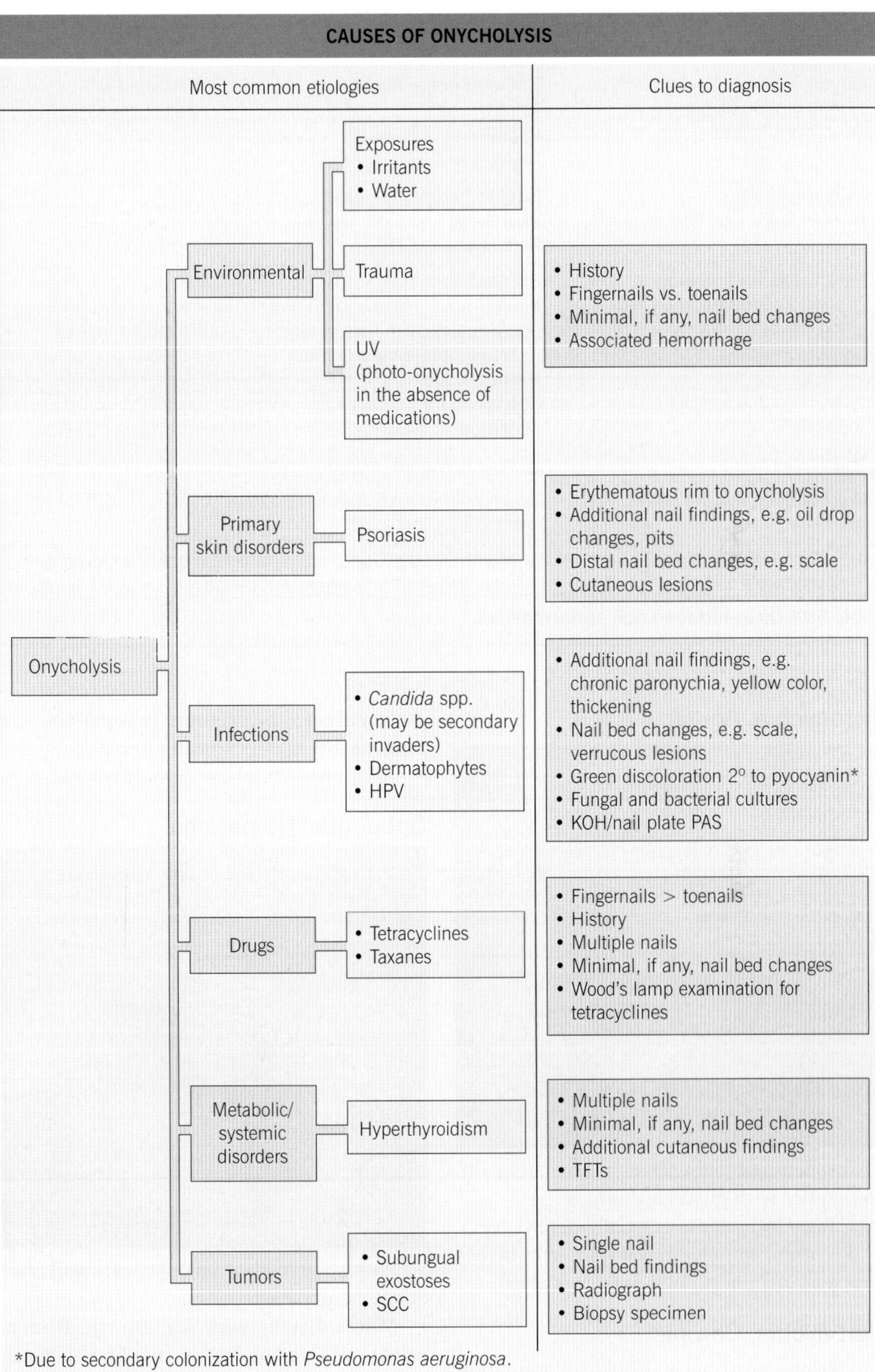

Fig. 58.3 Causes of onycholysis. TFTs, thyroid function tests.

DRUG-INDUCED NAIL ABNORMALITIES	
Nail abnormality	**Responsible agents**
Beau's lines and onychomadesis	Chemotherapeutic agents
Onycholysis/photo-onycholysis (see Fig. 58.3)	Chemotherapeutic agents, in particular taxanes Tetracyclines Psoralens NSAIDs
Melanonychia	Chemotherapeutic agents Psoralens Zidovudine (AZT)
Paronychia and periungual pyogenic granulomas (see Fig. 58.6)	Retinoids Antiretroviral drugs (e.g. indinavir, efavirenz, lamivudine) Epidermal growth factor receptor (EGFR) inhibitors (e.g. cetuximab, panitumumab) Methotrexate Capecitabine Sirolimus
True leukonychia	Chemotherapeutic agents
Nail thinning and brittleness	Chemotherapeutic agents Retinoids
Apparent leukonychia (e.g. Muehrcke's nails)	Chemotherapeutic agents, in particular polychemotherapy including anthracyclines, vincristine

Table 58.4 Drug-induced nail abnormalities.

Paronychia, Acute

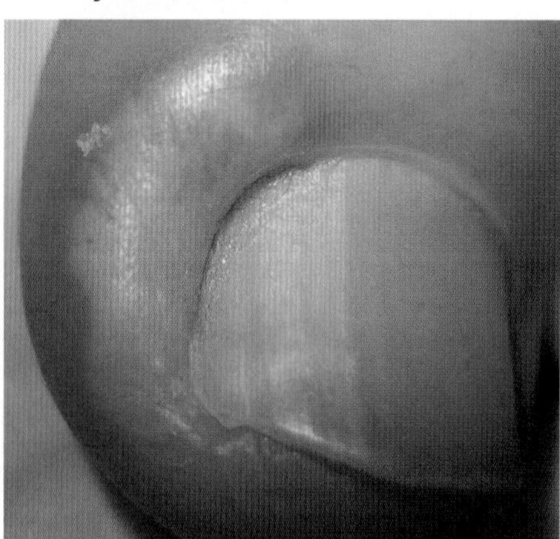

- Swollen nail fold with erythema and pain, sometimes with pustular drainage.
- Caused by bacteria, especially staphylococci.
- Recurrent episodes may be caused by herpes simplex virus infection (herpetic whitlow).

Paronychia, Chronic

- Chronic proximal nail fold inflammation with loss of cuticle (natural sealant).
- Exacerbated by exposure to water and irritants or overaggressive nail grooming.
- May have secondary *Candida* colonization.

Subungual Hematoma

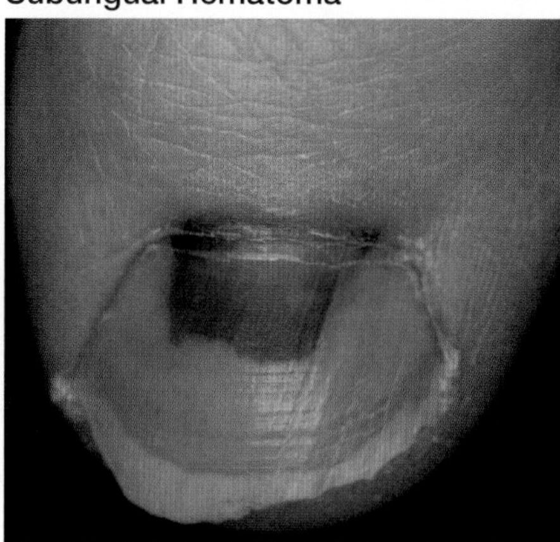

- Purple-red to black color beneath nail plate due to hemorrhage.
- Moves distally with nail growth; if more recent onset, a band of normal nail plate can be seen by pushing back the cuticle.
- Secondary to trauma.

True Leukonychia

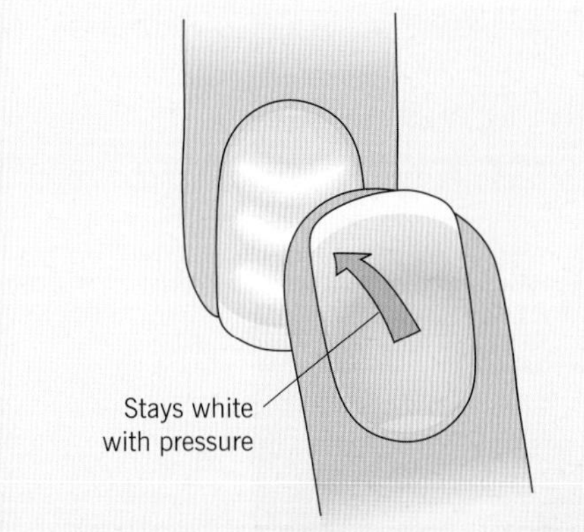

- White discoloration of nail that persists when pressure is applied.
- Punctate form, which is due to trauma, is the most common form.
- Less often, a linear or diffuse pattern is seen.
- Linear bands may be transverse (e.g. Mee's lines, trauma) or longitudinal (e.g. Darier disease).
- Diffuse variant may be inherited and occasionally associated with hearing loss.
- **DDx**: superficial white onychomycosis and apparent leukonychia.

Less Common Nail Findings

Beau's Lines

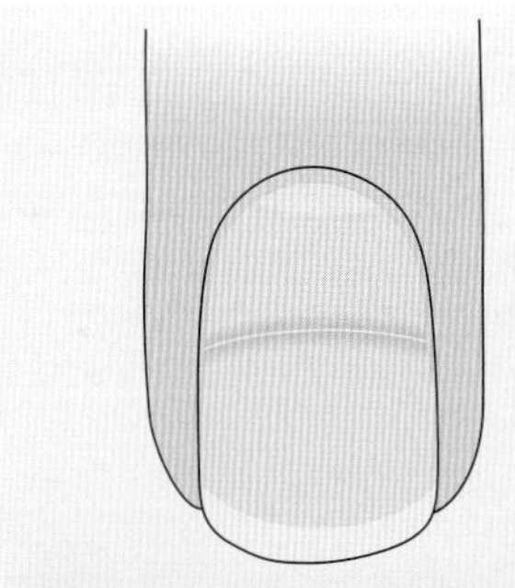

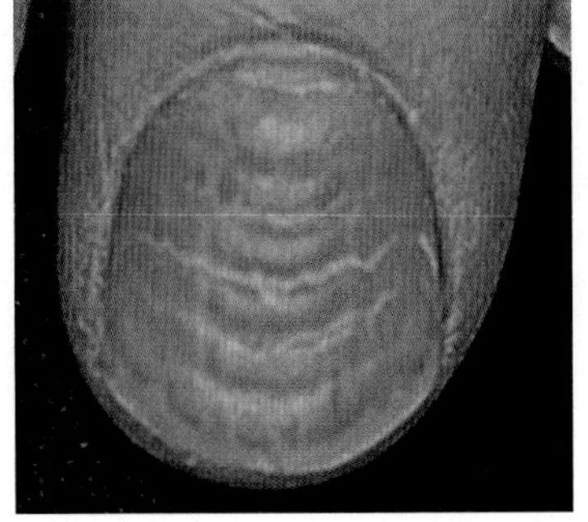

- Transverse depressions in the nail plate.
- Often secondary to trauma, especially when limited to a single digit.
- Consider systemic insult (e.g. high fever, chemotherapy) if multiple nails involved.

Dorsal Pterygium

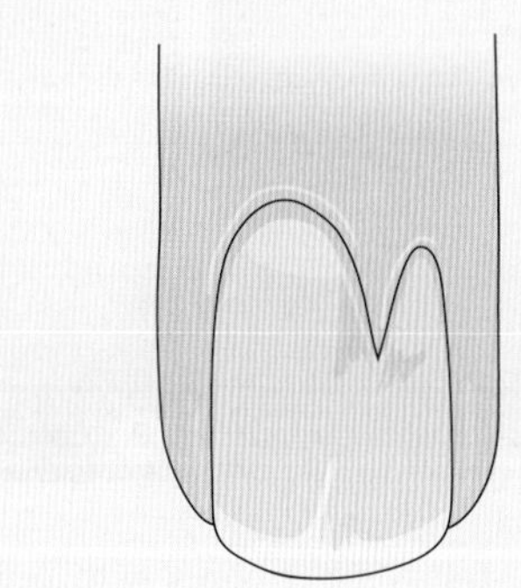

- Triangular extension of the proximal nail fold into the nail bed.
- Local loss of nail plate.
- Most commonly associated with lichen planus (see below); also seen in other disorders (e.g. dyskeratosis congenita).

Green Nail

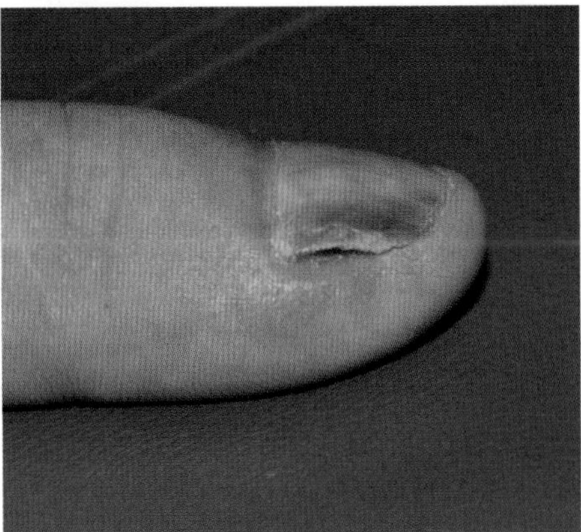

- Blue-green to green-black discoloration secondary to pyocyanin produced by *Pseudomonas aeruginosa*.
- Usually in association with onycholysis (creates a favorable moist environment).

Malalignment

- Lateral deviation of nail plate, often bilateral and congenital.
- Most commonly 1st toe(s).
- May result in ingrown toenails and nail thickening.

Median Nail Dystrophy (Tic Deformity)

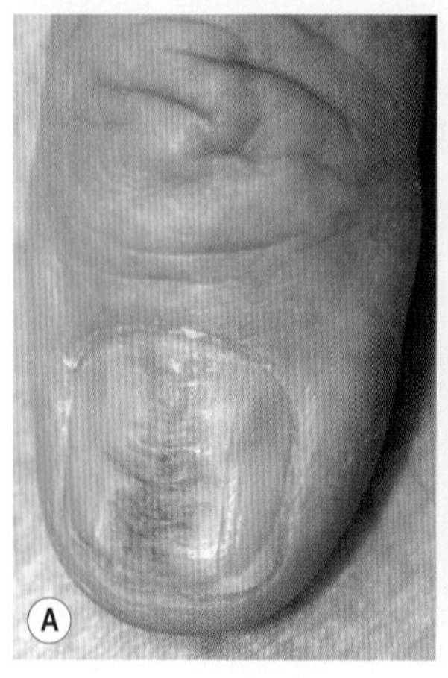

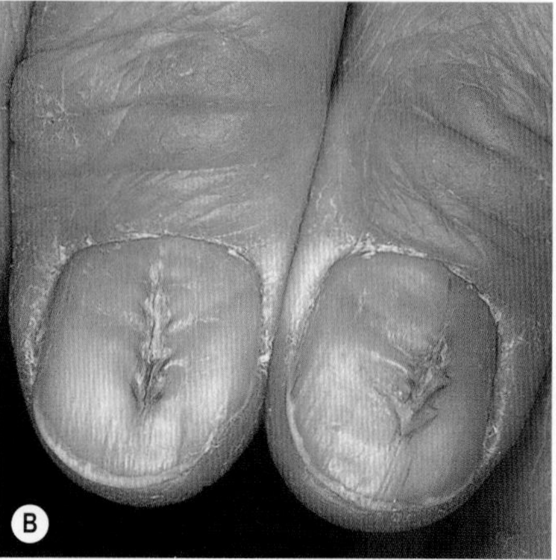

- Multiple transverse grooves with central longitudinal depression that resemble a washboard (**A**).
- Primarily thumbnail(s).
- Due to manipulation of skin overlying matrix.
- **DDx**: primarily median canaliform dystrophy of Heller which presents as a central longitudinal split with an inverted fir tree pattern (**B**).

Onychogryphosis

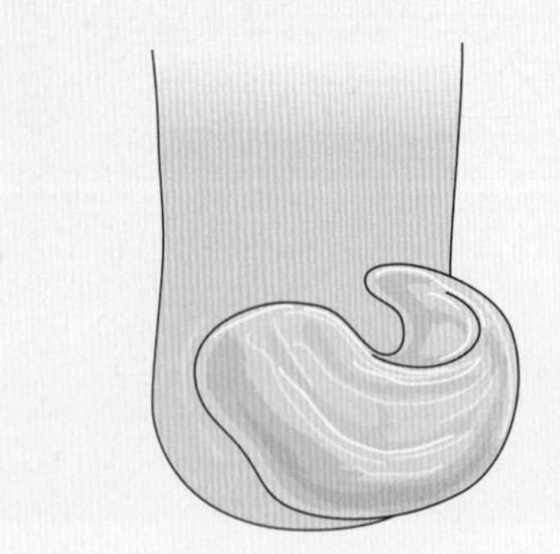

- Curling of nail plate leads to ram's horn appearance.
- Most commonly nail(s) of 1st toe(s).
- Affects elderly patients.

Onychomadesis (Nail Shedding)

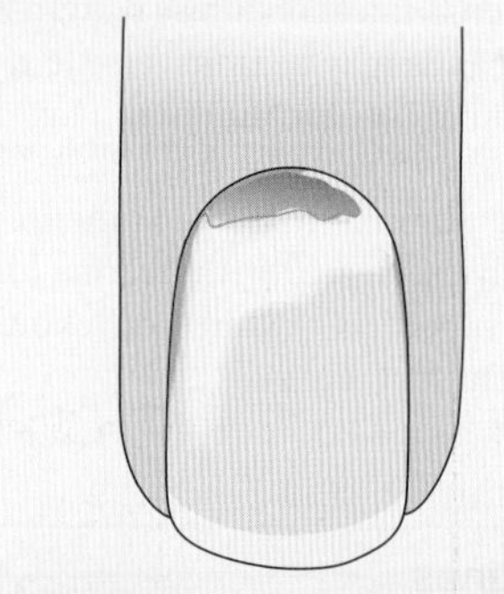

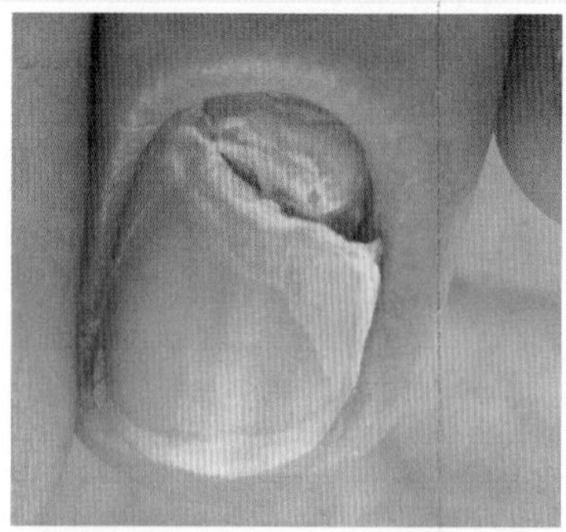

- Proximal detachment of nail plate.
- When single digit, often due to trauma.
- Consider systemic cause (e.g. post-viral, high fever, chemotherapy, post-erythroderma) if multiple nails involved; coxsackie infections are a common cause in children.

Subungual Exostosis

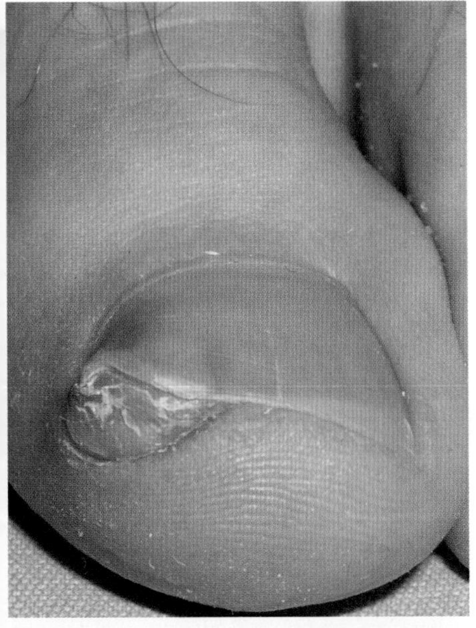

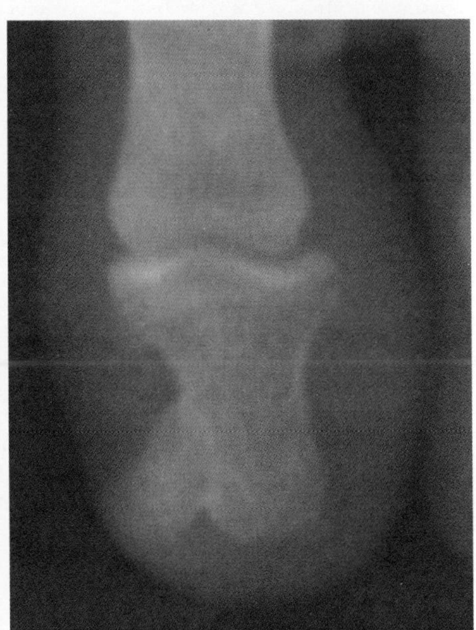

- Associated with onycholysis and tender subungual nodule.
- Diagnosis confirmed by X-ray.

Splinter Hemorrhages

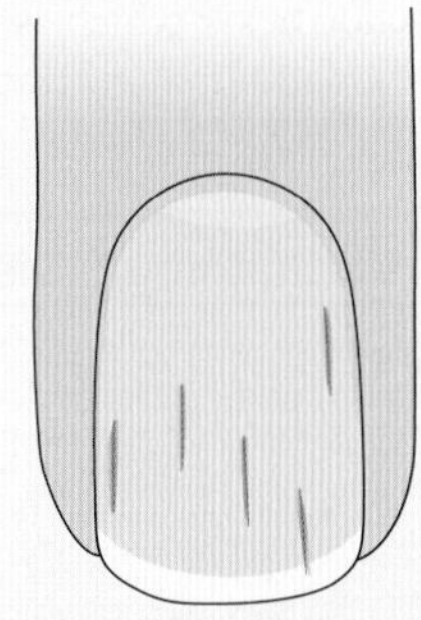

- Thin, longitudinal, dark-red subungual lines.
- Usually secondary to trauma.
- Can be seen in patients with psoriasis or endocarditis.
- Pattern reflects the longitudinal orientation of dermal blood vessels within the nail bed.

Trachyonychia

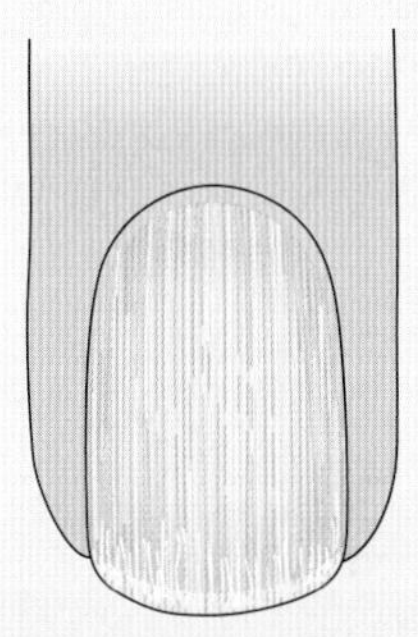

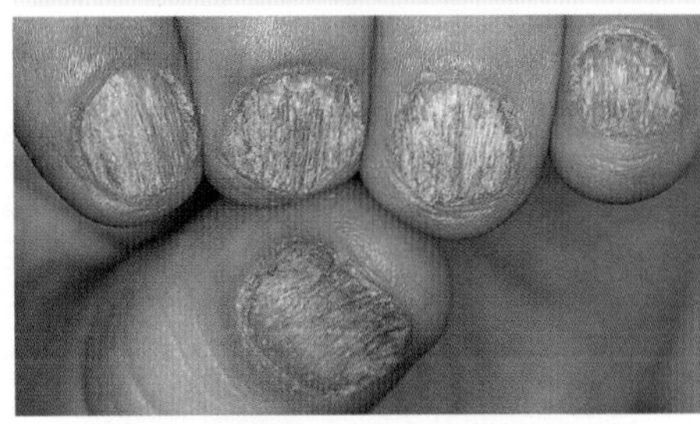

- Rough, "sandpaper" nails, often thin.
- Associated with alopecia areata or lichen planus >> psoriasis.

• May affect most or all nails, especially in children; often termed "20-nail dystrophy."

• **DDx:** onychorrhexis which is a common entity due to longitudinal ridging secondary to aging.

The Nail in Dermatologic Diseases

Alopecia Areata

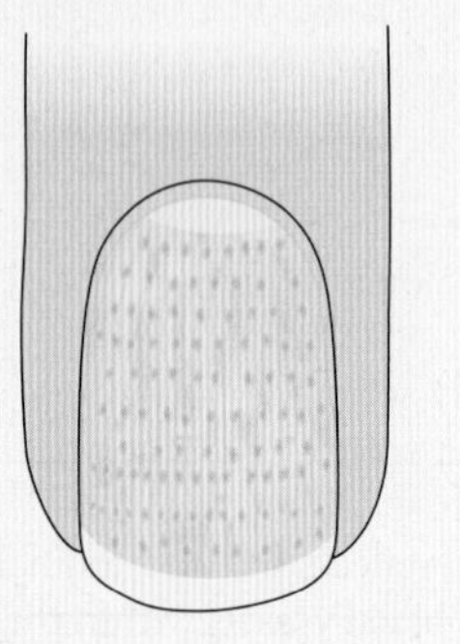

• Pitting, e.g. punctate depressions in nail plate, in a geometric or "scotch-plaid" pattern.

• Compared to psoriasis, pits are smaller and more numerous.

• Additional manifestations include trachyonychia > leukonychia or onychomadesis.

Darier Disease

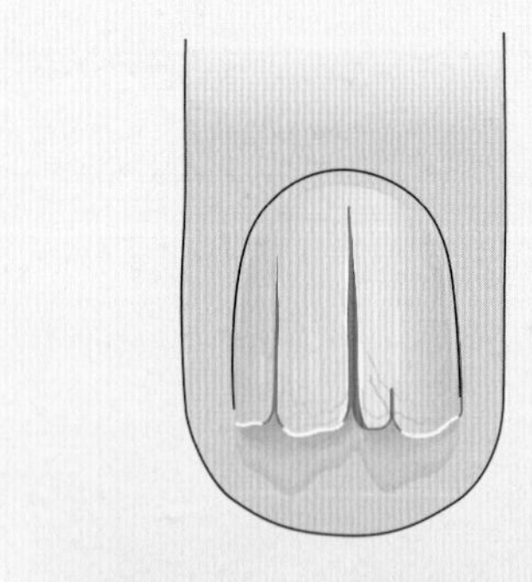

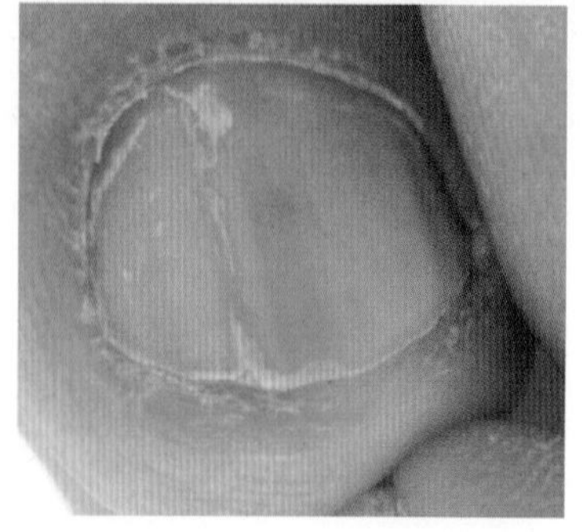

• Alternating longitudinal red and white streaks (i.e. longitudinal erythronychia and leukonychia).

• Distal fissuring (notches).

Lichen Planus (see Ch. 9)

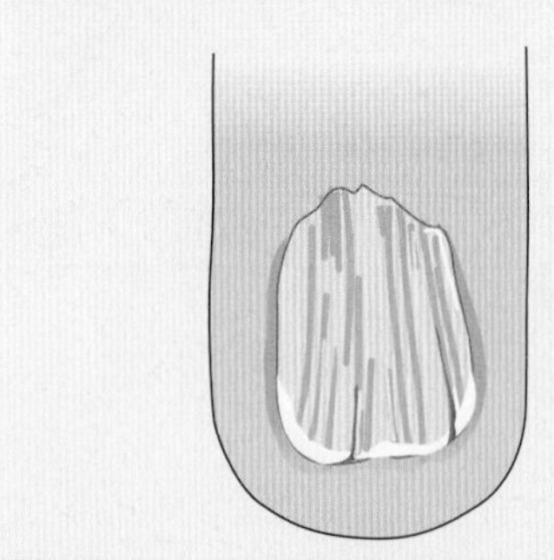

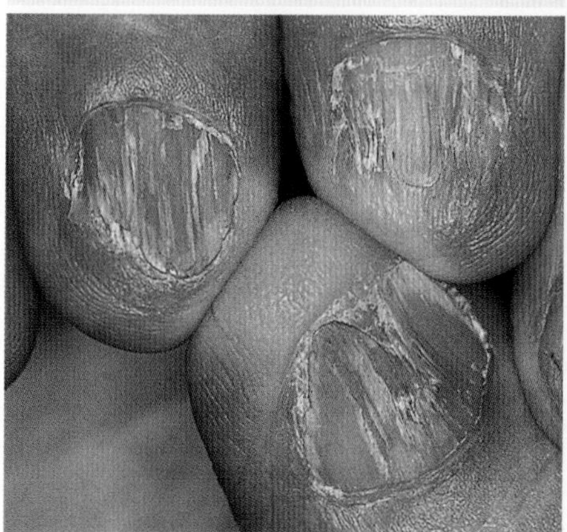

• Thinning of nail plate and atrophy, especially laterally.

• Additional clues include dorsal pterygium and trachyonychia (see above).

Psoriasis (see Ch. 6)

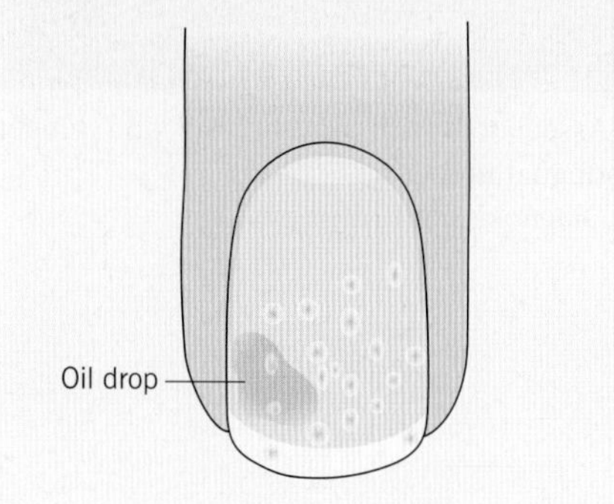

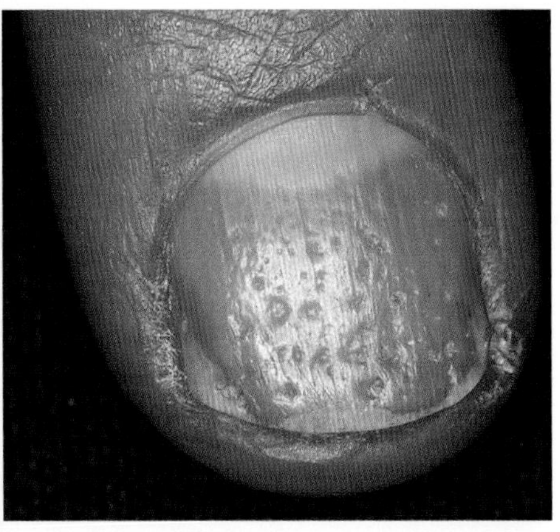

- Nail changes are often associated with arthritis and enthesitis.
- Pitting, punctate depressions in the nail plate, irregular in size and distribution.
- Oil drop changes which appear as irregular area of yellow-orange discoloration.
- Additional manifestations include yellowing, thickening and crumbling of the nail plate, onycholysis, subungual debris, splinter hemorrhages, paronychia, and rarely pustules (see next section).
- **DDx:** onychomycosis.

Pustular Psoriasis

- Pustules can form under the nail plate.
- May have lesions of psoriasis on the tips of the digits.

The Nail in Systemic Diseases

Examples, in addition to those below, are in Table 58.5.

Apparent Leukonychia

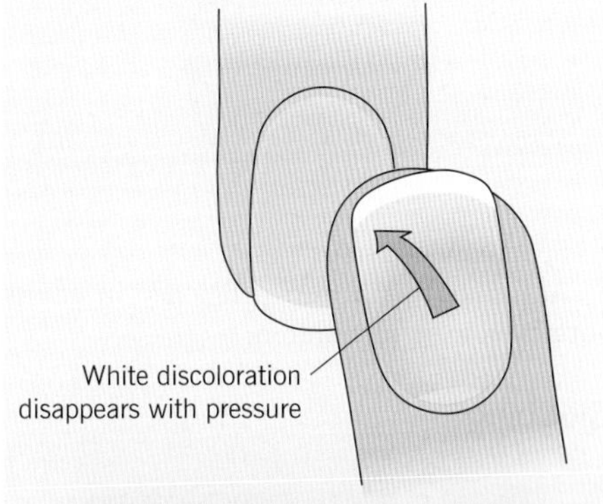

- Nail plate appears white due to alterations in nail bed (e.g. edema).
- Secondary to drugs or systemic disease (e.g. hypoalbuminemia leads to Muehrcke's lines).
- *Terry's nails*: only distal several millimeters of nail plate unaffected; associated with liver disease.
- *Lindsay's nails*: proximal half of nail is white and distal nail is red; associated with renal disease.

EXAMPLES OF NAIL CHANGES IN SYSTEMIC DISEASES AND GENODERMATOSES	
Nail finding	**Systemic or genetic disease**
Onycholysis	Hyperthyroidism
Splinter hemorrhages	Endocarditis
Beau's lines/onychomadesis	High fever Viral infection, e.g. coxsackie
Various, e.g. characteristic thickening ("door-wedge"), atrophy, partial to complete loss of nails, pterygium	Genodermatoses, e.g. pachyonychia congenita, hidrotic ectodermal dysplasia (see Fig. 52.10), dominant dystrophic epidermolysis bullosa, dyskeratosis congenita

Table 58.5 Examples of nail changes in systemic diseases and genodermatoses. Additional entities are discussed in more detail in the text.

Koilonychia

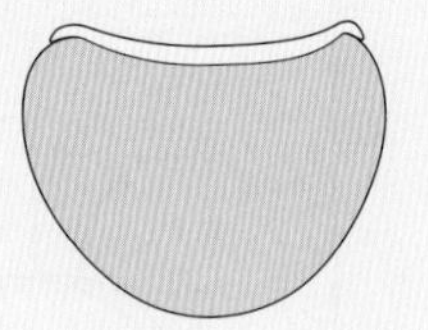

- Spoon-shaped nails.
- Associated with iron deficiency in adults but physiologic in children.

Clubbing

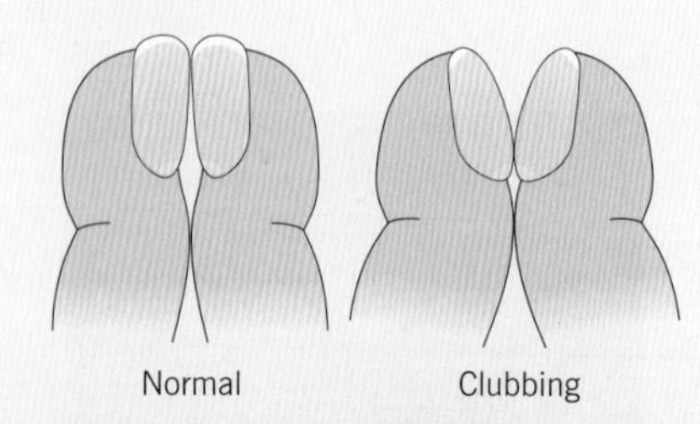

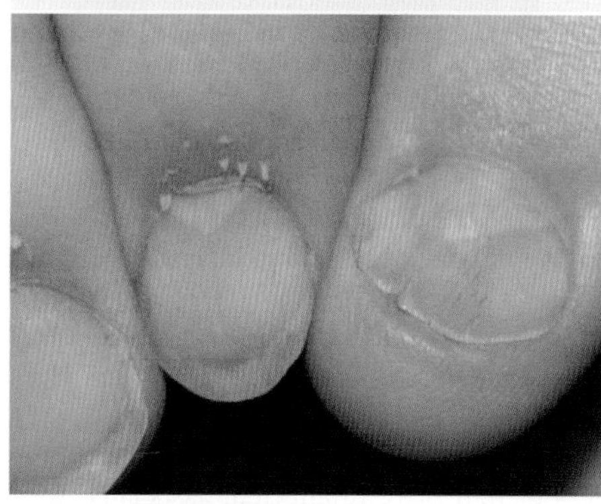

- Bulbous digits with watch-glass nails (>180° angle between proximal nail fold and nail).
- Most commonly seen in thyroid acropachy and in association with cardiovascular and bronchopulmonary disorders (e.g. interstitial lung disease).

Nail Patella Syndrome

- Hypoplasia of fingernails, greatest on the thumb, least on the fifth digit, triangular lunulae.
- Absent or hypoplastic patella; associated renal disease in up to 40%.

Proximal Nail Fold (Cuticular) Telangiectasias

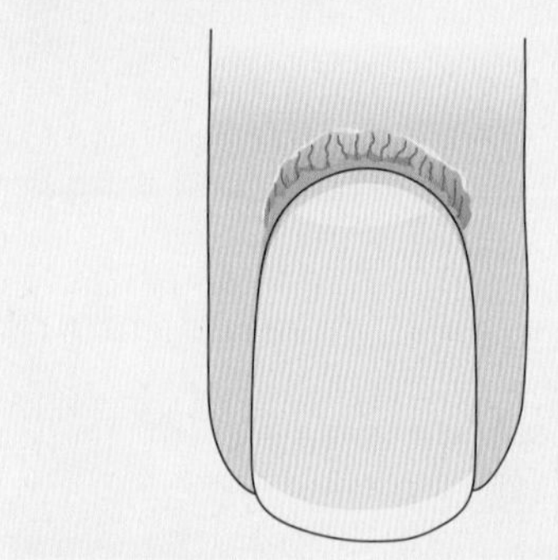

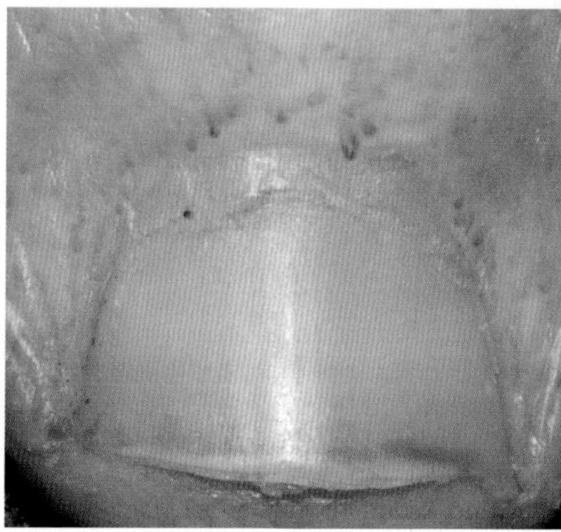

- Capillary prominence ± cuticular hemorrhages.
- Associated with lupus erythematosus and hereditary hemorrhagic telangiectasia.
- Also associated with dermatomyositis and systemic sclerosis, with a slightly different appearance of capillary dropout alternating with dilated capillary loops (see below).
- In dermatomyositis, ragged cuticles may also be present.
- In systemic sclerosis, ventral pterygium (loss of distal subungual space) may be seen.

Yellow Nail Syndrome

- Yellow coloration of all or most fingernails > toenails (see Fig. 45.1C).
- Loss of cuticle, onychomadesis, overcurvature of nail plate.
- Associated with lymphedema and bronchopulmonary disease.

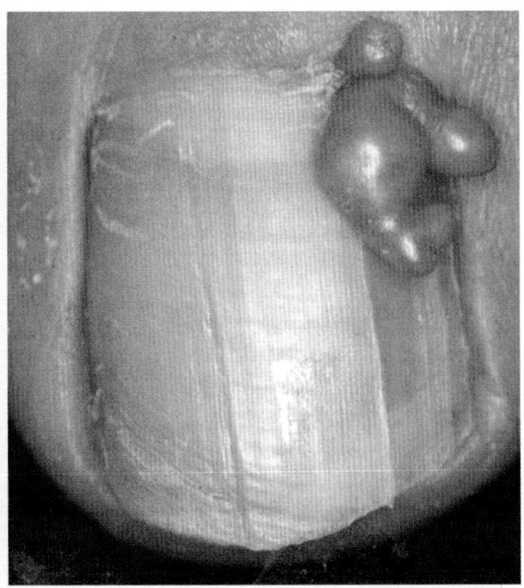

Fig. 58.4 Periungual fibroma producing a longitudinal groove due to matrix compression. *Courtesy, Antonella Tosti, MD.*

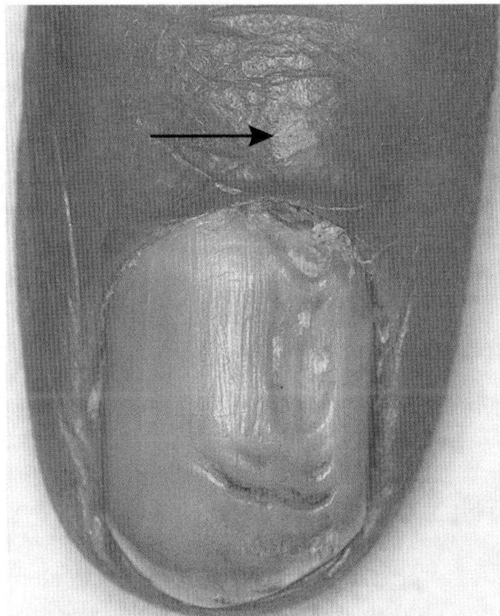

Fig. 58.5 Myxoid cyst. The longitudinal nail groove is a result of the compression of the nail matrix by the cyst (arrow). *Courtesy, Antonella Tosti, MD.*

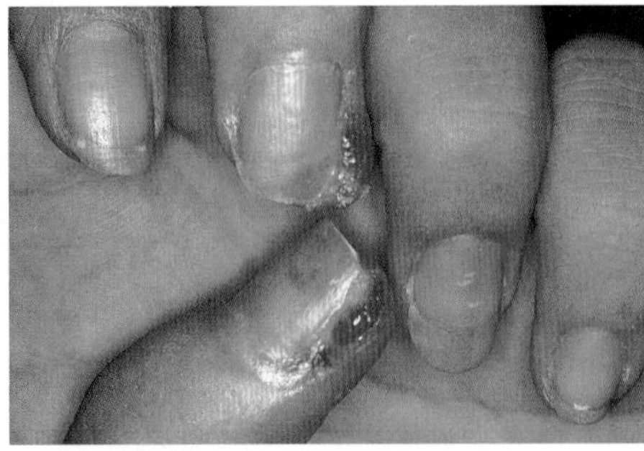

Fig. 58.6 Multiple periungual pyogenic granulomas in a patient taking indinavir. Similar lesions can be seen in patients receiving systemic retinoids or epidermal growth factor receptor inhibitors. *Courtesy, Antonella Tosti, MD.*

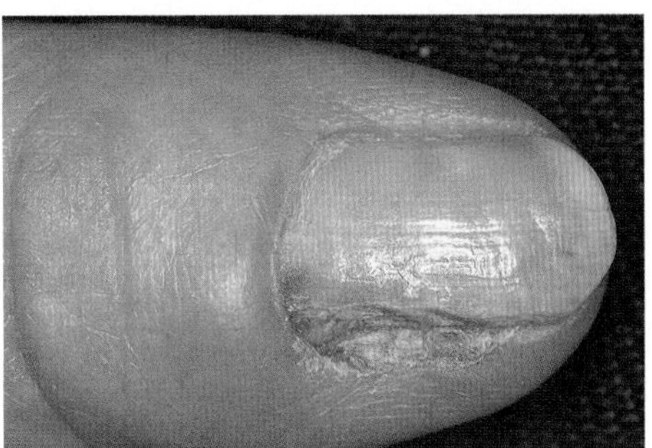

Fig. 58.7 Bowen disease. The lateral portion of the nail plate is absent. The nail bed shows hyperkeratosis with scaling and fissuring of the epithelium. *Courtesy, Antonella Tosti, MD.*

Tumors

- Various cysts, hyperplasias, and tumors may be seen on the distal digits, including fibromas (Fig. 58.4), myxoid cysts (Fig. 58.5, see Fig. 90.10), pyogenic granuloma (Fig. 58.6), glomus tumor (associated with paroxysmal pain) (see Ch. 94), Bowen disease (Fig. 58.7), keratoacanthoma (symptoms include pain, rapid growth), melanoma (signs include longitudinal melanonychia [see Fig. 58.2], Hutchinson's sign = pigmentation of proximal cuticle).

Additional figure details: onycholysis due to psoriasis; onychomadesis after an episode of acute paronychia; apparent leukonychia represents Muehrcke's lines; multiple Beau's lines were due to repeated cycles of systemic chemotherapy; proximal nail-fold telangiectasias and ragged cuticles due to dermatomyositis.

Additional courtesies: Antonella Tosti, Julie V. Schaffer, and Jean L. Bolognia.

For further information see Ch. 71 from *Dermatology, Fourth Edition*.

59 Oral Diseases

• In addition to common benign lesions such as bite fibromas and mucoceles, oral findings can represent clues to the diagnosis of skin disorders (e.g. lichen planus, early pemphigus vulgaris) or cutaneous signs of systemic disease (Table 59.1). Table 59.2 provides an overview of topical care for oral inflammatory conditions.
• Oral manifestations of infectious diseases (e.g. candidiasis, viral enanthems, findings associated with HIV infection) are covered in the chapters focused on these conditions.

Common Oral Mucosal Findings

Fordyce Granules

• "Free" sebaceous glands (i.e. not associated with hair follicles) evident in as many as 75% of adults (Fig. 59.1).
• Multiple 1- to 2-mm yellowish papules on the vermilion lips (upper > lower) and oral mucosa (especially buccal).

Geographic Tongue (Migratory Glossitis)

• Incidental finding on the dorsum of the tongue in ~2–3% of the population; may occasionally be associated with psoriasis, especially pustular variants.
• Well-demarcated areas of erythema and atrophy of the filiform papillae, surrounded by a whitish, hyperkeratotic serpiginous border (Fig. 59.2); lesions tend to migrate over time, may affect other oral sites, and are occasionally associated with a burning sensation.

Scrotal (Fissured) Tongue

• Asymptomatic finding that is occasionally associated with conditions such as granulomatous cheilitis (see below) and Down syndrome.
• Multiple grooves or furrows are present on the dorsal tongue, especially centrally (Fig. 59.3).

Hairy Tongue (Black Hairy Tongue)

• Reflects accumulation of keratin on the dorsum of the tongue; contributing factors may include poor oral hygiene, smoking, and a soft diet.
• Confluence of hairlike projections, which represent elongated papillae, with yellowish to brown-black discoloration (Fig. 59.4); may have exogenous staining from food, tobacco, or chromogenic bacteria (especially following antibiotic therapy); some patients report an unpleasant odor or taste.
• **DDx:** pigmented papillae of the tongue (in individuals with darkly pigmented skin).
• **Rx:** scraping or brushing the tongue.

Leukoedema

• Normal variant that is more often evident in smokers and individuals with darkly pigmented skin.
• Grayish-white, opalescent, sometimes "moth-eaten" appearance of the buccal > labial mucosa (Fig. 59.5); typically becomes less evident upon stretching.

Median Rhomboid Glossitis (Central Papillary Atrophy)

• Found in ~1% of adults, usually associated with local candidiasis.
• Well-demarcated diamond- or oval-shaped area of erythema and atrophy on the dorsum of the tongue (Fig. 59.6).
• **Rx:** clotrimazole troches or oral fluconazole (for dosage, see Table 64.5).

Periodontal and Dental Conditions with Dermatologic Relevance

Desquamative Gingivitis

• Clinical finding that can occur in several immune-mediated vesicular and erosive disorders (Fig. 59.7); favors women over 40 years of age.

SYSTEMIC DISEASES WITH ORAL MANIFESTATIONS	
Disorder	**Oral findings**
Primary systemic amyloidosis (see Ch. 39)	• Macroglossia, often with scalloped edges (due to dental impressions) or hemorrhagic papulonodules (see Fig. 39.3); xerostomia
Nutritional deficiencies (see Ch. 43)	• Atrophic glossitis (see text), stomatitis • *Scurvy*: gingival enlargement, hemorrhage and erosions (see Fig. 43.7B)
Inflammatory bowel disease	• *Crohn disease*: oral cobblestoning and ulcers (aphthous or linear; see Fig. 59.16), angular cheilitis, orofacial granulomatosis (see text) • *Pyostomatitis vegetans* (ulcerative colitis > Crohn): oral pustules and erosions in a "snail track-like" arrangement
Behçet disease (see Ch. 21)	• Aphthae (see text)
Sarcoidosis (see Ch. 78)	• Orofacial granulomatosis (see text), xerostomia, salivary gland enlargement
Sjögren syndrome (see Ch. 37)	• Xerostomia
Granulomatosis with polyangiitis (see Ch. 19)	• Gingival hemorrhage with a friable micropapular surface ("strawberry gums"; see Fig. 59.17)
Leukemia	• Hemorrhage due to thrombocytopenia, infections (viral, fungal, bacterial), gingival enlargement due to leukemic infiltration (especially in [myelo]monocytic forms)
Genodermatoses	• *Tuberous sclerosis complex*: oral fibromas, dental enamel pits • *Cowden syndrome*: oral papillomas favoring lips and tongue (see Fig. 45.3C and 52.1B) • *Multiple endocrine neoplasia type 2B*: mucosal neuromas – papulonodules favoring lips and anterior tongue (see Fig. 52.2B) • *Darier disease*: whitish papules and rugose plaques favoring palate and gingivae (see Fig. 48.8) • *Lipoid proteinosis*: diffuse infiltration or cobblestoned papules favoring lips and tongue/frenulum, xerostomia (see Fig. 40.4B) • *Chronic mucocutaneous candidiasis* (see Fig. 49.3A) • *Classic hyper-IgE syndrome*: retention of primary teeth, candidiasis • *Ectodermal dysplasias*: hypodontia, cone-shaped teeth • *Basal cell nevus syndrome*: odontogenic keratocysts of mandible > maxilla • *Gardner syndrome*: osteomas of maxilla and mandible • Peutz–Jeghers syndrome: brown macules on lips and oral mucosa (see Fig. 45.3B)

Table 59.1 Systemic diseases with oral manifestations.

• Diffuse gingival erythema with varying degrees of sloughing and erosion; frequently painful.

• Because desquamative gingivitis is often a manifestation of mucous membrane (cicatricial) pemphigoid and other autoimmune bullous disorders, evaluation should include routine histology plus direct and indirect immunofluorescence studies (see Ch. 23).

• **Rx:** treatment of underlying condition plus meticulous oral hygiene.

Gingival Enlargement (Hyperplasia, Overgrowth)

• Systemic medications and other causes of gingival enlargement are listed in Table 59.3.

• Drug-related gingival enlargement typically develops during the first year of

TOPICAL CARE FOR ORAL INFLAMMATORY CONDITIONS
Oral hygiene
Soft toothbrush Water pick, soft-tipped gum pick, or waxed tape-type dental floss to remove plaque Non-alcohol-based mouthwash Avoid trauma, e.g. sharp/rough dental restorations/appliances or biting cheeks
Topical anesthetics for erosions/ulcers
2% viscous lidocaine (to surface of ulcers or as swish & spit) "Magic mouthwash" with equal parts of: (1) 2% viscous lidocaine; (2) diphenhydramine 12.5 mg/5 ml; (3) magnesium and aluminum hydroxide plus sucralfate (Maalox®); consider adding dexamethasone elixir and/or nystatin suspension Dyclonine lozenges (e.g. Sucrets®) Benzocaine gel or lozenges
Topical anti-inflammatory medications
Corticosteroids, e.g. clobetasol 0.05% gel/ointment, fluocinonide 0.05% gel/ointment, triamcinolone 0.1% paste BID Dexamethasone elixir 0.5 mg/5 ml, swish and spit 5 ml BID–TID (leaving in mouth for 5 minutes)* Corticosteroid inhaler BID Tacrolimus 0.1% ointment BID Tacrolimus 1 mg capsule dissolved in 0.5–1 L of water, swish and spit 5 ml BID (leaving in mouth for ≥2 minutes)*
Prevention of secondary infection**
Clotrimazole 10 mg troches 4 times/day Nystatin suspension (400,000–6000,000 units), swish and swallow 4 times/day Chlorhexidine 0.12% oral rinse, swish and spit BID Dilute hydrogen peroxide (one part 3% solution, 2 parts water), swish and spit BID

**Especially for patients with more widespread involvement.*
***Consider for patients with extensive oral erosion/ulceration, especially if using topical or systemic immunosuppressive agents.*

Table 59.2 Topical care for oral inflammatory conditions.

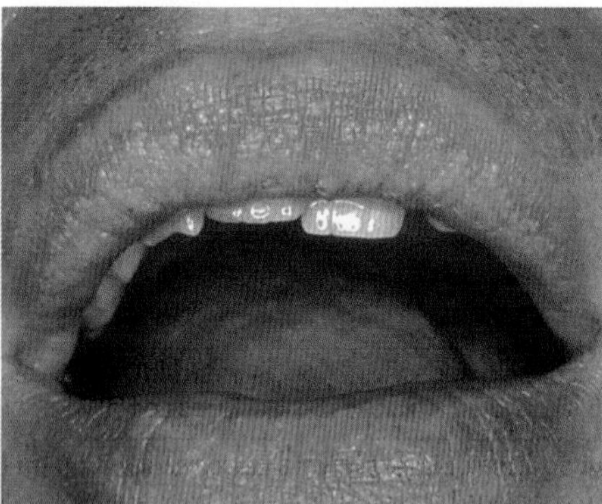

Fig. 59.1 Fordyce granules. Multiple yellowish 1- to 2-mm papules on the vermilion portion of the upper lip, representing "free" sebaceous glands. *Courtesy, Carl M. Allen, MD, and Charles Camisa, MD.*

administration and is first evident in the interdental papillae.

Dental Sinus

- Occurs in the setting of a chronic periapical abscess in a carious tooth.

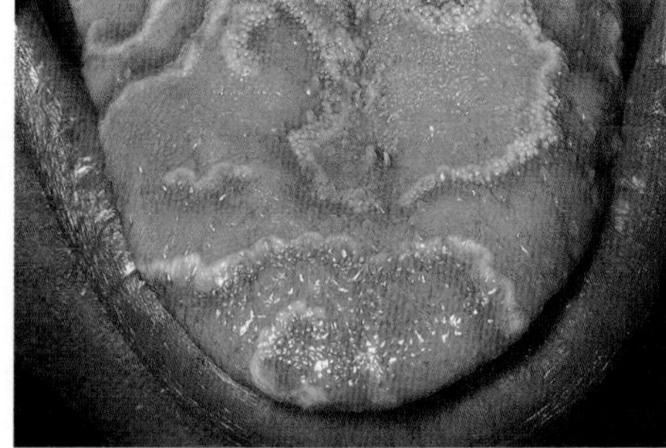

Fig. 59.2 Geographic tongue. A florid example, demonstrating well-delineated areas of erythema partially surrounded by white serpiginous borders. *Courtesy, Carl M. Allen, MD, and Charles Camisa, MD.*

- *Intraoral ("parulis")*: soft, nontender, erythematous papule on the alveolar process in the region of the affected tooth.
- *Cutaneous*: erythematous papule, often with an umbilicated or ulcerated center; found on the chin or submandibular region (mandibular teeth) > the cheek or upper lip (maxillary teeth) (Fig. 59.8).

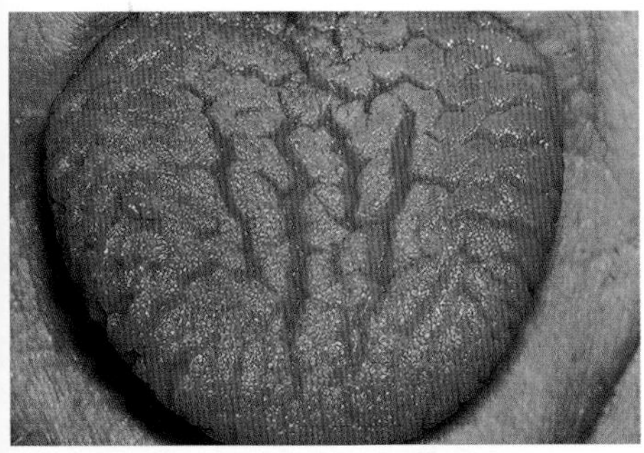

Fig. 59.3 Fissured tongue. Numerous asymptomatic furrows and grooves on the dorsal tongue. *Courtesy, Carl M. Allen, MD, and Charles Camisa, MD.*

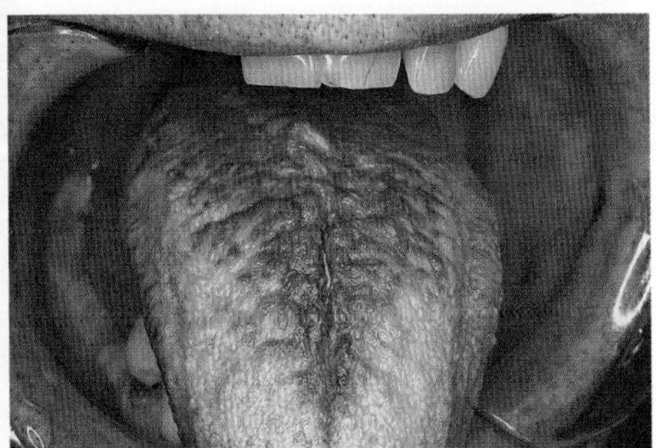

Fig. 59.4 Hairy tongue. The dorsum of the tongue exhibits marked accumulation of keratin and brown discoloration. *Courtesy, Carl M. Allen, MD, and Charles Camisa, MD.*

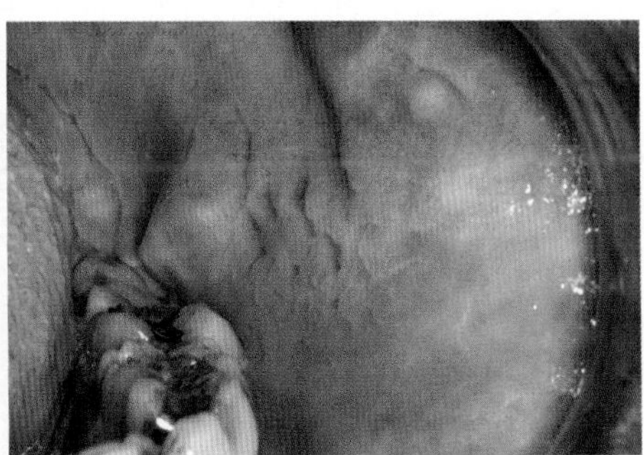

Fig. 59.5 Leukoedema. Diffuse grayish-white and wrinkled appearance of the buccal mucosa. These findings disappear when the cheek is stretched. *Courtesy, Carl M. Allen, MD, and Charles Camisa, MD.*

Sequelae of Trauma or Toxic Insults

Fibroma (Bite Fibroma)

- Results from reactive connective tissue hyperplasia in response to local trauma.
- Smooth pink papulonodule; most often located on the labial mucosa, especially of the lateral lower lip, or along the "bite line" of the buccal mucosa.
- **Rx:** if bothersome, excision with histologic evaluation to exclude a neoplastic condition.

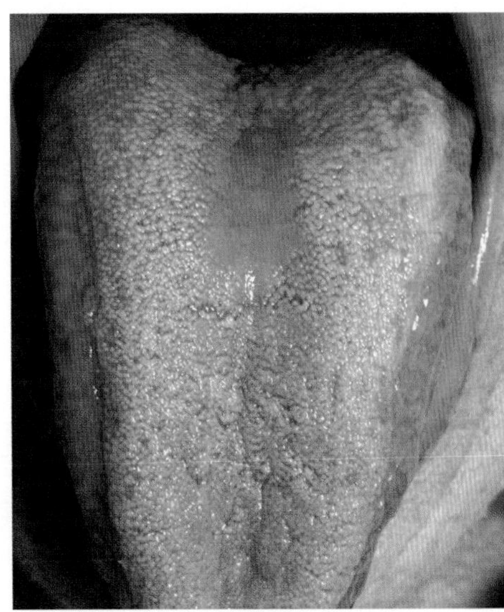

Fig. 59.6 Median rhomboid glossitis. On the dorsum of the tongue (anterior to the circumvallate papillae), there is a well-demarcated, smooth area with loss of the filiform papillae. *Courtesy, NYUDSC.*

Morsicatio Buccarum (Chronic Cheek Chewing)

- Characteristic mucosal changes related to habitual chewing or biting.
- Shaggy white mucosa, usually bilaterally in the buccal region along the "bite line" (Fig. 59.9).

Mucocele

- Translucent to bluish papule due to disruption of a minor salivary gland duct, most often located on the lower mucosal lip (Fig. 59.10; see Ch. 90).

Chemotherapy- and Radiation Therapy-Induced Mucositis

- Results from cytotoxic effects on the oral epithelium, especially in the setting of neutropenia; typically develops 4–7 days after administration of chemotherapy and ≥2 weeks after beginning radiation therapy.

DIFFERENTIAL DIAGNOSIS OF DESQUAMATIVE GINGIVITIS

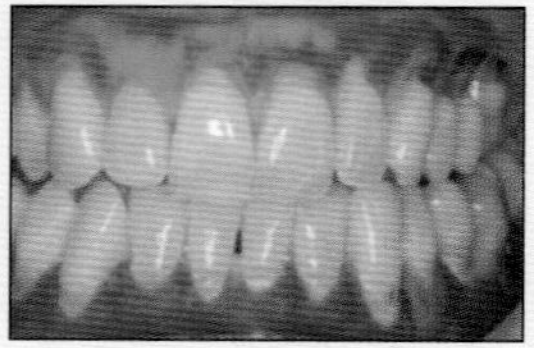

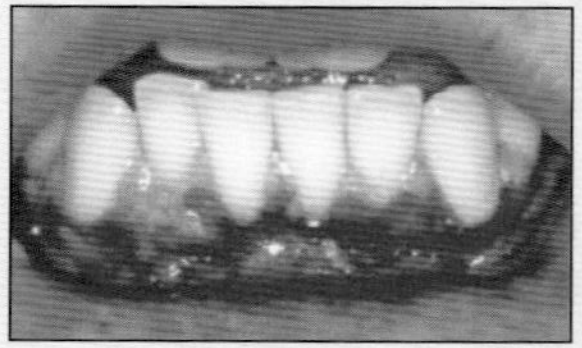

Differential diagnosis of desquamative gingivitis*

Lichen planus (LP) Lichenoid drug reaction Lupus erythematosus (LE) GVHD	Autoimmune bullous disorder – mucous membrane (cicatricial) pemphigoid, pemphigus vulgaris, paraneoplastic pemphigus > EBA, BP, LABD	Erythema multiforme, fixed drug eruption	Chronic ulcerative stomatitis	Contact dermatitis, allergic or irritant	Lichenoid contact stomatitis, lichenoid foreign body gingivitis
• Lacy white plaques (e.g. Wickham striae) of oral &/or other mucosae • Correct clinical setting for LE or GVHD • Appropriate medication history	• Erosions, ulcers & occasionally vesicles/ bullae of oral &/or other mucosae • Ragged ulcers → pemphigus; smooth but irregular ulcers → mucous membrane pemphigoid	• Erosions, ulcers & occasionally vesicles/ bullae of oral &/or other mucosae** • Recurrent episodes	• Clinically, resembles oral erosive LP, but asymmetric distribution of lesions & striae less sharply defined	• Need to look for unusual causes (e.g. nail polish in nail biters, sucking on metal objects)	• Lesions may result from exposure to cinnamon flavoring in food, beverage, and oral hygiene products; embedded particles from dentifrices and dental restorative materials in foreign body gingivitis

*Some entities may have cutaneous lesions.
**Erythema multiforme is more likely to affect other mucosal sites (e.g. genital, ocular).

Fig. 59.7 Differential diagnosis of desquamative gingivitis. If the gingivae are painful, hemorrhagic, and necrotic with punched-out interdental papillae, then

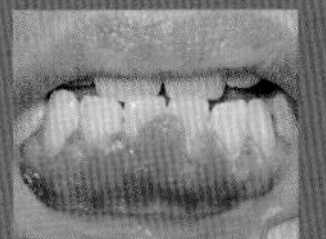

CAUSES OF GINGIVAL ENLARGEMENT (HYPERPLASIA, HYPERTROPHY)

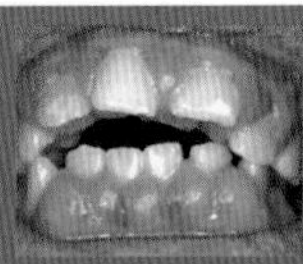

Systemic medications
• Phenytoin (~50%) > other anticonvulsants • Cyclosporine (~25%)* • Nifedipine (~25%) > other calcium channel blockers • Others – e.g. amphetamines, estrogens
Other etiologies
• Poor oral hygiene**, periodontal disease • Hormone-related – pregnancy, acromegaly • Orofacial granulomatosis (see text) • Granulomatosis with polyangiitis (friable "strawberry" gums) • Scurvy • Genetic disorders – e.g. tuberous sclerosis complex, Cowden syndrome, hereditary gingival fibromatosis • Malignancies – e.g. leukemia, Kaposi sarcoma • Deposition – e.g. primary systemic amyloidosis

**Consider substitution with oral tacrolimus.*
***Often contributes to gingival enlargement related to drugs and other factors.*

Table 59.3 Causes of gingival enlargement (hyperplasia, hypertrophy). *Insert images, courtesy, YDRSC.*

• Multiple erosions and/or ulcerations favor the gingivae, lateral tongue, and buccal mucosa; self-limited.
• **DDx:** herpetic or candidal infections (may be concomitant).
• **Rx:** topical anesthetics, analgesics, maintenance of oral hygiene; palifermin (recombinant human keratinocyte growth factor) can reduce severity but produces whitish discoloration of the dorsum of the tongue due to hyperkeratosis.

Cheilitis

• The differential diagnosis of cheilitis and clues to determining the etiology are outlined in Fig. 13.5; granulomatous cheilitis is discussed below.
• *Cheilitis glandularis*, seen primarily in men with actinic cheilitis and/or lip irritation, is characterized by tiny red macules on the lower labial mucosa at sites of inflamed salivary ducts.

Other Inflammatory Conditions

Aphthae (Aphthous Stomatitis; Canker Sores)

• Common condition characterized by recurrent oral ulcers, with a peak prevalence during the second and third decades of life; outbreaks may be triggered by trauma, psychological stress, or hormonal fluctuations.
• *Minor aphthae* (most frequent form): painful, round to ovoid, shallow ulcers that are usually <5 mm in diameter; feature a yellowish-white to gray pseudomembranous base, well-defined border, and prominent erythematous rim (Fig. 59.11); favor the buccal or labial mucosa and typically heal in 1–2 weeks without scarring.
• *Major aphthae*: larger (>1 cm), deeper ulcers that persist for up to 6 weeks; occasionally affect keratinized mucosa (e.g. dorsum of tongue, hard palate, attached gingiva) as well as non-keratinized mucosa, may heal with scarring, and are more common in HIV-infected individuals.

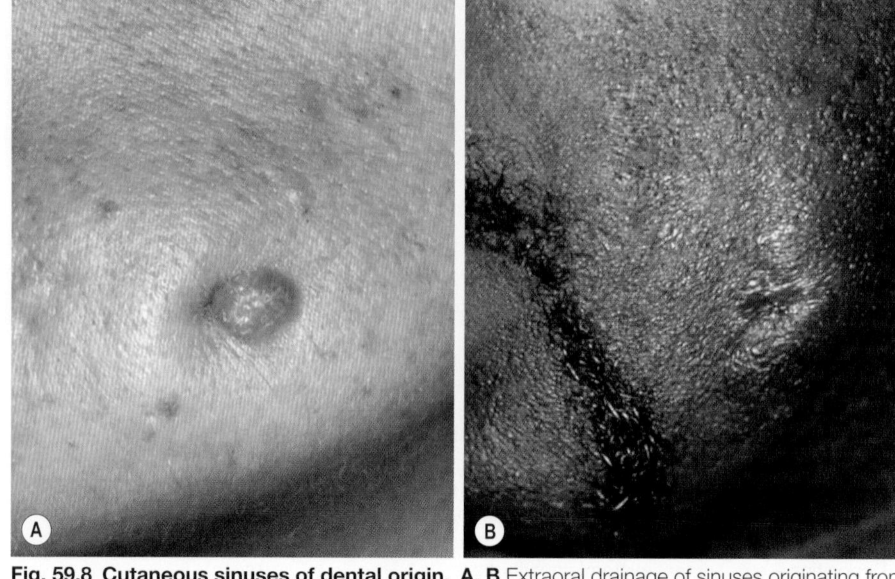

Fig. 59.8 Cutaneous sinuses of dental origin. A, B Extraoral drainage of sinuses originating from periapical dental abscesses within the mandible. These sinuses channel through the overlying skin. They may be mistaken for a pyogenic granuloma, cutaneous infection, or neoplasm. *A, Courtesy, Judit Stenn, MD; B, Courtesy, Carl M. Allen, MD, and Charles Camisa, MD.*

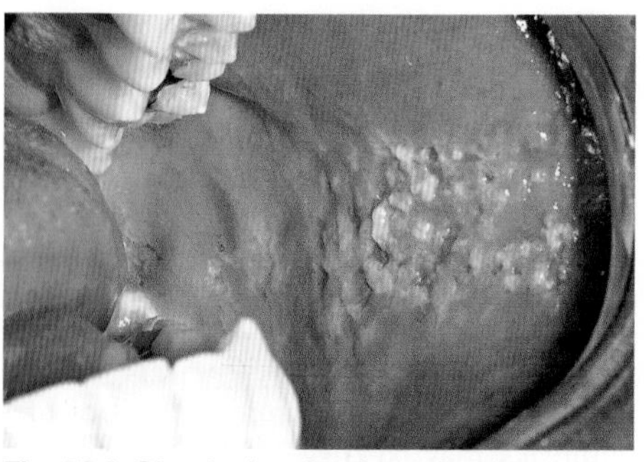

Fig. 59.9 Cheek chewing (morsicatio buccarum). Repetitive nibbling of the superficial layers of the epithelium resulted in these changes. Note that the characteristic shaggy, white lesion approximates the area where the upper and lower teeth meet. *Courtesy, Carl M. Allen, MD, and Charles Camisa, MD.*

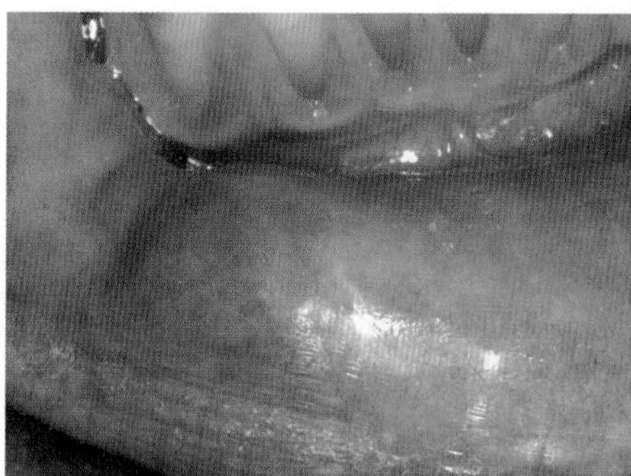

Fig. 59.10 Mucocele. Soft nodule with bluish hue in a typical location: lower lateral labial mucosa. *Courtesy, Carl M. Allen, MD, and Charles Camisa, MD.*

- *Herpetiform aphthae*: simultaneous development of numerous small lesions that tend to coalesce; tends to favor non-keratinized mucosa, unlike recurrent oral HSV, which favors keratinized mucosa.
- *Complex aphthosis*: frequent outbreaks of multiple (≥3) oral aphthae, or recurrent genital as well as oral aphthae, in the absence of Behçet disease (see Ch. 21).
- Recurrent aphthae can occur in the setting of systemic disorders such as inflammatory bowel disease, SLE, Behçet disease, cyclic neutropenia, and PFAPA (*p*eriodic *f*ever, *a*phthous stomatitis, *p*haryngitis and *a*denitis) syndrome (see Table 59.1).
- **DDx:** in addition to associated systemic conditions, may include HSV infection, trauma, and the disorders listed in Fig. 59.7.
- **Rx:** superpotent topical CS gel, CS inhaler, topical analgesics (see Table 59.2); if severe or frequent recurrences: colchicine, dapsone, thalidomide (the latter is especially helpful for major aphthae).

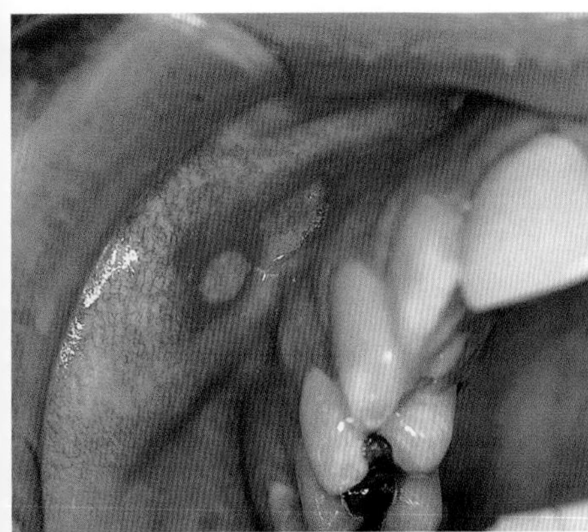

Fig. 59.11 Recurrent aphthous stomatitis. Shallow, creamy-white ulceration surrounded by an intensely red halo and located on non-keratinized mucosa, representing a classic presentation. *Courtesy, Carl M. Allen, MD, and Charles Camisa, MD.*

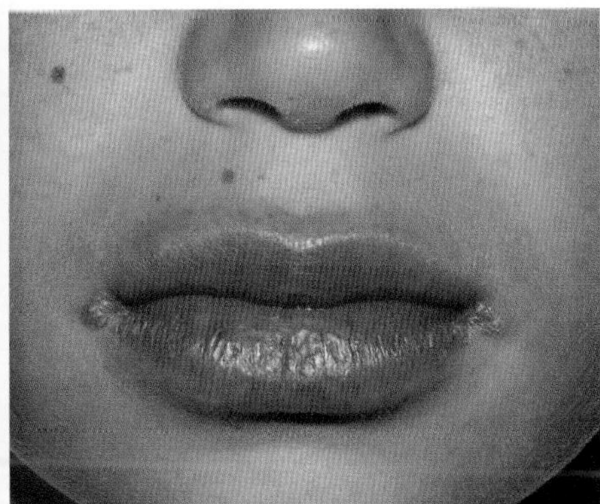

Fig. 59.12 Orofacial granulomatosis. Note the swelling of the lips (lower > upper) and angular cheilitis in this 10-year-old boy with Crohn disease. *Courtesy, Julie V. Schaffer, MD.*

Granulomatous Cheilitis and Other Forms of Orofacial Granulomatosis

- The term *orofacial granulomatosis* refers to non-infectious, non-necrotizing granulomatous inflammation of the lips, face, and/or oral cavity; this term includes isolated granulomatous cheilitis as well as manifestations of Crohn disease and sarcoidosis (see Table 59.1); usually develops during the second or third decade of life.
- *Granulomatous cheilitis* presents as diffuse swelling of the lip(s) (lower > upper or both) that can initially be intermittent (raising the possibility of angioedema) but is eventually persistent (Fig. 59.12); patients may have oral cobblestoning, recurrent aphthae, and gingival enlargement. The less frequent association with a scrotal tongue and/or facial nerve palsy is referred to as *Melkersson–Rosenthal syndrome.*
- **Rx:** intralesional CS, topical calcineurin inhibitors, dapsone, tetracyclines (given for several months), thalidomide, or TNF inhibitors (for severe disease); patients should be evaluated for Crohn disease and sarcoidosis.

Contact Stomatitis

- Irritant or allergic contact stomatitis can result from a variety of foods, food additives, materials used in dentistry, chewing on metal objects, and propylene glycol from vaping; in particular, cinnamon flavoring and dental amalgam ("silver" fillings) can lead to a lichenoid mucositis histologically.
- Shaggy white or erythematous areas, most often on the buccal mucosa or lateral tongue; lacy white streaks (resembling lichen planus) or erosions may be seen (Fig. 59.13).
- **Rx:** evaluation with patch testing and avoidance of offending agents, sometimes requiring replacement of amalgam with other materials.

Nicotine Stomatitis

- Presents as gray-white discoloration of the palate, often with umbilicated papules that represent inflamed salivary ducts (Fig. 59.14).

Atrophic Glossitis

- Manifestation of candidiasis and several nutritional deficiencies, e.g. vitamin B_{12} (pernicious anemia), folate, iron, niacin (pellagra), and riboflavin (see Ch. 43).
- Presents with a smooth, "beefy red" tongue (Fig. 59.15); involvement may initially be patchy but is eventually diffuse and may be associated with a burning sensation or sore mouth.

Oral Signs of Systemic Disease

- Systemic diseases that can present with oral findings are listed in Table 59.1 (Figs 59.16 and 59.17).

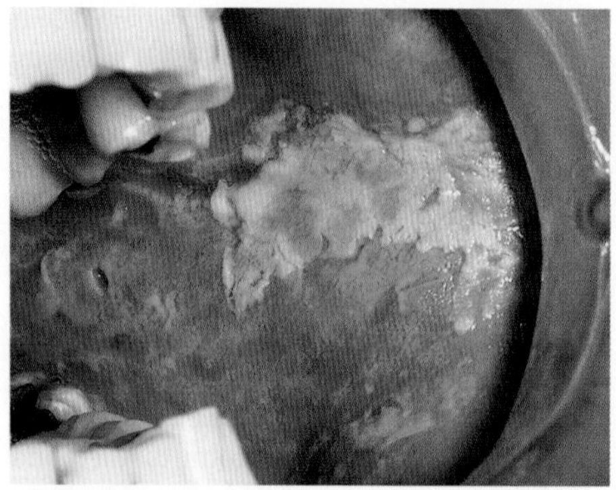

Fig. 59.13 Contact stomatitis from artificial cinnamon flavoring. Use of artificial cinnamon-flavored gum caused this shaggy, white keratotic lesion of the buccal mucosa. *Courtesy, Carl M. Allen, MD, and Charles Camisa, MD.*

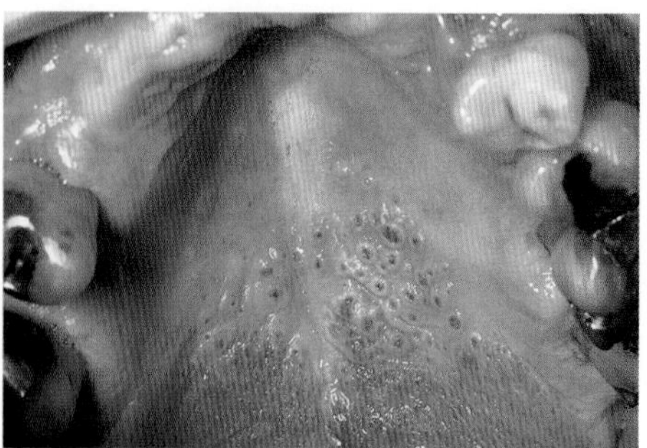

Fig. 59.14 Nicotine stomatitis. Gray-white palatal mucosa with numerous umbilicated papules representing inflamed palatal salivary glands. *Courtesy, Carl M. Allen, MD, and Charles Camisa, MD.*

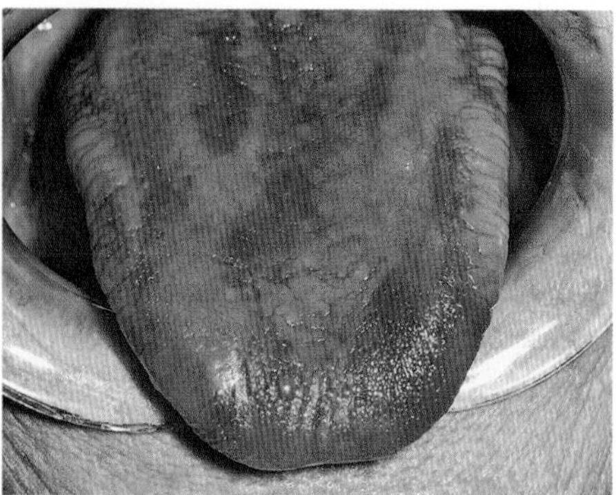

Fig. 59.15 Atrophic glossitis due to pernicious anemia plus candidiasis. Erythematous, atrophic tongue as a manifestation of pernicious anemia with a superimposed candidal infection. *Courtesy, Carl M. Allen, MD, and Charles Camisa, MD.*

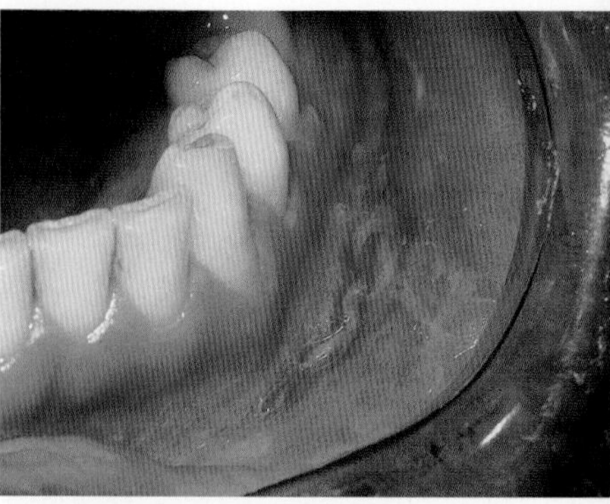

Fig. 59.16 Crohn disease. Linear ulceration of the mandibular vestibule is the classic oral manifestation of this disease. *Courtesy, Carl M. Allen, MD, and Charles Camisa, MD.*

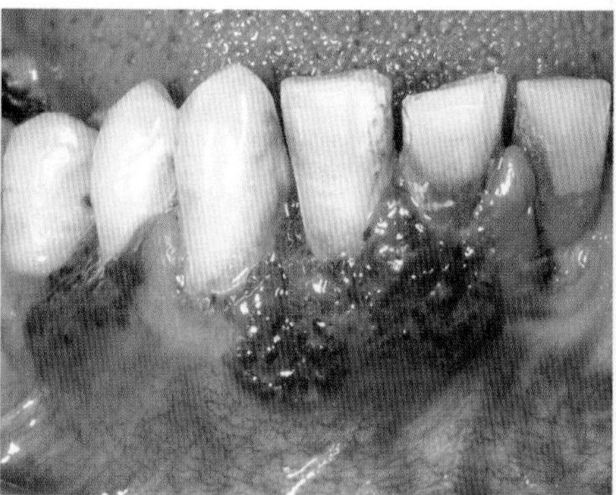

Fig. 59.17 Granulomatosis with polyangiitis – strawberry gums. The affected areas of the gingiva are red-purple, micropapular, and friable, with a resemblance to ripe strawberries. *Courtesy, Carl M. Allen, MD, and Charles Camisa, MD.*

Premalignant and Malignant Conditions

Leukoplakia and Erythroplakia

- *Leukoplakia* refers to a white patch or plaque on the oral mucosa that cannot be clinicopathologically characterized as a specific disease process; typically occurs in middle-aged and older adults (men > women), especially those who use tobacco ± alcohol, and is regarded as a premalignant condition for SCC.
  - Often a homogeneous white patch or plaque, but may be non-homogeneous and "speckled" (e.g. white flecks on a red base); usually has sharply demarcated borders (Fig. 59.18)

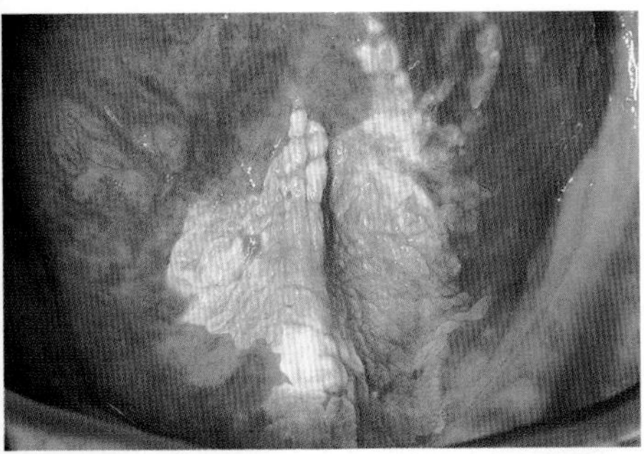

Fig. 59.18 Leukoplakia. Sharply demarcated, white plaque involving the ventral surface of the tongue and floor of the mouth. *Courtesy, Carl M. Allen, MD, and Charles Camisa, MD.*

- Similarly, *erythroplakia* is defined as a red intraoral patch or slightly elevated, velvety plaque that cannot be diagnosed as a particular disease; biopsies usually show more severe epithelial dysplasia than leukoplakia.
- Often affects the buccal mucosa, lower inner lip, floor of the mouth, and lateral or ventral tongue.
- The degree of histologic epithelial dysplasia influences the risk of transformation to SCC; non-homogeneous leukoplakia, erythroplakia, and lesions located on the floor of the mouth or lateral/ventral tongue also have higher malignant potential.
- **DDx** of leukoplakia: may include SCC, lichen planus, candidiasis, morsicatio buccarum (see above), and nicotine or contact stomatitis.
- After elimination of possible causative factors (e.g. tobacco use, candidiasis, irritation/trauma) for 2–6 weeks, persistent lesions should be biopsied.
- **Rx:** for leukoplakia with moderate to severe dysplasia or in high-risk sites and for erythroplakia – excision, cryosurgery, or laser ablation; all patients need longitudinal evaluation and should avoid carcinogenic habits.
- *Proliferative verrucous leukoplakia*, which tends to occur in women without traditional risk factors, is characterized by multifocal red and white patches that eventually develop a verrucous surface; difficult to treat and associated with high risk of transformation to SCC.

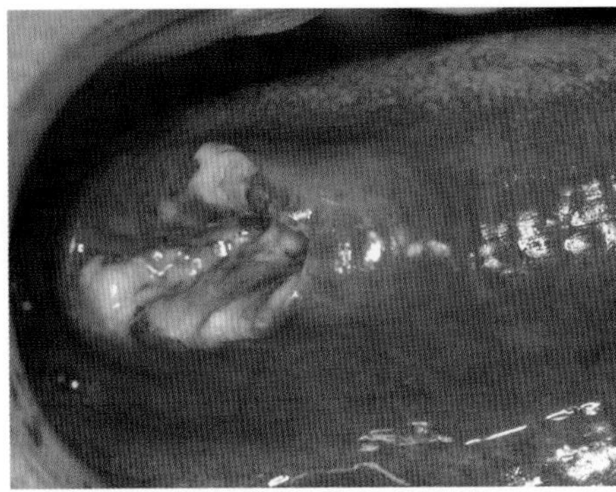

Fig. 59.19 Squamous cell carcinoma. Ulcerated, indurated, exophytic mass involving the right lateral border of the tongue, a typical presentation and site for this tumor. *Courtesy, Carl M. Allen, MD, and Charles Camisa, MD.*

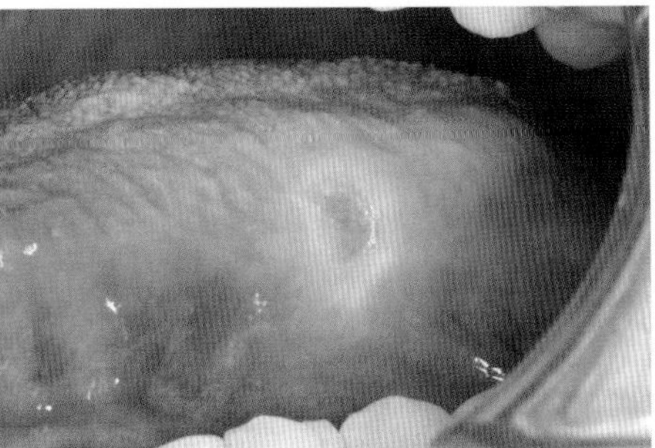

Fig. 59.20 Traumatic ulcer. This lesion on the lateral tongue demonstrates a yellow fibrinous base with a white hyperkeratotic border. Compare this to the oral SCC depicted in Fig. 59.19, which presented as an ulcerated, indurated mass. *Courtesy, Carl M. Allen, MD, and Charles Camisa, MD.*

Squamous Cell Carcinoma

- Most common malignancy of the oral cavity, favoring middle-aged and older men; risk factors include tobacco and alcohol use, HPV infection (see Ch. 66), and betel nut chewing.
- May present as an ulcer, exophytic mass, or area of induration; most often on the lateral or ventral tongue and floor of the mouth (Fig. 59.19).
- **DDx:** leukoplakia, traumatic ulcer (Fig. 59.20), salivary gland tumor, amelanotic melanoma.
- **Rx:** combinations of surgery, radiation therapy (especially if HPV-associated), and chemotherapy.
- *Verrucous carcinoma* (*oral florid papillomatosis*) is a low-grade variant of SCC that presents as slowly growing, exophytic papillomatous masses that favor the buccal mucosa and gingiva; **Rx:** excision, traditionally

avoiding radiation therapy due to a possible association with anaplastic transformation.

Melanoma

- Uncommon oral malignancy that favors middle-aged and older men; often diagnosed at a locally advanced stage.
- Pigmented (with findings similar to cutaneous melanoma; see Ch. 93) > amelanotic, with a predilection for the hard palate and maxillary gingivae.
- **DDx:** for pigmented lesions – foreign body tattoo (Fig. 59.21), blue nevus, oral melanotic macule, physiologic pigmentation.

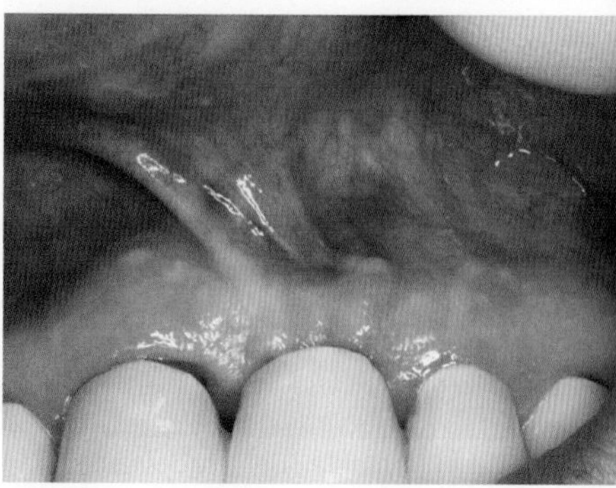

Fig. 59.21 Amalgam tattoo. Foreign body tattoos are the most common cause of acquired oral pigmentation, and most of them are due to implantation of dental amalgam. In this patient, the amalgam was used to seal the apices of endodontically treated teeth, resulting in tattooing of the maxillary vestibule. *Courtesy, Carl M. Allen, MD, and Charles Camisa, MD.*

For further information see Ch. 72 from *Dermatology, Fourth Edition*.

For additional online figures and tables visit www.expertconsult.com 

Anogenital Diseases 60

Introduction

- The anatomy (Fig. 60.1), normal cutaneous findings, and benign lesions of the anogenital area (Table 60.1) should be appreciated before addressing diseases in this area.
- A number of systemic diseases affect the anogenital area (Table 60.2).
- Cutaneous disorders of the anogenital area may be more difficult to diagnose than those involving other cutaneous sites, as typical features may not be present.
- A number of dermatologic conditions affect the anogenital region, including inflammatory (Table 60.3; Figs 60.2–60.6), bullous (Table 60.4; Fig. 60.7), infectious (Table 60.5; see Ch. 69), and premalignant and malignant conditions (Table 60.6; Figs 60.8–60.11).
- Pain and pruritus can be the presenting symptoms in a wide variety of anogenital diseases (Figs 60.12 and 60.13).
- Patients with anogenital disease should use soap substitutes and bland emollient ointments; irritants and potential allergens (e.g. flushable moist wipes, previous topical medications) should be avoided.
- Ointments are preferred over creams in this area because of less irritation and burning with application, as well as providing a better barrier to urine and feces.
- The anogenital region is an area of occlusion and more prone to adverse side effects from and increased absorption of topical agents (e.g. CS).
- High-potency topical CS are generally avoided because of the increased risk for atrophy and striae, but they are used with confidence in certain situations (e.g. lichen sclerosus, erosive lichen planus) for periods of up to 12 weeks once to twice yearly.
- Because of increased moisture, warmth, and occlusion, anogenital diseases have an increased risk of superimposed bacterial and fungal infections.
- Diseases that result in scarring of the anogenital region (e.g. lichen sclerosus, erosive lichen planus) carry an increased long-term risk of developing invasive SCC.

Intraepithelial Neoplasia

- The term *intraepithelial neoplasia* (*IN*) refers to a change within the anogenital epithelium that is premalignant, and as such has the potential to become an invasive SCC.
- IN has replaced older synonymous terms, such as genital Bowen disease, erythroplasia of Queyrat, and genital SCC *in situ*; use of the term leukoplakia with atypia is also not recommended.
- IN is further subdivided based on location: vulvar IN (VIN), penile IN (PIN), perianal IN (PaIN), and anal IN (AIN) (see Table 60.6), as well as the degree of atypia: 1, mild; 2, moderate; 3, severe.
- VIN is now classified as either *usual type* VIN associated with HPV infection (typically HPV types 16 and 18) or *differentiated type* VIN that can arise in the setting of lichen sclerosus or lichen planus.
- Recently recommended terminology that can replace or qualify IN: high-grade and low-grade squamous intraepithelial lesion.
- Bowenoid papulosis (BP) is a distinct clinical variant of IN that occurs in a younger (more sexually active) age group, is caused by the human papillomavirus (HPV subtypes 16 and 18), has a better prognosis, and sometimes spontaneously regresses (see Ch. 66).

Condyloma Acuminata

- See Ch. 66.

THE NORMAL VULVA

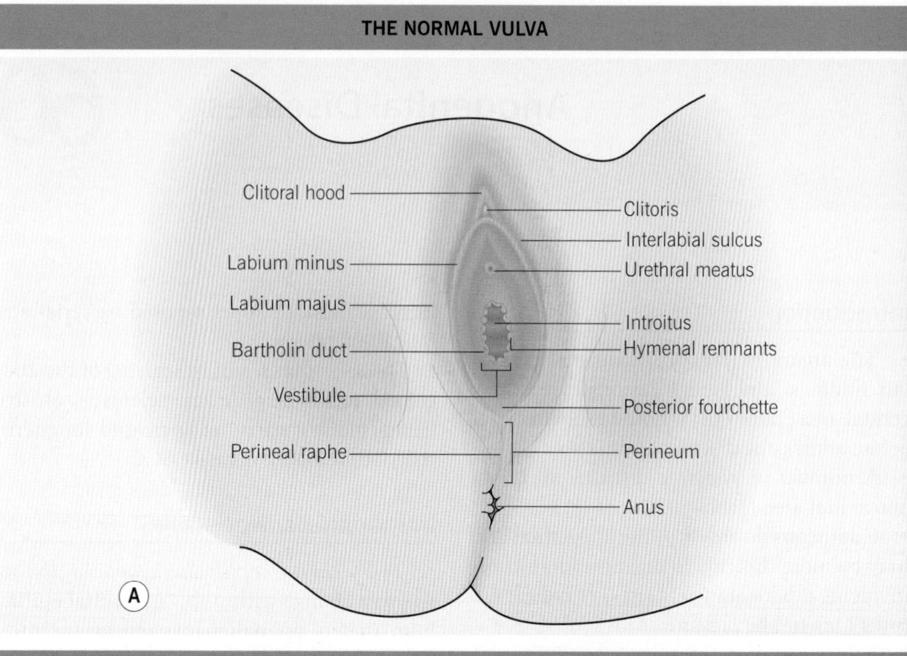

THE NORMAL PENIS, CIRCUMCISED AND UNCIRCUMCISED

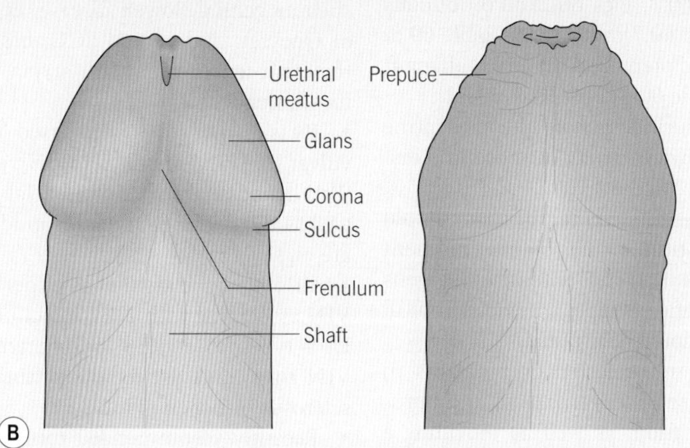

Fig. 60.1 Genital anatomy. A The normal vulva. **B** The normal penis, circumcised and uncircumcised.

Dysesthetic Genital Pain Syndromes

- Includes several regional pain syndromes in which clinical appearance of the involved anogenital region is normal despite the patient's experience of debilitating pain (Fig. 60.14); associated depression is common.
- *Localized vulvodynia* (vestibulodynia) occurs in young, sexually active females and is characterized by superficial dyspareunia and tenderness upon localized pressure within the vulvar vestibule.
- *Generalized* (dysesthetic) *vulvodynia/scrotodynia* is characterized by persistent burning pain that involves the entire vulva, scrotum, or penis, and may extend down the thighs.

NORMAL FINDINGS AND BENIGN LESIONS OF THE ANOGENITAL REGION	
Common	**Less common**
Epidermoid cysts	Fox–Fordyce disease
Open comedones	Syringomas
Pearly penile papules (see Fig. 95.7)	Idiopathic calcinosis of the scrotum
Vestibular papillomatosis	Urethral caruncle
Angiokeratomas (see Fig. 94.11)	Hidradenoma papilliferum
Seborrheic keratoses and acrochordons	
Melanocytic nevi and genital lentigines (see Fig. 92.2)	
Free sebaceous glands	

Table 60.1 Normal findings and benign lesions of the anogenital region. Papules in the anogenital region can also result from HPV infection, in particular condylomata acuminata and common warts (see Ch. 66).

SYSTEMIC DISEASES THAT MAY PRESENT IN THE ANOGENITAL REGION
• Inflammatory bowel disease, especially Crohn disease (see Ch. 45) • Nutritional dermatoses, e.g. acrodermatitis enteropathica, necrolytic migratory erythema, cystic fibrosis (see Ch. 43) • Langerhans cell histiocytosis (see Ch. 76) • Kawasaki disease (see Ch. 3) • Behçet disease – ulcers (see Ch. 45) • Infections (nonvenereal), e.g. recurrent toxin-mediated perineal erythema, Fournier gangrene • Infections (venereal) (see Ch. 69) • Drug reactions (see Chs 16 & 17), e.g. EM major, SJS, TEN; fixed drug eruption; toxic erythema of chemotherapy • Neutrophilic dermatoses, e.g. Sweet syndrome (see Ch. 21)

Table 60.2 Systemic diseases that may present in the anogenital region. EM, erythema multiforme; SJS, Stevens–Johnson syndrome; TEN, toxic epidermal necrolysis.

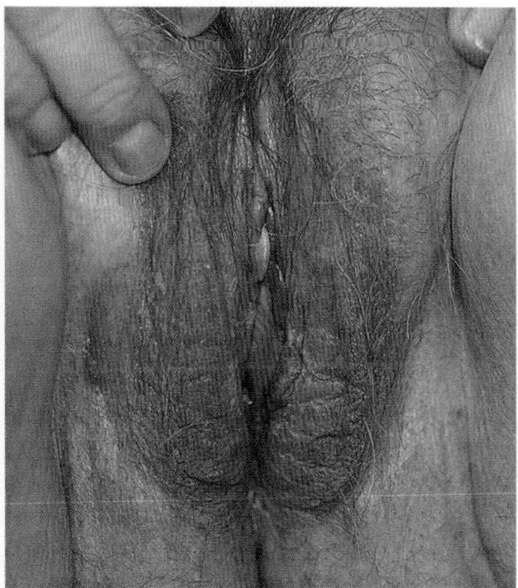

Fig. 60.2 Vulvar dermatitis. Lichenification is prominent. The underlying diagnosis was atopic dermatitis. *Courtesy, Susan M. Cooper, MD, and Fenella Wojnarowska, MD.*

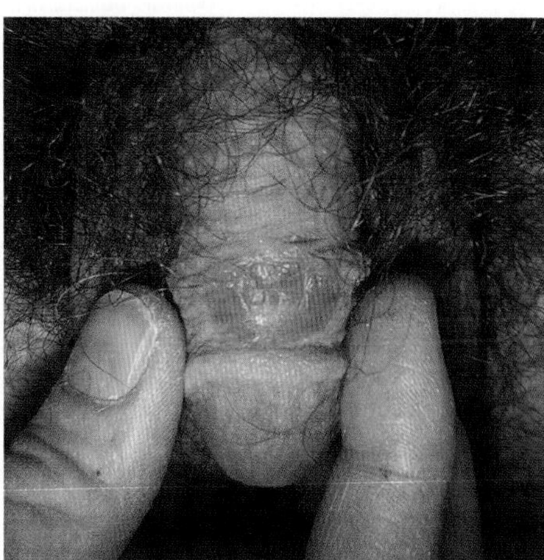

Fig. 60.3 Psoriasis of the penile shaft. Well-demarcated erythematous plaque with slight scale. Similar lesions can be seen in patients with reactive arthritis (formerly Reiter disease). *Courtesy, Jean L. Bolognia, MD.*

INFLAMMATORY DISORDERS WITH ANOGENITAL FEATURES		
Inflammatory disorder	**Anogenital features**	**Rx**
Anogenital dermatitis	• Female > male • Varied presentations, from mild erythema to significant lichenification (Fig. 60.2) • Unremitting itch/scratch cycle **Female:** perianal, labia majora, mons pubis **Male:** crura and scrotum	• Examine entire body for clues to etiology (e.g. seborrheic or atopic dermatitis) • Eliminate irritants/allergens • Break itch/scratch cycle with potent topical CS for several weeks and then taper • Oral antihistamines may help control pruritus • Consider patch testing
Psoriasis (including inverse psoriasis) (See Ch. 6)	• Perianal and intergluteal cleft fissuring; erythematous, smooth, well-demarcated plaques **Female:** labia majora and mons pubis **Male**: glans and shaft of penis (Fig. 60.3)	**Mild–moderate** • Moderate potency topical CS for 2–3 weeks with taper to less potent topical CS plus antifungal • Topical calcineurin inhibitors and vitamin D analogues (may sting) **Severe** (see Ch. 6)
Lichen sclerosus (LS)	See Fig. 60.4 and Ch. 36	See Ch. 36
Lichen planus (LP) (see Ch. 9)	• Intense pruritus common in all forms	**First-line** • Superpotent topical CS • For vaginal disease, CS foams, enemas, suppositories or ointments (± dilators) **Second-line** • Longer-term maintenance with superpotent topical CS or combined moderately potent CS/ antifungal/antibacterial preparations • Topical calcineurin inhibitors • Intralesional CS (hypertrophic) • Systemic antimalarials (e.g. hydroxychloroquine) • Systemic immunosuppressants (e.g. weekly methotrexate, mycophenolate mofetil) • Systemic antibiotics (e.g. minocycline ± nicotinamide) • Surgery to lyse adhesions
1. Classic	• Violaceous flat-topped papules and plaques; lacy white streaks **Female:** mons pubis and labia **Male:** glans and shaft of penis; often annular (Fig. 60.5A)	
2. Erosive	• Female > male • Erosions surrounded by white lacy pattern; prominent scarring/ adhesions (Fig. 60.5B) • Desquamative vaginitis with discharge; significant pain and dyspareunia • Usually severe oral involvement/ desquamative gingivitis • Increased risk for SCC	
3. Hypertrophic	• Hyperkeratotic white plaques on the vulva or shaft of penis (Fig. 60.5C) • Increased risk for SCC	
Zoon balanitis/vulvitis (plasma cell balanitis/vulvitis)	• Male (uncircumcised) > female • Pruritus and pain **Male:** glans penis (Fig. 60.6) • Erythematous discrete moist plaques with speckled appearance and orange hue • Involvement of adjacent surfaces produce "kissing lesions" **Female:** similar lesions involving vulva	• Circumcision curative • Topical CS if symptoms

Table 60.3 Inflammatory disorders with anogenital features. Porokeratosis ptychotropica is a rare disorder and can mimic anogenital dermatitis or inverse psoriasis. The DDx of these disorders includes the other entities listed in this table; consider infections, either primary or superimposed (see Table 60.5); less commonly bullous disorders (see Table 60.4); if nonhealing consider malignancy, most commonly SCC (see Table 60.6).

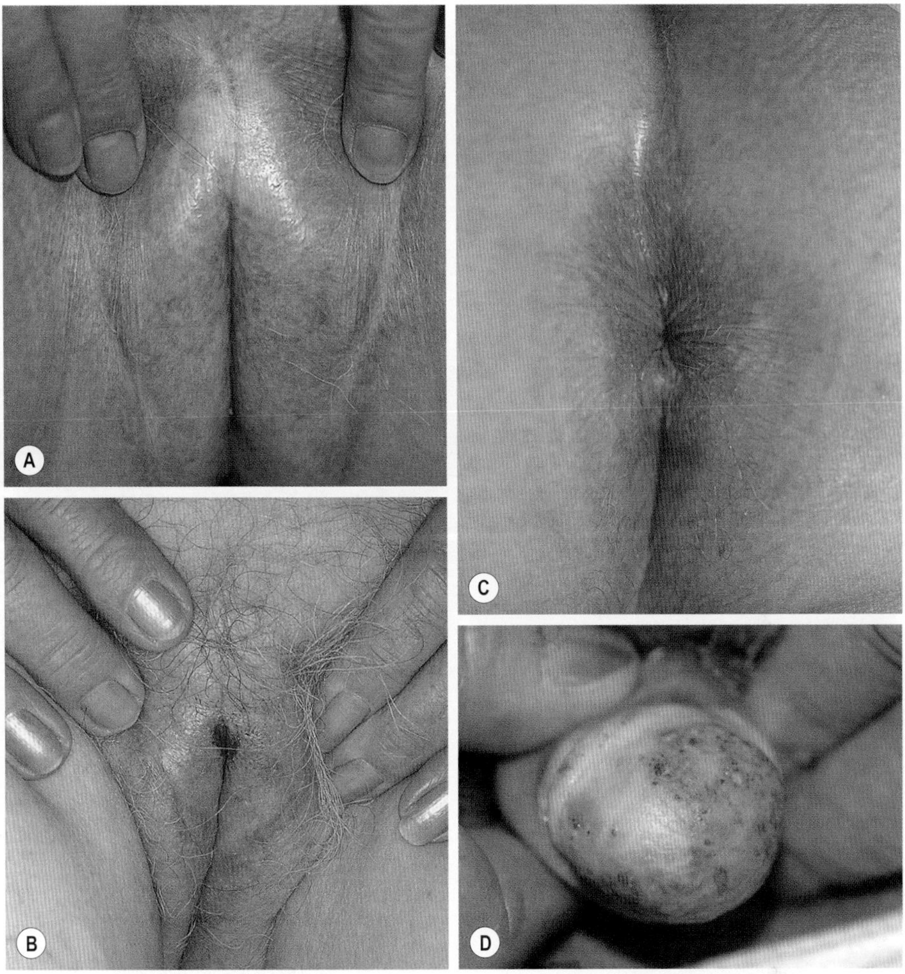

Fig. 60.4 Lichen sclerosus (LS). Typical involvement of the vulva demonstrating marked architectural change with the loss of the labia minora and midline fusion **(A)** and purpura **(B).** Perianal LS **(C)** and involvement of the penis **(D)** with an erythematous and white plaque on the glans. *A,C Courtesy, Susan M. Cooper, MD, and Fenella Wojnarowska, MD; B, Courtesy, Kalman Watsky, MD; D, Courtesy, Luis Requena, MD.*

- *Cyclical vulvovaginitis* is a recurrent vulvovaginitis, with or without a typical candidal discharge, that most often occurs premenstrually and is associated with superficial dyspareunia; often responds to prolonged course of oral antifungals.
- *Anodynia* is an anal/perianal regional pain syndrome in males and females that shares many features of the previously described entities.
- **Rx:** individualized and may include topical local anesthetics, oral tricyclic antidepressants, oral gabapentin, referral to a neurologist or specialized pain clinic (to exclude underlying neurologic disorder; see Ch. 4), acupuncture, or biofeedback.

For further information see Ch. 73 from *Dermatology, Fourth Edition*.

For additional online figures visit www.expertconsult.com 

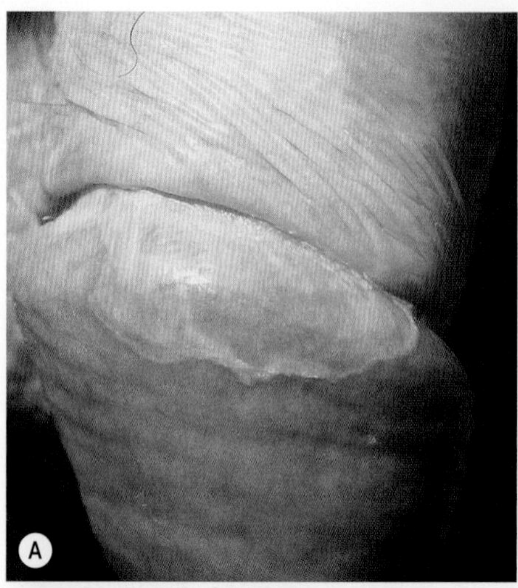

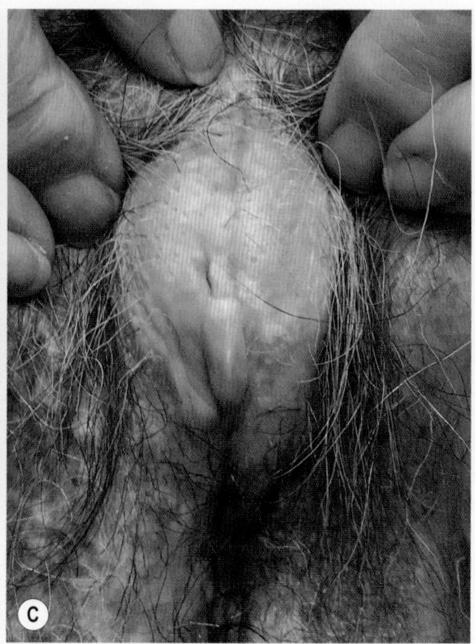

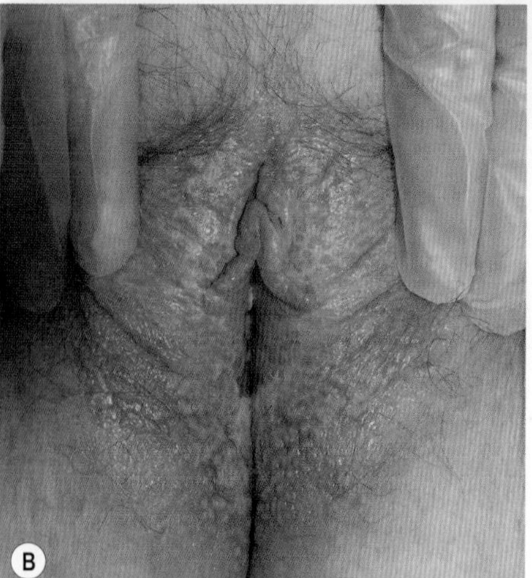

Fig. 60.5 Anogenital lichen planus. A Involvement of the penis with an annular band on the glans, a typical finding. **B** Erosive lichen planus of the vulva with fissures and an extensive white lacy pattern. **C** This patient with extensive hypertrophic lichen planus of the vulva and perineum had developed an invasive SCC. *A, Courtesy, R. Turner, MD; B, Courtesy, Susan M. Cooper, MD, and Fenella Wojnarowska, MD; C, Courtesy Karynne O. Duncan, MD.*

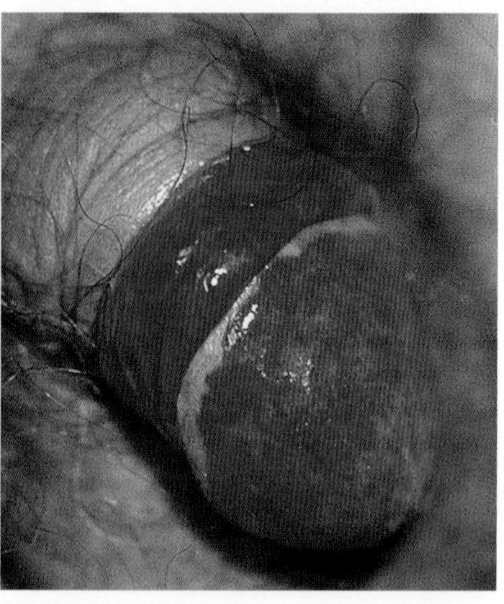

Fig. 60.6 Zoon balanitis. There are moist "kissing lesions" on adjacent surfaces of the glans and prepuce. *Courtesy, Susan M. Cooper, MD, and Fenella Wojnarowska, MD.*

<table>
<tr><th colspan="3">SELECTED BULLOUS DISORDERS WITH ANOGENITAL FEATURES</th></tr>
<tr><th>Bullous disorder</th><th>Anogenital features</th><th>Rx</th></tr>
<tr><td>Hailey–Hailey disease</td><td>See Ch. 48</td><td>See Ch. 48</td></tr>
<tr><td>Bullous pemphigoid (BP) (See Ch. 24)</td><td>• Mostly affects the elderly, but a localized vulvar variant is occasionally seen in children
• A vegetans form favors flexural sites
• Less likely than PV to involve mucosal sites</td><td rowspan="2">Mild
• Potent topical/intralesional CS
Severe
• Systemic CS
• Other systemic immunosuppressants
• Methotrexate (BP)
• Dapsone, cyclophosphamide (MMP)
• Dapsone or sulfapyridine (LABD)
• Mycophenolate mofetil, azathioprine (PV)</td></tr>
<tr><td>Mucous membrane (cicatricial) pemphigoid (MMP) (See Ch. 24)</td><td>• External genitalia and anus
Early: erosions, ulcerations, blisters (Fig. 60.7)
• Pain, pruritus, dysuria
Late: scarring prominent with related disability
• Phimosis, narrowing of vaginal introitus, anal stricture</td></tr>
<tr><td>Pemphigus vulgaris (PV) (See Ch. 23)</td><td>• Vagina, labia, anus, penis
• Widespread erosions; vegetative and papillomatous nodulo-plaques may develop (pemphigus vegetans)</td><td>See Ch. 23</td></tr>
</table>

Table 60.4 Selected bullous disorders with anogenital features. Acquired autoimmune bullous diseases are clinically difficult to differentiate from one another and require biopsies for H&E and DIF, as well as serum for IIF and/or ELISA. MMP can be clinically indistinguishable from erosive lichen planus in the anogenital area. The DDx (especially of PV) may include other causes of erosions (Table 60.7). Other blistering disorders, including LABD (linear IgA bullous dermatosis), epidermolysis bullosa acquisita (EBA), and paraneoplastic pemphigus can occur in the genital area (see Chs 23 and 24). DIF, direct immunofluorescence; IIF, indirect immunofluorescence.

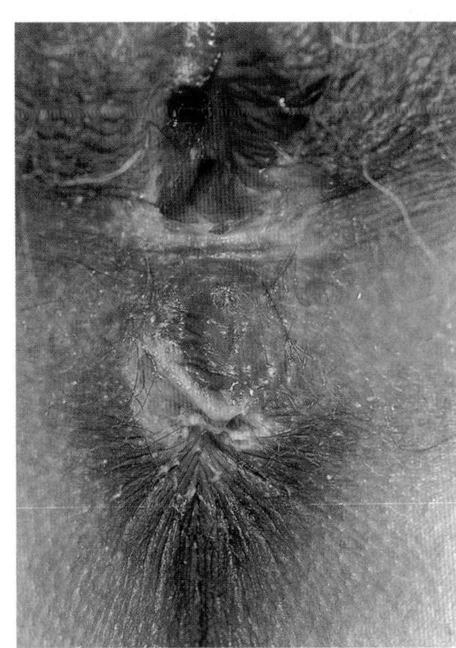

Fig. 60.7 Mucous membrane pemphigoid of the vulva. Ulcerations and scarring of the perianal area and perineum. Positive direct immunofluorescence with linear deposition of immunoreactants distinguished this from erosive lichen planus. *Courtesy, Susan M. Cooper, MD, and Fenella Wojnarowska, MD.*

INFECTIOUS (NONVENEREAL) DISORDERS WITH ANOGENITAL FEATURES			
Infectious (nonvenereal) disorder	**Anogenital features**	**Dx and DDx**	**Rx**
Candidiasis (See Ch. 64 and Figs 13.2 and 13.4)	• Favors the perianal area and inguinal crease, with sheet-like erythema, fissuring, erosions, and satellite pustules **Female** • Vulvar erythema, small fissures • Severe pruritus • Creamy-white vaginal discharge **Male** • Uncircumcised > circumcised • Balanitis or balanoposthitis • In the inguinal/scrotal folds, see erythema and focal white areas	• Many anogenital diseases may be misdiagnosed as a "yeast" infection or develop superimposed candidiasis • Confirm by microscopy (KOH preparation) and/or culture • If pustules, consider impetigo	• Address precipitating factors (e.g. diabetes mellitus, systemic antibiotics) **Mild** • Topical antifungal/anti-yeast agents • Vaginal anti-yeast suppositories • Single, oral dose of fluconazole 150 mg (vaginal candidiasis) **Severe** • Fluconazole 50–100 mg daily for 14 days **Recurrent (>3 episodes/year)** • Treat sexual partners • Oral fluconazole 150 mg weekly for 6 months • Clotrimazole vaginal 500 mg tablets weekly for 6 months • Oral itraconazole 200 mg, twice a day, once per month, for 6 months
Dermatophytosis (tinea cruris) (See Ch. 64 and Fig. 13.2)	• Chronic, slowly advancing, scaly, erythematous patches and thin plaques; ± pustules • Favors the groin (but scrotum often spared) with extension onto upper, medial thighs; medial buttocks • Tinea pedis and toenail onychomycosis often present	• Confirm with microscopy (KOH preparation)	**Mild** • Topical antifungals **Severe** • Oral terbinafine 250 mg daily for 2 weeks
Erythrasma (See Ch. 61 and Fig. 13.2)	• Well-defined, pink to red-brown, pigmented patches or thin plaques with fine diffuse scale and wrinkling • Favors flexural areas, such as groin and intergluteal cleft • Caused by *Corynebacterium minutissimum*	• Wood's lamp examination (coral pink fluorescence)	**Mild** • Antibacterial soaps • Topical 10–20% aluminum chloride • Topical 2% clindamycin, erythromycin **Severe** • Oral erythromycin for 5 days

INFECTIOUS (NONVENEREAL) DISORDERS WITH ANOGENITAL FEATURES			
Infectious (nonvenereal) disorder	**Anogenital features**	**Dx and DDx**	**Rx**
Perianal and vulvovaginal streptococcal infection (See Ch. 61 and Fig. 13.4)	• Children >> adults • Sharply demarcated, bright perianal erythema, extending 2–3 cm around the anal verge • Painful defecation or urination • Blood-streaked stools • Irritation or pruritus • Caused by group A β-hemolytic *Streptococcus* • May also involve the neck and inguinal regions, especially in children (streptococcal intertrigo) • May be preceded or accompanied by pharyngitis	• Diagnosis made with bacterial culture or rapid strep test of involved site • Also consider: candidiasis, irritant contact dermatitis, pinworm infection, child abuse, and early Kawasaki disease (if inguinal) • May trigger guttate psoriasis	• Oral cephalosporin, penicillin or erythromycin for 10–14 days • Follow with re-culture to exclude recurrence

Table 60.5 *Continued* **Infectious (nonvenereal) disorders with anogenital features.** Condylomata acuminata and venereal diseases are covered in Chapters 66 and 69, respectively. The DDx of these disorders includes the other entities listed in this table; they may be confused with the disorders listed in Tables 60.2 and 60.3 as well as superimposed upon them; topical medications can also lead to a superimposed contact dermatitis.

PREMALIGNANT AND MALIGNANT DISORDERS WITH ANOGENITAL FEATURES			
Premalignant and malignant disorders	**Anogenital features**	**Other**	**Rx**
Premalignant lesions			
• Vulvar intraepithelial neoplasia (VIN) • Penile intraepithelial neoplasia (PIN) • Perianal intraepithelial neoplasia (PaIN) • Anal intraepithelial neoplasia (AIN)	Varied presentations • Erythematous or pigmented, well-demarcated plaque (genital Bowen disease variant) • Verrucous white-gray plaque • Erosions • Nonhealing ulcer • Erythematous, shiny, velvety patch or plaque (erythroplasia of Queyrat variant) (Fig. 60.8)	Several etiologies/ predisposing factors • Oncogenic HPV (e.g. subtypes 16, 18, 31, 33) • Inflammatory, scarring conditions (e.g. lichen sclerosus, erosive lichen planus) • Uncircumcised male • Immunosuppression • HIV infection	• In conjunction with gynecologic or urologic oncologist • Long-term evaluation necessary, including anal and cervical cytology • Examine sexual partners • Varies from topical agents (e.g. imiquimod, 5-fluorouracil) to surgical excision, including Mohs surgery • Prevention: HPV vaccination
• Bowenoid papulosis	See Fig. 60.9 and Ch. 66	See Ch. 66	See Ch. 66
Malignant lesions			
• Invasive SCC	Varied presentations • Nonhealing ulcer or fissure • Erythematous plaque with heaped-up edges (Fig. 60.10) • Verrucous plaque • Nodule	• Most common anogenital tumor, but overall rare • Etiologies are similar to those listed for premalignant lesions	• Consult with gynecologic or urologic oncologist • First-line: surgical excision, including Mohs surgery • Second-line: XRT
• Extramammary Paget disease	• Slowly expanding erythematous plaque with demarcation between normal and involved skin; erosions and scale present (Fig. 60.11) • Favors vulva and perianal regions • Pruritus, burning, or asymptomatic	• Rare intraepithelial adenocarcinoma • More common in older females and Japanese males • May be primary or secondary to an underlying malignancy • Associated underlying visceral malignancy in 10–20% • Associated underlying adnexal adenocarcinoma in <5%	• Initial and periodic systemic evaluations for internal malignancy are necessary • Surgical excision vs. Mohs surgery • Combination therapy, e.g. topicals (see above), XRT, photodynamic therapy

Table 60.6 Premalignant and malignant disorders with anogenital features. Multiple biopsies may be necessary to make a diagnosis. The DDx of these disorders

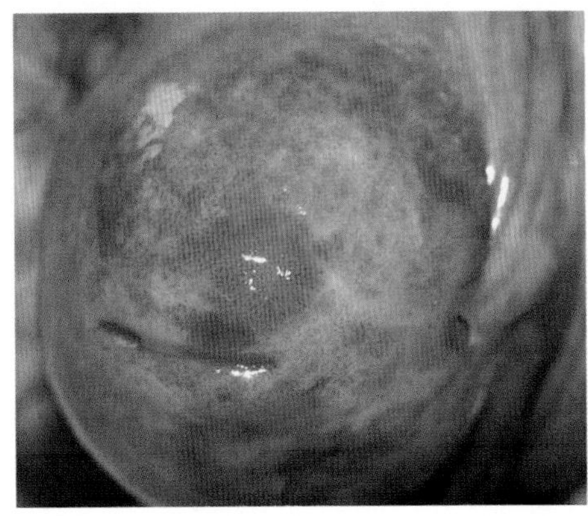

Fig. 60.8 Penile intraepithelial neoplasia (PIN). Persistent erythema not responding to topical steroids. *Courtesy, R. Turner, MD.*

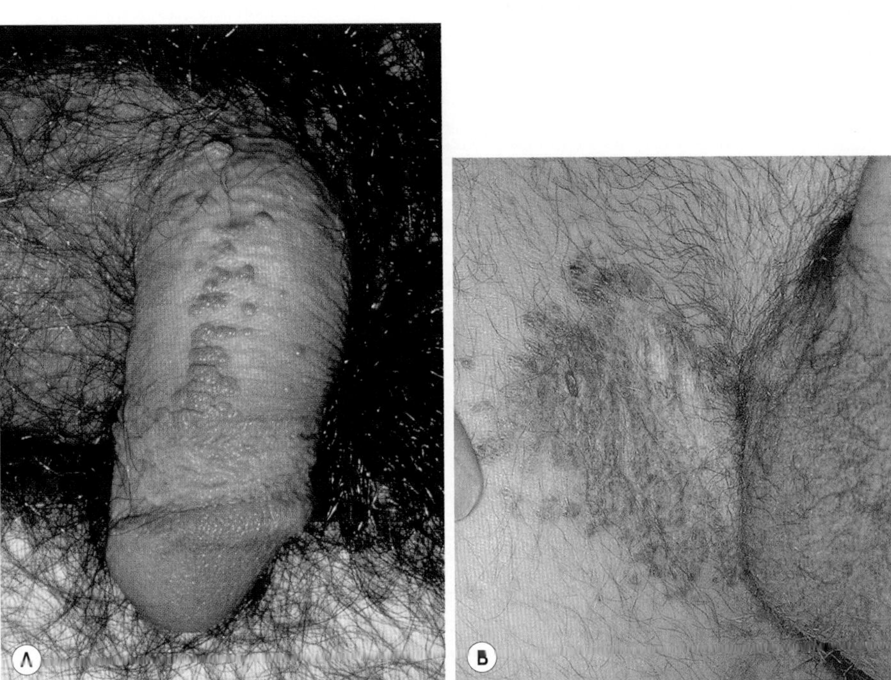

Fig. 60.9 Bowenoid papulosis variant of intraepithelial neoplasia. A Multiple red-brown to brown papules on the shaft of the penis. **B** Coalescence of red-brown to brown papules on the upper inner thigh. *A, Courtesy, YDRSC; B, Courtesy, Robert Hartman, MD.*

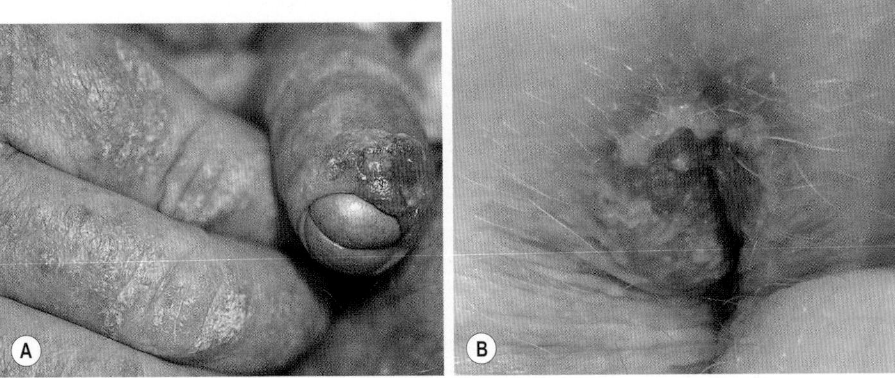

Fig. 60.10 Invasive squamous cell carcinoma. A Erythematous plaque on the foreskin in this patient with psoriasis who had received PUVA therapy without genital protection. **B** Erythematous, indurated plaque in another patient with non-HPV-related perianal SCC. *A, Courtesy, Susan M. Cooper, MD, and Fenella Wojnarowska, MD; B, Courtesy, Karynne O. Duncan, MD.*

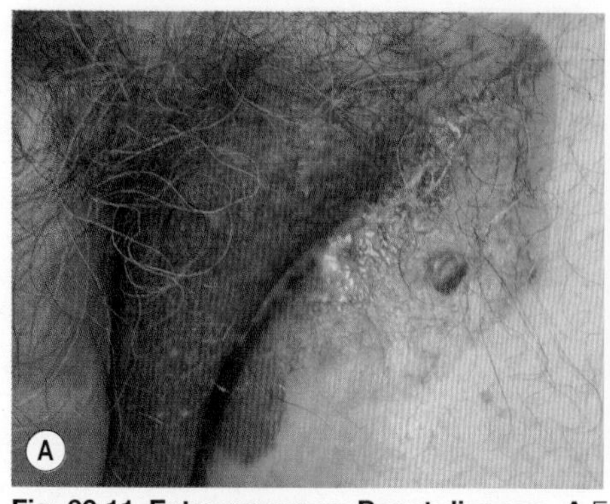

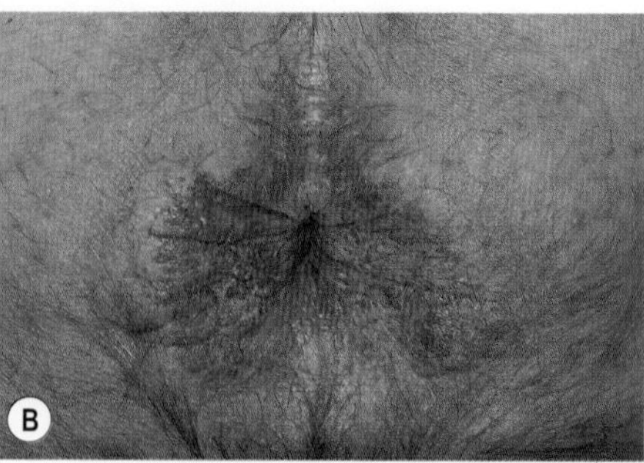

Fig. 60.11 Extramammary Paget disease. A Eroded erythematous plaque with exudate, especially in the inguinal crease. The patient refused any further evaluation and had never undergone colonoscopy or cystoscopy. **B** Well-demarcated perianal plaque with both erosions and scale, giving rise to a "strawberries and cream" appearance. *A, Courtesy, Kathryn Schwarzenberger, MD, and Jeffrey P. Callen, MD; B, Courtesy, Kalman Watsky, MD.*

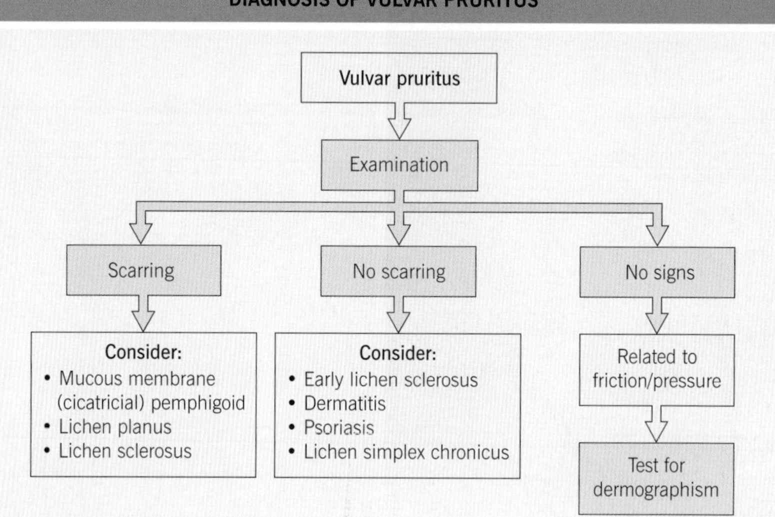

Fig. 60.12 Diagnosis of vulvar pruritus. *Courtesy, Susan M. Cooper, MD, and Fenella Wojnarowska, MD.*

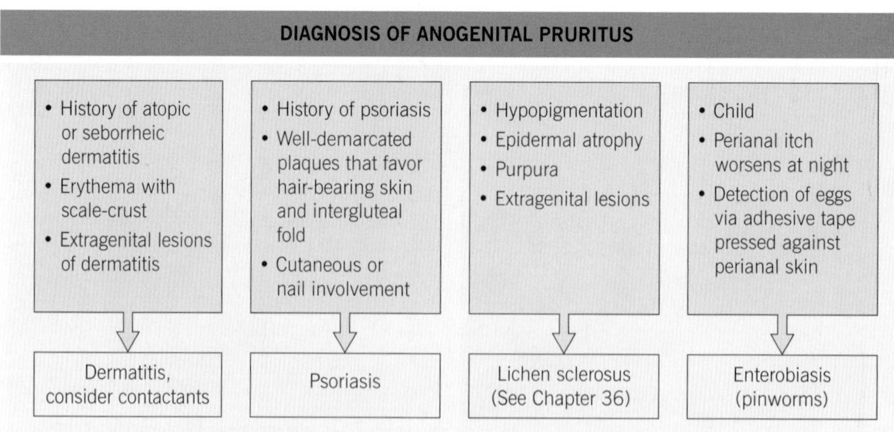

Fig. 60.13 Diagnosis of anogenital pruritus. Histologic evaluation may be required to confirm the clinical diagnosis (e.g. lichen sclerosus) or to exclude more unusual etiologies (e.g. extramammary Paget disease). Systemic contact dermatitis reactions in this region may also be very pruritic. *Courtesy, Susan M. Cooper, MD, and Fenella Wojnarowska, MD.*

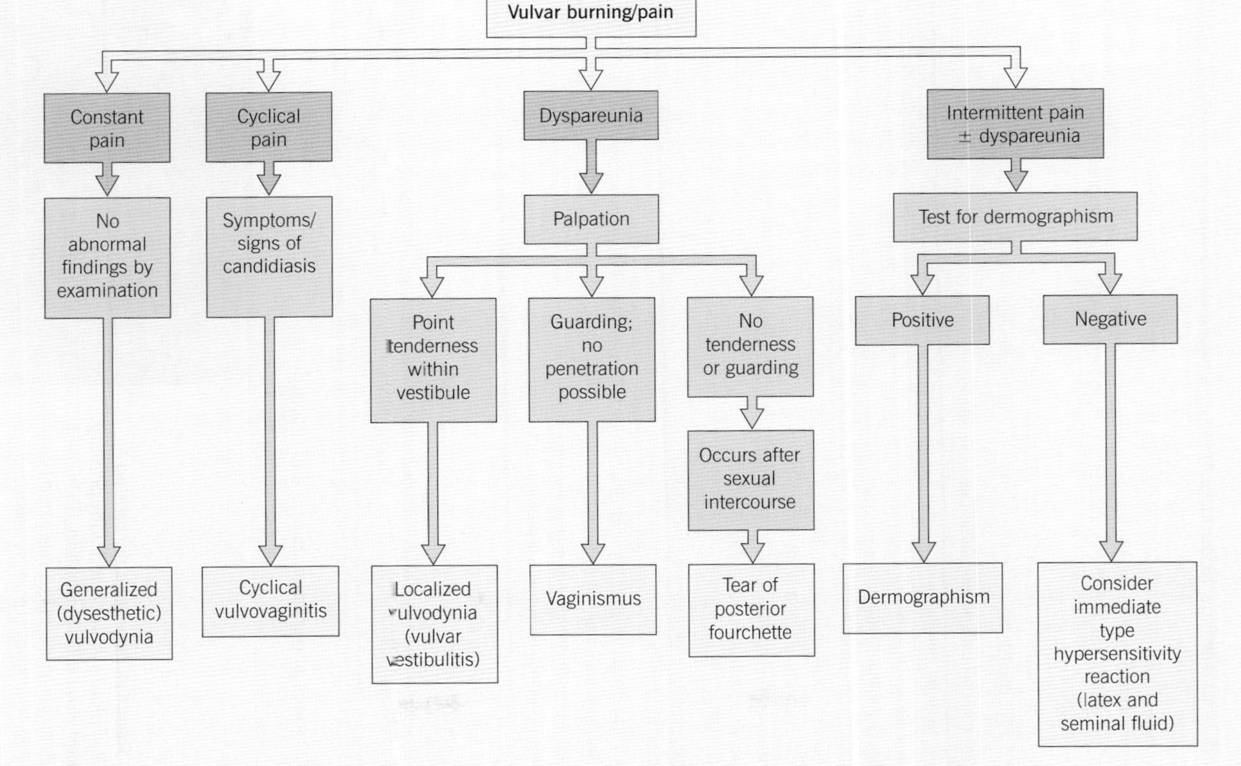

Fig. 60.14 Diagnosis of vulvar burning/pain in the setting of a normal-appearing vulva. *Courtesy, Susan M. Cooper, MD, and Fenella Wojnarowska, MD.*

CAUSES OF GENITAL EROSIONS AND ULCERATIONS
• Lichen sclerosus (see Fig. 36.9B) • Erosive lichen planus (see Fig. 60.5B) • Genital aphthae/aphthosis*
• Infection - Candidiasis (see Figs 13.2 and 13.4) - Impetigo (*Staphylococcus/Streptococcus*) - Herpes simplex viral infection (see Figs 67.2E and 67.6D) or herpes zoster - Primary syphilis, chancroid - Epstein–Barr virus (EBV; Fig. 60.15)**,†, cytomegalovirus†, *Mycoplasma*† - Tuberculosis
• Squamous cell carcinoma and other malignancies • Intraepithelial neoplasia
• Zoon plasma cell balanitis/vulvitis (see Fig. 60.6)
• Acquired bullous diseases - Pemphigus vulgaris - Bullous pemphigoid - Mucous membrane (cicatricial) pemphigoid (see Fig. 60.7) - Linear IgA bullous dermatosis - Epidermolysis bullosa acquisita - Erythema multiforme, Stevens–Johnson syndrome (see Fig. 16.7B) - Fixed drug eruption (see Fig. 17.10B) • Inherited bullous disease - Hailey–Hailey disease (see Fig. 13.2) - Epidermolysis bullosa
• Complex aphthosis due to Behçet disease or inflammatory bowel disease • Crohn disease (see Fig. 13.2) • Extramammary Paget disease (see Fig. 60.11) • Langerhans cell histiocytosis (see Fig. 76.1) • Necrolytic migratory erythema, acrodermatitis enteropathica (see Fig. 43.9) • Papular acantholytic dyskeratosis • Toxic erythema of chemotherapy (see Fig. 17.15A)
**Includes reactive non-sexually related acute genital ulcers, which can be triggered by a variety of viral and bacterial infections.* ***Diagnosed via EBV IgM antibodies or PCR; favors female children and adolescents.* *†Cause/trigger of reactive non-sexually related acute genital ulcers.*

Table 60.7 Causes of genital erosions and ulcerations.

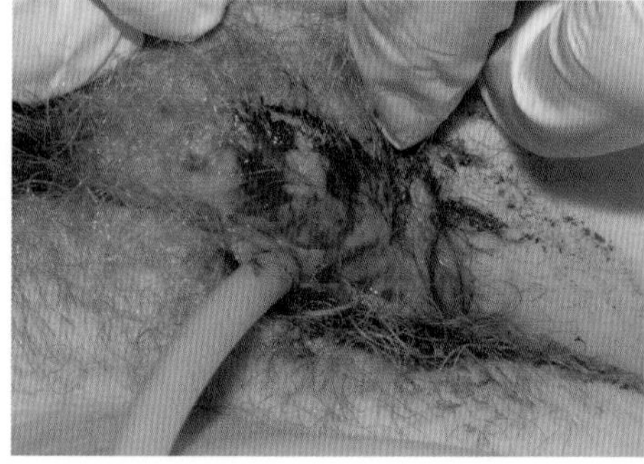

Fig. 60.15 Reactive non-sexually related acute genital ulcers associated with primary Epstein–Barr virus (EBV) infection. Extreme pain with urination required placement of a Foley catheter in this 13-year-old girl. EBV-related genital ulcers are often misdiagnosed as a genital herpes simplex viral infection. *Courtesy, Julie V. Schaffer, MD.*

Bacterial Diseases 61

The skin is normally colonized by hundreds of species of bacteria as part of the cutaneous microbiota (flora). These organisms help prevent skin infection by competing with pathogenic microorganisms.

Skin infection with bacteria may be a primary problem (e.g. impetigo) or a complication of another skin disease (e.g. atopic dermatitis) and may lead to multisystem dysfunction (e.g. toxic shock syndrome). Nomenclature of these diseases often reflects the site and the depth of infection – that is, from the stratum corneum to the subcutaneous tissue (Fig. 61.1) – as well as the suspected causative organism.

Gram-Positive Cocci

Staphylococcal and Streptococcal Skin Infections

Streptococcal infections may be complicated by acute post-streptococcal glomerulonephritis; this occurs in <1% of patients in high-income countries, but it remains a significant problem in low-income countries.

IMPETIGO

- Major organisms are *Staphylococcus aureus* and *Streptococcus pyogenes* (group A streptococci [GAS]).
- A very common, highly contagious bacterial infection. Occurs most commonly on the face or extremities of children, in particular around the nose and mouth (Fig. 61.2A). Usually the skin is eroded with overlying "honey-colored" crusts, but there is a bullous variant (Fig. 61.2B) that is often seen in the major body folds, e.g. axillae.
- The bullous variant is due to *S. aureus* and can be explained by local release of an exfoliative toxin that binds to desmoglein 1 and leads to dissolution (i.e. acantholysis) of the upper epidermis (see Ch. 23).
- Risk factors for infection: nasal carriage of *S. aureus* and breaks in the epidermal barrier, e.g. atopic dermatitis, arthropod bites, trauma, scabies.
- **DDx** of eroded lesions: insect bites, dermatitis (e.g. nummular, atopic), herpes simplex viral infection, prurigo simplex.
- **DDx** of bullae: bullous insect bites, thermal burns, herpes simplex viral infection, acute contact dermatitis, and occasionally autoimmune bullous dermatoses.
- **Rx:** local wound care (including soap), removal of crusts by soaking; for mild cases, topical mupirocin, retapamulin, ozenoxacin, or fusidic acid; for moderate to severe infections, oral antibiotics, the choice of which is dependent on prevalence of methicillin-resistant *S. aureus* (MRSA) in the local community (Table 61.1).

ECTHYMA

- Most commonly secondary to *Streptococcus pyogenes.*
- Ulceration with hemorrhagic crust that extends into the superficial dermis, i.e. is deeper than impetigo (Fig. 61.3); can heal with scarring.
- Often on the lower extremities, and risk factors include an edematous limb, arthropod bites, and a pre-existing ulceration.
- **DDx:** ulcers secondary to vasculitis or other etiology (e.g. cutaneous diphtheria; see Fig. 86.1); not to be confused with ecthyma gangrenosum which is due to septic emboli (see below).
- **Rx:** see Table 61.1.

BACTERIAL FOLLICULITIS

- *Staphylococcus aureus* is the most common cause, followed by Gram-negative bacteria; the latter can occur in patients with acne vulgaris on long-term antibiotic therapy; see Chapter 31 for *Pseudomonas* folliculitis.

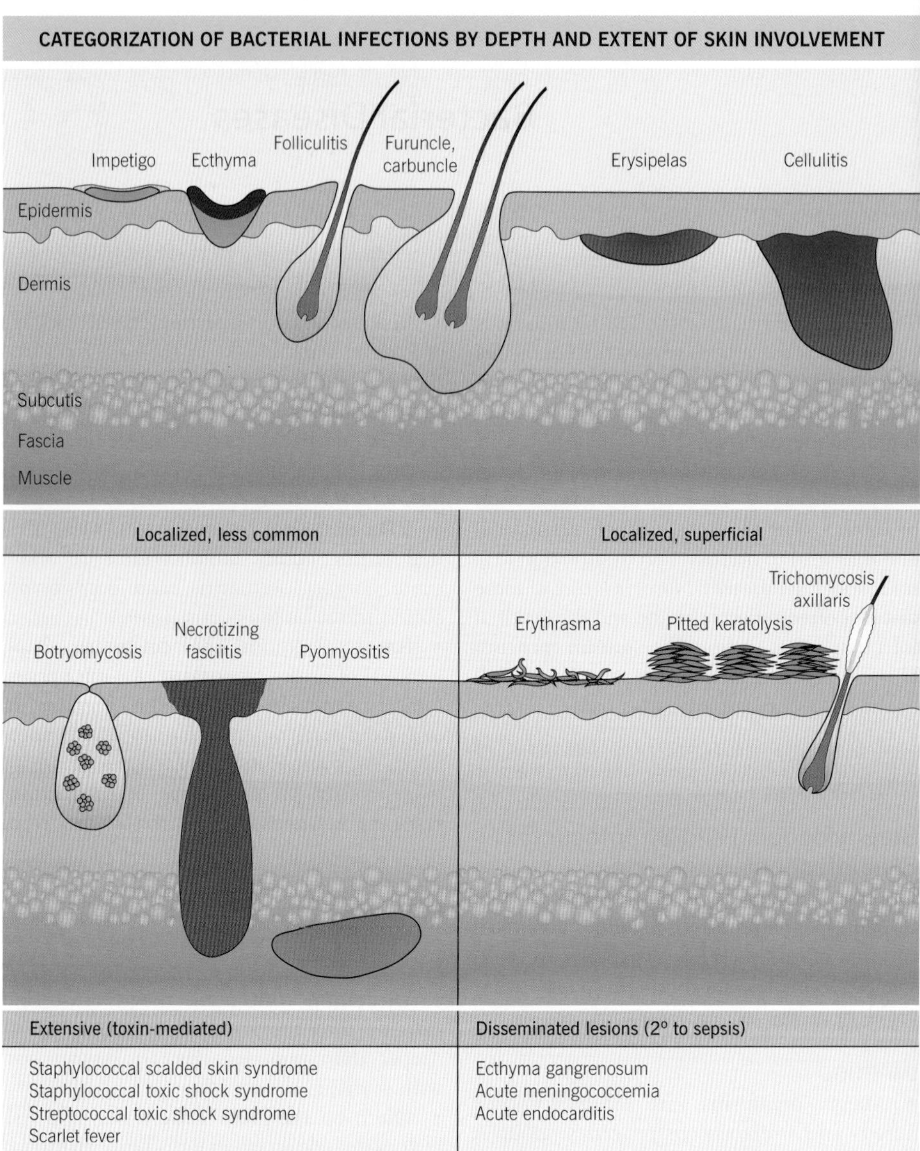

Fig. 61.1 Categorization of bacterial infections by depth and extent of skin involvement. More common, localized infections are depicted first; these infections are often secondary to *Staphylococcus aureus* or group A streptococci. *Adapted from "Common bacterial infections of the skin," American Academy of Dermatology.*

- Usually superficial, but occasionally deep, infection centered on hair follicles (see Fig. 61.1).
  - Superficial – 1- to 4-mm pustules on an erythematous base (see Fig. 31.2); centrally, a hair shaft may be noted
  - Deep – also referred to as sycosis – tender, erythematous papulonodules, often with a central pustule
- Commonly in the beard area, on the upper trunk, or on the buttocks and thighs; shaving can be an exacerbating factor.
- **DDx:** culture-negative (normal flora) folliculitis, acne vulgaris, folliculitis due to fungi (e.g. *Pityrosporum*), viruses (e.g. herpes simplex virus) or *Demodex* (Fig. 31.1); rosacea, chloracne, and pseudofolliculitis barbae.

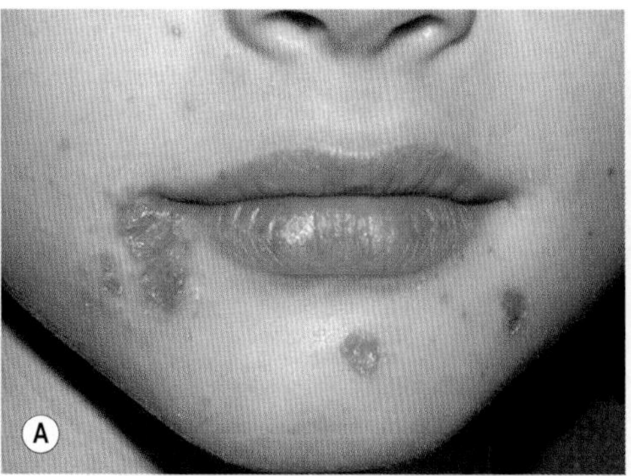

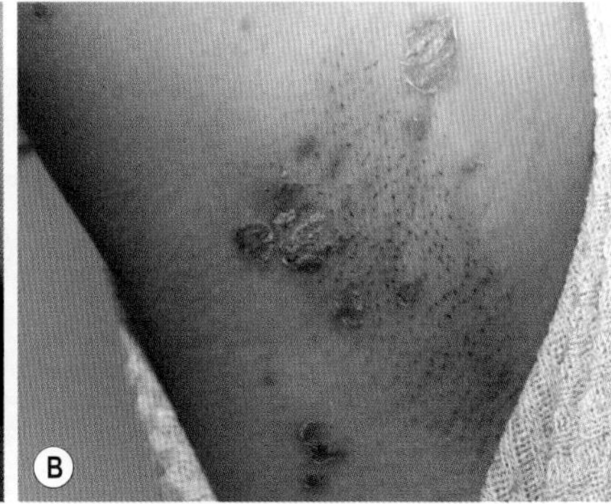

Fig. 61.2 Staphylococcal impetigo. A Honey-colored crusts on the chin and cheeks of a child with impetigo. **B** Superficial round to oval erosions with central thin crusting and a peripheral collarette due to bullous impetigo in the axilla. *A, Courtesy, Julie V. Schaffer, MD; B, Courtesy, Kalman Watsky, MD.*

- **Rx:** for superficial form – antibacterial washes (e.g. benzoyl peroxide, chlorhexidine) or topical gels (e.g. combination clindamycin /benzoyl peroxide); widespread staphylococcal folliculitis – oral antibiotics (see Table 61.1).

ABSCESSES, FURUNCLES, AND CARBUNCLES

- Abscesses are localized collections of pus. By definition, a furuncle is an abscess involving a hair follicle; involvement of multiple, adjacent follicles is termed a carbuncle (see Fig. 61.1).
- Most common organism is *S. aureus*, and this is the most frequent presentation for community-acquired MRSA (CA-MRSA).
- Clinically, furuncles appear as firm, tender, red nodules; carbuncles begin similarly but become larger in size and can develop multiple draining sinus tracts.
- Common locations for furuncles are the face, neck, axillae, buttocks, perineum, and thighs. Carbuncles often favor the trunk and thighs and heal with scarring.
- **DDx:** ruptured epidermoid cyst, hidradenitis suppurativa, and cystic acne.
- **Rx:** fluctuant lesions should be incised and drained. Administration of systemic antibiotics (see Table 61.1 for **Rx** options) reduces recurrence, even for small, isolated lesions and are indicated for: (1) furuncles around the nose, in the external auditory canal, or in other locations where drainage is difficult; (2) severe or extensive disease (e.g. multiple sites); (3) lesions with surrounding cellulitis/phlebitis or associated with signs or symptoms of systemic illness; (4) lesions not responding to local care; and (5) patients with concerning comorbidities or immunosuppression.

ERYSIPELAS

- Most commonly due to *Streptococcus pyogenes.*
- Represents infection of the superficial dermis along with significant lymphatic involvement; often on the face and neck or the leg.
- Presents as a well-defined area of hot, indurated, bright erythema that is painful and tender (Fig. 61.4); occasionally, there may be superimposed pustules, vesicles, bullae, or areas of hemorrhagic necrosis.
- Favors the young, debilitated, elderly, and limbs with edema or lymphedema.
- **DDx:** cellulitis, irritant contact dermatitis, early necrotizing fasciitis or herpes zoster, erysipeloid breast cancer, erysipeloid, Sweet syndrome, and if it involves the ear, chondritis.
- **Rx:** 10- to 14-day course of penicillin if due to *Streptococcus pyogenes*, with route depending on the severity and risk factors.

STREPTOCOCCAL INTERTRIGO, PERIANAL AND VULVOVAGINAL STREPTOCOCCAL INFECTION

- Sharply demarcated, bright red erythema, especially in young children (see Fig. 61.4 and Table 60.5).

EMPIRIC TREATMENT OF CUTANEOUS STAPHYLOCOCCAL AND STREPTOCOCCAL INFECTIONS IN ADULTS		
Organism/situation		**Suggested antibiotics**
Streptococci	Confirmed	• Amoxicillin 500 mg PO TID • Penicillin VK 500 mg PO four times a day
	Empiric treatment to cover both streptococci and staphylococci	• First-generation cephalosporin (see below) • Dicloxacillin 500 mg PO four times a day • Nafcillin or oxacillin 1–2 gm IV four times a day, if severe
Suspected MSSA (e.g. impetigo requiring systemic treatment or non-purulent cellulitis) or streptococci		• First-generation cephalosporin, e.g. cephalexin 250–500 mg PO three or four times a day • Dicloxacillin 250–500 mg PO four times a day • Amoxicillin-clavulanate 875/125 mg PO BID
Suspected CA-MRSA (e.g. furuncles/abscesses, purulent cellulitis, or infections that failed to respond to MSSA treatment) • Risk factors include participation in contact sports, other close interpersonal contact (e.g. military personnel), injection drug use		• Doxycycline 100 mg PO two times a day* • Trimethoprim-sulfamethoxazole 1 or 2 double-strength tablets PO twice a day* • Clindamycin 300–450 mg PO four times a day • Linezolid, tedizolid, delafloxacin
Suspected hospital-acquired MRSA (HA-MRSA) • Risk factors include recent contact with hospitals or health care facilities such as nursing homes or dialysis units		• See Suspected CA-MRSA
Penicillin-allergic patients		• Clindamycin (see above) • Clarithromycin 250 mg PO two times a day
Additional special considerations		• Furuncle/abscess: incision and drainage (without packing) is a key component of successful Rx • If recurrent infections, address carrier state: – Mupirocin 2% nasal ointment twice a day for 5 days – Mupirocin 2% cream to major body folds, e.g. axillae, groin, inframammary, as well as umbilicus – Wash body with chlorhexidine, bathe in dilute Clorox® (see Fig. 10.12A) once or twice a week, or use spray bottle with dilute Clorox® • Address fomites including sports equipment • Consider close human contacts or pets as source of infection

**Does not provide coverage of group A streptococci; if coverage of the latter is desired, a β-lactam is also prescribed.*

Table 61.1 Empiric treatment of cutaneous staphylococcal and streptococcal infections in adults. Treatment duration is usually 5–10 days, depending on the severity and clinical response. Initial choice of antibiotic is dependent on known resistance patterns in a given community. The contents of pustules or exudate (e.g. underlying a crust) should be sent for culture and sensitivities prior to beginning therapy. Quinolones and macrolides are not optimal for treatment of community-acquired methicillin-resistant *Staphylococcus aureus* (CA-MRSA) because resistance is common and may develop rapidly. MSSA, methicillin-sensitive *Staphylococcus aureus*.

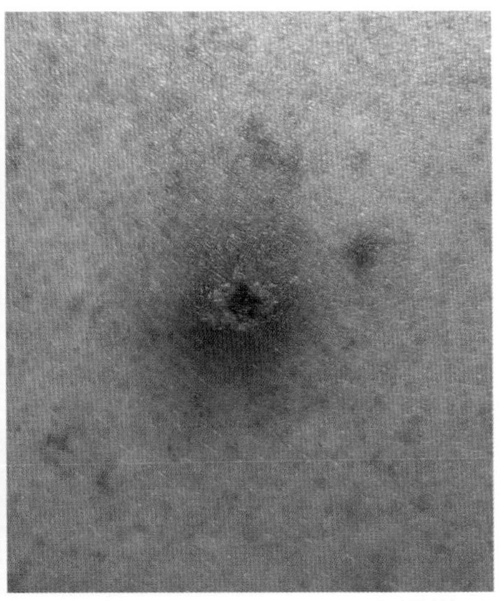

Fig. 61.3 Ecthyma. Ulceration with hemorrhagic crust due to infection with group A streptococci. *Courtesy, Karynne O. Duncan, MD.*

- **DDx:** outlined in Fig. 13.4 and Table 60.5.
- **Rx:** 7- to 10-day course of a first-generation cephalosporin (see Table 61.1) or penicillin.

CELLULITIS

- Most commonly due to *Streptococcus pyogenes* or *S. aureus*; in diabetics and immunocompromised hosts, other organisms (e.g. Gram-negative bacilli) may be the cause.
- In children, *Haemophilus influenzae* can be a cause of cellulitis, but its incidence has decreased since introduction of the *H. influenzae* vaccine.
- Infection of the deep dermis and sometimes the subcutaneous fat (see Fig. 61.1).
- Skin rubor (redness), calor (warmth), dolor (pain), and tumor (swelling) are present; more ill-defined borders than erysipelas and may have skip areas; can become bullous or necrotic (Figs 61.5 and 75.9).

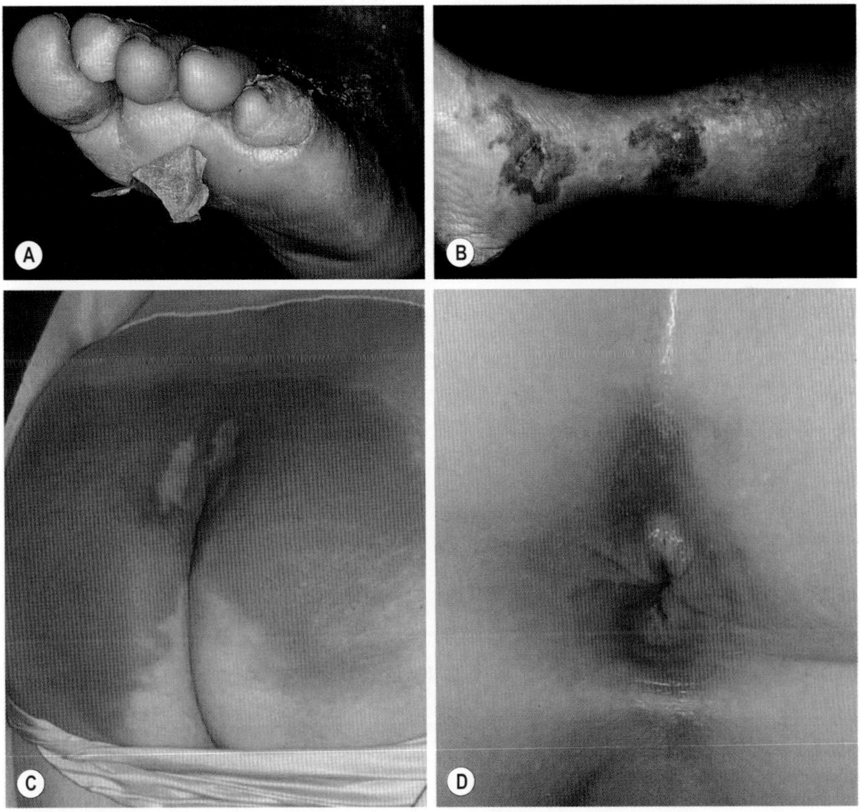

Fig. 61.4 Cutaneous manifestations of streptococcal infections. Prominent desquamation of the feet (**A**) following scarlet fever. Multiple areas of necrotic crusting and focal purulence due to streptococcal cellulitis (**B**). Sharply demarcated erythema of the buttocks (**C**) in erysipelas. Bright red erythema extending from the anal verge in a young boy with streptococcal perianal disease (**D**). *A, Courtesy, Eugene Mirrer, MD; B, YDRSC; C, Courtesy, Mary Stone, MD; D, Courtesy, Julie V. Schaffer, MD.*

- Systemic symptoms include fever, chills, and malaise; CBC usually shows leukocytosis and bandemia.
- Risk factors for cellulitis of the lower extremity include previous DVT, previous cellulitis with lymphangitis, chronic edema, and tinea pedis (especially in patients who have undergone saphenous venectomy).

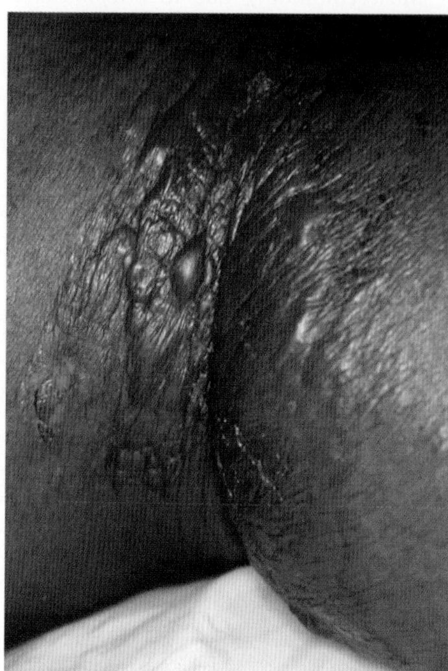

Fig. 61.5 Bullous cellulitis. Edema and confluent bullae. *Courtesy, YDRSC.*

- **DDx:** on the lower extremity, lipodermatosclerosis and stasis dermatitis (see Fig. 11.5); elsewhere, erysipelas and the early stage of necrotizing fasciitis, as well as causes of pseudocellulitis (Table 61.2).
- **Rx:** see Table 61.1.

BLISTERING DISTAL DACTYLITIS

- Secondary to GAS > *S. aureus*.
- Localized infection of the volar fat pad of a finger or, less often, a toe; occurs most commonly in children.
- Initially erythema and swelling of the skin, followed by development of one or more vesicles or bullae.
- **DDx:** herpetic whitlow, burn, acute paronychia, bullous impetigo, frictional bulla.
- **Rx:** drainage of blisters and systemic antibiotics (see Table 61.1).

BOTRYOMYCOSIS

- Most commonly caused by *S. aureus*, followed by *Pseudomonas* spp.
- Cutaneous and subcutaneous nodules that may have superimposed pustules, purulent discharge, or become ulcerative or verrucous; often in immunosuppressed hosts.

CAUSES OF "PSEUDOCELLULITIS"	
Infections and bites • Arthropod bite reactions (e.g. insect, spider) • Erythema migrans • Herpes zoster • Toxin-mediated erythema (e.g. recurrent toxin-mediated perineal erythema) **Neutrophilic dermatoses** • Sweet syndrome, neutrophilic panniculitis • Familial Mediterranean fever, other periodic fever syndromes **Drug reactions** • Fixed drug eruptions (especially non-pigmenting) • Vaccine/injection site reactions • Toxic erythema of chemotherapy (e.g. due to gemcitabine), neutrophilic eccrine hidradenitis*	**Other inflammatory disorders** • Allergic contact dermatitis (including airborne and dermal) • Phytophotodermatitis • Well syndrome • Panniculitis, e.g. lipodermatosclerosis, erythema nodosum • Thrombophlebitis • Angioedema • Interstitial granulomatous dermatitis, inflammatory granuloma annulare • Inflammatory morphea **Metabolic disorders** • Gout **Malignancy** • Erysipeloid skin metastases (especially breast carcinoma)

**Occasionally develops prior to onset of leukemia or due to infection.*

Table 61.2 Causes of "pseudocellulitis."

- Grains, representing macroscopic colonies of bacteria, are seen in biopsy specimens as well as the pustular discharge; grains are also seen in eumycotic and actinomycotic mycetoma (see Ch. 64) and actinomycosis (see below).
- Often develops at sites of trauma.
- **DDx:** ruptured epidermoid cyst, abscess, actinomycotic or eumycotic mycetoma, actinomycosis, and atypical mycobacterial or dimorphic fungal infection.
- **Rx:** surgical excision with debridement and/or antibiotic therapy based on pathogenic organism.

NECROTIZING FASCIITIS

- Usually represents polymicrobial infection with both anaerobes and aerobes; ~10% secondary to GAS; other organisms include community-acquired MRSA.
- Rapidly progressive necrosis of subcutaneous fat and fascia that leads to undermining and ulceration; may have a foul discharge and not bleed on incision.
- Risk factors include older age, diabetes mellitus, alcoholism, peripheral vascular disease, and immunosuppression.
- Initially may resemble cellulitis, but associated pain is often out of proportion to the clinical findings and may extend beyond the area of apparent involvement; additional clues include tense edema, blisters, crepitus, and a mottled violaceous or pale gray color reflecting impending necrosis (Figs 61.6 and 75.10).

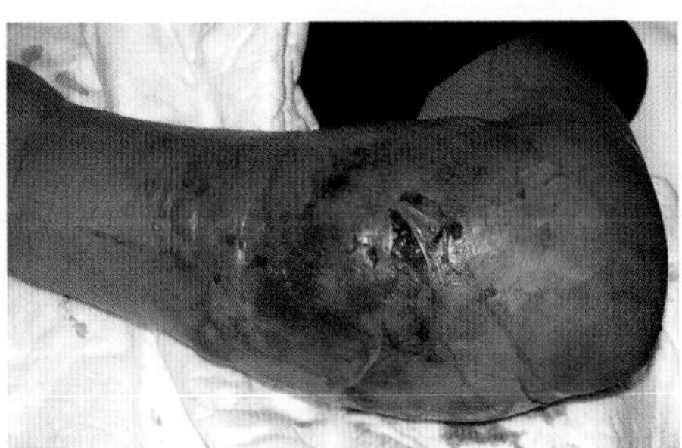

Fig. 61.6 Necrotizing fasciitis. Tense, woody edema of the forearm with purple-gray areas of necrosis and bullae with watery discharge. Intravenous drug use was a predisposing factor. *Courtesy, Luis Requena, MD.*

- Diagnosis requires a high index of suspicion; when anogenital, it is referred to as Fournier gangrene.
- Patients may have fever, chills, malaise, and leukocytosis.
- Dx: outlined in Fig. 61.7.
- **DDx:** cellulitis, trauma with hematoma, pyomyositis, clostridial myonecrosis, phlebitis.
- **Rx:** surgical debridement is the mainstay of therapy; broad-spectrum IV antibiotics.

PYOMYOSITIS

- Primary bacterial infection of skeletal muscle, most commonly with *S. aureus* (see Fig. 61.1); associated with immunosuppression, including HIV infection.

STAPHYLOCOCCAL SCALDED SKIN SYNDROME (SSSS)

- Secondary to *S. aureus*, phage group II strains, which produce exfoliative toxins that bind to desmoglein 1 and lead to dissolution (i.e. acantholysis) of the upper epidermis.
- More commonly seen in infants and children; occasionally, adults with chronic renal insufficiency can develop SSSS.
- Prodrome of malaise, fever, irritability, sore throat, and tender skin; purulent rhinorrhea or conjunctivitis may be present because the initial site of staphylococcal infection is usually extracutaneous.
- Tender erythema on the face and in intertriginous zones that generalizes to the remainder of the body over 1 or 2 days; due to the split in the upper epidermis, the skin becomes "wrinkled" and then sloughs over 3–5 days, leading to denuded areas; on the face, radial fissures with scale-crust develop around the mouth and eyes (Fig. 61.8; see Fig. 3.9).
- **DDx:** sunburn, drug reaction, Kawasaki disease (erythema often first appears in the groin), Stevens–Johnson syndrome/toxic epidermal necrolysis (SJS/TEN; usually affects older children and adults, has mucosal involvement, and nearly always drug-induced).
- **Rx:** hospitalization and IV anti-staphylococcal antibiotics (see Table 61.1).

TOXIC SHOCK SYNDROME (OTHER THAN STREPTOCOCCAL) (TSS)

- Secondary to *Staphylococcus aureus*, which produces an exotoxin, toxic shock syndrome toxin-1.

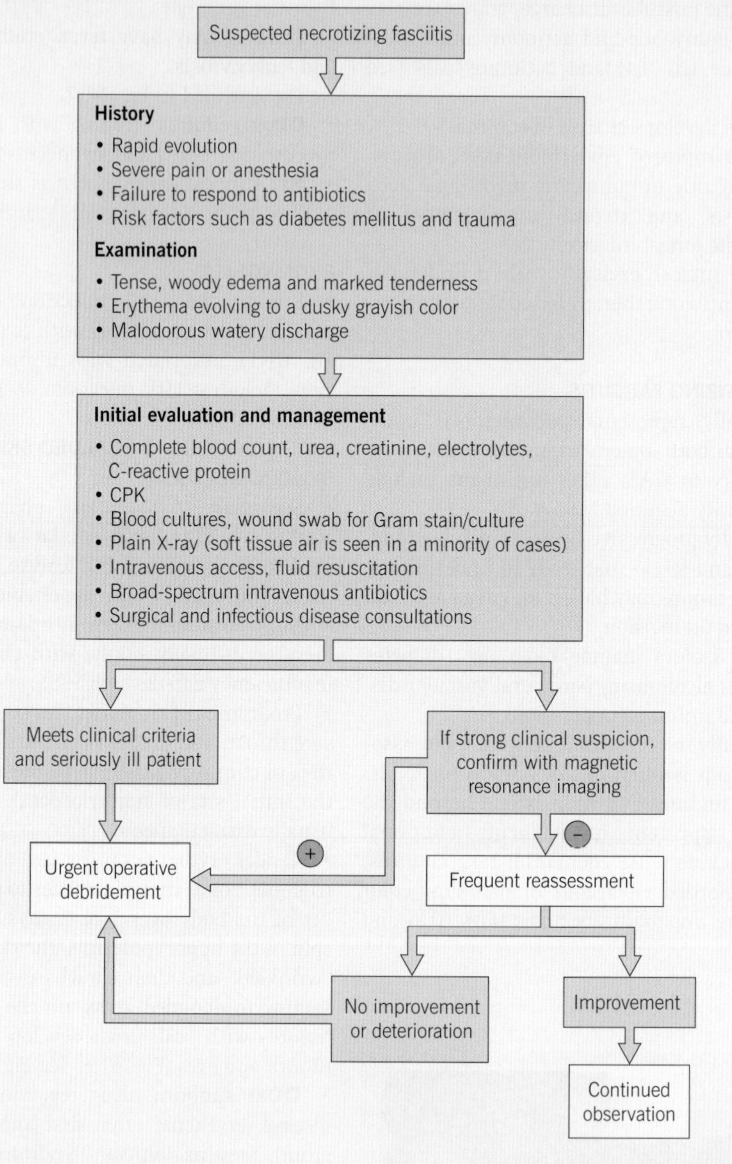

Fig. 61.7 Algorithm for assessment and treatment of suspected necrotizing fasciitis. CPK, creatine phosphokinase.

- Case definition of staphylococcal TSS is outlined in Table 61.3.
- Historically associated with menstruation and tampon use, but nowadays with surgical packing, meshes, and cutaneous infections (e.g. abscesses).
- Sudden onset of high fever, myalgias, vomiting, diarrhea, headache, and pharyngitis; hypotension is a key finding.
- Clinically, scarlatiniform changes initially appear on the trunk and then spread centrifugally; erythema and edema of the palms and

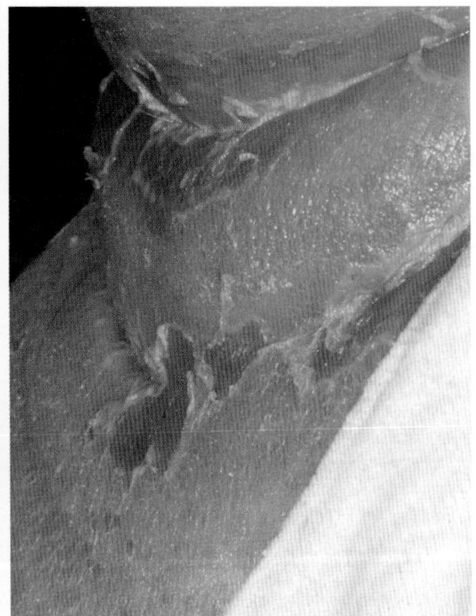

Fig. 61.8 Staphylococcal scalded skin syndrome. Extensive involvement on the neck with a wrinkled appearance of the erythematous skin in addition to peeling and multiple erosions. *Courtesy, Julie V. Schaffer, MD.*

soles can be followed by desquamation 1–3 weeks later.

- Mucous membrane findings: erythema, strawberry tongue, hyperemia of the conjunctivae (Fig. 61.9).
- **DDx:** streptococcal TSS, drug reaction plus hypotension from sepsis; in children, Kawasaki disease and scarlet fever.
- **Rx:** hospitalization and IV antibiotics (see Table 61.1).

STREPTOCOCCAL TOXIC SHOCK SYNDROME (STREPTOCOCCAL TSS)

- Secondary to GAS (especially M types 1 and 3), which produce exotoxins A and/or B.
- Case definition of streptococcal TSS is outlined in Table 61.3.
- Most common site of the associated streptococcal infection is the skin, e.g. cellulitis or necrotizing fasciitis.
- **Rx:** hospitalization and IV antibiotics (see Table 61.1).

SCARLET FEVER

- Secondary to GAS, which produce erythrogenic toxins types A, B, and C.
- Seen in children (ages 1–10 years), usually following streptococcal tonsillitis or pharyngitis.
- Sore throat, headache, malaise, chills, anorexia, nausea, and high fevers precede erythema of the neck, chest, and axillae that becomes generalized over 4–6 hours.
- The erythema blanches with pressure and is studded with tiny papules ("sunburn with goose pimples"); the cheeks are also flushed with circumoral pallor.
- Pastia lines (linear petechial streaks) are seen in major body folds, e.g. axillary, inguinal, antecubital.
- Desquamation of distal digits occurs after 7–10 days.
- Postinfectious sequelae include acute glomerulonephritis and rheumatic fever.
- **DDx** of palmoplantar desquamation: Kawasaki disease, TSS, and any preceding infection (including viral) with a high fever.
- **DDx** of exanthem: drug eruption, viral exanthem, early SSSS; a scarlatiniform eruption is also seen in TSS and Kawasaki disease.
- **Rx:** 10- to 14-day course of penicillin or amoxicillin.

BACTEREMIA/SEPTICEMIA

- Septic emboli can present as petechiae and purpura that may develop central pustules or hemorrhagic bullae; subcutaneous abscesses can also be seen.
- Endocarditis can be acute or subacute and caused by organisms including *S. aureus* and *Streptococcus* spp., respectively; cutaneous signs of endocarditis include splinter hemorrhages (see Ch. 58), Osler nodes, and Janeway lesions (see Table 18.2).

Gram-Positive Bacilli

Clostridial Skin Infections

- *Clostridia* spp. are Gram-positive bacilli that live on dead organic matter and can cause anaerobic cellulitis or myonecrosis (gas gangrene); they account for half of the normal skin microbiota.
- Anaerobic cellulitis.
  - Risk factors: trauma, diabetes mellitus, peripheral vascular disease, and injection drug use
  - Generally due to *Clostridium perfringens* > other anaerobic bacteria (e.g.

CASE DEFINITIONS FOR THE TOXIC SHOCK SYNDROMES	
Toxic shock syndrome (other than streptococcal)	
• Fever: temperature >102°F (or >38.9°C) • Rash: diffuse macular erythroderma • Desquamation: 1–2 weeks after the onset of illness (especially palms and soles) • Hypotension: systolic blood pressure <90 mmHg for adults (<5th percentile for children) • Involvement of three or more of the following organ systems:	
– Gastrointestinal – Muscular – Central nervous – Renal	– Hepatic – Mucous membranes (erythema) – Hematologic (platelets <100,000/mm^3)
• Negative results for the following tests (if done): – Blood and cerebrospinal fluid cultures (blood culture may be positive for *Staphylococcus aureus*) – Serologic tests for Rocky Mountain spotted fever, leptospirosis, measles	
Streptococcal toxic shock syndrome	
• Isolation of group A streptococci from a normally sterile site* (e.g. blood, cerebrospinal fluid, tissue biopsy, surgical wound) *or* • Isolation of group A streptococci from a nonsterile site† (e.g. throat, sputum, vagina, superficial skin lesion) *and* • Hypotension: systolic blood pressure <90 mmHg for adults (<5th percentile for children) *and* • Two or more of the following signs: – Renal impairment – Coagulopathy (platelets ≤100,000/mm^3 or disseminated intravascular coagulation) – Liver impairment – Acute respiratory distress syndrome – Generalized erythematous macular rash ± desquamation – Soft tissue necrosis (e.g. necrotizing fasciitis, myositis, gangrene)	

**Defined as a definite case.*
†Defined as a probable case, excluding any other possible etiology.

Table 61.3 Case definitions for the toxic shock syndromes. See https://ndc.services.cdc.gov/case-definitions/toxic-shock-syndrome-2011/ and https://ndc.services.cdc.gov/case-definitions/streptococcal-toxic-shock-syndrome-2010/ for details on the current case definitions.

Bacteroides); incubation period >3 days with a rapid course
  - Minimal visible skin changes; signs include crepitus and a thin, dark gray-brown, foul-smelling ("dirty dishwater") exudate; pain often absent or mild without symptoms of toxemia (e.g. tachycardia)

• Myonecrosis, in contrast to anaerobic cellulitis, has a shorter incubation period with a very rapid course; overlying skin has a dark yellow to bronze discoloration, sometimes with bullae or necrosis, and severe swelling; toxemia (e.g. hypotension) is generally present.

• **Rx:** early surgical debridement and empirical antibiotics (e.g. clindamycin plus a third-generation cephalosporin) until culture and sensitivities obtained.

Corynebacterium (and *Kytococcus*) Skin Infections

ERYTHRASMA

• Superficial, localized infection due to *Corynebacterium minutissimum.*

• Three major clinical variants:
  - Interdigital – the most common variant, characterized by chronic maceration with fissuring or scaling; needs to be distinguished from interdigital tinea pedis
  - Intertriginous – thin red-brown plaques in the axillae and groin/upper inner thigh that may be misdiagnosed as tinea cruris (see Table 60.5; Fig. 61.10)

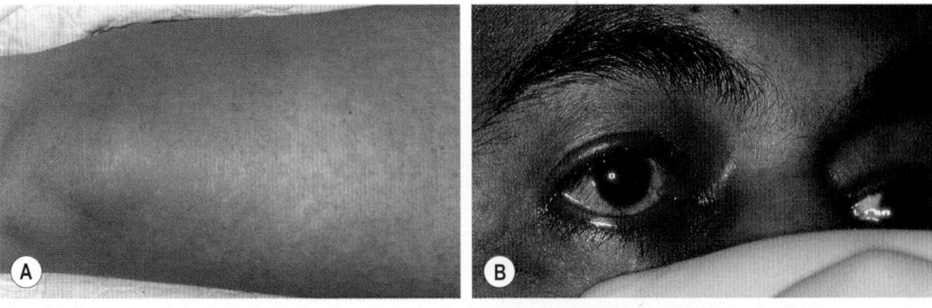

Fig. 61.9 Toxic shock syndrome due to *Staphylococcus aureus* infection. **A** Blotchy erythema is evident on the thigh. **B** Hyperemia of the conjunctiva is seen. *Courtesy, YDRSC.*

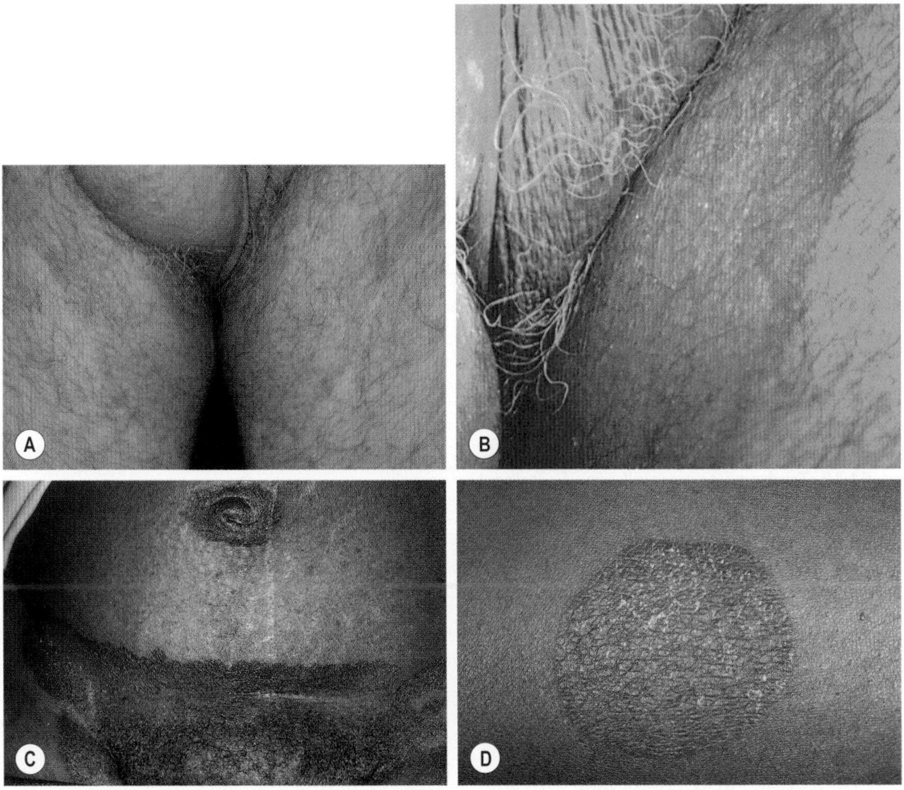

Fig. 61.10 Erythrasma. **A** Pink to brown scaly patches on the upper inner thighs. **B** Coral-red fluorescence upon illumination with a Wood's lamp. **C** Hyperpigmented plaques in the inguinal and periumbilical areas (intertriginous zones). **D** Well-demarcated, scaly, hyperpigmented plaque of disciform erythrasma. *A, B, Courtesy, Louis A. Fragola, Jr., MD; C, D, Courtesy, NYUDSC.*

  - "Disciform" – often on the trunk and diabetes mellitus is a risk factor (Fig. 61.10D)
- Bright, coral-red fluorescence with Wood's lamp examination (see Figs 61.10B and 13.2).
- **Rx:** topical clindamycin or erythromycin; prevent moisture accumulation with topical aluminum chloride 6–20% (axillae).

PITTED KERATOLYSIS

- Secondary to *Kytococcus sedentarius* (*Micrococcus sedentarius*) and *Corynebacterium* spp.
- Hyperhidrosis, prolonged occlusion, and increased surface pH are contributing factors; the latter plus bacterial infection lead to 1- to

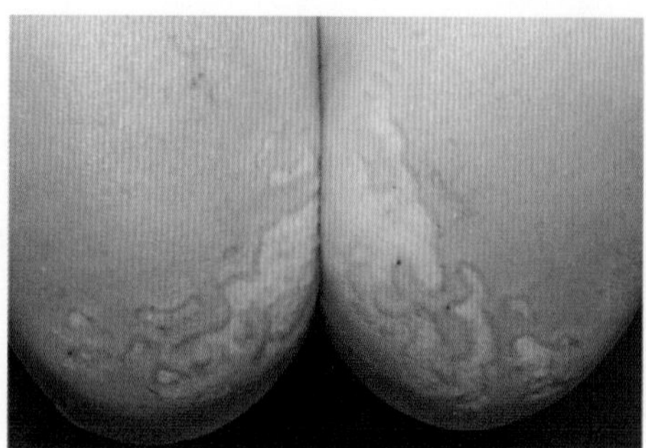

Fig. 61.11 Pitted keratolysis of the plantar surface of the foot. Multiple craters with decreased stratum corneum that favor pressure points on the plantar surface. *Courtesy, Kalman Watsky, MD.*

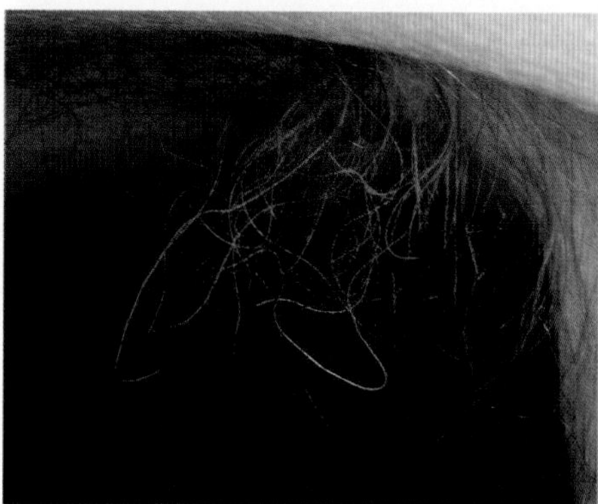

Fig. 61.12 Trichomycosis axillaris. Cylindrical sheaths and beading of the axillary hairs. A yellow color is seen most commonly. *Courtesy, YDRSC.*

3-mm crater-like depressions in the stratum corneum that may coalesce, with involvement of soles >> palms (Fig. 61.11).

- Often accompanied by a distinctive malodor.
- **Rx:** topical clindamycin or erythromycin; decrease eccrine sweat production with topical aluminum chloride 20%.

TRICHOMYCOSIS AXILLARIS

- Common disorder that may be clinically subtle; often accompanied by malodor.
- Hair shafts are ensheathed with adherent yellow > red or black concretions composed of organisms (Fig. 61.12); most common in the axillae and a cause of chromhidrosis (see Ch. 32).
- **DDx:** other causes of nodules on hair shafts (see Fig. 64.3).
- **Rx:** shaving of hair; topical antimicrobials (e.g. benzoyl peroxide, erythromycin) can help prevent recurrence.

CUTANEOUS ANTHRAX – CLINICAL CHARACTERISTICS
• Incubation period averages 7 days (range 1–12 days)
• A purpuric macule or papule develops in an exposed area (e.g. forearm, neck, chest, finger); the papule may resemble an insect bite and can be pruritic
• Within 48 hours of the lesion's appearance, a vesicle (1–3 mm) forms with surrounding non-pitting edema
• The central vesicle ulcerates and small vesicles may form around the ulcer
• The lesion becomes hemorrhagic and depressed, and a *painless*, black, necrotic eschar forms centrally with an increase in the surrounding erythema and edema
• The eschar dries, loosens, and sloughs over the next 1–2 weeks, with no permanent scar

Table 61.4 Cutaneous anthrax – clinical characteristics. *Adapted from Carucci JA, McGovern TW, Norton SA,* et al. *Cutaneous anthrax management algorithm. J. Am. Acad. Dermatol. 2002;47:766–769.*

Other Gram-Positive Skin Infections

ANTHRAX

- *Bacillus anthracis* causes inhalational, gastrointestinal, and cutaneous disease.
- Occurs most commonly in farmers and ranchers exposed to animals such as sheep, cows, horses, and goats; also secondary to exposure to hides from these animals (e.g. skins used for drums).
- Emerged as an agent of biological terrorism.
- Clinical characteristics of cutaneous disease are outlined in Table 61.4.
- **Rx** for cutaneous disease: fluoroquinolone (e.g. ciprofloxacin 500 mg PO twice daily) for 7–10 days or 60 days if also risk of inhalational disease.
- Prevention: vaccine (e.g. raxibacumab) for high-risk populations (e.g. military).

ERYSIPELOID

- Due to *Erysipelothrix rhusiopathiae*.
- Variants:
  - Localized cellulitis – infection due to traumatic inoculation; seen in individuals

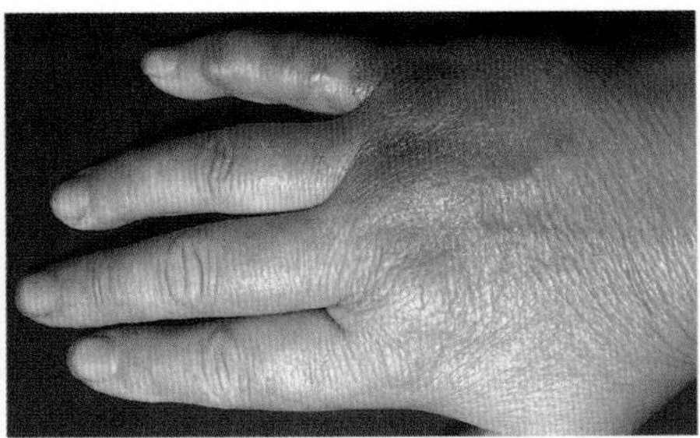

Fig. 61.13 Erysipeloid. Erythema and edema with vesicle formation on the hand and fifth digit. *Courtesy, NYUDSC.*

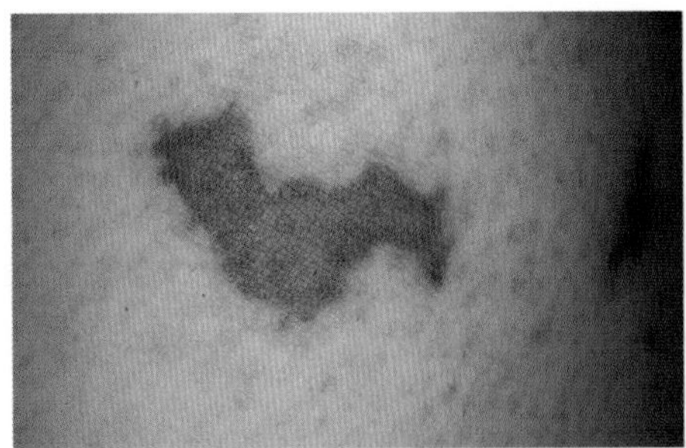

Fig. 61.14 Acute meningococcemia. Purpura with irregular outline and central gunmetal gray color. *Courtesy, Kalman Watsky, MD.*

who prepare fish and meat; the hand is a frequent site of involvement and the color is characteristically red-violet (Fig. 61.13)
  - Generalized – uncommon form; multiple pink plaques, usually in the setting of immunosuppression, with associated fever and arthralgias; blood cultures are generally negative

• **DDx** of localized form: cellulitis due to more common infectious agents (see above), atypical mycobacterial infection, early *Vibrio* infection.

• **Rx** for localized form: penicillin 500 mg PO four times a day for 7–10 days.

Gram-Negative Cocci

ACUTE MENINGOCOCCEMIA

• Systemic infection due to *Neisseria meningitides.*

• Primarily seen in young children (6 months to 1 year of age) and young adults in close quarters (e.g. dormitories, barracks).

• In most individuals, infection results in an asymptomatic carrier state.

• In acute meningococcemia, one-third to one-half of patients have skin lesions due to septic emboli, initially subtle petechiae that evolve into irregularly shaped purpura with a central gunmetal gray color that reflects necrosis (Fig. 61.14); Gram-negative cocci may be seen on Gram staining of lesional tissue.

• The septic lesions are to be distinguished from those due to disseminated intravascular coagulation (see Table 18.1).

• Additional systemic manifestations include fever, chills, hypotension, meningoencephalitis, pneumonia, pericarditis, and myocarditis.

• **Rx:** IV penicillin or ceftriaxone; vaccination is important for prevention.

CHRONIC MENINGOCOCCEMIA

• An indolent infection due to *Neisseria meningitides.*

• Recurrent episodes of fever, chills, night sweats, and arthralgias; skin lesions are polymorphous, e.g. pink macules and papules, nodules, petechiae/purpura; the skin lesions represent small vessel vasculitis without visible organisms by light microscopy, but PCR may be used to detect organisms.

• **Rx** as for acute meningococcemia; close contacts should be treated as well.

GONORRHEA & DISSEMINATED GONOCOCCAL INFECTION

See Chapter 69.

Gram-Negative Bacilli

Pseudomonal Infections

Green nail syndrome is discussed in Chapter 58.

GRAM-NEGATIVE TOE-WEB INFECTION

• Although *Pseudomonas aeruginosa* is the most common cause, other Gram-negative bacilli can be implicated (e.g. *Escherichia coli*, *Proteus mirabilis*).

• Risk factors are pre-existing tinea pedis and occlusion (e.g. tight-fitting shoes).

• Symptoms of burning and pain; signs include a malodorous exudate with a

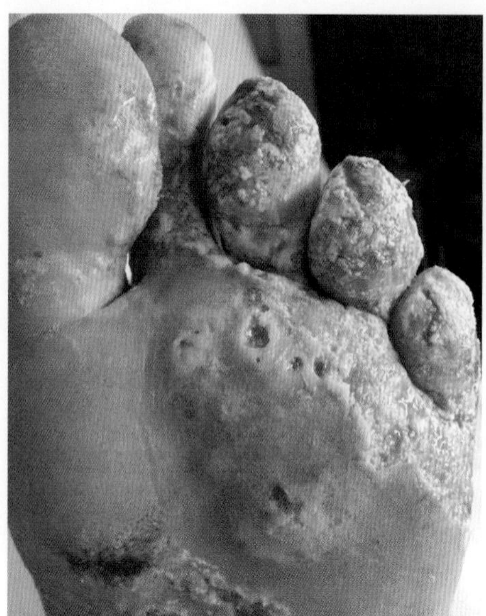

Fig. 61.15 Severe superficial infection of the skin with *Pseudomonas*. Note the macerated border, the erosions, and the moth-eaten appearance of the skin. Often represents secondary infection superimposed on interdigital tinea pedis. *Courtesy, Kalman Watsky, MD.*

blue-green tinge, a grape-juice odor, and a moth-eaten appearance of skin due to maceration and erosions (Fig. 61.15).

- In severe cases, there can be cellulitis.

OTITIS EXTERNA ("SWIMMER'S EAR")

- Swollen auditory ear canal with greenish purulent discharge.
- Extreme pain with manipulation of the pinna.
- **Rx:** antimicrobial drops (e.g. ofloxacin) with or without an ear wick, oral analgesics (e.g. NSAIDs).

PSEUDOMONAL FOLLICULITIS (HOT TUB FOLLICULITIS)

See Table 31.2.

PSEUDOMONAS HOT-FOOT SYNDROME

- Develops acutely on the soles of children and adolescents who are otherwise healthy after swimming in water with high concentrations of *Pseudomonas aeruginosa*.
- Painful and tender, red-purple, 1- or 2-cm nodules appear on the weight-bearing aspects of the feet (Fig. 61.16).
- Self-limiting and **DDx** is primarily idiopathic palmoplantar hidradenitis (Ch. 32).

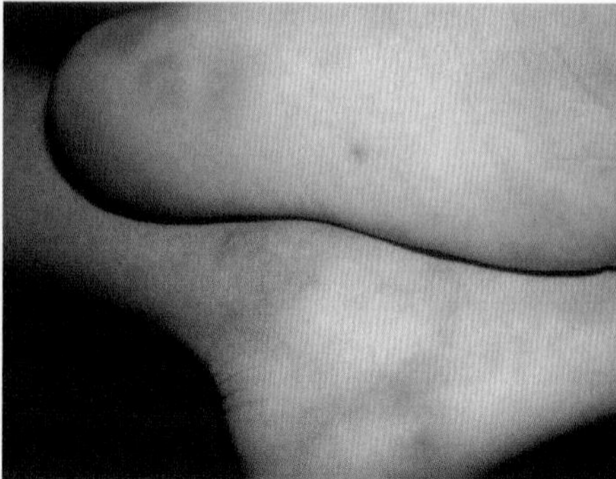

Fig. 61.16 *Pseudomonas* hot-foot syndrome. Tender erythematous nodules on the heel. *Courtesy, Justin J. Green, MD.*

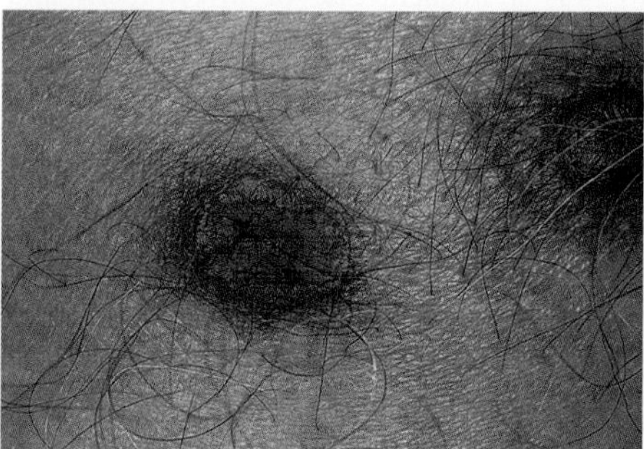

Fig. 61.17 Ecthyma gangrenosum. Embolic lesion of *Pseudomonas aeruginosa* on the chest. Note the necrotic center and inflammatory border. *Courtesy, YDRSC.*

CELLULITIS

- Clinical features are similar to those of cellulitis due to *S. aureus* (see above); can occur on the lower extremity in the setting of Gram-negative toe-web infection or on the external ear postoperatively.
- Sometimes, it can be difficult to distinguish soft tissue infection from colonization with *Pseudomonas*, particularly in chronic ulcers.

ECTHYMA GANGRENOSUM

- A sign of bacteremia or septicemia.
- Most commonly due to Gram-negative bacilli, including *Pseudomonas*, but can also be due to opportunistic fungi; primarily seen in immunocompromised hosts, especially those with prolonged neutropenia.
- A red-purple macule or patch that develops central necrosis; sometimes the necrosis is preceded by a hemorrhagic bulla; the number can vary from one to a dozen or more (Fig. 61.17).

- The most common location for ecthyma gangrenosum due to *Pseudomonas* is the groin.
- To establish the diagnosis, culture of tissue, obtained via sterile biopsy technique (see Fig. 2.10), is performed in combination with histopathology.

TREATMENT OF PSEUDOMONAL INFECTIONS

- For superficial infection (e.g. Gram-negative toe-web infection): 5% acetic acid soaks followed by application of a topical antibiotic (e.g. gentamicin, silver sulfadiazine); if minimal improvement or severe, oral fluoroquinolone.
- For severe or systemic infections: piperacillin/tazobactam or doripenem if penicillin-allergic; may be combined with an aminoglycoside antibiotic.

Diseases Caused by *Bartonella* Species

See Table 61.5.

Other Gram-Negative Skin Infections with Fever and Skin Findings

See Table 61.6, Table 61.7.

Spirochetes

LYME DISEASE

See Chapter 15.

SYPHILIS

See Chapter 69.

OTHER TREPONEMAL DISEASES

- Like syphilis, other treponemal diseases may have primary, secondary, and tertiary stages.
- Endemic syphilis.
  - Due to *Treponema pallidum endemicum*
  - Seen most commonly in Africa, the Arabian peninsula, and Southeast Asia
  - Children younger than the age of 15 years are most often affected
  - Primary lesion often missed
  - Secondary stage: macerated patches on lips, tongue, and pharynx; angular stomatitis; condyloma lata; generalized lymphadenopathy
  - Tertiary stage: gummas that can lead to destruction of the palate and nasal septum
- Pinta.
  - Due to *T. carateum*
  - Seen primarily in Central and South America
  - Primary stage: minute macules or papules with erythematous haloes, most commonly on the lower extremities, that develop into infiltrated plaques over several months
  - Secondary stage: smaller, variably pigmented (red, blue, black, or hypopigmented), scaly macules and papules that may coalesce; clustered near the initial primary lesion or generalized
  - Tertiary stage: symmetric, depigmented, vitiligo-like lesions that are atrophic or keratotic
- Yaws.
  - Due to *T. pallidum pertenue*
  - Seen in warm, humid, tropical climates
  - Children younger than the age of 15 years are most often affected
  - Primary: erythematous, infiltrated, painful papule, usually on the extremities; enlarges to become up to 5 cm in diameter and ulcerates; heals spontaneously over 3–6 months
  - Secondary: smaller lesions adjacent to orifices or adjacent to site of initial primary lesion (Fig. 61.18)
  - Tertiary: destructive skin lesions, palmoplantar thickening that can lead to difficulty with ambulation, chronic osteitis (sabre tibia)

Filamentous Bacteria

ACTINOMYCOSIS

- Most commonly due to *Actinomyces israelii*.
- Three major sites of involvement – cervical, pulmonary, and gastrointestinal.
- Skin involvement is most common with the cervical variant and is sometimes referred to as "lumpy jaw" due to irregular subcutaneous nodules; the latter can drain and the exudate contains grains (Fig. 61.19).
- **Rx:** penicillin.

ACTINOMYCOTIC MYCETOMA

- Most commonly due to *Nocardia* as well as *Actinomadura madurae*, *Actinomadura pelletieri*, and *Streptomyces somaliensis*; organisms are found in soil and on plant material (Table 61.8).

MAJOR HUMAN DISEASES CAUSED BY *BARTONELLA* SPECIES				
Species	**Disease**	**Vector**	**Epidemiology**	**Clinical features**
B. henselae	Cat-scratch disease	Cat flea (*Ctenocephalides felis*)*	Young people, <18 years of age	• Lymphadenopathy • Systemic symptoms (e.g. fever, malaise)
	Bacillary angiomatosis		Immunocompromised patients	• Bright red papules that can resemble pyogenic granulomas; lichenoid papules/plaques; subcutaneous nodules • Hepatic involvement (peliosis)
B. bacilliformis	Bartonellosis (Carrion disease, Oroya fever, verruga peruana)	Sand fly (*Lutzomyia verrucarum*)	Peru, Ecuador, and southwestern Colombia	• Oroya fever – fever, hemolytic anemia, secondary bacterial infections, e.g. *Salmonella* • Verruga peruana – erythematous patches with overlying bright red papules and nodules
B. quintana	Trench fever/"urban" trench fever	Human body louse (*Pediculus humanus corporis*)	Originally seen in World War I troops; today, associated with homelessness and poor hygiene	Relapsing fever
	Bacillary angiomatosis		See above	See above

**More commonly by a cat scratch or bite.*

Table 61.5 Major human diseases caused by *Bartonella* species. Treatment must be tailored to the particular presentation; commonly employed antibiotics include azithromycin, erythromycin, doxycycline, and/or rifampin. Therapy may be administered for up to 3 months.

SELECTED GRAM-NEGATIVE INFECTIONS THAT PRESENT WITH NONSPECIFIC SYSTEMIC SYMPTOMS (E.G. FEVER) AND SKIN FINDINGS				
Infection	**Common organism(s)**	**Transmission/other factors**	**Unique/characteristic findings**	**Skin findings**
Infection with *Vibrio vulnificus*	*Vibrio vulnificus*	Raw seafood or exposure of cutaneous wounds to infected sea water, primarily in warmer climates; patients at risk are middle-aged men with chronic liver disease or diabetes		Hemorrhagic bullae with cellulitis
Tularemia	*Francisella tularensis*	Infected rabbits; deerfly or tick (e.g. *Amblyomma americanum*) as vector	May show sporotrichoid pattern	Ulcers, lymphadenopathy
Glanders	*Burkholderia mallei*	Direct contact with infected animals (horses, mules, donkeys)	Sporotrichoid (lymphocutaneous) pattern	Nodule, pustule, or vesicle surrounded by erythema
Plague	*Yersinia pestis*	Contaminated food, water, or raw milk; fleas can be the vector	Bubonic form can have a sporotrichoid pattern	• Bubonic form due to inoculation: wound becomes a pustule or ulcer with painful regional lymphadenopathy • Septicemic form: emboli present as vesicles, carbuncles, petechiae, or purpura
Melioidosis	*Burkholderia pseudomallei*	Contact with contaminated soil or water; ingestion or inhalation; sexual intercourse; fleas can be the vector		Abscesses, granulomatous lesions, purpura, pustules, urticaria, ecthyma gangrenosum

Table 61.6 Selected Gram-negative infections that present with nonspecific systemic symptoms (e.g. fever) and skin findings. *Continued*

SELECTED GRAM-NEGATIVE INFECTIONS THAT PRESENT WITH NONSPECIFIC SYSTEMIC SYMPTOMS (E.G. FEVER) AND SKIN FINDINGS				
Infection	**Common organism(s)**	**Transmission/other factors**	**Unique/characteristic findings**	**Skin findings**
Rat-bite fever (Haverhill fever)	*Streptobacillus moniliformis*	Close contact with infected rodents or contaminated food, water, or raw milk (Haverhill fever)	Migratory polyarthritis in 50% of patients that mimics rheumatoid arthritis	Acral palmoplantar eruption of macules, papules, petechiae, vesicles, pustules, with secondary crusts
Brucellosis	*Brucella abortus*	Consumption of unpasteurized milk products	Malodorous perspiration	• Erythema nodosum • Vasculitis
Typhoid fever	*Salmonella typhi*	Contact with infected persons	Rose spots	• Rose spots – 2–8 mm pink, blanching papules, often in clusters of 5–15 on the anterior trunk • Erythema multiforme, Sweet syndrome, hemorrhagic bullae, pustules
Malacoplakia (malakoplakia)	*Escherichia coli* (less commonly *Pseudomonas* or other bacteria)	Immunocompromised hosts	Michaelis–Gutmann bodies: intracytoplasmic concretions within large histiocytes	Most commonly perianal abscesses or ulcers
Rhinoscleroma	*Klebsiella rhinoscleromatis*	Endemic to Central Europe, India, Egypt, other countries (e.g. Indonesia)	Intracellular bacteria within large histiocytes (Mikulicz cells)	Rhinitis that progresses to granulomatous nodules and scarring of nose and upper respiratory tract

Table 61.6 *Continued* **Selected Gram-negative infections that present with nonspecific systemic symptoms (e.g. fever) and skin findings.**

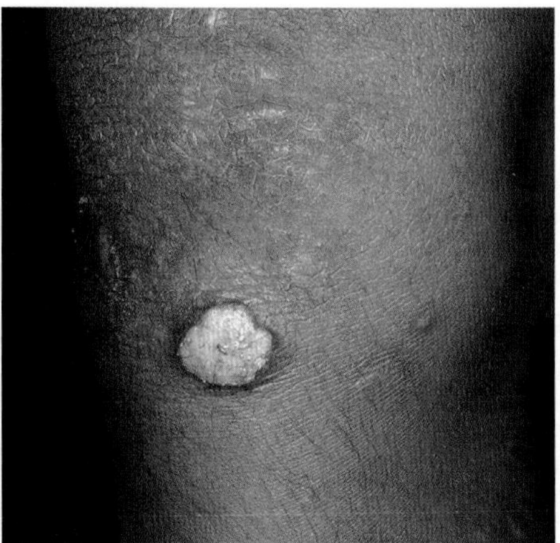

Fig. 61.18 Cutaneous yaws on the knee of an adolescent from Indonesia. *Courtesy, Peter Ehrnstrom, MD.*

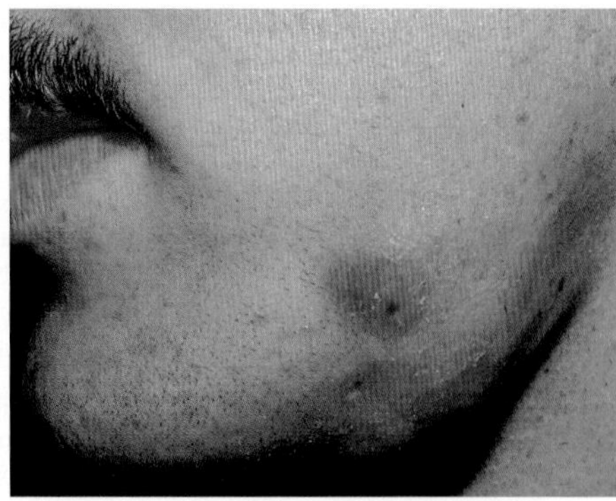

Fig. 61.19 Cervicofacial actinomycosis or "lumpy jaw" with soft tissue swelling and draining ulcerated nodules. The discharge contained sulfur granules, a term used when the grains are yellow in color. *Courtesy, M. Joyce Rico, MD.*

RISK FACTORS FOR *VIBRIO VULNIFICUS* INFECTION
Acquisition of infection
Cutaneous exposure to contaminated seawater and/or shellfish
• Exposure to warm coastal salt water (April–October in temperate climates) • Handling shellfish • New injury to the skin or a pre-existing wound predisposes to a primary cutaneous infection, which can lead to cellulitis, necrotizing fasciitis, and/or septicemia in susceptible hosts (see below)
Consumption of contaminated raw/undercooked seafood
• Classically raw oysters, but also found in clams, crabs, and other shellfish • Leads to an acute gastrointestinal illness in immunocompetent individuals and septicemia in susceptible hosts (see below)
Underlying medical conditions that predispose to severe infections
Liver disease

• Hemochromatosis or iron overload in the setting of thalassemia
  – *V. vulnificus* is ferrophilic and requires higher levels of iron than other pathogens
  – Patients have decreased hepcidin antibacterial activity
• Alcoholic cirrhosis or chronic hepatitis

Diabetes mellitus
• Peripheral neuropathy predisposes to cutaneous wounds that serve as a portal of entry
Gastrointestinal disease
• Peptic ulcer disease   – Antacid use may lead to increased survival of *V. vulnificus* • Gastrointestinal surgery
Immunosuppression
• HIV infection • Leukemia or lymphoma • Treatment with corticosteroids, chemotherapy, and other immunosuppressive agents
Chronic kidney disease

Table 61.7 Risk factors for *Vibrio vulnificus* infection. Infections are most common in men >40 years of age.

FOUR MAJOR CLINICAL FORMS OF CUTANEOUS NOCARDIOSIS	
Primary	
Actinomycotic mycetoma	• Half of all cases of actinomycotic mycetoma are due to *Nocardia* species* • Traumatic inoculation causes a painless nodule that enlarges, suppurates, and drains via sinus tracts • Purulent discharge contains grains • The foot is the usual site of involvement • May involve underlying muscle and bone
Lymphocutaneous	• Occurs days to weeks after trauma • Appears as a persistent crusted pustule or abscess, often resistant to shorter courses of antibiotics • Ascending lymphatic streaks, a sporotrichoid pattern of papulonodules, and tender palpable lymph nodes may be seen
Superficial cutaneous	• Traumatic implantation of foreign objects (including soil and gravel) into the skin • The diagnosis is based on a high index of suspicion, lack of response to routine antibiotic treatment, and laboratory results
Secondary	
Pulmonary/ systemic	• Subcutaneous abscesses of the chest wall • Pustules, nodules, cutaneous fistulae • Almost universally fatal if left untreated • Most commonly caused by *Nocardia asteroides*

**In Mexico and Central and South America,* N. brasiliensis *is the etiologic agent of 90% of actinomycotic mycetomas, whereas in the United States, most mycetomas are caused by true fungi.*

Table 61.8 Four major clinical forms of cutaneous nocardiosis. Rx: sulfonamides are the drugs of choice for primary cutaneous nocardiosis, with minocycline being an alternative for sulfonamide-allergic patients. Duration of treatment is at least 6–12 weeks for localized disease in immunocompetent hosts. Surgical excision may be required for deep abscesses.

- **DDx:** distinguishing this entity from eumycotic mycetoma requires culture of grains or tissue; prior to the return of tissue or grain culture results, a presumptive diagnosis can be made based on the diameter of the filaments or hyphae composing the grains in biopsy specimens.

NOCARDIOSIS

See Table 61.8.

For further information see Ch. 74 from *Dermatology, Fourth Edition*.

For additional online figures and tables visit www.expertconsult.com 

Mycobacterial Diseases 62

Key Points

- Mycobacteria are the etiologic agents of three major types of infection:
  - Leprosy – *Mycobacterium leprae*
  - Tuberculosis – *Mycobacterium tuberculosis*
  - Atypical or nontuberculous infections – e.g. *Mycobacterium marinum, Mycobacterium chelonae* (Tables 62.1 and 62.2)

Leprosy

- Slowly progressive disease characterized by granuloma formation in nerves and the skin.
- Affects all ages, but bimodal peak distribution – ages 10–15 years and 30–60 years.
- Currently, the highest reported prevalence is in the South Sudan (Fig. 62.1), with high incidence in Brazil, India, and Indonesia.
- Spread of leprosy is dependent on: (1) a contagious person (predominantly through nasal/oral droplets); (2) a susceptible person; and (3) close/intimate contact.
- Incubation period averages 4–10 years.
- Degree of immunity is reflected in clinical findings (Table 62.3; Figs 62.2–62.4) and histopathologic features; the latter range from macrophages containing numerous bacilli (globi) in lepromatous leprosy to granulomas without organisms in tuberculoid leprosy.
- Nerves are often affected, particularly ones close to the surface of the skin (Fig. 62.5); sensations of pain, temperature, and/or touch should be evaluated within skin lesions.
- Sequelae of leprosy can be disfiguring (Figs 62.6 and 62.7).

MYCOBACTERIA THAT CAUSE CUTANEOUS DISEASE		
Group and pigment	**Rate of growth**	**Examples of pathogens**
Slow growers		
Photochromogens*	2–3 weeks	*M. kansasii, M. marinum, M. simiae*
Scotochromogens†	2–3 weeks	*M. scrofulaceum, M. szulgai, M. gordonae, M. xenopi*
Nonchromogens‡	2–3 weeks	*M. tuberculosis, M. avium, M. intracellulare, M. chimaera, M. ulcerans, M. haemophilum, M. bovis*§
Rapid growers	3–5 days	Examples include *M. fortuitum, M. chelonae, M. abscessus***
Noncultured (to date)		*M. leprae*

**Capable of yellow pigment formation upon exposure to light.*
†Capable of yellow pigment production without light exposure.
‡Incapable of pigment production.
§Including bacillus Calmette–Guérin.
***Including M. abscessus subsp. massiliense and M. abscessus subsp. bolletii.*

Table 62.1 Mycobacteria that cause cutaneous disease. Modified classification of Runyon from: *Hautmann G, Lotti T. Atypical mycobacterial infections of the skin. Dermatol Clin 1994;12:657–68; Yates VM, Rook GAW. Mycobacterial infections. In: Burns T, Breathnach S, Cox N, Griffiths C (eds). Rook's Textbook of Dermatology, 7th edn. London: Blackwell Science, 2004;28.1–39; Neves RG, Pradinaud R. Micobacterioses atípicas. In: Neves RG, Talhari S (eds). Dermatologia Tropical. Rio de Janeiro: Medsi, 1995:283–90.*

IMPORTANT FEATURES OF ATYPICAL MYCOBACTERIA		
Mycobacteria	**Clinical features**	**Clinical setting**
M. marinum	• See text	Found in the environment
M. fortuitum, M. chelonae, M. abscessus	• Infected tattoos and post-pedicure lower extremity furuncles • Infected surgical sites	Can occur in immuno-competent hosts
M. ulcerans	• Often infects children • Can form large ulcers • May require surgical Rx as responds poorly to antibiotic therapy	
M. avium intracellulare M. kansasii	• Skin lesions rare	Found in the environment
M. scrofulaceum	• Classically causes lymphadenopathy	Often develops in immunocompromised hosts

Table 62.2 Important features of atypical mycobacteria. Disseminated skin lesions are an HIV-defining criterion, most commonly due to *M. avium intracellulare* or *M. kansasii*.

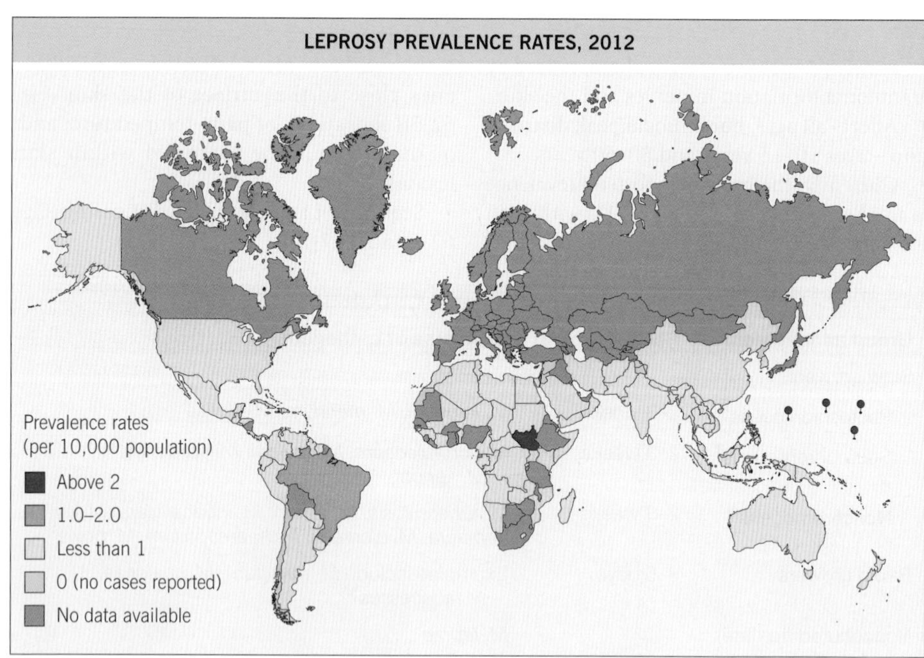

Fig. 62.1 Leprosy prevalence rates, 2012. The World Health Organization (WHO) has achieved its goal of a prevalence rate of less than 1 case per 10,000 persons in all but a few countries. *From World Health Organization,* https://www.who.int/lep/situation/Leprosy_PR_2011.pdf?ua=1.

CLASSIFICATION OF LEPROSY: RIDLEY–JOPLING AND OPERATIONAL

Operational	Multibacillary, >5 skin lesions		Paucibacillary, 1–5 skin lesions	
Ridley–Jopling*	Lepromatous leprosy (LL)	Borderline leprosy (BL)	Tuberculoid leprosy (TT)	Indeterminate (I)
Clinical findings				
Cellular immunity	Least (Th2 CD4$^+$ T-cell response) →		Greatest (Th1 CD4$^+$ T-cell response)	
Type of lesions	Macules, papules, and plaques and sometimes diffuse infiltration of the skin	Macules, papules, and plaques with variable induration	Infiltrated thin plaques with raised edges, often hypopigmented	Macules, often hypopigmented
Distribution	Symmetric; favors face, buttocks, lower extremities	Tendency to symmetry	Localized, asymmetric	Variable
Definition	Vague, difficult to distinguish normal versus affected skin	Less well-defined borders	Well-defined, sharp borders	Not always defined
Sensation	Not affected	Diminished	Absent	Impaired
Bacilli in skin lesions	←			Usually none detected

Disease states intermediate between LL and TT include borderline LL, mid-borderline leprosy, borderline TT, and indeterminate.

Table 62.3 Classification of leprosy: Ridley–Jopling and operational. Adapted from A Guide to Leprosy Control, 2nd ed. Geneva: World Health Organization, 1988;27–8.

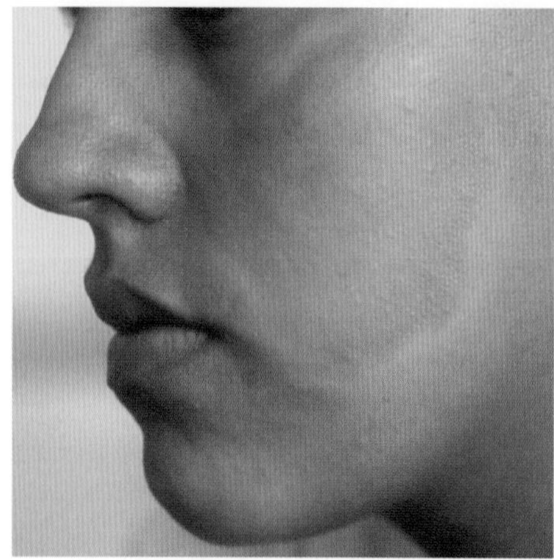

Fig. 62.2 Tuberculoid leprosy. Large annular lesion on the cheek with a red-brown color and rim of hypopigmentation. *Courtesy, Marcia Ramos-e-Silva, MD.*

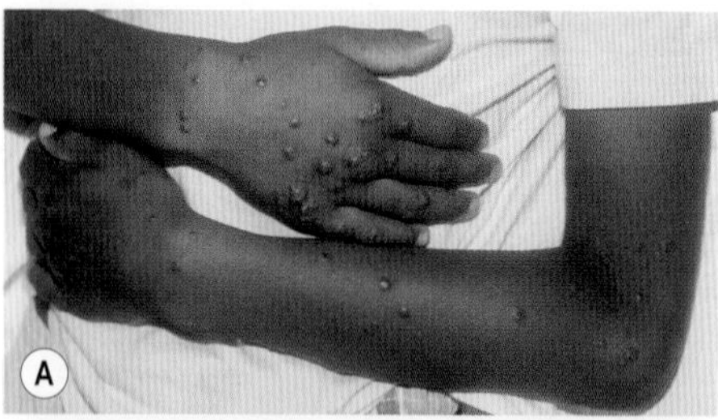

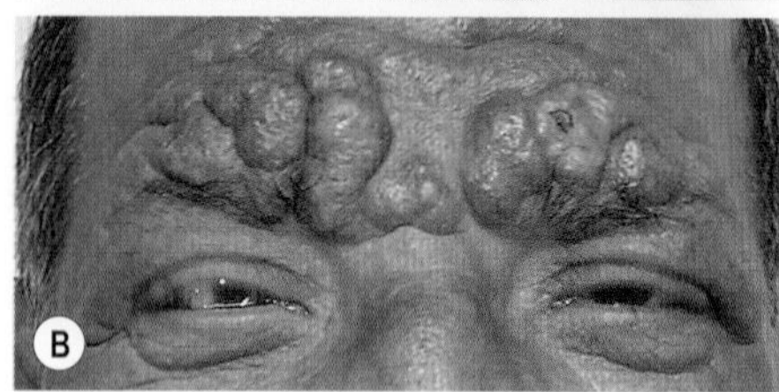

Fig. 62.3 Lepromatous leprosy. A Numerous erythematous papules and nodules on the forearms and hands. **B** Infiltrated nodules coalescing on the forehead with leonine facies and madarosis. Note the ocular involvement. *Courtesy, Marcia Ramos-e-Silva, MD.*

- Reactive states that can involve the skin may develop, especially following institution of antimicrobial treatment.
  - Type 1 (reversal reaction) – acute inflammation of cutaneous lesions (Fig. 62.8A) and nerves; appears rapidly due to a change in the immunologic state of the patient; in the case of upgrading, subclinical lesions can become clinically apparent

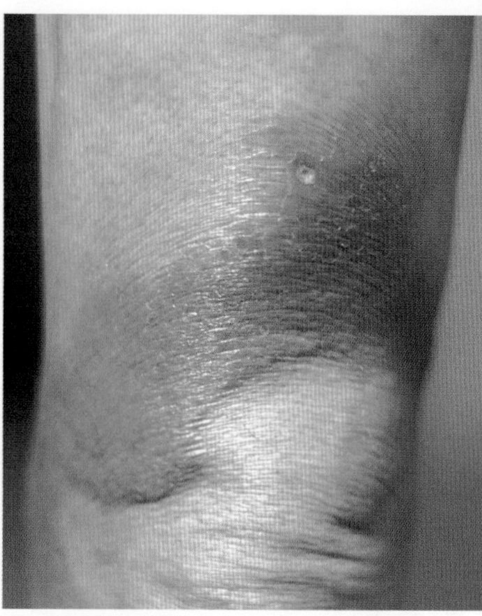

Fig. 62.4 Borderline leprosy. Erythematous, arcuate lesions with ill-defined outer borders and well-demarcated inner borders. *Courtesy, Marcia Ramos-e-Silva, MD.*

  - Type 2 (vasculitis) – formation of immune complexes in the setting of an excessive humoral immune reaction, leading to the appearance of cutaneous lesions, particularly erythema nodosum leprosum (Fig. 62.8B)
- **DDx:** outlined in Table 62.4.
- **Rx** for adults: multibacillary leprosy – rifampin 600 mg PO once a month, dapsone 100 mg PO daily, and clofazimine 300 mg PO once a month plus 50 mg PO daily for 12 months; paucibacillary leprosy – rifampin 600 mg PO once a month and dapsone 100 mg PO daily for 6 months; single lesion – one-time dose of rifampin 600 mg, ofloxacin 400 mg, and minocycline 100 mg; prednisone for type 1 (reversal) reactions; thalidomide for type 2 reactions. Second-line antimicrobials include moxifloxacin, clarithromycin, and rifapentine.

Cutaneous Tuberculosis (TB)

- Cutaneous lesions reflect mode of exposure and the degree of immunity.
- Exogenous exposure (inoculation).
  - Tuberculous chancre – seen in previously uninfected persons; 2–4 weeks after inoculation, a painless, firm, red-brown

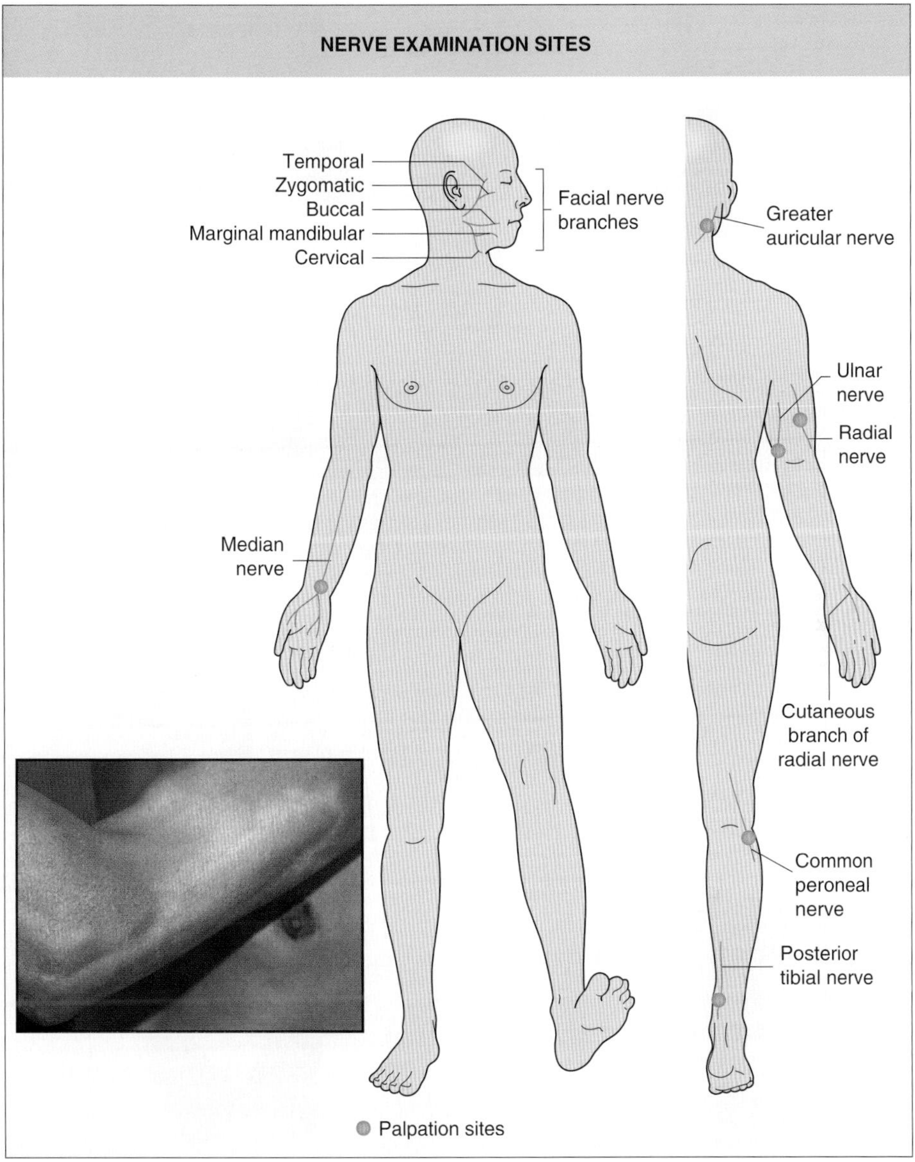

NERVE EXAMINATION SITES

Temporal
Zygomatic
Buccal
Marginal mandibular
Cervical
Facial nerve branches
Greater auricular nerve
Ulnar nerve
Radial nerve
Median nerve
Cutaneous branch of radial nerve
Common peroneal nerve
Posterior tibial nerve
Palpation sites

Fig. 62.5 Nerve examination sites.

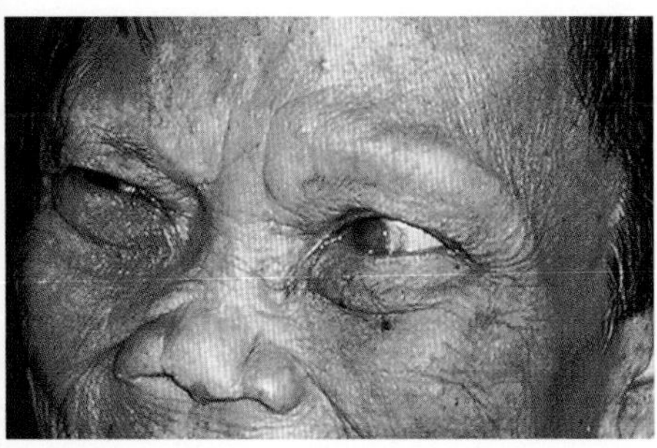

Fig. 62.6 Sequelae of leprosy. The patient has madarosis, a saddle nose, and blindness in the left eye. *Courtesy, Evangeline Handog, MD.*

papulonodule appears that ulcerates centrally; generally heals within 3–12 months

- TB verrucosa cutis – secondary to inoculation in persons with moderate to high immunity to *M. tuberculosis*; asymptomatic, wart-like papule that gradually enlarges (Fig. 62.9); may heal spontaneously after several years

- Endogenous spread of infection.
  - Some degree of cellular immunity (TST/PPD [tuberculin skin test] usually positive)

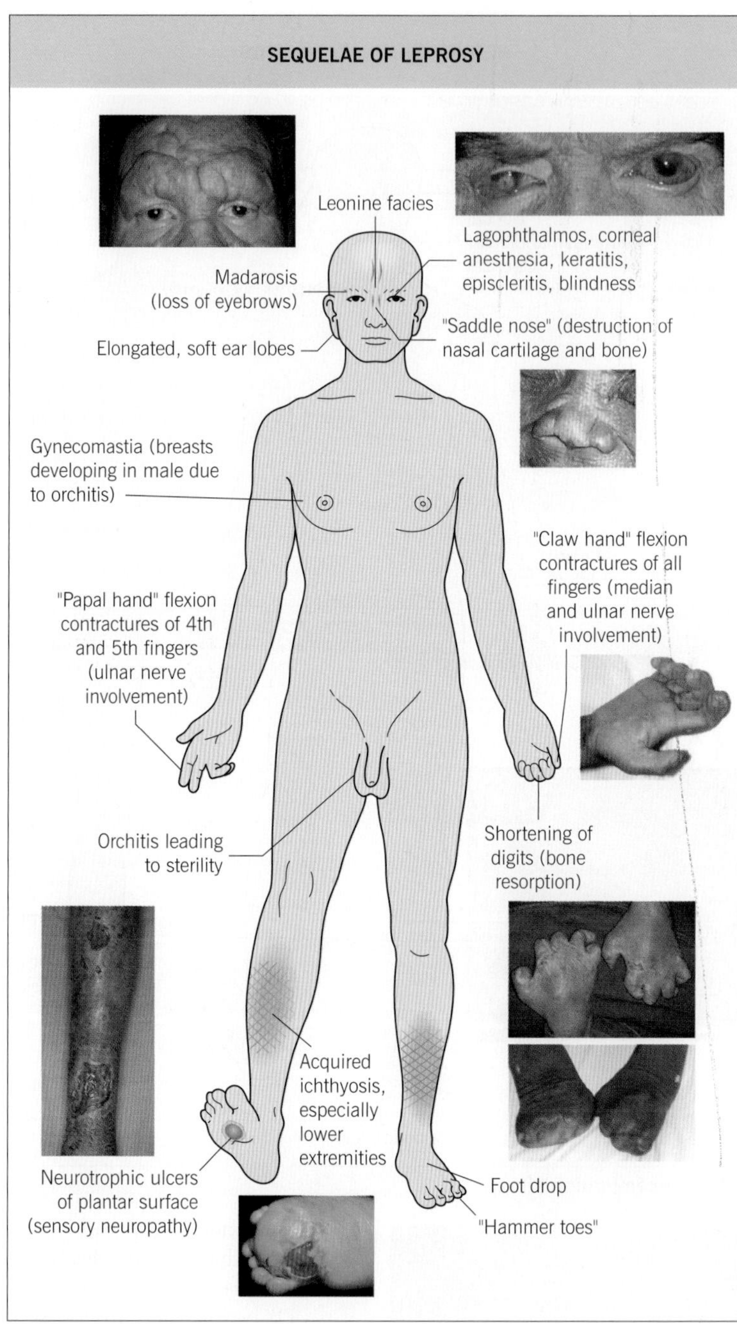

Fig. 62.7 Sequelae of leprosy. *Insets, Courtesy, Louis A. Fragola, Jr., MD, and Joyce Rico, MD.*

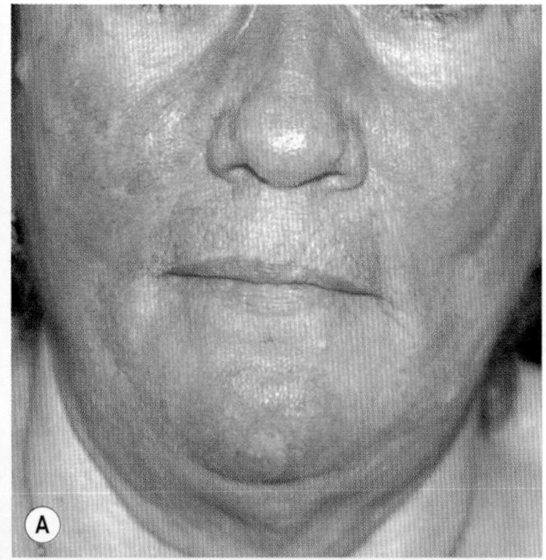

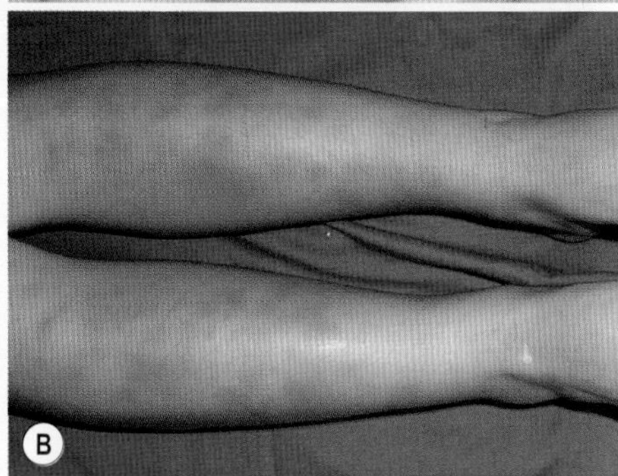

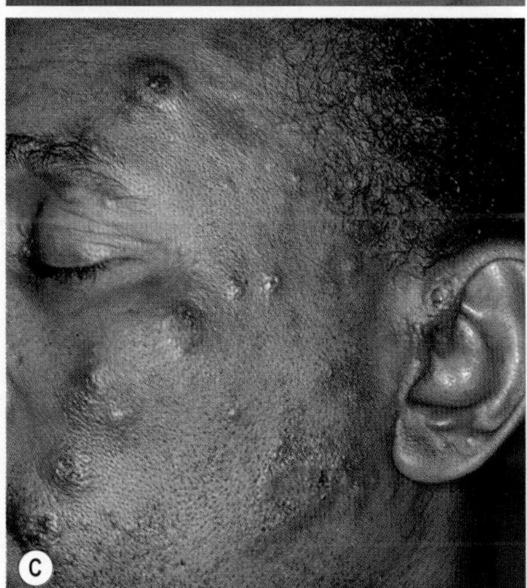

Fig. 62.8 Leprosy reactions. A Type 1 "upgrading" reaction with lupus erythematosus-like facial involvement in a "butterfly" distribution with marked inflammation. **B** Erythema nodosum leprosum, a type 2 reaction, presenting with erythematous nodules on the legs. **C** Type 2 reaction presenting with red facial papulonodules due to immune complex-mediated small vessel vasculitis in a patient with lepromatous leprosy. *A,B, Courtesy, Marcia Ramos-e-Silva, MD; C, Courtesy, Louis A. Fragola, Jr., MD.*

- Scrofuloderma – firm, subcutaneous nodules that become fluctuant; may ulcerate or drain via sinus tracts that heal as tethered scars; represents spread of infection from underlying disease (e.g. in bones and lymph nodes, often cervical; Fig. 62.10).
- Lupus vulgaris – typically a red-brown plaque that can expand with central scar formation (Fig. 62.11); as with other granulomatous skin diseases such as sarcoidosis, pressure (diascopy) results in a yellow-brown color; represents direct extension or hematogenous/lymphatic spread of infection.
  - Impaired cellular immunity (TST/PPD usually negative)
- Orificial TB – autoinoculation of skin or mucosa adjacent to an orifice draining an active tuberculous infection (Fig. 62.12); occurs in patients with advanced internal TB.
- Miliary TB – small erythematous papules that develop central crusting and may resemble a viral exanthem or pityriasis lichenoides et varioliformis acuta (PLEVA); secondary to hematogenous spread from a primary lung focus.
- Tuberculous gumma – firm subcutaneous nodule or fluctuant swelling that often ulcerates; seen in the setting of hematogenous dissemination.
- Tuberculids (cutaneous immune reactions to *M. tuberculosis*).
  - Papulonecrotic tuberculid – widely distributed, dusky red papules or papulopustules, sometimes with central crusts; favors the extremities and may resemble PLEVA (Fig. 62.13)
  - Lichen scrofulosorum – small pink to yellow-brown perifollicular papules with scale, often in clusters on the trunk
  - Erythema induratum, a form of panniculitis – subcutaneous nodules that may ulcerate; favors the posterior calves (see Ch. 83)
- Confirmation of diagnosis: tuberculin skin test (TST/PPD) or IFN-γ release assays (e.g. QuantiFERON-TB Gold [In-Tube]) or testing of tissue with polymerase chain reaction for *M. tuberculosis* DNA; advantages and disadvantages of the first two tests are outlined in Table 62.5.
- **Rx:** pending sensitivities, an example of an initial multidrug regimen includes rifampin, isoniazid, pyrazinamide, and ethambutol.

DIFFERENTIAL DIAGNOSIS OF LEPROSY		
Hypopigmented lesions		• Mycosis fungoides, including the hypopigmented variant • Sarcoidosis, but hypopigmented variant is usually more papulonodular • Postinflammatory hypopigmentation
Circinate (annular) plaques		• Mycosis fungoides and other forms of cutaneous lymphoma • Sarcoidosis • Psoriasis • Interstitial granulomatous dermatitis • Granuloma annulare • Tinea corporis
Infiltrated plaques/nodules		• Lymphoma • Sarcoidosis • Other infections (dimorphic fungal, tuberculous) • For DDx of leonine facies, see Table 38.1
Neurologic findings		• Peripheral neuropathy due to other disorders (e.g. diabetes mellitus, vasculitis)
Deforming acral features		• Systemic sclerosis • Tabes dorsalis • Dupuytren contracture
Type 1 reaction		• Acute lupus erythematosus • Cellulitis • Drug reactions • Misdiagnosed as worsening of disease as subclinical lesions may become apparent
Type 2 reaction		• Sweet syndrome • Medium-vessel vasculitis • Panniculitides, e.g. erythema nodosum* • Infections, including other mycobacterial, bacterial, dimorphic fungal, and other opportunistic fungal

**Lesions favor the shins and are longer-lived than erythema nodosum leprosum lesions, which are widespread, appear in crops and then resolve relatively rapidly.*

Table 62.4 Differential diagnosis of leprosy.

Atypical Mycobacteria

• Found in the natural environment (water, wet soil, vegetation, cold-blooded animals [e.g. fish], dairy products, human feces).

• Skin infections most commonly arise via traumatic inoculation; other routes include surgical or cosmetic procedures (e.g. liposuction, tattooing) and exposure to contaminated water (e.g. soaking distal lower extremities prior to pedicure; see Table 62.2).

• Clinically, pustules, plaques, or nodules develop that may become keratotic or centrally ulcerated.

• A sporotrichoid or lymphocutaneous pattern (linear arrangement of lesions along draining lymphatics) may be seen (Figs 62.14–62.16).

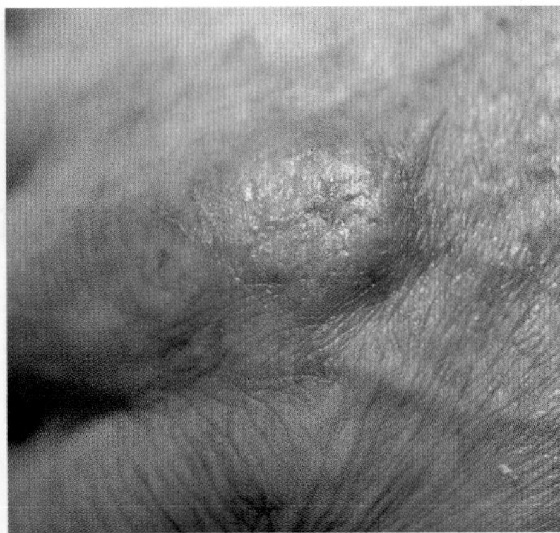

Fig. 62.9 Tuberculosis verrucosa cutis. A wart-like papule at the site of exogenous inoculation in a patient with immunity against *M. tuberculosis*. *Courtesy, YDRSC.*

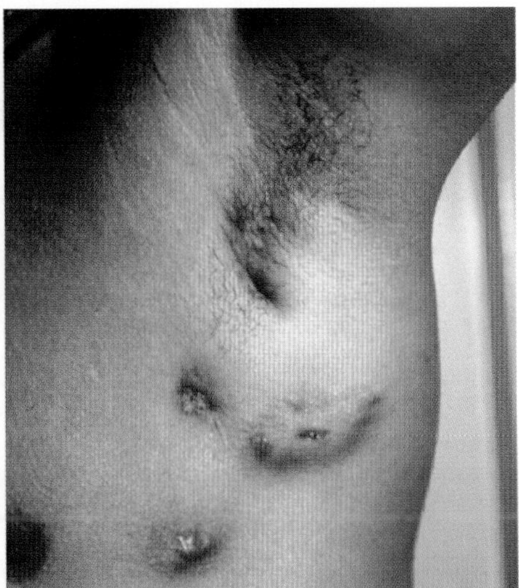

Fig. 62.10 Scrofuloderma. Plaques and nodules with central ulceration as well as resultant scarring with retraction. *Courtesy, YDRSC.*

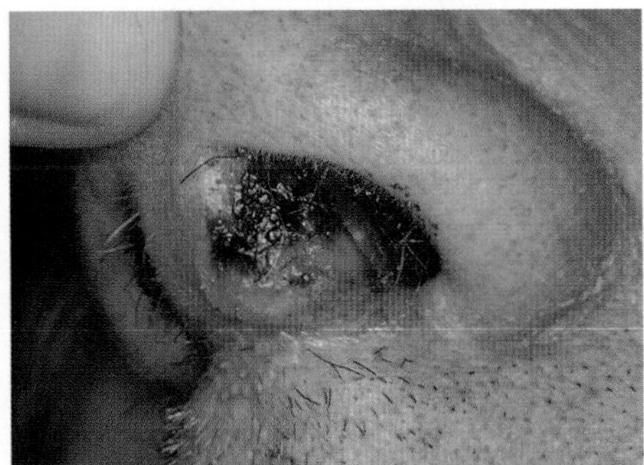

Fig. 62.12 Orificial tuberculosis. A non-healing ulcer of the nasal mucosa. *Courtesy, Louis A. Fragola, Jr., MD.*

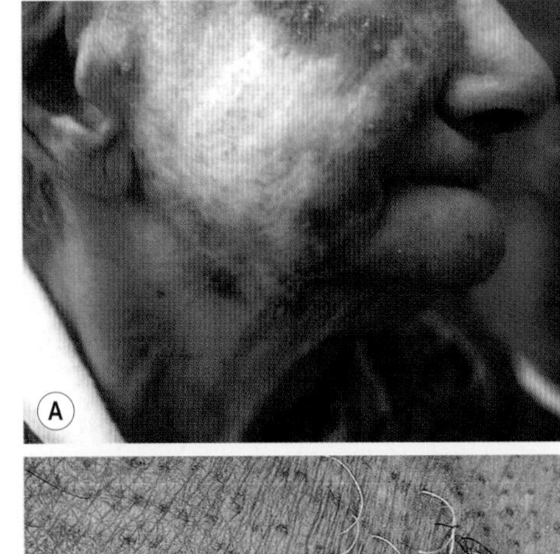

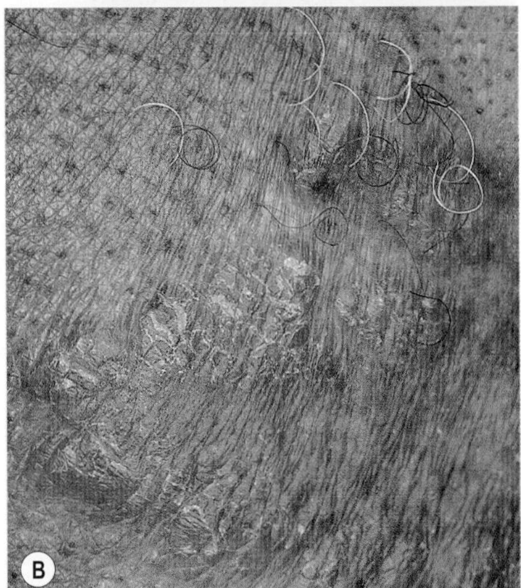

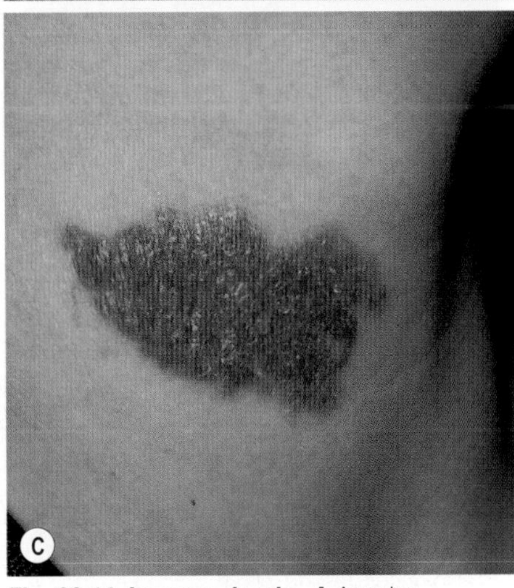

Fig. 62.11 Lupus vulgaris. A Annular granulomatous plaque with central scarring. **B** Two dull red-brown plaques with papular borders, scale and central clearing. **C** Violet-brown plaque on the neck. *A, Courtesy, Marcia Ramos-e-Silva, MD; B, Courtesy, YDRSC; C, Courtesy, Eugene Mirrer, MD.*

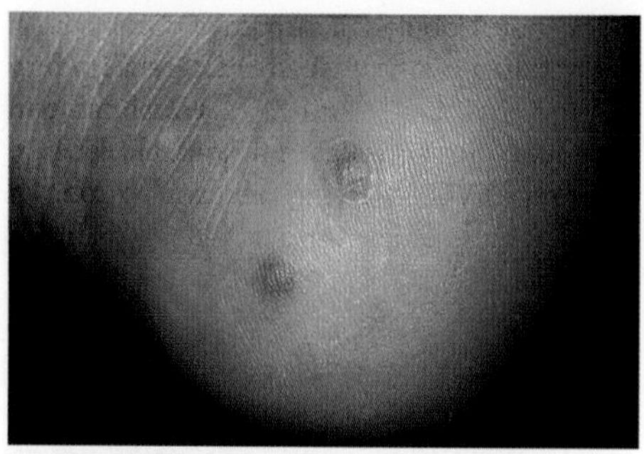

Fig. 62.13 Papulonecrotic tuberculid. Erythematous papules and papulopustules on the heel. *Courtesy, YDRSC.*

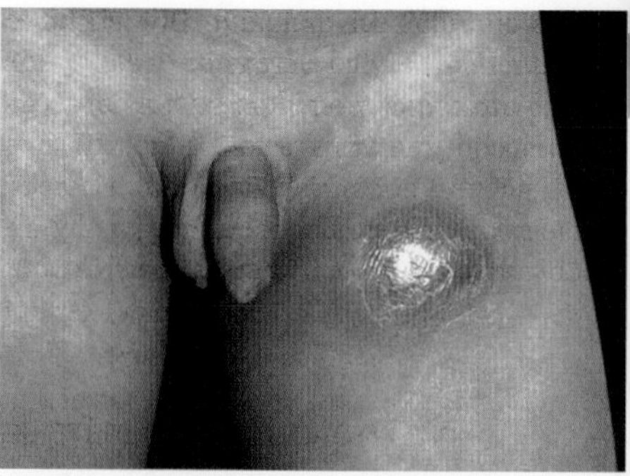

Fig. 62.14 Suppurative lymphadenitis due to *Mycobacterium fortuitum* infection. The inoculation chancre was on the foot. *From Azulay RD, Neves RG, Estrella RR, et al. Complexo primario cutaneoganglionar por Mycobacterium fortuitum. AMB Rev Assoc Med Bras. 1974;20:177–81. Courtesy, Rubem Azulay, MD.*

ADVANTAGES AND DISADVANTAGES OF IFN-γ RELEASE ASSAYS AND TUBERCULIN SKIN TESTING		
	Tuberculin skin test	**IFN-γ release assays**
Advantages	Does not require a laboratory Relatively low cost	Requires a single patient visit Results can be available within 24 hours Prior BCG vaccination does not cause a false-positive result Does not boost responses measured by subsequent tests
Disadvantages	Requires two patient visits Results not available for 48 hours Prior BCG vaccination can cause a false-positive result May boost responses in subsequent tests Infections with non-tuberculous mycobacteria may lead to a false-positive result	Requires laboratory processing within 16 hours (for QuantiFERON®-TB Gold [In-Tube]) or 8 hours (for T-SPOT®.TB; time limit of 30 hours if use T-cell Xtend®) Relatively high cost Infections with some non-tuberculous mycobacteria (e.g. *M. kansasii*, *M. szulgai*, and *M. marinum*) may lead to a false-positive result
Situations where preferable	Children <5 years of age	Patient groups that historically have low rates of returning for a second visit (e.g. homeless persons, drug users) Individuals who have received BCG

Table 62.5 Advantages and disadvantages of interferon-γ (IFN-γ) release assays and tuberculin skin testing. Both types of tests may be negative in patients with early active tuberculosis. Indeterminate IFN-γ release assay results due to failure of the internal positive control (i.e. a "low mitogen" response) are more common in immunocompromised individuals and young children. Indeterminate results due to inappropriately high IFN-γ levels in the negative control ("high nil") can also occur. Testing with a second method after an initial negative test may be useful when the risk of infection/progression is high or when there is clinical suspicion of active tuberculosis. The QuantiFERON®-TB Gold (In-Tube) test directly measures IFN-γ levels, whereas the T-SPOT®.TB test determines the number of IFN-γ-producing T cells; both use a peripheral blood sample. BCG, bacille Calmette–Guérin.

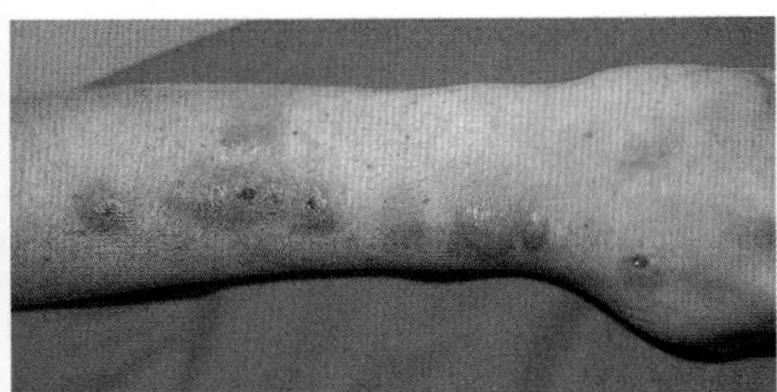

Fig. 62.15 Complication of injection of methanol extraction residue (MER) of bacille Calmette–Guérin (BCG), an attenuated strain of *Mycobacterium bovis*. Nodules, some of which have ulcerated, are arranged in a linear "lymphatic" pattern in a patient with a high-risk extremity melanoma who had received an injection of MER of BCG as adjuvant immunotherapy. *Courtesy, YDRSC.*

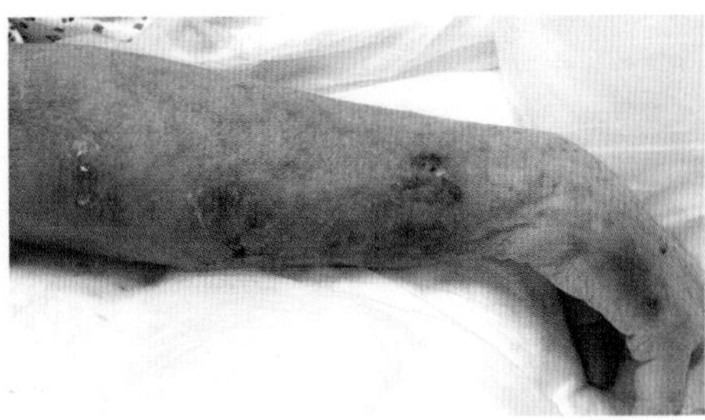

Fig. 62.16 *Mycobacterium avium* complex cellulitis in a patient on chronic CS for rheumatoid arthritis. Note the sporotrichoid (lymphocutaneous) pattern of the coalescing nodules with abscess formation. *Courtesy, YDRSC.*

- Disseminated infection can occur in immunocompromised hosts.
- *Mycobacterium marinum* infection is seen most frequently in the United States.
  - Found in aquatic environments, including fish tanks and swimming pools
  - Bluish-red inflammatory nodule or pustule that may ulcerate; over time, can develop additional lesions in a sporotrichoid pattern (Fig. 62.17)
- **DDx:** other infections with sporotrichoid spread (e.g. sporotrichosis, nocardiosis) (see Table 64.7).
- **Rx:** pending sensitivities, empiric treatment of infection with *M. marinum* is clarithromycin, and additional antibiotics include minocycline and rifampin; localized infection with *M. ulcerans* or *M. scrofulaceum* can be excised; more disseminated disease usually requires a multidrug regimen for at least 3–6 months.

For further information see Ch. 75 from *Dermatology, Fourth Edition*.

For additional online figures and tables visit www.expertconsult.com 

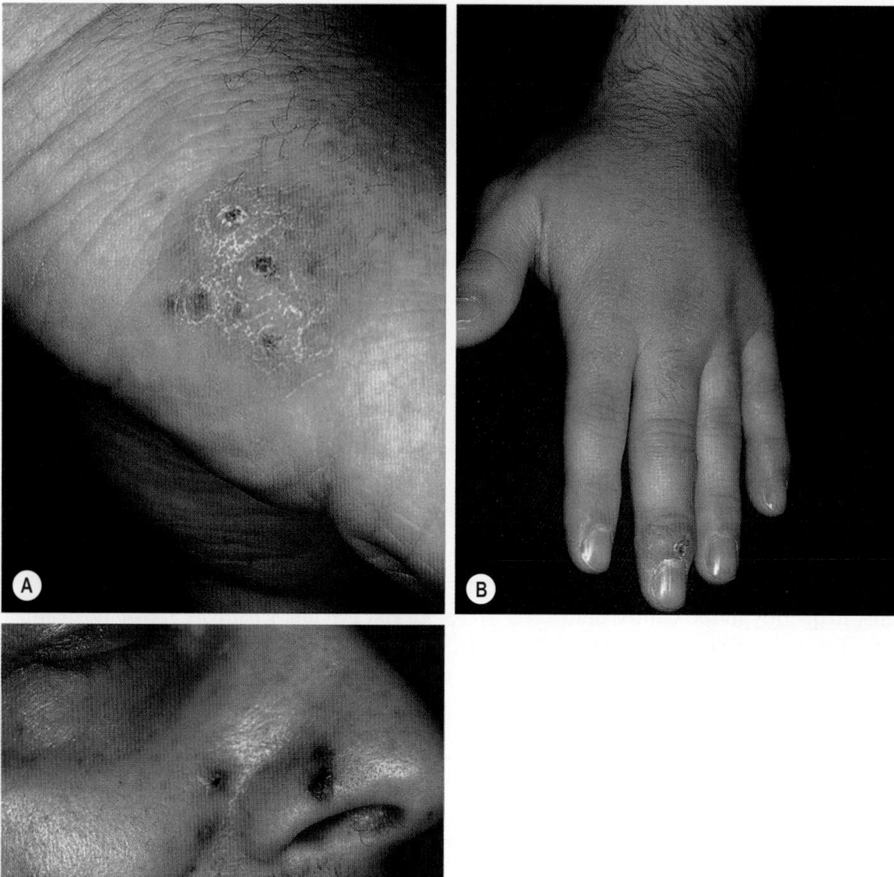

Fig. 62.17 *Mycobacterium marinum* infections. A range of presentations, including an erythematous plaque with scale-crust at the inoculation site on the lateral hand (**A**), a sporotrichoid pattern with the inoculation site on the distal third finger (**B**), and disseminated necrotic lesions on the face of an immunocompromised patient (**C**). *Courtesy, YDRSC.*

Rickettsial Diseases 63

Rickettsial infections often have cutaneous manifestations that can vary from nonspecific maculopapular eruptions to an eschar at the site of inoculation (by the vector) to petechiae and retiform purpura (Table 63.1). These Gram-negative bacteria reside within an arthropod – tick, flea, mite, or louse – during a portion of their life cycle and are transmitted to humans while feeding, either via saliva or via feces (Table 63.2). As a result, rickettsial diseases exhibit both seasonality and geographic diversity.

Rickettsia and *Orientia* spp. target endothelial cells of multiple organs, including the skin, whereas *Ehrlichia*, *Anaplasma*, and *Coxiella* spp. target monocytes or neutrophils, neutrophils, and macrophages, respectively.

Rocky Mountain Spotted Fever (RMSF)

- Due to transmission of *Rickettsia rickettsia* by the bite of a tick, most commonly *Dermacentor* spp. (Fig. 63.1); the incubation period is 2–14 days (mean, 7 days) following the bite.
- Highest incidence in the south Atlantic and south central states (Fig. 63.2), not the Rocky Mountain states, with peak incidence from late spring to the end of summer (tick season).
- Begins as a subtle cutaneous eruption with pink to erythematous macules then papules, initially in acral sites (e.g. wrists, ankles); over time central petechiae develop and lesions become more widespread (Figs 63.3–63.6).
- In the majority of patients, the skin findings are preceded by a fever (for 3–5 days), myalgias, and severe headache; some patients also develop nausea and vomiting and a change in mental status; if not treated appropriately, acute renal failure, hypotension, and coma can ensue, with a mortality rate of up to 25%.
- Dx: biopsy of petechial papule or eschar followed by PCR and/or immunohistochemistry (Table 63.3); serologic results are not helpful in the acute setting.
- **DDx:** viral exanthem (e.g. enterovirus, EBV, measles, parvovirus B19, dengue virus; see Fig. 68.1), other rickettsial spotted fevers (similar eruption but more likely to have an inoculation eschar; see Table 63.1), typhus (several forms), ehrlichiosis, morbilliform drug reaction; when severe and purpuric, meningococcemia, other thrombotic vasculopathies, vasculitis, hemorrhagic fevers.
- **Rx:** begun empirically; doxycycline or tetracycline represents first-line therapy, even in children (Table 63.4).

Typhus – Epidemic and Endemic (Murine)

- While the vector differs for epidemic (human body louse) versus endemic (flea) typhus, spread of the infection involves deposition of feces onto the skin followed by scratching into the skin, rubbing into mucous membranes, or inhalation.
- The eruption often begins in the axillae and then becomes more widespread, with relative sparing of the face; individual lesions are similar to those seen in RMSF.
- **DDx** and **Rx:** see section on RMSF.

Rickettsialpox

- Most often occurs in urban areas.
- Within 48 hours, a papulovesicle (then eschar) develops at the site of the bite of the mouse mite (Fig. 63.7A); fever, myalgias, and headache appear 1–2 weeks later followed soon thereafter by a cutaneous eruption.
- The eruption has a widespread distribution that includes the face, but the number of lesions is usually limited, i.e. ~20–40;

DERMATOLOGIC MANIFESTATIONS OF RICKETTSIAL INFECTIONS				
Disease	**Rash incidence (%)**	**Appearance of rash after onset of illness**	**Characteristics**	**Eschar (%)**
Rocky Mountain spotted fever, Brazilian spotted fever	90	3–5 days	Early macules, later papules; petechiae in 50% of cases; retiform purpura in severe disease	<1
Rickettsialpox	100	2–3 days	Early macules and papules; later papulo-vesicles and crusts	90
Rickettsia parkeri rickettsiosis	80	2–4 days	Macules, papules, often vesicles	100
Boutonneuse fever and related conditions	95	3–5 days	Early macules, later papules	50
North Asian tick typhus and related conditions	100	4–5 days	Macules and papules	75
Queensland tick typhus	90	2–6 days	Macules, papules, and vesicles	75
Flinders Island spotted fever	85	A few days	Early macules and pap-ules, later (in some patients) petechiae	50
Japanese spotted fever	100	A few days	Early macules, later (in some patients) petechiae	90
Flea-borne spotted fever	80	A few days	Macules and papules; occasionally pustules	15–20
African tick bite fever	50	2–5 days	Generally relatively few lesions; macules, often vesicles	90, often multiple
R. aeschlimannii infection	50	Not known	Macules, papules	100
Tick-borne lymphadenopathy	5	Not reported	Macules, papules	100
Epidemic louse-borne typhus	50–100	4–5 days	Early macules, later papules; petechiae	None
Brill–Zinsser disease	50	4–6 days	Macules, papules	None
Flying squirrel typhus	65	2–8 days	Macules, papules	None
Murine (endemic) typhus	80	5 days	Early macules, later papules	None
Scrub typhus	50	4–6 days	Early macules, later papules	60–90
Human monocytic ehrlichiosis	40	Median, 5 days	Macules, papules, occasionally petechiae	None
Ehrlichia muris-like agent ehrlichiosis	10	Not reported	Not reported	None
Anaplasmosis (human granulocytic anaplasmosis)	≤5	Not reported	Erythematous eruption on neck/chest; petechiae or purpura	None
Q fever	Rare	Associated with chronic infection	Macules, papules, pal-pable purpura; rarely erythema nodosum	None

Table 63.1 Dermatologic manifestations of rickettsial infections. Skin findings have not been described in patients with *Ehrlichia ewingii* ehrlichiosis. *Courtesy, David H. Walker, MD.*

EPIDEMIOLOGY OF RICKETTSIAL INFECTIONS			
Agent	**Disease**	**Transmission**	**Geographic distribution**
Rickettsia rickettsii	Rocky Mountain spotted fever, Brazilian spotted fever	**Bite of tick:**	
		Dermacentor variabilis (Fig. 63.1)	Eastern two-thirds and Pacific Coast of US
		D. andersoni	Rocky Mountain states
		Rhipicephalus sanguineus	Southwestern US; northern Mexico; Brazil
		Amblyomma cajennense, A. aureolatum, A. imitator, A. sculptum	Mexico; Central and South America
Rickettsia akari	Rickettsialpox	**Bite of mouse mite:**	
		Liponyssoides sanguineus	North America; Eurasia
Rickettsia parkeri	*Rickettsia parkeri* rickettsiosis (maculatum disease, American tick bite fever)	**Bite of tick:**	
		Amblyomma maculatum, A. americanum	North America
		A. triste	South America
Rickettsia conorii (4 subspecies)	Boutonneuse fever (Mediterranean spotted fever), Indian and Israeli tick typhus, Astrakhan spotted fever	**Bite of tick:**	
		Rhipicephalus sanguineus	Southern Europe; Africa; western and southern Asia
		Rh. pumilio	Southern Russia
Rickettsia sibirica	North Asian and Siberian tick typhus, lymphangitis-associated rickettsiosis	**Bite of tick:**	
		Dermacentor nuttallii, D. silvarum, Haemaphysalis concinna, Hyalomma asiaticum, other species	Eurasia and Africa
Rickettsia australis	Queensland tick typhus	**Bite of tick:**	
		Ixodes holocyclus	Eastern Australia
Rickettsia honei	Flinders Island spotted fever	**Bite of tick:**	
		Bothriocroton hydrosauri, other species	Australia and Nepal (Flinders Island is located between Tasmania and mainland Australia)
Rickettsia japonica	Japanese spotted fever	**Bite of tick:**	
		Vector status not established for ticks that carry the agent (*Haemaphysalis flava, H. longicornis, Ixodes ovatus, Dermacentor taiwanensis*)	Japan; eastern Asia

Table 63.2 Epidemiology of rickettsial infections. *Continued*

EPIDEMIOLOGY OF RICKETTSIAL INFECTIONS			
Agent	**Disease**	**Transmission**	**Geographic distribution**
Rickettsia felis	Flea-borne spotted fever	**By flea**:	
		e.g. *Ctenocephalides felis*	Worldwide
Rickettsia africae	African tick bite fever	**Bite of tick**:	
		Amblyomma hebraeum	Southern Africa
		A. variegatum	Central, eastern, and western Africa; Caribbean islands
Rickettsia aeschlimannii	*Rickettsia aeschlimannii* disease	**Bite of tick**:	
		Hyalomma marginatum	Africa
Rickettsia slovaca, *R. raoultii*, or *Candidatus Rickettsia rioja*	Tick-borne lymphadenopathy, *Dermacentor*-borne necrosis and lymphadenopathy (DEBONEL)	**Bite of tick** (usually on the scalp):	
		Dermacentor marginatus, *D. reticularis*	Europe
Rickettsia prowazekii	Epidemic louse-borne typhus	**Feces of human body louse** (*Pediculus humanus* var. *corporis*)	South America; Africa; Eurasia
	Brill–Zinsser disease	**None (recrudescence of latent infection)**	
	Flying squirrel typhus	**Contact with flying squirrel** (*Glaucomys volans*) and its fleas and lice	North America
Rickettsia typhi	Murine (endemic) typhus	**Feces of fleas:** *Xenopsylla cheopis* *Ctenocephalides felis*	Worldwide North America
Orientia tsutsugamushi	Scrub typhus	**Bite of larval trombiculid mites:**	
		Leptotrombidium deliense, *L. fletcheri*, *L. scutellare*, *L. arenicola*	Southern and eastern Asia; islands of the southwestern Pacific and Indian Oceans; northern Australia
		e.g. *L. pallidum*	Japan; Korea; Russian Far East
		e.g. *L. scutellare*	China; Malaysia
		e.g. *L. deliense, L. fletcheri*, *L. arenicola*	Tropical regions
Ehrlichia chaffeensis	Human monocytic ehrlichiosis	**Bite of tick**:	
		Amblyomma americanum (Fig. 63.1), *Dermacentor variabilis*	Southeastern and south central US

Table 63.2 *Continued* **Epidemiology of rickettsial infections.**

EPIDEMIOLOGY OF RICKETTSIAL INFECTIONS			
Agent	**Disease**	**Transmission**	**Geographic distribution**
Ehrlichia muris-like (EML) agent	EML agent ehrlichiosis	**Bite of tick:**	
		Ixodes scapularis	Upper midwestern US
Ehrlichia ewingii	*Ehrlichia ewingii ehrlichiosis*	**Bite of tick**:	
		Amblyomma americanum	Southeastern and south central US
Anaplasma phagocytophilum	Human granulocytic anaplasmosis	**Bite of tick**:	
		Ixodes scapularis (Fig. 63.1)	Northern US
		I. pacificus	Far western US
		I. ricinus, I. persulcatus	Eurasia
Coxiella burnetii	Q fever	**Aerosol** of infected products of parturition of ruminants (e.g. sheep, cattle, goats), cats, and other animals*	Worldwide

**Less common means of transmission include ingestion of contaminated dairy products and tick bites (e.g. Dermacentor spp.).*

Table 63.2 *Continued* **Epidemiology of rickettsial infections.** Additional tick-borne infections include Pacific Coast tick fever (*Rickettsia philipii*, type strain "Rickettsia 364D"), Far Eastern spotted fever (*Rickettsia heilongjiangenesis*), *Rickettsia massiliae* rickettsiosis, and *Candidatus Neoehrlichia mikurensis* infection. *Courtesy, David H. Walker, MD.*

the individual macules and papules develop central vesicles and hemorrhagic crusts (Fig. 63.7B).

- **DDx:** varicella and disseminated zoster, other vesicular viral exanthems (e.g. Coxsackie), pityriasis lichenoides et varioliformis acuta (PLEVA), bullous insect bite reactions, scabies.
- **Rx:** tetracycline or doxycycline (dosages in Table 63.4).

Ehrlichiosis

- The primary vector for ehrlichiosis is the lone star tick *Amblyomma americanum* (Figs 63.1 and 63.8), with the white-tailed deer serving as a major reservoir.
- In addition to fever, headache, and myalgias, patients with human monocytic ehrlichiosis (HME) can develop meningoencephalitis and acute respiratory distress syndrome, with overwhelming disease in immunocompromised hosts.
- Mucocutaneous lesions appear an average of 5 days into the illness of HME and vary from a widespread morbilliform eruption to petechiae favoring the palms and soles to vesicular; occasionally palpable purpura due to small vessel vasculitis can occur.
- Dx: PCR of blood, with intracytoplasmic macrocolonies of bacteria sometimes noted in peripheral blood smears.
- **DDx:** see sections on RMSF and rickettsialpox (if vesicular).
- **Rx:** see Table 63.4.

Anaplasmosis (Human Granulocytic Anaplasmosis)

- Cutaneous manifestations are rare (<5% of patients), but patients may have concurrent signs and symptoms of Lyme borreliosis and/or babesiosis because all three infections are transmitted by *Ixodes* ticks, e.g. *I. scapularis* in the northeastern United States (see Fig. 63.8).
- The illness is usually not as severe as HME and patients may have peripheral neuropathy.
- **Rx:** see Table 63.4.

For further information see Ch. 76 from *Dermatology, Fourth Edition*.

For additional online figures visit www.expertconsult.com 

COMPARISON OF *IXODES SCAPULARIS*, *AMBLYOMMA AMERICANUM*, AND *DERMACENTOR VARIABILIS*, BY LIFE STAGE

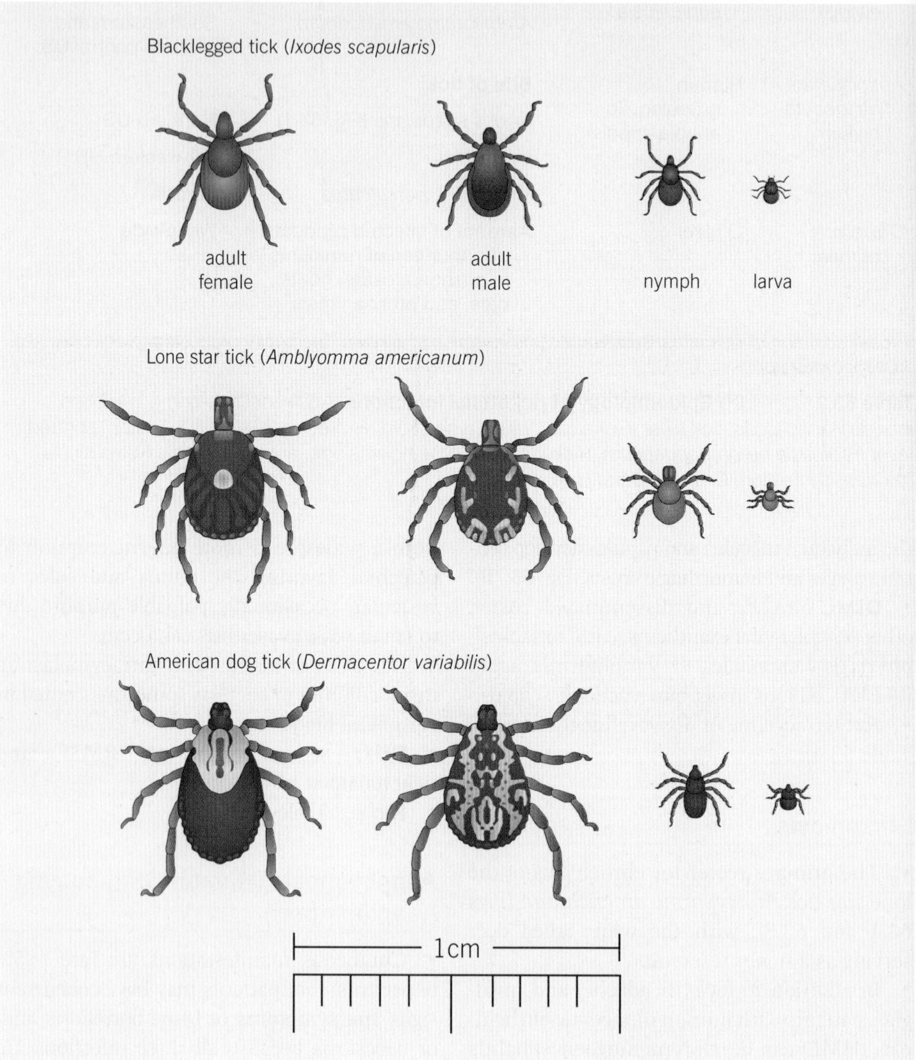

Blacklegged tick (*Ixodes scapularis*)

adult female | adult male | nymph | larva

Lone star tick (*Amblyomma americanum*)

American dog tick (*Dermacentor variabilis*)

1cm

Fig. 63.1 Comparison of *Ixodes scapularis* (blacklegged tick), *Amblyomma americanum* (lone star tick), and *Dermacentor variabilis* (American dog tick), by life stage. *From Chapman, A. S., et al. MMWR Recomm Rep 2006;55:1–27.*

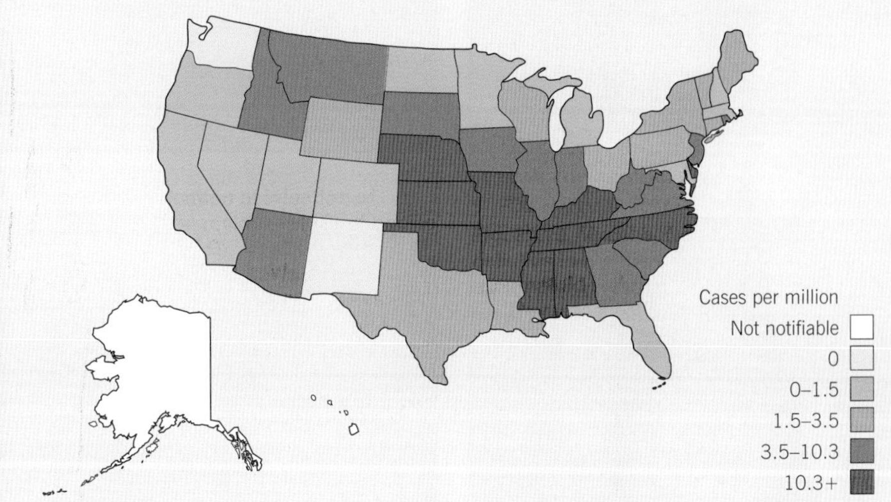

Fig. 63.2 Annual reported incidence (per million persons) for spotted fever rickettsiosis (SFR) in the United States, 2016. As of 2010, cases of RMSF are reported under the category of SFR, along with *Rickettsia parkeri* rickettsiosis, Pacific Coast tick fever, and rickettsialpox. *From* www.cdc.gov/rmsf/stats/#reportsurv.

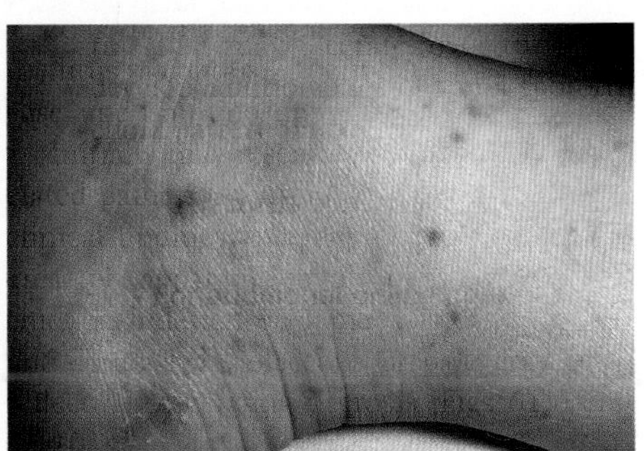

Fig. 63.3 Rocky Mountain spotted fever. The cutaneous lesions often first appear on the ankles and wrists. These are nonblanching due to hemorrhage within the skin. *Courtesy, Philippe Berbis, MD.*

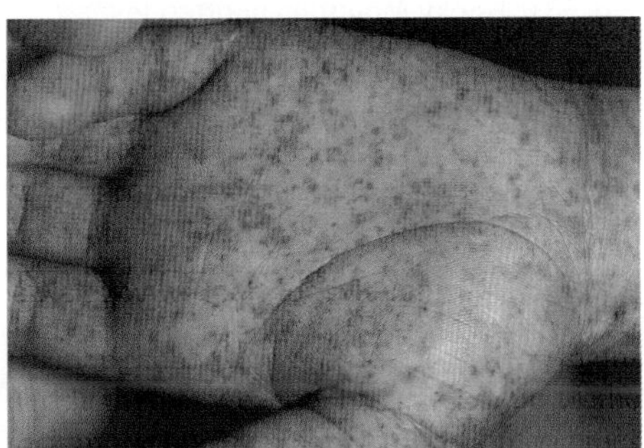

Fig. 63.4 Rocky Mountain spotted fever. Petechiae on the palms and soles often develop relatively later in the disease course. *Courtesy, Ronald Rapini, MD.*

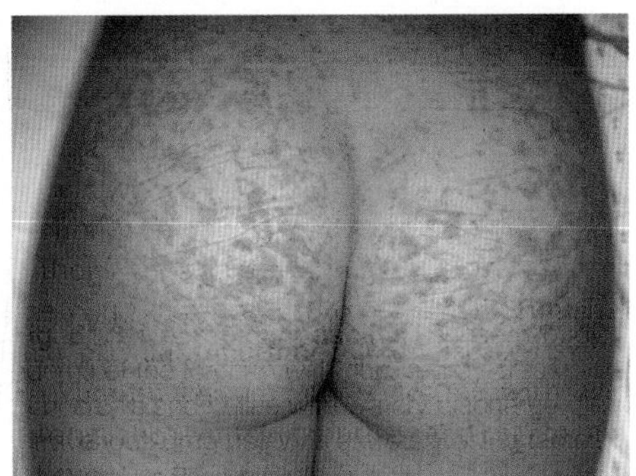

Fig. 63.5 Rocky Mountain spotted fever. Petechiae are present within erythematous papules and plaques on the buttocks. Some of the lesions have a retiform pattern. *Courtesy, YDRSC.*

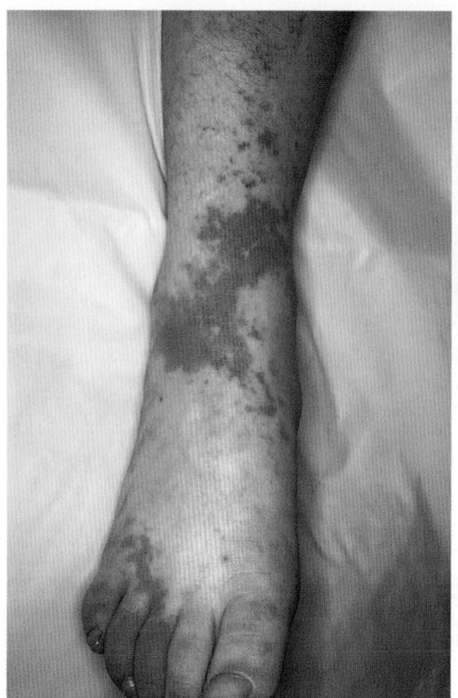

Fig. 63.6 Rocky Mountain spotted fever. Retiform purpura on the distal lower extremity in a patient with more severe disease. *Courtesy, YDRSC.*

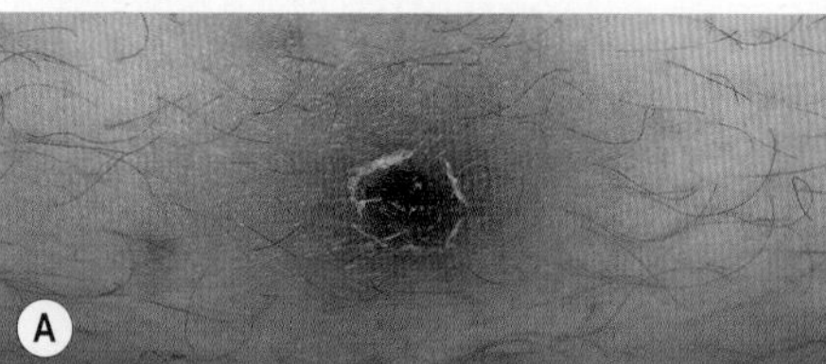

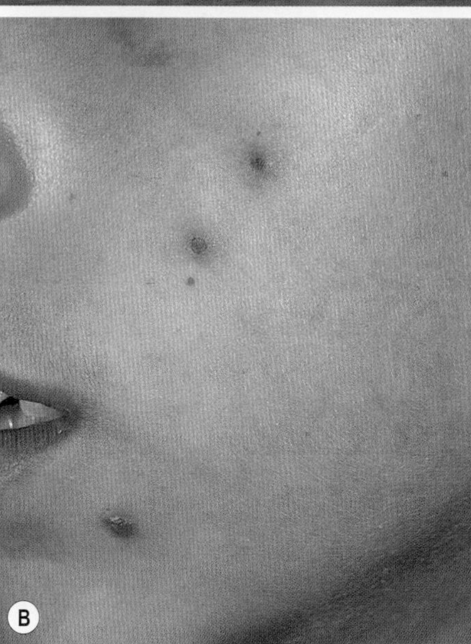

Fig. 63.7 Rickettsialpox. A Eschar at the site of the mite bite. **B** Scattered papules with central hemorrhagic crusts. *A, B, Courtesy, NYUDSC.*

EVALUATION OF SUSPECTED CUTANEOUS LESION(S) OF A SPOTTED FEVER, INCLUDING RMSF, VIA REAL-TIME PCR
• Contact the state health department to assist (required if utilizing the CDC) • 4- to 5-mm skin biopsy of a fresh but developed lesion (e.g. in the case of a spotted fever, a maculopapular lesion with pinpoint hemorrhage) that includes the center of the lesion • Appropriate treatment for <24 hours does not appear to alter sensitivity • Appropriate treatment for ≥72 hours often results in a negative test • Fresh, non-frozen tissue preferred with placement of skin biopsy inside sterile urine container on gauze moistened with sterile saline (transport overnight with cold packs) (see Fig. 2.10B) • PCR can be done on frozen tissue (transport overnight with dry ice)

Table 63.3 Evaluation of suspected cutaneous lesion(s) of a spotted fever, including Rocky Mountain spotted fever (RMSF), via real-time PCR. These recommendations are those of the Centers for Disease Control and Prevention (CDC) (https://www.cdc.gov/ncezid/dvbd/pdf/Collection-Submission-Skin-Biopsy-Specimens-Rickettsial-Disease.pdf). Cell culture isolation from fresh tissue can also be done.

TREATMENT OF RICKETTSIAL DISEASES				
	Medication	**Adult dose**	**Pediatric dose**	**Treatment duration**
• First choice for virtually all rickettsial infections in both children and adults*	Doxycycline	100 mg PO or IV twice daily	2.2 mg/kg (max. 100 mg) PO or IV twice daily	Until ≥3 days after defervescence, for a minimum total course of 5–7 days†
• Alternative for non-life-threatening rickettsial infections in pregnant women	Chloramphenicol‡	500 mg IV every 6 hours	Not recommended	Until ≥3 days after defervescence, for a minimum total course of 5–7 days†
• Alternative for non-life-threatening HME or HGA in pregnant women • Alternative for resistant scrub typhus	Rifampin	300 mg PO twice daily	10 mg/kg (max. 300 mg) twice daily	Until ≥3 days after defervescence, for a minimum total course of 7–10 days
• First choice for scrub typhus in pregnant women and potentially in children • Alternative for mild rickettsioses (e.g. early boutonneuse fever) during pregnancy or in children	Azithromycin§	500 mg PO daily	10 mg/kg PO daily	3 days

*With the exception of infections in pregnant women, although doxycycline administration during pregnancy can be considered in life-threatening situations when the suspicion of RMSF or other severe rickettsioses is high; other tetracyclines are also effective for rickettsial infections.
†Recommended by the CDC; others recommend a 10-day course.
‡May be associated with gray baby syndrome when administered late in the third trimester of pregnancy.
§Clarithromycin may also be considered.

Table 63.4 Treatment of rickettsial diseases. Empiric treatment with an appropriate agent should be initiated immediately when a diagnosis of Rocky Mountain spotted fever (RMSF), human monocytic ehrlichiosis (HME), human granulocytic anaplasmosis (HGA), or another potentially severe rickettsiosis is suspected clinically.

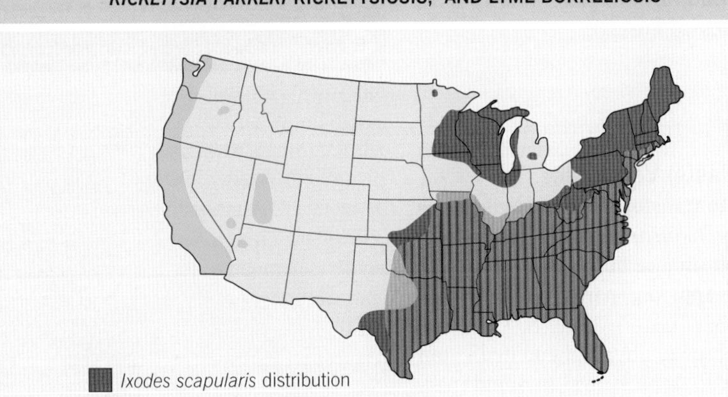

Fig. 63.8 Approximate distribution in the United States of vector tick species for human monocytic ehrlichiosis, human granulocytic anaplasmosis, *Rickettsia parkeri* rickettsiosis, and Lyme borreliosis. It has been postulated that *Amblyomma maculatum*, which is classically found primarily along the Atlantic and Gulf coasts, has a range as broad as that of *Amblyomma americanum*. *From Chapman, A. S., et al. MMWR Recomm Rep 2006;55:1–27.*

64 Fungal Diseases

Key Points

- Cutaneous fungal diseases can be broadly divided into two groups:
  - Superficial – limited to the stratum corneum, hair, and/or nails
  - Deep – dermal and/or subcutaneous
- Superficial fungal infections can be further subdivided into:
  - Non-inflammatory – most commonly tinea versicolor, but includes tinea nigra and piedra
  - Inflammatory – primarily infections due to dermatophytes (*Trichophyton*, *Microsporum*, *Epidermophyton*; e.g. tinea corporis, tinea cruris) or *Candida* spp. (e.g. cutaneous candidiasis of the groin)
- Deep fungal infections are often secondary to implantation (e.g. sporotrichosis, chromo(blasto) mycosis, eumycetoma) or hematogenous spread of an underlying systemic infection (e.g. cryptococcosis, coccidioidomycosis).
- Opportunistic pathogens (e.g. *Aspergillus*, *Mucor*) can lead to systemic infection in immunosuppressed hosts.

Superficial Fungal Infections

Tinea (Pityriasis) Versicolor

- Secondary to transformation of *Malassezia* spp., especially *M. furfur*, from the yeast form to the hyphal form (see Fig. 2.1A).
- *Malassezia* spp. are part of the normal flora.
- Multiple, brown (hyperpigmented), tan (hypopigmented), or pink, oval to round macules, patches, or thin plaques; there is often coalescence of lesions centrally with scattered lesions at the periphery.
- Associated scale may be subtle but becomes more obvious with gentle scratching or stretching of the skin.
- Most commonly develops on the upper trunk and shoulders, but can also involve flexural sites such as the antecubital fossae, submammary folds, and groin (Fig. 64.1); in children more frequently than adults, there can also be facial involvement.

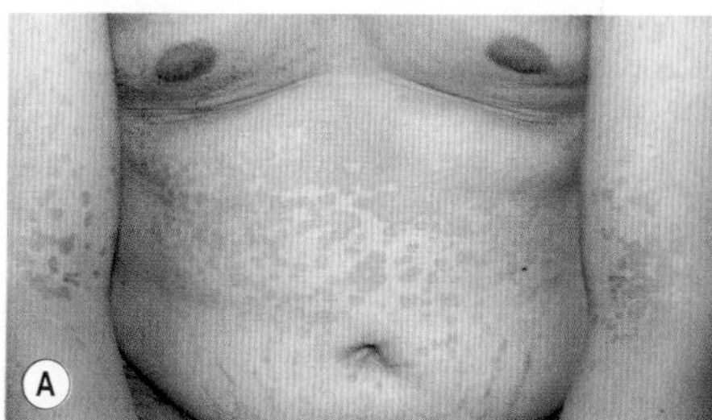

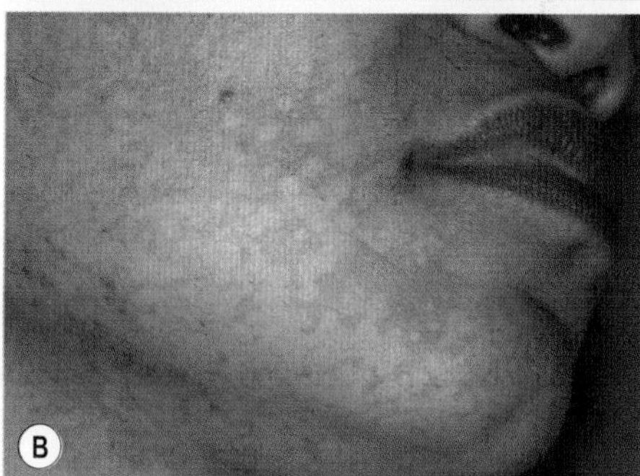

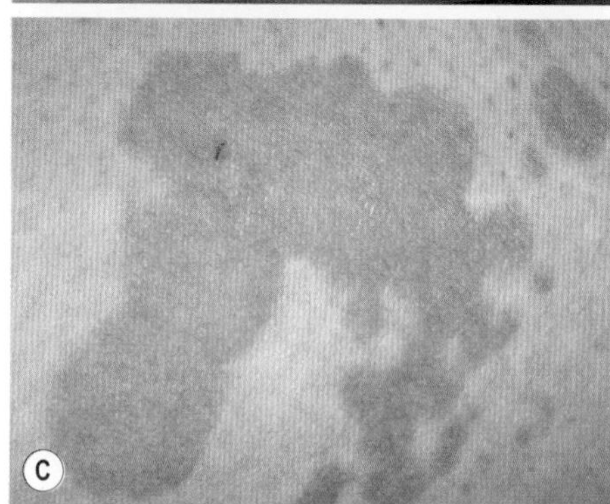

Fig. 64.1 Tinea (pityriasis) versicolor. **A** Hyperpigmented variant. **B** Hypopigmented variant on the face. **C** Coalescing pink lesions with fine scale. *A, B, Courtesy, Kalman Watsky, MD; C, Courtesy, Boni E. Elewski, MD and Roderick J. Hay, MD.*

TREATMENT OF TINEA (PITYRIASIS) VERSICOLOR	
Initial therapy (often combination)	**Topical** • Application of antifungal shampoo for 10 minutes to 1 hour weekly to twice weekly for 2–4 weeks • Selenium sulfide shampoo, 1% (OTC) or 2.5% • Ketoconazole shampoo, 1% (OTC) or 2% • Imidazoles, e.g. ketoconazole 2% cream daily to BID × 2 weeks • Apply several hand-widths beyond clinically visible lesions
	Oral • Fluconazole 200–400 mg PO once weekly × 2–3 doses
Maintenance therapy (tinea versicolor commonly recurs)	**Examples of topical regimens** • Treat previously affected sites with topical imidazole daily for 2 weeks prior to anticipated sun exposure (temperate climates) • Apply antifungal shampoo (see above) 1–2 times every month (tropical climates)

Table 64.1 Treatment of tinea (pityriasis) versicolor.

- Often first noticed in the summer, and a suntan accentuates the hypopigmented variant.
- **DDx:** postinflammatory hypopigmentation and idiopathic macular hypomelanosis (if hypopigmented); confluent and reticulated papillomatosis of Gougerot and Carteaud (if hyperpigmented; see Ch. 89).
- **Rx:** outlined in Table 64.1.
- Following appropriate **Rx**, the associated hypopigmentation may persist for months until there is repigmentation or fading of the suntan.

Tinea Nigra, Black Piedra, and White Piedra

- Typically seen in tropical areas.
- Tinea nigra:
  - Most commonly due to infection with *Hortaea werneckii*, a pigmented fungus found in soil
  - Brown, sharply marginated macule or patch; most commonly on the palms (Fig. 64.2)
  - **Rx:** keratolytic agents (e.g. salicylic acid 6% cream) and topical antifungals (e.g. terbinafine 1% cream)
- Black piedra and white piedra are characterized by the formation of nodules on hair shafts (Table 64.2; Fig. 64.3).

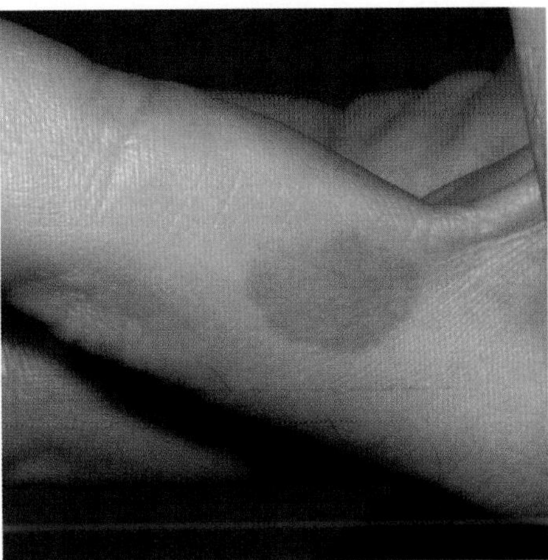

Fig. 64.2 Tinea nigra. Single, sharply demarcated brown macule on the finger. *Courtesy, Frank Samarin, MD.*

Dermatophytoses (Tinea Infections)

- The names of dermatophyte infections consist of the word "tinea" followed by the Latin name for the involved body site; examples are tinea pedis (foot) and tinea cruris (groin) (Fig. 64.4).
- Due to fungi of three genera – *Trichophyton*, *Microsporum*, and *Epidermophyton* – that invade only keratinized tissue (stratum corneum, hair, and nails):
  - With the exception of tinea capitis, *Trichophyton rubrum* and *T. mentagrophytes* are the most common pathogens
  - *Trichophyton mentagrophytes* (previously *T. mentagrophytes* var. *mentagrophytes*) is acquired from animals (zoophilic); *T. interdigitale*

(previously *T. mentagrophytes* var. *interdigitale* [anthropophilic]) is spread human-to-human

- Transmission occurs via close contact with infected humans or domestic animals, occupational or recreational exposure (e.g. locker rooms), and contact with contaminated clothing, furniture, or brushes; the latter inanimate objects serve as fomites.
- More commonly seen in adults, with the exception of tinea capitis, which occurs more often in children.
- The classic presentation is an erythematous, annular lesion with an active, scaly border; superficial pustules may also be present (Fig. 64.5).
- Occasionally, vesicles may develop, especially in tinea pedis or manuum due to *T. mentagrophytes*.
- Dx: KOH ± fungal culture of skin scrapings (see Fig. 2.1) as well as hairs and nails, in the case of tinea capitis and tinea unguium, respectively.
- Important variants:
  - *Tinea incognito* refers to atypical clinical presentations, often due to inappropriate treatment with potent topical CS or combination topical therapies that contain CS; lesions may lack scale or be minimally inflamed (Fig. 64.6)
  - *Majocchi granuloma* is characterized by erythematous papules or pustules within an area of tinea corporis; the papules represent sites of hair shaft invasion, usually due to *T. rubrum*; often seen in women with tinea pedis who shave their legs or in immunosuppressed patients (see Fig. 31.4A; Fig. 64.7)

EXAMPLES OF SPECIFIC TYPES OF DERMATOPHYTOSES

- Tinea pedis (Fig. 64.8; **DDx**, see Table 13.1):
  - Most commonly due to *T. rubrum* or *T. interdigitale* and *T. mentagrophytes* > *Epidermophyton floccosum*
  - Four major types: (1) interdigital – erythema, scaling, and maceration in the web spaces, especially the two lateral web spaces, which have the most occlusion; can be accompanied by fissures as well as superimposed bacterial infection; (2) moccasin – diffuse scaling and erythema that extends onto the lateral aspect of the feet;

COMPARISON OF BLACK AND WHITE PIEDRA		
	White piedra	**Black piedra**
Nodule color	White (occasionally red, green, or light brown)	Brown to black
Nodule firmness	Soft	Hard
Nodule adherence to the hair shaft	Loose	Firm
Typical anatomic location	Face, axillae, and pubic region (occasionally scalp)	Scalp and face (occasionally pubic region)
Favored climate	Tropical	Tropical
Causative organism	*Trichosporon beigelii*	*Piedraia hortae*
KOH examination of "crush prep" of cut hair shafts	Non-dematiaceous hyphae with blastoconidia and arthroconidia (see Fig. 2.17A)	Dematiaceous hyphae with asci and ascospores (sexual reproduction)
Culture on Sabouraud's agar	Moist, cream-colored, yeast-like colonies*	Slow-growing, dark green to dark brown-black colonies
Treatment	Clip affected hairs, wash affected hairs with antifungal shampoo	Clip affected hairs, wash affected hairs with antifungal shampoo

**Growth inhibited by cycloheximide.*

Table 64.2 Comparison of black and white piedra. *From Elewski B. The superficial mycoses, the dermatophytoses, and select dermatomycosis. In: Elewski BE, editor. Cutaneous Fungal Infections. Massachusetts: Blackwell Science; 1998.*

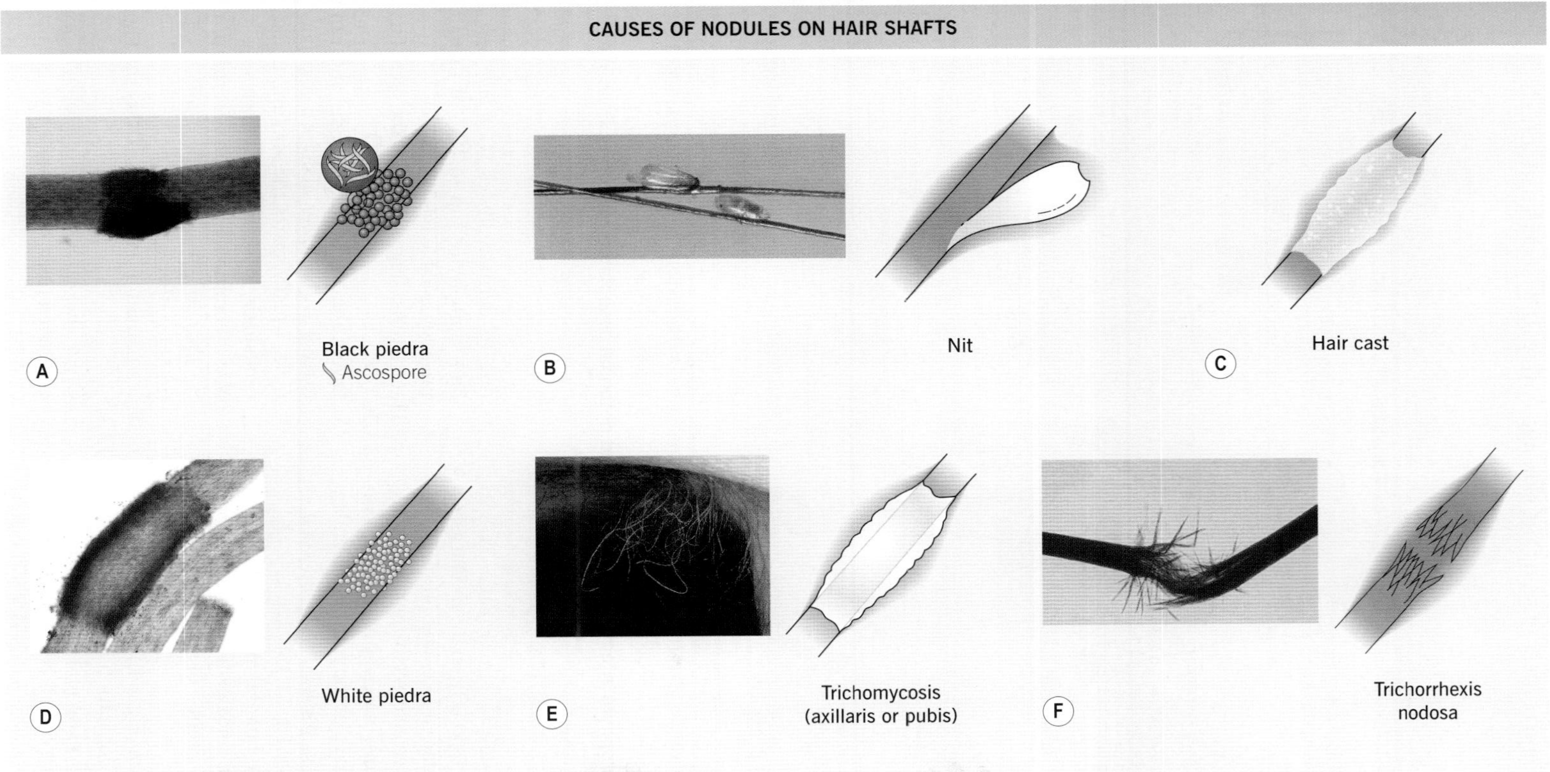

CAUSES OF NODULES ON HAIR SHAFTS

A

Black piedra

Ascospore

B

Nit

C

Hair cast

D

White piedra

E

Trichomycosis (axillaris or pubis)

F

Trichorrhexis nodosa

Fig. 64.3 Causes of nodules on hair shafts. *A inset, From Bonifaz, A. Tinea versicolor, tinea nigra, white piedra, and black piedra. Clinics in Dermatology, 2010-03-01, Volume 28, Issue 2, pp. 140–5, Copyright © 2010 Elsevier Inc. ISSN: 0738-081X. Fig. 11; D inset, Courtesy, YDRSC.*

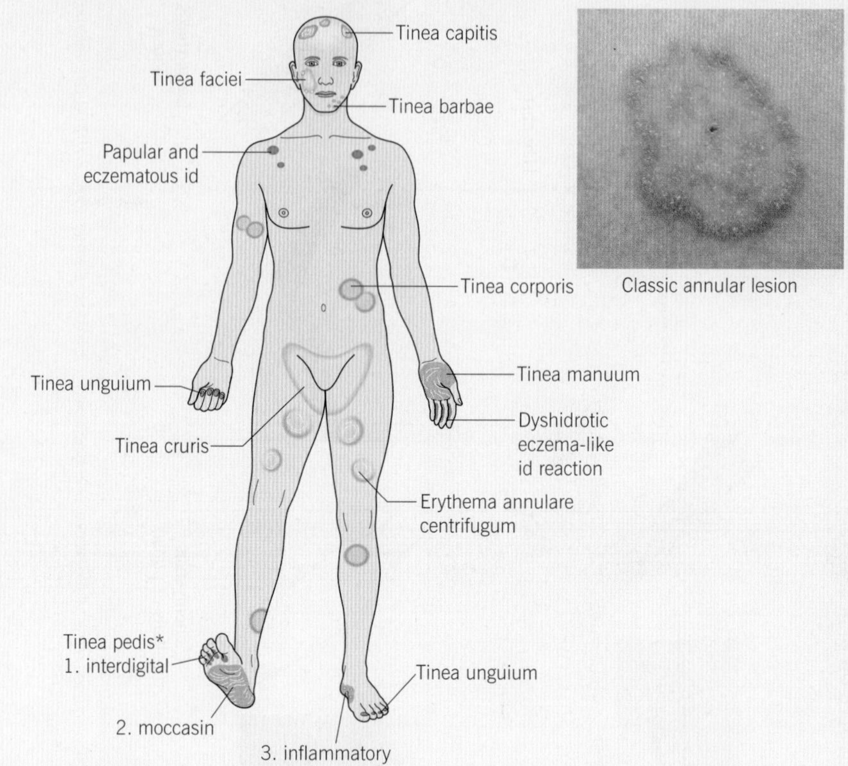

Fig. 64.4 Dermatophyte infections of the skin and potential associated reactions. Erythema annulare centrifugum is a reaction pattern that can be idiopathic or associated with tinea infections (see Ch. 15).

(3) in inflammatory (vesicular) – vesicles and bullae, especially on the medial aspect of the plantar surface; and (4) ulcerative, which is often an exacerbation of interdigital tinea pedis, especially in immunocompromised and diabetic patients. Secondary bacterial (e.g. pseudomonal) infection is common (see Fig. 61.15)

- Consider use of oral antifungal medications if the tinea pedis fails to respond to topical agents or is severe (Table 64.3)

- Tinea unguium (Fig. 64.9):
  - Dx: KOH preparation and/or fungal culture of nail plate and subungual scale, PAS-staining of nail clippings
  - Of note, *onychomycosis* is a more general term that includes nail infections due to dermatophytes, *Candida* spp., and saprophytes (up to 10% of toenail infections; Table 64.4)
- Tinea cruris (Fig. 64.10; **DDx**, see Fig. 13.2):
  - Favors the upper inner thighs and can extend to the lower abdomen and buttocks; usually spares the scrotum, unlike candidiasis; associated with tinea pedis
  - Most commonly due to *T. rubrum* > *Epidermophyton floccosum* > *T. mentagrophytes*
- Tinea manuum (Fig. 64.11; **DDx**, see Fig. 13.1):
  - Often due to same dermatophyte as associated tinea pedis
  - Can be unilateral ("one hand, two feet syndrome"; see Fig. 64.8A)

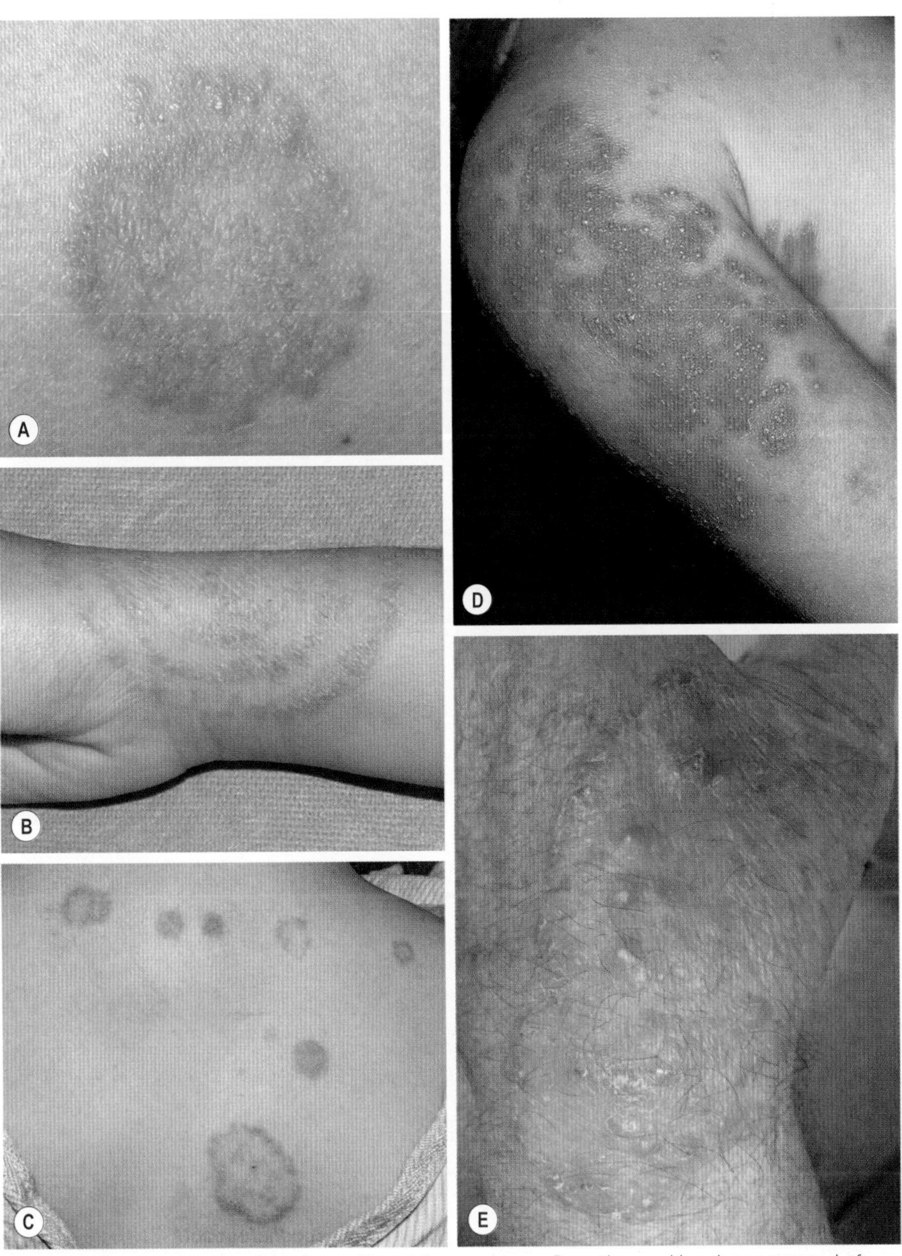

Fig. 64.5 Tinea corporis. A Lesions with subtle annular configuration and border composed of individual, slightly scaly papules. **B** Scaly concentric rings on the arm. **C** Multiple annular and circinate lesions of various sizes on the upper back. **D** Pustules within multiple figurate lesions on the upper arm. **E** Against the diagnosis of folliculitis, all of the pustules are contained within the pink plaque.
A, B, D, Courtesy, Julie V. Schaffer, MD; C, Courtesy, Kalman Watsky, MD; E, Courtesy, Karynne O. Duncan, MD.

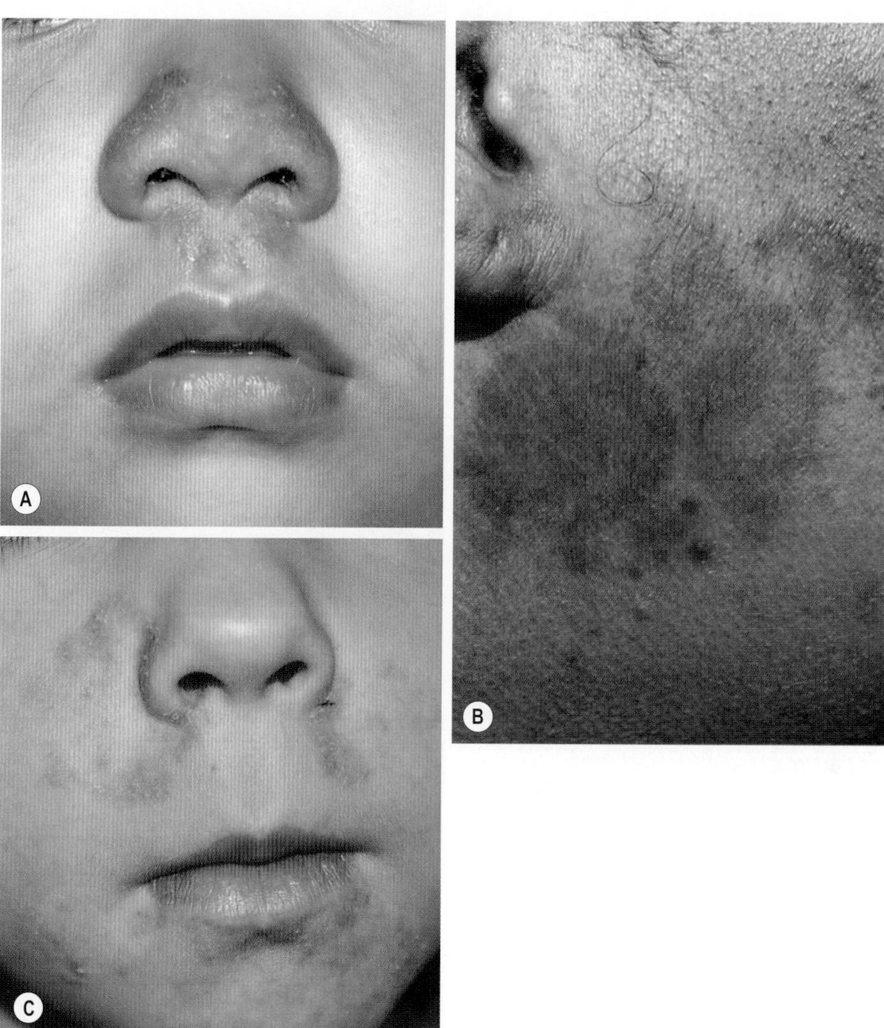

Fig. 64.6 Tinea faciei and tinea incognito. A Area of erythema and scale on the nose and philtrum of a young child. **B** Hyperpigmented lesions with subtle arcuate and annular configurations in a woman with darkly pigmented skin. There is minimal scale following the use of topical CS ("tinea incognito"). The clue to application of topical CS is the relative hypopigmentation as compared with the more medial cheek. **C** Child with pink papules, a few tiny pustules, and thin annular and arcuate scaly plaques in a perinasal and perioral distribution. These clinical findings could be mistaken for periorificial dermatitis. *A, Courtesy, Julie V. Schaffer, MD; B, Courtesy, Kalman Watsky, MD; C, Courtesy, Antonio Torrelo, MD.*

– Tinea unguium of the involved hand is a clinical clue

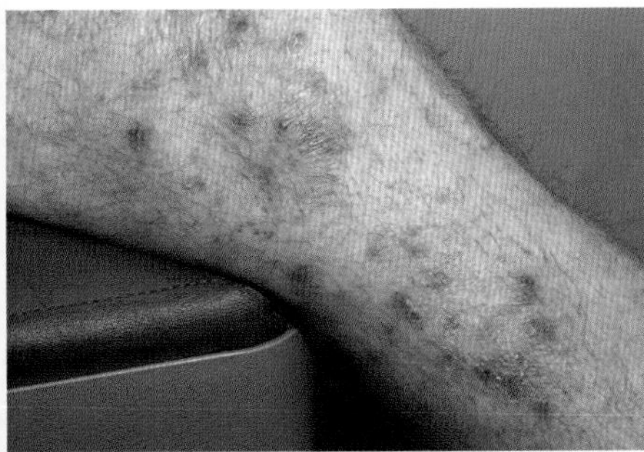

Fig. 64.7 Nodular perifolliculitis (Majocchi granuloma). Perifollicular inflammation and follicular pustules on the leg due to *Trichophyton rubrum*. A few of the lowermost papules have a granulomatous appearance. *Courtesy, Kalman Watsky, MD.*

- Tinea faciei (see Fig. 64.6):
  - Misdiagnosis is common and application of topical CS is a typical history, often leading to tinea incognito
  - An arciform shape with pustules in the border points to the diagnosis
- Tinea barbae (Fig. 64.12; see Fig. 31.7):
  - Often secondary to a zoophilic dermatophyte – i.e. acquired from an animal, e.g. *T. mentagrophytes* (small mammals) and *T. verrucosum* (cattle)
  - Favors postpubertal males
  - Invasion of hair shafts and intense inflammation with follicular pustules and abscess formation; can resemble a kerion
- Tinea capitis (Fig. 64.13):
  - Occurs more frequently in children
  - In the United States as well as other

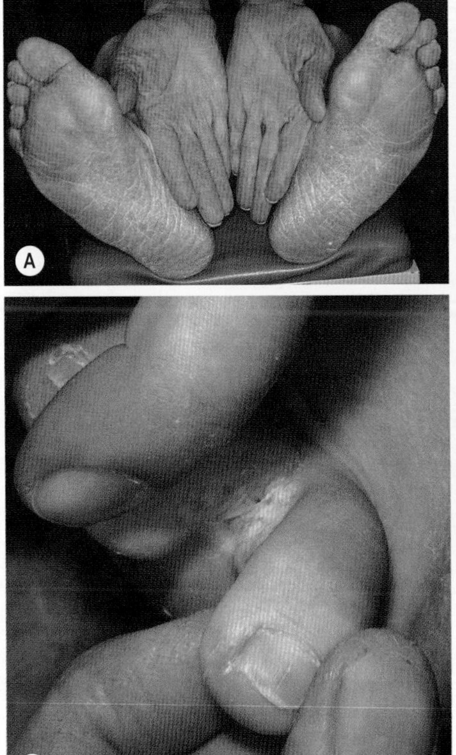

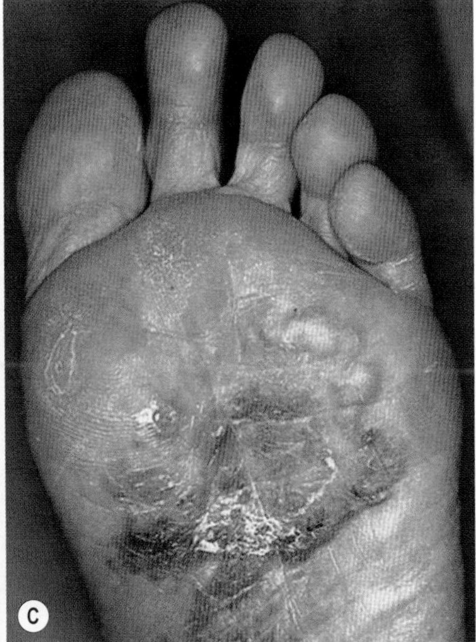

Fig. 64.8 Tinea pedis. Diffuse scaling in the moccasin type **(A),** maceration between the third and fourth toes in the interdigital form **(B),** and erythema, scale-crust, and bullae in the inflammatory form **(C)**. The patient in **(A)** also has involvement of the right hand (i.e. one hand–two feet tinea). *A, C, Courtesy, YDRSC; B, Courtesy, Jean L. Bolognia, MD.*

THERAPEUTIC REGIMENS FOR DERMATOPHYTOSES				
Topical medications				
Twice daily for 2–4 weeks • Allylamines (e.g. terbinafine 1% cream, naftifine 1% gel) • Imidazoles (e.g. econazole 1% cream, sulconazole 1% solution) • Hydroxypyridinones (e.g. ciclopirox 0.77% cream or gel)				
Oral medications				
	Fluconazole	**Griseofulvin**	**Itraconazole***	**Terbinafine**
Tinea corporis and pedis (moccasin type)/tinea manuum (*adults*)**	150–200 mg/ week × 2–6 weeks	500–1000 mg/day (microsize) or 375–750 mg/day (ultra-microsize) × 4 weeks	200–400 mg/day × 1 week	250 mg/day × 1–2 weeks
Majocchi granuloma	Terbinafine is used most commonly Doses as above × 2–8 weeks (or until all lesions cleared)			
Tinea corporis and pedis (moccasin type)/tinea manuum (*children***)	6 mg/kg/ week × 2–6 weeks	15–20 mg/kg/ day (microsize suspension) × 4 weeks	3–5 mg/kg/day (maximum 400 mg) × 1 week	Daily dosing as for tinea capitis (see below) × 2 weeks
Tinea unguium (*adults*)	Toenail ± fingernail involvement			
	200–450 mg/ week until nails are clear	1–2 gm/day (microsize) or 750 mg/ day (ultra-microsize) until nails are normal†	200 mg/day × 12 weeks or 200 mg BID × 1 week per month for 3–4 consecutive months	250 mg/day × 12 weeks
	Fingernail involvement only			
	200–450 mg/ week until nails are clear	1–2 gm/day (microsize) or 750 mg/ day (ultra-microsize) until nails are normal†	200 mg/day × 6 weeks or 200 mg BID × 1 week per month for 2 consecutive months	250 mg/day × 6 weeks
Tinea capitis (*adults*)‡	6 mg/kg/ day × 3–6 weeks	10–15 mg/kg/day (ultra-microsize; usually maximum 750 mg/day) × 6–8 weeks	5 mg/kg/day (maximum 400 mg) × 4–8 weeks	250 mg/day × 3–4 weeks§
Tinea capitis (*children*)‡	6 mg/kg/ day × 3–6 weeks	20–25 mg/kg/day (microsize suspension) × 6–8 weeks	5 mg/kg/day (maximum 400 mg) × 4–8 weeks	If available (not in U.S.), granules 125 mg (<25 kg), 187.5 mg (25–35 kg), or 250 mg (>35 kg) × 3–4 weeks§

**Not approved in the United States for use in children.*
***In general, the shorter courses and lower doses tend to be used for tinea corporis.*
†No longer commonly used for this indication.
‡Combined with 2.5% selenium sulfide shampoo or ketoconazole 2% shampoo; "id" reaction should not be confused with a medication allergy.
§Not recommended for Microsporum canis, unless given at double-dose.

Table 64.3 Therapeutic regimens for dermatophytoses.

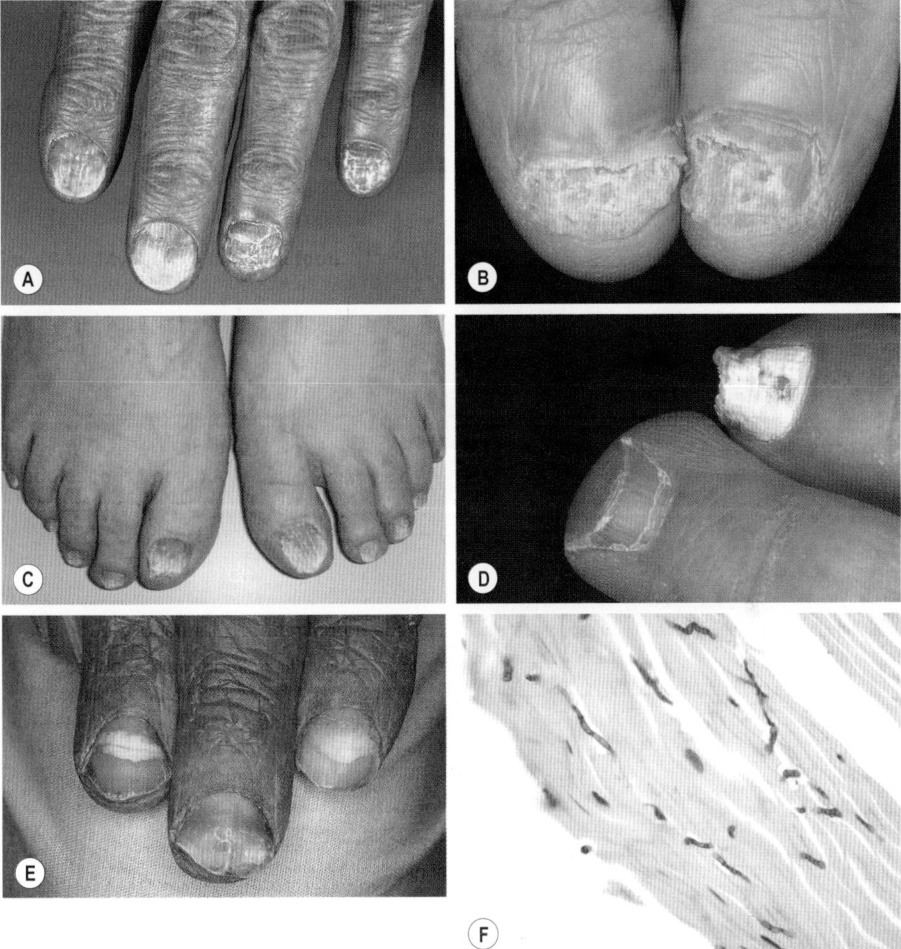

Fig. 64.9 Tinea unguium. Onycholysis, yellowing, crumbling, and thickening of the fingernails **(A)**, thumb nails **(B)**, and toenails **(C)** in the distal/lateral subungual variant. Diffuse **(D)** white discoloration of the toenail in the superficial white variant. **E** Proximal white subungual onychomycosis of the second and fourth fingernails in an HIV-infected patient. Hyphae within a formalin-fixed, PAS-stained nail plate **(F)**. *A, D, Courtesy, Jean L. Bolognia, MD; B, Courtesy, Louis A. Fragola, Jr., MD; C, Courtesy, Boni E. Elewski, MD and Roderick J. Hay, MD; E, From Callen, J. et al. Dermatological Signs of Systemic Disease, 5th Edition. Elsevier, 2016, ISBN: 9780323358293, Fig. 29.14; F, Courtesy, Mary Stone, MD.*

regions such as the United Kingdom, *T. tonsurans* is the most common pathogen; for example, in the United States, it causes >95% of tinea capitis; *T. tonsurans* favors those with afrocentric hair

- Tinea capitis due to *T. tonsurans* can be more difficult to diagnose because the clinical findings may be subtle with only seborrheic dermatitis-like scaling of the scalp, minimal alopecia, and no fluorescence by Wood's lamp examination (in contrast to ectothrix infection due to *M. canis*)
- Multiple spores (conidia) within or surrounding hair shafts, referred to as endothrix or ectothrix tinea capitis, respectively, cause fragility and breakage of hair, leading to areas of alopecia (see Figs 2.2 and 2.3)
- In addition to alopecia, clinical clues include pustules, scale, and crusting; occasionally, there is formation of a kerion (see Fig. 64.13E) or development

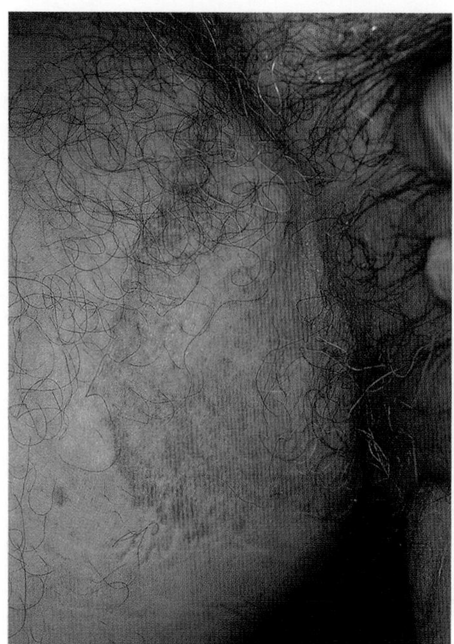

Fig. 64.10 Tinea cruris. Note the arciform erythematous border on the upper inner thigh. *Courtesy, YDRSC.*

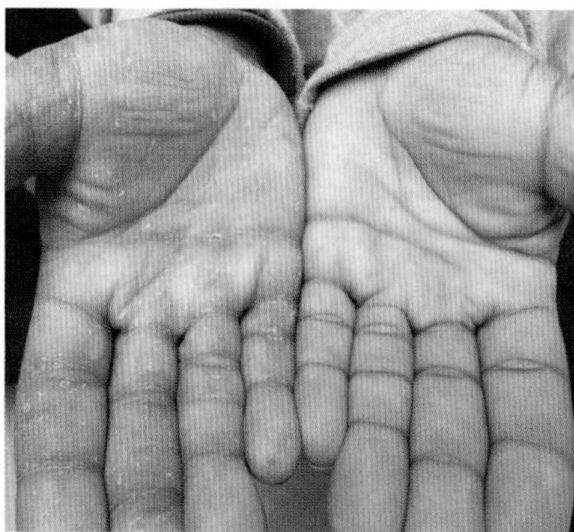

Fig. 64.11 Tinea manuum. Multiple collarettes of scale reminiscent of keratolysis exfoliativa on one palm. *Courtesy, Boni E. Elewski, MD and Roderick J. Hay, MD.*

of posterior cervical and posterior auricular lymphadenopathy

- A type of tinea capitis seen in the Mediterranean basin and Middle East is favus, in which there are keratotic masses that contain hyphae and keratin (Fig. 64.14)

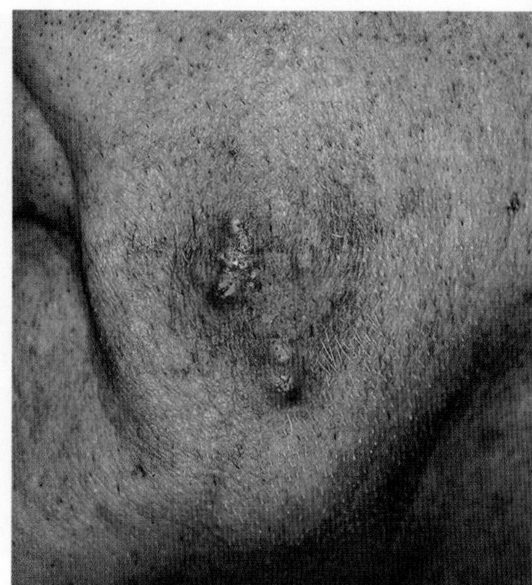

Fig. 64.12 Tinea barbae. More superficial form due to *Trichophyton rubrum*. Several follicular pustules are seen. *Courtesy, Jean L. Bolognia, MD.*

- **Rx:** oral treatment is required; for children, an adequate dose of griseofulvin is 20–25 mg/kg/day (microsized suspension) × 6–8 weeks; combination therapy with 2.5% selenium sulfide or 2% ketoconazole shampoo is recommended to kill spores and reduce transmission; see Table 64.3 for additional oral therapies

• Id reactions (see Ch. 11) can occur in the setting of dermatophyte infections; two of the more common examples are as follows (see Fig. 64.4):

- Dyshidrotic eczema-like papules and vesicles of the palms and fingers seen in association with tinea pedis
- Pruritic papules favoring the upper trunk in the setting of tinea capitis, often following the initiation of appropriate therapy

• Erythema annulare centrifugum may also be present in association with tinea pedis (see Ch. 15 and Fig. 64.4).

• **DDx:** outlined in Table 64.4.

• **Rx:** outlined in Table 64.3.

Candidal Infections

Superficial Mucocutaneous Candidal Infections

• Most commonly due to *Candida albicans* or *C. tropicalis*.

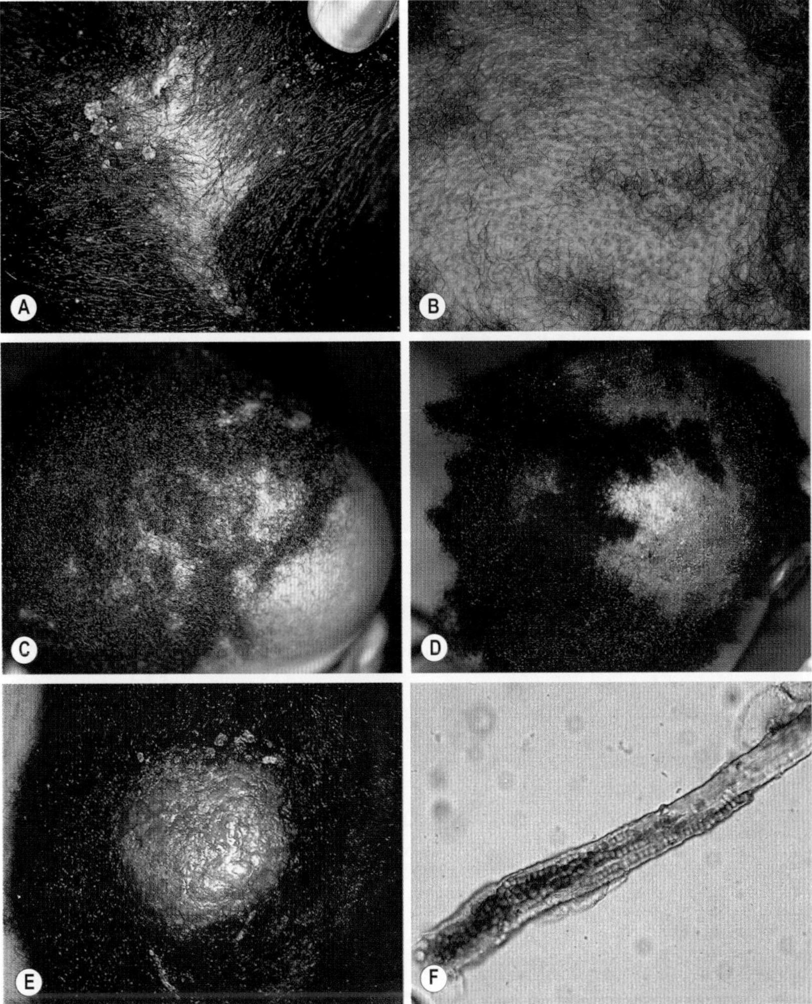

Fig. 64.13 Tinea capitis. The range of clinical presentations of tinea capitis due to *Trichophyton tonsurans*, from mild scalp scaling **(A)** to patchy alopecia with black dots **(B)** or scale **(C)** to large areas of alopecia with pustules and scale-crust **(D). E** Kerion formation due to *T. tonsurans*. There is a boggy plaque that can be misdiagnosed as a bacterial abscess. **F** Microscopic examination of involved hairs demonstrates an endothrix pattern (KOH–chlorazol black stain). *A, C, D–F, Courtesy, YDRSC; B, Courtesy, Louis A. Fragola, Jr., MD.*

- Wide spectrum of clinical presentations, from diaper dermatitis in infants (see Fig. 13.4) to intertrigo (see Table 60.5 and Fig. 13.2) to chronic mucocutaneous candidiasis (see Ch. 49).
- Mucosal:
  - Oral candidiasis (thrush) presents as a white exudate resembling cottage cheese; risk factors include diabetes mellitus, treatment with broad-spectrum antibiotics, use of inhaled CS, dentures, and immunosuppression; common in otherwise healthy neonates and infants
  - Additional forms: intraoral erythematous patches and adherent white plaques, glossitis, angular cheilitis (see Fig. 13.5), and vulvovaginitis and balanitis (see Ch. 60)
- Cutaneous:
  - Most common presentation is an erosive, erythematous patch with satellite pustules in an intertriginous zone (inframammary, axillary, inguinal,

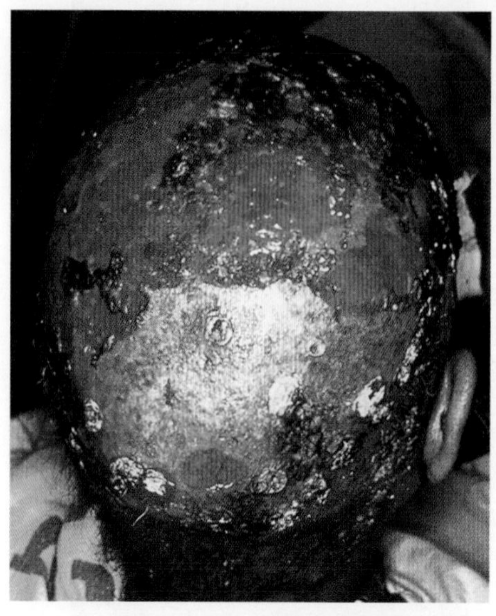

Fig. 64.14 Favus due to *Trichophyton schoenleinii*. Scarring alopecia with erosions and several scutula on the occipital scalp. The latter represent masses of keratin plus fungi. *Courtesy, Israel Dvoretzky, MD.*

DIFFERENTIAL DIAGNOSIS OF DERMATOPHYTE INFECTIONS	
Tinea corporis	• Dermatitis (atopic, nummular, contact, stasis, seborrheic [petaloid]) • Tinea versicolor • Pityriasis rosea • Erythema annulare centrifugum • Annular psoriasis • Parapsoriasis • Subacute cutaneous lupus erythematosus • Granuloma annulare (lacks scale) • Impetigo
Tinea capitis	• Alopecia areata • Trichotillomania • Seborrheic dermatitis (unusual in prepubertal populations) • Psoriasis • Tinea amiantacea • If pustules, pyoderma and folliculitis • If scarring, other scarring alopecias (e.g. lichen planus)
Tinea unguium	• Onychomycosis due to saprophytes (e.g. *Fusarium*); primarily toenails • Candidal onychomycosis (ridging, yellow discoloration, and onycholysis primarily of fingernails; often there is concurrent paronychia) • Psoriasis • Chronic trauma
Tinea faciei	• Dermatitis (seborrheic, contact, atopic, perioral) • Rosacea • Lupus erythematosus • Acne vulgaris • Annular psoriasis (children)
Tinea barbae	• Folliculitis (e.g. culture-negative, staphylococcal, herpetic; see Fig. 31.1) • Acne vulgaris, rosacea • Dermatitis (e.g. seborrheic, contact)
Tinea pedis (see also Fig. 13.1 and Table 13.1)	If interdigital: • Erythrasma • Gram-negative toe-web infection

Table 64.4 Differential diagnosis of dermatophyte infections.

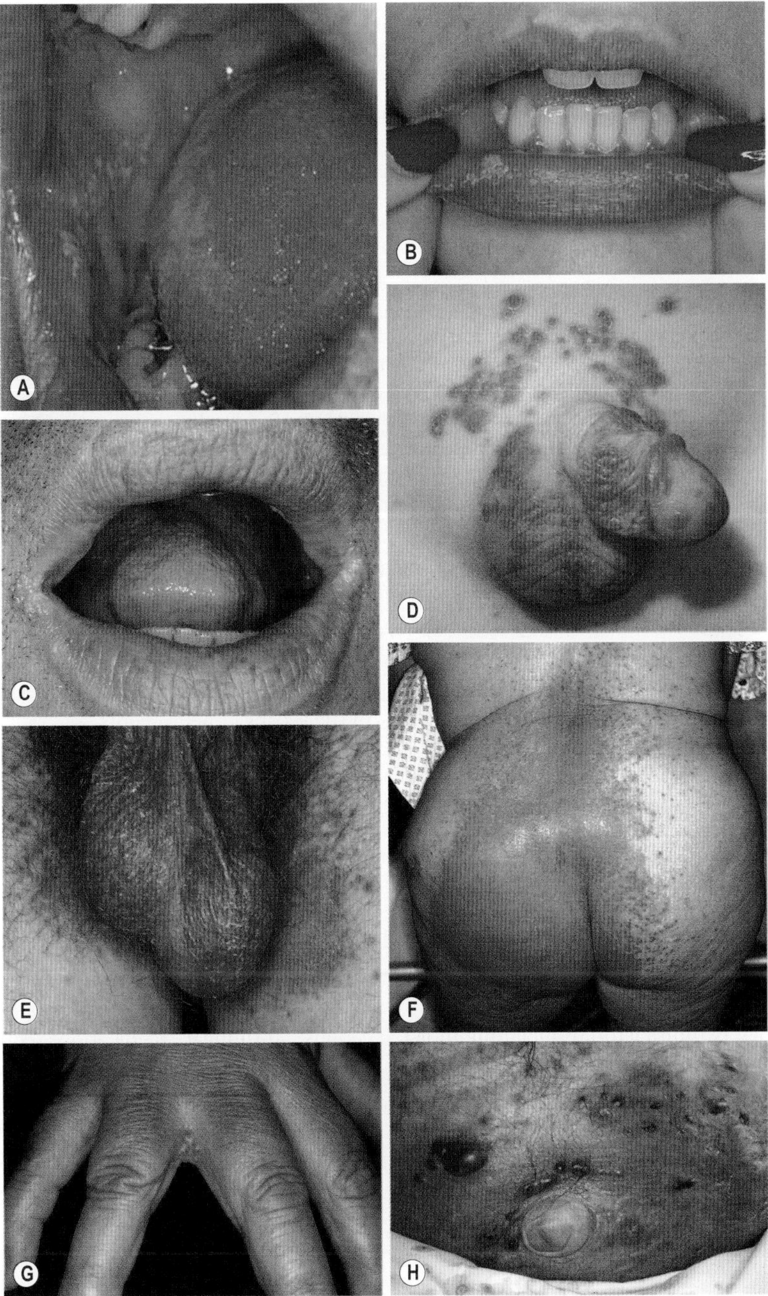

Fig. 64.15 Mucocutaneous candidiasis. **A** Thrush with "cottage cheese"-like exudate on the buccal mucosa. **B** Candidal cheilitis with white plaques of the vermilion lip. **C** Angular cheilitis (perlèche). **D** Candidiasis of the suprapubic area, scrotum and penis in a young boy. Note the collarettes of scale on the coalescing, brightly erythematous papules. **E** Candidiasis of the scrotum and medial thighs with beefy red erythema, scale, and satellite papules. **F** This infection occurred in a hospitalized patient with diabetes mellitus who was receiving broad-spectrum antibiotics. Note the multiple satellite lesions. **G** Erosio interdigitalis blastomycetica in the classic location between the third and fourth fingers. **H** Dermal candidiasis in an immunosuppressed patient. *A, Courtesy, Judit Stenn, MD; B, Courtesy, Kalman Watsky, MD; C, D, Courtesy, Louis A. Fragola, Jr., MD; E, G, Courtesy, Eugene Mirrer, MD; F, Courtesy, YDRSC; H, Courtesy, Boni E. Elewski, MD and Roderick J. Hay, MD.*

TREATMENT OF MUCOCUTANEOUS CANDIDIASIS	
Candidiasis	**Treatment**
Mucosal (continue treatment for 7–14 days after clinical resolution)	Immunocompetent patient • Clotrimazole 10 mg troche five times daily • Nystatin 100,000 units/ml suspension: 4–6 ml swish and swallow four times daily (adults and children); 1 ml in each cheek four times daily (infants) Immunocompromised patient *OR* failure to respond to topical **Rx** • Oral fluconazole 200 mg PO on day 1, then 100–200 mg PO daily
Cutaneous	If mild, topical treatment • Imidazoles (e.g. ketoconazole 2% cream) or other topicals (e.g. ciclopirox cream) twice daily for 2 weeks or until resolved If moderate to severe *OR* fails to respond to topical **Rx** • Fluconazole 50–100 mg daily for 14 days *OR* • Fluconazole 150 mg PO weekly for 2–4 weeks *Chronic mucocutaneous candidiasis* • Fluconazole 400–800 mg PO daily for 4–6 months • May require lifelong suppressive treatment with fluconazole 200 mg PO daily

Table 64.5 Treatment of mucocutaneous candidiasis.

beneath a pannus; Fig. 64.15), on the scrotum, or in the diaper area of infants (see Fig. 13.4)
  - Predisposing factors for cutaneous infection – similar to oral candidiasis plus hyperhidrosis with occlusion
- **DDx** of candidal intertrigo: see Chapter 13.
- **Rx:** outlined in Table 64.5.
- **Rx** of candidal intertrigo or balanitis: outlined in Table 60.5.

Perianal Pseudoverrucous Papules (Granuloma Gluteale Infantum)

- Etiology is multifactorial, including moist occlusion, irritation from urine and stool, and candidal infection.
- Seen primarily in infants but also in older individuals with urinary and fecal incontinence.
- Erythematous papules and nodules, as well as erosions, develop in the anogenital region.
- When the lesions become erosive, some clinicians use the term Jacquet diaper dermatitis or erosive papulonodular dermatosis.
- **DDx:** outlined in Fig. 13.4.

Congenital Candidiasis

Congenital candidiasis is discussed in Chapter 28.

Systemic Candidiasis

- Generally affects immunosuppressed hosts in the setting of neutropenia.
- Clinical features are outlined in Table 64.6.
- Although the skin lesions represent septic emboli, blood cultures may be negative; as a result, skin biopsy for tissue culture and histology can play a critical role.

Deep Fungal Infections

Deep mycoses are treated with oral or intravenous antifungal medications, often for an extended period of time (e.g. 6 months). Culture results direct therapy, but initial empiric treatment is often started based on the clinical presentation plus histologic findings (e.g. itraconazole 200–400 mg/day for chromo(blasto)mycosis).

Dermal/Subcutaneous

CHROMO(BLASTO)MYCOSIS

- Commonly due to several species of dematiaceous fungi – *Fonsecaea pedrosoi*, *F. compacta*, *F. monophora*, *Phialophora verrucosa*, *Cladophialophora carrionii*, and *Rhinocladiella aquaspersa* – that are found in soil and decaying wood.
- Follows trauma and implantation of the fungus into the skin.

CUTANEOUS FEATURES OF COMMON OPPORTUNISTIC MYCOSES	
Mycosis	**Common cutaneous presentations**
Systemic candidiasis* • *Candida albicans* • *C. tropicalis* (frequent skin lesions) • Other *Candida* spp. (e.g. *C. glabrata*, *C. auris*)	• Firm erythematous papules and nodules, often with a pale center • Lesions can be hemorrhagic, especially in the setting of thrombocytopenia • Ecthyma gangrenosum-like lesions • Occasionally, the lesions are nonspecific, i.e. purpuric macules
Aspergillosis* • *Aspergillus flavus* • *A. fumigatus* Serum assays to screen high-risk patients • Galactomannan (more specific, lower sensitivity) • 1,3-D-glucan (less specificity)	• Primary cutaneous – Necrotic papulonodules – May be associated with an intravenous catheter site, burns, trauma, or surgical wounds • Secondary cutaneous (septic emboli from disseminated infection) – Necrotic papulonodules and ecthyma gangrenosum-like lesions – Associated with the final stages of AIDS
Zygomycosis* • *Mucor* • *Rhizopus* • *Absidia*	• Ecthyma gangrenosum-like lesions, cellulitis, facial edema (commonly unilateral due to contiguous spread of sino-orbital disease), necrotic papulonodules, plaques, large hemorrhagic crusts on the face • May be associated with an intravenous catheter site (primary cutaneous) • Also associated with poorly controlled diabetes mellitus
Cryptococcosis† • *Cryptococcus neoformans*	• Molluscum contagiosum-like lesions, ulceration, cellulitis
Phaeohyphomycosis*,† • *Alternaria* • *Exophiala* • *Phialophora*	• Subcutaneous cysts, ulcerated plaques, necrotic papulonodules
Hyalohyphomycosis*,‡ • *Fusarium* • *Talaromyces* • *Paecilomyces*	• Umbilicated or necrotic papules, pustules, abscesses, cellulitis, subcutaneous nodules • *Fusarium* infection can begin with a periungual focus
Trichosporonosis (e.g. *Trichosporon* spp.)	• Papulovesicles, purpuric papules, necrotic papulonodules

**With the use of prophylactic voriconazole, posaconazole, and isavuconazole in high-risk oncology patients (e.g. neutropenic patients with hematologic malignancies), the incidence of disseminated candidiasis, systemic aspergillosis, and mucormycosis (psoaconazole and isavuconazole) have declined in these individuals.*
†Especially in the setting of AIDS; also histoplasmosis, coccidioidomycosis, penicilliosis, and sporotrichosis.
‡Less common infections.

Table 64.6 Cutaneous features of common opportunistic mycoses.

• Expanding, verrucous plaque, usually on an extremity (Fig. 64.16); central scarring can occur.
• More common in tropical and subtropical regions.
• Diagnostic histologic finding – round, pigmented bodies with internal septations that are said to resemble copper pennies, also referred to as sclerotic bodies or Medlar bodies.

MYCETOMA (MADURA FOOT)

• Two major subtypes: (1) actinomycotic mycetoma – secondary to filamentous bacteria, especially *Nocardia* and *Actinomyces* (see Ch. 61); and (2) eumycotic mycetoma – caused by true fungi, e.g. *Madurella mycetomatis*, *Pseudallescheria boydii.*
• Contracted from trauma and implantation of fungus into the skin (Fig. 64.17A).
• Most common site is the distal lower extremity but can also be seen in other sites, such as the distal upper extremity, trunk, and scalp.
• Clinical triad of draining sinuses, grains (macroscopic colonies of organisms; see Ch. 61), and edema (Fig. 64.18). Grains can also

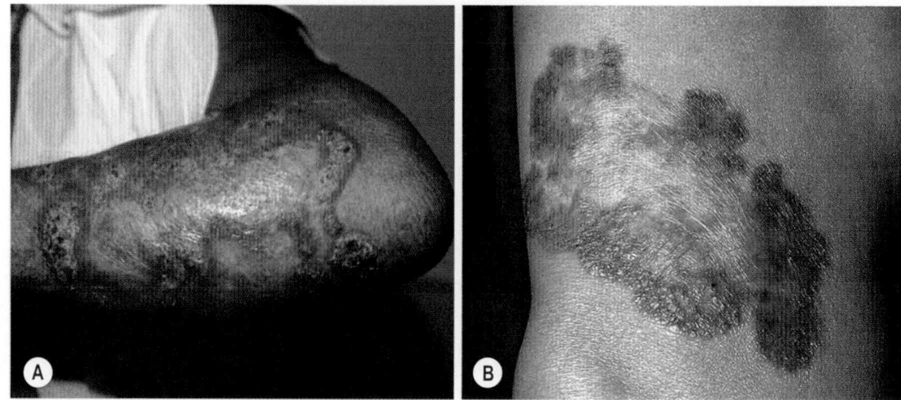

Fig. 64.16 Chromo(blasto)mycosis. Annular and figurate plaques due to central clearing and scarring with a verrucous surface on the arm **(A)** and a more granulomatous appearance on the leg **(B)**. *Courtesy, USCDRSC.*

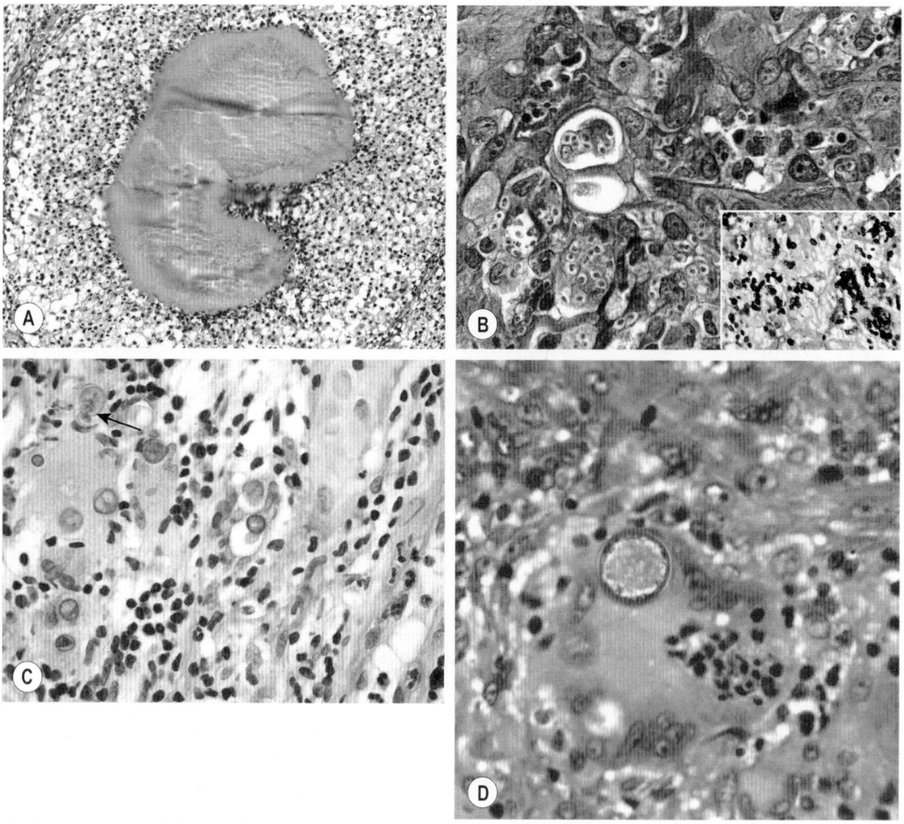

Fig. 64.17 Histologic features of selected deep fungal infections. A Eumycetoma with formation of a grain, which represents tightly packed colonies of fungal organisms. **B** Histoplasmosis – *Histoplasma capsulatum* yeast forms are present within macrophages and giant cells, highlighted with a methenamine silver stain (inset). **C** Blastomycosis – budding yeast forms in the dermis, several of which are within a giant cell (PAS stain). Note the single, broad-based budding (arrow). **D** Coccidioidomycosis – an endospore-containing spherule within a giant cell. *A, Courtesy, Lorenzo Cerroni, MD; B, Courtesy, C. Massone, MD; C, Courtesy, Mary Stone, MD; D, Courtesy, Jennifer McNiff, MD.*

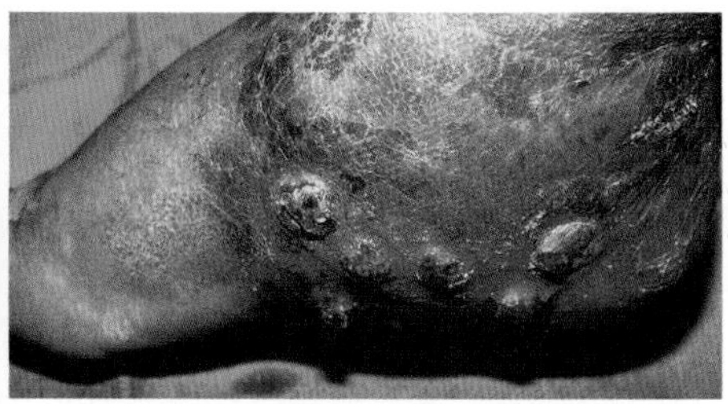

Fig. 64.18 Mycetoma (Madura foot). Note the soft tissue swelling of the foot as well as multiple nodules with pustular discharge. *Courtesy, USCDRSC.*

INFECTIOUS CAUSES OF A LYMPHOCUTANEOUS ("SPOROTRICHOID") PATTERN
Most common • Atypical mycobacteria, especially *Mycobacterium marinum*, but also other species (e.g. *M. chelonae*, *M. kansasii*) • Sporotrichosis
Unusual • Nocardiosis • Pyogenic bacteria (e.g. *Staphylococcus aureus*, *Streptococcus pyogenes*) • *Pseudallescheria boydii*
Rare (in high-income countries) • Leishmaniasis • Tularemia* • Tuberculosis* • Dimorphic fungi (other than *Sporothrix schenckii*) • Opportunistic fungi in immunocompromised hosts (e.g. *Fusarium*, *Alternaria* spp.) • Glanders (*Burkholderia mallei*)* • Cat scratch disease* • Anthrax • Cowpox • *Acanthamoeba* spp.

*Often ulceroglandular.

Table 64.7 Infectious causes of a lymphocutaneous ("sporotrichoid") pattern. There are also noninfectious causes, such as lymphoma, Langerhans cell histiocytosis, and in-transit metastases. In addition, perineural spread of leprosy can mimic a lymphocutaneous pattern.

be seen in botryomycosis and actinomycosis (see Ch. 61).

• **Rx:** excision of more localized lesions; for larger areas of involvement as well as pre- and postoperatively, long-term course (i.e. 6 months or longer) of oral antifungal medication (e.g. itraconazole 400 mg PO daily × 3 months followed by 200 mg PO daily for 9 months).

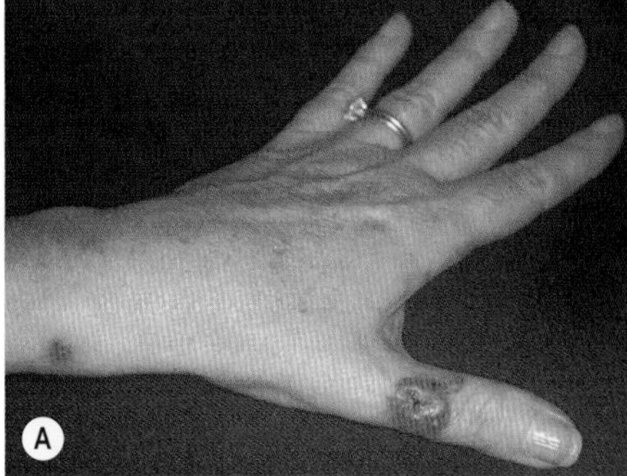

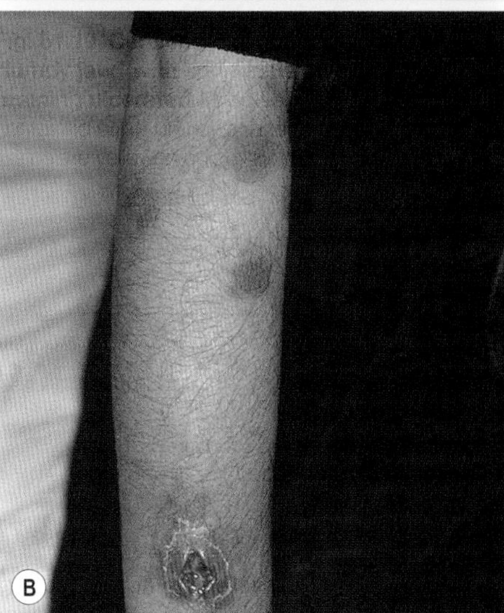

Fig. 64.19 Lymphocutaneous (sporotrichoid) pattern. A An eroded nodule on the thumb, representing the primary lesion, with a secondary lesion along the lymphatics due to sporotrichosis. **B** Ulcerated nodule on the extensor forearm with multiple more proximal nodules due to nocardiosis in a patient with lymphoma who was receiving systemic CS. *A, Courtesy, YDRSC; B, Courtesy, Jean L. Bolognia, MD.*

SPOROTRICHOSIS

• Secondary to organisms of the genus *Sporothrix* (e.g. *Sporothrix schenkii*), which are dimorphic, i.e. a yeast at 37°C (human body) and a mold at 25°C (soil).

• Worldwide distribution; present in soil and sphagnum moss.

• Most common presentation is a lymphocutaneous or "sporotrichoid" pattern (~75% of patients) that initially presents as a papule or nodule at the site of inoculation; this is followed by the appearance of papulonodules along the draining lymphatics (Fig. 64.19; Table 64.7).

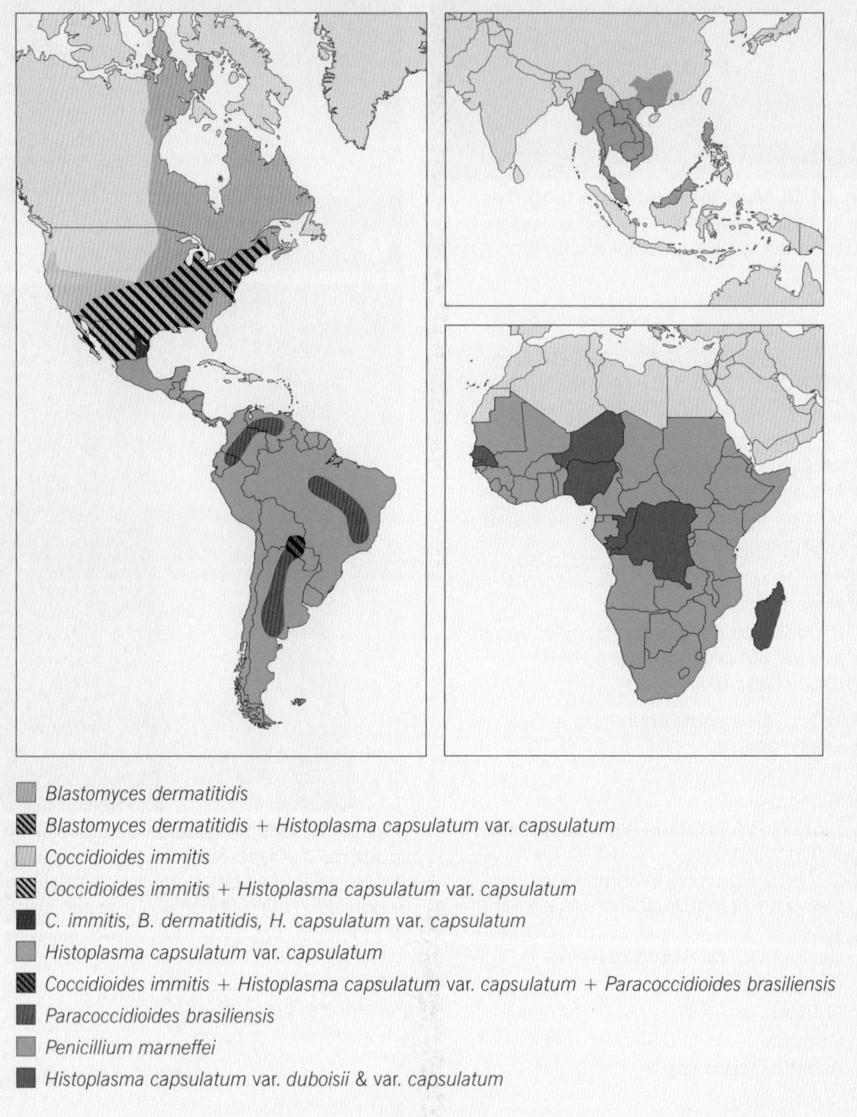

Fig. 64.20 Major geographic distribution of dimorphic fungi. *Histoplasma capsulatum* var. *capsulatum* is also endemic along river basins in some areas of India, Southeast Asia, and Australia. *Courtesy, Braden A. Perry, MD.*

- Less common variants: (1) a fixed, ulcerated plaque on the face in someone with prior exposure, a form prevalent in Brazil due to transmission by infected cats; and (2) cutaneous dissemination (e.g. papulonodules) from a systemic infection.

Systemic (Unless Primary Inoculation into Skin)

BLASTOMYCOSIS

- Due to *Blastomyces dermatitidis*, a dimorphic fungus; yeast form displays broad-based budding (see Fig. 64.17C).

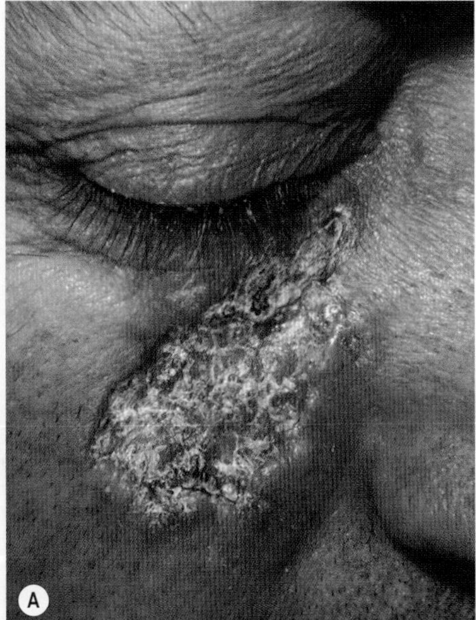

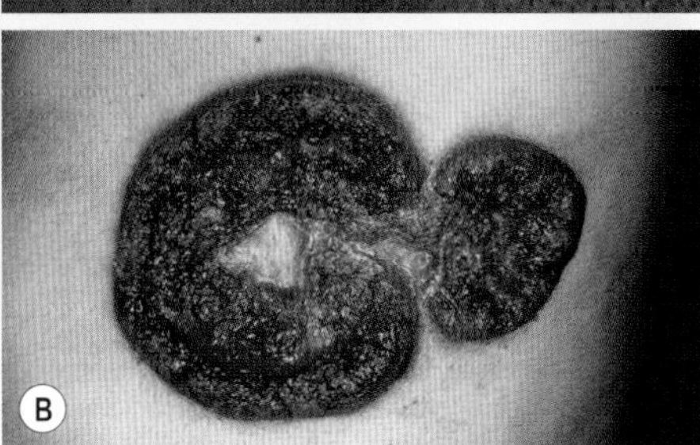

Fig. 64.21 Blastomycosis. A Facial plaque with scale-crust and a border with a granulomatous appearance. **B** Well-demarcated plaques with erosions, central scarring, and black crusting. *A, Courtesy, Louis A. Fragola, Jr., MD; B, Courtesy, Paul Lucky, MD.*

- Endemic to the southeastern United States and other areas of North America (Fig. 64.20).
- Contracted via inhalation, with the skin, bones, and genitourinary tract being the most common sites of secondary infection.
- Cutaneous lesions can vary from papulopustules to verrucous plaques with crusted borders (Fig. 64.21).

COCCIDIOIDOMYCOSIS

- Due to *Coccidioides immitis*, a dimorphic fungus that forms arthrospores in the soil and spherules within the skin (see Fig. 64.17D).
- Endemic to the southwestern United States (see Fig. 64.20).

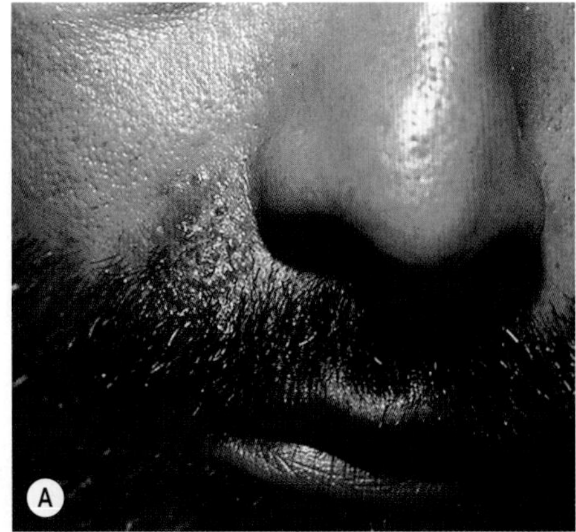

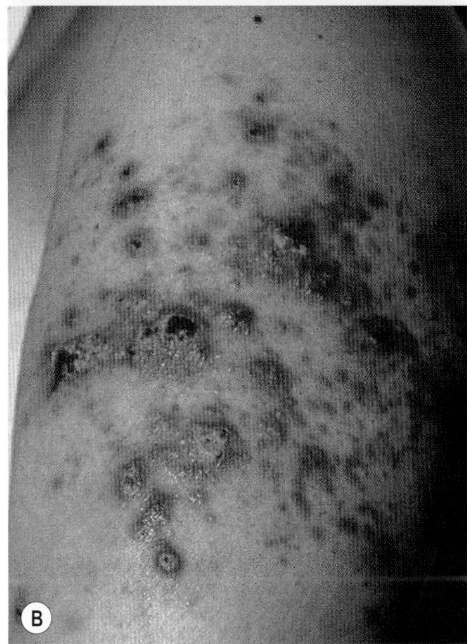

Fig. 64.22 Coccidioidomycosis. Moist erythematous plaque on the face **(A)** and multiple papules and suppurative nodules on the arm **(B)** in two patients living in the southwestern United States. *Courtesy, USCDRSC.*

- Contracted via inhalation, with disseminated disease more common in African-Americans, Mexicans, and immunocompromised hosts.
- Cutaneous manifestations: lesions vary from papules to pustules, abscesses, and plaques with sinus tracts (Fig. 64.22).
- Non-infectious hypersensitivity reactions include toxic erythema, erythema multiforme, and erythema nodosum.
- Molluscum contagiosum-like lesions may be seen in HIV-infected persons.

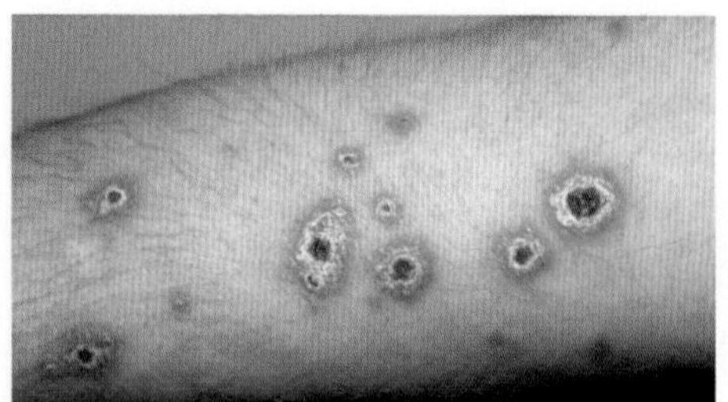

Fig. 64.23 Histoplasmosis. Papules and nodules with scale-crust in a patient with AIDS. *Courtesy, USCDRSC.*

CRYPTOCOCCOSIS

- Molluscum contagiosum-like lesions may be seen in HIV-infected patients and other immunocompromised hosts (see Fig. 64.25G), in addition to ulcers and cellulitis (see Fig. 64.25F).

HISTOPLASMOSIS

- Due to *Histoplasma capsulatum* var. *capsulatum*, a dimorphic fungus (see Fig. 64.17B).
- Endemic to the southeastern and central United States and many other countries with reservoirs in birds, including fowl, and bats (see Fig. 64.20).
- Disease contracted through inhalation or, rarely, implantation.
- Immunocompetent hosts: oral ulcers in up to 75% of patients; occasionally cutaneous papulonodules.
- Immunosuppressed hosts: oral ulcers and multiple papules or plaques (Fig. 64.23), including ones that resemble molluscum contagiosum.

PARACOCCIDIOIDOMYCOSIS

- Due to *Paracoccidioides brasiliensis*, a dimorphic fungus that displays multiple narrow-based buds in tissue, including the skin.
- Endemic to South America.
- Disease contracted via inhalation, with dissemination primarily to lymph nodes > oropharynx > adrenal glands > spleen and gastrointestinal tract, in addition to the skin.
- Cutaneous lesions are primarily periorificial and associated with involvement of the oral mucosa; verrucous and ulcerative plaques are seen (Fig. 64.24).

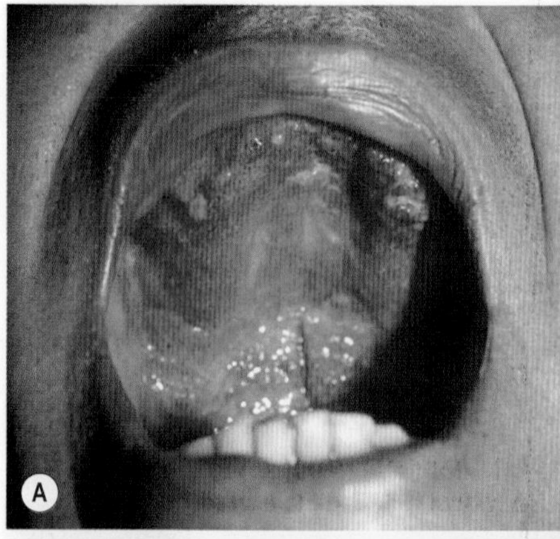

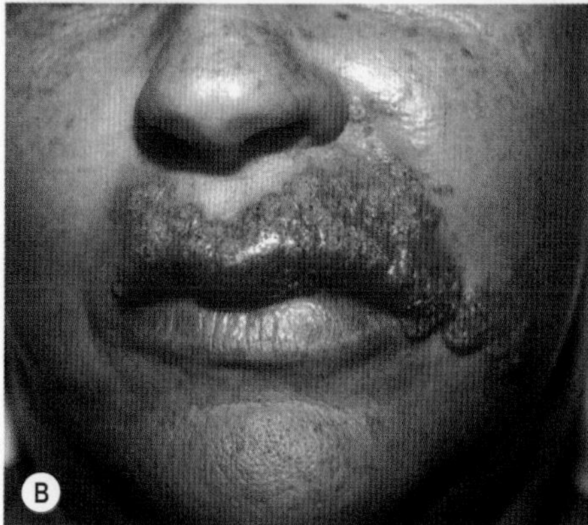

Fig. 64.24 Paracoccidioidomycosis. Ulcerated plaques on the palate (**A**) and verrucous granulomatous red-brown plaques with crusting involving the perioral region and upper lip (**B**). *Courtesy, Marcia Ramos-e-Silva, MD, PhD.*

OPPORTUNISTIC PATHOGENS

See Table 64.6 and Fig. 64.25.

For further information see Ch. 77 from *Dermatology, Fourth Edition*.

For additional online figures and tables visit www.expertconsult.com 

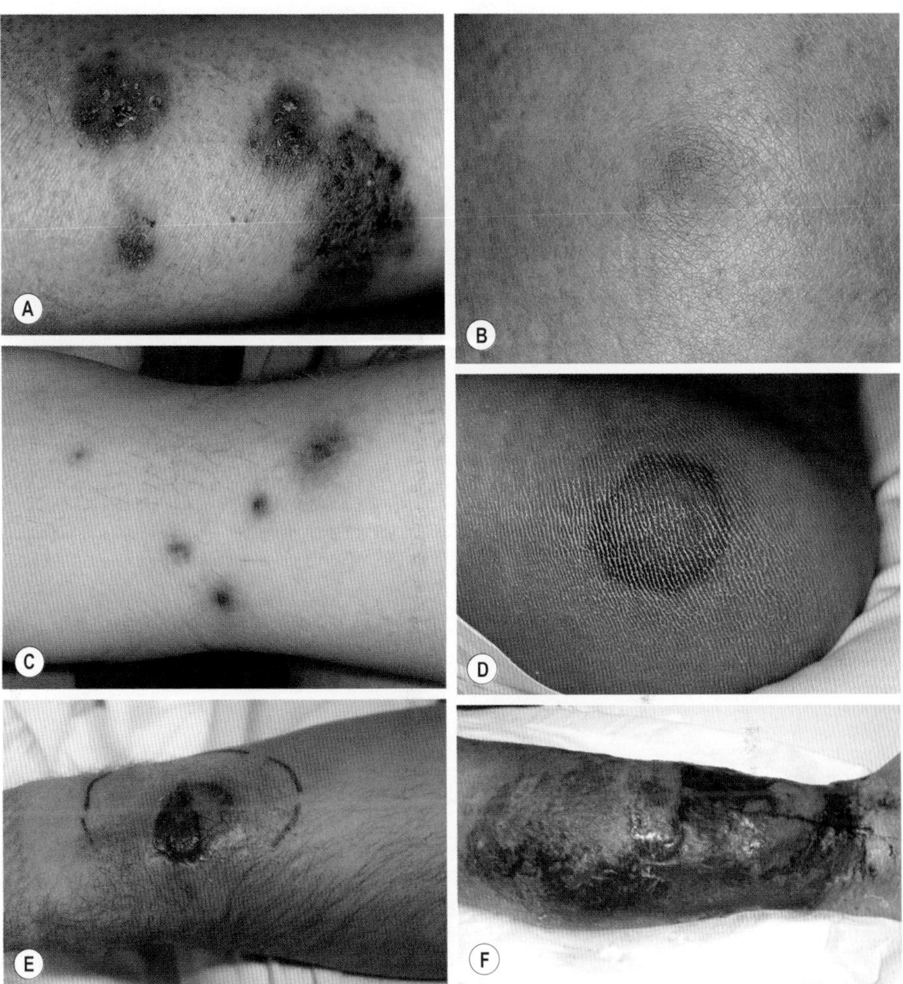

Fig. 64.25 Clinical findings of opportunistic fungal infections in immunocompromised hosts. Primary cutaneous aspergillosis characterized by hyperpigmented plaques with brown-black scale-crusts at the site of intravenous catheters on the arm (**A**); firm pink papulonodule due to disseminated candidiasis (**B**); erythematous papulonodules with central purpura, vesiculation and/or crusting in a leukemic patient with disseminated fusariosis (**C**); necrotic hemorrhagic bulla due to embolus of *Aspergillus flavus* (**D**); cellulitis with large areas of necrosis due to *Rhizopus* (**E**) and *Cryptococcus neoformans* (**F**). *Continued*

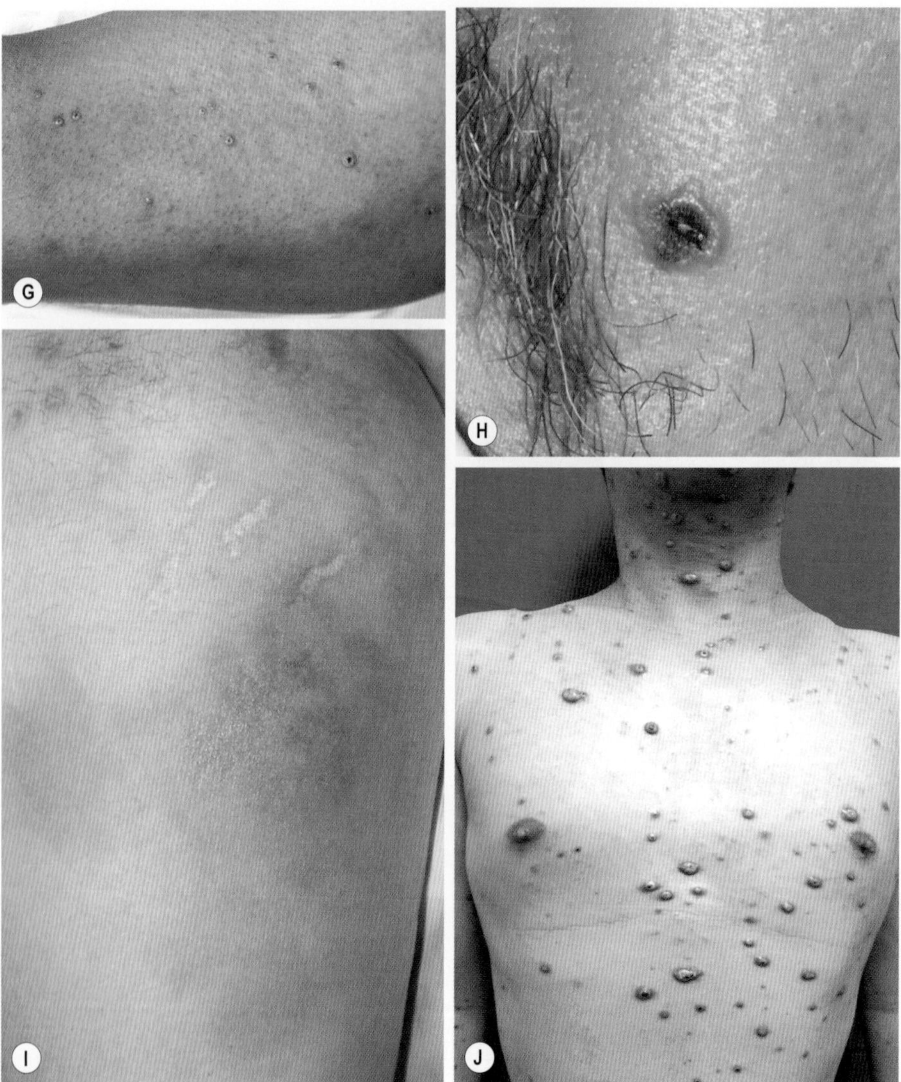

Fig. 64.25 *Continued* **Clinical findings of opportunistic fungal infections in immunocompromised hosts.** Disseminated cryptococcosis presenting with lesion(s) resembling molluscum contagiosum (**G**); and a basal cell carcinoma (**H**); cryptococcal cellulitis (**I**); numerous papules and nodules with central umbilication and crusting in disseminated *Talaromyces (Penicillium) marneffei* infection (**J**). *A, B, D, E, Courtesy, YDRSC; C, F–I, Courtesy, Boni E. Elewski, MD and Roderick J. Hay, MD; J, Courtesy, Evangeline Handog, MD and the Dermatology Department, Research Institute for Tropical Medicine.*

Cutaneous Manifestations of HIV Infection

65

There are a number of cutaneous disorders that point to the diagnosis of HIV infection. For some, it is the mere presence of the skin disease, whereas for others, the disease is extensive or proves recalcitrant to therapy (Table 65.1; Figs 65.1–65.14). As HIV infection is associated with immunosuppression, the clinical presentation of various infectious diseases is often reminiscent of that observed in individuals whose immunocompromised state is due to medications (e.g. CS plus chemotherapy) or underlying diseases (e.g. acute leukemia).

In HIV-infected patients, several cutaneous diseases (e.g. disseminated coccidioidomycosis, Kaposi sarcoma) are AIDS-defining conditions (see who.int/hiv/pub/guidelines/HIVstaging150307.pdf), whereas others such as oral hairy leukoplakia and seborrheic dermatitis can serve as early clues to the infection, i.e. when there are >400 CD4$^+$ cells/mm^3.

Epidemiology

- With the advent of antiretroviral therapy (ART), HIV infection/AIDS has become a chronic disease.
- High-risk groups still include commercial sex workers, men who have sex with men (MSM), and intravenous drug users, but heterosexual transmission has become a significant mode of transmission.
- Approximately 70% of individuals living with HIV infection are in sub-Saharan Africa.

Exanthem of Primary HIV Infection (Acute Retroviral Syndrome)

- Follows an incubation period of 3–6 weeks, but the latter may be shorter if infection acquired hematogenously.
- Morbilliform eruption (40–80% of patients) appears in the setting of peak viremia; accompanied by orogenital ulcerations (5–20%)

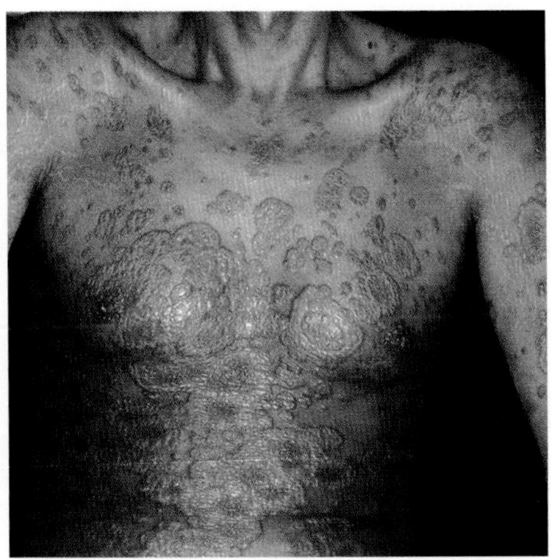

Fig. 65.1 Severe psoriasis in a patient with AIDS. Both sudden acute exacerbations and treatment resistance can be observed.

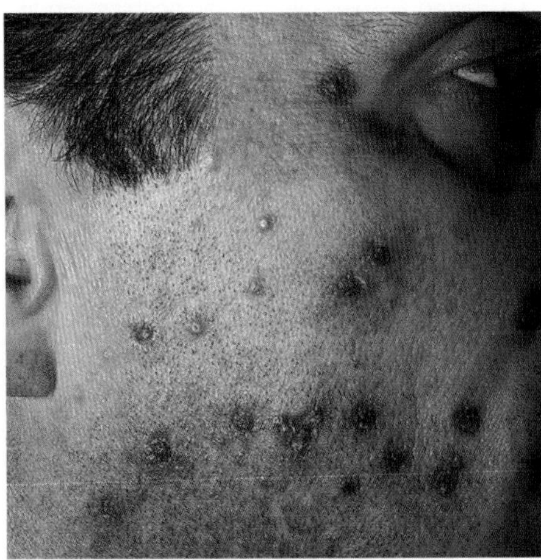

Fig. 65.2 Eosinophilic folliculitis. Due to associated pruritus, follicular papules are often excoriated; lesions favor the head and upper trunk. *Courtesy, Clay J. Cockerell, MD.*

MUCOCUTANEOUS DISORDERS ASSOCIATED WITH HIV INFECTION
Inflammatory disorders
When severe, recalcitrant, or of sudden onset, consider HIV infection
• Seborrheic dermatitis (e.g. face, scalp)
• Psoriasis vulgaris (Fig. 65.1)
• Reactive arthritis (previously referred to as Reiter disease)
Alone raises the possibility of HIV infection
• Eosinophilic folliculitis (Fig. 65.2; Ch. 31)*
• Pityriasis rubra pilaris type VI, with follicular spines & acne conglobata
Infectious diseases and infestations*
When severe and/or recalcitrant, consider HIV infection
• Human papilloma virus infections (warts), including acquired epidermodysplasia verruciformis-like lesions (Ch. 66)
• Molluscum contagiosum, numerous, coalescent, and/or giant-sized, especially in adults (Fig. 65.3)
• Dermatophyte infections (Ch. 64)
Alone raises the possibility of HIV infection
• Syphilis (Fig. 65.4) and other sexually transmitted infections (e.g. chancroid; Ch. 69)
• Bacillary angiomatosis (Fig. 65.5)
• Botryomycosis ("grains" within the dermis composed of *Staphylococcus*, *Pseudomonas*)
• Disseminated mycobacterial infections (tuberculous and nontuberculous; Fig. 65.6)
• Chronic oral and anogenital herpes simplex (Fig. 65.7) or disseminated HSV
• Herpes zoster, especially if multi-dermatomal, disseminated, verrucous or chronic, but can have classic presentation (see Fig. 67.11A)
• Oral hairy leukoplakia due to EBV infection (Fig. 65.8)
• Anogenital and oral ulcers, verrucous plaques or morbilliform eruption due to CMV (Ch. 67)
• Kaposi sarcoma due to HHV-8 infection (Fig. 65.9; Chs 67 and 94)
• Oropharyngeal candidiasis (thrush; Fig. 65.10; Ch. 64)
• Proximal subungual onychomycosis
• Disseminated cryptococcosis (Fig. 65.11; Ch. 64)
• Disseminated dimorphic fungal infections (e.g. coccidioidomycosis, histoplasmosis, penicilliosis)
• Crusted scabies (Norwegian scabies; Fig. 65.12)
• Disseminated or necrotic cutaneous leishmaniasis
Other
• Papular pruritic eruption of HIV (Fig. 65.13)
• Xerosis and acquired ichthyosis
• Major aphthae (Fig. 65.14); acute necrotizing ulcerative stomatitis with gingivitis or periodontitis
• Porphyria cutanea tarda, often in association with hepatitis C
• Facial hyperpigmentation, idiopathic or due to photolichenoid drug eruption
• Linear telangiectasias of the chest
• Trichomegaly of the eyelashes and change in texture of scalp hair (e.g. curly -> fine and straight)
• *Demodex* folliculitis
• Cutaneous lesions of non-Hodgkin lymphoma
• Anal intraepithelial neoplasia/anal carcinoma
• Acral persistent papular mucinosis; atypical variants of granuloma annulare

**In particular when there is no known cause of immunosuppression.*

Table 65.1 Mucocutaneous disorders associated with HIV infection.

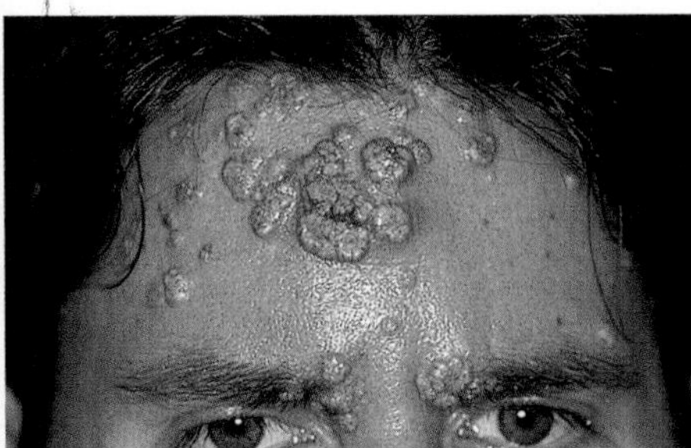

Fig. 65.3 Molluscum contagiosum in the setting of HIV infection. Large lesions due to coalescence of individual papules. The face is a common location.

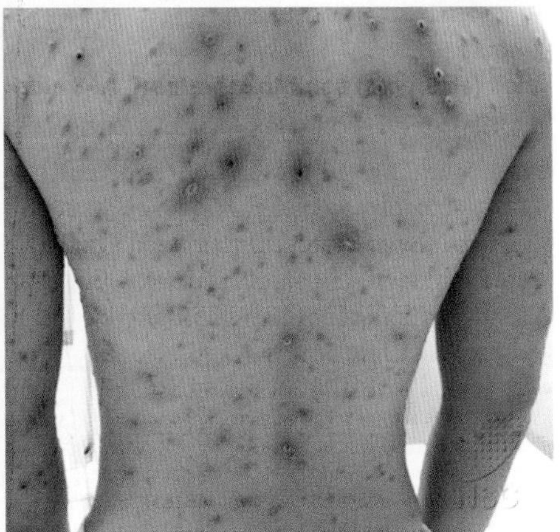

Fig. 65.4 Secondary syphilis presenting as lues maligna. This HIV-positive man had a fever, headache, arthralgias, and myalgias together with this widespread eruption of pustules and crusted papulonodules. *Courtesy, Singapore National Skin Centre.*

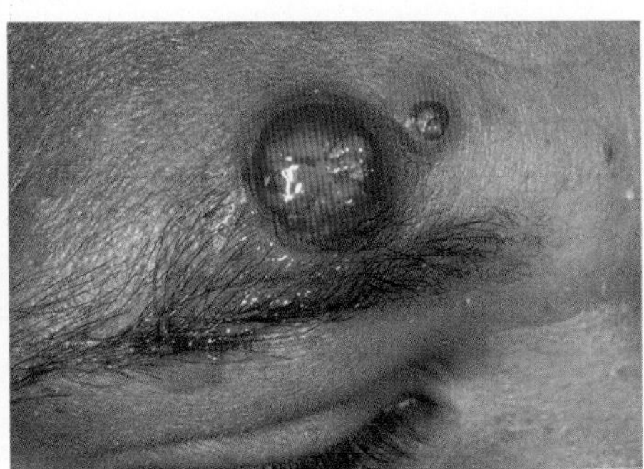

Fig. 65.5 Bacillary angiomatosis. Lesions can resemble vascular tumors or pyogenic granulomas and are a reflection of infection with *Bartonella henselae* or *B. quintana*. *Courtesy, NYUDSC.*

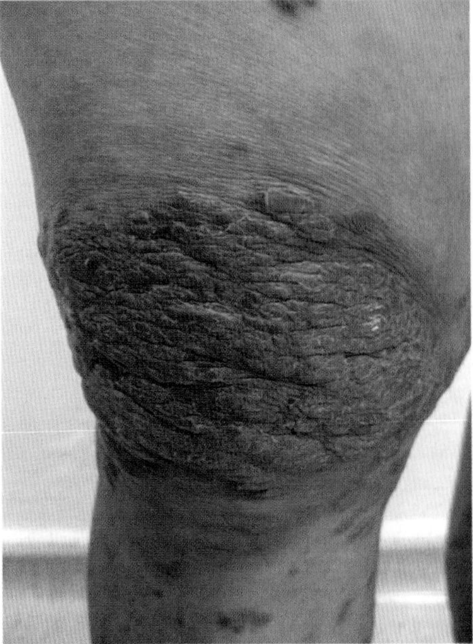

Fig. 65.6 *Mycobacterium haemophilum* infection. This HIV-positive man with a CD4$^+$ T-cell count of 350/mm^3 presented with a 4-month history of slowly enlarging, thick plaques on his extremities. The lesions resolved over six months with antimicrobial therapy that included ciprofloxacin, clarithromycin, and ethambutol. *Courtesy, Singapore National Skin Centre.*

as well as fever, fatigue, headache, pharyngitis, arthralgia, myalgia, lymphadenopathy, night sweats and a decrease in circulating CD4$^+$ T cells.

- While the cutaneous eruption usually lasts 4–5 days, the constitutional symptoms can last from a few days to a few months.
- **Dx:** detection of viral RNA by PCR and/or p24 antigen in the plasma; assays for anti-HIV-1 antibodies are less reliable as they may be negative, especially early on in the course of the disease.

Immune Reconstitution Inflammatory Syndrome (IRIS)

- Those disorders that can "flare" or "worsen" due to an increase in the ability to mount an inflammatory response following the institution of ART are outlined in Table 65.2 (Fig. 65.15).

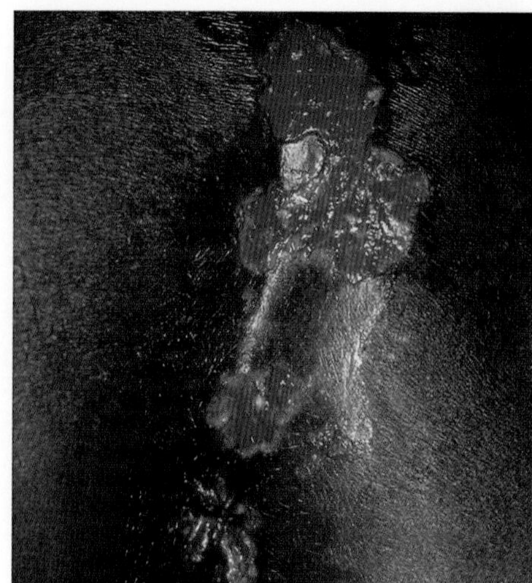

Fig. 65.7 Chronic ulcerative herpes simplex viral infection in an HIV-infected patient. These slowly enlarging ulcers of the buttocks and perianal area have a characteristic scalloped border. *Courtesy, YDRSC.*

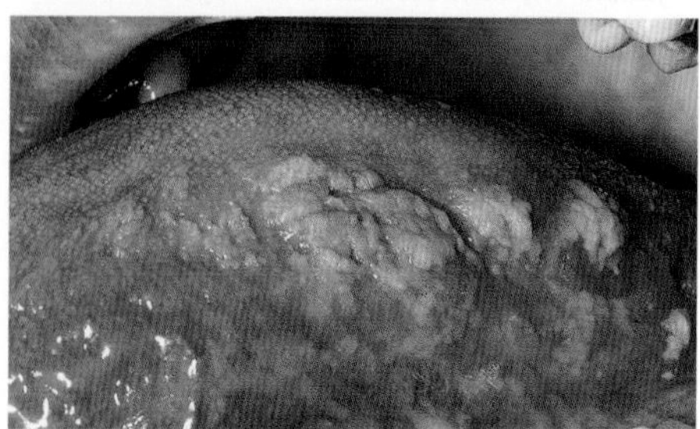

Fig. 65.8 Oral hairy leukoplakia. Shaggy white keratotic plaques along the lateral aspect of the tongue. A corrugated pattern is often seen. *Courtesy, Charles Camisa, MD.*

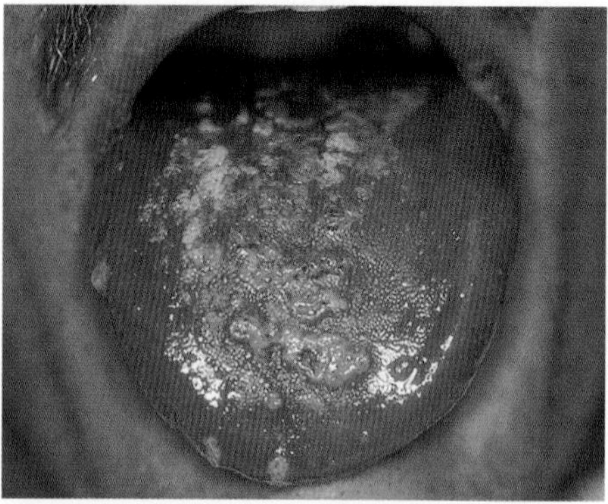

Fig. 65.10 Both oral candidiasis and oral herpes viral infection involving the tongue. The white plaques represent the former, whereas the circular and scalloped areas of detached epithelium represent the latter. Either of these infections, and especially their combination, points to immunosuppression and the possibility of HIV infection.

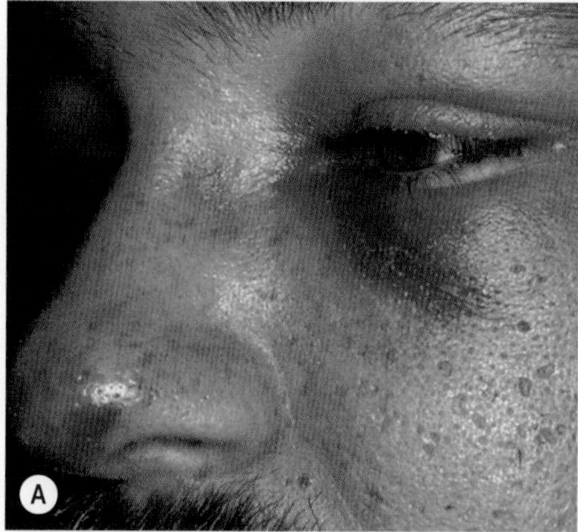

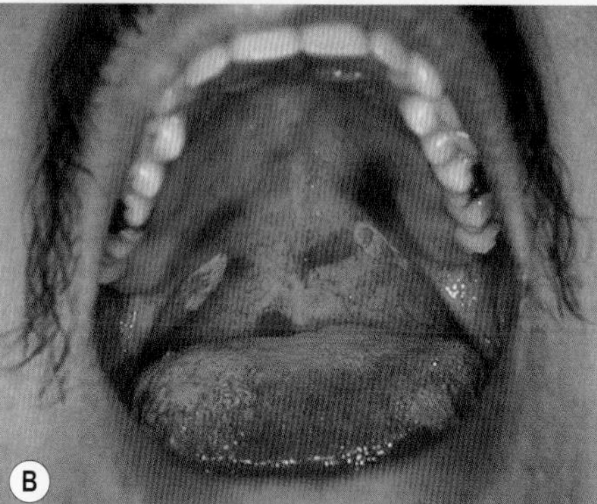

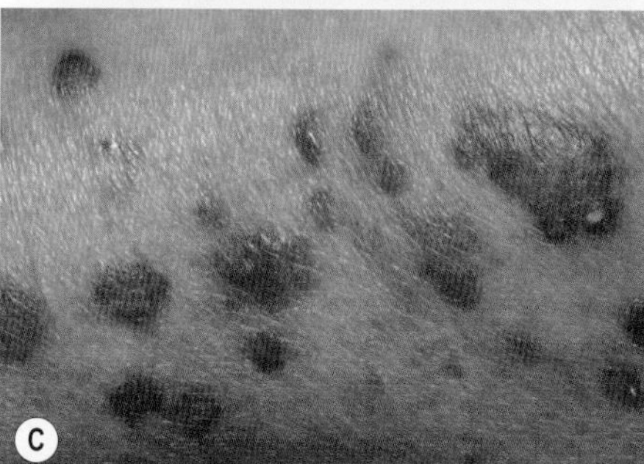

Fig. 65.9 Kaposi sarcoma in the setting of AIDS. Violaceous papules and plaques involving the face **(A),** palate **(B),** and an extremity **(C).** The patient also has oral candidiasis. *A, B, Courtesy, YDRSC; C, Courtesy, Thomas Horn, MD.*

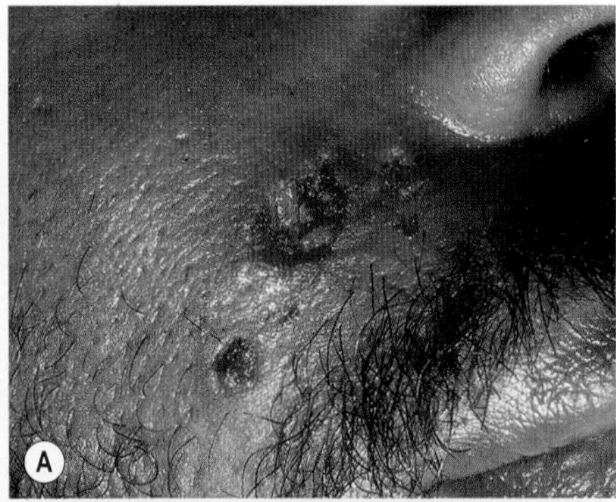

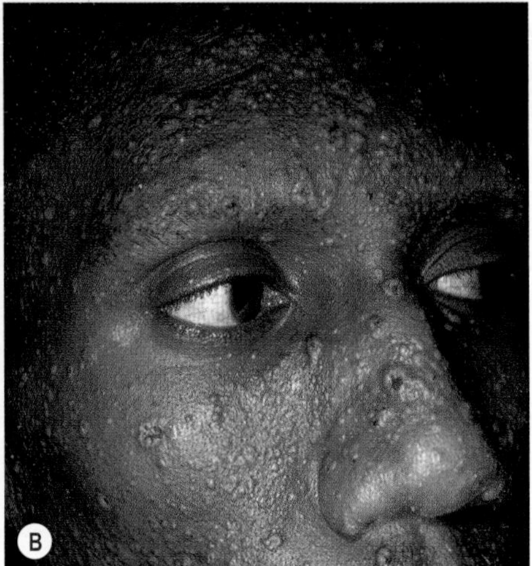

Fig. 65.11 Disseminated cryptococcosis in the setting of AIDS. A Several ulcers with rolled borders. **B** Numerous molloscum contagiosum-like lesions. Microscopic examination and culture of either dermal scrapings or a biopsy specimen confirm the diagnosis. *A, Courtesy, YDRSC; B, Courtesy, NYUDSC.*

- It is noteworthy that depending on the patient, some of these disorders improve rather than "worsen" in the setting of ART, e.g. Kaposi sarcoma.

Antiretroviral Therapy (ART)

- Recommended for all HIV-infected individuals, irrespective of CD4 count.
- For naive patients, first-line therapy consists of *dual* NRTIs (nucleoside reverse transcriptase inhibitors) plus an integrase inhibitor while second-line therapy consists of *dual* NRTIs plus either an NNRTI (non-nucleoside reverse transcriptase inhibitor) or a ritonavir-boosted protease inhibitor. In low- and middle-income countries, the first-line regimen can consist of *dual* NRTIs plus an NNRTI.
- Table 65.3 (Figs 65.16 and 65.17) outlines the mucocutaneous side effects of these antiretroviral drugs (Fig. 65.18); such reactions can lead to the discontinuation of the incriminated medication.
- When taken daily, pre-exposure prophylaxis (PrEP) reduces the risk of contracting HIV infection, e.g. a >90% reduction if due to sexual exposure. However, reduced use of condoms leads to an increase in sexually transmitted infections.

For further information see Ch. 78 from *Dermatology, Fourth Edition*.

For additional online figures and tables visit www.expertconsult.com 

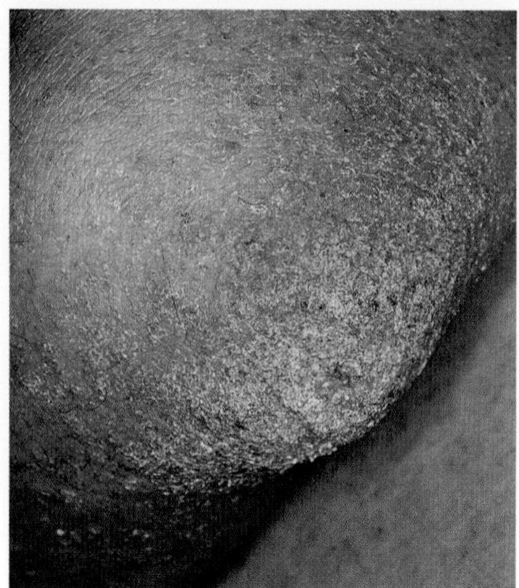

Fig. 65.12 Crusted scabies in the setting of HIV infection. Crusted scabies is often misdiagnosed as dermatitis, but these scale-crusts are teeming with mites. This form of the disease was previously referred to as Norwegian scabies. *Courtesy, YDRSC.*

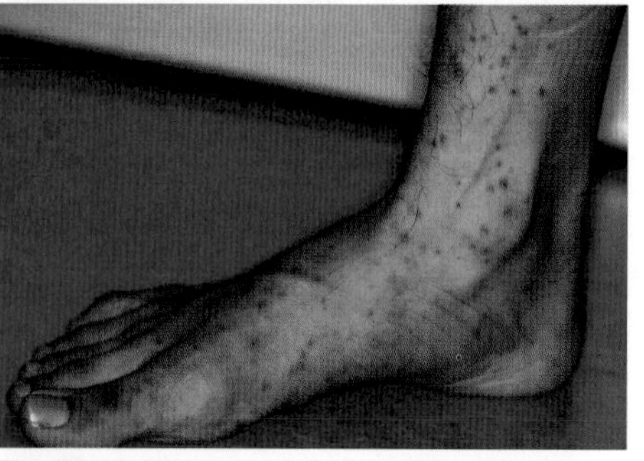

Fig. 65.13 HIV-associated pruritic papular eruption. This eruption is characterized by extremely pruritic erythematous papules and a predilection for the extremities. It is thought to represent a hypersensitivity reaction to arthropod antigens. *Courtesy, Singapore National Skin Centre.*

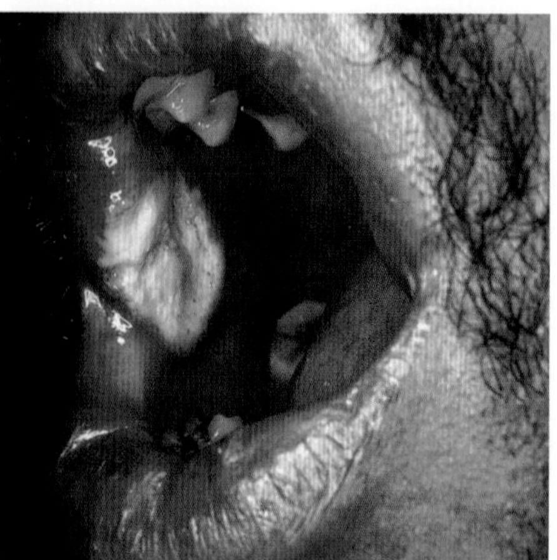

Fig. 65.14 Major aphthae in a patient with AIDS. Resolution of these oral ulcers may require thalidomide. *Courtesy, YDRSC.*

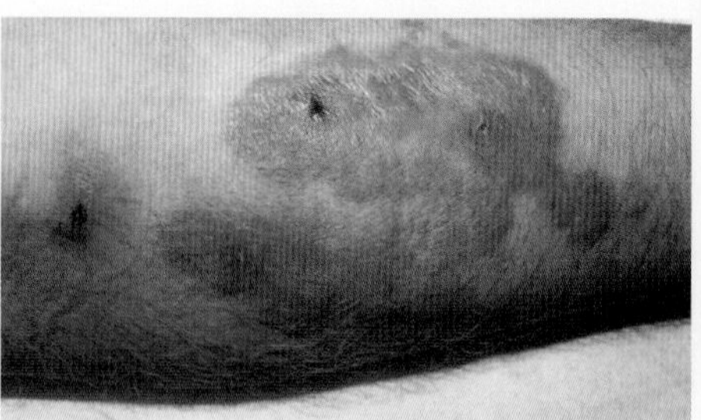

Fig. 65.15 Exacerbation of leprosy due to immune reconstitution inflammatory syndrome (IRIS) following institution of ART. *Courtesy, Beatriz Trope, MD, PhD.*

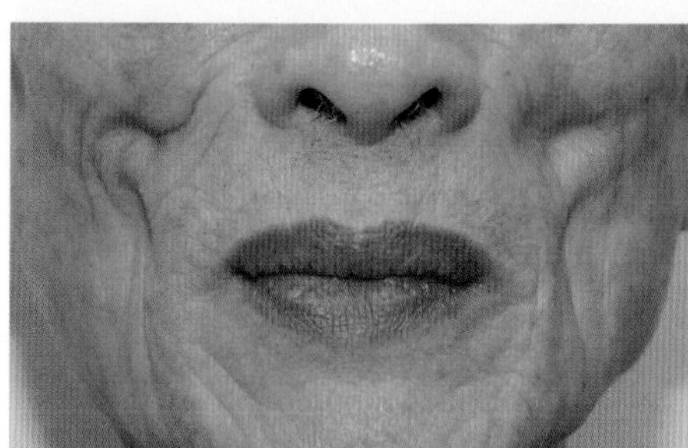

Fig. 65.16 HIV/ART-associated lipodystrophy. Marked indentation of the medial cheeks due to lipoatrophy is a characteristic finding, as is a decrease in subcutaneous fat of the extremities and an increase in abdominal fat (central obesity). *Courtesy, Priya Sen, MD.*

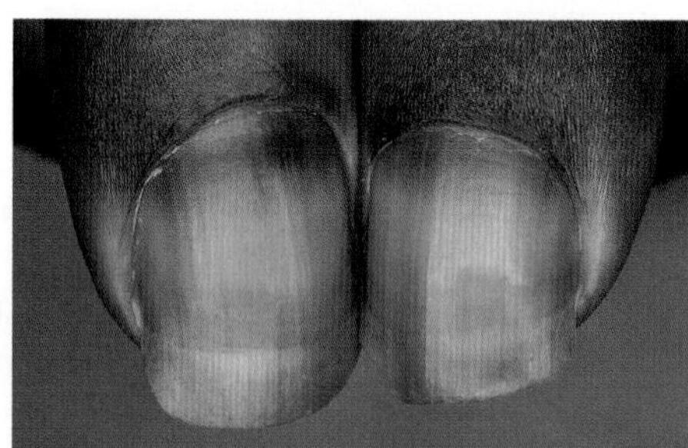

Fig. 65.17 Zidovudine-associated melanonychia. Patients receiving zidovudine (AZT) may develop longitudinal streaks, horizontal bands, or diffuse hyperpigmentation as well as oral and cutaneous hyperpigmentation. *Courtesy, YDRSC.*

CUTANEOUS DISEASES THAT CAN "FLARE" DUE TO THE IMMUNE RECONSTITUTION INFLAMMATORY SYNDROME (IRIS)
Infections
• *Mycobacterium tuberculosis* • *Mycobacterium leprae* (Fig. 65.15) • *Mycobacterium avium* complex and other species • Herpes simplex virus 1 and 2 • Varicella–zoster virus • Epstein–Barr virus (e.g. oral hairy leukoplakia) • Cytomegalovirus • Human papillomavirus • Molluscum contagiosum virus • *Candida* spp. • Dermatophytes • *Cryptococcus* spp. • *Histoplasma capsulatum*, *Penicillium marneffei* • *Demodex*, *Malassezia* spp. (e.g. folliculitis) • *Leishmania* spp.
Inflammatory disorders
• Psoriasis, seborrheic dermatitis • Pityriasis rubra pilaris • Granuloma annulare • Sarcoidosis • Foreign body reactions (granulomatous) • Eosinophilic folliculitis • Acne vulgaris, rosacea • Papular pruritic eruption • Lupus erythematosus (systemic, discoid, tumid), relapsing polychondritis • Alopecia areata • Dyshidrotic eczema • Mid-dermal elastolysis
Neoplasms
• Kaposi sarcoma • Non-Hodgkin lymphoma • Multiple eruptive dermatofibromas

Table 65.2 Cutaneous diseases that can "flare" due to the immune reconstitution inflammatory syndrome (IRIS). IRIS can also occur in other settings of immunosuppression (e.g. solid organ transplants, TNF administration).

CUTANEOUS SIDE EFFECTS OF ANTIRETROVIRAL THERAPY (ART)

Type of skin reaction	NRTIs/NtRTIs	NNRTIs	Protease inhibitors	Integrase inhibitors	CCR5 inhibitors	Fusion inhibitors
Injection site reaction						
Morbilliform eruption	Emtricitabine* / Abacavir**	Nevirapine> etravirine, efavirenz	Atazanavir, fosamprenavir^ > darunavir^, tipranavir^ > lopinavir			
DRESS (DIHS)	**Abacavir****	**Etravirine, efavirenz** / **Nevirapine**	Atazanavir, darunavir^, fosamprenavir^, tipranavir^, lopinavir	Rare	Rare	Rare
SJS/TEN	Rare	Rare / Nevirapine > efavirenz, etravirine	Rare	Rare		
Lipodystrophy (also insulin resistance and elevated TTGs)	d4T, ddI	Efavirenz	Fig. 65.16			
Paronychia, excessive periungual granulation tissue	Lamivudine		Indinavir			
Xerosis			Indinavir			
Hyperpigmentation of skin and nails	AZT (Fig. 65.17), emtricitabine (palmoplantar)					

**Palmoplantar eruption.*

***Associated with HLA-B*5701 allele.*

^Sulfonamide-like structure and should be used cautiously in patients with sulfonamide allergy.

Table 65.3 Cutaneous side effects of antiretroviral therapy (ART). In general, patients with HIV infection have an increased risk of developing drug-induced morbilliform eruptions and toxic epidermal necrolysis, e.g. to sulfonamides. Bold = most common; dark-colored cells = common; light-colored cells = less common. A whole cell that lacks specific drug names refers to that class of drugs, whereas in subdivided cells, it refers to the remainder of that class of drugs. AZT, zidovudine; CCR5, CC-chemokine receptor 5; NNRTIs, non-nucleoside reverse transcriptase inhibitors; NRTIs/NtRTIs, nucleoside/nucleotide reverse transcriptase inhibitors; SJS, Stevens–Johnson syndrome; TEN, toxic epidermal necrolysis; TTGs, triglycerides.

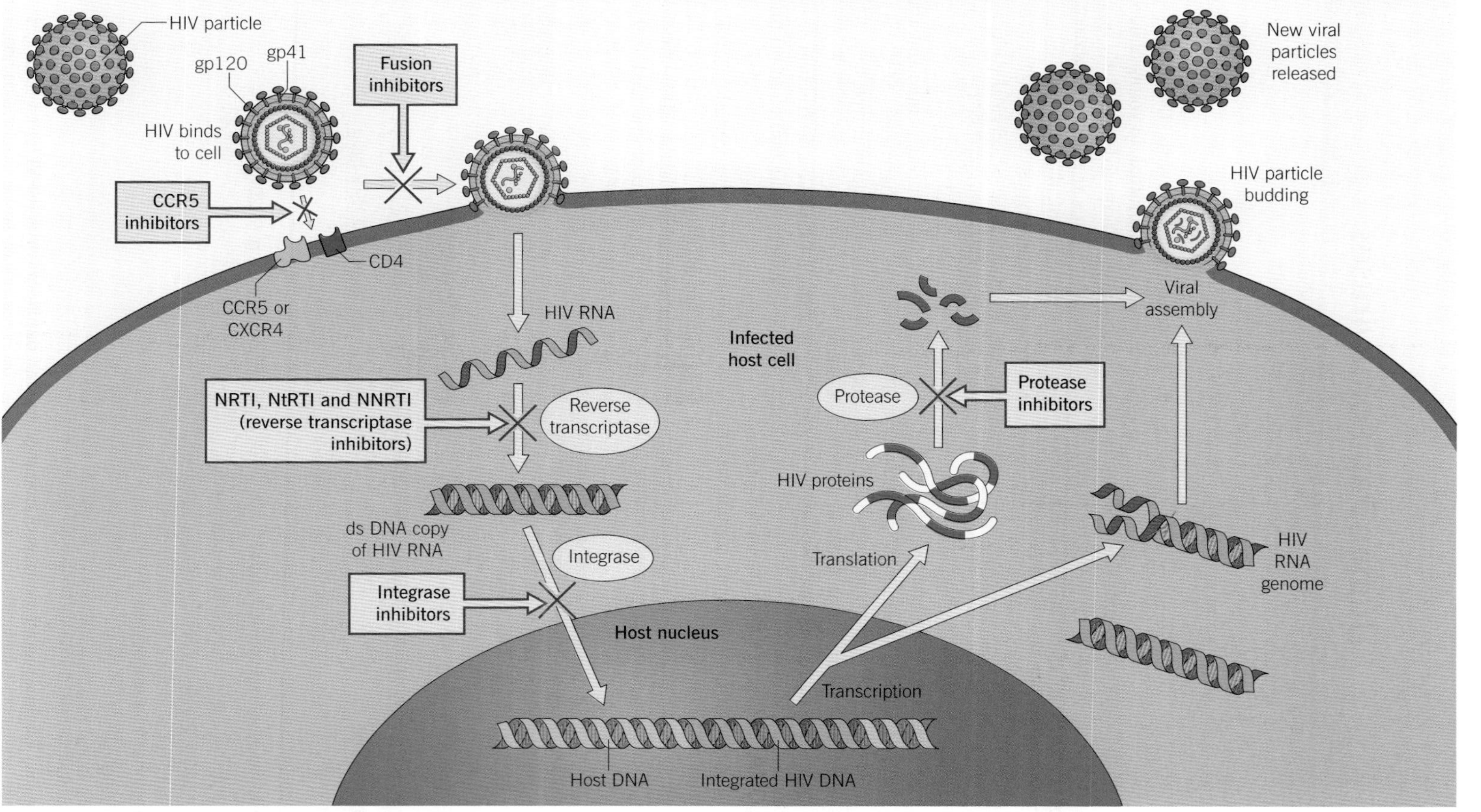

Fig. 65.18 Replication of HIV within CD4+ lymphocyte and target sites of antiretroviral drugs. CCR5, CC-chemokine receptor 5; NRTI, nucleoside reverse transcriptase inhibitor; NtRTI, nucleotide reverse transcriptase inhibitor; NNRTI, non-nucleoside reverse transcriptase inhibitor.

66 Human Papillomaviruses

Key Points

- Human papilloma viruses (HPV) comprise a large group of at least 200 genotypes of DNA viruses that infect the skin and mucosa.
- Different genotypes cause different skin lesions (Table 66.1).
  - Clinical variants differ as to anatomic location, morphology, histopathology, and HPV subtype; correlation of clinical and histopathologic findings is particularly important for bowenoid papulosis and verrucous carcinoma in order to prevent over- or undertreatment, respectively
- Nongenital warts:
  - Transmitted via person-to-person contact or contact with contaminated surfaces/objects
  - Prevalence of 20% in schoolchildren
  - A third or more self-regress within 1–2 years
  - Numerous warts or persistent/progressive warts should prompt consideration of immunosuppression, defects in cellular immunity, or other syndromes (e.g. HIV infection, epidermodysplasia verruciformis, WHIM syndrome [see Ch. 49])
- Anogenital infection with HPV:
  - Sexually transmitted; in young children may also be acquired perinatally or via the same routes as nongenital warts
  - May be subclinical
- High-risk HPV types, especially 16 and 18, are a major cause of cervical cancer as well as cutaneous (periungual SCC) and other mucosal intraepithelial neoplasias or SCCs, in particular vaginal, vulvar, penile, and anal; HPV-associated oropharyngeal SCC is a recently identified specific subtype.
- **Rx**:
  - If desired, focuses on destruction of visible lesions or induction of an immune response
  - Effective targeted antiviral treatments are not available
- Prevention: prophylactic HPV vaccines (e.g. Gardasil®9) are recommended in both genders from ages 9 to 45.

Common Warts (Verrucae Vulgares)

- Any site, but commonly on the fingers, dorsal hands, and/or sites prone to trauma (Figs 66.1 and 66.2).

CLINICAL MANIFESTATIONS OF COMMON HUMAN PAPILLOMAVIRUS (HPV) TYPES	
Skin lesions	**Frequently detected HPV type**
Common, palmar, plantar, myrmecial warts	1, 2 > 27, 57
Flat warts	3, 10
Epidermodysplasia verruciformis	5*, 8* > others (e.g. 9, 20)
Condylomata acuminata (anogenital warts)	6, 11
High-grade squamous intraepithelial neoplasia (cervical lesions, bowenoid papulosis, erythroplasia of Queyrat)	16, 18, 31, 33 > others (e.g. 35)
Cervical cancer	16, 18

**Oncogenic, like HPV types 16, 18.*

Table 66.1 Clinical manifestations of common human papillomavirus (HPV) types. In clinical practice, subtyping is generally only performed routinely on Papanicolaou smears. Subtyping does not usually change management of cutaneous lesions.

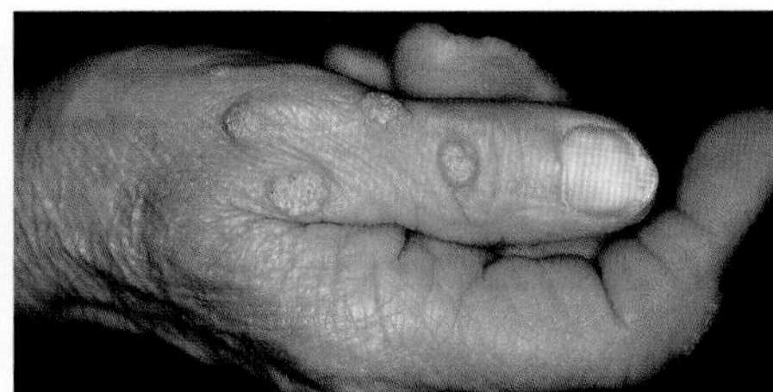

Fig. 66.1 Verrucae vulgares (common warts). *Courtesy, A. Geusau, MD.*

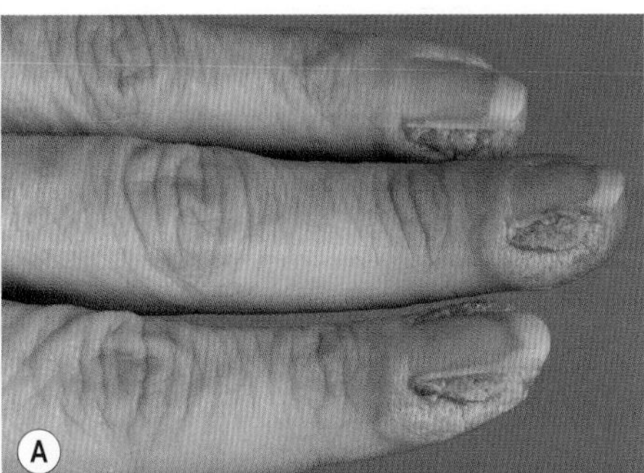

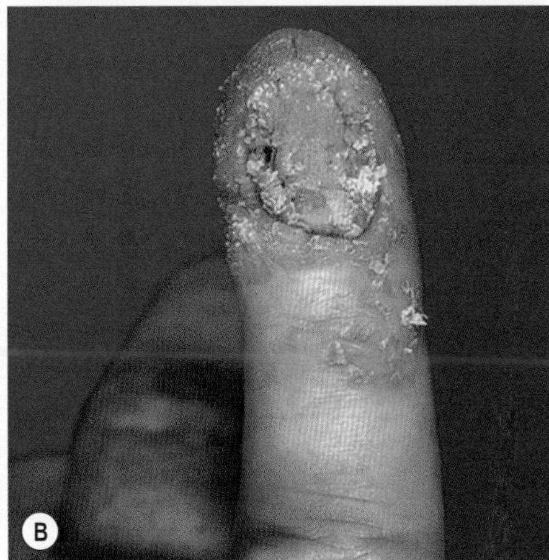

Fig. 66.2 Periungual common warts. Destruction of the nail matrix and bed can lead to partial **(A)** or complete **(B)** absence of the nail plate. Bowen disease may be considered in the differential diagnosis, especially for a single, recalcitrant digital wart. *A, B, Courtesy, Reinhard Kirnbauer, MD, and Petra Lenz, MD.*

- Hyperkeratotic, exophytic or dome-shaped papules or plaques with punctate black dots (hemorrhage in the stratum corneum) that may require paring to see (Fig. 66.3).
- Histopathology: papillomatosis, acanthosis, hypergranulosis; epidermal keratinocytes have haloes around their nuclei (koilocytes).

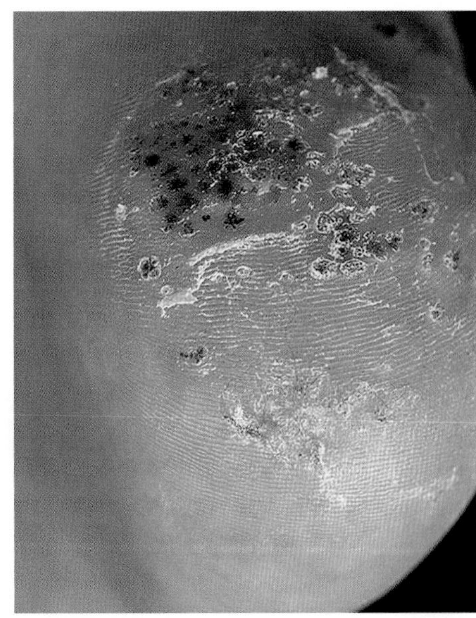

Fig. 66.3 Verrucae plantares (plantar warts). The photo was taken after shaving of the hyperkeratotic surface; the black dots represent intracorneal hemorrhage. *Courtesy, Reinhard Kirnbauer, MD, and Petra Lenz, MD.*

- **DDx:** seborrheic keratosis, actinic keratosis, cutaneous horn, SCC (especially periungual), trichilemmoma, Spitz nevus.
- **Rx:** outlined in Fig. 66.4; may regress spontaneously within 1–2 years; may be difficult to eradicate.

Plantar/Palmar Warts

- Thick, exo- and endophytic hyperkeratotic papules and plaques (Fig. 66.5); coalescence of lesions can lead to extensive areas of involvement referred to as mosaic warts.
- May see sloping sides and a central depression (the term *myrmecia* is used because it can resemble an anthill); tender with pressure (Fig. 66.6).
- **DDx:** corns (clavi; see Ch. 74), punctate palmoplantar keratoderma (see Table 47.1), arsenical keratoses, SCC, amelanotic melanoma.
- **Rx:** overlaps with Rx of common warts (see Fig. 66.4).

Flat Warts (Verrucae Planae)

- Commonly on the dorsal hands, arms, and face, as well as the legs (exacerbated by shaving).
- Skin-colored to pink or brown (sometimes hypopigmented in darker skin), minimally

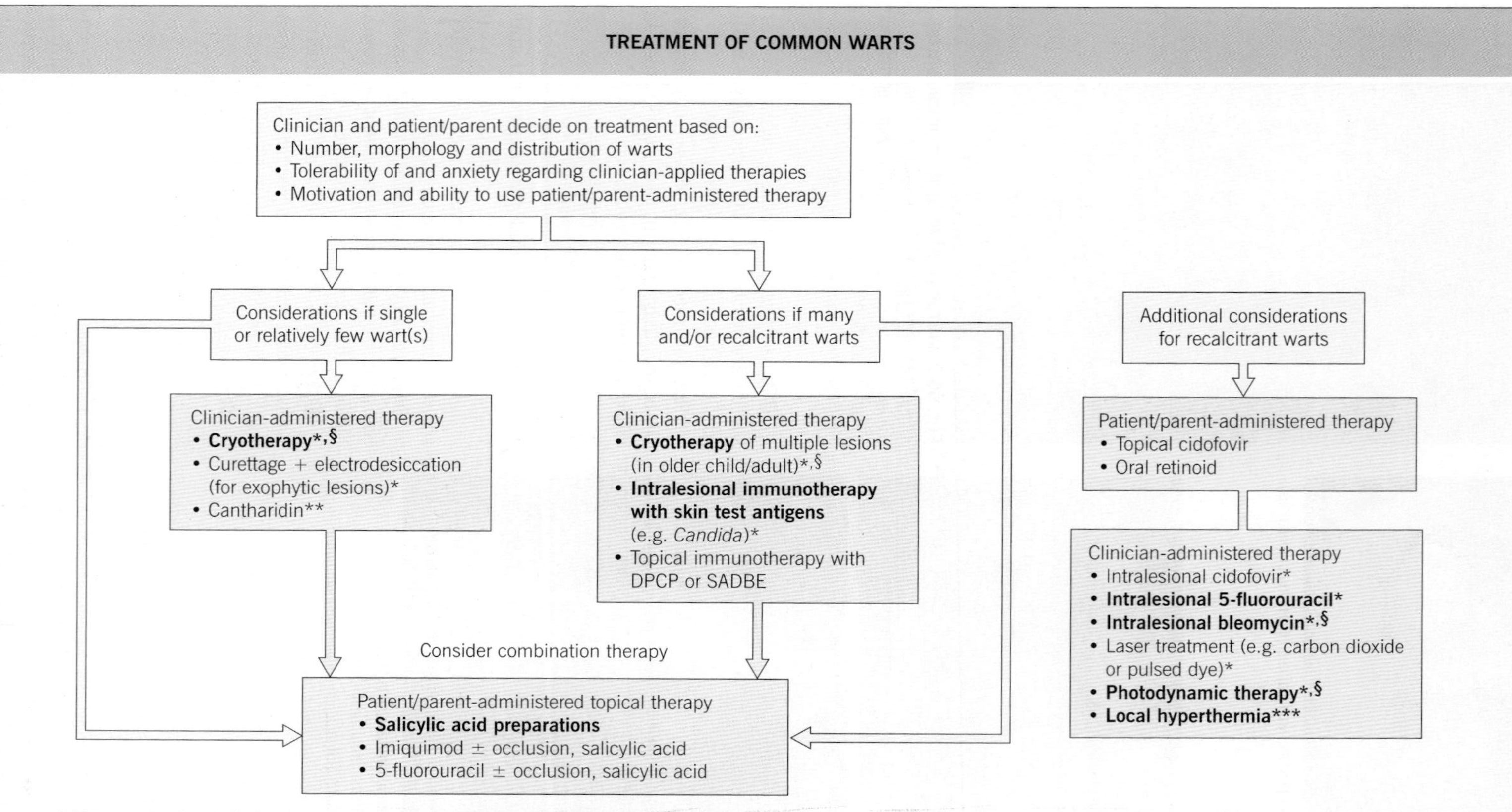

Fig. 66.4 Treatment of common warts.

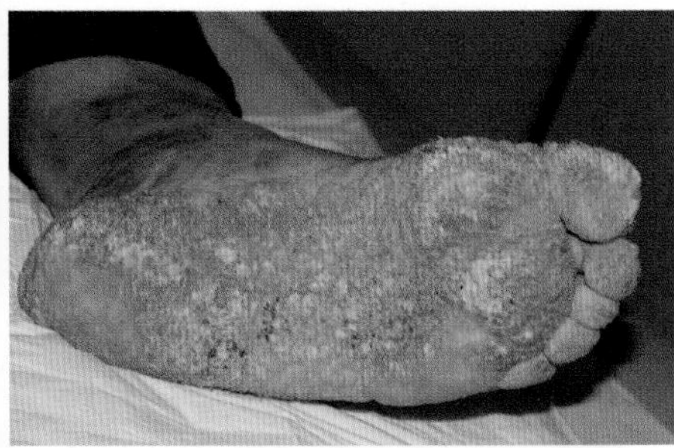

Fig. 66.5 Extensive and chronic verrucosis of the sole in a patient with hepatic cirrhosis due to alcoholism. HPV-27 DNA was isolated from the lesions. *Courtesy, Reinhard Kirnbauer, MD, and Petra Lenz, MD.*

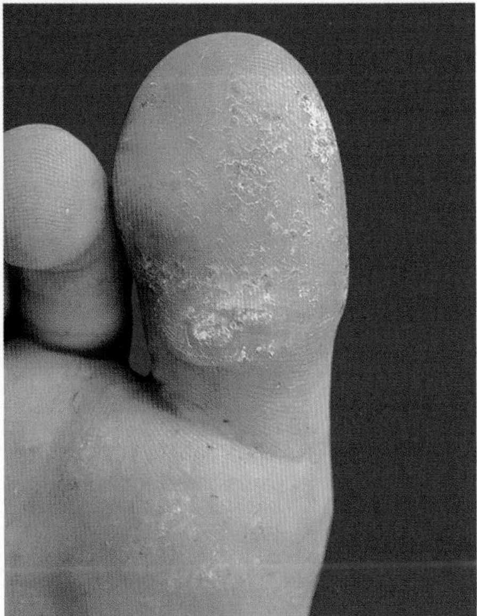

Fig. 66.6 Myrmecial wart. The wart at the base of the distal phalanx of the hallux is painful due to deep endophytic growth; in addition, there are confluent plaques of superficial warts (mosaic warts). *Courtesy, Reinhard Kirnbauer, MD, and Petra Lenz, MD.*

elevated papules; the surface is smooth and often flat-topped (Fig. 66.7).

- **DDx:** small seborrheic keratoses, common warts, Gottron papules of dermatomyositis, lichen nitidus, lichen planus, acrokeratosis verruciformis (see Ch. 48), epidermodysplasia verruciformis (see below).
- **Rx:**
  - If a few lesions, destructive or ablative therapies (e.g. cryosurgery, trichloroacetic acid; see Fig. 66.4)
  - If numerous, topical application of irritants (e.g. retinoids), immunotherapy (see Fig. 66.4), topical 5-fluorouracil

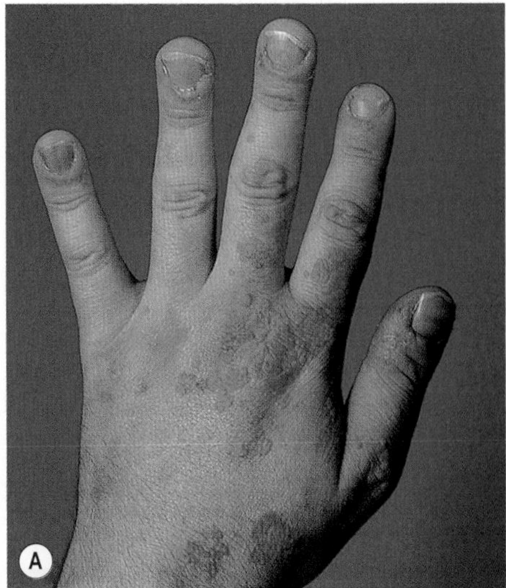

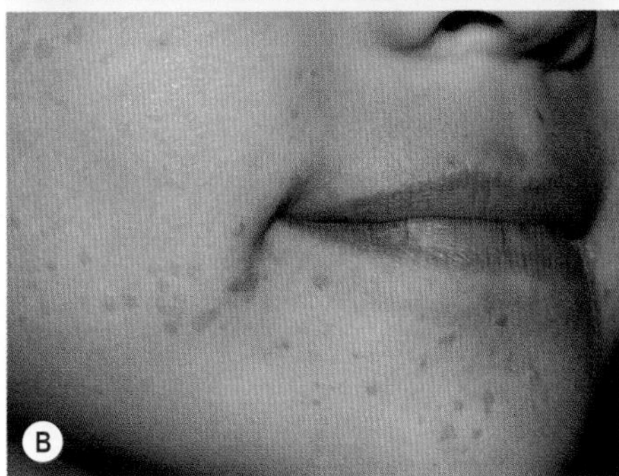

Fig. 66.7 Verrucae planae (flat warts). Multiple skin-colored or pink **(A)** to brown **(B)** smooth-surfaced, flat-topped papules. These lesions are typically caused by HPV-3 or -10. *A, Courtesy, Reinhard Kirnbauer, MD, and Petra Lenz, MD; B, Courtesy, Julie V. Schaffer, MD.*

Oral Warts

- Buccal, gingival, and labial mucosae as well as tongue and hard palate (Fig. 66.8).
- Small, soft, mucosal-colored to white, slightly elevated papillomatous papules.
- **DDx:** bite fibroma, early SCC, leukoedema, Heck disease (focal epithelial hyperplasia; multiple white to pink sessile papules; secondary to HPV types 13 and 32), verrucous proliferative leukoplakia, white sponge nevus.

Condylomata Acuminata

- Involve primarily the anogenital region.
- Range from discrete, sessile, smooth-surfaced papillomas to large cauliflower-like lesions (Figs 66.9 and 66.10).
- Skin-colored to pink to brown.

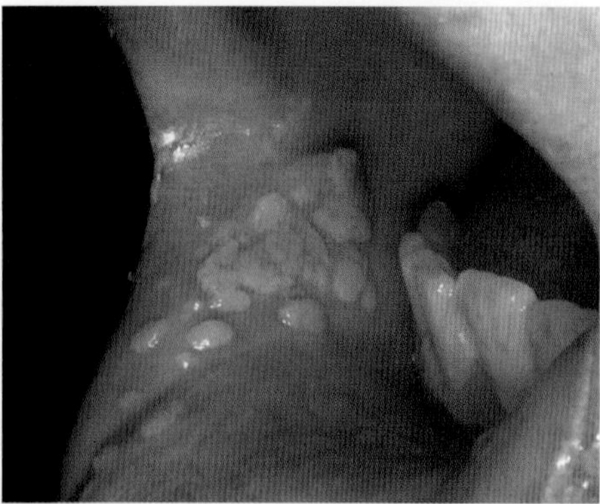

Fig. 66.8 Oral warts. Papillomas of the labial mucosa in a 6-year-old child. *Courtesy, Reinhard Kirnbauer, MD, and Petra Lenz, MD.*

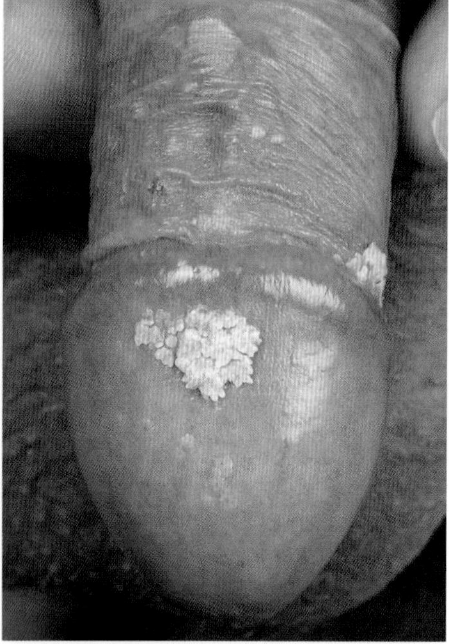

Fig. 66.9 Penile condylomata acuminata (genital warts). Both sessile and exophytic warts are present. *Courtesy, Reinhard Kirnbauer, MD, and Petra Lenz, MD.*

- If present in children, especially those >3 years of age, the possibility of sexual abuse should be considered (see Ch. 75).
- **DDx:** seborrheic keratosis, skin tag, molluscum contagiosum, bowenoid papulosis, SCC, pearly penile papules (see Ch. 95), free sebaceous glands, condyloma lata of secondary syphilis.
- **Rx:** outlined in Fig. 66.11.

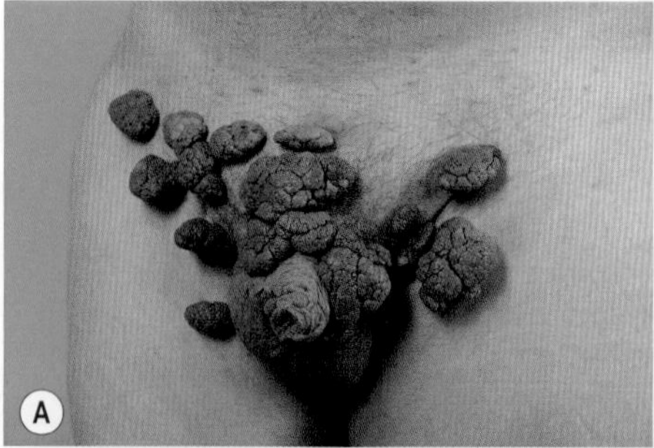

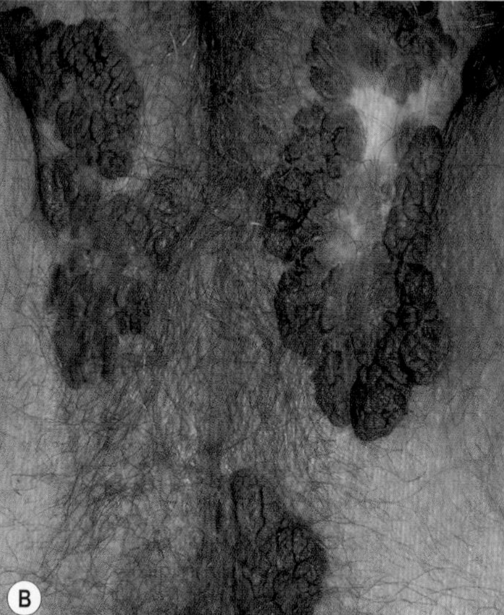

Fig. 66.10 Condylomata acuminata. **A** Large, exophytic, broad-based or peduculated papillomas in a healthy 15-year-old boy. **B** Confluent lesions forming hyperpigmented plaques in the perineal region and along the inguinal fold. A depigmented scar is seen at the site of treatment with liquid nitrogen. *A,B, Courtesy, Reinhard Kirnbauer, MD, and Petra Lenz, MD.*

Bowenoid Papulosis (Intraepithelial Neoplasia-3; High-Grade Squamous Intraepithelial Lesion)

- Similar to condylomata acuminata, primarily in the anogenital region.
- Multiple pink to red-brown smooth to warty papules or plaques (Figs 66.12 and 66.13; see Fig. 60.9).
- Histopathology: numerous mitoses scattered throughout the epidermis (which distinguishes it from condyloma acuminatum); keratinocytes may show less atypia than in an SCC.
- **Rx:** outlined in Fig. 66.11.

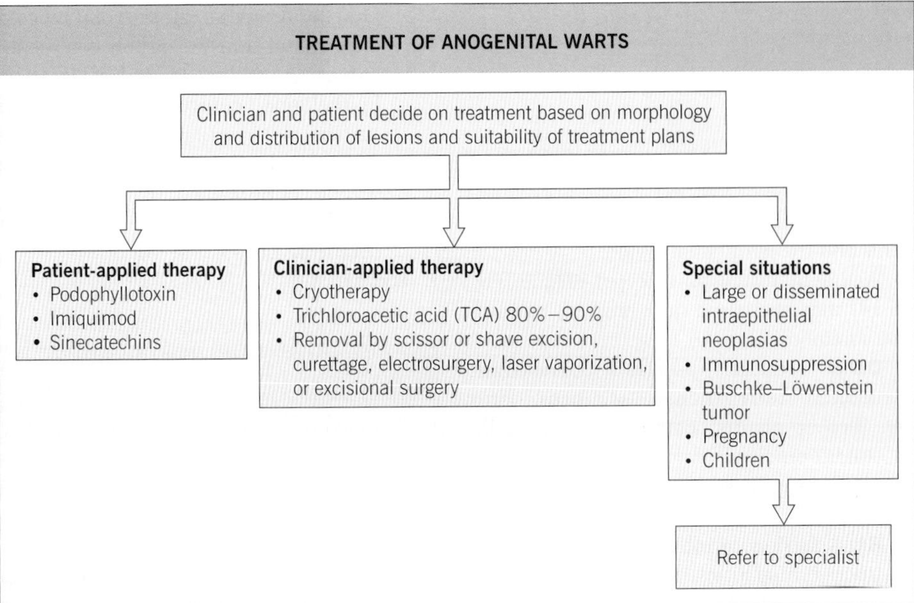

Fig. 66.11 Treatment of anogenital warts. TCA, trichloroacetic acid. *Courtesy, Reinhard Kirnbauer, MD, and Petra Lenz, MD.*

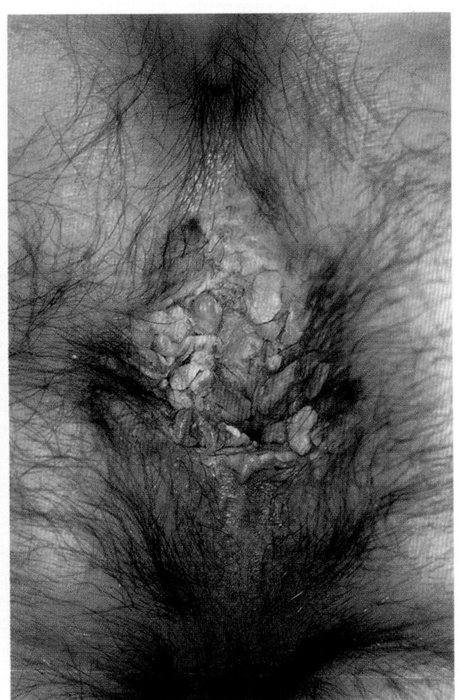

Fig. 66.12 Bowenoid papulosis of the anus positive for high-risk mucosal HPV in a man who had sex with men. Histology revealed high-grade anal intraepithelial neoplasia (AIN). *Courtesy, Reinhard Kirnbauer, MD, and Petra Lenz, MD.*

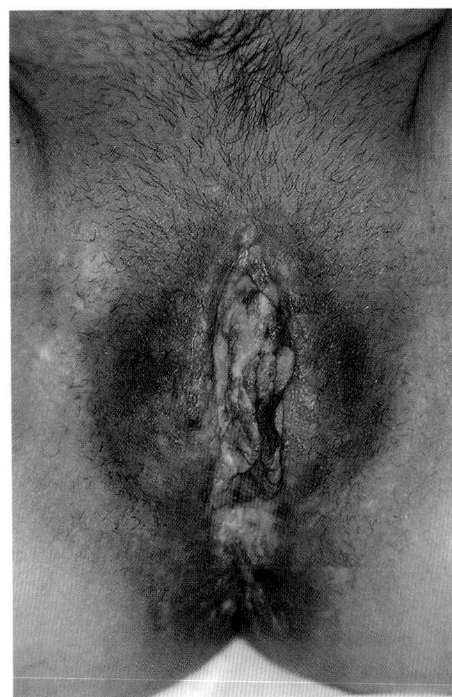

Fig. 66.13 Bowenoid papulosis of the vulva with histopathologic features of vulvar intraepithelial neoplasia (VIN). Extensive red-brown or whitish papules and plaques containing high-risk mucosal HPV in an HIV-positive patient. Analogous high-grade squamous intraepithelial lesions (HSIL) were present perianally (AIN) and on the cervix (CIN). *Courtesy, Reinhard Kirnbauer, MD, and Petra Lenz, MD.*

Squamous Cell Carcinoma *In Situ* (Intraepithelial Neoplasia-3 or High-Grade Squamous Intraepithelial Lesion *If Anogenital*; Bowen Disease *If Periungual*; Historically Erythroplasia of Queyrat *If Penile*)

- Favors the glabrous skin of the vulva or penis and the periungual region.
- Well-demarcated pink to red plaque (Fig. 66.14) that over time may progress to invasive carcinoma (Fig. 66.15).
- **DDx:** dermatitis, psoriasis, Rx-resistant periungual wart, lichen sclerosus, erosive lichen planus, candidiasis especially in uncircumcised male, extramammary Paget disease, Zoon balanitis, amelanotic melanoma.
- **Rx:** excision, Mohs surgery, or other destructive modalities depending on patient/lesion characteristics; imiquimod with careful re-evaluation.

Verrucous Carcinoma

- Low-grade malignancy that is locally invasive and destructive, but rarely metastasizes; lesions can attain a large size when left untreated.
- Major types:
  - Buschke–Löwenstein tumor (Fig. 66.16) – anogenital region; fistulas and/or abscesses may be present
  - Oral florid papillomatosis – oral mucosa or perinasal sinuses – pebbly confluence of whitish papillomas
  - Epithelioma cuniculatum – plantar surface – irregularly shaped, well-demarcated, verrucous nodule, often several centimeters in diameter
  - Papillomatosis cutis carcinoides – other cutaneous sites
- **Rx:** excision.

Epidermodysplasia Verruciformis (EDV)

- Cutaneous infection with particular HPV types in patients with an inherited predisposition (mutations in *TMC6* [*EVER1*], *TMC8* [*EVER2*]) or acquired immunosuppression (e.g. HIV infection); see Table 66.1.
- Widespread lesions that begin to appear during childhood (inherited form), with a predisposition for sun-exposed areas.
- Lesions vary in color from white to pink to brown and can resemble flat warts or tinea versicolor (Fig. 66.17).
- Distinctive histopathology with expanded gray-blue cytoplasm within the keratinocytes of the upper stratum spinosum.
- Increased risk of SCC, especially in sun-exposed areas.
- **Rx:** difficult (similar to that for flat warts), sun protective measures, address immunosuppression in acquired cases.

For further information see Ch. 79 from *Dermatology, Fourth Edition*.

For additional online figures visit www.expertconsult.com 

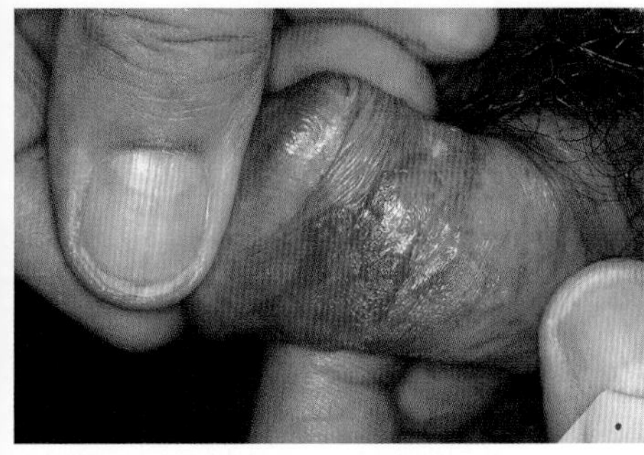

Fig. 66.14 Erythroplasia of Queyrat. A well-demarcated velvety plaque of the prepuce positive for high-risk HPV; histology detected a high-grade penile intraepithelial neoplasia (PIN). *Courtesy, Reinhard Kirnbauer, MD, and Petra Lenz, MD.*

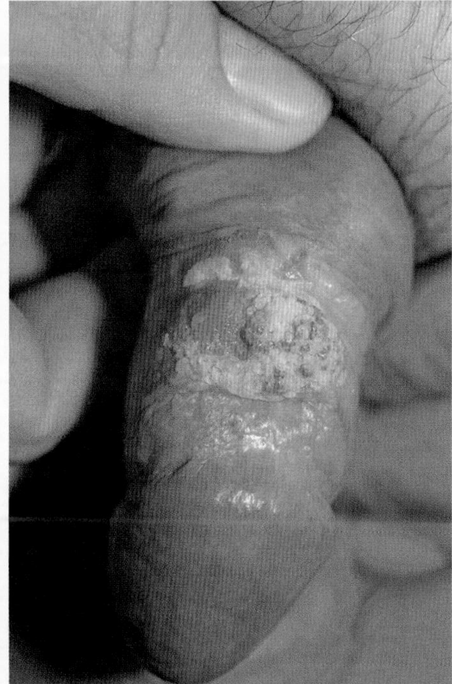

Fig. 66.15 Invasive squamous cell carcinoma of the penis. It developed over more than a decade from a papular lesion of the prepuce. HPV-16 and -51 DNAs were detected by RT-PCR. *Courtesy, Reinhard Kirnbauer, MD, and Petra Lenz, MD.*

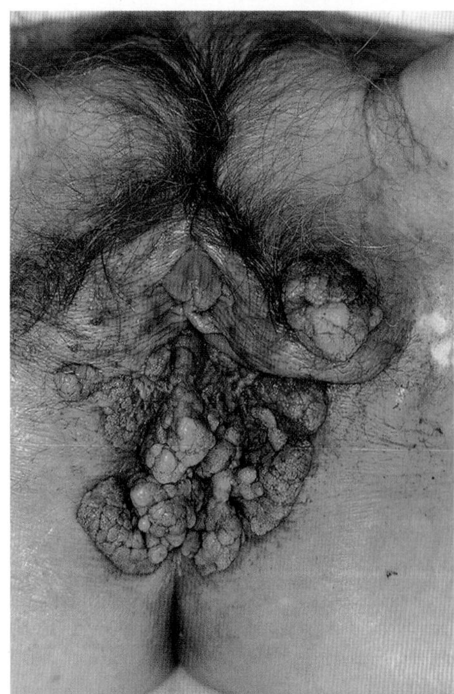

Fig. 66.16 Giant condylomata acuminata (Buschke–Löwenstein tumor). Cauliflower-like, deeply infiltrating giant condylomata acuminata in an older woman. *Courtesy, Reinhard Kirnbauer, MD, and Petra Lenz, MD.*

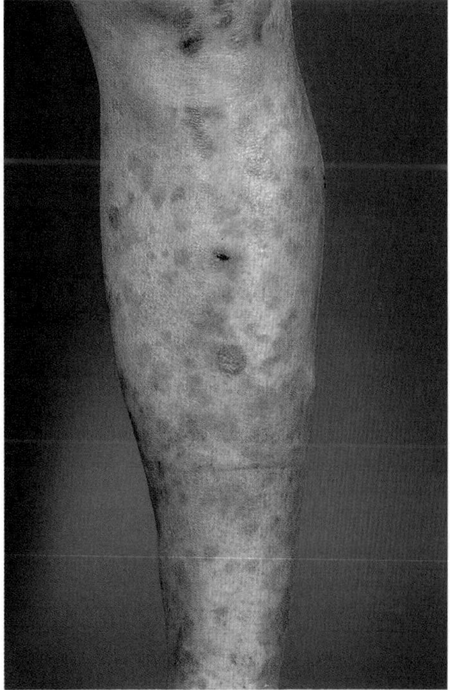

Fig. 66.17 Epidermodysplasia verruciformis. Generalized erythematous macules and plaques are seen. Lesions tested positive for HPV-8 and -36. *Courtesy, Reinhard Kirnbauer, MD, and Petra Lenz, MD.*

67 Human Herpesviruses

General

- Human herpesviruses (HHV) are a family of double-stranded DNA viruses (8 members) with a lipid envelope.
- All share the ability to establish lifelong latency in their host following primary infection.
- Basic pathogenesis of HHV infections involves a sequence of primary infection, establishment of latency, reactivation, and recurrent (secondary) infection.
- Clinical presentations depend on the host's age, anatomic location, immune status, and ethnicity (e.g. EBV).
- Spread of infection is usually the result of contact with bodily secretions containing the virus.
- Asymptomatic shedding of virus is common.

Herpes Simplex Viruses (HSV-1/HHV-1 and HSV-2/HHV-2)

- Ubiquitous pathogens that produce primarily orolabial (HSV-1 > HSV-2) and genital infections (HSV-2 > HSV-1) characterized by recurrent vesicular eruptions (Table 67.1).
- *Transmission* can occur during both symptomatic and asymptomatic periods of viral shedding.
- *Reactivation* can occur either spontaneously or due to an appropriate stimulus (e.g. stress, UVR, fever, tissue trauma, or immunosuppression).
- A wide range of clinical presentations exists, with asymptomatic infection being the most common.
- In ***primary infection***:
  - Onset is usually 3–7 days after exposure
  - *Generalized prodrome* (before the onset of mucocutaneous lesions) of tender lymphadenopathy, fever, and malaise; localized pain, burning, and tenderness
  - Initial lesions: small round vesicles on an erythematous base; often painful or burning; the grouping of these vesicles is a clue to the diagnosis; vesicles may become umbilicated or pustular, followed by erosions or ulcerations with hemorrhagic crusts, often with a scalloped border; lesions resolve over 2–6 weeks (Fig. 67.1)
- In ***reactivation infection***:
  - *Localized prodrome* of dysesthesia (e.g. burning/tingling, pain, pruritus) and tenderness
  - Mucocutaneous lesions similar as in primary but fewer in number, less severe, and shorter duration (Fig. 67.2)
- In addition to the classic orolabial and genital infections, HSV can cause other infections (Table 67.2; Figs 67.3–67.7).
- **DDx** and Dx: see Table 67.1.
- **Rx:** outlined in Table 67.3.

Varicella–Zoster Virus (VZV or HHV-3)

- **Primary varicella infection (chickenpox)**
  - Usually self-limited in otherwise healthy children but more severe with more numerous lesions and a greater risk for complications in adults (including pregnant women) and immunocompromised individuals (Table 67.4; Fig. 67.8)
- **Herpes zoster (shingles) – reactivation of VZV**
  - Incidence, severity, and risk of complications increase significantly with age and immunosuppression due to a decline in specific cell-mediated immune response to VZV
  - Reactivation results in a sensory neuritis and painful neuralgia, followed by a

MAJOR CLINICAL FEATURES OF CLASSIC HERPES SIMPLEX VIRUS (HSV) OROLABIAL AND GENITAL INFECTIONS			
Mucocutaneous HSV infection	**Primary infection***	**Reactivation infection***	**DDx**
Orolabial HSV (HSV1 > HSV2) Latency is established in the neuronal cells of dorsal root ganglia, especially trigeminal	• Asymptomatic infection most common • Gingivostomatitis primarily in children <10 years of age (see Fig. 67.1A) • Pharyngitis and mononucleosis-like syndrome in young adults • Dysphagia and drooling may occur	• Favors vermilion border of lips (see Fig. 67.2B) and occurs less commonly in the perioral region and cheek (see Fig. 67.2A), nasal mucosa, and hard mucosa (i.e. mucosa overlying bone) such as the hard palate and gingivae • In immunocompromised hosts, can see on the soft mucosa, e.g. buccal mucosa and soft palate	**Vermilion lips/perioral** • Impetigo • Coxsackie infection (also intraoral) • EM major or SJS (also intraoral) **Intraoral** • Aphthous stomatitis • Pharyngitis (e.g. EBV)/herpangina • Drug-induced mucositis
Genital HSV (HSV2 > HSV1) Latency is established in the neuronal cells of dorsal root ganglia, especially sacral	• Seropositive persons often report no history of primary genital infection • Frequently presents with excruciatingly painful erosive balanitis, vulvitis, or vaginitis • In **males** typically involves the glans or shaft of the penis • In **females** can also involve cervix, buttocks (see Fig. 67.1D), and perineum with associated dysuria, urinary retention, and inguinal lymphadenopathy (see Fig. 67.1C)	• Usually a subclinical presentation • Typically a limited number of grouped vesicles* occur on the genitalia or buttocks (especially in females) (see Fig. 67.2C,D) • Frequency of recurrence correlates with the severity of the primary infection	• Trauma • EBV- or CMV-related ulcers • Aphthae • Syphilitic chancre • Chancroid • Lymphogranuloma venereum • Granuloma inguinale
Diagnosis is made at the bedside by either (1) performance of a Tzanck smear (see Fig. 2.7; results in minutes); DFA or PCR (results in hours); or viral culture (results in days) or (2) performing a skin biopsy for H&E staining (see Fig. 2.6; results in days). *In immunocompromised hosts it is prudent to request testing for HSV-1, HSV-2, and VZV, as clinical presentations are often atypical.*			

For the description of typical lesions, see text; occasionally, intact vesicles are not seen but rather grouped ulcerations with hemorrhagic crusts predominate.

Table 67.1 Major clinical features of classic herpes simplex virus (HSV) orolabial and genital infections. In the United States, ~50% of adults are seropositive for HSV-1 and ~12% are seropositive for HSV-2. Treatment is outlined in Table 67.3. EM, erythema multiforme; SJS, Stevens–Johnson syndrome.

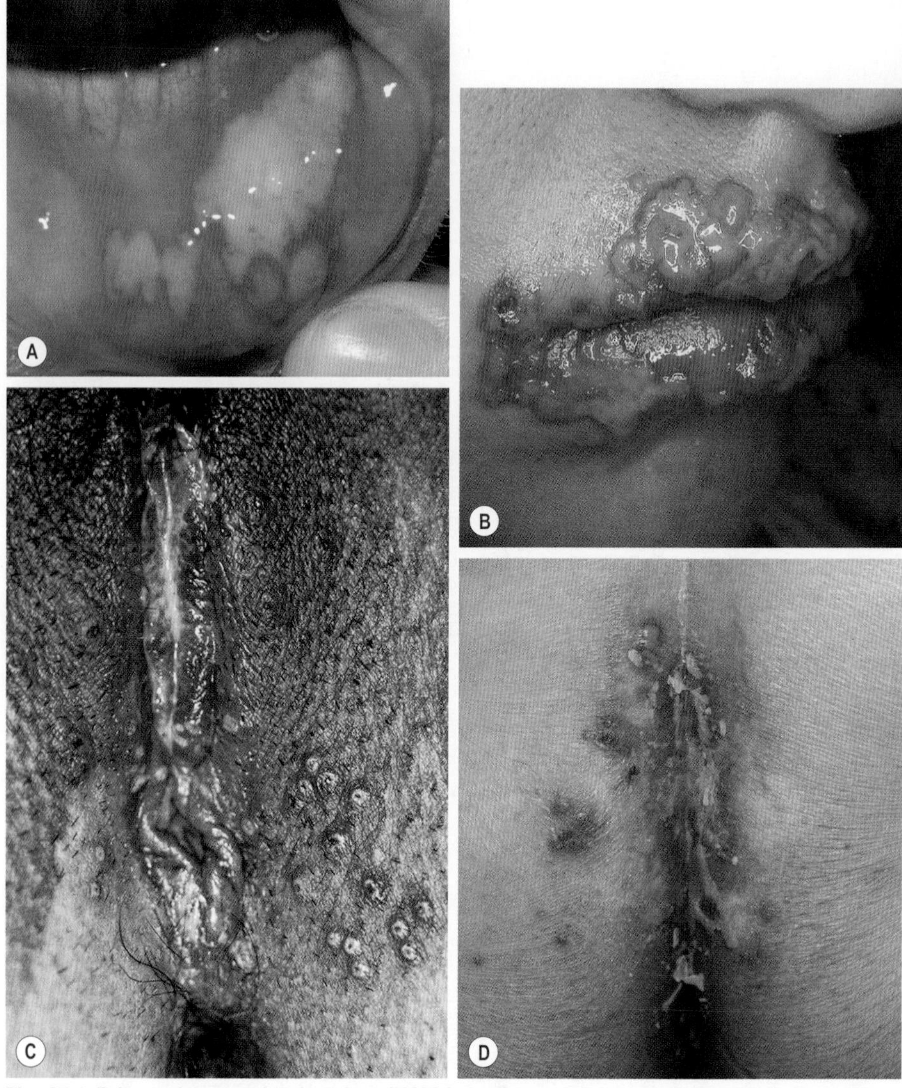

Fig. 67.1 Primary herpes simplex virus (HSV) infections. A Primary herpes gingivostomatitis due to HSV-1 in a child. Note the coalescing lesions with scalloped borders. **B** HSV-2 infection in a teenager (primary vs non-primary initial infection). Note the scalloped borders. **C** Primary genital HSV infection. In addition to 1- to 2-mm hemorrhagic crusts, there are perifollicular vesiculopustules. **D** Grouped vesicles and erosions in the gluteal cleft. *A, Courtesy, Julie V. Schaffer, MD; B, Courtesy, Jean L. Bolognia, MD; C, Courtesy, Stephen K. Tyring, MD; D, Courtesy, Kalman Watsky, MD.*

dermatomal vesicular eruption; clinical course is outlined in Table 67.4 (Figs 67.9–67.11)
- Exposure of a susceptible person to an individual with chickenpox or zoster can lead to primary varicella but not zoster
- **Rx:** early antiviral treatment (within 72 hours of the onset of the first vesicle) is ideal, but initiation after 72 hours but within 7 days may also be helpful (see Table 67.3)
- **Selected complications of herpes zoster:**

1. Disseminated zoster
- Defined as >20 vesicles outside the area of the primary or adjacent dermatomes
- Implies viremia and an increased risk for visceral or CNS involvement (see Table 67.4)
- Requires intravenous acyclovir

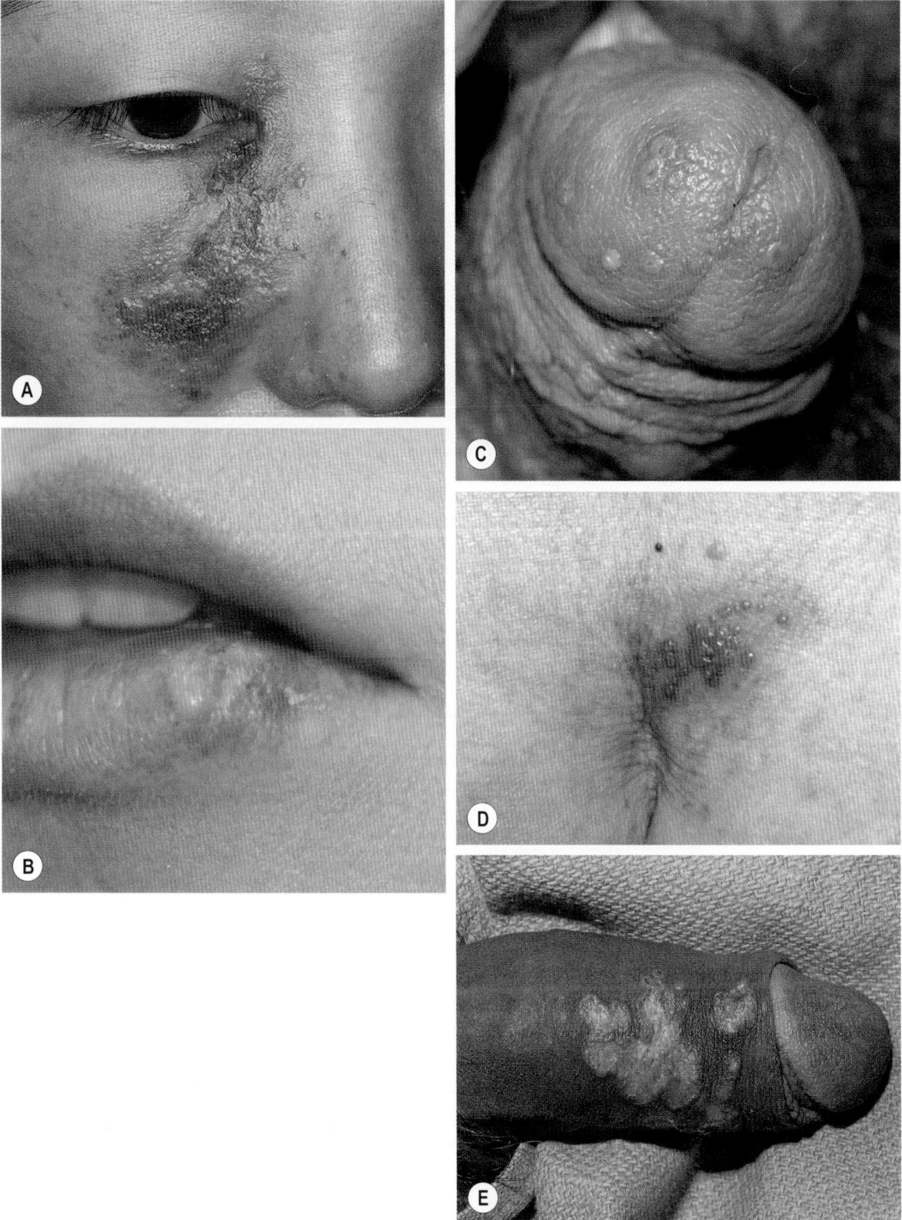

Fig. 67.2 Reactivation of herpes simplex virus (HSV) infections. A Recurrent HSV-1 infection on the cheek. Occasionally such lesions are misdiagnosed as cellulitis or bullous impetigo. **B** Recurrent herpes labialis (cold sore, fever blister). **C, D** Intact grouped vesicles and/or vesiculopustules with an erythematous base on the penis (**C**) and above the gluteal cleft (**D**). The buttock is a common location in women. **E** Healing ulcerations with scalloped borders on the penis. *A, C, D, Courtesy, Kalman Watsky, MD; B, Courtesy, Stephen K. Tyring, MD; E, Courtesy, Joseph L. Jorizzo, MD.*

MAJOR CLINICAL FEATURES OF OTHER HERPES SIMPLEX VIRUS (HSV) INFECTIONS	
HSV infection	**Major clinical features**
Eczema herpeticum (Kaposi varicelliform eruption [KVE])	• Widespread eruption of HSV, usually occurring in association with skin conditions that disrupt the epidermal barrier (e.g. atopic dermatitis, burns, Darier disease) (see Fig. 67.3); DDx includes infections with coxsackievirus or *Streptococcus*
Herpetic whitlow	• HSV infection of the digit(s) (Fig. 67.4); most often seen in children; in the past was common in health-care workers who did not wear gloves
Herpes gladiatorum	• Occurs in contact sports (e.g. wrestling) (see Fig. 67.5)
HSV folliculitis	• Uncommon; most often seen in patients who shave with a blade razor (e.g. herpes sycosis in the beard region) or in immunocompromised hosts (see Fig. 31.4B)
HSV in immunocompromised hosts (e.g. HIV (+), solid organ and hematopoietic stem cell transplant recipients, leukemia and lymphoma patients)	• May present with chronic or atypical mucocutaneous presentations (e.g. multiple sites; disseminated lesions; verrucous, exophytic or pustular lesions; see Fig. 67.6) • Most common presentation is a chronic, enlarging ulceration; in the buttock area may be misdiagnosed as a pressure ulcer (see Fig. 67.6D)
Ocular HSV	• Most often acquired in newborns during the vaginal birthing process • *Primary infection:* typically presents as unilateral or bilateral keratoconjunctivitis, eyelid edema, tearing, photophobia, chemosis, and preauricular lymphadenopathy; with *recurrent infection* usually unilateral and may be confused with a contact dermatitis or periocular cellulitis • Potential complications: corneal ulceration, scarring • Pathognomonic finding: branching, dendritic lesions of the corneal epithelium
Neonatal HSV	• Greatest risk of transmission (30–50%) from infected mother to neonate is among women with first episode of genital HSV near the time of delivery; lowest risk (<3%) is among women with recurrent genital HSV • Significant morbidity and mortality in affected infants, especially if disseminated disease • Clinical presentations vary (see Fig. 67.7 and see Ch. 28)
Herpes encephalitis	• *No* cutaneous manifestations • Most common cause of sporadic, fatal viral encephalitis in the U.S.

Table 67.2 Major clinical features of other herpes simplex virus (HSV) infections. Treatment is outlined in Table 67.3.

2. **Post-herpetic neuralgia (PHN) and post-herpetic itch (PHI)**
   - Affects 10–20% of patients; incidence and severity increase with age
   - Characterized by persistent pain, dysesthesia (PHN) or pruritus (PHI) along the affected dermatome for weeks to years after the resolution of the eruption
   - **Rx:** gabapentin, tricyclic antidepressants (e.g. amitriptyline, nortriptyline); topical agents (e.g. lidocaine patch, capsaicin); oral analgesics (e.g. ibuprofen, opioids)
   - Note that opioids are typically ineffective or even aggravating in patients with PHI

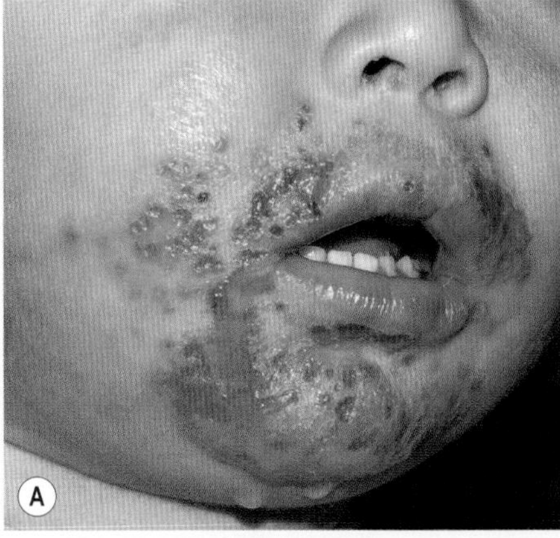

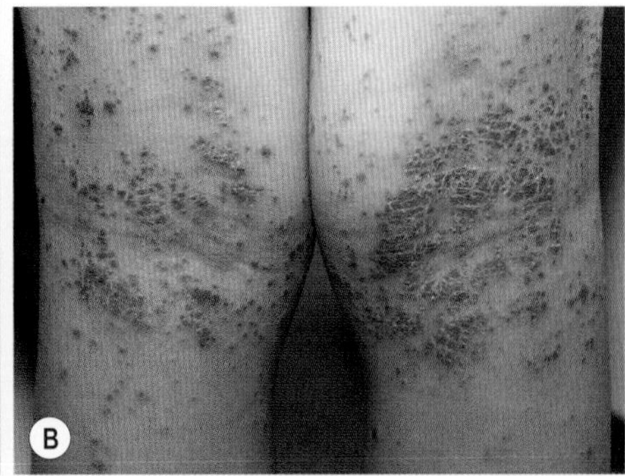

Fig. 67.3 Eczema herpeticum. A Monomorphic, punched-out erosions with a scalloped border in this infant with a history of facial atopic dermatitis. **B** Monomorphic, small hemorrhagic crusts and erosions coalescing in the popliteal fossae, an area of pre-existing atopic dermatitis. *A, Courtesy, Julie V. Schaffer, MD; B, Courtesy, Kalman Watsky, MD.*

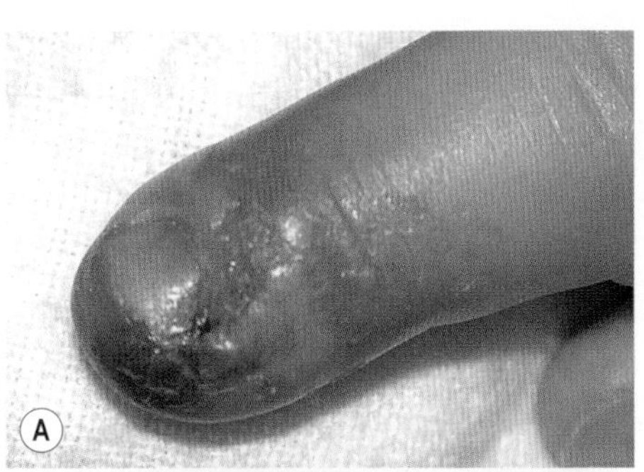

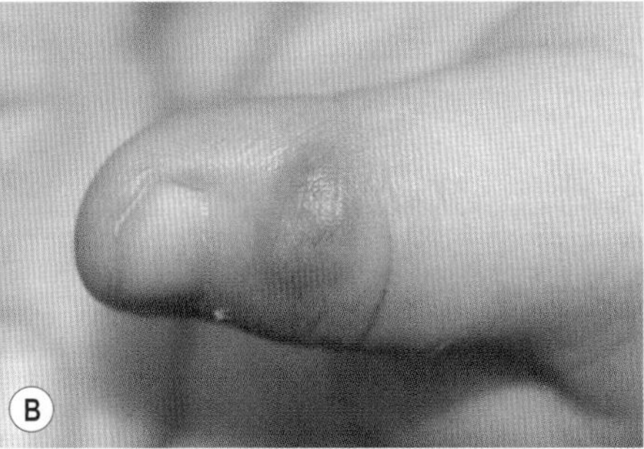

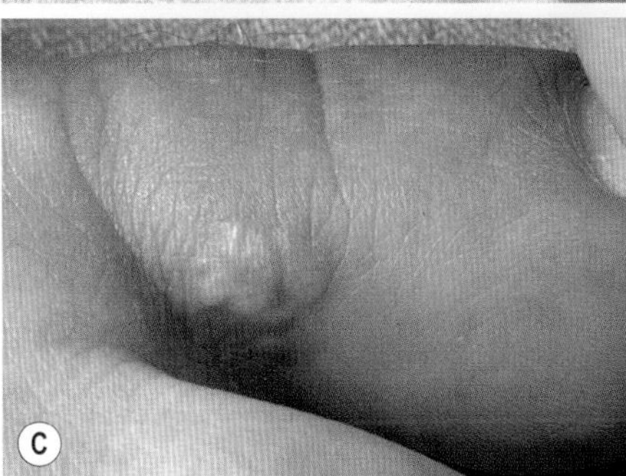

Fig. 67.4 Herpetic whitlow. A Coalescing vesicles and erosions on the distal finger of a child. **B** An edematous, erythematous plaque with relatively subtle central vesicle formation on the thumb of a child. **C** Grouped vesicles on the toe of an adult. Herpetic whitlow is sometimes misdiagnosed as cellulitis or blistering dactylitis, or, depending on the distribution, paronychia. *A, Courtesy, YDRSC; B, Courtesy, Stephen K. Tyring, MD; C, Courtesy, Louis A. Fragola, Jr, MD.*

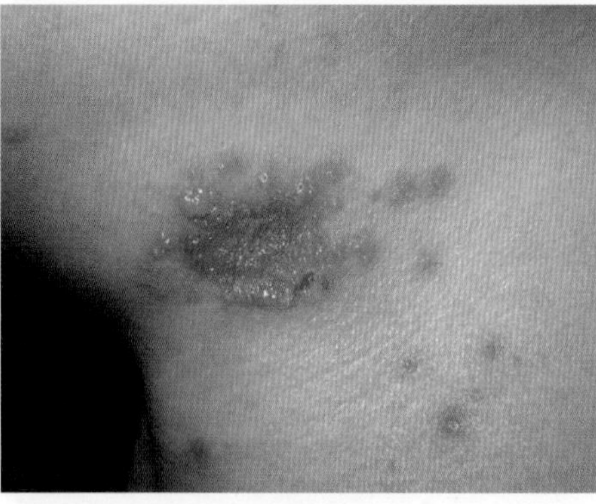

Fig. 67.5 Herpes gladiatorum. Grouped vesicles and erosions on the neck of a high school wrestler. *Courtesy, Louis A. Fragola, Jr., MD.*

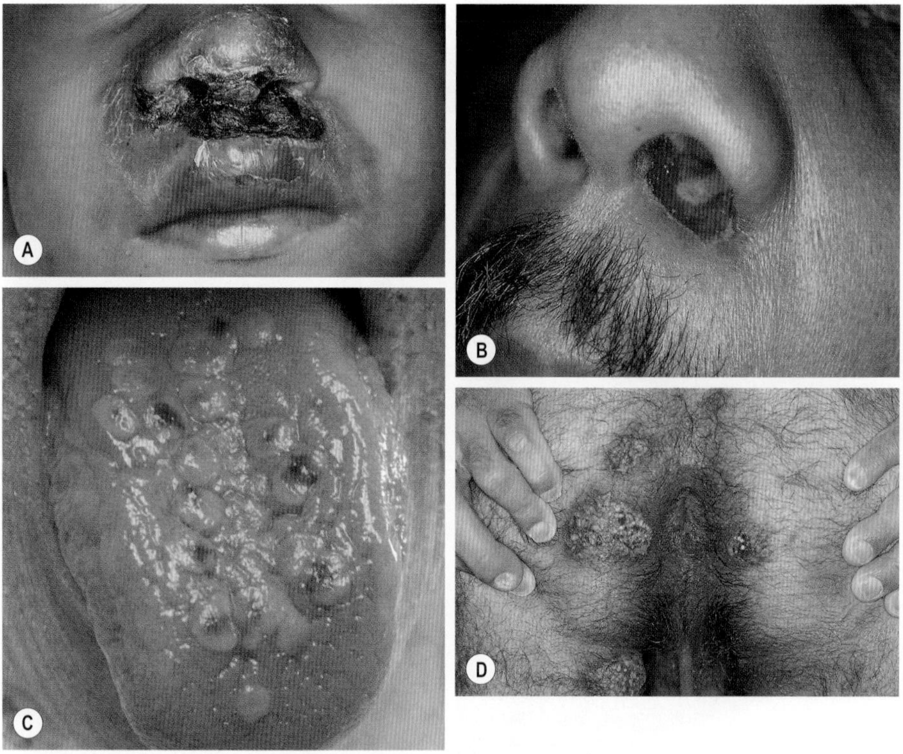

Fig. 67.6 Herpes simplex viral infections in immunocompromised hosts. A Enlarging ulcerations in a child with acute lymphocytic leukemia who was presumed to have a *Rhizopus* infection, and **(B)** in a young man with AIDS. **C** Coalescence of eroded, yellow-white papules and plaques on the tongue. **D** Chronic perianal ulcerations in an HIV-infected male. *A–C, Courtesy, YDRSC; D, From Callen JP, Jorizzo JL, et al. Dermatological Signs of Internal Disease, 4th edn.; Saunders/Elsevier, 2009.*

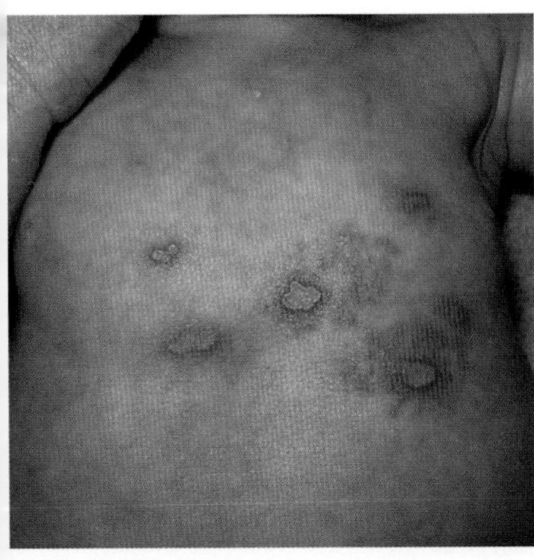

Fig. 67.7 Neonatal herpes. Grouped papulovesicles with an erythematous base on the chest. Note the scalloped borders in areas of coalescence. *Courtesy, Frank Samarin, MD.*

ANTIVIRAL THERAPY FOR HERPES SIMPLEX VIRUS AND VARICELLA–ZOSTER VIRUS	
Disease context	**Drug and dosage**
Herpes simplex infections	
Orolabial herpes* (recurrence)	*Topical* Docosanol: 5×/d until healed Penciclovir: 1% cream applied q2 h while awake × 4 days Acyclovir: 5% ointment applied q3 h/6 times/day × 7–10 days Acyclovir + hydrocortisone: 5%/1% cream applied 5×/d × 5 days Acyclovir mucoadhesive tablet: 50 mg single application in the canine fossa on the side affected *Oral** Acyclovir**: 400 mg PO TID × 7–10 days Famciclovir: 1.5 gm PO × 1 dose Valacyclovir: 2 gm PO BID × 1 day
Genital herpes (first episode)	Acyclovir: 200 mg PO 5×/d × 10 days or 400 mg PO TID × 10 days Famciclovir: 250 mg PO TID × 10 days Valacyclovir: 1 gm PO BID × 10 days
Genital herpes (recurrence)	Acyclovir: 400 mg PO TID × 5 days or 800 mg PO BID × 5 days or 800 mg PO TID × 2 days Famciclovir: 1 gm PO BID × 1 day or 500 mg PO × 1 dose then 250 mg PO BID × 2 days or 125 mg PO BID × 5 days Valacyclovir: 500 mg PO BID × 3 days or 1 gm PO daily × 5 days
Chronic suppression	Acyclovir: 400 mg PO BID Famciclovir: 250 mg PO BID Valacyclovir: 500 mg PO daily for <10 outbreaks/year or 1 gm PO daily for ≥10 outbreaks/year
Neonatal	Acyclovir: 20 mg/kg IV q8 h × 14–21 days
Immunocompromised	*Recommend use until all mucocutaneous lesions are healed* Acyclovir: 400 mg PO 5×/d or 5 mg/kg (if age ≥12 y) to 10 mg/kg (if age <12 y) IV q8 h Famciclovir**: 500 mg PO BID Valacyclovir**: 1 gm PO BID

Table 67.3 Antiviral therapy for herpes simplex virus and varicella–zoster virus. Topical antiviral agents should be applied using a finger with intact skin. *Continued*

ANTIVIRAL THERAPY FOR HERPES SIMPLEX VIRUS AND VARICELLA–ZOSTER VIRUS	
Disease context	**Drug and dosage**
Eczema herpeticum/Kaposi varicelliform eruption**	*Recommend use for 10–14 days or (especially if immunocompromised) until all mucocutaneous lesions are healed* Acyclovir: 15 mg/kg (400 mg max) PO 3–5×/d or, if severe, 5 mg/kg (if age ≥12 y) to 10 mg/kg (if age <12 y) IV q8 h Famciclovir: 500 mg PO BID Valacyclovir: 1 gm PO BID
Genital herpes, recurrent in the setting of HIV infection	*Recommend use until all mucocutaneous lesions are healed* Acyclovir**: 400 mg PO TID Famciclovir: 500 mg PO BID Valacyclovir**: 1 gm PO BID
Chronic suppression in the setting of HIV infection	Acyclovir**: 400–800 mg PO BID–TID Famciclovir**: 250–500 mg PO BID Valacyclovir: 500 mg PO BID
Acyclovir-resistant HSV in immunocompromised patients	Foscarnet: 40 mg/kg IV q8–12 h × 2–3 weeks (or until all lesions are healed) Cidofovir: 1% cream or gel daily × 2–3 weeks or (for severe disease) 5 mg/kg IV weekly × 2 weeks then every other week (together with probenecid)
Varicella–zoster virus infections	
Varicella	Acyclovir: 20 mg/kg (800 mg max) PO 4×/d × 5 days Valacyclovir†: 20 mg/kg (1 gm max) PO TID × 5 days
Herpes zoster	Acyclovir: 800 mg PO 5×/d × 7–10 days Famciclovir: 500 mg PO TID × 7 days Valacyclovir: 1 gm PO TID × 7 days
Immunocompromised patient or disseminated disease	Acyclovir: 10 mg/kg (500 mg/m^2) IV q8 h × 7–10 days *or until cropping has ceased* (depending on the setting, consider continuing until lesions are healed)

**Indications for and efficacy of antiviral treatment for initial episodes of orolabial herpes in immunocompetent adults have not been defined, but the regimens used for initial genital episodes can be considered in individuals with severe disease; acyclovir 15 mg/kg (200 mg max) PO 5×/day ×7 days (initiated within 3 days of disease onset) has been shown to be beneficial in young children with primary herpes gingivostomatitis.*
***Not specifically FDA-approved for this indication.*
†FDA-approved for ages 2–17 years; pharmacies can compound valacyclovir tablets into an oral suspension (25 or 50 mg/ml).

Table 67.3 *Continued* **Antiviral therapy for herpes simplex virus and varicella–zoster virus.** d, day; h, hours; q, every.

3. **Ocular involvement (see Fig. 67.9H)**
   - Occurs in ~10% of patients, with 20–70% developing ocular disease (occasionally blindness)
   - Due to VZV reactivation in the first division of the trigeminal nerve (V_1)
   - Clues to its diagnosis include lesions in the V_1 distribution (see Fig. 67.10), which may be accompanied by unilateral eye pain or conjunctivitis
   - *Hutchinson sign* is the presence of vesicles at the tip, side, or bridge of the nose, indicating involvement of the nasociliary branch of the trigeminal nerve, which also innervates the cornea
   - Initial and longitudinal evaluation by ophthalmology is required
4. **Ramsay–Hunt syndrome (herpes zoster oticus)**
   - Due to VZV reactivation in the geniculate ganglion
   - Clues to its diagnosis: vesicles in the ear canal, tongue, and/or hard palate
   - Patients may have severe ear pain, acute facial nerve paralysis, and/or taste loss of the anterior two-thirds of the tongue
   - If the vestibulocochlear nerve is also affected, may have tinnitus, hearing loss, or vertigo
   - Consider referral to otolaryngology

VZV infection	Major clinical features	Complications (also see text)	DDx
Primary infection*: Varicella (chickenpox) Latency is established in the neuronal cells of dorsal root ganglia ~98% of adults worldwide are seropositive	• 11- to 20-day incubation period • *Generalized prodrome* of mild fever, malaise, and myalgia, followed by an eruption of erythematous, pruritic macules and papules that develop central vesicles ("dew drops on a rose petal") and then evolve into pustules and crusts (see Fig. 67.8); lesions heal over 7–10 days • Favors scalp and face first, with progression to trunk, extremities, and sometimes oral mucosa (see Fig. 67.8D) • *Hallmark:* lesions in all stages of development (see Fig. 67.8A-C) • Affected individual is contagious via airborne droplets and contact with vesicular fluid (until all lesions have crusted over) • *Breakthrough varicella:* seen in previously immunized persons; characterized by a much milder course and often an atypical presentation, e.g. only a few papules or papulovesicles	***Immunocompetent host*** **Most common:** secondary bacterial infection (especially staphylococcal and streptococcal), scarring **Less common**: pneumonia **Rare**: CNS (e.g. Reye syndrome, encephalitis); glomerulonephritis; optic neuritis; hepatitis **Congenital varicella**: associated with multiple fetal abnormalities as well as cutaneous scarring ***Immunocompromised host*** • Significant morbidity and mortality with more extensive, atypical eruptions (e.g. hemorrhagic, purpuric) and an increased likelihood of CNS and visceral involvement (lung, liver)	• Vesicular viral exanthems (e.g. coxsackievirus, ECHO) • PLEVA • Disseminated HSV† • Rickettsialpox • Drug eruption • Scabies • Insect bites
Reactivation infection: Zoster (shingles)**	• *Localized (dermatomal) prodrome* of intense pain and dysesthesia, with subsequent development of cutaneous lesions • Painful grouped vesicles on erythematous bases, developing within a sensory dermatome (see Figs 67.9 and 67.10) • Most often on the trunk > face, neck, scalp, extremity • Typically self-limited in children and young adults • Occasionally localized dysesthesia but no cutaneous eruption ("*zoster sine herpete*")	***Immunocompetent host*** • Postherpetic neuralgia (~10–15%) • Local: secondary bacterial infection; scarring; motor paralysis • Systemic (see below): occasionally pneumonitis • Ophthalmic zoster (see Fig. 67.9H) • Ramsay–Hunt syndrome ***Immunocompromised host*** (see Fig. 67.11) • More severe and unusual presentations (e.g. persistent and verrucous lesions or postherpetic hyperhidrosis) • Disseminated disease • Visceral involvement: pneumonitis; meningoencephalitis; hepatitis	• Zosteriform HSV • Localized contact dermatitis • Bacterial skin infection (e.g. bullous impetigo, cellulitis)
Diagnosis is outlined in Table 67.1			

Prevention is now a major focus: In the United States, all eligible children are recommended to receive the two-dose, live-attenuated VZV vaccine. Varicella IgG (VIG) given to immunocompromised hosts with first-time exposure; VIG given to neonates whose mothers became infected shortly before birth.

***Prevention is now a major focus in the United States and United Kingdom; in 2017 the FDA approved a two-dose, adjuvanted recombinant VZV vaccine for individuals 50 years of age or older (efficacy is ~91–97%).*

†Especially in immunocompromised hosts.

Table 67.4 Major clinical features of varicella–zoster virus (VZV) infections. Treatment is outlined in Table 67.3. ECHO, enteric cytopathic human orphan; PLEVA, pityriasis lichenoides et varioliformis acuta.

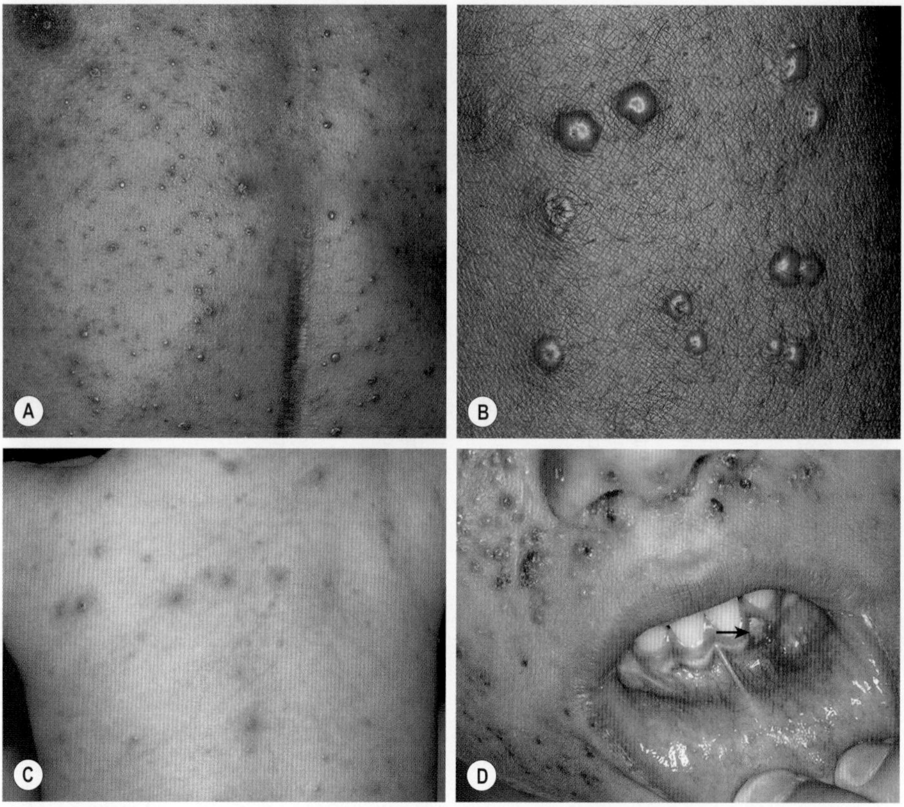

Fig. 67.8 Primary varicella–zoster virus (VZV) infection (varicella or chickenpox). A–C Lesions in different stages of evolution, including vesicles, pustules, and hemorrhagic crusts. Vesicles often develop central umbilication. **D** Oral lesions can also occur (arrow). *A, B, Courtesy, Robert Hartman, MD; C, Courtesy, Julie V. Schaffer, MD; D, Courtesy, Judit Stenn, MD.*

Epstein–Barr Virus (EBV or HHV-4)

- Table 67.5 and Figs 67.12 and 67.13.

Cytomegalovirus (CMV or HHV-5)

- Table 67.6 and Fig. 67.14.

Human Herpesvirus 6 and 7 (HHV-6 and HHV-7)

- Table 67.7 and Fig. 67.15.

Human Herpesvirus 8 (Kaposi Sarcoma-Associated Herpesvirus [KSHV])

- Table 67.8 and Fig. 67.16.

For further information see Ch. 80 from *Dermatology, Fourth Edition*.

For additional online figures and tables visit www.expertconsult.com 

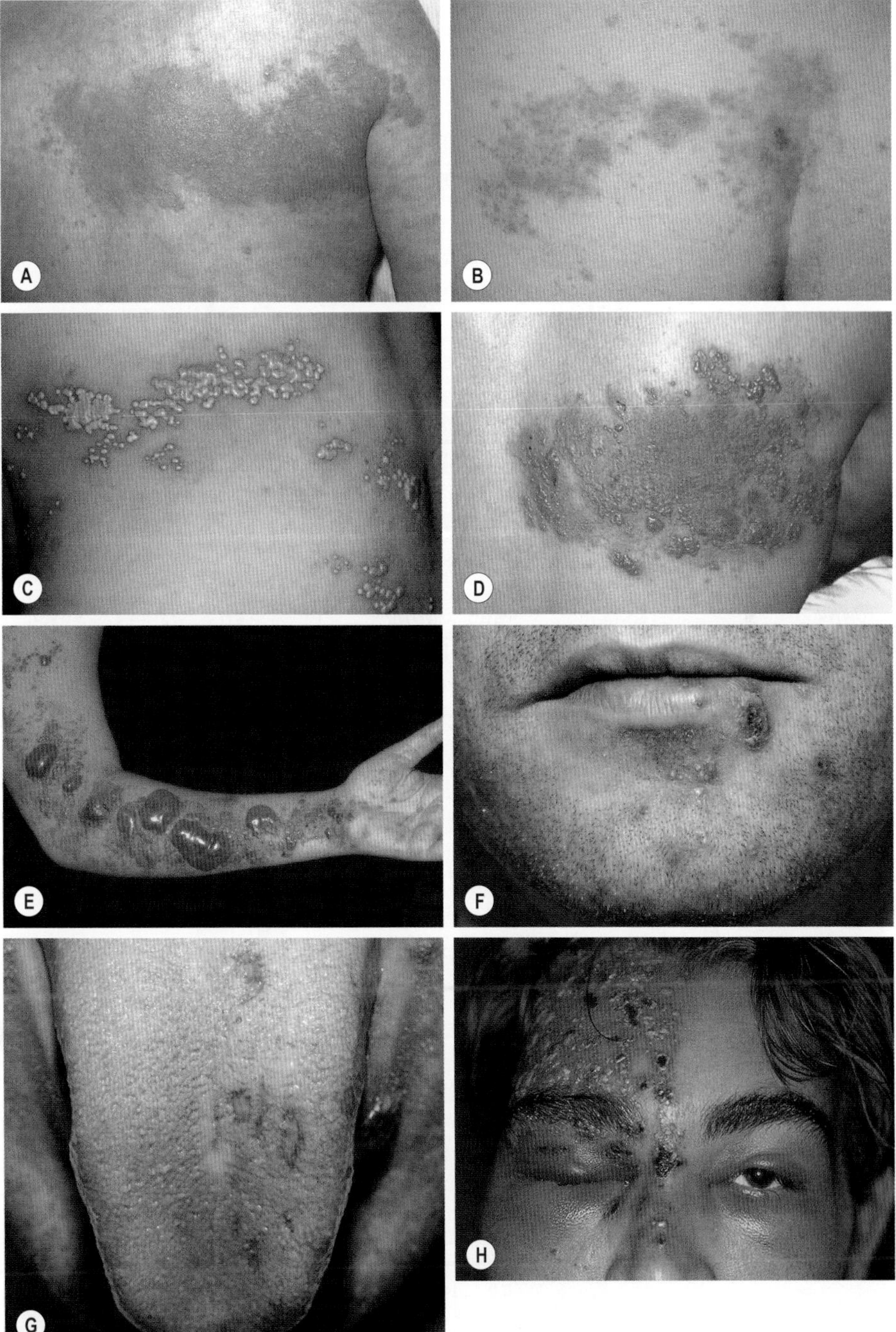

Fig. 67.9 Herpes zoster (shingles) infection. A, B Erythematous, edematous plaques with early vesicle formation. Note the perifollicular accentuation **(B). C**, **D** Later stages of evolution with prominent pustule formation **(C)** and a dusky purple color associated with older vesicles **(D). E** Bullous variant on the flexor arm. **F–H** Facial herpes zoster. **F** In the distribution of V_3, grouped pustules on the left side of the chin and hemorrhagic crusting of the lower lip, with one lesion extending past the midline. This could be mistaken for an acneiform eruption or impetigo. **G** In the same patient, erosions are present on the left side of the tongue. The anterior two-thirds of the tongue is innervated by the facial nerve (VII; taste) as well as V_3 (sensory). **H** Ophthalmic zoster (V_1) with sharp midline demarcation of erythema and crusts on the forehead as well as contralateral periorbital edema. *A, D, E, H, Courtesy, YDRSC; B, Courtesy, Jean L. Bolognia, MD; C, Courtesy, Louis A. Fragola, Jr., MD; F, G, Courtesy, Kalman Watsky, MD.*

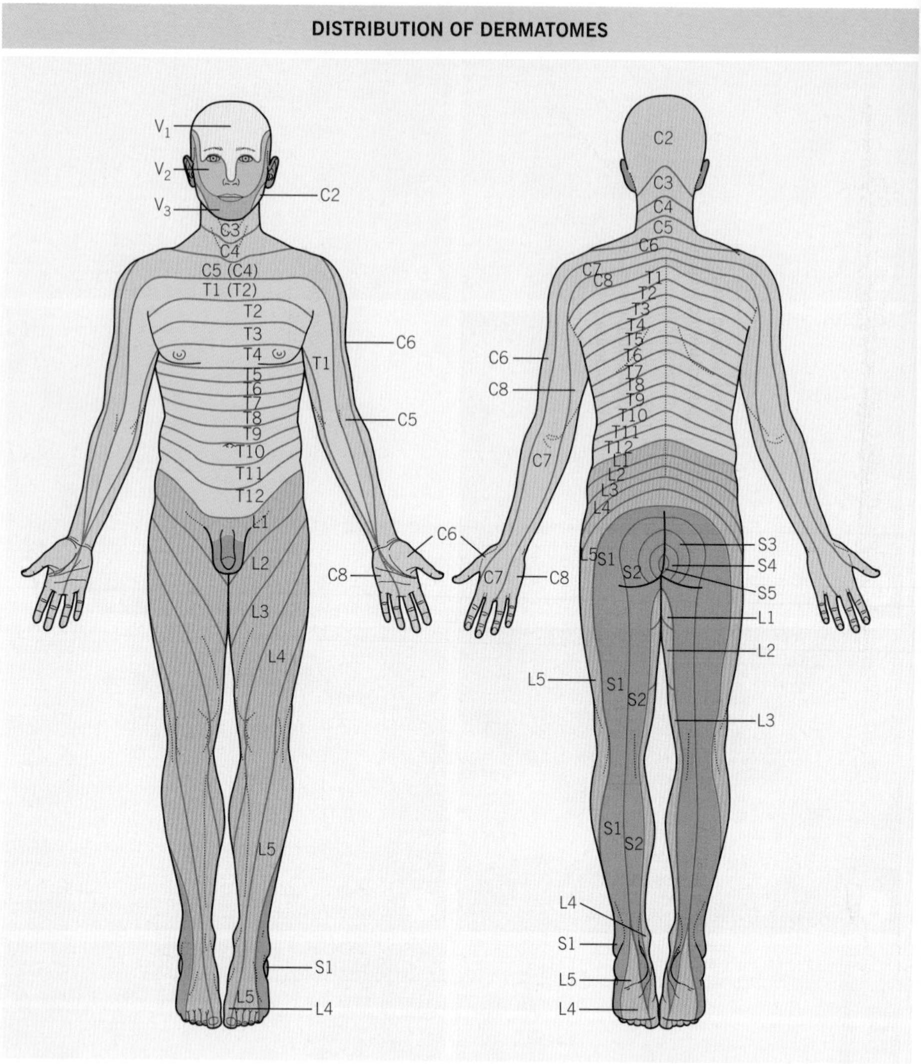

DISTRIBUTION OF DERMATOMES

Fig. 67.10 Distribution of dermatomes.

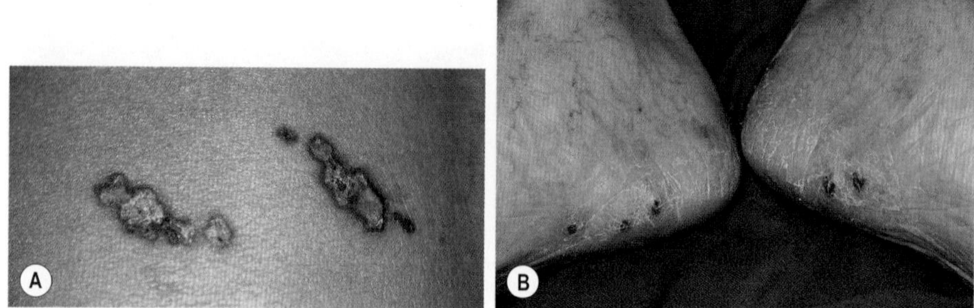

Fig. 67.11 Herpes zoster (shingles) in immunocompromised hosts. A Chronic verrucous zoster in an HIV-infected patient. **B** Disseminated cutaneous zoster with multiple violet-black papules on the feet. Patients with disseminated cutaneous skin lesions should be evaluated for possible CNS or visceral involvement, e.g. hepatic, pulmonary, especially if they are immunocompromised. *Courtesy, YDRSC.*

MAJOR CLINICAL FEATURES OF EPSTEIN–BARR VIRUS (EBV) INFECTIONS			
EBV infection	**Major clinical features**	**Complications**	**DDx**
Primary infection*: Infectious mononucleosis (IM) Latency is established in B lymphocytes ~95% of adults worldwide are seropositive	• Long, 30- to 50-day incubation period; usually asymptomatic in children, but symptomatic in adolescents and young adults • *Generalized prodrome* of headache, malaise, fatigue • *Classically,* ~80% present with triad of fever, pharyngitis, and lymphadenopathy • *Other clinical findings*: exudative tonsillitis, splenomegaly (50%), lymphocytosis with atypical lymphocytes, mild hepatitis • *Cutaneous eruption:* onset ~day 4 and lasts several days; most often a faint, nonspecific exanthem on trunk and proximal extremities, with spread to face and forearms • Occasionally eyelid, palatal, and cutaneous petechiae • Less often genital ulcers (see Fig. 67.12), Gianotti–Crosti syndrome, urticaria > erythema multiforme, erythema nodosum	**Common, *not* serious:** antibiotic-induced hypersensitivity reaction (most often with penicillins or cephalosporins); this is not a true allergic reaction and typically safe for that patient to take the antibiotic in the future (see Fig. 67.13) **Rare, but serious**: splenic rupture, especially post-traumatic; airway and oral compromise from oropharyngeal lymphoid tissue swelling **Other**: severe hepatitis; thrombocytopenia; hemolytic anemia; glomerulonephritis; CNS (e.g. encephalitis, aseptic meningitis)	**Oro-cutaneous** • Primary CMV, HHV-6, or HIV infections • Drug eruption (e.g. DRESS/DIHS) **Pharyngitis** • Group A *Streptococcus* infection **Other** • Acute viral hepatitis • Lymphoma • Toxoplasmosis
Reactivation infection: EBV lymphoproliferative disorders**	***In United States***: B-cell lymphoma; lymphoproliferative disorders in immunocompromised hosts (e.g. solid organ transplant recipients; HIV (+) infection; and taking immunosuppressive medications, classically methotrexate and/or infliximab in the setting of rheumatoid arthritis) ***Worldwide***: Hydroa vacciniforme, necrotic hypersensitivity to mosquito bites, African (endemic) Burkitt lymphoma, nasopharyngeal carcinoma		• Other cutaneous and systemic lymphomas (see Chs 97–99)

Diagnosis of suspected* ***primary EBV infection* *is confirmed by a positive heterophile antibody test ("Monospot" test); if the heterophile antibody test is negative but IM is still suspected (e.g. early in the course of disease [≤6 weeks]) or in younger children (<2 years), then consider: repeat heterophile antibody testing, EBV-specific serologies, and/or EBV DNA levels.*

Diagnosis of a suspected* ***EBV lymphoproliferative disorder *is confirmed by the presence of elevated circulating EBV DNA levels.*

Table 67.5 Major clinical features of Epstein–Barr virus (EBV) infections. Treatment of primary EBV infection is primarily supportive; treatment of EBV lymphoproliferative disorders is focused on reversing the host's immunosuppressed state, if possible.

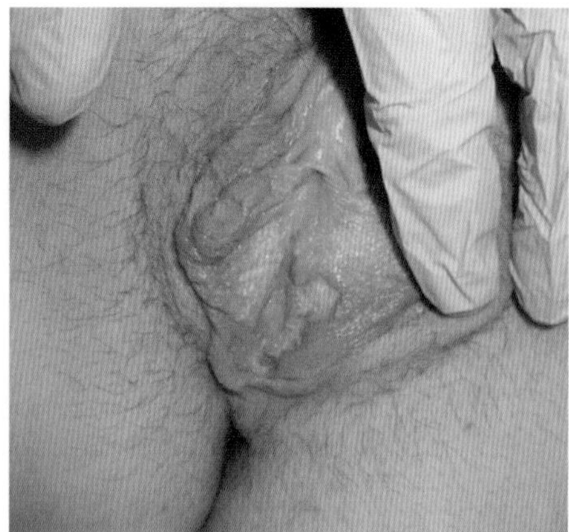

Fig. 67.12 Vulvar ulcers associated with primary EBV infection. EBV-related genital ulcers, which are most common in adolescent girls, are often misdiagnosed as genital herpes simplex infection and in some patients represent a variant of aphthosis. *Courtesy, YDRSC.*

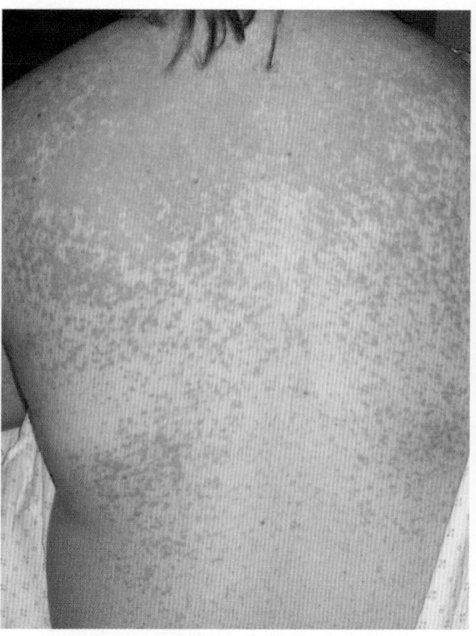

Fig. 67.13 Ampicillin-induced eruption in a patient with infectious mononucleosis due to Epstein–Barr virus infection. Erythematous macules and papules have become confluent on the upper trunk. *Courtesy, YDRSC.*

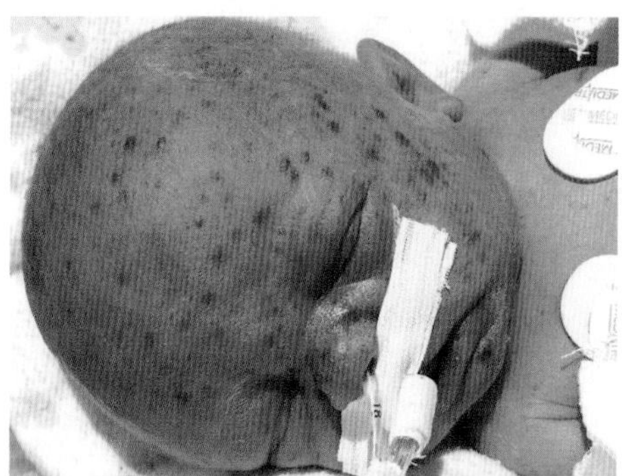

Fig. 67.14 TORCH syndrome due to cytomegalovirus. Multiple firm, red-violet papules of dermal erythropoiesis. *Courtesy, Mary S. Stone, MD.*

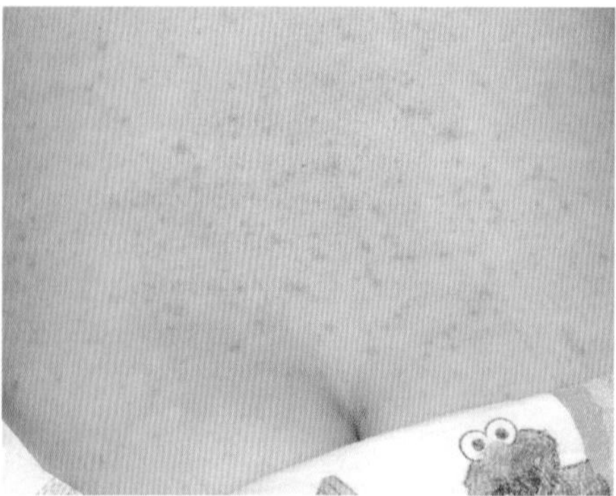

Fig. 67.15 Exanthem subitum (roseola infantum). Small pink-red macules and papules developed on the trunk and neck of this 9-month-old boy during defervescence of a high fever that lasted 5 days. *Courtesy, Julie V. Schaffer, MD.*

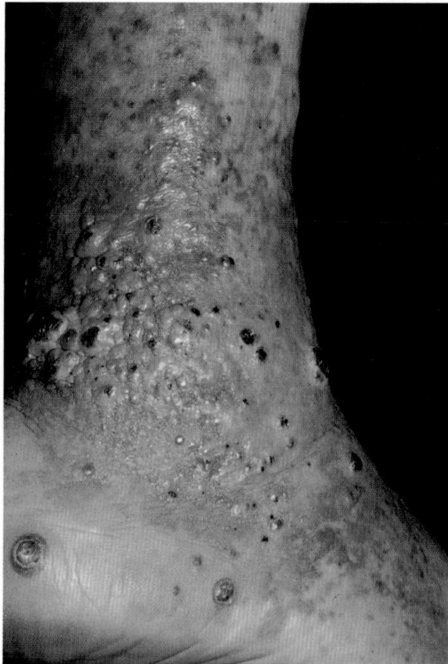

Fig. 67.16 Classic Kaposi sarcoma. Multiple red-violet nodules with hemorrhagic crusting and plaques on the ankle and foot. *Courtesy, Joyce Rico, MD.*

MAJOR CLINICAL FEATURES OF CYTOMEGALOVIRUS (CMV) INFECTIONS

CMV infection*	Major clinical features	Complications	DDx of skin lesions
Primary infection Latency is established primarily in monocytes and macrophages ~40–100% of adults are seropositive	• 4–8 week incubation period **Immunocompetent hosts** • >90% are subclinical and in children > adults • Occasionally (adults > children) presents as a mononucleosis-like syndrome; usually less severe, no exudative tonsillitis, and heterophile antibody (–); in those patients, ~33% have a morbilliform or petechial eruption **Congenital and neonates** • ~5–10% of infected neonates present with jaundice, IUGR, thrombocytopenia, chorioretinitis, and petechiae or the papules of extramedullary hematopoiesis ("blueberry muffin" lesions) (see Fig. 67.14) **AIDS patients** • Chorioretinitis, esophagitis, colitis, pneumonitis • Rarely, chronic perineal and lower extremity ulcerations **Organ transplant recipients** • Gastrointestinal involvement and pneumonitis	**Immunocompetent hosts:** rarely colitis, encephalitis, myocarditis, and anterior uveitis **Congenital and neonates:** congenital deafness; intellectual disability **AIDS patients:** blindness	**Immunocompetent hosts** • Other mononucleosis-like syndromes (e.g. EBV, HHV-6, toxoplasmosis) • Morbilliform drug eruption • Other causes of petechiae (see Ch. 18) **Congenital and neonates** • Other causes of TORCH
Reactivation infection	• May result from reactivation of latent CMV (greatest risk in immunosuppressed hosts) or from reinfection with a novel exogenous strain of CMV • Overall rare in immunocompetent hosts • Clinical presentations are similar to those described in primary CMV infections		

**Diagnosis is made via various techniques: (1) serologies (e.g. IgM and IgG antibodies); (2) various molecular amplification techniques (e.g. PCR); (3) cultures (helpful to determine if drug resistance is present); (4) CMV antigenemia assays (helpful in immunosuppressed hosts); (5) biopsy of cutaneous lesions (e.g. ulcerations) may show characteristic findings of enlarged endothelial cells with prominent intranuclear inclusions ("owl's eyes").*

Table 67.6 Major clinical features of cytomegalovirus (CMV) infections. Treatment of uncomplicated CMV infection in immunocompetent hosts is primarily supportive; treatment in immunocompromised hosts or in those with complicated infections involves systemic therapy (e.g. intravenous ganciclovir, oral valganciclovir, cidofovir, foscarnet). Prevention is possible by matching CMV serologies between donor and transplant recipients. IUGR, intrauterine growth retardation; TORCH, toxoplasmosis, other agents, rubella, cytomegalovirus, herpes simplex virus.

MAJOR CLINICAL FEATURES OF HUMAN HERPESVIRUS 6 AND 7 (HHV-6 AND HHV-7) INFECTIONS			
Infection	**Primary infection**	**Reactivation infection**	**DDx**
HHV-6* Latency is established in T lymphocytes ~70–90% of adults are seropositive	• Usually acquired between 6 months and 2 years of age • ~30% of children develop observable clinical manifestations • Febrile seizures may occur in infants **Clinical presentations** ***Exanthem subitum (roseola, sixth disease)*** • 3–5 days of high fever followed by cutaneous eruption as fever fades (see Fig. 67.15) • Discrete circular "rose red," 2- to 5-mm macules or maculopapules, often surrounded by a white halo • Enanthem of red papules on soft palate (Nagayama spots) • Late, may see palpebral edema ***Febrile syndrome without a cutaneous eruption*** ***Mononucleosis-like syndrome in adults***	**Seen primarily in immunosuppressed hosts** • Fever, cutaneous eruption, hepatitis, pneumonitis, bone marrow suppression, encephalitis, colitis • Also implicated in DRESS/DIHS syndrome and possibly pityriasis rosea	***Exanthem subitum*** • Other viral exanthems (see Ch. 68); Kawasaki disease (if fever persists after appearance of eruption) ***Mononucleosis-like syndrome*** • EBV, CMV, toxoplasmosis
HHV-7** Latency is established in T lymphocytes ~85% of U.S. adults are seropositive	• Usually acquired in the first 5 years of life, peaking at about age 3 years • Usually asymptomatic • Can cause *exanthem subitum*, but is less common than HHV-6 • Potential complications include febrile seizures and acute hemiplegia	• Implicated in DRESS/DIHS syndrome and possibly pityriasis rosea	• See above, under *exanthem subitum*

**Diagnosis of HHV-6 is clinical in most cases of classic exanthema subitum in children; laboratory investigation with serologies and seroconversion data (e.g. IgM and IgG antibodies and titers) or detection of HHV-6 DNA in clinical/tissue specimens is reserved for atypical presentations and complications or in immunosuppressed hosts.*
***Serologic tests and quantitative PCR may be useful for immunosuppressed hosts.*

Table 67.7 Major clinical features of human herpesvirus 6 and 7 (HHV-6 and HHV-7) infections. No definitive treatment is available.

MAJOR CLINICAL FEATURES OF HUMAN HERPESVIRUS 8 (HHV-8) INFECTIONS		
HHV-8 infection	**Major clinical features**	**DDx**
Primary infection Latency is established in B lymphocytes and vascular endothelial cells	**Children** • Fever and morbilliform eruption **Men who have sex with men (MSM)** • New-onset lymphadenopathy, fatigue, diarrhea, and a localized cutaneous eruption **Immunosuppressed hosts (e.g. solid organ transplant recipients, HIV (+) infection)** • Fever, splenomegaly, lymphoid hyperplasia, pancytopenia • Occasionally rapid-onset KS	
Reactivation infection	**Kaposi sarcoma (KS) (four subtypes)** • Cutaneous lesions progress through stages as red, brown, or violaceous papules, plaques, and nodules 1. ***Classic KS*** (see Fig. 67.16) • Indolent; primarily seen in elderly males of Mediterranean and Jewish descent; favors the lower extremities 2. ***African-endemic KS*** • Seen in equatorial Africa; primarily in children and young adults; more aggressive than classic KS; may disseminate to lymph nodes, bone, or skin 3. ***Iatrogenic immunosuppression-associated KS*** • Most often seen in solid organ transplant recipients; similar to AIDS-related KS; may be acquired from the donor or transplanted tissue; typically regresses with reduction of immunosuppression medications or a change to sirolimus 4. ***AIDS-related KS*** • Typically presents with more widely distributed lesions on the skin and internally (e.g. lungs, GI tract); can improve with ART treatment, but can also flare as part of IRIS **Primary effusion lymphoma** • B-cell lymphoma **Multicentric Castleman disease** • Lymphoproliferative disorder characterized by fever, hepatosplenomegaly, and massive lymphadenopathy	**KS (lower extremity)** • Acroangiodermatitis (pseudo-KS) • Lymphoma • Ecchymoses **KS (more widespread distribution)** • Bacillary angiomatosis • Ecchymoses • Other vascular tumors and hyperplasias (see Ch. 94) • Lymphoma
The optimal serologic assay for diagnosis of HHV-8 is not known; when cutaneous lesions are present, a skin biopsy for histochemical analysis for LANA-1 can be diagnostic.		

HHV-8 is also known as Kaposi sarcoma (KS)-associated herpesvirus. Treatment of KS involves reconstitution of the host's immune system (e.g. decrease immunosuppressive therapy, ART, change to sirolimus); systemic and intralesional chemotherapy; radiation therapy; cryotherapy.

Table 67.8 Major clinical features of human herpesvirus 8 (HHV-8) infections. IRIS, immune reconstitution inflammatory syndrome.

68 Other Viral Diseases

Viral infections frequently have cutaneous manifestations, especially in children. This chapter covers classic childhood exanthems, poxvirus infections, and several other viral infections with characteristic skin findings. *Nonspecific viral exanthems*, typically presenting with blanchable erythematous macules and papules in a widespread distribution, are also common in children infected with enteroviruses (see below) and a variety of respiratory viruses, generally resolving spontaneously within a week. Fig. 68.1 outlines clinical features to consider when evaluating a patient with a morbilliform ("maculopapular") exanthem, and Chapter 3 addresses considerations in patients with fever and a rash. HIV, human papillomavirus, and herpesvirus (including infectious mononucleosis and roseola infantum) infections are discussed in Chapters 65–67.

Enterovirus Infections

- Non-polio enteroviruses (e.g. coxsackieviruses, echoviruses) are single-stranded RNA picornaviruses with a worldwide distribution; they cause a variety of exanthems, enanthems, and systemic manifestations.
- Spread via fecal–oral (e.g. swimming pools, ingestion of oysters) and respiratory routes, with an incubation period of 3–6 days; most common in the summer and fall in temperate climates, favoring young children.
- *Hand-foot-and-mouth disease* (HFMD; in the United States, coxsackievirus A16 and A6 > others) features oval vesicles on the hands and feet (palms/soles > dorsally) and buttocks plus an erosive stomatitis (e.g. tongue, buccal mucosa, palate, tonsils), often associated with fever and malaise (Fig. 68.2A–C); onychomadesis occasionally occurs 1–2 months later.
- Coxsackievirus A6 infection can produce a more widespread vesiculobullous exanthem favoring the perioral area > oral mucosa, extremities > trunk, and areas of previous dermatitis ("eczema coxsackium") or injury as well as the classic sites of HFMD (Fig. 68.2D–F; see Fig. 3.6B–D).
- *Herpangina* presents with fever and oropharyngeal erosions, but usually no exanthem.
- The diverse spectrum of enteroviral exanthems also includes morbilliform, scarlatiniform, Gianotti–Crosti syndrome-like, petechial, and pustular eruptions (see Fig. 3.6A); eruptive pseudoangiomatosis is an uncommon manifestation.
- Organ systems that can be affected by enteroviral infections include the respiratory (upper > lower) and gastrointestinal tracts, liver, CNS (meningitis > encephalitis; especially with enterovirus 71), eyes (hemorrhagic conjunctivitis), joints, muscles, and heart.
- Spontaneous resolution typically occurs within 1–2 weeks.

Measles (Rubeola)

- Incidence has decreased dramatically since introduction of a live vaccine for this single-stranded RNA paramyxovirus in 1963; however, measles outbreaks still occur in both low- and high-income countries, often because of unfounded fears of vaccination.
- Highly contagious and spread by respiratory droplets, with an incubation period of 10–14 days.
- Prodrome of fever, cough, coryza, and conjunctivitis (the 3 Cs), followed in 2–4 days by the appearance of pathognomonic Koplik spots (gray-white papules on the buccal mucosa).
- An exanthem develops 3–5 days after the onset of symptoms, with erythematous macules and papules spreading cephalocaudally from the forehead, hairline, and behind the ears to the trunk and extremities (Fig. 68.3); after 5 days, the eruption fades in the order it appeared.

1. Exclude other causes

- Drug reaction
- Kawasaki disease
- Bacterial infections, e.g. group A β-hemolytic streptococcal, *Arcanobacterium haemolyticum**, meningococcemia (if petechiae), ehrlichiosis, leptospirosis, rickettsioses, syphilis
- Other viral exanthems, e.g. due to HIV seroconversion (see Ch. 65), COVID-19, chikungunya fever, dengue, and infections with Zika, Barmah Forest, and Ross River viruses

2. Specific features

Clinical signs and symptoms		Viruses								
		Measles (rubeola)	**Rubella**	**Parvovirus B19**	**HHV-6 or-7**	**Epstein–Barr virus**	**Adenovirus**	**Enterovirus**	**Cytomegalo-virus**†	**West Nile virus**
Exanthem	Cephalocaudad spread	✓	✓							
	Rose-pink macules		✓		✓	✓	✓	✓	✓	
	Red cheeks; reticulate or lacy			✓						
	Punctate lesions on extremities									✓
	Rash starts as fever subsides				✓					
	Most prominent following antibiotics					✓			✓	
	Petechiae	✓		✓		✓	✓	✓	✓	
Enanthem	Gray–white papules, buccal mucosa (Koplik)	✓								
	Red macules, soft palate (Forschheimer)		✓							
	Red papules, soft palate/uvula (Nagayama)				✓					
	Uvulo-palatoglossal junctional ulcers				✓					
	Painful erosions, esp. of posterior pharynx			✓				✓		
	Pharyngitis					✓	✓	✓		
Lymph-adenopathy	Generalized	✓				✓				✓
	Localized: occipital, posterior auricular		✓							
	Localized: cervical					✓		✓	✓	
Musculoskeletal	Arthralgias/arthritis		✓	✓		✓		✓	✓	✓
	Muscle weakness									✓
Eye	Conjunctivitis	✓	✓				✓	✓		✓
Liver/spleen	Hepatosplenomegaly	✓				✓			✓	
CNS	Encephalitis (E) ± Meningitis (M)	✓(E)	✓(E)		✓(E**)		✓(E,M)	✓(E,M)	✓(E)	✓(E,M)
Lungs	Pneumonia	✓					✓	✓		
Heart	Myocarditis	✓	✓					✓		
3. Laboratory tests		Serology; Virus isolation NP; PCR	Serology; Virus isolation NP/U/CSF; PCR	Serology; PCR	Serology; PCR	Heterophile antibody; Serology; Atypical lymphocytosis; PCR	Antigen detection T/S; Virus isolation NP; Serology; PCR	Virus isolation T/S/V; Serology; PCR	Antigen detection, PCR Blood[ab]; Virus isolation U[b]; Serology	Serology also CSF; PCR

Serology; Virus isolation; xxxxxx (PCR) Polymerase chain reaction assay; Antigen detection; Heterophile antibody; Atypical lymphocytosis

CSF = Cerebrospinal fluid
NP = Nasopharyngeal
V = Vesicle fluid
U = Urine
T = Throat
S = Stool

Notes: [a] Immunocompromised host [b] Immunocompetent host

Fig. 68.1 Approach to the patient with a presumed morbilliform or macular/papular viral exanthem. *Gram-positive rod; may result in severe pharyngitis and scarlatiniform exanthem in adolescents and young adults. †Intracellular inclusions in endothelial cells are another finding. **Usually febrile seizures.

- Complications include otitis media, pneumonia, and encephalitis; subacute sclerosing panencephalitis occasionally develops 5–10 years later.
- *Atypical measles* in the setting of partial immunity features high fevers, cough, and a variable exanthem that may be vesicular, petechial, or associated with acral edema.
- **Rx:** vitamin A administration for children with acute disease; prevention via vaccination.

Rubella (German Measles)

- Incidence has markedly declined since introduction of a live vaccine for this single-stranded RNA togavirus in 1969.
- Spread via respiratory droplets, with an incubation period of 16–18 days.
- Mild prodrome of fever, headache, and upper respiratory symptoms, followed in 1–5 days

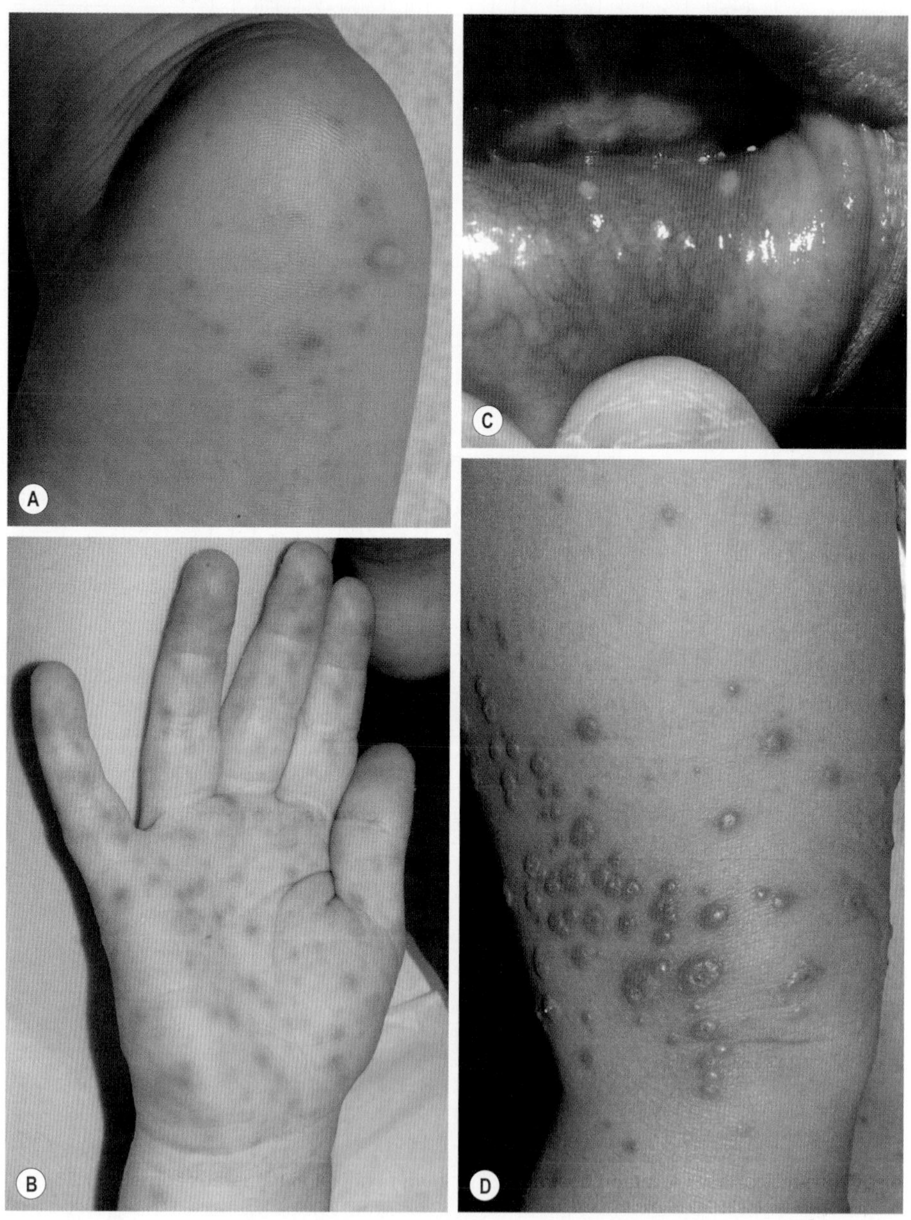

Fig. 68.2 Hand-foot-and-mouth disease (HFMD). A Oval vesicle and erythematous macules on the plantar surface. **B** Multiple erythematous macules on the palm, some with a dusky appearance reminiscent of erythema multiforme. **C** Small oval erosions on the buccal mucosa resembling aphthae. **D** Coxsackievirus A6 infection presenting as vesicles and papulovesicles in a widespread distribution including the thigh. *Continued*

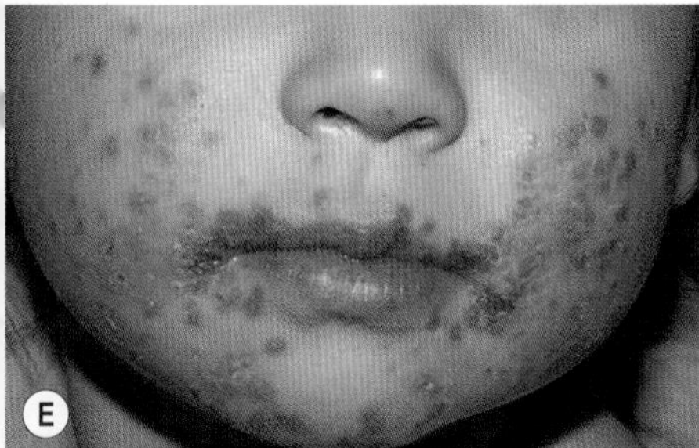

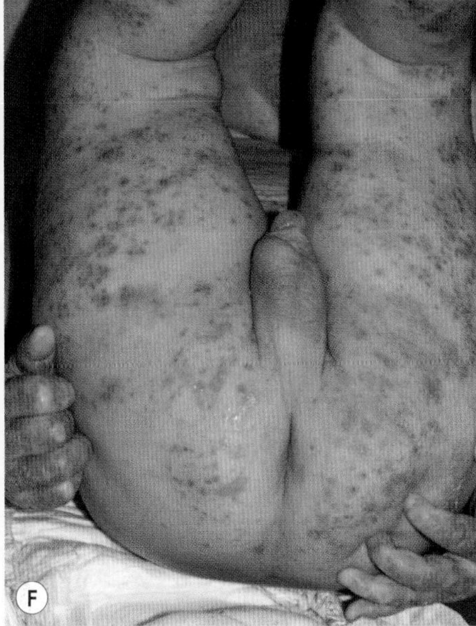

Fig. 68.2 *Continued* **Hand-foot-and-mouth disease (HFMD).** Coxsackievirus A6 infection presenting as: perioral monomorphic crusted lesions resembling eczema herpeticum (**E**); and more extensive "eczema coxsackium" in a toddler with atopic dermatitis (**F**). *A, B, D–F, Courtesy, Julie V. Schaffer, MD; C, Courtesy, Kalman Watsky, MD.*

by an eruption of erythematous macules and papules that spreads downward from the face and lasts ~3 days; Forchheimer spots (red or petechial macules on the soft palate) and tender lymphadenopathy (especially occipital and posterior auricular) are characteristic findings.

- Although usually self-limited, complications include arthralgias/arthritis (especially in adolescent girls and women), thrombocytopenia, and encephalitis.
- *Congenital rubella syndrome*, most common with maternal infection in the first 16 weeks of pregnancy; can result in cataracts, deafness, congenital heart defects, and microcephaly; a "blueberry muffin baby" presentation occasionally occurs (see Fig. 67.14).

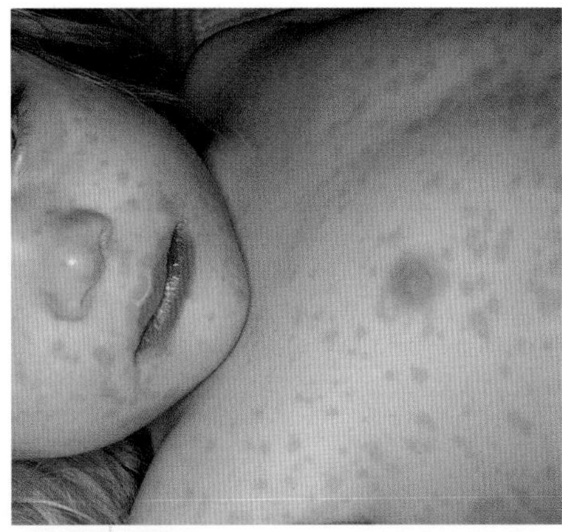

Fig. 68.3 Measles. Pink macules and minimally elevated papules. *Courtesy, Louis A. Fragola, Jr., MD.*

Parvovirus B19 Infection (Erythema Infectiosum, Fifth Disease, "Slapped Cheek Disease")

- Single-stranded DNA virus with tropism for erythroid progenitor cells; found worldwide.
- Transmitted via respiratory secretions and blood products as well as vertically from mother to fetus, with an incubation period of 4–14 days; peak incidence in the winter and spring, favoring children 4–10 years of age.
- A mild prodrome (e.g. low-grade fever, myalgias, headache) is followed in 7–10 days by bright red, macular erythema on the cheeks; a few days later, a lacy, reticulated pattern of erythematous macules and papules may appear on the extremities > trunk, lasting 1–3 weeks and fluctuating in intensity (with flares upon sun exposure and overheating) (Fig. 68.4).
- *Papular–purpuric gloves and socks syndrome* (parvovirus B19 > other viruses) features painful acral edema, erythema, and petechiae/purpura (especially on the palms and soles; Fig. 68.5).
- More widespread petechial eruptions and an enanthem (petechiae, erosions) can also occur.
- Complications include arthritis/arthralgias favoring small joints of the hands (especially in young adults) and aplastic

anemia > pancytopenia in susceptible individuals (e.g. with red blood cell disorders or immunosuppression).

- *Fetal parvovirus B19 infection* may lead to self-limited anemia, hydrops fetalis (extensive edema), or miscarriage/stillbirth (2–6%, especially if in first half of pregnancy).
- **Rx:** NSAIDs for arthropathy, RBC transfusions for severe aplastic crises, serial fetal ultrasonography for infections during the first two trimesters of pregnancy.

Unilateral Laterothoracic Exanthem (Asymmetric Periflexural Exanthem of Childhood)

- A consistent causative infectious agent has not been identified.
- Most often occurs in the spring and favors preschool-aged children.
- Morbilliform or eczematous eruption that begins unilaterally (axilla > trunk or thigh) and then spreads to contralateral sites (Fig. 68.6).
- Often pruritic and may be preceded by upper respiratory or gastrointestinal symptoms.
- **DDx:** allergic contact dermatitis, eczematous reaction to molluscum contagiosium, pityriasis rosea, scabies; eruptions with a more widespread distribution may overlap with Gianotti–Crosti syndrome.
- Resolves spontaneously, usually within 3–8 weeks.
- **Rx:** topical CS are often of limited benefit.

Gianotti–Crosti Syndrome (Papular Acrodermatitis of Childhood)

- Associated with a variety of infectious triggers, most often Epstein–Barr virus, hepatitis B virus (outside the United States), and vaccines.
- Most common in the spring and early summer, favoring young children.
- Often preceded by a low-grade fever and/or upper respiratory symptoms.
- Rapid onset of monomorphic, skin-colored to pink-red, edematous papules > papulovesicles in a symmetric distribution on the extensor surfaces of the extremities, buttocks, and face (Fig. 68.7); pruritus, purpuric lesions, and extension to the trunk occasionally occur.
- **DDx:** inflammatory response to molluscum contagiosum, id reaction (e.g. due to allergic contact dermatitis to nickel), papular

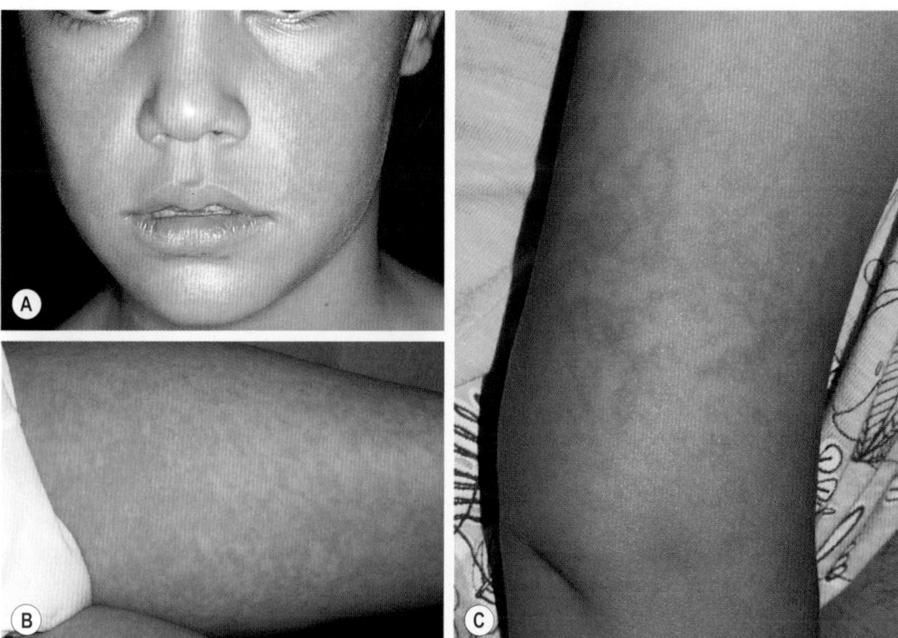

Fig. 68.4 Erythema infectiosum. Bright macular erythema on the cheeks, with characteristic sparing of periorificial areas **(A)**. Lacy, reticulated erythematous eruption on the thigh **(B)** and arm **(C)** during the second stage of the exanthem. *A, Courtesy, Louis A. Fragola, Jr., MD; B, C Courtesy, Julie V. Schaffer, MD.*

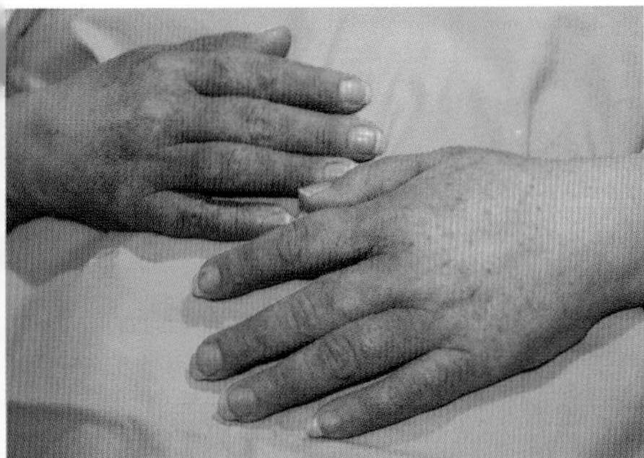

Fig. 68.5 Papular–purpuric gloves and socks syndrome. Erythema and edema with associated petechiae and small purpuric papules on the dorsal aspect of the fingers and hands. *Courtesy, Luis Requena, MD.*

urticaria, another viral exanthem (e.g. coxsackievirus A6), drug eruption, scabies.

- Resolves spontaneously, usually within 3–8 weeks (longer than a classic viral exanthem); laboratory evaluation for specific viral agents can be performed if indicated by clinical findings and geographic region.
- **Rx:** topical CS are often of limited benefit.

Molluscum Contagiosum (MC)

- Common cutaneous infection caused by a poxvirus.
- Spread by skin-to-skin contact >> fomites (e.g. towels), favoring young children but also occurring via sexual contact in adults; larger and more numerous lesions may be seen in immunocompromised hosts, especially those with HIV infection.
- Firm, skin-colored to pink papules with a waxy surface and central umbilication; predilection for the skin folds (e.g. axillae, neck, groin), lateral trunk, thighs, buttocks, genitals, and face (Fig. 68.8).
- Inflammatory reactions frequently occur, including eczematous dermatitis (diffuse or nummular) in the skin surrounding MC lesions, furuncle-like inflammation of individual MC lesions, and a Gianotti–Crosti syndrome-like eruption of pruritic erythematous papules favoring the elbows and knees (see Fig. 68.8B–F).
- **DDx** (in addition to above): *multiple lesions* – verrucae, condyloma acuminata, papular eczema; *solitary to few lesions* – juvenile xanthogranuloma or Spitz nevus in a child, BCC in an adult; *in immunocompromised*

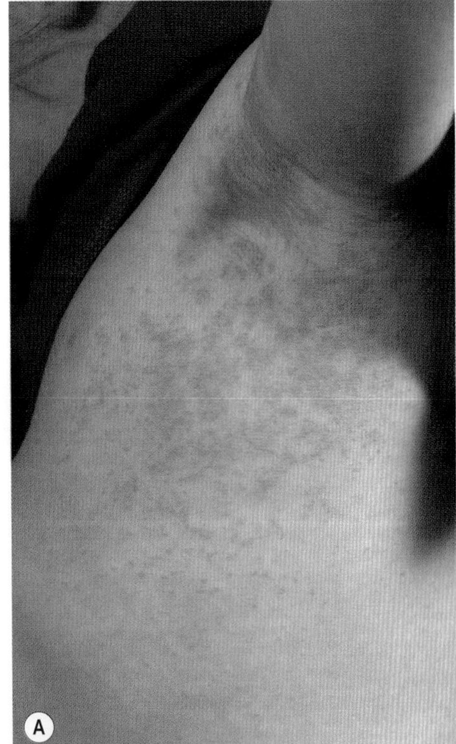

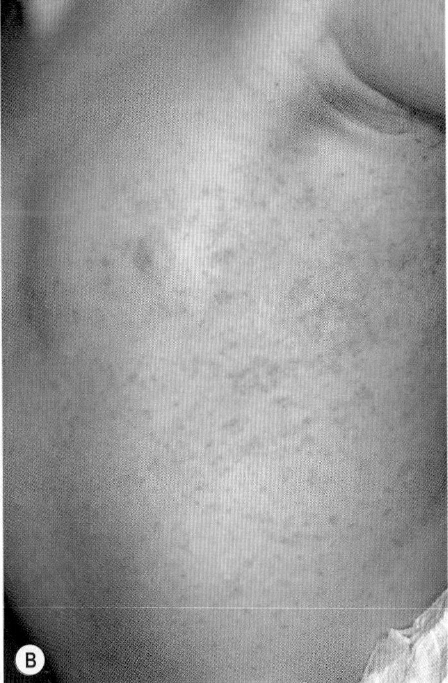

Fig. 68.6 Unilateral laterothoracic exanthem. Erythematous macules and papules involving the left axilla and upper flank **(A)** and a slightly more extensive distribution on the left lateral trunk **(B)**. *Courtesy, NYUDSC.*

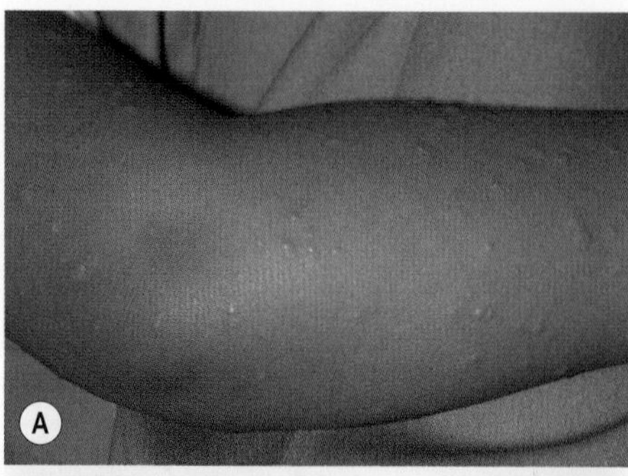

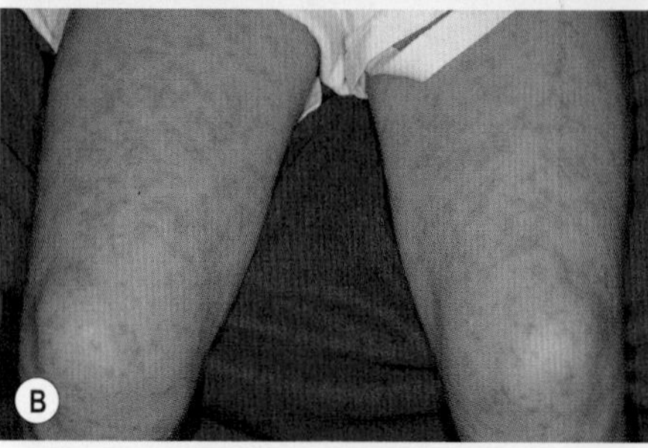

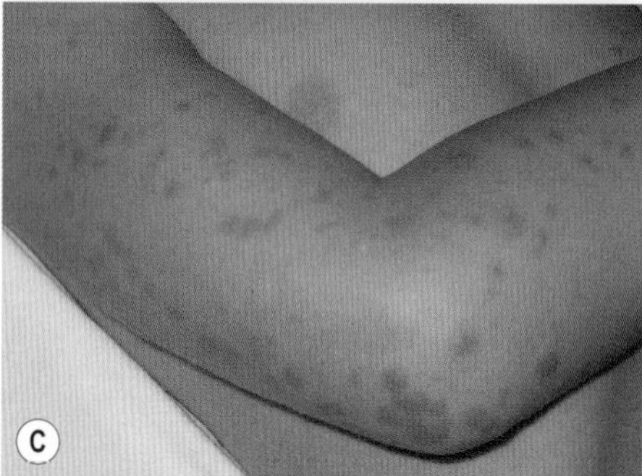

Fig. 68.7 Gianotti–Crosti syndrome. **A** Monomorphic, small erythematous papules on the elbow. **B** A more exuberant eruption of coalescing edematous, erythematous papules on the thighs and knees. **C** Larger edematous, erythematous papules on the elbow.
A, C, Courtesy, YDRSC; B, Courtesy, Anthony Mancini, MD.

hosts – cryptococcosis, histoplasmosis, other dimorphic fungal infections.

- Microscopic evaluation following curettage of lesional contents or biopsy shows large, round intracytoplasmic inclusion bodies (see Ch. 2); dermoscopy can identify a characteristic yellow-white, lobular central structure surrounded by a "crown" of blood vessels.
- Resolves spontaneously over months to several years in immunocompetent children, with larger numbers of lesions often developing in those with atopic dermatitis.
- **Rx:** options are listed in Table 68.1.

Other Poxvirus Infections

- The most historically significant poxvirus infection was smallpox, which has been responsible for millions of human deaths; the world was declared free of smallpox in 1980, although two reference collections remain (in the United States and Russia) and it is feared that smallpox could be exploited for bioterrorism.
- The clinical manifestations of smallpox and varicella are compared in Table 68.2, and selected poxvirus infections and complications of smallpox vaccination are presented in Figs 68.9 and 68.10 and Table 68.3.

Hemorrhagic Fevers and Other Viral Infections with Cutaneous Manifestations

- *Hemorrhagic fevers*: group of zoonotic viral infections with nonspecific cutaneous manifestations that include petechiae, purpura, and mucosal hemorrhage; although overall most common in Africa and South America (e.g. Ebola, Marburg, and yellow fever viruses), some have a worldwide distribution (e.g. hantavirus).
- Cutaneous manifestations of coronavirus disease 2019 (COVID-19 [SARS-CoV-2]) include urticarial, morbilliform, papulovesicular, erythema multiforme-like, chilblains-like, and purpuric eruptions; livedo reticularis/racemosa and retiform purpura (primarily in severely ill adults) and a multisystem inflammatory syndrome in children (MIS-C) with mucocutaneous findings similar to Kawasaki disease (see Ch. 3) may also occur.
- Cutaneous manifestations of hepatitis A, B, and C infections are listed in Table 68.4.
- Major features of other viral infections with cutaneous findings are presented in Table 68.5.

For further information see Ch. 81 from *Dermatology, Fourth Edition*.

For additional online figures and tables visit www.expertconsult.com

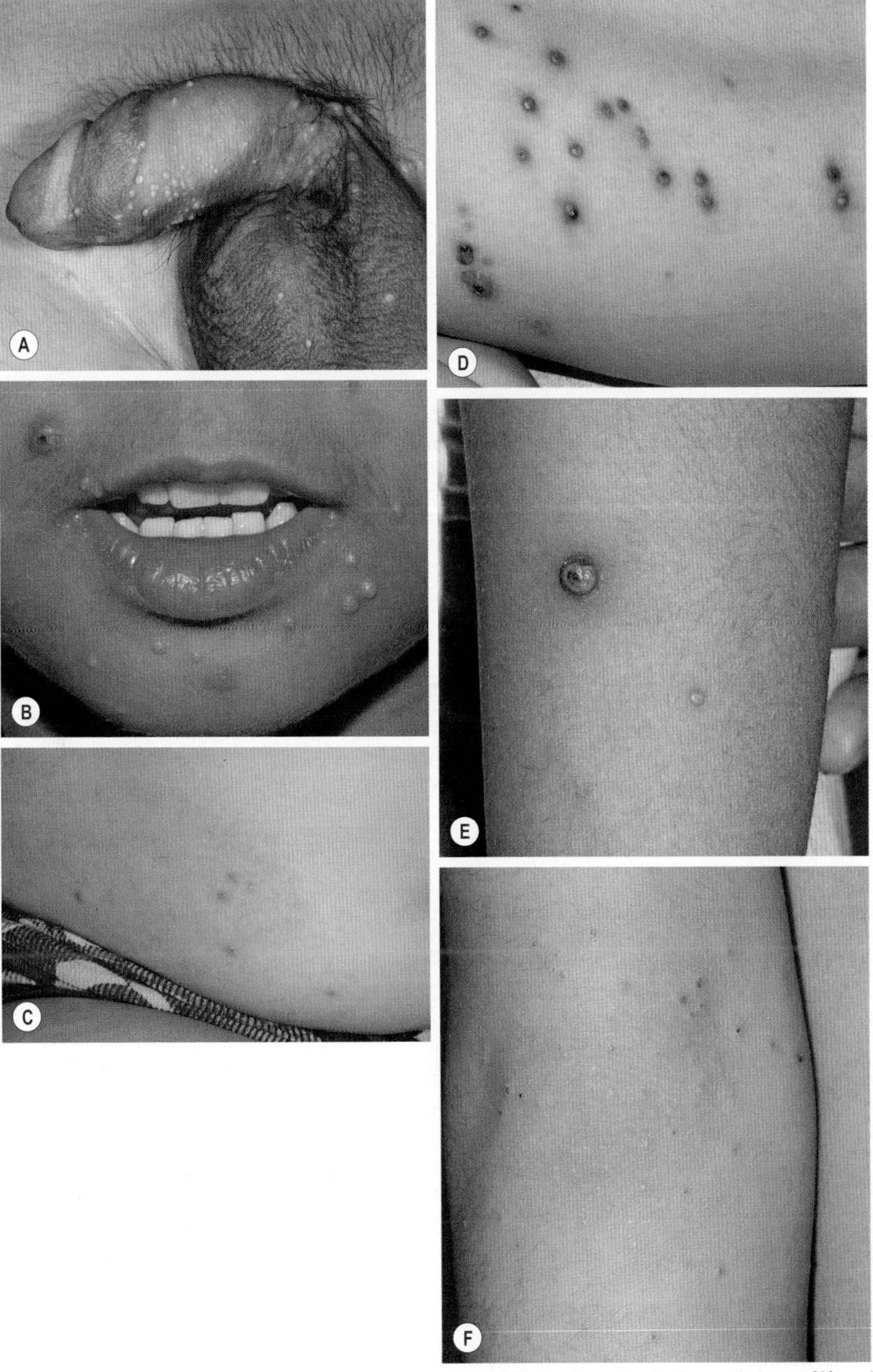

Fig. 68.8 Molluscum contagiosum. Multiple pearly, umbilicated papules in the genital area **(A)** and on the face **(B)**; note the inflamed lesion on the right cheek. Inflammatory reactions are a sign of the host immune response to the virus. **C** Inflamed lesions surrounded by "molluscum dermatitis." **D, E** Pustular presentations of inflamed molluscum. Cultures revealed only normal skin flora. **F** Monomorphic eruption of pruritic pink papules with crusting on the elbow. These reactive lesions were also present on knees of this child with molluscum contagiosum on the trunk. *A, C, Courtesy, Anthony Mancini, MD; B, D–F, Courtesy, Julie V. Schaffer, MD.*

TREATMENT OF MOLLUSCUM CONTAGIOSUM
No direct therapy
Spontaneous involution in immunocompetent patients (mean duration ~1 year) Treatment of associated dermatitis with a topical CS can prevent autoinoculation from scratching
Physical modalities
Curettage* (1) or manual extraction (3) Cryotherapy (2) Electrodesiccation* (3)
Topical therapy
Cantharidin (1) Podophyllotoxin (1) Retinoids (3) Trichloroacetic acid (1)

**Discomfort can be minimized by prior application of a topical anesthetic (e.g. lidocaine 4–5% cream).*

Table 68.1 Treatment of molluscum contagiosum. Other options include topical sinecatechins, KOH 5–10% solution, other irritants (e.g. retinoids), intralesional immunotherapy with *Candida* antigen, pulsed dye laser, and (for extensive lesions) systemic medications (e.g. oral cimetidine or [in immunosuppressed patients] intravenous cidofovir). Imiquimod was found to be ineffective in two large randomized controlled trials. Key to evidence-based support: (1) prospective controlled trial; (2) retrospective study or large case series; (3) small case series or individual case reports.

COMPARISON OF VARICELLA/DISSEMINATED ZOSTER TO SMALLPOX

	Varicella/disseminated zoster	Smallpox
Prodrome	None or mild fever and malaise	Fever ≥101°F/38.3°C for 1–4 days prior to rash onset, plus malaise, headache, backache and/or abdominal pain
Distribution of lesions	Initially on face/scalp; trunk > distal extremities May have an enanthem	Concentrated on face and limbs; can progress to involve entire body surface Oropharyngeal lesions often precede cutaneous eruption
Stage of lesions	Different stages occur simultaneously in any one area of the skin (nonsynchronous)	Adjacent lesions are all at same stage of development (synchronous)
Types of lesions	Superficial papules, vesicles, and pustules	Papulovesicles → firm, deep-seated pustules with a tendency to confluence
Course	Lesions appear in crops over a 3-day period	Lesions spread over 1–2 weeks Crusting develops over 1 week
Scarring	Rare in uncomplicated cases	Common and marked

Table 68.2 Comparison of varicella/disseminated zoster to smallpox.

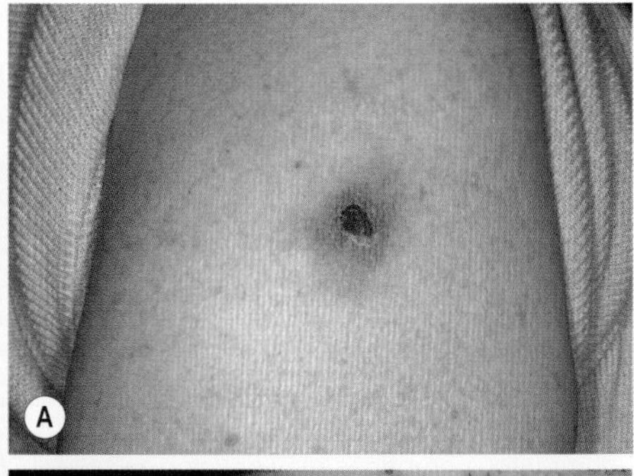

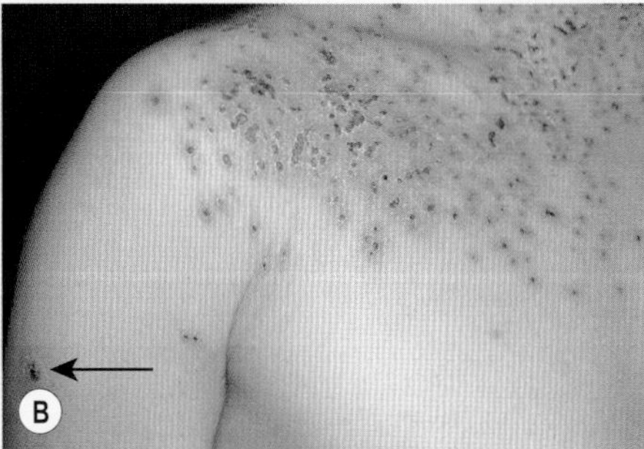

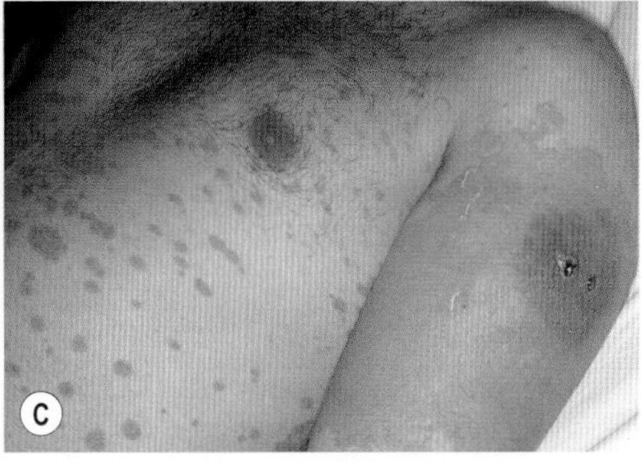

Fig. 68.9 Smallpox vaccine. A Crusted papule at the site of vaccination, 14 days following administration. **B** Eczema vaccinatum in a patient with atopic dermatitis. Spread from the vaccination site (arrow) to areas of eczema. **C** Erythema multiforme-like reaction associated with marked erythema and edema at the vaccination site. *A, Courtesy, Anthony J. Mancini, MD, and Ayelet Shani-Adir, MD; B, C, Courtesy, Louis A. Fragola, Jr., MD.*

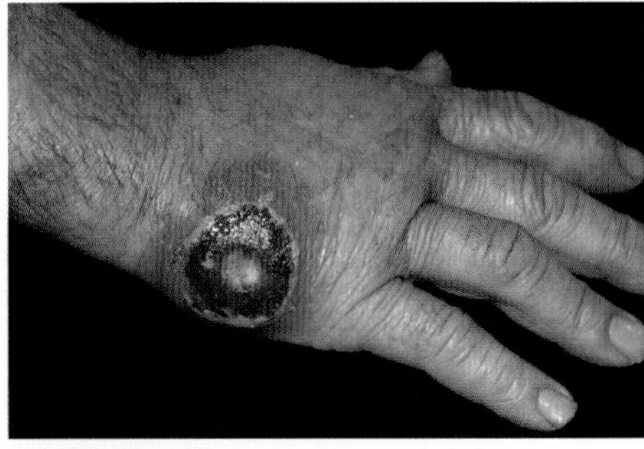

Fig. 68.10 Orf. Erythematous nodule with oozing and central ulceration on the dorsal aspect of the hand. *Courtesy, Luis Requena, MD.*

SELECTED POXVIRUS INFECTIONS	
Disease/virus (genus; host)	**Major features**
Smallpox/variola (*Orthopoxvirus*; only humans)	• Theoretically eradicated; respiratory transmission, 7- to 17-day incubation period • See Table 68.2 for clinical findings* • Complications: panophthalmitis, arthritis, encephalitis
Vaccinia (*Orthopoxvirus*; used as vaccine in humans)	• Currently used for smallpox vaccination in the military and first responders • Papule at vaccination site (e.g. deltoid or thigh) → vesiculopustules → crust (Fig. 68.9A) → scar, occasionally with satellite lesions; fever and LAN are common, and urticarial or exanthematous eruptions may develop 1–3 weeks postvaccination • Possible adverse events* – Superinfection of the vaccination site or lymph nodes – Inadvertent autoinoculation or contact transmission – Generalized or progressive vaccinia (especially in immunocompromised hosts) – Eczema vaccinatum (e.g. in patients with atopic dermatitis) (Fig. 68.9B) – Postvaccination nonviral pustulosis or erythema multiforme (Fig. 68.9C) – Ocular vaccinia, myo/pericarditis, postvaccinial CNS disease
Monkeypox (*Orthopoxvirus*; monkeys, rodents)	• Primarily in Africa; cutaneous inoculation or respiratory transmission, 10- to 12-day incubation period • Malaise and fever, then nonsynchronous eruption of papules (few to >100) → vesiculopustules → crusts → scars, favoring face and extremities (often on palms/soles); LAN and respiratory symptoms • Smallpox vaccination protective
Cowpox (*Orthopoxvirus*; cats > rodents > cattle)	• Primarily in Europe and Central Asia; 7-day incubation period • At site of contact (usually hands or face) with infected animal: papule → vesicle → pustule → crusted eschar → scar; often fever and LAN • Occasionally generalized in patients with atopic dermatitis
Orf (*Parapoxvirus*; sheep, goats, reindeer)	• At-risk occupations: shepherds, veterinarians, butchers • On hands (Fig. 68.10) following contact with infected animal (especially perioral area and udder of ewes): papule (1 to few) → targetoid lesion → nodule (weeping then dry with black dots then papillomatous) → regression without scar; ± fever and LAN, and erythema multiforme may occur 10–14 days later • Diagnosis often made histologically
Milker's nodules (bovine papular stomatitis)/paravaccinia (*Parapoxvirus*; cattle)	• At-risk occupations: dairy farmers, ranchers, butchers, veterinarians • Lesions on hands virtually identical to orf (see above)

**Additional information (e.g. diagnostic criteria, algorithms, case definitions) is available at http://www.cdc.gov/smallpox/index.html.*

Table 68.3 Selected poxvirus infections. Real-time PCR is currently the diagnostic method of choice. Other poxviruses that occasionally lead to skin lesions (single or few) in humans include *deer-associated parapoxvirus* (eastern United States; reported in deer hunters) and *tanapox* (equatorial Africa; endemic in nonhuman primates, likely arthropod vector). LAN, lymphadenopathy.

CUTANEOUS MANIFESTATIONS OF HEPATITIS A, B, AND C INFECTIONS	
Acute urticaria (A, B, C) Serum sickness-like reaction (B, C) Gianotti–Crosti syndrome (B > A, C) Small vessel vasculitis (B, C > A) Cryoglobulinemic vasculitis (C > B > A) Urticarial vasculitis (B, C) Polyarteritis nodosa (classic – B, cutaneous – C) Livedo reticularis (C)	Necrolytic acral erythema (C) Porphyria cutanea tarda (B, C) Pruritus (B, C > A) Lichen planus – especially erosive oral disease (C) Sarcoidosis (with interferon and/or ribavirin therapy; C > B) Erythema multiforme (B, C) Erythema nodosum (B > C)

Table 68.4 Cutaneous manifestations of hepatitis A, B, and C infections.

ADDITIONAL SELECTED VIRAL INFECTIONS WITH CUTANEOUS FINDINGS		
Viral infection (family)	**Geography/primary source of infection**	**Major features**
Dengue (Flaviviridae)	Caribbean, Mexico, Central and South America, Africa, Asia (especially tropics)/ mosquitoes	• 3- to 10-day incubation period → variable fever, headache (especially retro-orbital), myalgias, vomiting* • ~50% of patients: macular erythema of head, neck, and upper trunk, followed by morbilliform eruption with islands of sparing and often petechiae*
West Nile (Flaviviridae)	Africa, Europe, Asia, North > South America, Australia/ mosquitoes that feed on infected birds	• 5- to 14-day incubation period → fever, headache, myalgias > meningo-encephalitis, flaccid paralysis • ~25% of patients: exanthem with erythematous macules/papules, often punctate and favoring extremities
Zika (Flaviviridae)	Caribbean, Mexico, Central and South America, Africa, Pacific Islands, Asia (especially tropics)/ mosquitoes, sexual contact, mother to fetus, blood products	• 2- to 14-day incubation period → symptomatic in ~20% of patients: fever, arthralgias, headache, conjunctivitis, morbilliform exanthem (often pruritic, may involve palms/soles) • Risk of fetal microcephaly with maternal infection
Chikungunya (Togaviridae)	Asia, Indian and Pacific islands, Africa, Europe, Americas/mosquitoes	• 1- to 14-day incubation period → fever, headache, myalgias/arthralgias • ~50% of patients: acrofacial erythema/edema, morbilliform exanthem; occasionally ulcers (genital, intertriginous, oral), vesiculobullae, and postinflammatory hyperpigmentation (freckle-like, flagellate, or diffuse)
Trichodysplasia spinulosa (viral-associated trichodysplasia) (Polyomaviridae)	Worldwide**	• Numerous erythematous to skin-colored, spiny papules favoring the mid face and ears; ± alopecia or leonine facies

**Severe dengue (including dengue hemorrhagic fever and shock syndrome), which is more common in children and following repeat infection with a second virus serotype, features marked thrombocytopenia with bleeding, plasma leakage leading to shock and respiratory distress, and organ impairment.*
***In solid organ transplant recipients or patients receiving chemotherapy for a hematologic malignancy.*

Table 68.5 Additional selected viral infections with cutaneous findings. Other viruses with limited geographic distributions have prominent skin findings, e.g. Barmah Forest virus in Australia.

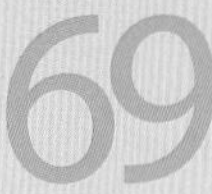

69 Sexually Transmitted Infections

In this chapter, five sexually transmitted infections (STIs) are covered – syphilis, gonorrhea, chancroid, lymphogranuloma venereum (LGV), and granuloma inguinale. Additional more common STIs including herpes simplex infections, mollusca contagiosa, condyloma acuminata, pubic lice, and HIV infection are discussed in Chapters 67, 68, 66, 71, and 65, respectively. When one STI is present, a search for others is indicated.

Syphilis (Lues)

- Etiologic agent is the spirochete *Treponema pallidum*; the infection is divided into four phases: primary, secondary, latent, and tertiary (Fig. 69.1), in addition to a congenital form.
- Syphilis is currently 7–10 times more common in men than in women in the United States and the incidence has been rising, especially in men, over the past 15 years; the highest rates are in Black and Hispanic individuals and in men who have sex with men (MSM); there is an increased risk of transmission of HIV infection in those with ulcers due to syphilis as well as chancroid or herpes simplex viral infection.
- One or more ulcers, usually anogenital, characterize *primary syphilis* and are referred to as chancres (Fig. 69.2); the ulcers are painless (unless secondarily infected) and upon palpation the base is firm; regional lymphadenopathy may be present (Fig. 69.3).
- *Secondary syphilis* reflects hematogenous dissemination and the skin lesions vary from macular to papulosquamous and from annular to granulomatous (Figs 69.4 and 69.5; see Fig. 65.4); mucosal involvement is common and includes mucous patches, split papules at the angles of the mouth and condyloma lata (Fig. 69.6); usually accompanied by constitutional symptoms (Table 69.1).
- *Tertiary syphilis* is preceded by a latent phase that can last for years (Fig. 69.7); the skin and mucous membranes, as well as the bones, develop gummas (Fig. 69.8), with cardiovascular syphilis and neurosyphilis representing the major causes of death in those who remain untreated.
- *In utero* infection of a fetus can occur, primarily during the secondary or latent phases, leading to congenital syphilis or stigmata (Tables 69.2 and 69.3); the cutaneous lesions of early congenital syphilis are similar to those of secondary syphilis (Fig. 69.9), but they may be bullous; additional findings include a bloody or purulent nasal discharge ("snuffles"), perioral and perianal fissures, and osteochondritis.
- Dx: darkfield microscopic examination (serous exudate from primary or secondary lesions); anti-cardiolipin antibodies (*r*apid *p*lasma *r*eagin [RPR] or *V*enereal *D*isease *R*esearch *L*aboratory [VDRL] assay): ~80%+ in primary and 99%+ in secondary; anti-*T. pallidum* (TP) antibodies (*m*icro*h*em*a*gglutination assay [MHA-TP] or *f*luorescent *t*reponemal *a*ntibody *abs*orption [FTA-ABS]: ~90%+ in primary and 99%+ in secondary.
- A false-positive VDRL can occur in pregnant women and in association with a number of disorders including antiphospholipid antibody syndrome, LE, lymphoma, and drug abuse as well as infections (e.g. endemic treponematoses, borreliosis, malaria), while a false-positive FTA-ABS can occur in patients with LE, HIV infection, hypergammaglobulinemia, endemic treponematoses, and borreliosis.
- **DDx:** see Table 69.4.
- **Rx:** see Table 69.5 for treatment of primary, secondary, and early latent syphilis; patients with symptoms or signs suggesting neurologic disease should have CSF analysis and HIV-infected patients are at increased risk for

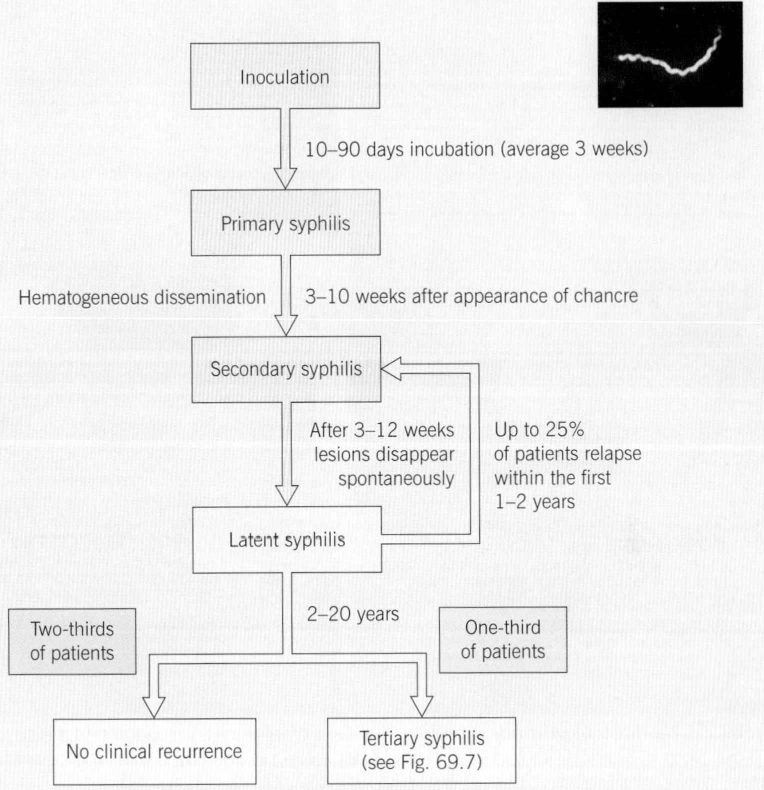

Fig. 69.1 Natural history of untreated syphilis. Chancres spontaneously resolve after a few weeks (see Fig. 69.3). In the group of patients with no recurrence, the rapid plasma reagin (RPR) becomes negative in 50% and remains positive in 50%. *Adapted from Rein MF, Musher DM. Late syphilis. In: Rein MF (Ed.), Atlas of Infectious Diseases, Vol. V: Sexually Transmitted Diseases. New York: Current Medicine, 1995:10.1–10.13. Inset figure: Adapted from Morse SA, et al. Atlas of Sexually Transmitted Diseases and AIDS, 3rd ed. London: Mosby; 2003.*

neurosyphilis; for treatment of late latent, ocular, tertiary, and congenital syphilis as well as neurosyphilis, see www.cdc.gov/std/treatment or download the CDC STD Tx Guide App; a fourfold decrease in the antibody titer based on the RPR or VDRL assay is indicative of successful treatment.

Gonorrhea

- The etiologic agent is *Neisseria gonorrhoeae* and the primary infection is usually genital but can be anal, rectal, or oropharyngeal; gonorrhea is acquired primarily via sexual contact and the incubation period is 2–5 days.
- While acute urethritis in men accompanied by a purulent discharge is the most common clinical presentation, the manifestations of gonorrhea are varied (Fig. 69.10; Table 69.6); asymptomatic infections are common in women and when the rectum or pharynx is the site of infection.
- In disseminated gonococcal infection, often referred to as the arthritis–dermatosis syndrome, a limited number of acral inflammatory pustules appear due to septic vasculitis, along with fever, arthralgia, and tenosynovitis (Fig. 69.11); risk factors include menstruation and deficiencies of the late components of complement (C5–C9; see Ch. 49).

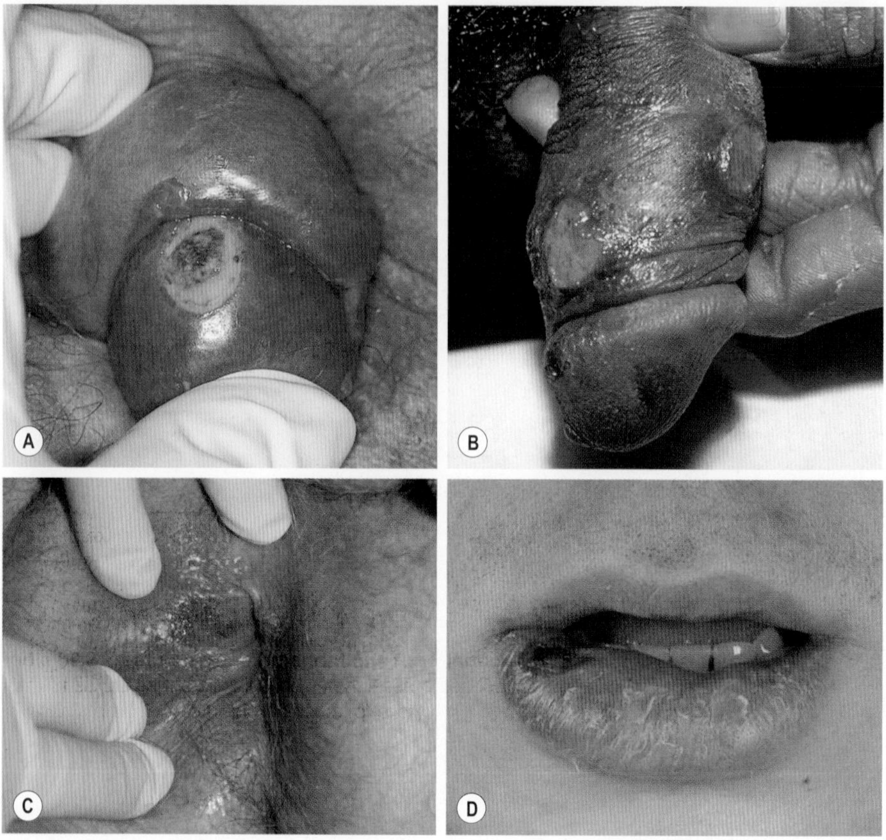

Fig. 69.2 Chancres of primary syphilis. The lesions are firm to palpation and are occasionally multiple. Sites of chancres include the penis **(A, B),** perianal area **(C),** and lip **(D)**, as well as the fingers, cervix, and breast. *A, C, D, Courtesy, Angelika Stary, MD; B, Courtesy, YDRSC.*

CLINICAL MANIFESTATIONS OF SYPHILIS

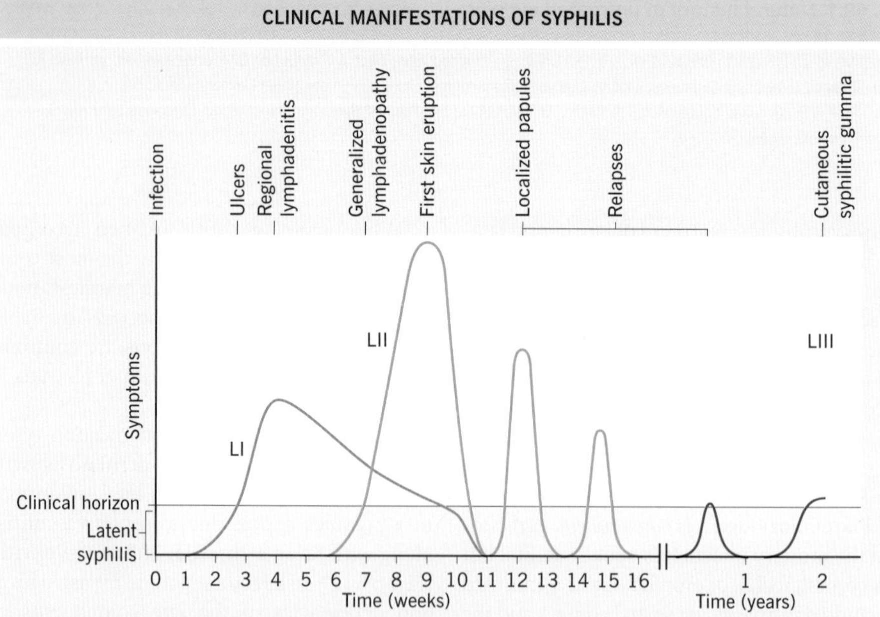

Fig. 69.3 Clinical manifestations of syphilis. LI, primary syphilis (lues); LII, secondary syphilis (lues); LIII, tertiary syphilis (lues). *Adapted from Fritsch P, Zangerle R, Stary A. Venerologie. In: Fritsch P (Ed.), Dermatologie und Venerologie. Berlin: Springer, 1998:865–86.*

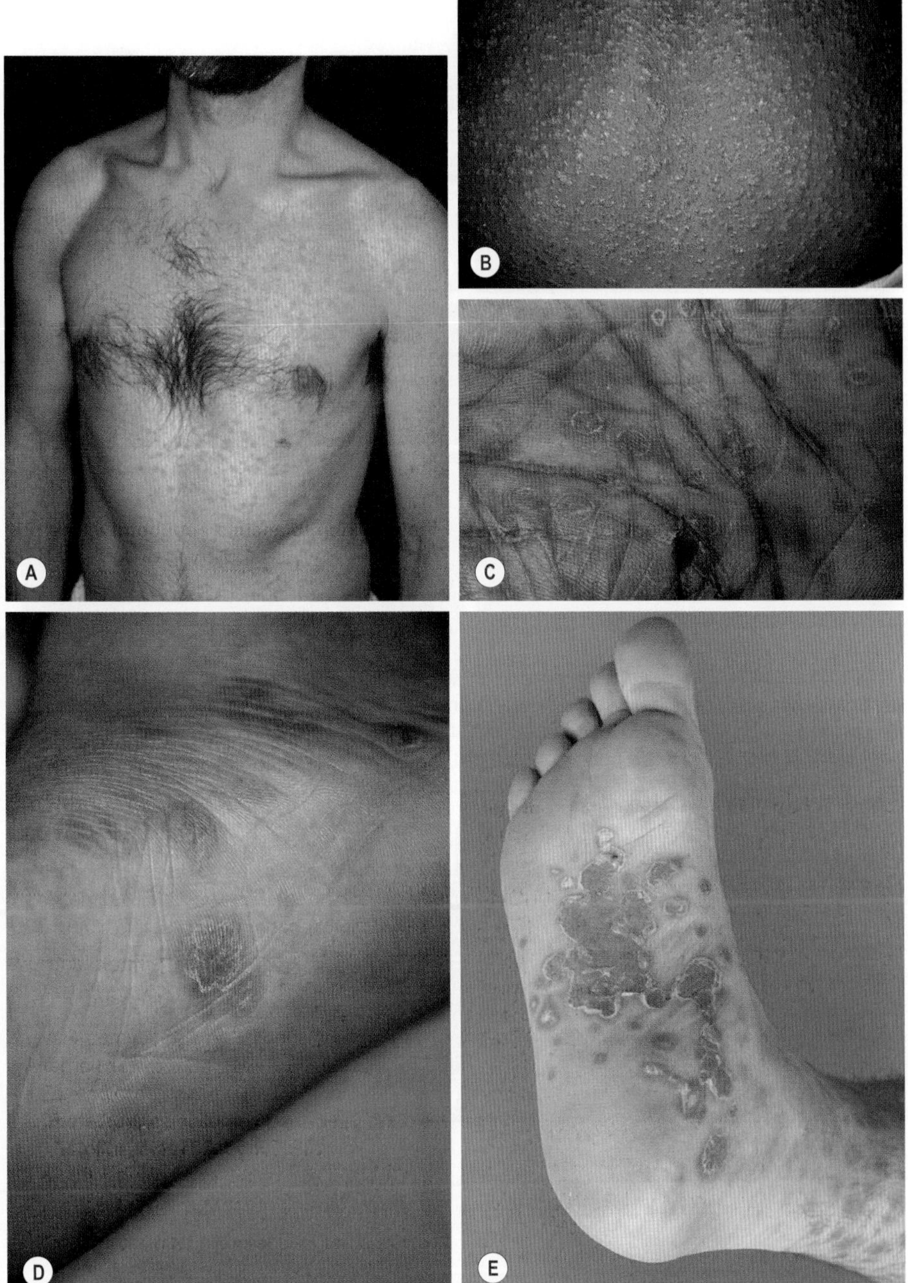

Fig. 69.4 Secondary syphilis – cutaneous manifestations. Widespread exanthem of pink papules **(A)** and generalized papulosquamous lesions **(B)**. Lesions on the palms **(C)** and soles **(D, E)** can have a collarette of scale; in patients with more darkly pigmented skin, these lesions may have a copper color. *A–D, Courtesy, YDRSC; E, Courtesy, Angelika Stary, MD.*

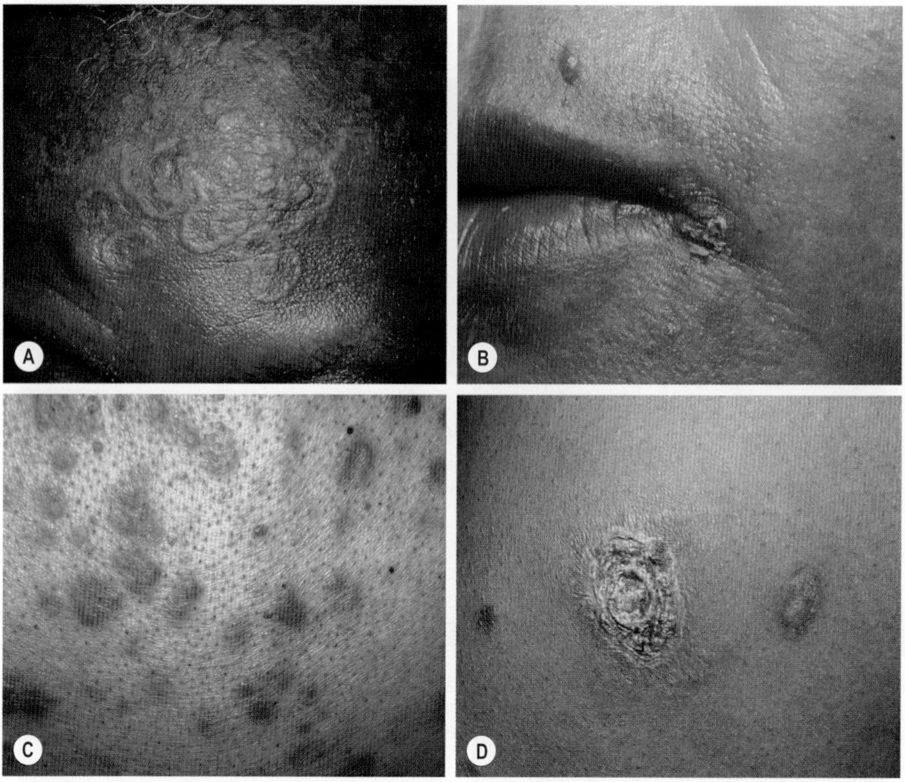

Fig. 69.5 Less common manifestations of secondary syphilis. **A** Annular plaques with central hyperpigmentation on the forehead. **B** Split papule at the oral commissure. **C** Granulomatous nodules and plaques. **D** Necrotic lesion with scale-crust in a patient with AIDS. *A–C, Courtesy, YDRSC; D, Courtesy, Judit Stenn, MD.*

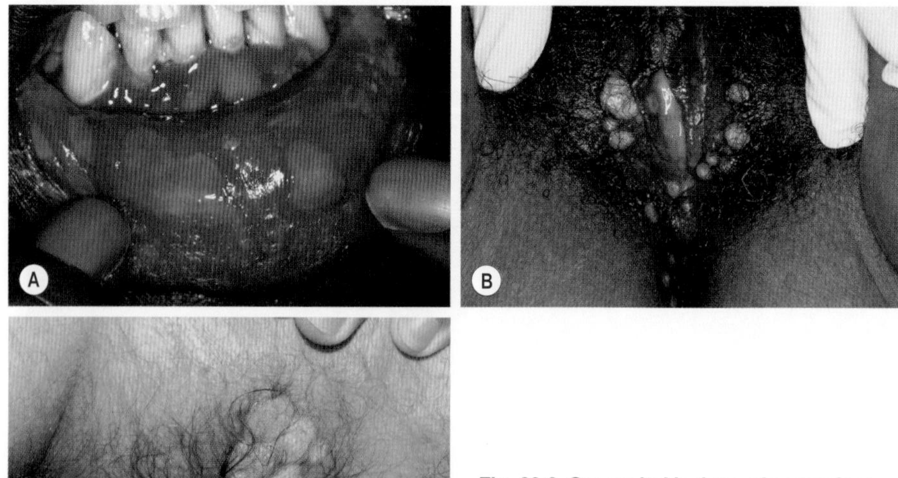

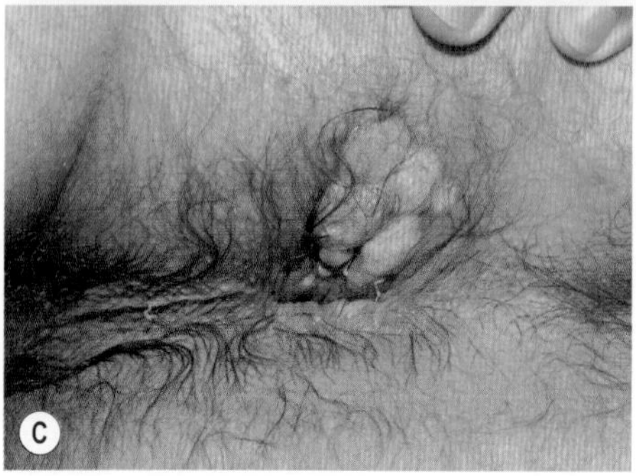

Fig. 69.6 Orogenital lesions of secondary syphilis. Oral lesions can vary from small superficial ulcers to mucous patches **(A)**. Condylomata lata in the vulvar **(B)** and perianal **(C)** areas may be misdiagnosed as HPV infection (i.e. condylomata acuminata). *A, B, Courtesy, YDRSC; C, Courtesy, Angelika Stary, MD.*

CLINICAL FEATURES OF SECONDARY SYPHILIS
• **Prodromal symptoms and signs** • Weight loss • Low-grade fever • Malaise • Headache (meningeal irritation) • Sore throat • Conjunctivitis (iridocyclitis) • Arthralgia (periostitis) • Myalgias, bone pain • Hepatosplenomegaly (mild hepatitis)
• **Generalized lymphadenopathy with indolent enlargement of lymph nodes** (50–85%)
• **Skin manifestations** • *Early* (10%): generalized eruption; non-pruritic, roseola-like, discrete macules, initially distributed on the flanks and shoulders • *Late* (70%): generalized maculopapular and papulosquamous eruptions; more infiltrated lesions, often copper-colored; annular plaques on the face; corymbose arrangement (satellite papules around a larger central lesion); occurs in successive waves and is polymorphic • *Localized syphilids* (specific infiltrations of treponemes; positive darkfield examination): – palms and soles: symmetric papules and plaques with a collarette of scale (collarette of Biett) – anogenital area: condylomata lata – seborrheic area: "corona veneris" along the hairline • *Hypopigmented macules*, mainly on the neck (postinflammatory; "necklace of Venus")
• **Manifestations involving mucous membranes** (30%) • Syphilitic perlèche, split papules • Mucous patches: "plaques muqueuses" in the oropharynx (equivalent to condylomata lata in the genital area) • Syphilitic sore throat: inflammation of the whole pharynx
• **Patchy alopecia** (7%): "moth-eaten" localized areas of hair loss; toxic telogen effluvium

Table 69.1 Clinical features of secondary syphilis. *Courtesy, Angelika Stary, MD.*

CLINICAL MANIFESTATIONS OF LATE SYPHILIS

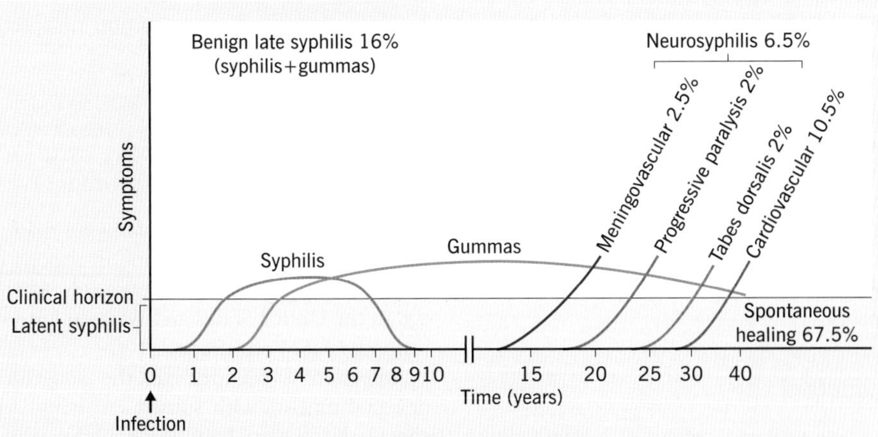

Fig. 69.7 Clinical manifestations of late syphilis. Gummas occur most commonly in the skin (70%) and less often in the bones (10%) or mucous membranes (10%). In neurosyphilis, both endarteritis and direct invasion of the brain parenchyma can occur. Tabes dorsalis presents with painful paresthesias of the limbs, ataxia, and Argyll Robertson pupils. *Adapted from Fritsch P, Zangerle R, Stary A. Venerologie. In: Fritsch P (Ed.), Dermatologie und Venerologie. Berlin: Springer, 1998:865–86.*

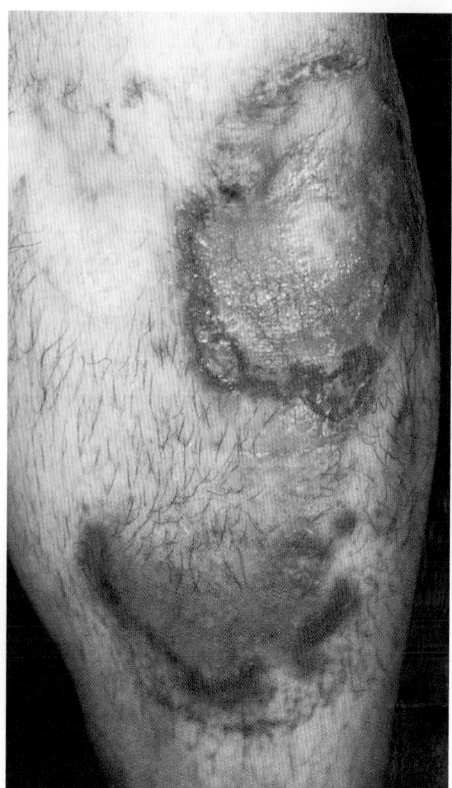

Fig. 69.8 Cutaneous gummas of tertiary syphilis. Arciform, erythematous eroded plaques with central scarring. *Courtesy, NYUDSC.*

MOTHER-TO-CHILD TRANSMISSION OF UNTREATED SYPHILIS AND ITS CONSEQUENCES
Risk
• Infection of the mother from conception to 7th month of pregnancy: transmission in nearly 100% (often fetal demise or severe congenital syphilis) • Infection at least 2 years before pregnancy: reduced risk of transmission to 50% • Infection during 7th, 8th, or early 9th month: reduced risk of transmission • Infection 3–6 weeks before labor: no placental transmission; risk of perinatal transmission
Consequences of infection
• Spontaneous abortion (second or third trimester) (10%) • Stillbirth (10%) • Infant death (20%) • Congenital syphilis (20%) • Healthy child (40%)

Table 69.2 Mother-to-child transmission of untreated syphilis and its consequences. *Courtesy, Angelika Stary, MD.*

• Dx: stained smears of urethral and cervical exudates or cutaneous pustules; culture, PCR, or DNA hybridization of samples from any site of infection.

• **DDx:** for urethral or cervical discharge, other infections, in particular *Chlamydia trachomatis*; for the cutaneous lesions due to gonococcemia, other infectious emboli, small vessel vasculitis, and neutrophilic dermatoses.

• **Rx:** see Table 69.7. Resistance to multiple antibiotics, including ciprofloxacin, is of concern.

Chancroid

• The etiologic agent is *Haemophilus ducreyi*; this infection occurs more commonly in Africa and South Asia (Fig. 69.12), and it has a male:female ratio of 10:1.

• After an incubation period of 3–10 days, painful genital ulcers, usually multiple, develop in conjunction with tender inguinal lymphadenitis (usually unilateral; Fig. 69.13); the base of the ulcer is purulent and soft, as opposed to the induration of syphilitic chancres.

• Dx: stained smears and culture (on special media) of ulcer exudate; PCR.

• **DDx:** see Table 69.8.

• **Rx:** see Table 69.9.

Lymphogranuloma Venereum (LGV)

• The etiologic agent is *Chlamydia trachomatis* serovars L1–L3; endemic in regions of Africa, Asia, and South America; elsewhere, e.g. in the United States and Western Europe, primarily MSM are affected.

• Infection is acquired via the anogenital or rectal mucosa with subsequent lymphatic spread, leading to lymphadenopathy which is usually unilateral (Fig. 69.14); ~50% of patients develop a herpetiform lesion at the initial site of infection that heals

STIGMATA OF CONGENITAL SYPHILIS
Cutaneous
• Rhagades (radial periorificial [mouth, nose, eyes, anus] scars at sites of previous fissures)
Dental
• Hutchinson teeth – peg-shaped, notched permanent incisors* • Mulberry molars – multiple rounded rudimentary cusps on the permanent first molars • Caries due to defective enamel
Skeletal
• Saddle nose – depression of the nasal root due to destruction of cartilage/bone • Frontal bossing of Parrot ("Olympian brow") • Hypoplastic maxilla, relatively prominent mandible • High palatal arch ± perforation • Higouménakis sign – thickening of the medial clavicle • Scaphoid scapulae • Saber shins – anterior tibial bowing • Clutton joints – painless synovitis and effusions of the knees
Other
• Eighth nerve deafness* • Interstitial keratitis leading to corneal ulcers and opacities*

Components of Hutchinson's triad.

Table 69.3 Stigmata of congenital syphilis. These findings represent the delayed consequences of inflammation at the sites of infection. *Courtesy, Angelika Stary, MD.*

spontaneously, following an incubation period of 3–12 days; the subsequent clinical manifestations are outlined in Table 69.10.

- Dx: detection of *Chlamydia*-specific DNA by PCR from affected tissues.
- **DDx:** see Table 69.8.
- **Rx:** see Table 69.9.

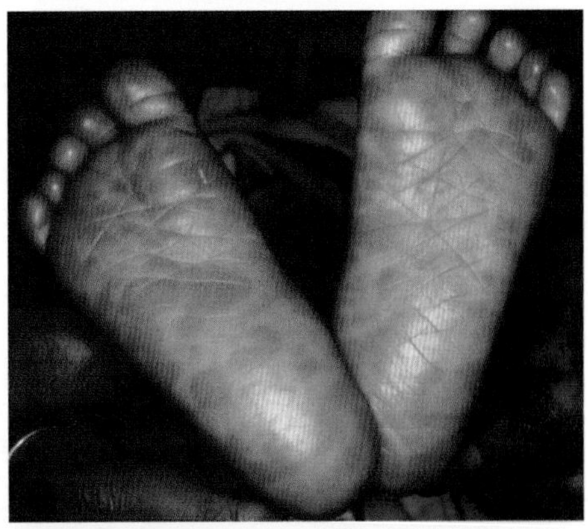

Fig. 69.9 Congenital syphilis. Red-brown plaques on the plantar surface, reminiscent of secondary syphilis in adults. Laboratory diagnosis includes identification of treponemes by darkfield microscopy and/or detection of 19S antibodies by the FTA-ABS-19S-IgM test (90% sensitivity) or spirochetemia by PCR.

Granuloma Inguinale (Donovanosis)

- The etiologic agent is *Klebsiella granulomatis* (previously named *Calymmatobacterium granulomatis*), and the majority of infections occur in southern Africa, Southeast Asia, and northern Australia; histologically, "parasitized" macrophages with intracellular organisms (Donovan bodies) are seen.
- Clinically, an initial small papulonodule in the anogenital region ulcerates and then enlarges following an incubation period of up to 1 year (usually ~15–20 days); the base of the ulcer is often quite vascular with a foul-smelling drainage (Fig. 69.15).
- Dx: detection of Donovan bodies in smears of tissue scrapings or touch preps of biopsy specimens (see Ch. 2).
- **DDx:** see Table 69.8.
- **Rx:** see Table 69.9.

For further information see Ch. 82 from *Dermatology, Fourth Edition*.

For additional online figures visit www.expertconsult.com 

DIFFERENTIAL DIAGNOSES FOR SYPHILIS
Primary syphilis
Other causes of genital ulcers should be considered: • Genital trauma • Entities in Tables 69.8 and 60.7 (e.g. genital herpes, lichen planus, reactive non-sexually related acute genital ulcers [multiple etiologies including EBV]) • Fixed drug eruption • Ulcerative genital carcinoma (e.g. squamous cell carcinoma) • Behçet disease
Secondary syphilis
• Cutaneous: pityriasis rosea, guttate psoriasis, viral exanthems, lichen planus, pityriasis lichenoides chronica, primary HIV infection, drug eruption, nummular eczema, folliculitis • Mucous membranes: lichen planus; chronic aphthae; hand, foot, and mouth disease; herpangina; perlèche • Condylomata lata: warts due to HPV, bowenoid papulosis, squamous cell carcinoma
Tertiary syphilis
• Cutaneous: lupus vulgaris, chromoblastomycosis, dimorphic fungal infections, leishmaniasis, lupus erythematosus, mycosis fungoides, sarcoidosis, tumors, venous ulcer

Table 69.4 Differential diagnoses for syphilis. *Courtesy, Angelika Stary, MD.*

TREATMENT RECOMMENDATIONS FOR EARLY SYPHILIS (PRIMARY, SECONDARY, AND EARLY LATENT [ACQUIRED <1 YEAR PREVIOUSLY])
Recommended
• Benzathine penicillin, 2.4 million units* IM as a single dose - *or* - • Procaine penicillin, 1.2 million units IM daily for 10 days#
Alternative regimens for penicillin-allergic patients‡
• Doxycycline, 200 mg daily (100 mg PO BID preferred over a single 200-mg dose) for 14 days - *or* - • Tetracycline, 500 mg PO qid for 14 days - *or* - • Ceftriaxone, 1–2 gm IM or IV daily for 10–14 days - *or* - • Azithromycin, 2 gm PO as a single dose§
Pregnancy
Recommended
• Benzathine penicillin, 2.4 million units IM weekly for two doses
In the case of penicillin allergy

• Desensitization to penicillin - *or* -
• Alternative regimens**
  • Azithromycin, 500 mg daily for 10 days - *or* -
  • Ceftriaxone, 1 gm IM or IV daily for 10–14 days

**In children, 50,000 U/kg IM up to the adult dose.*
#Alternative treatment regimen in the World Health Organization (WHO) guidelines (www.who.int/reproductivehealth/publications/rtis/syphilis-treatment-guidelines/en/) and the guidelines of the International Union against Sexually Transmitted Infections (IUSTI) (www.iusti.org/sti-information/guidelines/).
‡Limited data; desensitization to penicillin is recommended when compliance is an issue.
§Resistance reported; not recommended in men who have sex with men and pregnant women.
***Limited data; not recommended by the CDC but included in the WHO and European Branch of the International Union against Sexually Transmitted Infections (IUSTI) guidelines.*

Table 69.5 Treatment recommendations for early syphilis (primary, secondary, and early latent [acquired <1 year previously]). A Jarisch–Herxheimer reaction characterized by the acute onset of fever, headache, and myalgias can occur upon treatment of early syphilis. See the Centers for Disease Control and Prevention (CDC) guidelines (http://www.cdc.gov/std/treatment) or download the CDC STD Tx Guide App. h, hours; qid, four times daily.

CLINICAL MANIFESTATIONS OF GONORRHEA		
Disseminated infection	Local extension	Direct mucosal infection
• Arthritis • Fever • Tenosynovitis • Acral cutaneous pustules • Scalp abscesses* • Endocarditis • Meningitis	• Prostatitis • Vesiculitis • Epididymitis • Salpingitis • Oophoritis • Pelvic inflammatory disease	• Urethritis • Cervicitis • Proctitis • Pharyngitis • Vulvovaginitis (children) • Ophthalmia neonatorum

In neonates at sites of fetal scalp monitor electrodes.

Table 69.6 Clinical manifestations of gonorrhea. Both urethritis and cervicitis lead to a purulent discharge. *Courtesy, Angelika Stary, MD.*

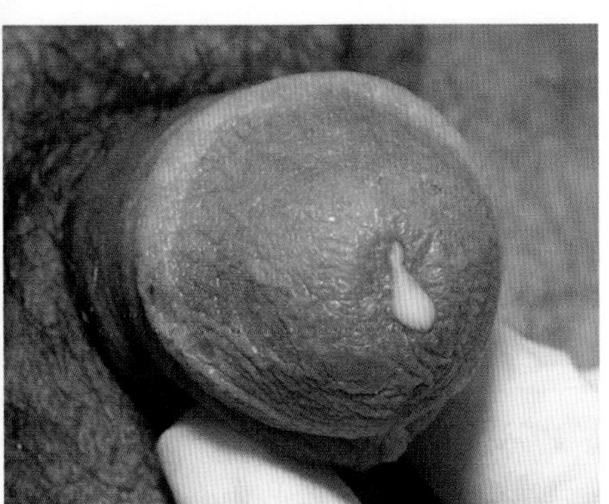

Fig. 69.10 Gonococcal urethritis with a purulent urethral discharge.

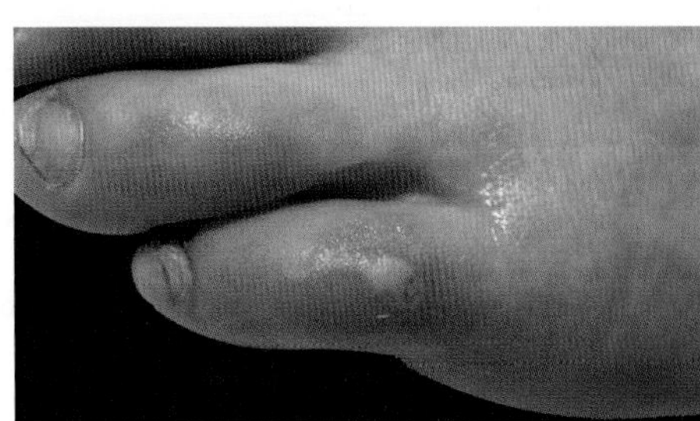

Fig. 69.11 Gonococcemia (arthritis–dermatosis syndrome). Pustule with surrounding erythema on the toe. *Courtesy, Angelika Stary, MD.*

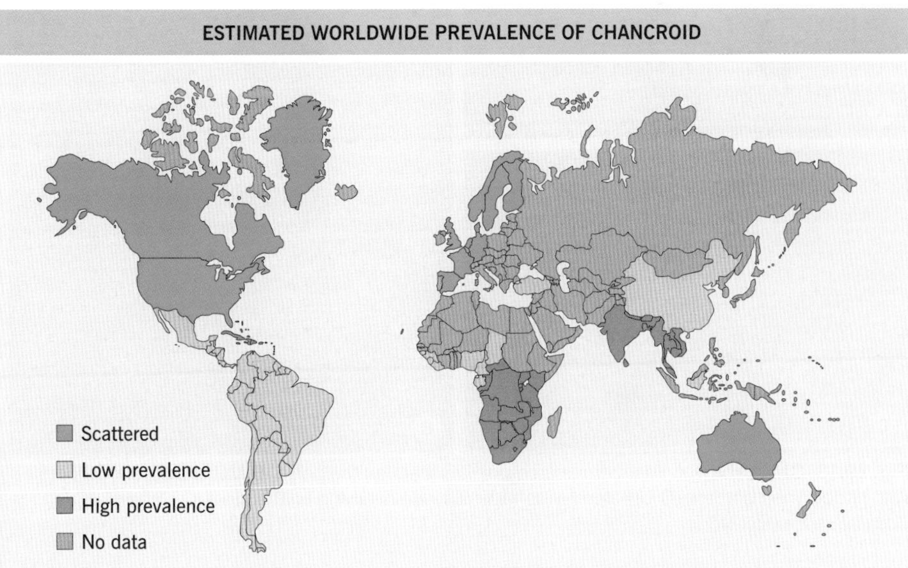

Fig. 69.12 Estimated worldwide prevalence of chancroid. *Adapted from Ronald A. Chancroid. In: Mandell GL (Ed.-in-Chief), Rein MF (Ed.), Atlas of Infectious Diseases: Vol. 5. Sexually Transmitted Diseases. New York: Current Medicine, 1995:16.1–10.*

TREATMENT RECOMMENDATIONS FOR GONOCOCCAL INFECTIONS
Uncomplicated gonococcal infections of the urethra, cervix, rectum or pharynx
Recommended regimen
• Ceftriaxone, 500 mg IM in a single dose, PLUS doxycycline 100 mg PO BID x 7 days*
Alternative regimens (urethra, cervix, rectum)
• Gentamicin, 240 mg IM in a single dose, PLUS azithromycin 2 gm PO in a single dose • Cefixime, 800 mg PO in a single dose, PLUS doxycycline 100 mg PO BID x 7 days*
Disseminated gonococcal infection
Recommended regimen
• Ceftriaxone, 1 gm IM or IV q24h, PLUS azithromycin 1 gm PO in a single dose • 24–48 hours after substantial clinical improvement and guided by antimicrobial susceptibility testing, can switch to oral agent (e.g. cefixime 400 mg PO BID) to complete at least 1 week of therapy
Alternative regimens
• Cefotaxime or ceftizoxime, 1 gm IV q8h, PLUS azithromycin 1 gm PO in a single dose • Switch to oral agents as above

*If *Chlamydia* not excluded, add doxycyline or during pregnancy add azithromycin 1 g in a single dose; dose of ceftriaxone is 1 gm IM if patient weighs ≥150 kg.

Table 69.7 Treatment recommendations for gonococcal infections. Examination and treatment of sexual partners is also indicated. Recommendations are based on the CDC guidelines (www.cdc.gov/std/treatment). h, hours; q, every.

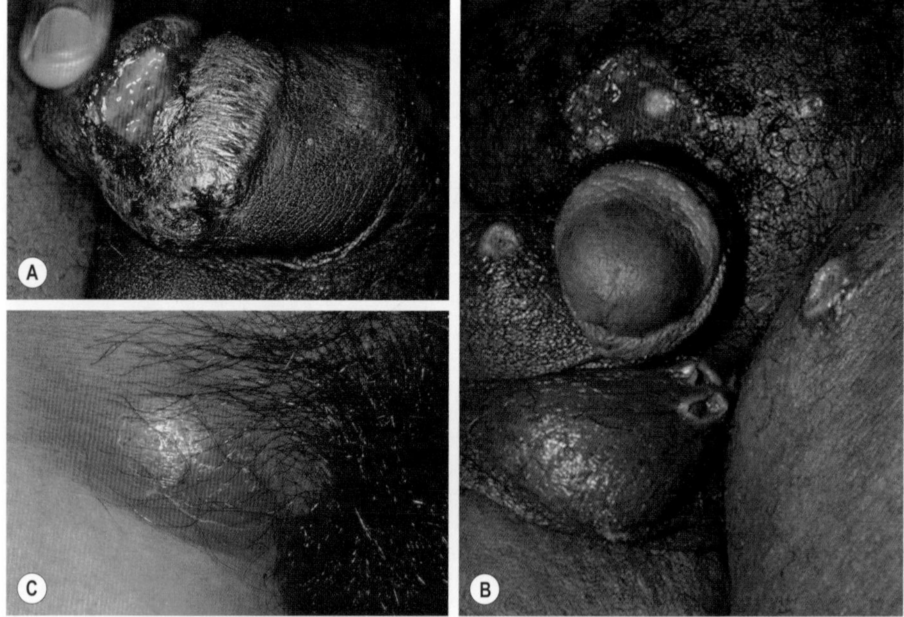

Fig. 69.13 Chancroid. A Well-demarcated painful ulcers on the penis. **B** Multiple purulent ulcers with undermined borders. **C** Unilateral lymphadenitis with overlying erythema. *A, C, Courtesy, YDRSC; B, Courtesy, Joyce Rico, MD.*

INFECTIOUS CAUSES OF GENITAL ULCER DISEASE				
Disease	**Incubation time**	**Clinical lesion**	**Diagnosis**	**Organism**
Genital herpes	3–7 days	Vesicles, erosions, ulcers; history of herpes infection; painful	PCR, culture, DFA, Tzanck (if vesicles)	HSV 2 > 1
Primary syphilis	10–90 days, average 3 weeks	Non-purulent; usually single ulcer; indurated; relatively painless	Darkfield microscopy, serology, PCR	*Treponema pallidum*
Chancroid	3–10 days	Purulent; often multiple ulcers; soft, undermined edges; painful	Culture, PCR	*Haemophilus ducreyi*
LGV	3–12 days	Transient ulcer; indurated; painless	PCR, culture, serology	*Chlamydia trachomatis* serovars L1–L3
Donovanosis	2–12 weeks	Chronic ulcer; indurated, beefy red, friable	Smears, histology	*Klebsiella (Calymmatobacterium) granulomatis*

Table 69.8 Infectious causes of genital ulcer disease. LGV, lymphogranuloma venereum.
Courtesy, Angelika Stary, MD.

TREATMENT REGIMENS FOR CHANCROID, LGV, AND GRANULOMA INGUINALE
Chancroid
• Azithromycin, 1 gm PO, single dose - *or* - • Ceftriaxone, 250 mg IM, single dose - *or* - • Ciprofloxacin, 500 mg PO BID for 3 days*,† - *or* - • Erythromycin base, 500 mg PO QID for 7 days†
LGV
• Recommended: doxycycline, 100 mg PO BID • Alternative and in case of pregnancy: erythromycin base, 500 mg PO QID **Duration for both regimens:** at least 3 weeks
Granuloma inguinale
*Recommended***
• Azithromycin, 1 gm PO once weekly - *or* - 500 mg PO daily Alternative** • Doxycycline, 100 mg po BID – *or* – • Trimethoprim–sulfamethoxazole, 1 double-strength (160 mg/800 mg) tablet PO BID - *or* - • Ciprofloxacin, 750 mg PO BID - *or* - • Erythromycin base, 500 mg PO QID **Duration for all regimens:** until all lesions completely healed (at least 3 weeks)

**Contraindicated for pregnant or lactating women.*
†Worldwide, isolates with intermediate resistance.
***For any of the regimens, the addition of an aminoglycoside (e.g. gentamicin 1 mg/kg iv q8h) should be considered if lesions do not respond within the first few days of therapy.*

Table 69.9 Treatment regimens for chancroid, LGV, and granuloma inguinale. Examination and treatment of sexual partners is also indicated. LGV, lymphogranuloma venereum; QID, four times daily.
Courtesy, Angelika Stary, MD.

CLINICAL MANIFESTATIONS OF LYMPHOGRANULOMA VENEREUM
Initial manifestations: 3–12 days
• Papule • Erosion or ulcer • Herpetiform vesicle • Nonspecific urethritis or cervicitis
Inguinal syndrome: 10–30 days up to 6 months
• Regional lymphadenopathy (mostly inguinal and femoral; also perirectal, deep iliac) • Overlying erythema • Constitutional symptoms • Eruption of buboes • Pelvic inflammatory disease (PID), back pain
Ano-genito-rectal syndrome: months to years
• Proctocolitis • Hyperplasia of intestinal and perirectal lymphatic tissue • Perirectal abscesses • Ischiorectal and rectovaginal fistulas • Anal fistulas • Rectal strictures and stenoses
Other manifestations
• Urethro-genito-perineal syndrome • Peno-scrotal elephantiasis • Erythema nodosum • Submaxillary or cervical lymphadenopathy associated with oropharyngeal lesions

Table 69.10 Clinical manifestations of lymphogranuloma venereum. *Courtesy, Angelika Stary, MD.*

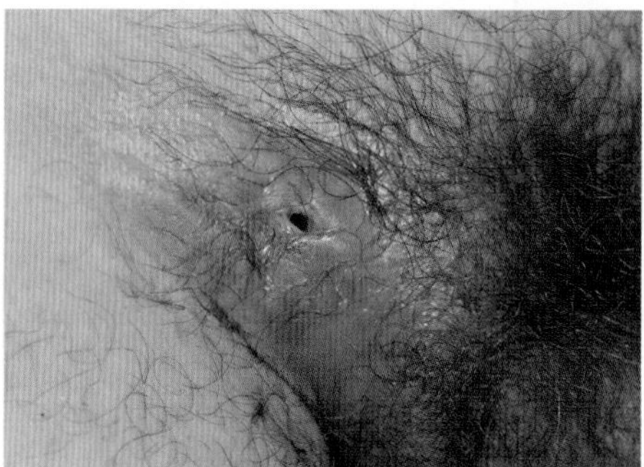

Fig. 69.14 Lymphogranuloma venereum. Inguinal bubo that has ruptured and drained. *Courtesy, Angelika Stary, MD.*

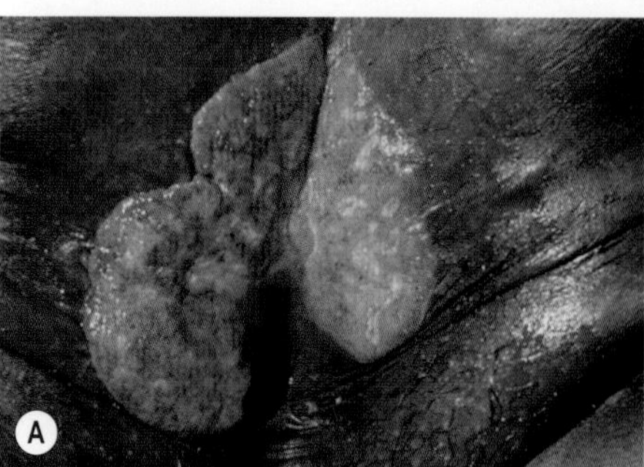

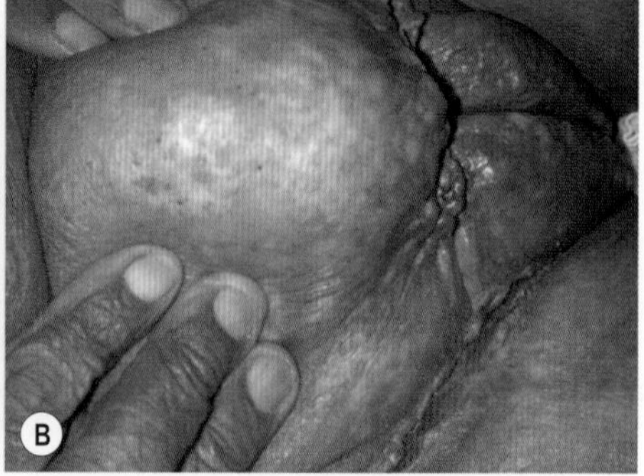

Fig. 69.15 Granuloma inguinale (donovanosis). A Large ulcers with a characteristic "beefy" appearance. **B** The vulva is the most common site of involvement in women with granulomatous plaques as well as ulcerations. *A, Courtesy, Joyce Rico, MD; B, Courtesy, Francisco Bravo, MD.*

Protozoa and Worms 70

Leishmaniasis

- Three major forms: (1) cutaneous (Fig. 70.1); (2) mucocutaneous (Fig. 70.2); and (3) visceral (e.g. liver, spleen).
- Caused by more than 15 different species of *Leishmania* (Table 70.1).
- Vector = sandfly (*Phlebotomus* and *Lutzomyia* spp.) (Fig. 70.3).
- Disease seen worldwide but endemic in areas of Asia, Africa, Latin America, and the Mediterranean basin (Fig. 70.4).
- Cutaneous disease affects skin only and is commonly a papule that expands and ulcerates (Fig. 70.5); pattern may be sporotrichoid (Fig. 70.6; see Table 64.7), disseminated, or diffuse (Fig. 70.7); lesion(s) may heal spontaneously (Fig. 70.8).
- Mucocutaneous form, often due to *Leishmania brasiliensis*, involves mucosal (e.g. nose, lips, oropharynx) sites as well as the skin.
- Visceral leishmaniasis (kala-azar) affects the bone marrow, spleen, and liver and is commonly due to *Leishmania donovani*; symptoms include fever, cough, lymphadenopathy, and hepatosplenomegaly; post-kala-azar dermal leishmaniasis (Fig. 70.9) may follow treatment.
- **Rx:** for an isolated or limited number of lesions, conservative therapy (e.g. observation, heat, cryotherapy), topical paromycin, or intralesional pentavalent antimonial; for more extensive disease, IV or IM pentavalent antimonial (sodium stibogluconate, meglumine antimonate), oral miltefosine.

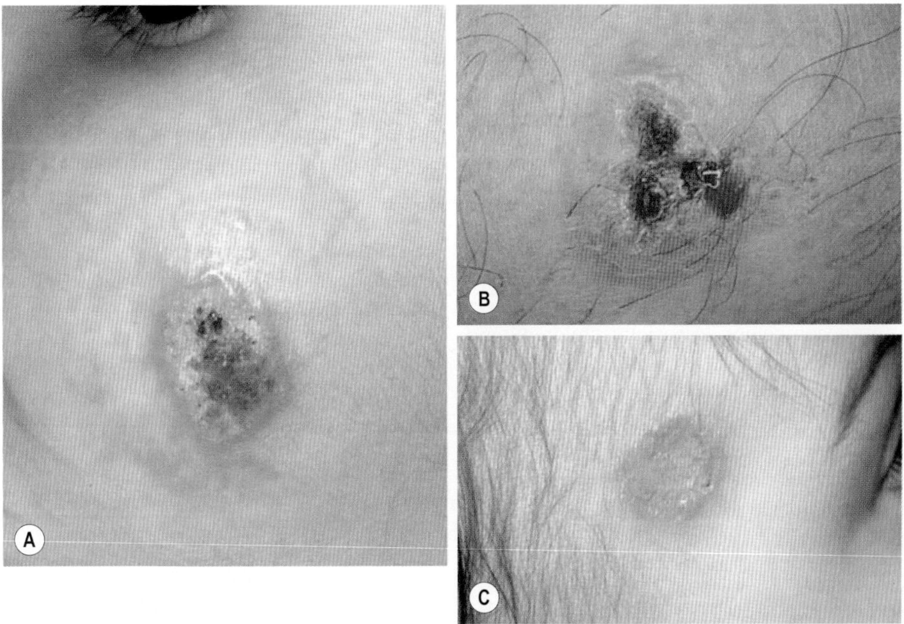

Fig. 70.1 Variable presentations of cutaneous leishmaniasis. Ulcerated plaques with rolled border **(A)** and central crusting **(A, B)**. Plaque with translucent borders containing telangiectasias and central scarring **(C).** Cutaneous leishmaniasis is sometimes mistaken for a basal cell carcinoma in adults. *A, C, Courtesy, Julie V. Schaffer, MD; B, Courtesy, YDRSC.*

FOUR MAJOR SPECIES OF *LEISHMANIA* THAT CAUSE CUTANEOUS DISEASE		
Complex	**Species**	**Major geographic distribution**
Leishmania tropica	*L. major*	Arid areas of Africa (north and south of the Sahara), Middle East, Central Asia
	L. tropica	Eastern Mediterranean region, Middle East, Central Asia
Leishmania mexicana	*L. mexicana*	Mexico, Central America
Leishmania braziliensis	*L. braziliensis**	Central and South America

**Can also cause mucosal leishmaniasis or visceral leishmaniasis in immunocompromised individuals.*

Table 70.1 Four major species of *Leishmania* that cause cutaneous disease.

• For assistance in diagnosis and treatment, helpful sources of information include the Centers for Disease Control and World Health Organization.

Amebiasis

• Protozoan infection (*Entamoeba histolytica*) that most commonly causes colitis; fecal–oral spread.
• Occasionally presents in the skin with necrotic ulcers that can resemble pyoderma gangrenosum or verrucous plaques that resemble squamous cell carcinoma or condyloma acuminatum.
• Skin involvement generally secondary to extension of rectal amebiasis to perianal or perigenital skin or extension of a liver abscess to skin of abdominal wall.
• **Rx:** for *Entamoeba histolytica*, metronidazole; other treatments include diloxanide, tinidazole.

Free-Living Ameba

• *Balamuthia mandrillaris* can infect immunocompetent (especially children) and immunocompromised patients; the typical cutaneous lesion is a slow-growing indurated plaque on the central face with eventual hematogenous spread to the central nervous system.
• *Acanthamoeba* spp. can cause cutaneous papulonodules and encephalitis in immunocompromised patients.

Trypanosomiasis – American (Chagas disease)

• *Trypanosoma cruzi* carried by reduviid (kissing) bugs.

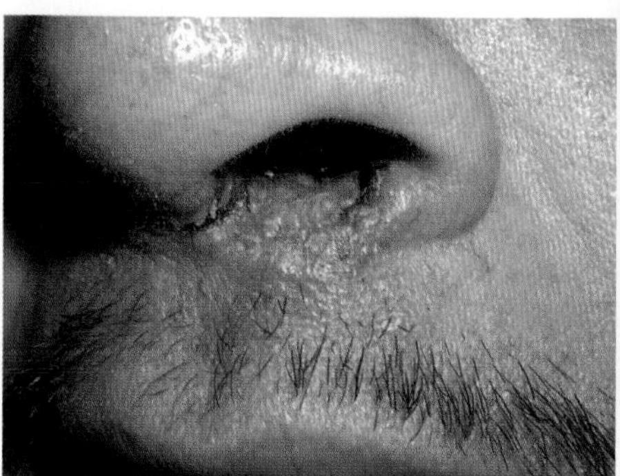

Fig. 70.2 Mucocutaneous leishmaniasis. Ulceration and induration of the nasal vestibule extending onto the cutaneous lip due to *Leishmania braziliensis*. *Courtesy, Kalman Watsky, MD.*

• Endemic in areas of Central and South America.
• Systemic disease that can affect the autonomic nervous system, gastrointestinal tract, and heart.
• Primary acute phase: local erythema and edema at inoculation site ± regional lymphadenopathy; when periorbital, termed Romaña sign (Fig. 70.10).
• Chronic phase seen after years to decades: congestive heart failure, arrhythmias, including heart block, megacolon, megaesophagus.

Trypanosomiasis – African

• Vector = tsetse fly.
• Found in both West (*Trypanosoma brucei gambiense*) and East (*Trypanosoma brucei rhodesiense*) Africa.
• Skin findings: trypanosomal chancre (localized bite reaction; Fig. 70.11) and annular erythematous eruption with fever.

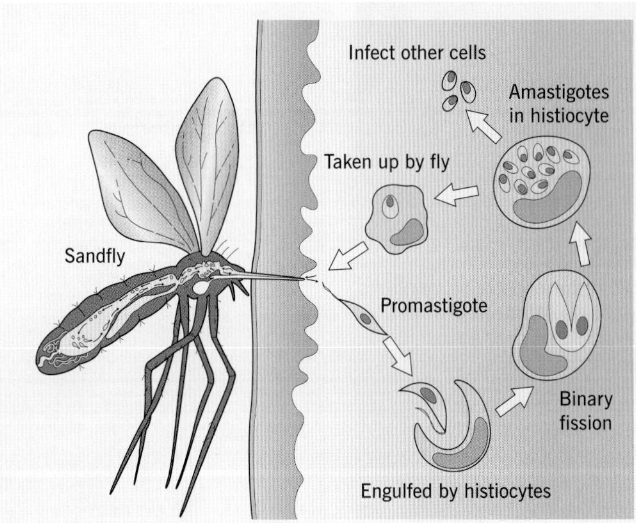

Fig. 70.3 Life cycle of *Leishmania* species. Promastigotes develop within the gut of the sandfly and then migrate to the proboscis.

DISTRIBUTION OF CUTANEOUS LEISHMANIASIS

Leishmania braziliensis complex
Leishmania mexicana complex

Leishmania major

Leishmania tropica

Leishmania aethiopica

*Leishmania infantum**

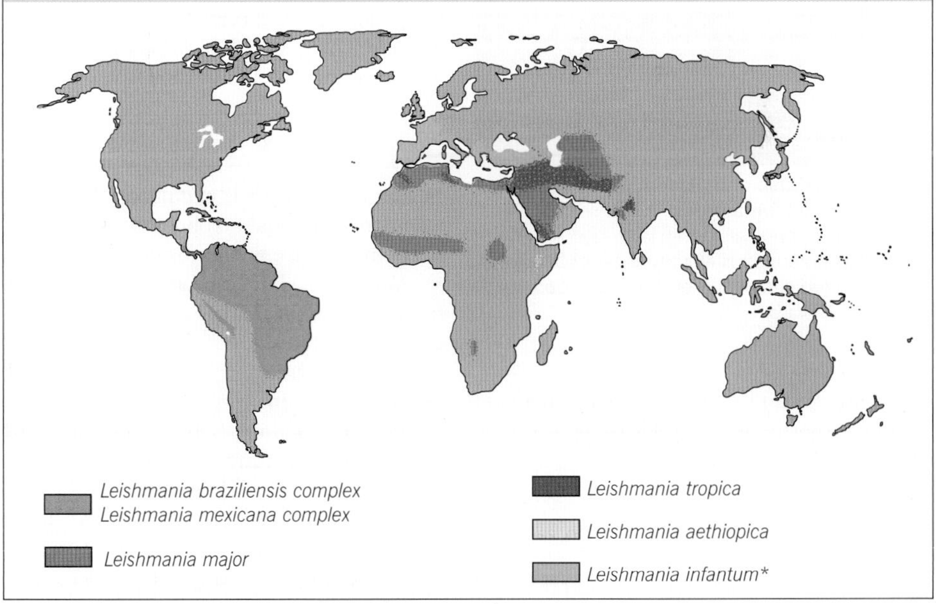

Fig. 70.4 Distribution of cutaneous leishmaniasis. *The *L. infantum* subspecies in Central and South America was previously known as *L. chagasi*. *Adapted with permission from Davidson RN, Leishmaniasis. In Cohen J, Powderly WG (Eds.), Infectious Diseases. Edinburgh, UK: Mosby, 2004.*

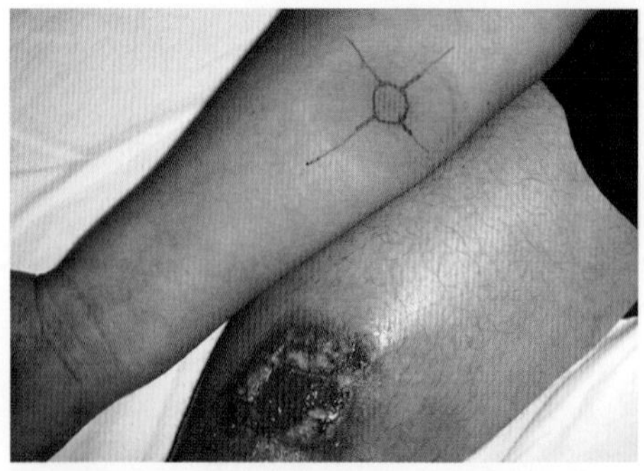

Fig. 70.5 Ulcerative cutaneous leishmaniasis on the leg and a positive Montenegro test. This expanding ulcer could be misdiagnosed as pyoderma gangrenosum. *Courtesy, Omar P. Sangüeza, MD.*

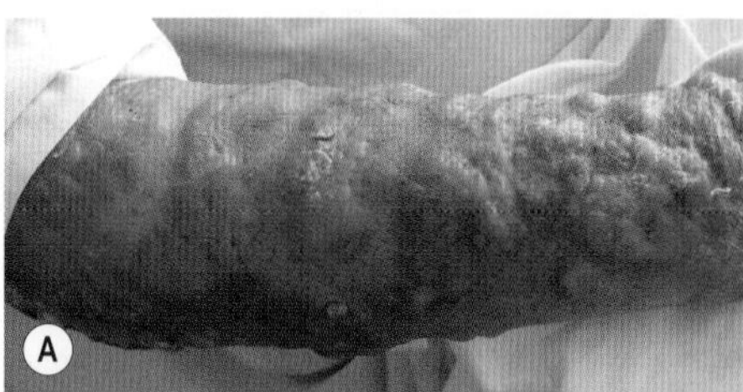

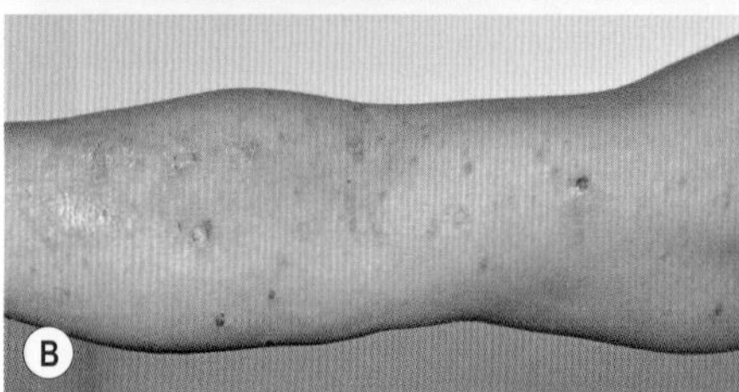

Fig. 70.7 Diffuse and disseminated cutaneous leishmaniasis. A Diffuse cutaneous leishmaniasis presenting with large nodules that resemble lepromatous leprosy. **B** Small papules in disseminated cutaneous leishmaniasis. *Courtesy, Francisco G. Bravo.*

• Winterbottom's sign – enlargement of nodes of posterior cervical triangle – classic finding in West African form.

Toxoplasmosis

• Worldwide infection secondary to *Toxoplasma gondii*; oocytes present in cat feces or infected meat.
• Rare skin involvement; congenital infections present with necrotic or hemorrhagic papules on the trunk ('T' in TORCH complex).

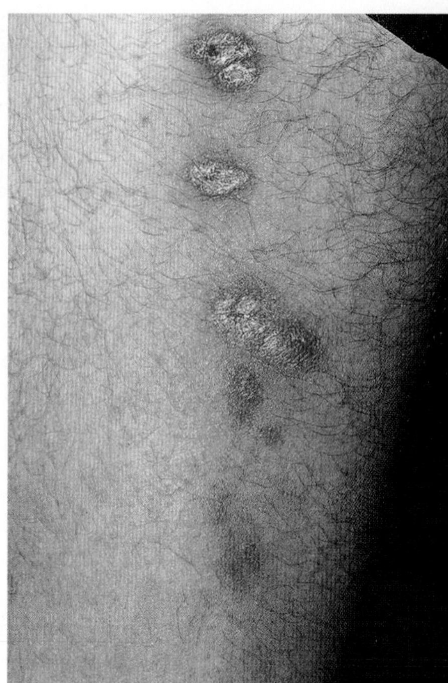

Fig. 70.6 Sporotrichoid form of cutaneous leishmaniasis. *With permission from Tyring S, Lupi O, Hengge U (Eds.), Tropical Dermatology. Oxford: Churchill Livingstone, 2005.*

• Common presentations include cervical lymphadenitis or chorioretinitis.
• Tissue cysts may lead to recrudescence in immunosuppressed individuals.

Cutaneous Larva Migrans

• Secondary to larvae of *animal* (e.g. usually wild/domestic dogs/cats) hookworms (intestinal nematodes), e.g. *Ancylostoma braziliense.*
• Worldwide, but especially common in tropical/subtropical areas and the southwestern United States.
• Larvae in infected soil, including sand, penetrate the skin.
• Pruritic, inflamed, serpiginous tracks are produced by migrating organisms (Fig. 70.12); migration averages 1–2 cm/day.
• Most common locations are the lower extremities, especially the feet, and buttocks, due to walking and sitting at the beach.
• **DDx:** not to be confused with larva currens (secondary to *Strongyloides*; see Table 70.2).
• Disease is self-limited but treatment can include oral albendazole or ivermectin; topical thiabendazole for localized disease.

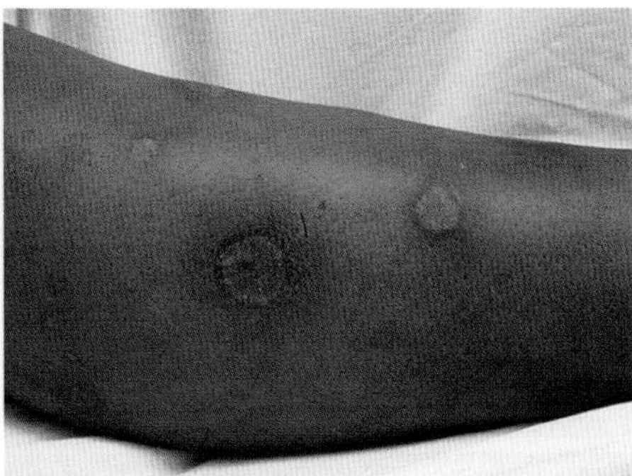

Fig. 70.8 Scars secondary to previous cutaneous leishmaniasis. Circular scars at previous sites of cutaneous leishmaniasis are often the only sign of a prior infection. *Courtesy, Omar P. Sangüeza, MD.*

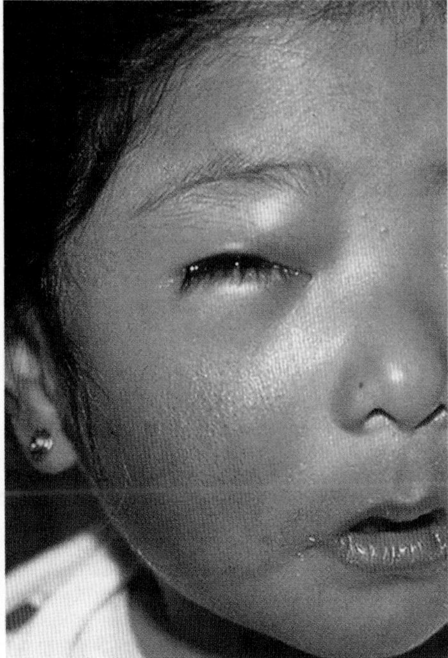

Fig. 70.10 Chagas disease. Young child with unilateral periorbital edema characteristic of this disease (Romaña sign) when the conjunctiva is the portal of entry. *Courtesy, Omar P. Sangüeza, MD.*

Onchocerciasis

- Secondary to *Onchocerca volvulus*, a tissue-dwelling nematode.
- Vector = black fly (*Simulium*).
- Endemic in Africa, Yemen, and some areas of Central and South America; near fast-flowing rivers.
- Skin findings: subcutaneous nodules containing adult worms (onchocercomas),

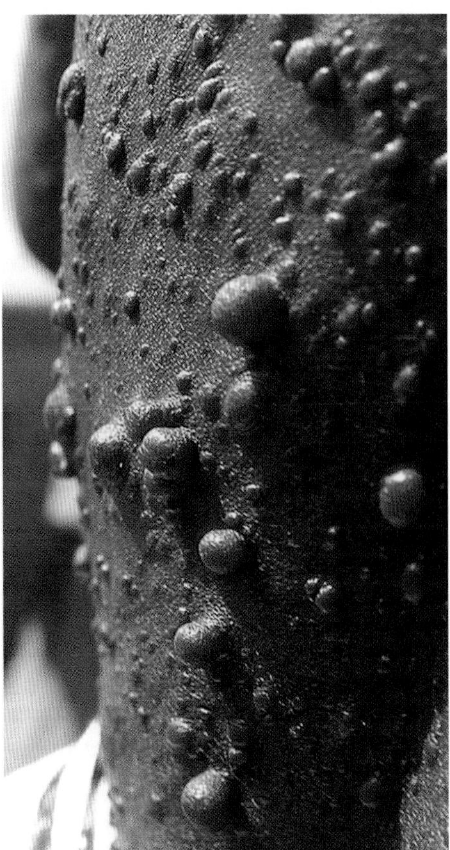

Fig. 70.9 Post-kala-azar dermal leishmaniasis. Nodules of various sizes, some pedunculated, are seen in this patient who had been treated for kala-azar over a period of 6 months, 20 years previously. *With permission from Peters W, Pasvol G. Tropical Medicine and Parasitology, 6th edition, London, Mosby, 2007.*

pruritic papular dermatitis, depigmented, lichenified skin, especially over the shins (sowda) (Fig. 70.13).

- Chronic ocular involvement leads to sclerosing keratitis, iridocyclitis, and ultimately blindness, hence the name river blindness.
- **Rx:** oral ivermectin (single dose – nonendemic areas; repeated doses – endemic areas); sometimes doxycycline is subsequently added to sterilize adult female worms.

Filariasis

- Tissue nematodes (*Wuchereria bancrofti* or *Brugia malayi/B. timori*) infect the lymphatic system.
- Vector = mosquito (*Culex, Anopheles, Aedes* spp.).

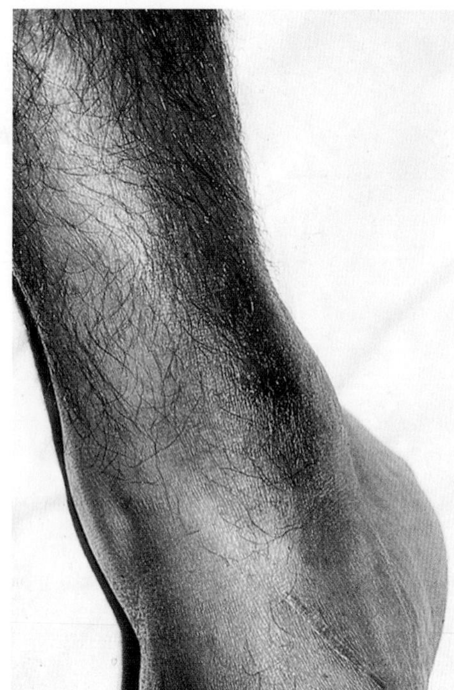

Fig. 70.11 Trypanosomal chancre. The bite reaction, the earliest clinical lesion, is known as a "trypanosomal chancre." It resembles a boil but is usually painless. Fluid aspirated from the nodule contains actively dividing trypanosomes. This reaction is seen more commonly in *T. b. rhodesiense* than in *T. b. gambiense* infection. *With permission from Peters W, Pasvol G, Tropical Medicine and Parasitology, 6th ed. London: Mosby, 2007.*

- Endemic in tropical and subtropical regions of India, the Americas, and Africa.
- Acute form: lymphangitis and orchitis.
- Chronic form: lymphedema, elephantiasis (the enlarged limb becomes indurated with skin folds and overlying verrucous changes), hydrocele, chyluria.
- Complicated by recurrent cellulitis.

Schistosomiasis

- Trematode (fluke) infection secondary to three major species with specific geographic distributions (Africa – *Schistosoma hematobium*, Asia – *S. japonicum*, South America – *S. mansoni*); intermediate host is the freshwater snail; organisms penetrate skin.
- Variants of cutaneous disease – cercarial dermatitis (transient erythema, urticaria, or pruritic papules), Katayama fever (systemic allergic reaction with urticaria, fever, chills, sweats, headache, peripheral eosinophilia).
- Chronic fibro-occlusive disease in the liver (*S. japonicum*), intestine (*S. mansoni*), or urinary tract (*S. hematobium*).

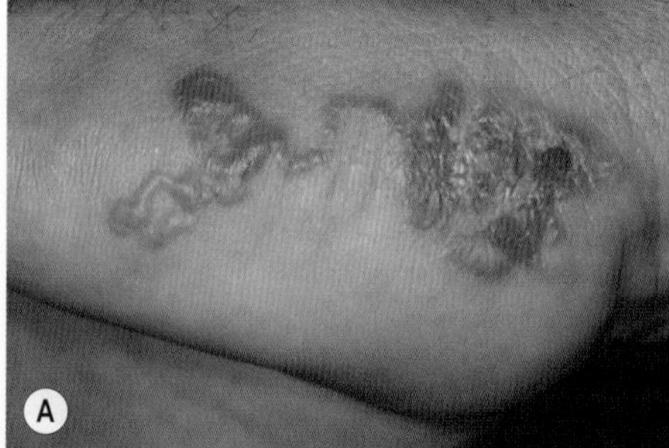

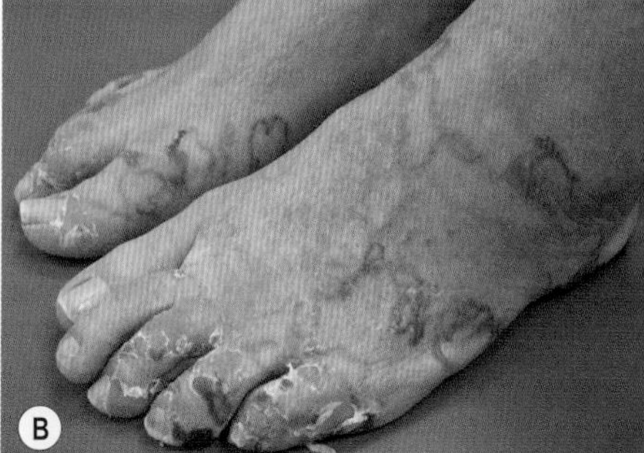

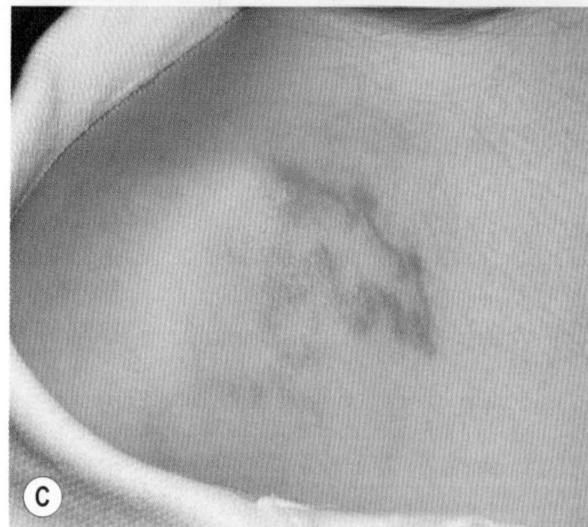

Fig. 70.12 Cutaneous larva migrans. Note the characteristic serpiginous erythematous tracks on the lateral foot **(A)**, both feet **(B),** and the shoulder **(C)**. Vesiculation and crusting **(B)** are sometimes seen. *B, Courtesy, Peter Klein, MD; C, Courtesy, Julie V. Schaffer, MD.*

Swimmer's Itch

- Cercariae of >20 species of *animal* schistosomes (e.g. *Ornithobilharzia*) can penetrate skin and cause swimmer's itch.

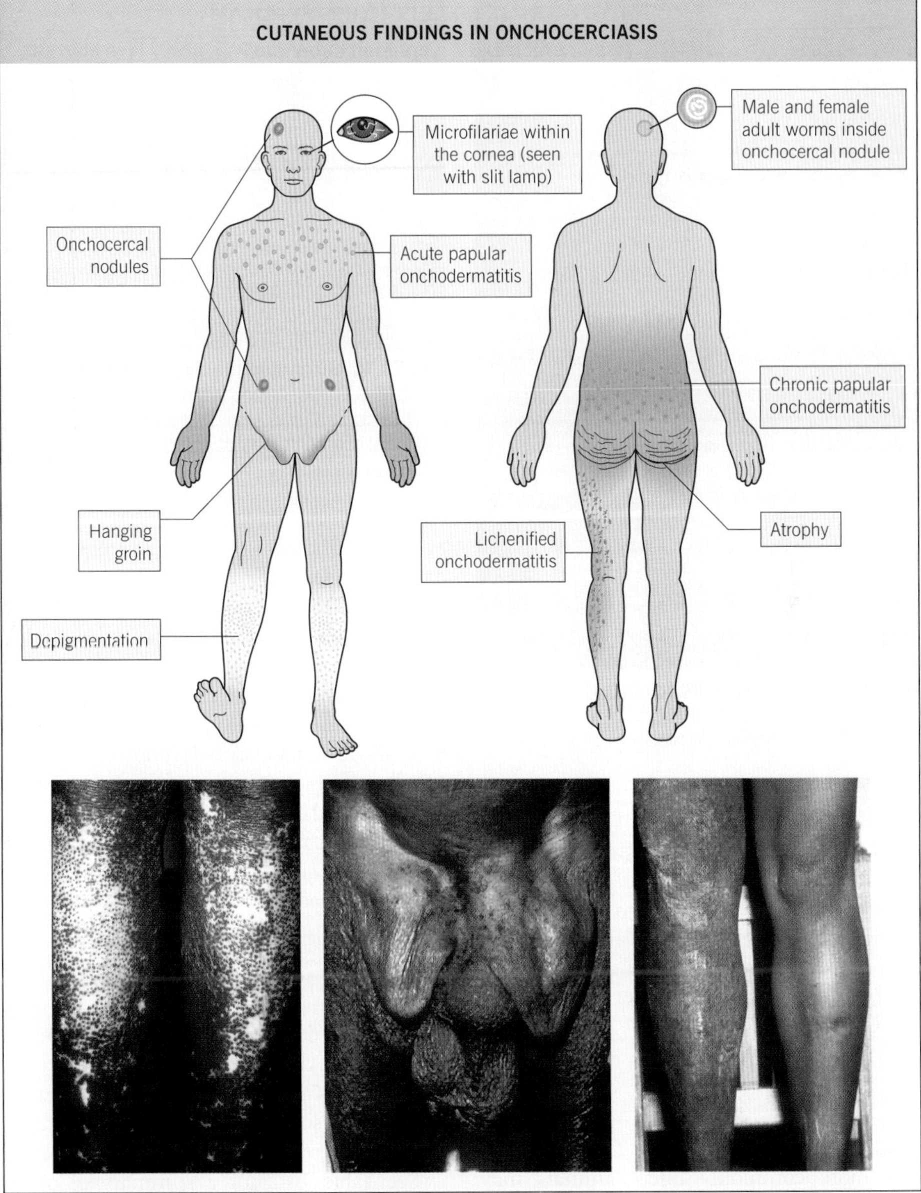

Fig. 70.13 Cutaneous findings in onchocerciasis. Photos: left, depigmentation with perifollicular sparing ("leopard" skin); middle, hanging groin due to chronic lymphatic obstruction and lymph node involvement; right, lichenified onchodermatitis ("sowda"). *Insets, courtesy, David O. Freeman, MD.*

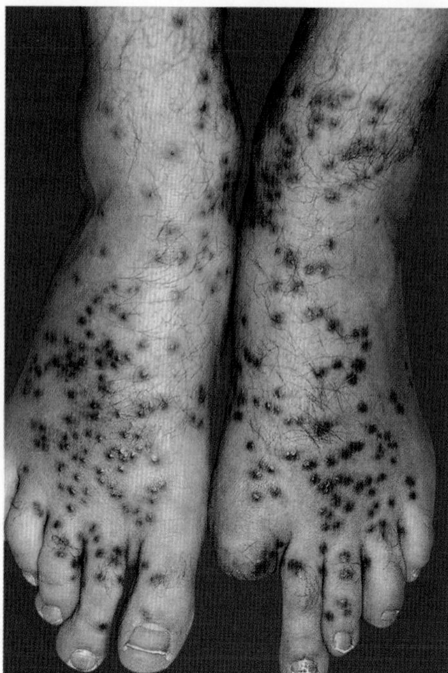

Fig. 70.14 Swimmer's itch. Numerous edematous dark red papules on the feet and ankles. *Courtesy, Kalman Watsky, MD.*

- Worldwide; endemic to the Great Lakes.
- Erythematous papules on exposed skin (Fig. 70.14).
- Self-limited (7–10 days).
- Not to be confused with seabather's eruption (secondary to *Linuche, Edwardsiella* spp.), which affects areas under the swimsuit (see Ch. 72).

Cysticercosis

- Cestodes (tapeworms; e.g. *Taenia solium*) that more commonly infect animals may infect humans; spread from ingestion of contaminated meat or fecal–oral spread.

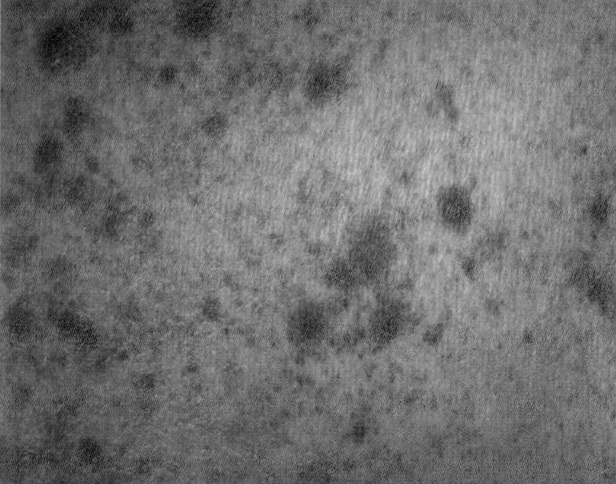

Fig. 70.15 Strongyloidiasis hyperinfection. Multiple purpuric lesions (sometimes referred to as "thumbprint" purpura) on the abdomen of an immunocompromised patient. *Courtesy, Jean L. Bolognia, MD.*

- Skin findings: small, asymptomatic papulonodules.
- May have systemic involvement of the brain, eye, heart, muscles, or peritoneal cavity.

Echinococcosis

- Cestode (tapeworm *Echinococcus*) that usually infects dogs; spread from ingestion of contaminated dog feces.
- Human may be an intermediate host and develop liver or lung hydatid cysts.
- Rarely leads to urticaria, asthma, or anaphylaxis.

Gnathostomiasis

- Due to ingestion of raw or poorly cooked freshwater fish (e.g. ceviche) and eels or frogs that contain larvae of *Gnathostoma* spp. (nematodes).
- Transient subcutaneous swellings that may be pruritic are due to migration of the larvae.

See Table 70.2 for a summary of other major parasitic worms that cause skin findings.

For further information see Ch. 83 from *Dermatology, Fourth Edition*.

For additional online figures visit www.expertconsult.com 

OTHER MAJOR PARASITIC WORMS THAT CAUSE CUTANEOUS MANIFESTATIONS IN HUMANS					
Disease	**Organism**	**Distribution**	**Mode of spread**	**Skin findings**	**Systemic findings**
Enterobiasis (pinworms), intestinal nematode	*Enterobius vermicularis*	Widespread and high prevalence, especially in countries within temperate zones	Ingestion of eggs	Perianal and perineal pruritus	Restlessness Asymptomatic in most patients
Ancylostomiasis (human hookworms), intestinal nematode	*Ancylostoma duodenale*, *Necator americanus*	Tropical and subtropical distribution	Percutaneous via contact with infective larvae in soil	Dermatitis ("ground itch") at the site of larval entry	Iron deficiency anemia, GI symptoms, Loeffler syndrome, eosinophilia
Strongyloidiasis, intestinal nematode	*Strongyloides stercoralis*	Occurs worldwide, especially in tropical areas; in cooler climates found in warm humid deep mines	Percutaneous via contact with infective larvae; occasionally ingestion of larvae Autoinfection via penetration of perianal skin Hyperinfection in immunocompromised patients, due to penetration of intestinal mucosa	Generalized or localized urticarial eruption beginning perianally and extending to the buttocks, thighs, and abdomen (larva currens) "Thumbprint" purpura in hyperinfection (Fig. 70.15)	Diarrhea, duodenitis, eosinophilia, pulmonary symptoms Symptoms more severe in immunocompromised patients
Loiasis, tissue nematode	*Loa loa*	West and central Africa	Transmitted by bite of tabanid flies of the genus *Chrysops* (mango flies) carrying infective larvae Mature in connective tissue	Transient localized subcutaneous edema (Calabar swellings), often of the hands, wrists and forearms; represent tracts of migrating adult worms; associated with pruritus and pain	Conjunctivitis (due to movement of adult worms under conjunctiva), eosinophilia, renal disease

Table 70.2 Other major parasitic worms that cause cutaneous manifestations in humans. *Continued*

OTHER MAJOR PARASITIC WORMS THAT CAUSE CUTANEOUS MANIFESTATIONS IN HUMANS					
Disease	**Organism**	**Distribution**	**Mode of spread**	**Skin findings**	**Systemic findings**
Dirofilariasis, tissue nematodes of animals	*Dirofilaria immitis* (dog heartworms); *D. tunuis* (filaria of raccoons); *D. repens* (filaria of dogs and cats); *D. ursi* (filaria of bears)	*D. immitis* occurs worldwide; *D. tunuis* in southeast US; *D. repens* in Europe and Asia; *D. ursi* in North America and Japan	Transmitted by mosquitoes carrying infective larvae Do not mature in humans	*D. tunuis*, *D. repens*, and *D. ursi* cause small painful subcutaneous nodules with or without inflammation	*D. immitis* causes nodules in the lungs
Dracunculiasis (guinea worm), tissue nematode	*Dracunculus medinensis*	Africa, particularly Ghana and the Sudan	Ingestion of infected water fleas of the genus *Cyclops* in drinking water Migrate from intestine to subcutaneous tissue, usually of the legs	Papulonodule then blister and/or ulceration, usually of the lower extremity; calcified nodules	Anaphylactic shock, rheumatic symptoms
Trichinosis, tissue nematode	*Trichinella spiralis*	Widespread in temperate zones	Ingestion of encysted larvae from raw/undercooked animal meat, usually pork	Periorbital edema in severe infection, splinter hemorrhages	Most infections are subclinical Heavy infection also leads to fever, enteritis, myositis, and eosinophilia; occasionally myocarditis and encephalitis
Sparganosis, larval stage of tapeworms of dogs and cats, cestode	*Spirometra*	Sporadic in most countries, seen most frequently in the Far East	Ingestion of larvae in intermediate hosts (e.g. snakes, frogs, fish) Occasionally following application of frogs to eyes as poultice	Painless small subcutaneous nodules at sites of larval proliferation Edema if periorbital involvement	Rarely, pulmonary or CNS involvement

Table 70.2 *Continued* **Other major parasitic worms that cause cutaneous manifestations in humans.**

Infestations 71

Scabies

- Infestation by *Sarcoptes scabiei* var. *hominis*, a mite that lives within the stratum corneum of human skin (Fig. 71.1).
- Transmission is primarily by direct contact with an infested person and occasionally by fomites (e.g. clothing); incubation period may be up to 6 weeks; in some tropical regions, scabies can infest the majority of individuals in a community.
- Asymptomatic infestation by scabies is not uncommon ("carriers" of scabies).
- In symptomatic cases, pruritus is severe, often worse at night or after a hot shower; secondary bacterial infections (e.g. staphylococcal, streptococcal) may occur. Post-streptococcal glomerulonephritis can be a significant issue in countries with endemic scabies and poor resources.
- Skin lesions are variable and include erythematous papules with scale-crust, small patches of eczema, excoriations, vesicles (especially acrally in infants), and nodules; the classic burrow – a thread-like, grayish-white, wavy, 1- to 10-mm linear structure – favors acral sites (Figs 71.2–71.4).
- Clinical confirmation is by mineral oil examination of skin scrapings (see Ch. 2) or dermoscopy (see Fig. 71.3).
- Usually <100 mites, but often no more than 10–15, living on an infested individual (Fig. 71.5); there may be thousands of mites in crusted scabies (thick scale, especially acrally, with minimal inflammation), which affects immunocompromised hosts, those with altered skin sensation, and sometimes the elderly (Fig. 71.6).
- In general, the mites live off the body ≤3 days; if accompanied by sloughed skin, as in crusted scabies, the duration may be longer.
- **DDx:** arthropod bites, including bites of animal mites (e.g. *Cheyletiella*); diseases associated with generalized pruritus (e.g. atopic dermatitis; see Table 4.1); in infants, infantile acropustulosis (may also occur following successful treatment of scabies), incontinentia pigmenti.
- **Rx:** see Table 71.1:
  - Two overnight applications of a topical antiscabetic medication, 1 week apart, to the entire body surface from the neck down to the toes; in infants, the elderly, and the immunocompromised, need to include the face and scalp
  - Permethrin 5% cream is the preferred topical agent
  - Oral ivermectin (200–400 mcg/kg given on days 1 and 8) is increasingly replacing topical medications, especially when large groups of individuals are affected as in a nursing home
  - All clothing and bedding should be washed in hot water and dried with high heat, or stored in a bag for 10 days (3 days after the second treatment)
  - All family members and close contacts should be treated simultaneously, even if asymptomatic

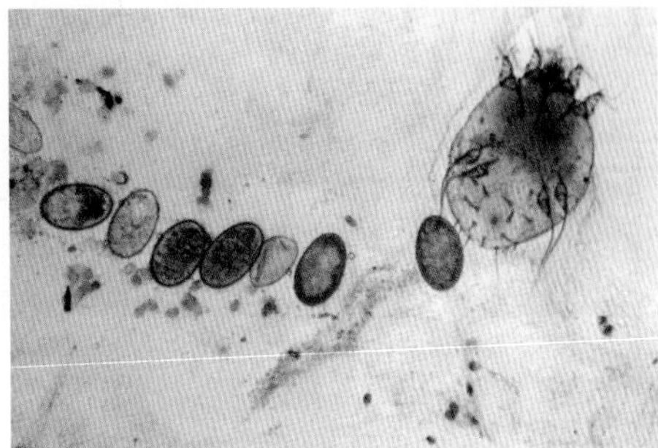

Fig. 71.1 Female scabies mite with eggs and scybala in skin scrapings. Note the mite's flattened, oval body and eight legs. *Courtesy, YDRSC.*

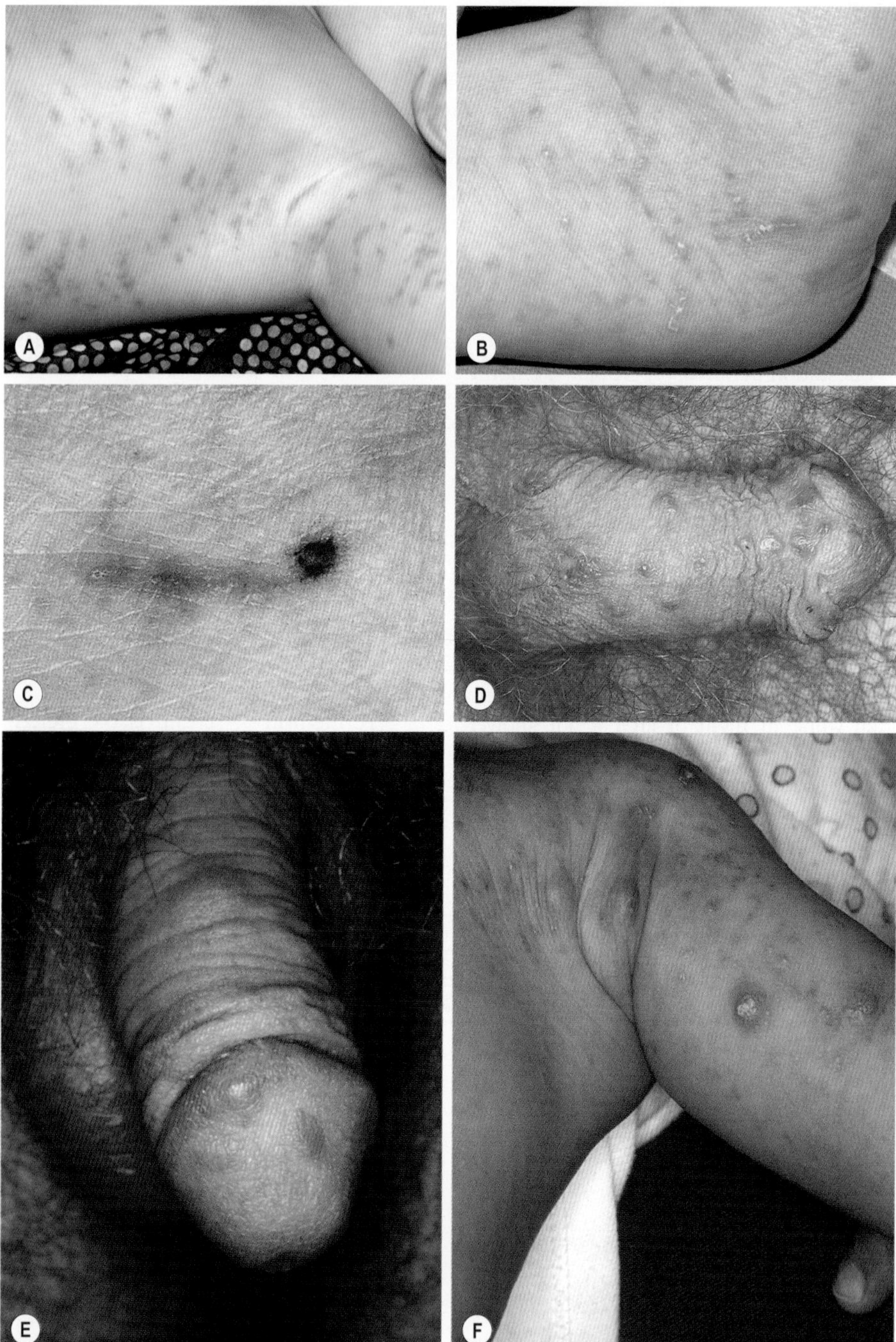

Fig. 71.2 Scabies. A, B Erythematous papules, linear burrows, areas of crusting and acral vesiculopustules in two infants with scabies. **C** Close-up of a linear burrow. **D, E** Penile involvement with erythematous papules and nodules. **F** Nodular scabies in an infant. *A, B, Courtesy, Julie V. Schaffer, MD; C, Courtesy, USCDRSC; D, Courtesy, YDRSC; E, Courtesy, Robert Hartman, MD; F, Courtesy, Kalman Watsky, MD.*

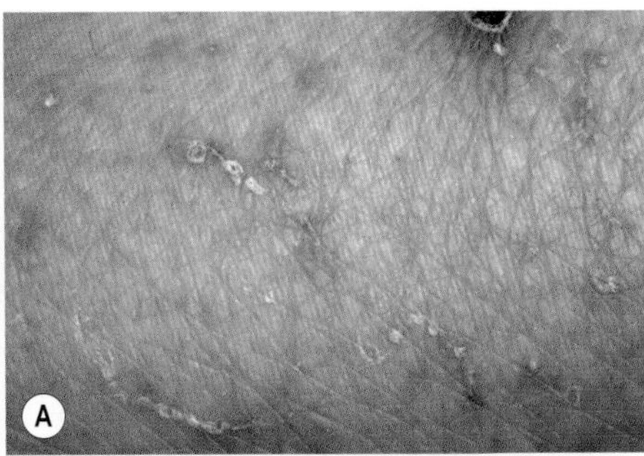

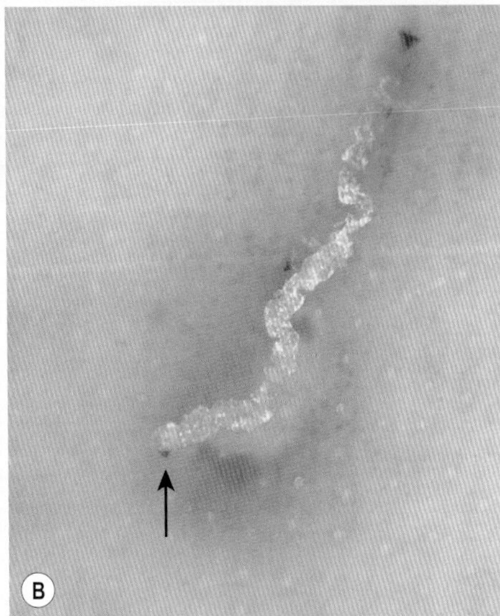

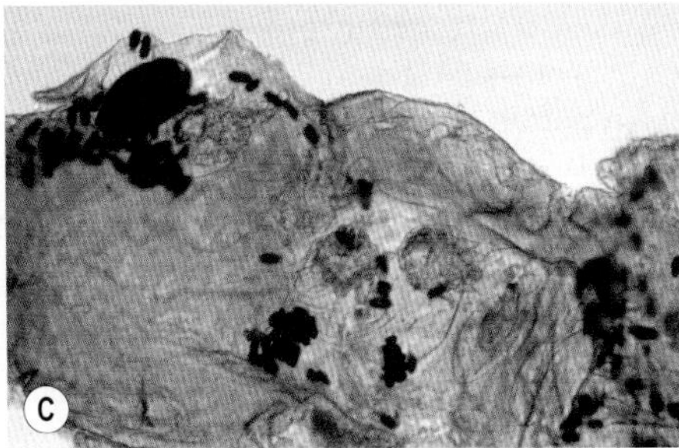

Fig. 71.3 Scabietic burrows and microscopy of a skin scraping from a patient with scabies. **A** Classic scabietic burrows – wavy, white, thread-like linear structures 1–10 mm in length. Burrows are highest yield in terms of isolating mites via skin scraping. **B** Dermoscopy can aid in identifying mites. By dermoscopy, a characteristic "jet with contrail" structure can be identified corresponding to the anterior part of the mite (arrow) and the burrow behind it. **C** Four mites, eggs, and scybala are present. The mites blend in with the background scale, making them difficult to see. *A, C, Courtesy, YDRSC; B, Courtesy, Iris Zalaudek, MD.*

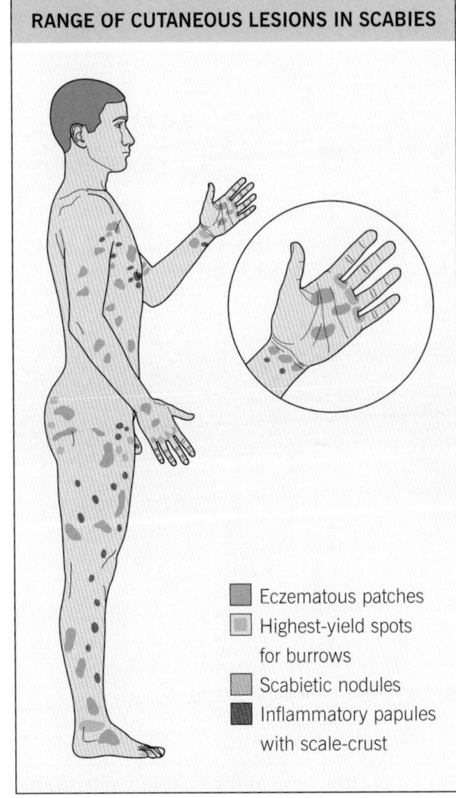

Fig. 71.4 Range of cutaneous lesions in scabies. Typical sites affected by scabies are highlighted. In infants and the elderly or immunocompromised, all surfaces can be involved, including the scalp and face.

- Pruritus and cutaneous lesions often last 2–4 weeks after successful treatment, but patients may feel relief within 3 days
- Once the diagnosis is established and initial treatment has been administered, topical corticosteroids (mild to moderate strength) can be used for symptomatic relief
- In crusted scabies, additional measures are necessary (e.g. combined and/or repeated treatments, cutting of nails, longer storage of clothing, vacuuming upholstery)

Head Lice (Pediculosis Capitis)

- Secondary to *Pediculus capitis*, a blood-sucking, six-legged insect that lays its eggs near the base of the hairs on the scalp (Fig. 71.7); the casing remains after the egg

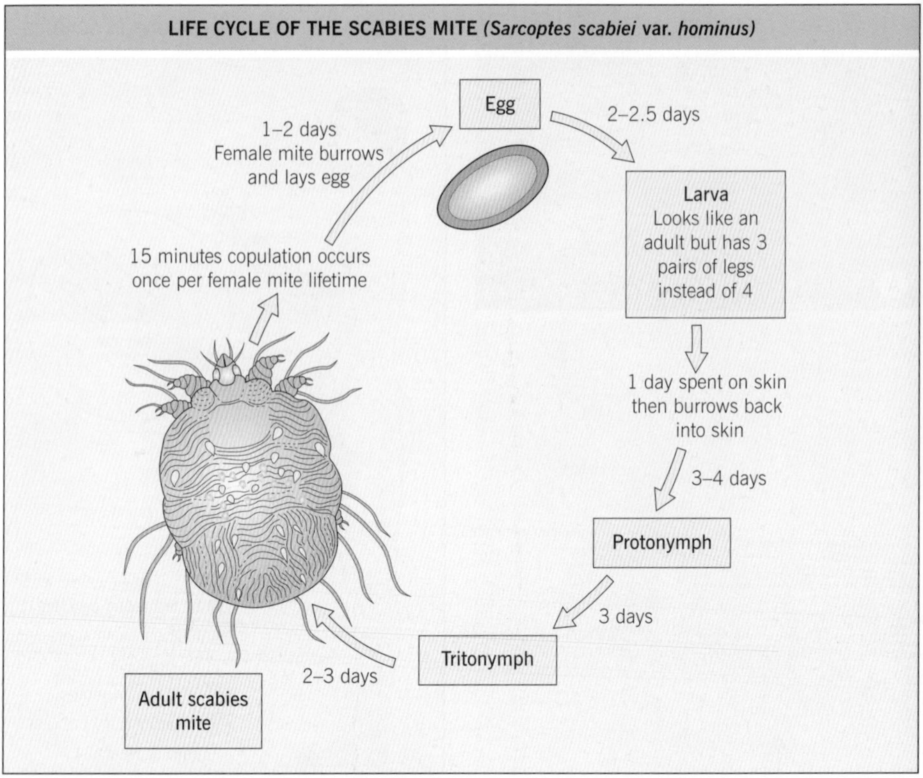

LIFE CYCLE OF THE SCABIES MITE *(Sarcoptes scabiei* var. *hominus)*

Egg

2–2.5 days

Larva
Looks like an adult but has 3 pairs of legs instead of 4

1 day spent on skin then burrows back into skin

3–4 days

Protonymph

3 days

Tritonymph

2–3 days

Adult scabies mite

15 minutes copulation occurs once per female mite lifetime

1–2 days
Female mite burrows and lays egg

Fig. 71.5 Life cycle of the scabies mite (*Sarcoptes scabiei* var. *hominus*).

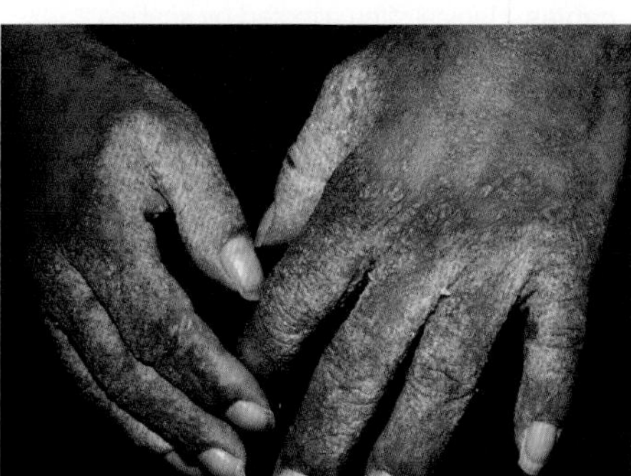

Fig. 71.6 Crusted scabies. Asymptomatic hyperkeratosis of the hands, which may be misdiagnosed as hand dermatitis. This disorder was previously referred to as Norwegian scabies. *Courtesy, Joyce Rico, MD.*

hatches and migrates outward with growth of the hair shaft.

- Transmission is by direct contact with an infested person or fomites (e.g. hats, brushes).
- Pruritus is variable.
- In addition to the presence of lice and eggs, there may be erythema, scaling, and excoriations of the head and neck region; occasionally there is a secondary pyoderma.
- Diagnosis is generally made by visual examination, followed by microscopic inspection and the detection of 0.8 mm eggs or their casings attached to scalp hairs ("nits"); high-yield locations include hairs above the ears and the lower occipital scalp (Fig. 71.8).
- **DDx** of scalp pruritus: seborrheic dermatitis, psoriasis, atopic dermatitis.
- **DDx** of nits: hair casts, dandruff, hair gel, and other causes of hair shaft nodules (see Fig. 64.3).
- **Rx:** outlined in Table 71.2. Most schools have a no-nit policy which requires mechanical removal of nits.

Crab Lice (Pediculosis Pubis)

- Secondary to *Phthirus pubis*, a bloodsucking, six-legged insect that lives on the terminal hairs of the pubic region, beard, eyelashes, axillae, and perianal region.

TOPICAL AND ORAL TREATMENTS FOR SCABIES					
Treatment	**Administration on days 1 and 8**	**Concerns**	**Efficacy and resistance**	**Use in infants**	**FDA pregnancy category**
Permethrin cream (5%)	Topically overnight	Allergic contact dermatitis in individuals with sensitivity to formaldehyde	Good, but some signs of resistance developing	FDA approved for infants ≥2 months of age	B
Ivermectin (available as 3 mg tablets)	Oral dose of 200–400 mcg/kg	Potential CNS toxicity in infants and young children	Excellent	Safety not established for children weighing <33 pounds (15 kg) or breast-feeding mothers	C (but generally not recommended for scabies in pregnant women)

Table 71.1 Topical and oral treatments for scabies. All treatments should be given on two separate occasions, 1 week apart. Other topical therapies are sometimes utilized, based on availability, but suffer from inferior efficacy and toxicities, e.g. lindane (CNS toxicity), sulfur 5–10%, and crotamiton.

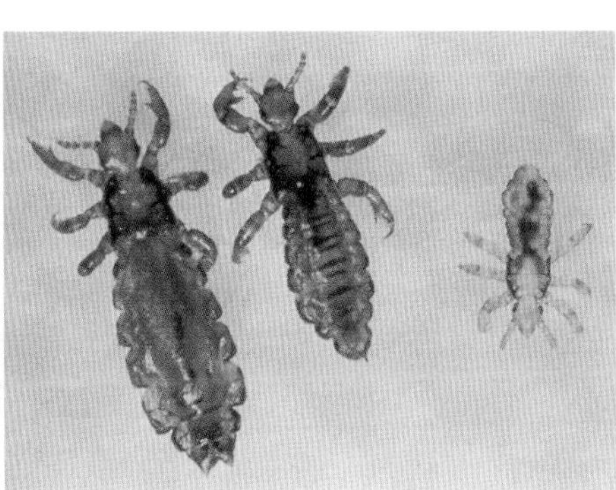

Fig. 71.7 Head louse family. From left to right: female, male, and nymph. *With permission from Taplin D, Meinking TL. Infestations. In: Schachner LA, Hansen RC (Eds.), Pediatric Dermatology, 4th edn. Edinburgh, UK: Mosby, 2011:1141–1180.*

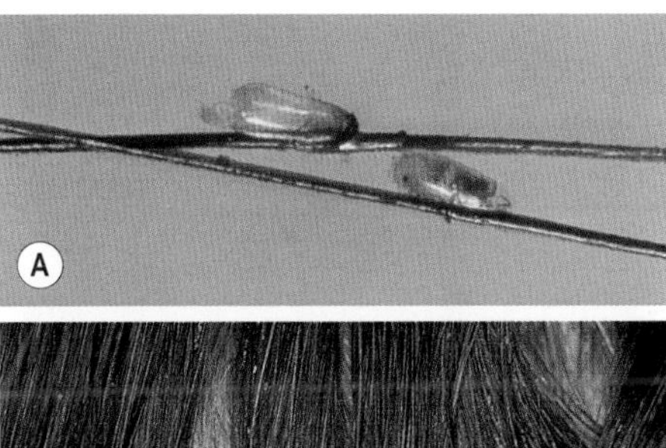

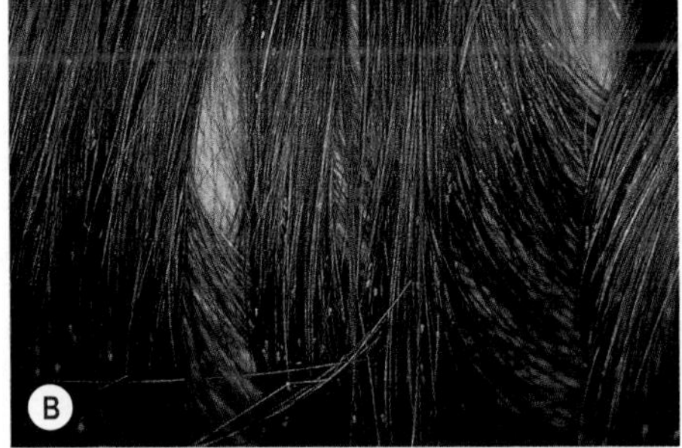

Fig. 71.8 Head lice. A The head louse egg or nit is 0.8 mm in length. **B** Head lice nits on hair. *With permission from Taplin D, Meinking TL. Infestations. In: Schachner LA, Hansen RC (Eds.), Pediatric Dermatology, 4th edn. Edinburgh, UK: Mosby, 2011:1141–1180.*

- While body and head lice are similar in appearance, crab lice are shorter and broader, thus actually resembling crabs (Fig. 71.9).
- Transmission is by direct contact (may be sexual) or occasionally via contaminated clothing, towels, or bedding.
- May coexist with other STIs; pruritus is common.
- In addition to lice that are attached to hairs or moving about the surface of the skin (Fig. 71.10A), hemorrhagic crusts, perifollicular erythema, and macula caerulea (asymptomatic slate-gray to blue macules on the trunk and thighs) may be seen; secondary bacterial infection may also occur.

TOPICAL AND ORAL TREATMENTS FOR HEAD LICE			
Treatment	**Administration on days 1 and 8**	**Concerns**	**Efficacy and resistance**
Permethrin cream rinse or lotion (1%)*	Topical application for 10 minutes to clean, dry hair	None	Poor–fair; resistance common
Pyrethrins (0.33%) synergized with piperonyl butoxide (4%), various formulations*	Topical application for 10 minutes to dry hair	Allergic reactions in individuals with sensitivity to chrysanthemums, ragweed, and related plants	Poor–fair; resistance common
Ivermectin lotion (0.5%)^	Topical application for 10 minutes to dry hair	Ocular irritation	Good; no resistance noted to date
Benzyl alcohol lotion (5%)^	Topical application for 10 minutes to dry hair	Potential skin irritation	Fair–good; no resistance noted to date
Spinosad cream rinse (0.9%)^	Topical application for 10 minutes to dry hair	None	Good; no resistance noted to date
Malathion lotion or gel (0.5%)**	Topical application for 8–12 hours to dry hair (Ovide® and gel products with isopropyl alcohol base are effective at 20 minutes)	Flammable isopropyl alcohol base; burning or stinging at sites of eroded skin	Excellent (in United States); resistance noted in United Kingdom and France, but to date not in United States
Ivermectin (available as 3 mg tablets)	Oral dose of 200–400 mcg/kg	Potential CNS toxicity; not recommended for children weighing <33 pounds (15 kg), breast-feeding mothers, or pregnant women (category C)	Excellent; no resistance noted to date

**Over-the-counter products.*
***Approved for individuals ≥6 years of age; pregnancy category B.*
^Approved for individuals ≥6 months of age; pregnancy category B.

Table 71.2 Topical and oral treatments for head lice. In general, treatments should be given on two separate occasions, 1 week apart, with the exception of a single application for ivermectin lotion or abametapir 0.74% lotion, an ovicidal metalloproteinase inhibitor. Carbaryl shampoo (0.5%), lindane shampoo (1%), and permethrin cream (5%) are sometimes used, but generally have inferior efficacy. Dimethicone (4%) is a silicone oil that can be applied for 15 minutes or overnight. AirAllé® is an FDA-cleared medical device that uses hot air to treat head lice via dehydration of their eggs, and, to a lesser degree, hatched lice.

- If the infestation involves the eyelashes, feces can accumulate at the base of the hairs and at the inferior margin of the lower eyelid (Fig. 71.10B).
- **DDx:** other causes of genital pruritus; nits must be distinguished from other causes of hair nodules (see Fig. 64.3).
- **Rx:** see Table 71.3.

Body Lice (Pediculosis Corporis)

- Secondary to infestation of clothing and humans by *Pediculus humanus* var. *corporis*, a bloodsucking six-legged insect.
- Associated with overcrowding, poor hygiene, poverty, wars, and natural disasters.

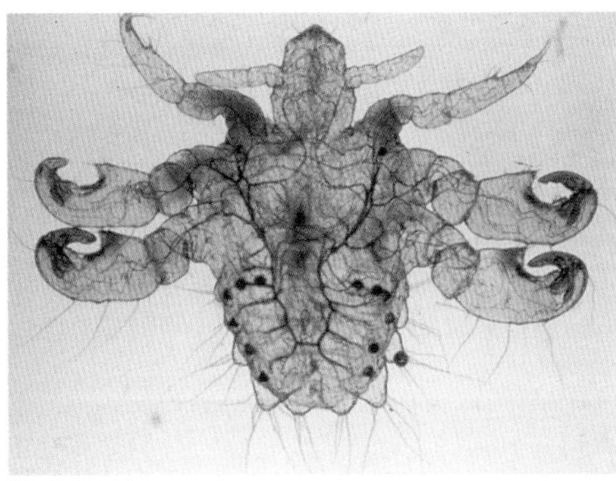

Fig. 71.9 Adult crab louse. The shape is shorter and broader than that of head and body lice. *Courtesy, Tony Burns, MD.*

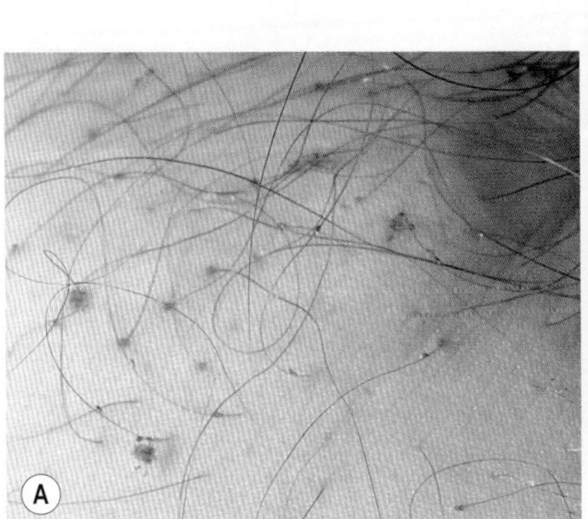

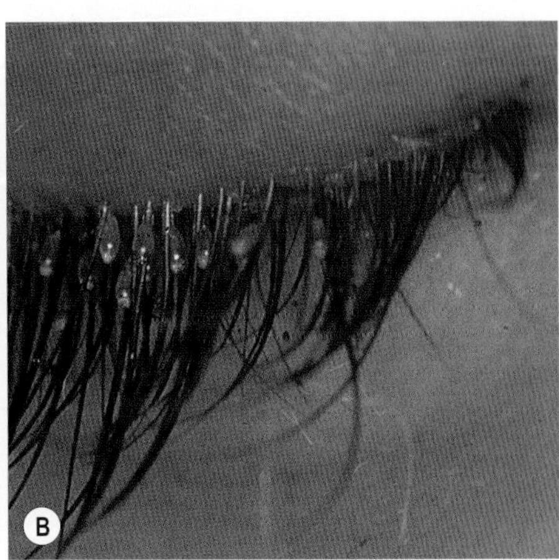

Fig. 71.10 Crab lice. A Both adult crab lice and nits are evident on pubic hairs. **B** Crab lice nits and feces on the eyelashes. *A, Courtesy, Louis A. Fragola, Jr., MD; B, With permission from Taplin D, Meinking TL. Infestations. In: Schachner LA, Hansen RC (Eds.), Pediatric Dermatology, 4th edn. Edinburgh, UK: Mosby, 2011:1141–1180.*

TOPICAL AND ORAL TREATMENTS FOR CRAB LICE		
Treatment	**Administration on days 1 and 8**	**Efficacy**
Permethrin (1%) cream rinse or synergized pyrethrin shampoo*	Topical application for 10 minutes to clean, dry hair	Fair
Permethrin cream (5%)	Topical application for 8–12 hours	Good
Ivermectin (available as 3 mg tablets)	Oral dose of 250 mcg/kg	Excellent

**Over-the-counter products.*

Table 71.3 Topical and oral treatments for crab lice. All crab lice treatments should be given on two separate occasions, 1 week apart. Lindane shampoo (1%) is occasionally used but has inferior efficacy.

- Body lice can transmit epidemic typhus (*Rickettsia prowazekii*), trench fever (*Bartonella quintana*), and relapsing fever (*Borrelia recurrentis*).
- Severe pruritus common, especially on the back, waist, shoulders, and neck.
- Body lice and nits are primarily found in clothing seams (Fig. 71.11).

- **DDx:** bites from other arthropods and other causes of generalized pruritus (e.g. amphetamine use; see Tables 4.1 and 4.2); systemic diseases associated with pruritus (e.g. hepatic or renal impairment).
- **Rx:** incinerate clothing and bedding if possible; otherwise wash and dry with high heat; in epidemics, mass delousing with dusting powders (e.g. DDT).

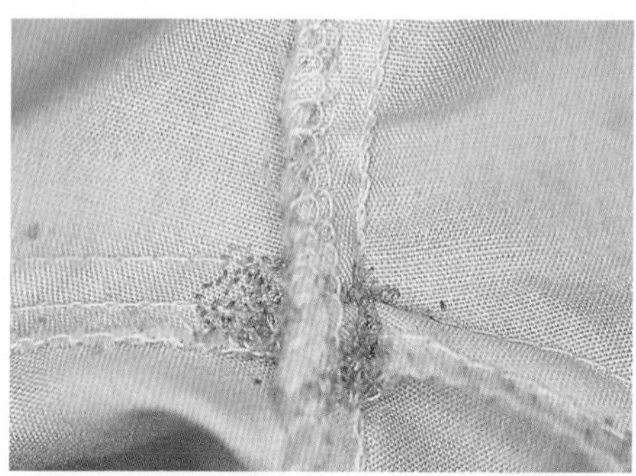

Fig. 71.11 Body lice eggs in the seams of clothing. *Courtesy, YDRSC.*

Tungiasis

- Secondary to the burrowing flea, *Tunga penetrans*.
- Endemic in Central and South America, Caribbean Islands, Africa, Pakistan, and India.
- Pregnant female flea burrows into the skin, especially on the feet of individuals who do not wear shoes or wear only flip-flops (Fig. 71.12).

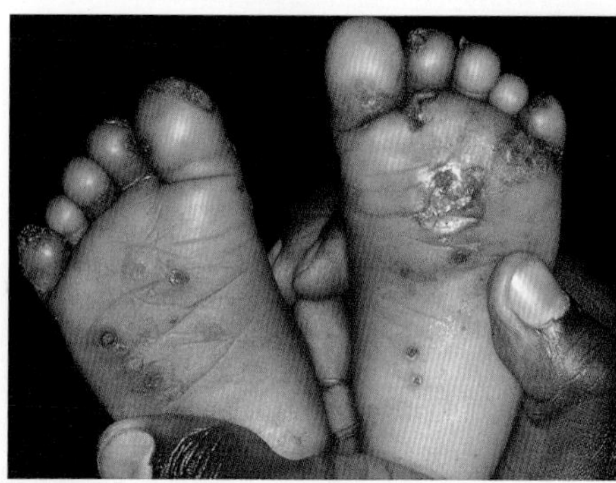

Fig. 71.12 Tungiasis in a child. *Courtesy, Terri L. Meinking, MD, Craig N. Burkhart, MD, and Craig G. Burkhart, MD.*

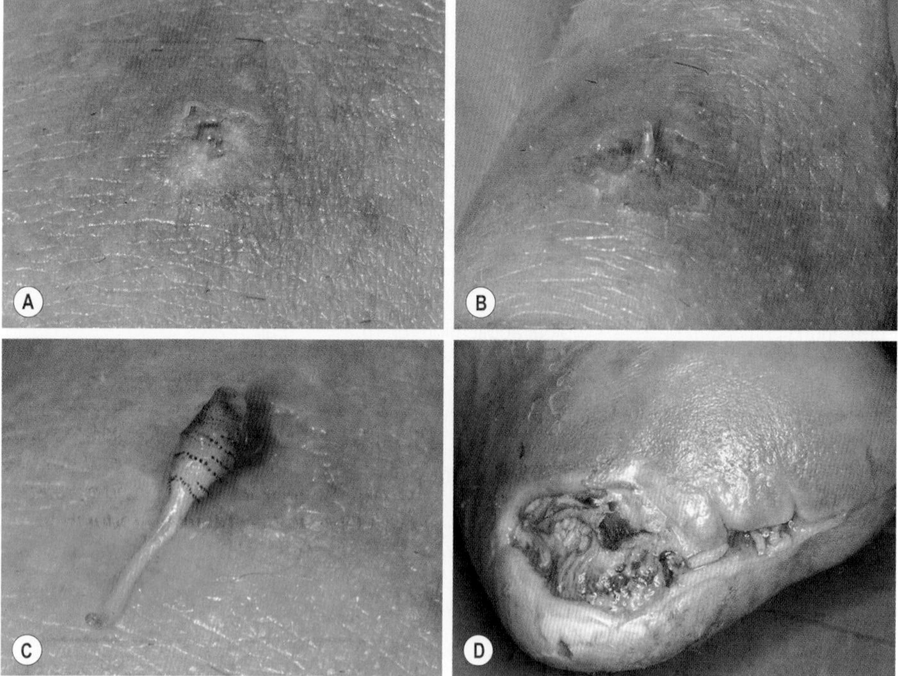

Fig. 71.13 Cutaneous myiasis. Furuncular myiasis presenting as a papulonodule with a central punctum (**A**) through which the larva's posterior end, which contains respiratory spiracles, may protrude (**B**). Note the characteristic appearance of the extracted botfly larva, with parallel rows of dark spines and hooks (**C**). **D** Wound myiasis in an amputation stump. *A–C, Courtesy, Edward W. Cowen, MD, MHSc; D, Courtesy, Louis A. Fragola, Jr., MD.*

- First sign is a small black dot that becomes a whitish papule and then a 1- or 2-cm nodule with surrounding erythema; there may be multiple lesions.
- Rarely, tetanus, gangrene, or autoamputation may result.
- **DDx:** myiasis, persistent arthropod bite reaction, cercarial dermatitis, pyoderma, wart, squamous cell carcinoma.
- **Rx:** removal of the flea; tetanus prophylaxis should be considered.
- Prevention: wear shoes and avoid sitting on sandy beaches in endemic areas.

Cutaneous Myiasis

- Infestation of skin by fly larvae; furuncular myiasis presents as a boil-like lesion, most commonly secondary to *Dermatobia hominis* (human botfly) and *Cordylobia anthropophaga* (tumbu fly); wound myiasis is most often due to *Cochliomyia hominivorax* or *Chrysomya bezziana* (Fig. 71.13).
- Complications may occur, especially when the sinuses, nasal cavity, or scalp are involved.
- **DDx** for furuncular myiasis: ruptured cyst, abscess, furunculosis, and foreign body reaction.
- **Rx:** excision or removal of larvae for furuncular myiasis; debridement and irrigation for wound myiasis; consider oral ivermectin if oral/ocular involvement. As myiasis can be a portal of entry for *Clostridium tetani*, vaccination of affected individuals should be considered.
- Prevention: insect repellent, including on the scalp; ironing all line-dried items will kill eggs of the tumbu fly.

For further information see Ch. 84 from *Dermatology, Fourth Edition*.

For additional online figures visit www.expertconsult.com 

72 Bites and Stings

Insects

• The bite of any insect can lead to a local cutaneous reaction whose intensity can vary depending on the individual's level of sensitivity; the typical presentation is a 2- to 8-mm, erythematous urticarial papule in an exposed area (Fig. 72.1); lesions are often multiple and can be grouped (Fig. 72.2).

• Secondary changes consisting of excoriations may be present; less often, vesicles or bullae develop at the site of bites (Fig. 72.3).

• Bite reactions typically resolve over 5–10 days; occasionally, patients develop persistent bite reactions that on biopsy may be diagnosed as pseudolymphoma (see Ch. 99).

• Postinflammatory hyperpigmentation is common, especially in patients with darkly pigmented skin.

• Secondary infection is a potential complication, most commonly from staphylococci or streptococci.

• Exaggerated bite reactions can be seen in patients with chronic lymphocytic leukemia; rarely, hypersensitivity reactions to mosquito bites that become necrotic can be associated with EBV infection (see Ch. 67).

• Anaphylaxis with urticaria and angioedema is generally due to stings from hymenopterids (bees, wasps, hornets, and fire ants) (Fig. 72.4).

• Insects may be vectors of infectious diseases (Table 72.1).

• Bites can trigger papular urticaria, especially in children, in which edematous papules are more widespread and longer-lasting; some of the lesions can represent reactivation.

• Prevention: insect repellents (e.g. DEET), mosquito netting, and protective or permethrin-treated clothing; Table 72.2.

• **Rx:** anti-pruritic topical agents (e.g. pramoxine, calamine), topical CS ± occlusion; for persistent lesions, intralesional CS (e.g. triamcinolone 5 mg/ml).

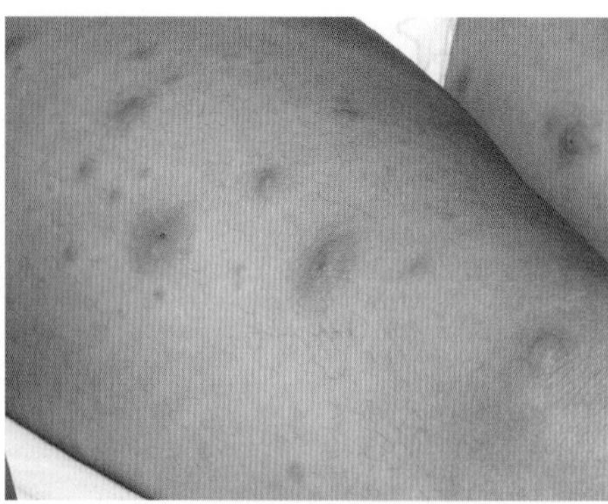

Fig. 72.1 Mosquito bite reactions. This patient has excoriated edematous papules and papulovesicles. When both insect repellent and sunscreen are used, the latter should be applied first. *Courtesy, Julie V. Schaffer, MD.*

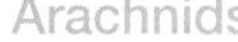

Arachnids

Hard Ticks

• Site of the tick bite can become papular, nodular, bullous, or plaque-like; expanding lesion suggests possible erythema migrans.

• Attached ticks may go unnoticed (e.g. scalp, groin); occasionally the attached tick is misinterpreted as a "new mole."

• Ticks are important disease vectors, especially in the nymphal stage (Table 72.3; see Fig. 63.1); tick control measures are important for public health (see Fig. 63.8 for geographic distribution of vector tick species).

• Removal of ticks should be performed carefully by grasping the protruding end of the tick as close to the skin surface as possible and firmly pulling away from the attachment site with fine-tipped tweezers.

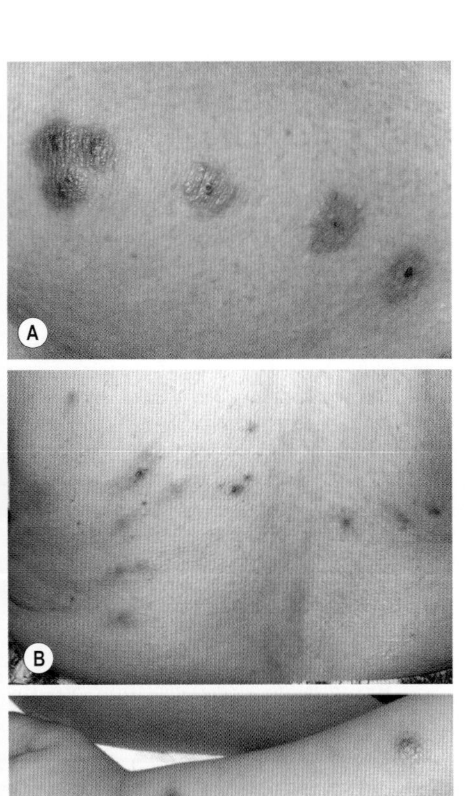

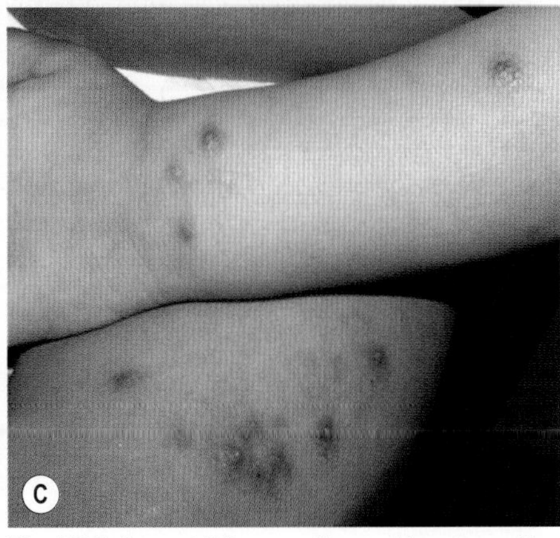

Fig. 72.2 Insect bite reactions. Linear, pruritic papules with central crusts demonstrating the "breakfast, lunch, and dinner" sign (**A**) that is characteristic of, but not specific to, bedbug bite reactions. Bedbug bite reactions are typically pink, edematous papules in linear to arcuate arrays with central punctum or excoriation (**B, C**). Residual hyperpigmentation following bug bite reactions is common in individuals with darker skin types and can persist for months. *A, Courtesy, Antonio Torrelo, MD; B, Courtesy, Kalman Watsky, MD; C, Courtesy, Julie V. Schaffer, MD.*

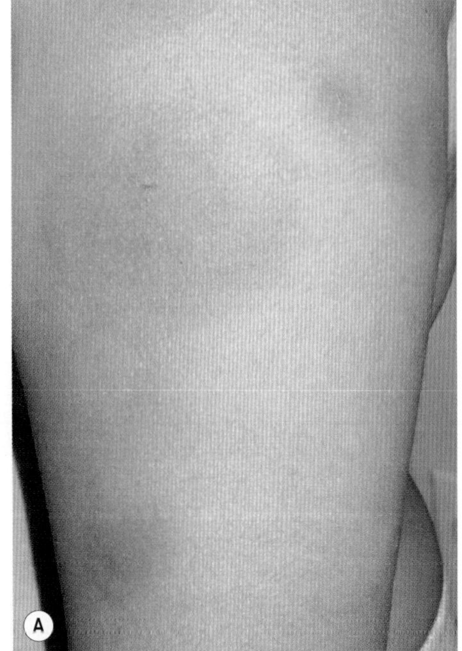

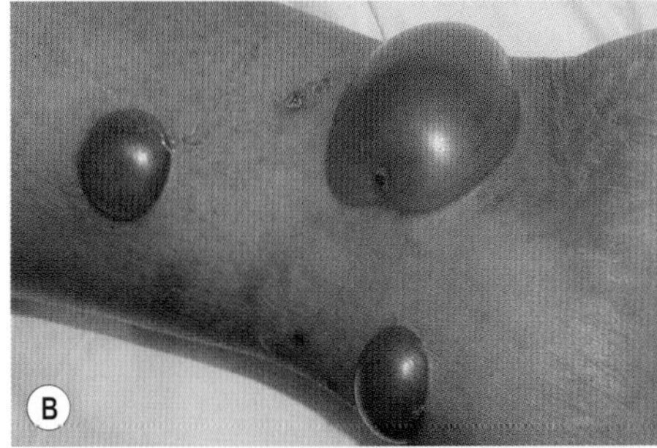

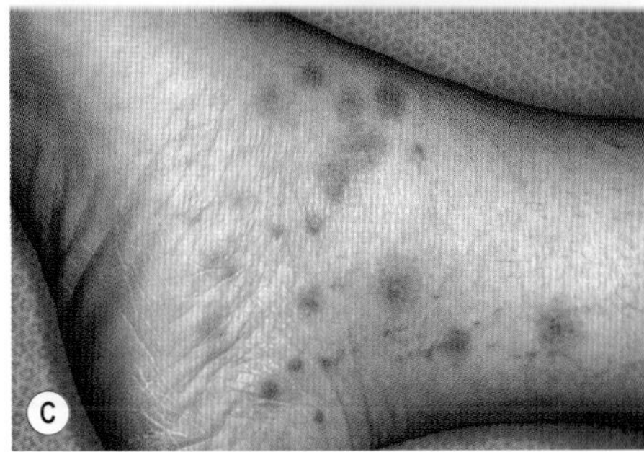

Fig. 72.3 Spectrum of insect bite reactions. Sometimes patients develop large, erythematous, edematous plaques **(A)**, frank bullae **(B),** or purpuric lesions that may be mistaken for leukocytoclastic vasculitis (**C**). *A, B, Courtesy, Julie V. Schaffer, MD; C, Courtesy Jean L. Bolognia, MD.*

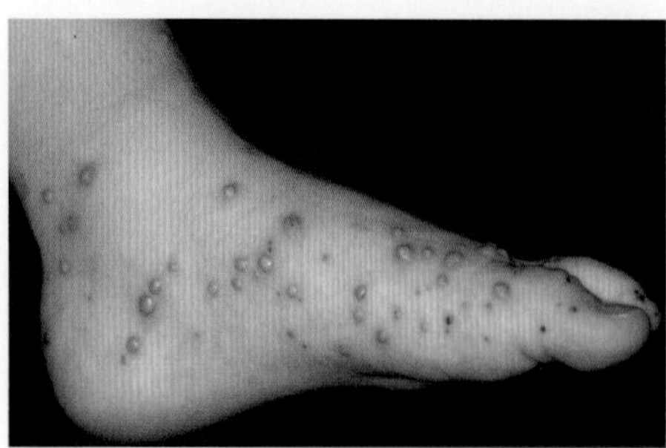

Fig. 72.4 Fire ant bites presenting as clusters of sterile pustules on the foot. *Courtesy, Dirk M. Elston, MD.*

- Prevention: permethrin repellent can be sprayed on clothing or other fabrics; protective clothing.
- **Rx** of persistent tick bite reactions: potent topical CS, intralesional CS, or even excision in severe cases; doxycycline is recommended in suspected cases of Rocky Mountain spotted fever (10-day course; see Ch. 63) or Lyme disease (14- to 21-day course).

Mites

- Thousands of species; parasitize humans as well as animals and plants.
- Human mites include *Demodex folliculorum* and *D. brevis* (may lead to folliculitis and exacerbate rosacea) and *Sarcoptes scabiei*, which causes scabies (see Ch. 71); these mites complete their life cycle on humans.
- *Cheyletiella* mites ("walking dandruff") are found on small mammals (e.g. cats, dogs) and may cause papulovesicular lesions in humans (Fig. 72.5); similar lesions can be seen in individuals exposed to avian mites.
- Chigger mites in Asia are vectors for scrub typhus; in other regions they lead to multiple bite reactions that tend to favor the buttocks and anogenital region.
- House mouse mites are vectors for rickettsialpox.

Spiders

- Black widow spider (*Latrodectus mactans* is the primary species in the United States):
  - Bites lead to acute pain and edema
  - Systemic symptoms may include an acute abdomen or rhabdomyolysis
  - **Rx:** if severe reaction, emergency medical treatment
- Brown recluse spider (*Loxosceles reclusa* is the predominant species in the United States) (Fig. 72.6):
  - Bites can cause dermonecrosis (sphingomyelinase D is the major toxin) which begins with erythema and/or vesiculation that becomes dusky, sometimes with bullae formation and eventual necrosis (Fig. 72.7)
  - Rarely, systemic findings of shock, hemolysis, renal insufficiency, and disseminated intravascular coagulation
  - **Rx:** rest, ice, and elevation are the mainstays of treatment

Dog and Cat Bites

- Infection of bite sites is common, especially with streptococci, staphylococci, *Pasteurella multocida*, *Capnocytophaga canimorsus*, and anaerobes (e.g. *Fusobacterium*).
- **Rx:** broad-spectrum antibiotics (e.g. amoxicillin–clavulanate) to cover the above organisms; depending on clinical setting, consider rabies vaccine/immunoglobulin and tetanus booster.

Marine Stings/Injuries

- Vary from dermatitis (secondary to contact with sea anemone, coral, or sponges) to foreign body reactions (e.g. to embedded sea urchin spines) to acute reactions (e.g. erythematous, urticarial or hemorrhagic streaks secondary to jellyfish stings; Fig. 72.8).
- Complications include secondary bacterial infection (e.g. *Staphylococcus aureus*);

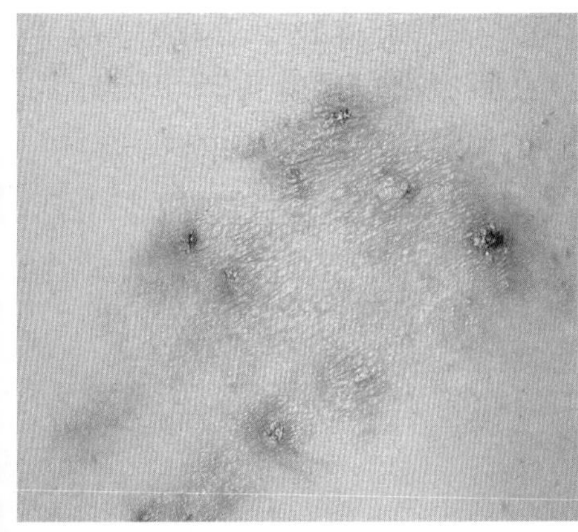

Fig. 72.5 *Cheyletiella* bites. These mites are non-burrowing and are found on cats, rabbits, and dogs. *Courtesy, Dirk M. Elston, MD.*

DISTRIBUTION IN THE US OF SPIDERS THAT MAY CAUSE DERMONECROTIC REACTIONS

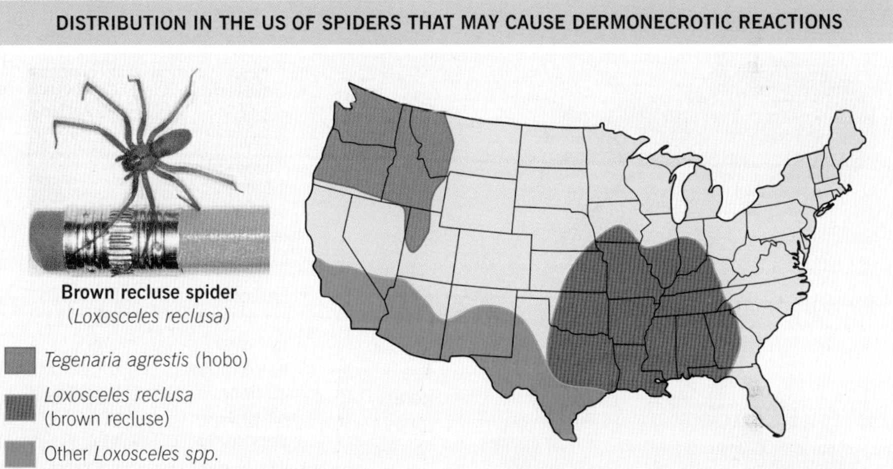

Fig. 72.6 Distribution in the United States of spiders that may cause dermonecrotic reactions. *Adapted from Sams HH, Dunnick CA, Smith ML, et al. Necrotic arachnidism. J Am Acad Dermatol 2001;44:561–73.*

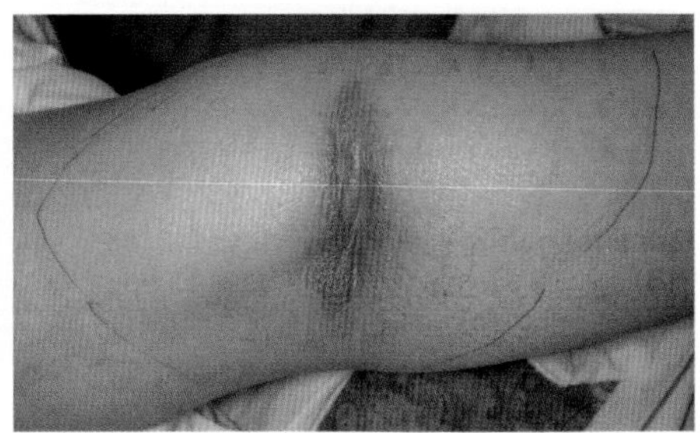

Fig. 72.7 Dermonecrotic spider bite reaction. Note the central dusky necrosis. The patient was initially misdiagnosed with cellulitis and hospitalized after failure to respond to oral antibiotic therapy. *Courtesy, YDRSC.*

MAJOR INSECTS OF DERMATOLOGIC SIGNIFICANCE			
Insect, size of an adult (length)	**Example(s)**	**Lesional clues**	**Vector of:**
Bedbugs, ~5–8 mm	*Cimex lectularius,* species most commonly found in the United States	• Lesions noted upon awakening • Bites often in groups of 2 or 3	
Triatome reduviids, ~1–3 cm	*Triatoma dimidiata, Rhodnius prolixus*	• Painless bites with delayed erythema, edema, and pruritus • Unilateral eyelid swelling (Romaña sign), a conjunctival reaction to infected feces	American trypanosomiasis (bugs defecate as they eat and infectious feces are rubbed into the wound)
Fleas*, ~2–10 mm	• *Pulex irritans* (human flea; shown here) • *Ctenocephalides felis* (often found on dogs) • *Xenopsylla cheopsis* (oriental rat flea)	• Lesions often limited to lower extremities as fleas jump but cannot fly • Wider distribution if an infested pet is held, groomed, or shares bed	• Endemic (murine) typhus, primarily oriental rat flea • Flea-borne spotted fever and plague, primarily oriental rat flea
Fire ants, 2–6 mm	*Solenopsis invicta*	Clusters of sterile pustules (Fig. 72.4), sometimes in rosettes	
Blister beetles, ~1–2.5 cm	*Epicauta occidentalis*	Vesicles/bullae result from secreted cantharidin	

*See Chapter 71 for information on *Tunga penetrans*, a burrowing flea.

Table 72.1 Major insects of dermatologic significance. *Photographs: inset 1, courtesy, YDRSC; insets 2, 3, courtesy, Dirk M. Elston, MD.*

TREATMENT AND PREVENTION OF MAJOR INSECTS OF DERMATOLOGIC SIGNIFICANCE	
Bedbugs	• Extermination
Triatome reduviids	• Elimination of hiding spots/ breeding grounds (e.g. cracked stone walls) • Extermination
Fleas	• Treat infested animals (e.g. fipronil, methoprene) • Treat house with insecticide
Fire ants	• Eradication of fire ant mounds

Table 72.2 Treatment and prevention of major insects of dermatologic significance.

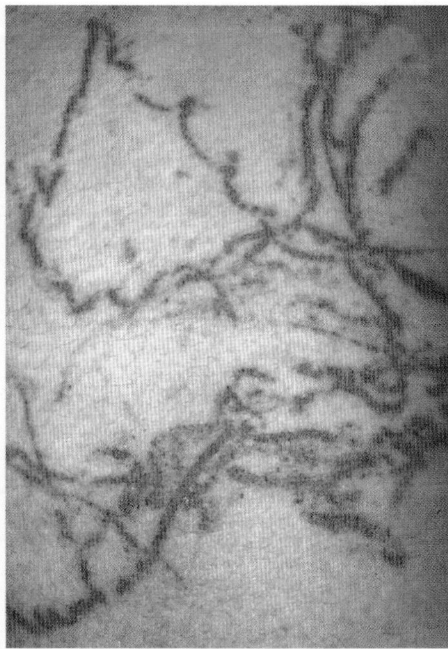

Fig. 72.8 Jellyfish sting. Painful red papules and papulovesicles in multiple linear streaks. *Courtesy, Joyce Rico, MD.*

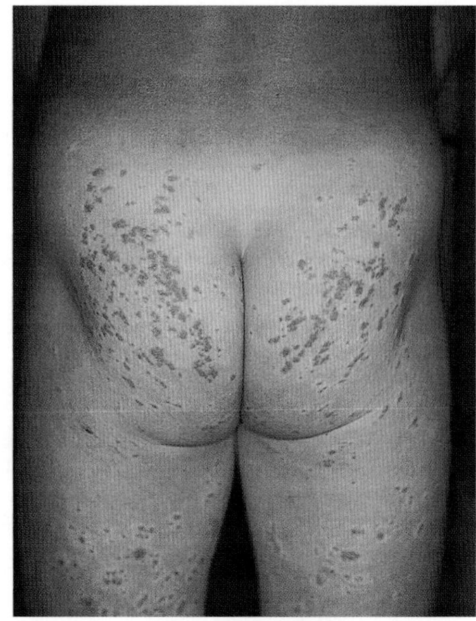

Fig. 72.9 Seabather's eruption. Edematous pink papules in the same distribution as the bathing trunks. *Courtesy, Kalman Watsky, MD.*

Vibrio vulnificus infections with hemorrhagic bullae more common in patients with liver disease.

- **Rx:** for acute marine envenomations – soaking in hot water to denature venom proteins; for symptoms of delayed reactions or dermatitis – topical CS; for foreign body reactions – removal of foreign material.
- Seabather's eruption:
  - Pruritic papules, localized to the bathing suit area and intertriginous areas (Fig. 72.9)
  - Secondary to a variety of stinging larvae, e.g. *Linuche unguiculata* (jellyfish), *Edwardsiella lineata* (sea anemone)

For further information see Ch. 85 from *Dermatology, Fourth Edition*.

For additional online figures and tables visit www.expertconsult.com 

MAJOR TICKS OF DERMATOLOGIC SIGNIFICANCE		
Tick	**Example/distribution**	**Vector of:**
Ixodes 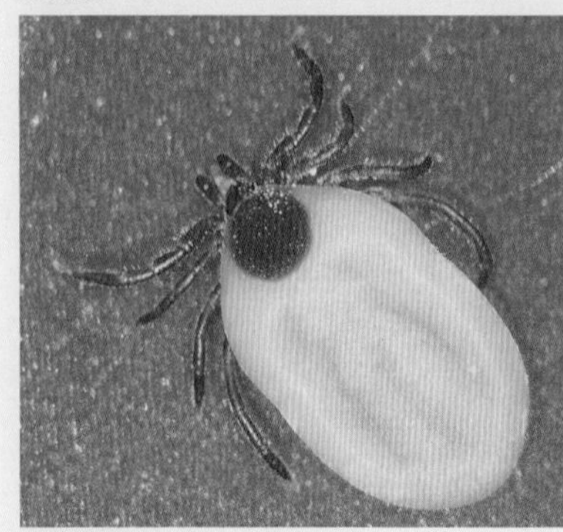	• *Ixodes scapularis* (black-legged tick; shown here), United States: eastern and mid-Atlantic states, Great Lakes region • *Ixodes pacificus* (western black-legged tick), western United States • *Ixodes ricinus*, Europe • *Ixodes persulcatus*, Eurasia	• Lyme disease • Babesiosis • Human granulocytic anaplasmosis • Other borrelial and rickettsial infections, e.g. Japanese spotted fever • Powassan encephalitis
Amblyomma 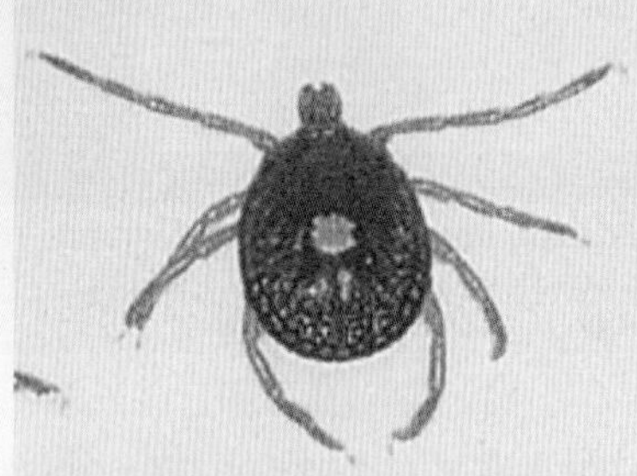	• *Amblyomma americanum* (lone star tick; shown here), United States: from Texas to Iowa and Connecticut • *Amblyomma maculatum*, U.S. Gulf Coast	• Human monocytic ehrlichiosis • *Ehrlichia ewingii* infection • Southern tick-associated rash illness (STARI) • Occasionally, rickettsial diseases are transmitted by *Amblyomma* species • Tularemia
Dermacentor 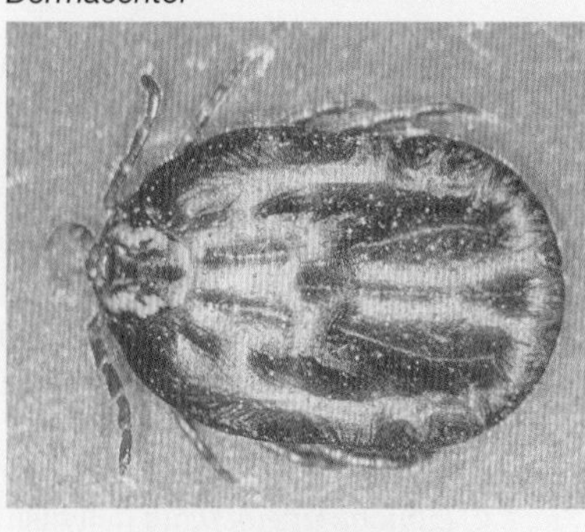	• *Dermacentor variabilis* (shown here), most of United States, except Rocky Mountain states • *Dermacentor andersoni*, United States: Rocky Mountain states • *Dermacentor reticulatus*, Europe	• Rocky Mountain spotted fever (United States) • Colorado tick fever • Tularemia • Other rickettsial infections (especially Europe, Asia); also Pacific Coast tick fever (*Rickettsia philipii*, type strain "Rickettsia 364D") • Ehrlichiosis • Occasionally, human monocytic ehrlichiosis and Q fever
Rhipicephalus (brown dog tick) 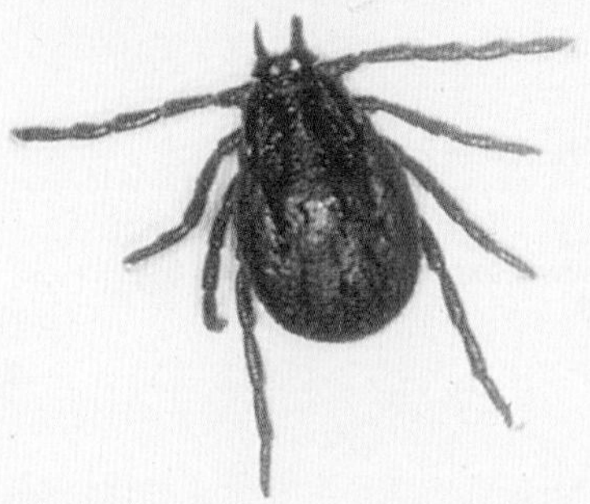	Southwestern United States and Mexico	• Boutonneuse fever • Occasionally Rocky Mountain spotted fever

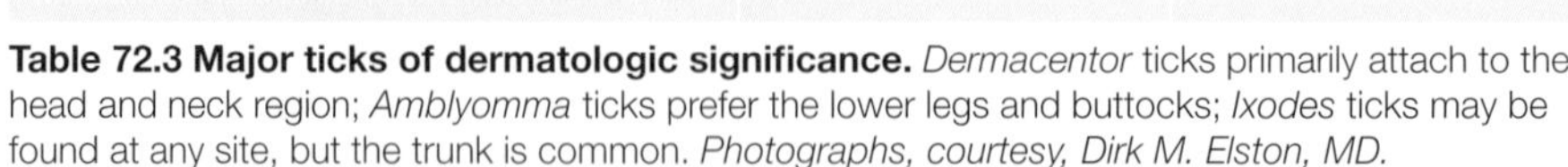
Table 72.3 Major ticks of dermatologic significance. *Dermacentor* ticks primarily attach to the head and neck region; *Amblyomma* ticks prefer the lower legs and buttocks; *Ixodes* ticks may be found at any site, but the trunk is common. *Photographs, courtesy, Dirk M. Elston, MD.*

Photodermatoses 73

Photo Facts

• The UV radiation (UVR) emitted by the sun is arbitrarily subdivided based on wavelength into UVA (400–320 nm), UVB (320–290 nm), and UVC (290–200 nm).
• More than 95% of UVR that reaches the earth's surface is UVA.
• UVA, but not UVB, can penetrate through glass windows.
• The penetration of UVR into the skin is wavelength-dependent (Fig. 73.1).
• Principles and formulations of sunscreens are discussed in the Appendix.

Cutaneous Effects of UVR Exposure: Acute

• The visible short-term effects of UVR include sunburn and tanning; in addition, it leads to vitamin D synthesis, epidermal hyperplasia, proinflammatory responses, and immunosuppression.
• **Sunburn** = inflammation + erythema; UVC (absorbed by ozone) > UVB > UVA in potential to cause sunburn.
• **MED** = "minimal erythema dose" = the lowest dose of UVR capable of inducing erythema (sunburn) in a given individual.

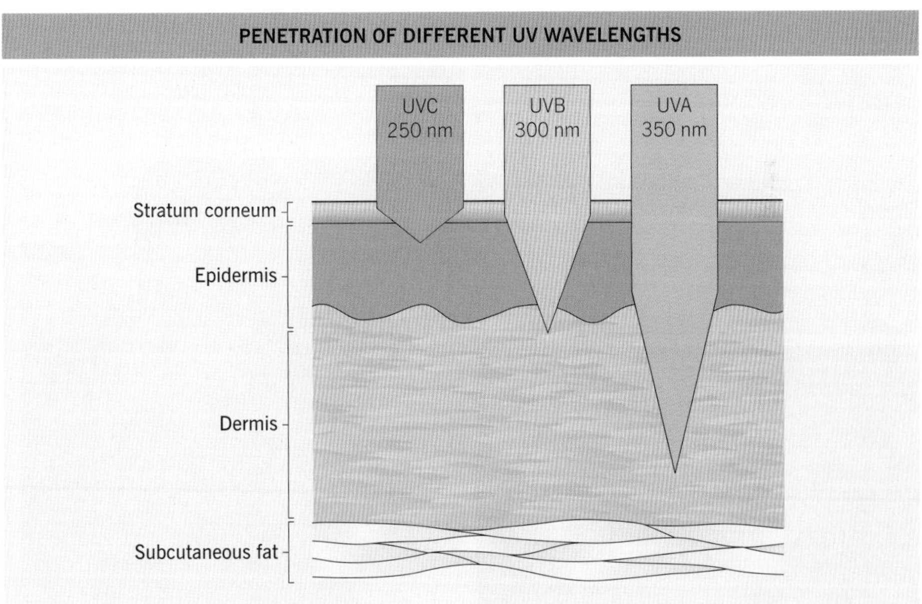

Fig. 73.1 Depth of penetration of different wavelengths of UV light into human skin. Depth of penetration varies greatly with the thickness of the different skin layers and their composition (e.g. melanin content). The beginning of the wedge-shaped portion of the penetration symbol represents a decrease to approximately one-third of the incident energy density, and the tip of the symbol represents a decrease to approximately 1%. Figure not drawn to scale.

- Typically, a UVB-induced sunburn appears within 30 minutes to 8 hours of sufficient exposure, peaks at 12–24 hours, and diminishes over hours to days with desquamation.
- **Tanning** occurs as a biphasic response to UVR and is wavelength-dependent.
  - –**"Immediate pigment darkening"** occurs during and immediately after exposure and is most prominent with UVA
  - –**"Delayed tanning"** usually results from UVB exposure and peaks about 3 days after sun exposure
- A "UVA-induced tan," such as from the use of tanning beds, provides 5–10 times less protection from subsequent UVR exposure than does a "UVB-induced tan," most likely because UVB also induces epidermal hyperplasia.

Cutaneous Effects of UVR Exposure: Chronic

- The visible long-term effects of UVR include **photoaging** and **photocarcinogenesis.**
- Cutaneous signs of photoaging are pictured in Fig. 73.2 and also include solar lentigines, sunburn lentigines, and ephelides; in more darkly pigmented skin, small seborrheic keratoses, melasma, and dyspigmentation may be seen.

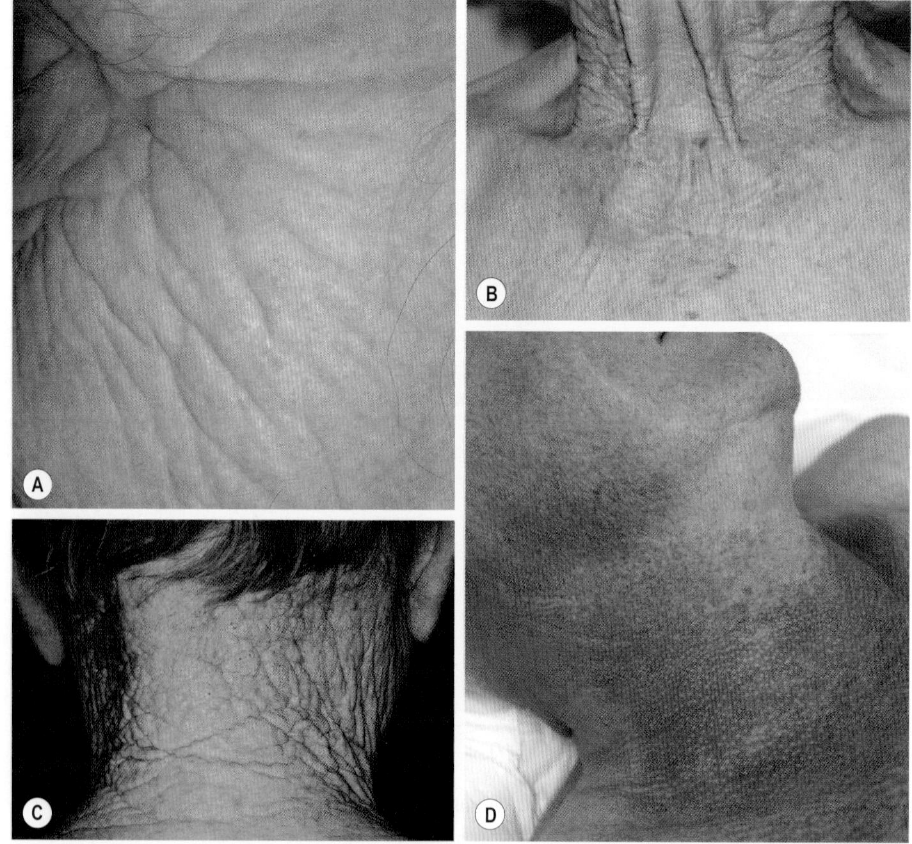

Fig. 73.2 Cutaneous signs of significant photoaging. A, B Solar elastosis of the cheek (**A**) and neck and V of the chest (**B**) with the characteristic yellow discoloration, thickening and furrowing of the skin. **C** Cutis rhomboidalis nuchae with deep furrowing of the posterior neck. **D** Poikiloderma of Civatte with sparing of the submental region and follicular skin. *Continued*

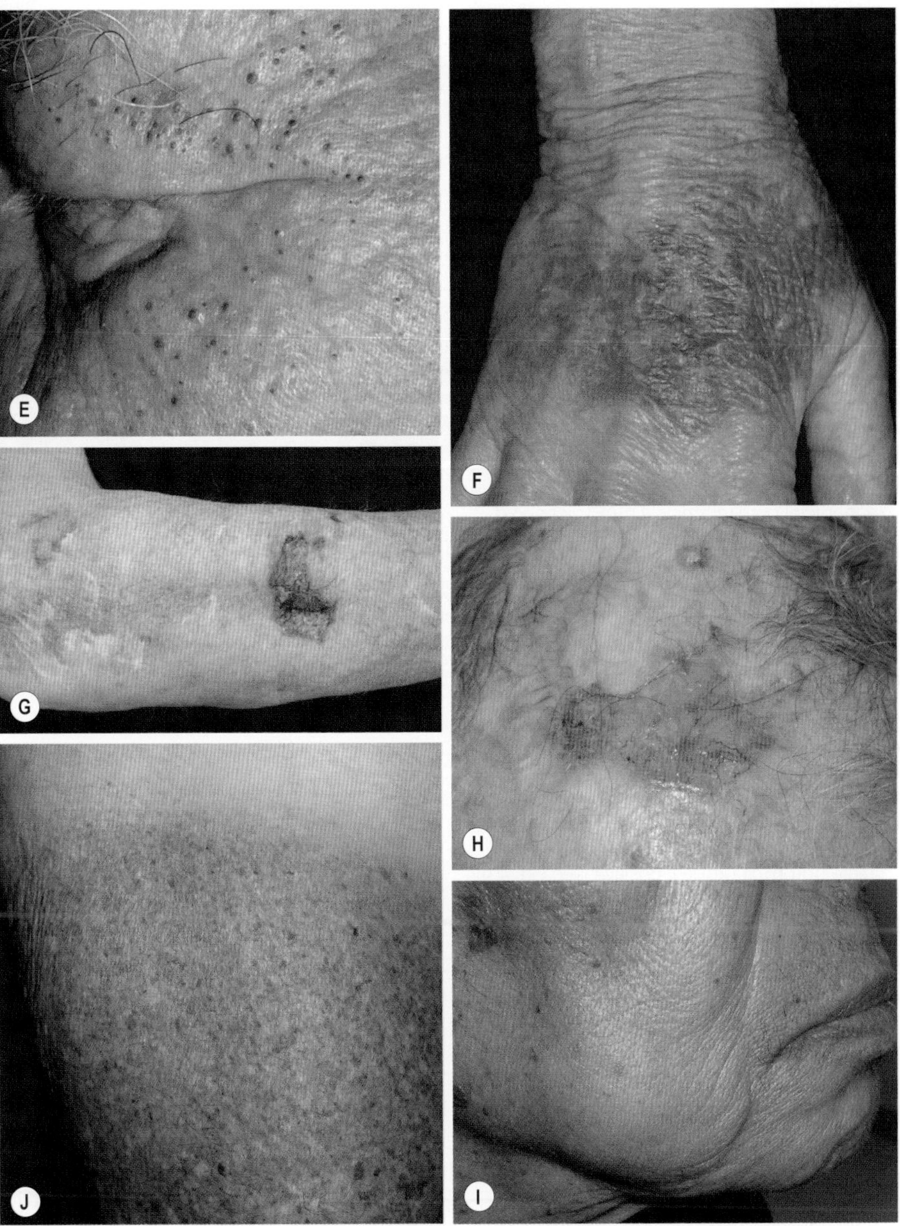

Fig. 73.2 *Continued* **Cutaneous signs of significant photoaging. E** Multiple open comedones of the malar region in Favre–Racouchot syndrome. **F** Brown discoloration of the dorsal hand due to hemosiderin deposits from recurrent solar purpura. **G** Skin tear due to fragility of atrophic photodamaged skin (dermatoporosis) and pseudoscars from previous tears. **H** Erosive pustular dermatosis of the bald scalp. **I** Photoaging in a 93-year-old African-American woman, demonstrating fine wrinkling and numerous tiny seborrheic keratoses. **J** Sharp demarcation on the thigh of solar lentigines and the dyspigmentation of photodamaged skin. The patient consistently wore spandex shorts. *A, E, I Courtesy, Henry Lim, MD; B, Courtesy, Kalman Watsky, MD; C, Courtesy, YDRSC; D, F, G, J, Courtesy, Jean L. Bolognia, MD; H, Courtesy, Harvey Lui, MD.*

CLASSIFICATION OF THE MORE COMMON PHOTODERMATOSES
Idiopathic, probably immunologically mediated photodermatoses (Table 73.2)
• Polymorphous light eruption (PMLE) • Actinic prurigo • Hydroa vacciniforme • Chronic actinic dermatitis (CAD) • Solar urticaria
Photoaggravated dermatoses (Table 73.2)
• Atopic dermatitis • Seborrheic dermatitis > psoriasis • Lupus erythematosus, dermatomyositis • Rosacea • Grover disease (transient acantholytic dermatosis) • Other: erythema multiforme, bullous pemphigoid, pityriasis rubra pilaris, Darier disease, GVHD, disseminated actinic superficial porokeratosis (DSAP), lichenoid keratoses
Chemical- and drug-induced photosensitivity (Table 73.3)
Inherited disorders characterized by defective DNA repair or chromosomal instability (Table 73.5)

Table 73.1 Classification of the more common photodermatoses. In some patients, clinicopathologic correlation (e.g. routine histopathology of a skin biopsy specimen), laboratory evaluation (e.g. ANA; anti-SSA/Ro, -SSB/La antibodies; plasma porphyrins, followed by complete porphyrin profile if positive [see Ch. 41]), and phototesting or photopatch testing (see Fig. 73.16) are required to make a diagnosis.

• Chronic UVR is responsible for development of actinic keratoses, squamous cell carcinoma, basal cell carcinoma, and cutaneous melanoma (see Chs 88 and 93).

Photodermatoses

• The photodermatoses are classified into four broad categories (Table 73.1) and are discussed in Table 73.2 (Figs 73.3–73.11), Table 73.3 (Figs 73.12–73.13), and Table 73.5 (Fig. 73.14).

• Clues to the diagnosis of various photodermatoses are outlined in Fig. 73.15.

• Of all the photodermatoses, polymorphous light eruption (PMLE) is the most common, followed by photoaggravated dermatoses; drug-induced photosensitivity is also a common disorder.

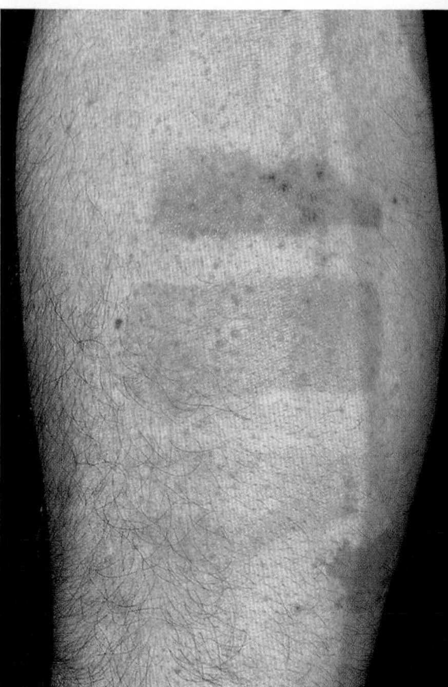

Fig. 73.3 Photoaggravated atopic dermatitis induced by solar stimulator. This was the appearance 24 hours after irradiation. *Courtesy, John L. M. Hawk, MD.*

• *Phototoxicity* results from direct tissue and cellular injury following UVR-induced activation of a phototoxic agent; resembles a sunburn (Table 73.4).

• *Photoallergy* is a delayed-type hypersensitivity response that requires both a photoallergen (usually topical) and UVR exposure; resembles eczema (Table 73.4).

• Photosensitivity to some medications (e.g. methotrexate [see Fig. 73.13], 5-fluorouracil, retinoids) does not require UVR activation of the drug.

• It is important to recognize photodistributed versus photoprotected areas on the body; sparing of certain sites, including behind the ears, under the chin, the upper eyelids, and the nasolabial folds, is a clue to a photodistributed eruption (Fig. 73.17).

• Some patients may have no cutaneous findings at the time of the visit and the diagnosis is based on historical information, in particular those with PMLE and solar urticaria.

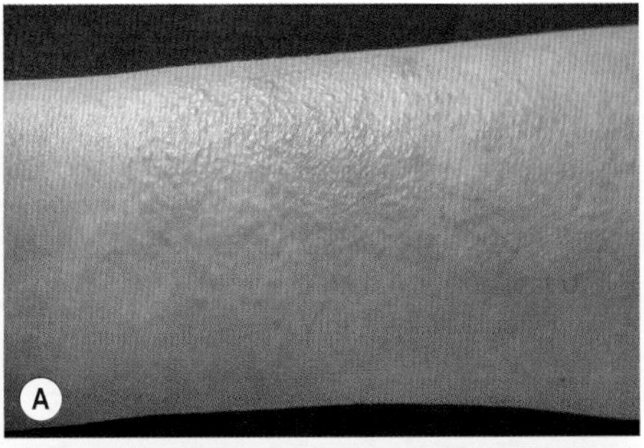

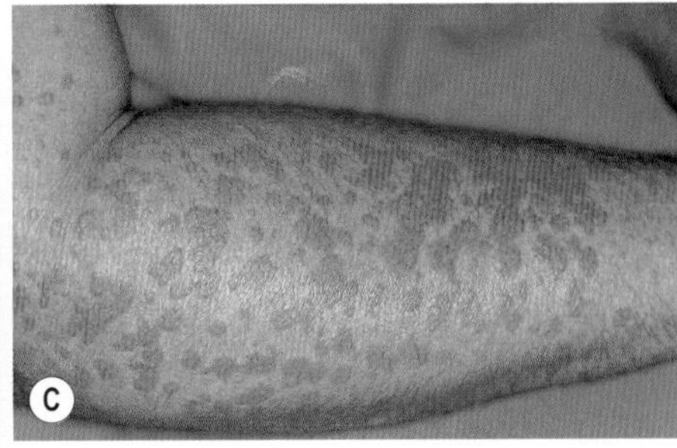

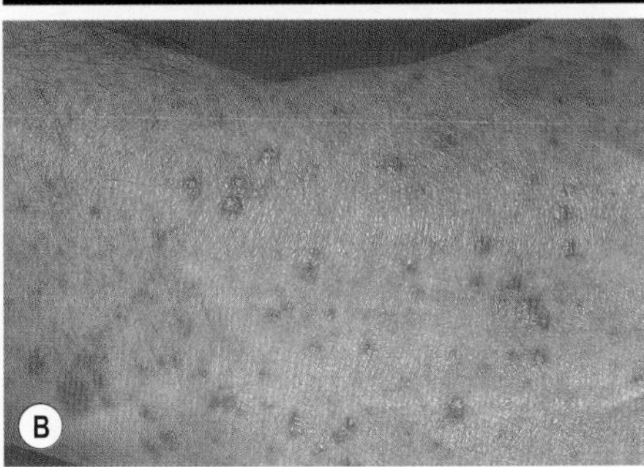

Fig. 73.4 Polymorphous light eruption (PMLE) of the upper extremity. A Small pink edematous papules that are coalescing into plaques on the forearm of an Asian patient. **B** Scattered discrete papulovesicles. **C** Larger and more pronounced edematous papules and plaques. *A, Courtesy, Henry W. Lim, MD and Cheryl F. Rosen, MD; B, Courtesy, NYUDSC; C, Courtesy, YDRSC.*

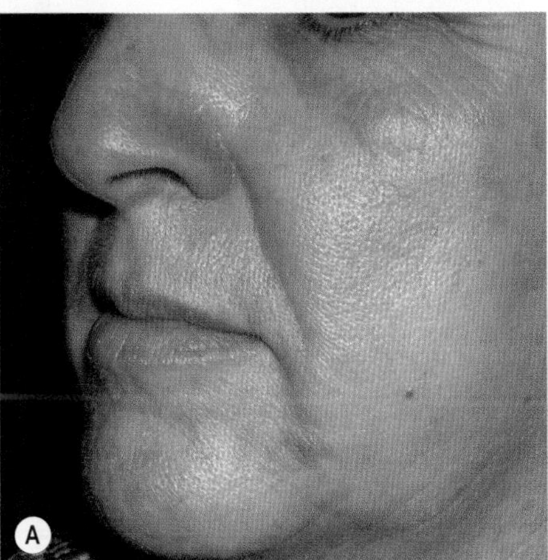

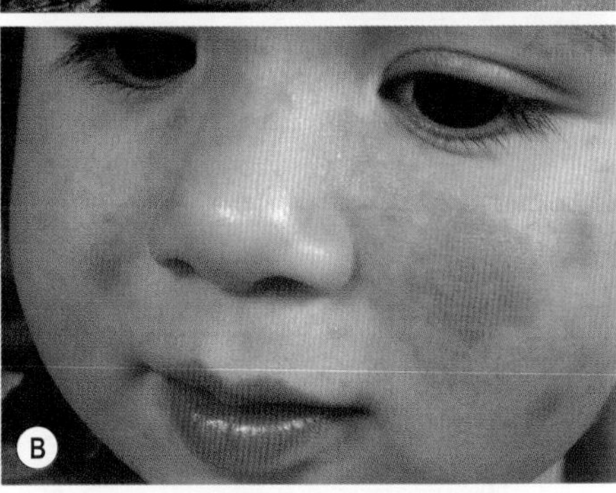

Fig. 73.5 Polymorphous light eruption (PMLE) of the face. A Larger erythematous patch on the nose as well as erythematous plaques on the malar eminence and chin. **B** Edematous erythematous plaques on the cheek in a young child. *A, Courtesy, Henry W. Lim, MD and Cheryl F. Rosen, MD; B, Courtesy, NYUDSC.*

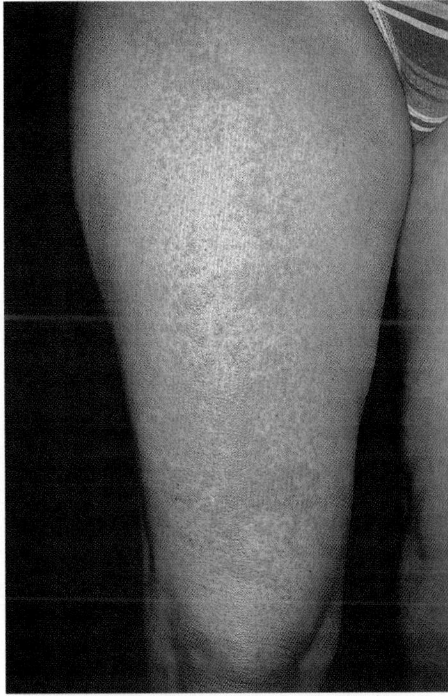

Fig. 73.6 Polymorphous light eruption (PMLE) of the thigh. Edematous papules becoming confluent into plaques. *Courtesy, Jean L. Bolognia, MD.*

CLINICAL FEATURES OF THE IDIOPATHIC, PROBABLY IMMUNOLOGICALLY MEDIATED PHOTODERMATOSES AND PHOTOAGGRAVATED DERMATOSES			
Photodermatosis (action spectrum)	**Clinical features**	**DDx**	**Rx**
Polymorphous light eruption (PMLE) Figs 73.4–73.6 (UVB and UVA; rarely visible light)	• **Onset:** one to several hours after sun exposure; appears primarily in spring and early summer, but initial episode may follow intense sun exposure (e.g. trip to the tropics in the winter) • **Duration:** lesions last days; tends to diminish or cease with repeated sun ("hardening" phenomenon) • **Clinical:** lesions seen on sun-exposed skin (extensor forearms > dorsal hands > face and neck > other areas); typically, recurrences have a similar appearance in a given individual • Symmetric, pruritic, skin-colored to red, various-sized papules and/or papulovesicles that often coalesce into larger plaques • Confluent erythema or edema may be seen on the face • "Juvenile spring eruption" is a clinical variant seen most often in boys, presenting as papulovesicles on the helices of the ears	• LE (lasts weeks to months) • Solar urticaria (more rapid onset and resolution) • Photoaggravated atopic or seborrheic dermatitis (eczematous) • Erythema multiforme • EPP (painful) • Parvovirus infection • In children also consider rare entities in Table 73.5	**Mild:** photoprotection*, topical CS **Severe** • Short course of antimalarials (e.g. hydroxychloroquine 5–6.5 mg/kg/day [ideal body weight] for 4–8 weeks) • "Hardening" via phototherapy (may lead to flare requiring oral CS)
Actinic prurigo Fig. 73.7 (UVR: UVA + UVB)	• **Onset:** childhood; flares within hours of sun exposure • **Duration:** lesions are chronic and persistent throughout childhood, but often fade in adolescence • **Clinical:** seen most commonly in Native Americans; females > males • Typically involves sun-exposed skin (e.g. face/nose, distal limbs), but with time can involve non-exposed skin • Pruritic, erythematous papules and nodules with hemorrhagic crusts and lichenification • Fine, linear or pitted scars may be seen on the face as lesions resolve • Cheilitis, conjunctivitis	• Photoaggravated atopic dermatitis • Photoallergic contact dermatitis • PMLE (resolves more quickly) • Scabies, arthropod bites • Prurigo nodularis	**Mild:** photoprotection*, topical CS or CIs **Moderate–severe** • Antimalarials • "Hardening" phototherapy as for PMLE **Recalcitrant:** thalidomide, azathioprine, cyclosporine

Table 73.2 Clinical features of the idiopathic, probably immunologically mediated photodermatoses and photoaggravated dermatoses. *Continued*

CLINICAL FEATURES OF THE IDIOPATHIC, PROBABLY IMMUNOLOGICALLY MEDIATED PHOTODERMATOSES AND PHOTOAGGRAVATED DERMATOSES			
Photodermatosis (action spectrum)	**Clinical features**	**DDx**	**Rx**
Hydroa vacciniforme (HV) Figs 73.8 and 73.9 (Primarily UVA)	• **Onset:** childhood; flares within hours of sun exposure • **Duration:** active lesions last weeks; may resolve during adolescence or early adulthood • **Clinical:** males > females • Typically presents on sun-exposed skin (e.g. face, dorsal hands) as symmetric, pruritic or painful, erythematous macules and papules that progress to vesicles/bullae with central umbilication and hemorrhagic crusts • Resolves with varioliform scarring • Severe form features ulcerated nodules, a more widespread distribution, systemic findings (e.g. fever, hepatosplenomegaly, high circulating EBV DNA load and NK cells), and a high risk of hemophagocytic syndrome/lymphoma • Patients with HV should be screened for active EBV infection	• Overlaps with EBV-related necrotic hypersensitivity to mosquito bites • HSV, VZV • LE, dermatomyositis • Cutaneous porphyrias • Lymphoma • Histopathology, along with *in situ* hybridization for EBV RNA within lymphocytes, is very helpful in the diagnosis of HV	• Often refractory to therapy, as no effective medication is available for underlying EBV infection **Mild:** photoprotection*, beta-carotene, fish oil, antimalarials **Severe:** thalidomide, azathioprine, cyclosporine, hematopoietic stem cell transplant (if progression to lymphoma)
Chronic actinic dermatitis (CAD) Fig. 73.10 (UVB > UVA; occasionally visible light)	• **Onset:** older age at onset (>50 years) • **Duration:** persistent for years; typically, ~10% of cases resolve within 5 years, ~20% by 10 years, and 50% by 15 years • **Clinical:** males > females; darker phototypes • Presents on sun-exposed skin (initially with sharp cut-off at lines of clothing) as pruritic, eczematous papules and plaques with lichenification • Occasionally pseudolymphomatous papules, plaques, and erythroderma are seen • There is often a coexisting allergic contact dermatitis to plants (e.g. daisies)	• Photoaggravated dermatoses (e.g. atopic dermatitis) • Photoallergic contact dermatitis • Photoallergic drug • LE • Mycosis fungoides	**Mild:** photoprotection*, topical CS and CIs, and avoid relevant contact allergens and drugs **Severe/recalcitrant:** cyclosporine, azathioprine, mycophenolate mofetil, low-dose PUVA

Table 73.2 *Continued* **Clinical features of the idiopathic, probably immunologically mediated photodermatoses and photoaggravated dermatoses.** *Continued*

CLINICAL FEATURES OF THE IDIOPATHIC, PROBABLY IMMUNOLOGICALLY MEDIATED PHOTODERMATOSES AND PHOTOAGGRAVATED DERMATOSES			
Photodermatosis (action spectrum)	**Clinical features**	**DDx**	**Rx**
Solar urticaria Fig. 73.11 (UVA, visible light, rarely UVB; this action spectrum may change over the years)	• **Onset:** within 5–10 minutes of sun exposure; often older age at onset (30s–40s) • **Duration:** lesions typically resolve over 1–2 hours; ~15% of cases resolve within 5 years and ~25% by 10 years • **Clinical:** females > males • Seen on sun-exposed skin only, favoring the upper chest and outer arms • Individual lesions look like typical urticaria and cause pruritus, burning > pain • 20–50% of affected individuals also have atopic dermatitis • Several clinical variants exist, e.g. severe, anaphylactoid attacks; fixed; delayed; and drug-induced	• Other urticarias (not solely photodistributed) • EPP (childhood, pain) • PMLE (more delayed onset and lasts longer) • LE	**Mild:** photoprotection* is recommended but often not helpful because of visible light induction; oral antihistamines **Moderate–severe** • Graduated exposure to UVA, PUVA **Recalcitrant:** antimalarials, omalizumab, cyclosporine, plasmapheresis, IVIg
Photoaggravated dermatoses See Table 73.1 for list of disorders and Fig. 73.3 (UVA, UVB)	• **Onset:** usually flares within hours of sun exposure, but sometimes delayed a day or more • **Duration:** days to months • **Clinical:** exacerbation of underlying skin condition in sun-exposed and sometimes non-sun-exposed areas	• Sweat-aggravated dermatoses • PMLE • CAD	• Photoprotection* and treat the underlying dermatosis

**Photoprotection generally includes avoidance of sun, sun-protective clothing, broad-spectrum sunscreens, hats, sunglasses; for UVA-sensitive disorders, must also caution about protection from UVR received while driving or through glass windows; zinc- and titanium dioxide-based sunscreens are best for visible light-sensitive disorders.*

Table 73.2 *Continued* **Clinical features of the idiopathic, probably immunologically mediated photodermatoses and photoaggravated dermatoses.** CAD, chronic actinic dermatitis; CI, calcineurin inhibitor; EPP, erythropoietic protoporphyria; PMLE, polymorphous light eruption.

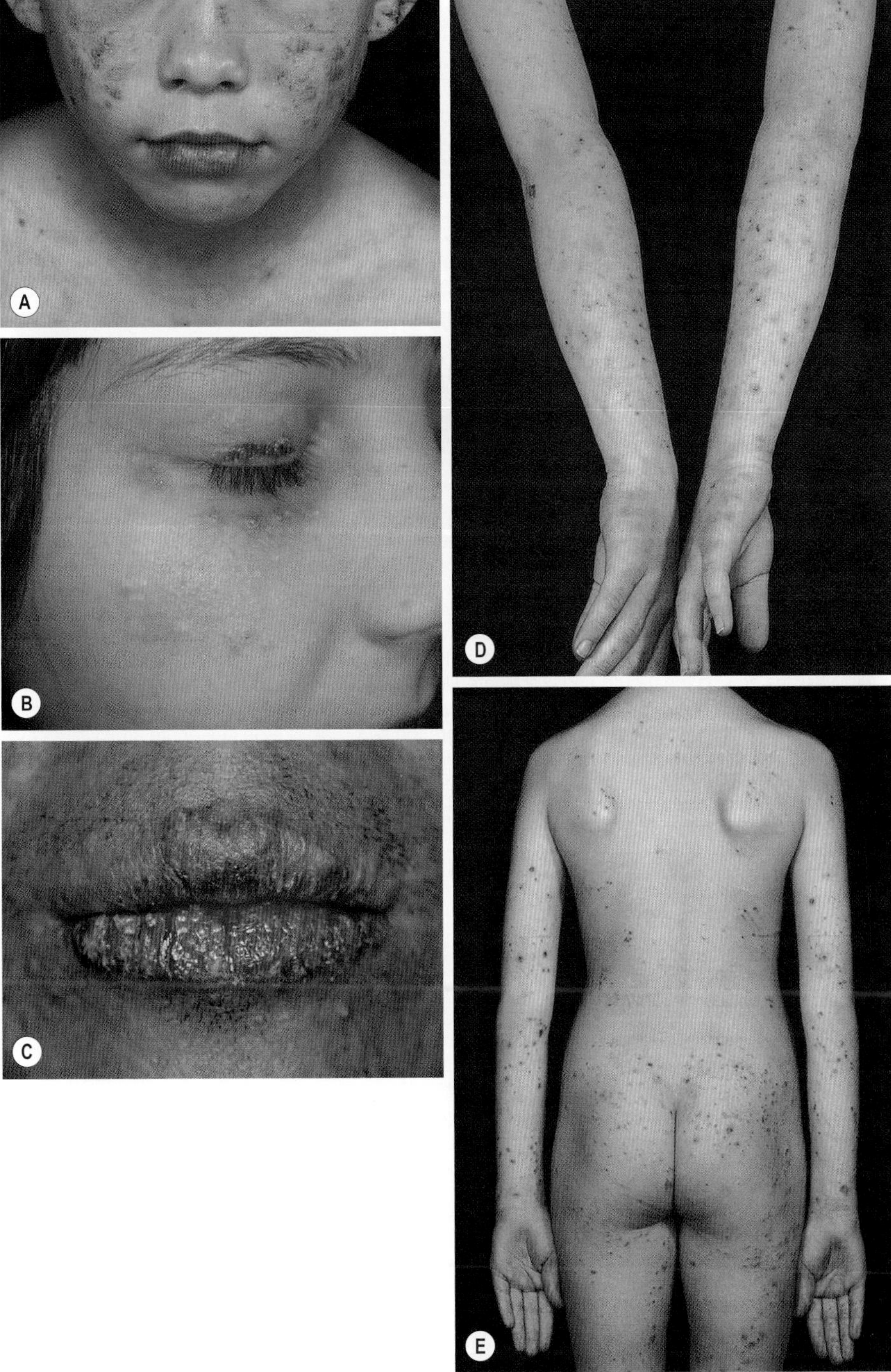

Fig. 73.7 Actinic prurigo. A The clinical features, including a photodistribution and worsening in the summer, are somewhat suggestive of polymorphous light eruption, but the lesions were persistent, and the HLA type was that seen in association with actinic prurigo. Note the involvement of the ears. **B** Multiple papules on the upper cheek, several of which have central crusts. A linear excoriation is seen on the lower portion of the upper eyelid. **C** The cheilitis is more severe on the lower vermilion lip. On the upper lip, chronic inflammation has led to blurring of the border between vermilion lip and the cutaneous lip. **D** The crusted papules are more dense on the distal arms. **E** This patient with severe actinic prurigo has involvement of the buttocks as well as sun-exposed sites. *A, D, E, Courtesy, John L. M. Hawk, MD; B, Courtesy, Henry W. Lim, MD and Cheryl F. Rosen, MD; C, Courtesy, Jean L. Bolognia, MD.*

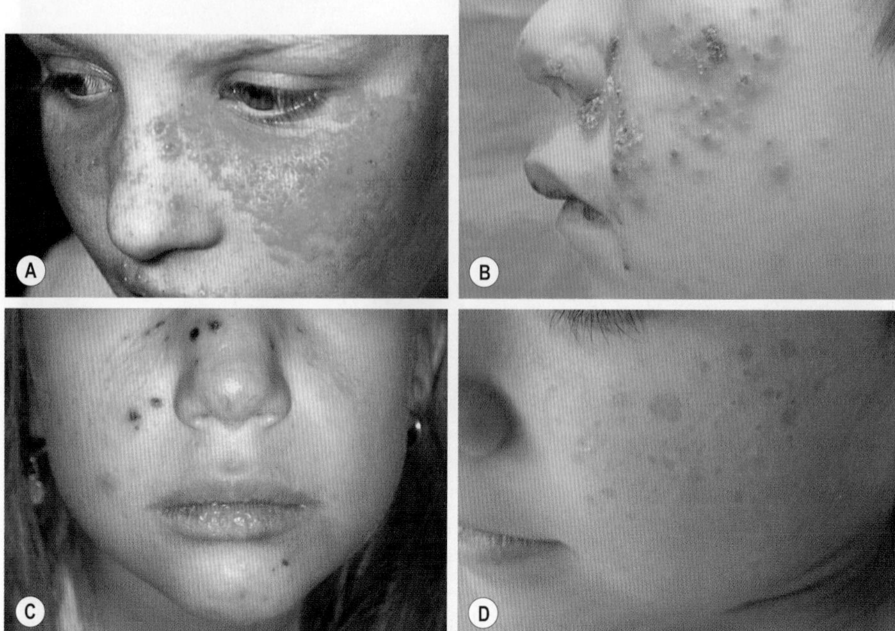

Fig. 73.8 Hydroa vacciniforme. A There is an early, polymorphous light eruption-like appearance, but with vesicles around the mouth and umbilicated lesions on the nose. **B** Papulovesicles with crusting on the nose, cheeks and lips appeared a few days after sun exposure. **C** Hemorrhagic crusts are admixed with varioliform scars; the latter are the sequelae of repeated acute attacks. Note the scaling and erosions of the lower vermilion lip. **D** Varioliform scars and postinflammatory hyperpigmentation on the cheek. *A, Courtesy, John L. M. Hawk, MD; B, D, Courtesy, Tor Shwayder, MD; C, Courtesy, Jean L. Bolognia, MD.*

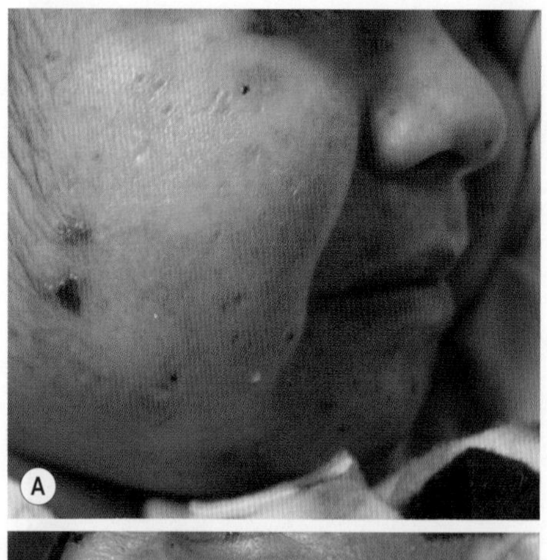

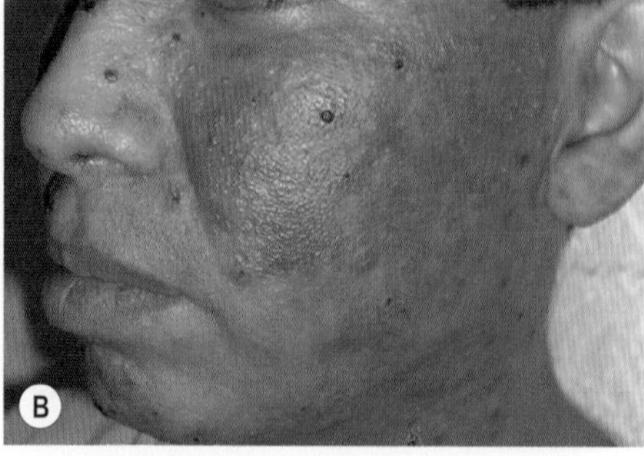

Fig. 73.9 EBV-associated hydroa vacciniforme-like eruption. A This Hispanic child had >50,000 copies of EBV DNA/100,000 WBCs as well as EBV RNA within skin lesions by *in situ* hybridization; he subsequently died of lymphoma. Note the facial edema, erythema, papulovesicles, hemorrhagic crusts, and varioliform scars. **B** Extensive involvement of the face by erythematous edematous plaques with hemorrhagic crusts at sites of vesiculation. *A, Courtesy, Richard Antaya, MD; B, Courtesy, Henry W. Lim, MD and Cheryl F. Rosen, MD.*

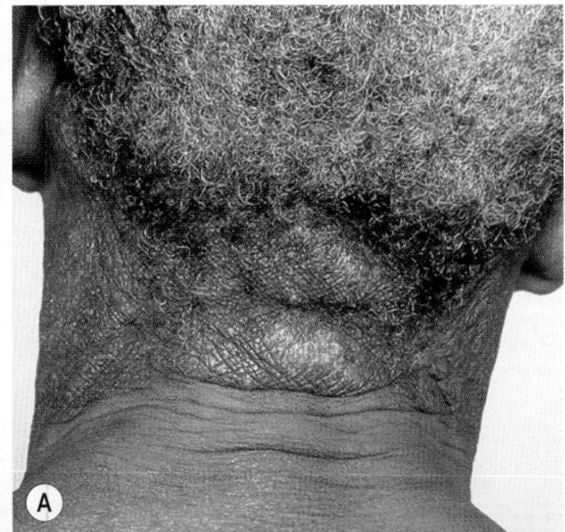

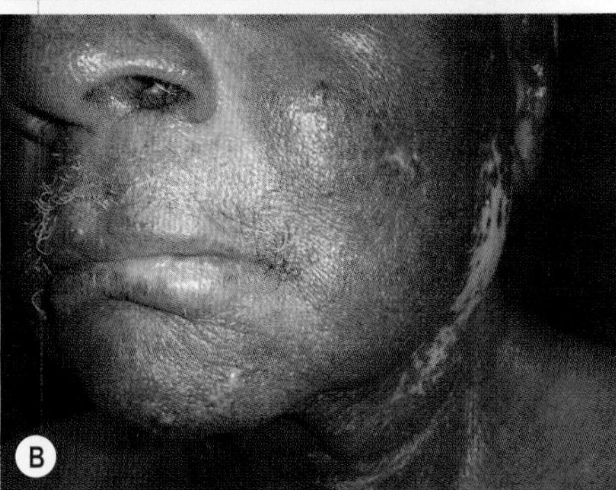

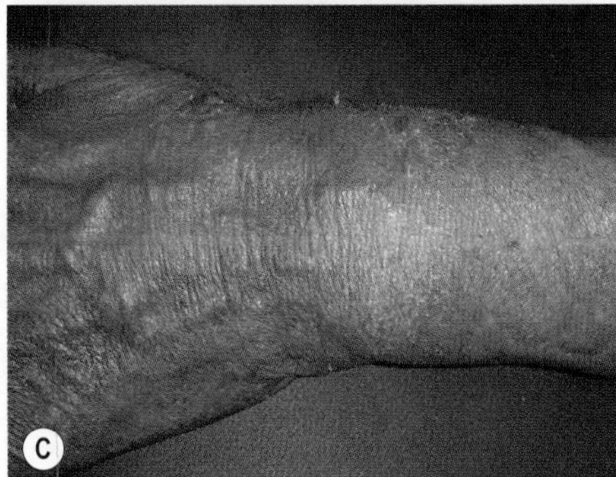

Fig. 73.10 Chronic actinic dermatitis (CAD). **A** Chronic eczematous changes of the posterior neck with lichenification and a sharp cut-off at the collar in a patient with phototype V skin. **B** Lichenification and hyperpigmentation in sun-exposed sites with areas of depigmentation. Note the sparing of sun-protected areas (i.e. nasolabial fold and shoulder). **C** Chronic eczematous changes of the dorsal hand and wrist with associated hyperpigmentation and scaling. Note the sharp cut-off at the distal forearm. *Courtesy, Henry Lim, MD.*

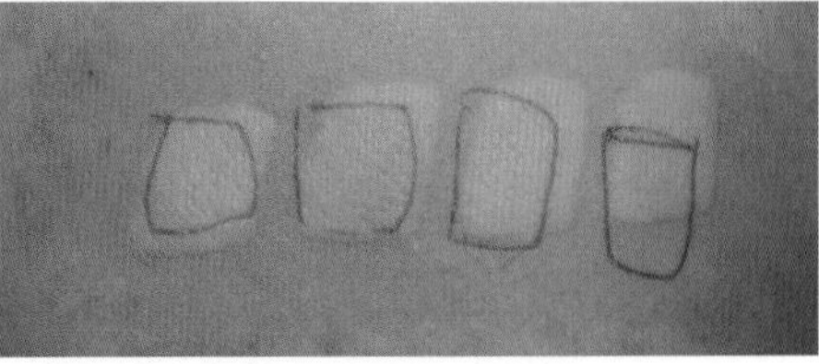

Fig. 73.11 Solar urticaria. Wheal and flare responses within minutes of exposure to UVB irradiation in a patient undergoing phototesting. *Courtesy, John L. M. Hawk, MD.*

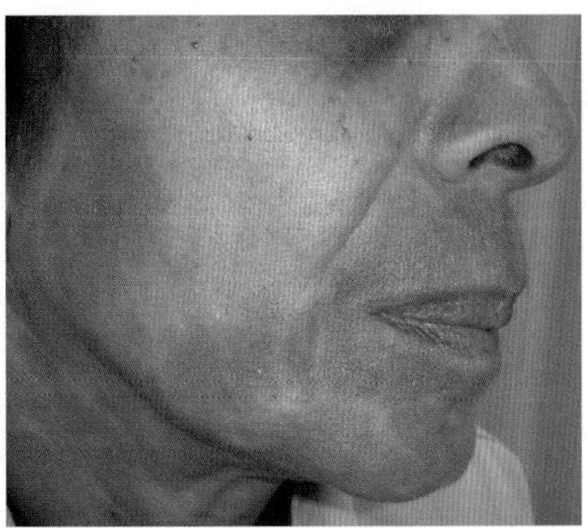

Fig. 73.12 Drug-induced photosensitivity and hyperpigmentation. Gray-brown patches involving the sun-exposed skin of a patient receiving diltiazem. *Courtesy, Henry Lim, MD.*

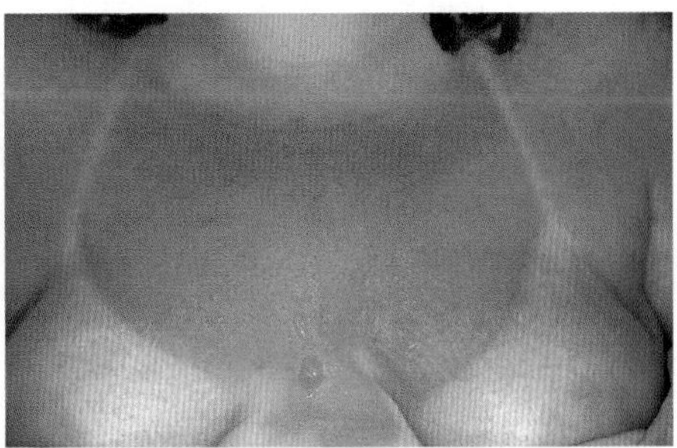

Fig. 73.13 Phototoxic reaction in a patient receiving methotrexate. The erythema and bullae are obviously limited to sun-exposed sites and resemble an exaggerated sunburn. Patients on methotrexate can also experience a "sunburn-recall" phenomenon. *Courtesy, YDRSC.*

CHEMICAL- AND DRUG-INDUCED PHOTOSENSITIVITY		
Disorder and etiology	**Clinical features**	**DDx/evaluation**
Exogenous		
Phototoxicity • Phototoxic drug reaction to systemic medication > phototoxic contact dermatitis to topical medication or chemical (Table 73.4) • Requires exposure to drug or chemical plus exposure to UVR (UVA > UVB)	• **Onset:** hours after sun exposure • **Clinical**: Typically presents as an exaggerated sunburn reaction; associated burning or stinging; when severe, vesicles and/or bullae develop; resolves with desquamation and hyperpigmentation • Other skin findings may include: 1. Photo-onycholysis (e.g. tetracyclines, psoralens) (Ch. 58) 2. Pseudo-PCT (e.g. NSAIDs) (Ch. 41) 3. Lichenoid eruption (e.g. thiazide diuretics [see Fig. 17.12], quinidine)* 4. Slate-gray hyperpigmentation (e.g. amiodarone, diltiazem [see Fig. 73.12], tricyclic antidepressants)	• Sunburn • LE • Photoallergy (see below) • Airborne contact dermatitis • EPP • Solar urticaria **Evaluation** • If persistent despite discontinuation of suspected drug or chemical, consider phototesting and photopatch testing (Fig. 73.16)
Phytophotodermatitis (Ch. 12) • Phototoxic reaction due to exposure to plants ("phyto") that contain a phototoxin plus exposure to UVA • Most commonly due to furocoumarins found in limes, celery, and false Bishop's weed	• **Inflammatory reaction** (onset usually within 1 day): initially erythematous streaks, often with vesicles or bullae, reflecting exposure to the plant or its juice; painful, non-pruritic; configuration may be unusual, depending on the type of exposure • **Delayed pigmentary reaction:** hyperpigmented streaks (occasionally appear without a preceding inflammatory phase); may last months to years	• Allergic contact dermatitis to plants, e.g. poison ivy or poison oak; distribution includes sites that are exposed to the environment but not the sun, e.g. inner arms • May be confused with child abuse

Table 73.3 Chemical- and drug-induced photosensitivity. *Continued*

CHEMICAL- AND DRUG-INDUCED PHOTOSENSITIVITY		
Disorder and etiology	**Clinical features**	**DDx/evaluation**
Photoallergy • Photoallergic contact dermatitis to topical medication or chemical > photoallergic drug reaction to systemic medication • Requires exposure to drug or chemical plus UVR (Table 73.4)	• **Onset:** first exposure: 7–10 days; subsequent: minutes to hours • **Clinical:** pruritic, eczematous eruption**;** occasionally vesicles and bullae	• Allergic contact dermatitis • Photoaggravated dermatosis (e.g. atopic dermatitis) • Airborne contact dermatitis • Phototoxicity **Evaluation** • If persistent despite discontinuation of suspected topical medication or systemic drug, consider phototesting and photopatch testing; photopatch testing is positive, whereas phototoxicity is negative (see Fig. 73.16)
Endogenous		
Erythropoietic protoporphyria (EPP) (Ch. 41)		
Porphyria cutanea tarda (PCT) (Ch. 41)		

Lichenoid drug eruptions, including photolichenoid drug eruptions, are discussed in Chapter 9.

Table 73.3 *Continued* **Chemical- and drug-induced photosensitivity.** Treatment of phototoxic and photoallergic reactions includes discontinuation of the offending agent or medication, photoprotection, symptomatic care, and occasionally topical or oral CS if severe. Photoprotection generally includes avoidance of sun, sun-protective clothing, broad-spectrum sunscreens, hats, and sunglasses; for UVA-sensitive disorders, must also caution about protection from UVR received while driving or through glass windows; zinc-and titanium dioxide-based sunscreens are best for visible light-sensitive disorders. EPP, erythropoietic protoporphyria; PCT, porphyria cutanea tarda.

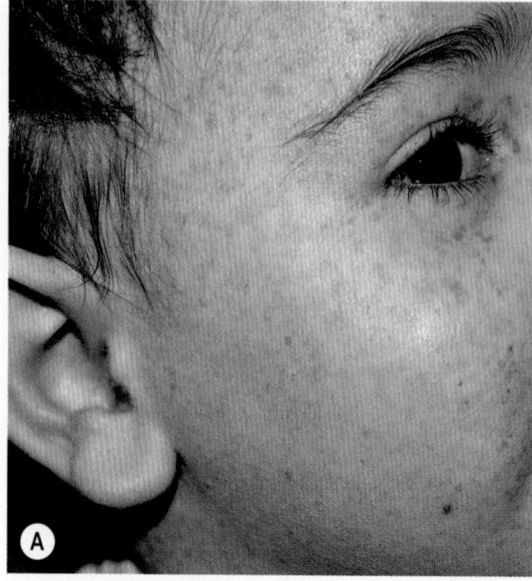

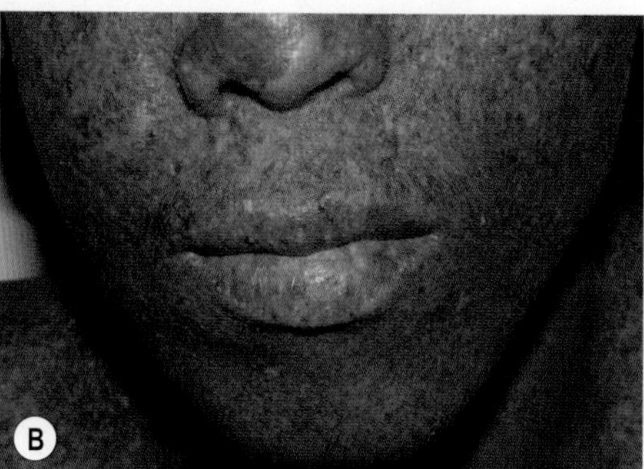

Fig. 73.14 Xeroderma pigmentosum. A Multiple solar lentigines on the face and a history of photosensitivity in this four-year-old child. **B** A 17-year-old boy with skin phototype V who has hyper- and hypopigmentation admixed with scarring, lentigines, and seborrheic as well as actinic keratoses. Note the squamous cell carcinoma *in situ* of the lower lip in association with severe actinic cheilitis. *A, Courtesy, Antonio Torrelo, MD; B, Courtesy, Julie V. Schaffer, MD.*

Grover Disease (Transient Acantholytic Dermatosis)

- Although referred to as transient, is often persistent; thought to result from a combination of photodamage and sweating.
- Occurs primarily in middle-aged males > females as pruritic, often crusted, skin-colored to pink papules and papulovesicles on the trunk, primarily in sun-exposed areas (see Fig. 48.2 and Fig. 73.18).
- **Rx:** difficult but may include low- to mid-potency topical CS and avoidance of exacerbating factors (e.g. heat, friction, sun exposure).

For further information see Ch. 87 from *Dermatology, Fourth Edition*.

For additional online figures and tables visit www.expertconsult.com 

COMMON PHOTOTOXIC AND PHOTOALLERGIC AGENTS	
Common phototoxic agents	**Common photoallergic agents**
• Antiarrhythmics Amiodarone Quinidine • Anti-fibrotic agents Pirfenidone • Triazole antifungals Voriconazole* • Antimicrobials Quinolones (e.g. ciprofloxacin, sparfloxacin, nalidixic acid) Sulfonamides Tetracyclines (e.g. doxycycline*, demeclocycline) • Calcium channel blockers Diltiazem (see Fig. 73.12) • Diuretics Furosemide Thiazides* • Nonsteroidal anti-inflammatory drugs Nabumetone Naproxen Piroxicam • Phenothiazines Chlorpromazine Prochlorperazine • Photodynamic therapy agents Aminolevulinic acid Methyl aminolevulinate • Psoralens (e.g. 5-, 8-methoxypsoralen) • St. John's wort (hypericin) • Sulfonylureas • Tar (topical) • Targeted therapies Vemurafenib*	**Topical agents** • Sunscreens (e.g. oxybenzone [benzophenone-3], octocrylene) • Fragrances 6-Methylcoumarin Musk ambrette Sandalwood oil • Antimicrobial agents Bithionol Chlorhexidine Fenticlor Hexachlorophene • Nonsteroidal anti-inflammatory drugs Diclofenac Ketoprofen • Phenothiazines Chlorpromazine Promethazine **Systemic agents** • Antiarrhythmics Quinidine • Antimalarials Quinine • Antifungals Griseofulvin • Antimicrobials Quinolones (e.g. enoxacin, lomefloxacin) Sulfonamides • Nonsteroidal anti-inflammatory drugs Ketoprofen Piroxicam**

**Also cause accelerated photocarcinogenesis.*
***Often have positive patch test to thimerosol.*

Table 73.4 Common phototoxic and photoallergic agents.

CLINICAL FEATURES OF SELECTED INHERITED PHOTOSENSITIVITY DISORDERS ASSOCIATED WITH DEFECTIVE DNA NUCLEOTIDE EXCISION REPAIR OR CHROMOSOMAL INSTABLILITY	
Inherited disorder	**Clinical features**
Defective DNA nucleotide excision repair	
Xeroderma pigmentosum (XP) (Fig. 73.14)	• Photosensitivity, xerosis, early onset lentigines (about age 2 years) and dyspigmentation • BCCs, SCCs, cutaneous melanomas in sun-exposed areas; median age of NMSC onset is 9 years & for melanomas, 22 years • Photophobia, keratitis, corneal opacification • Increased incidence of intraoral and ocular malignancies as well as CNS tumors • Neurologic abnormalities (e.g. hyporeflexia, deafness, seizures)
Cockayne syndrome (CS)	• Photosensitivity, pigmented macules, thinned skin, alopecia, nail clubbing, acral edema, prominent ears, dental caries • Progressive signs of premature aging • Cachectic dwarfism, microcephaly, hypogonadism, deafness, intellectual impairment • No increase in malignancies
Chromosomal instability	
Bloom syndrome	• More common in Ashkenazi Jews • Presents in first few weeks of life with malar erythema and telangiectasias, exacerbated by sun exposure • Café-au-lait macules with adjacent hypopigmented macules • Growth delay, short stature, normal intelligence, recurrent infections • Increased incidence of internal malignancies (e.g. leukemia)
Rothmund–Thomson syndrome	• Presents in first few months of life with photodistributed erythema, edema, and vesicles on cheeks and face • Later develop poikiloderma on dorsal extremities and buttocks • Acral keratoses, short stature and radial ray defects • Increased risk of SCC and osteosarcoma • Normal immune function and intelligence

Table 73.5 Clinical features of selected inherited photosensitivity disorders associated with defective DNA nucleotide excision repair or chromosomal instability. All of these diseases are rare and inherited in an autosomal recessive fashion. Another photosensitivity disorder due to hereditary defects in DNA repair is trichothiodystrophy (TTD; see Table 46.1).

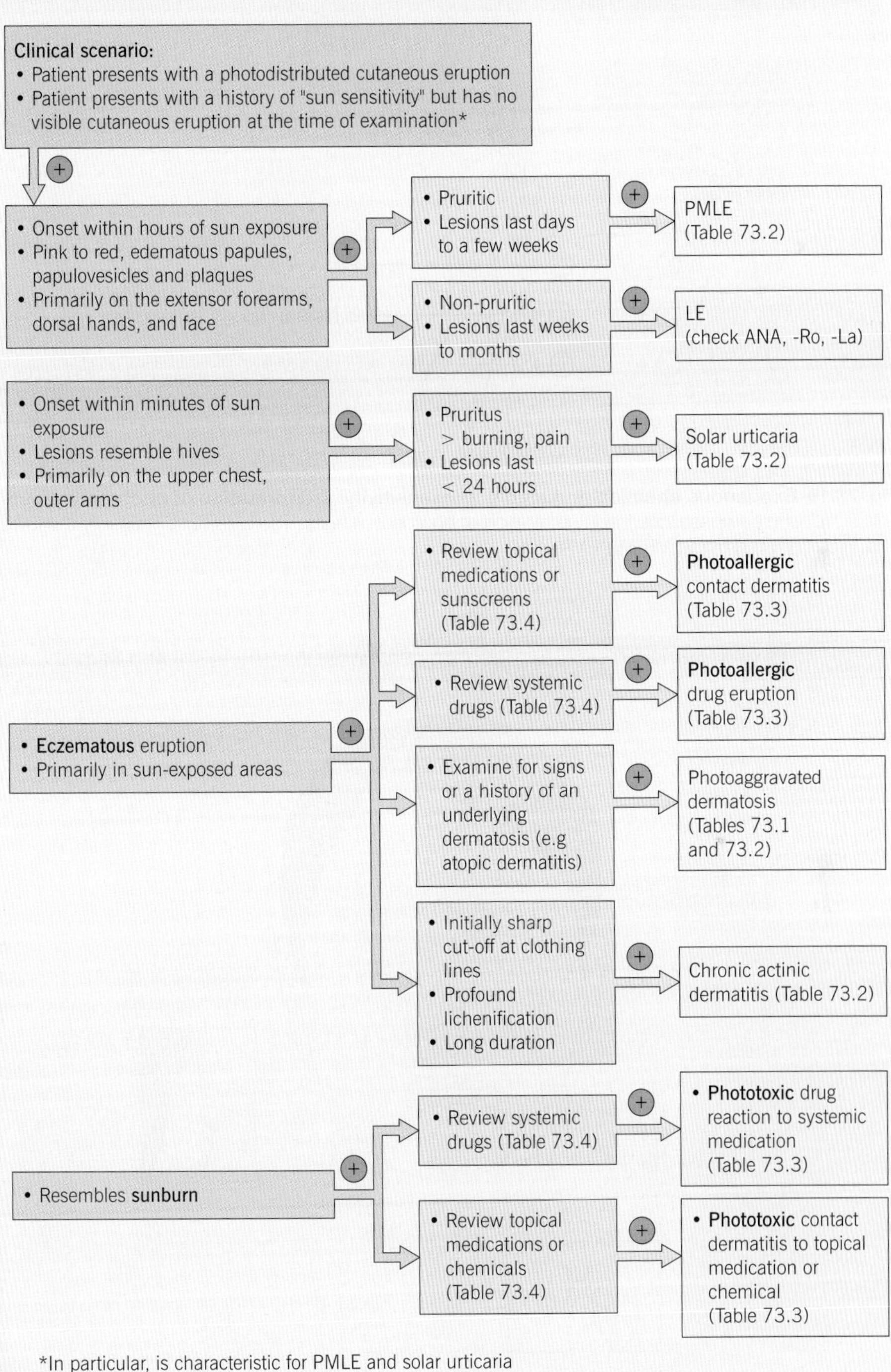

Fig. 73.15 Clues to the diagnosis of specific photodermatoses in adults. PMLE, polymorphous light eruption.

EXOGENOUS CHEMICAL-INDUCED PHOTOSENSITIVITY: INTERPRETATION OF PHOTOPATCH TESTS

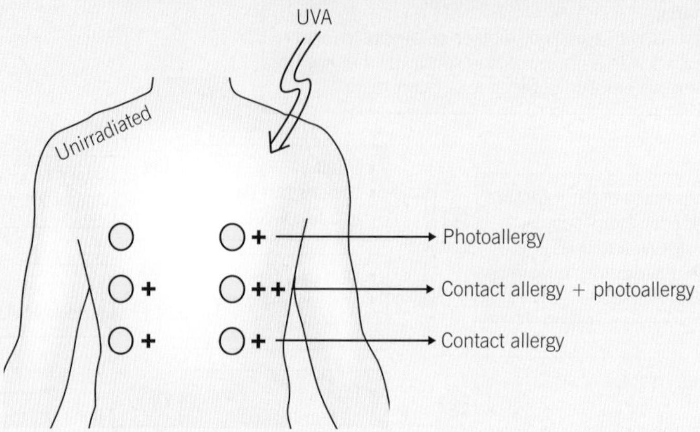

Fig. 73.16 Exogenous chemical-induced photosensitivity: interpretation of photopatch tests. This schematic demonstrates the interpretation of photopatch tests. The UVA dose is usually the lower of 5 J/cm^2, or 50% of the MED to UVA.

SITES OF SPARING IN PHOTODISTRIBUTED DERMATOSES OF THE HEAD AND NECK

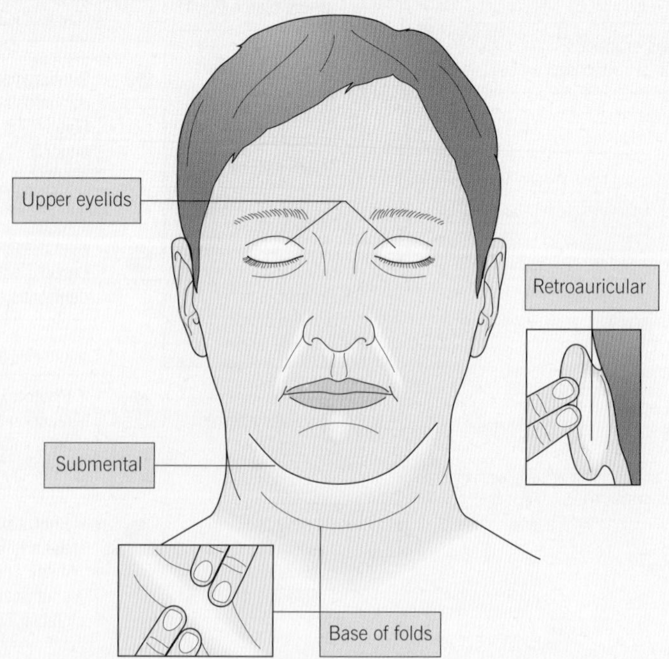

Fig. 73.17 Sites of sparing in photodistributed dermatoses of the head and neck (e.g. chronic actinic dermatitis and photoallergic dermatitis). Relatively sun-protected sites include the upper eyelids, nasolabial folds, retroauricular areas, submental region, and deepest portion of skin furrows. In airborne contact dermatitis, these areas may be involved.

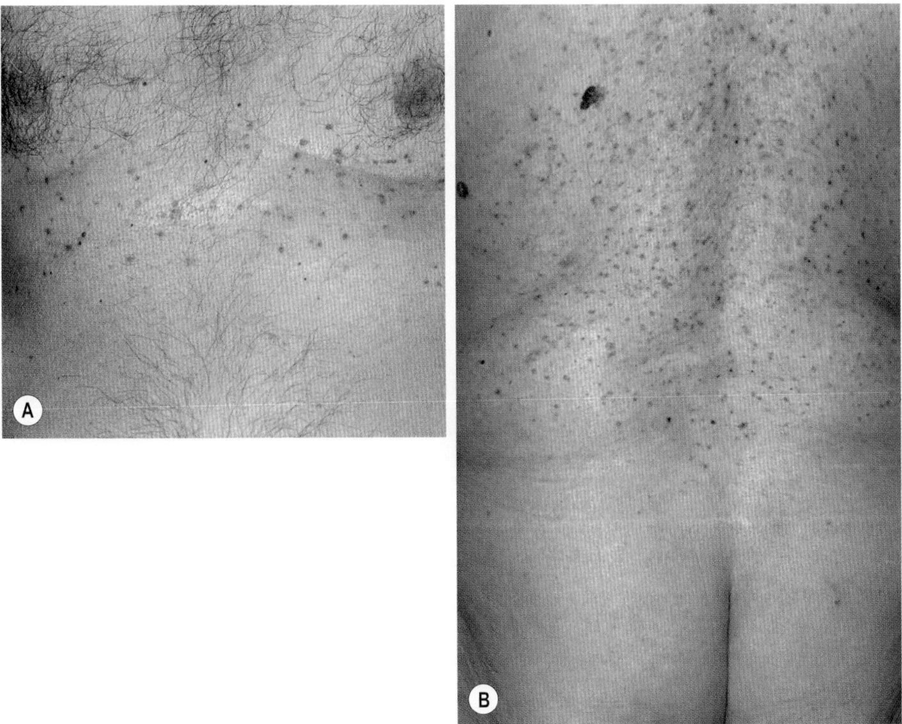

Fig. 73.18 Grover disease. Crusted papules of the trunk **(A)** and obvious sparing of the sun-protected skin of the buttocks **(B)** in this patient with significant photodamage.
Courtesy, Jean L. Bolognia, MD.

74 Environmental and Sports-Related Skin Diseases

Cutaneous Injury Due to Heat Exposure

Thermal Burns

- Traumatic injury to the skin caused by an external heat source (Fig. 74.1).
- The depth of the burn injury depends on the temperature of and the amount of contact time with the heat source as well as the thickness of the affected skin.
- The *burn depth* determines the severity and classification of the injury, its potential for healing, and need for surgical intervention (Table 74.1).
- An exact classification of the burn injury may not be possible upon initial presentation and may take up to 3 weeks to determine; burns may be deeper than initially suspected when occurring on thinner skin (e.g. in pediatric and elderly patients; on ears, volar forearms, medial thighs, and perineum).
- The *extent of burn injury* is expressed as a percentage of the body surface area (BSA) involved and is essential for guiding therapy and determining a patient's disposition (e.g. hospital admission for a partial-thickness burn involving >10% BSA in an individual 10–50 years of age).

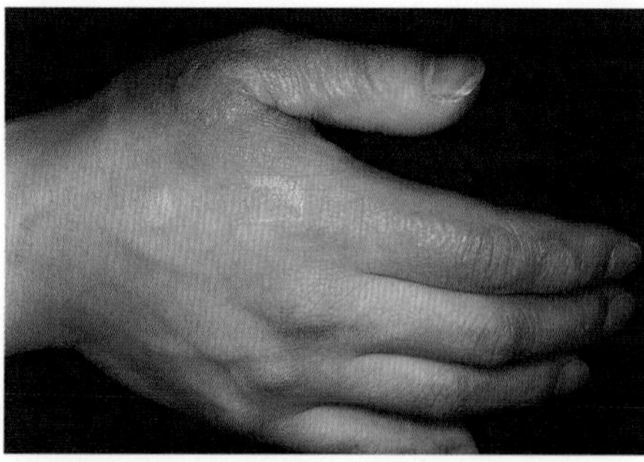

Fig. 74.1 Thermal burn. This superficial partial-thickness burn is characterized by bullae that contain serous fluid. *Courtesy, Kalman Watsky, MD.*

- The most accurate method for estimating BSA involvement in adults and children is the Lund–Browder chart (https://www.remm.nlm.gov/LundBrowder.pdf); the "rule of nines" method is perhaps more expeditious in adults, but it cannot be used for children (Fig. 74.2).
- General principles of treatment are outlined in Table 74.1.

Erythema Ab Igne

- Localized areas of reticulated erythema and hyperpigmentation due to chronic exposure to heat that is below the threshold for a thermal burn.
- Multiple heat sources have been implicated (Table 74.2).
- Most commonly seen in the lumbosacral region (due to heating pads applied to relieve pain from degenerative spinal disease); more recently seen on the anterior thighs from heated batteries in laptop computers.
- In long-standing erythema ab igne (latency period ≥30 years) there is an associated risk of malignant degeneration, resulting in thermal keratoses and SCC.
- *Early lesions*: asymptomatic, initially transient, blanchable macular erythema in a broad, reticulated pattern that corresponds to the venous plexus; size and shape approximates that of the heat source (Fig. 74.3A).
- *Later lesions*: dusky reticulated hyperpigmentation; lesions are fixed and no longer blanchable (Fig. 74.3B).
- *End stage*: may become keratotic and bullae may appear.
- **DDx:** livedo reticularis, cutis marmorata, poikiloderma (e.g. due to CTCL, dermatomyositis, several genodermatoses); the latter has a tighter net-like pattern.
- **Rx:** remove the heat source; if applicable, identify and treat the underlying source of pain.

CLASSIFICATION AND TREATMENT OF THERMAL BURNS		
Type	Depth	Clinical features / Treatment*
FIRST DEGREE (Superficial)	Epidermis only	• Pain, tenderness • Dry, erythema, no blistering • Blanches with pressure • Heals without scar in 3–6 days
		• No specific treatment needed • Aloe vera**, sun protection
SECOND DEGREE (Partial thickness – superficial) (**Fig. 74.1**)	Epidermis and superficial dermis	• Severe pain and tenderness • Serous or hemorrhagic bullae, deep rubor, erosion and exudation • Blanches with pressure • Heals in 7–21 days with mild but variable scarring
		• Daily dressing changes with topical antibiotic (e.g. silver sulfadiazine¶, silver nitrate¶¶, mafenide acetate, mupirocin) and gauze until re-epithelialization occurs*** • Sun protection
SECOND DEGREE (Partial thickness – deep)	Epidermis and most of dermis destroyed, including deep follicular structures	• Intense pain but reduced sensation (pressure only) • Deep red to pale and speckled in color • Does not blanch with pressure • Serosanguinous bullae (easily unroofed), erosions • May appear devitalized initially • Prolonged healing time (>21 days) • Hypertrophic scars and marked wound contracture
		• Surgical intervention¶¶¶
THIRD DEGREE (Full thickness)	Full-thickness epidermal and dermal destruction	• Sensation to deep pressure only • Dry, hard, waxy white to gray or charred black in color • Does not blanch with pressure • Small lesions heal with significant scarring • Most require surgical correction
		• Surgical intervention¶¶¶
FOURTH DEGREE	Extends through the skin into fascia, muscle, bone, and/or joints	• Sensation to deep pressure only • Does not heal unless surgical intervention • Potentially life-threatening
		• Surgical intervention¶¶¶

Clinical features are given in the first row of each type and **Treatment*** in the second.

Table 74.1 Classification and treatment of thermal burns.

Footnotes to Table 74.1:

**General principles of treatment include removal of the heat source; assessment and treatment of cardiopulmonary issues; cool compresses; pain control; cleaning of the wound (soap and water) and removal of foreign material; prevention of infection; tetanus prophylaxis; and creation of a proper wound healing environment.*

***May act as an anti-inflammatory agent and decrease levels of thromboxane, but can cause allergic contact dermatitis.*

****A basic dressing may include a first layer of a nonadherent gauze (e.g. Adaptic or Xeroform), a second layer of dry gauze, and an outer layer of wrapped gauze.*

¶Extensive use/percutaneous absorption may cause leukopenia, pseudoeschar, and argyria.

¶¶Potential for argyria.

¶¶¶Serial excisions; skin substitutes.

ASSESSING THE EXTENT OF BODY SURFACE AREA (BSA) INVOLVEMENT IN BURN INJURIES: RULE OF NINES

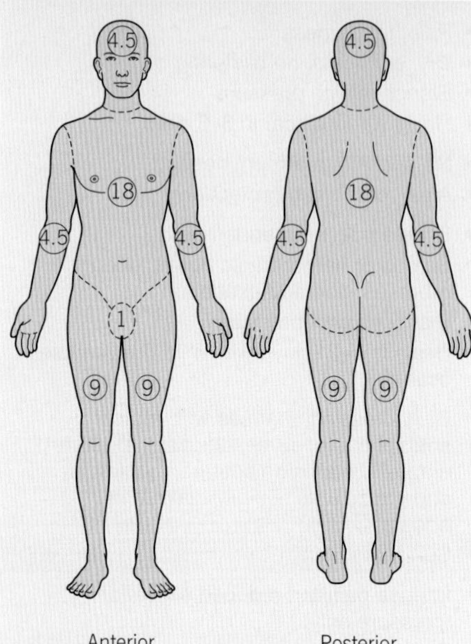

Fig. 74.2 Assessing the extent of body surface area (BSA) involvement in burn injuries: rule of nines. In adults, an estimate of burn extent is often based on this surface area distribution chart. Infants and children have a relatively increased head:trunk surface area ratio and this chart is ineffective for them. Note that the palm is ~1% of BSA and can be used for estimating patchy areas. These estimates are also used for primary cutaneous disorders. Only partial- and full-thickness burns are considered in BSA measurements. The most accurate method of estimating the BSA involvement of burn injury in adults and children is with the Lund–Browder chart (https://www.remm.nlm.gov/LundBrowder.pdf).

Burns Associated with MRI and Fluoroscopy

MRI

- MRI may produce first-, second-, or third-degree burns due to metal or wire contact with skin, creating a closed-loop conduction system.
- The shape and size of the burns are determined by the conductor causing the injury (e.g. circular burns under ECG electrodes).

FLUOROSCOPY

- Fluoroscopy, especially when performed repeatedly in patients with cardiovascular disease, may result in radiation-induced injury (radiodermatitis).
- This radiodermatitis may be acute, but with time continued changes can develop, e.g. hair loss, desquamation, permanent erythema, and ulceration (Fig. 74.4).

HEAT SOURCES REPORTED TO CAUSE ERYTHEMA AB IGNE

- Heating pads
- Hot water bottles
- Electric stove/heater
- Open fires
- Coal stoves
- Peat fires
- Wood stoves
- Sauna belt
- Prolonged hot bathing
- Steam radiators
- Heated car seats
- Heated reclining chairs
- Heating blanket
- Hot bricks
- Infrared lamps
- Microwave popcorn
- Laptop computer*

Anterior thighs >> abdomen

Table 74.2 Heat sources reported to cause erythema ab igne. *Courtesy, Michael L. Smith, MD.*

Cutaneous Injury Due to Cold Exposure

Frostbite

- Can occur when the skin temperature drops below about −2°C (28°F).
- Tissue freezing, vasoconstriction, and inflammatory mediator release are key features of its pathophysiology.
- There are four categories of severity based on depth of tissue injury; these are only recognizable upon rewarming (Fig. 74.5).
- Symptomatically, early erythema, edema, and numbness are replaced by marked hyperemia and pain.
- **Rx:** rapid rewarming in a warm water bath is the cornerstone of treatment, followed by appropriate wound care.

Pernio (Chilblains)

- An abnormal inflammatory response to cold, damp, non-freezing conditions.

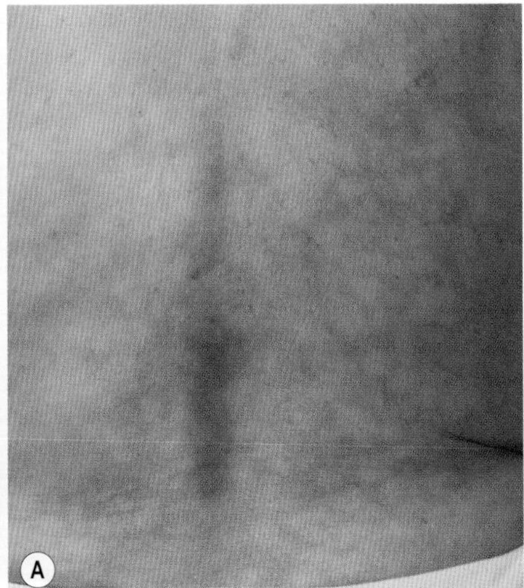

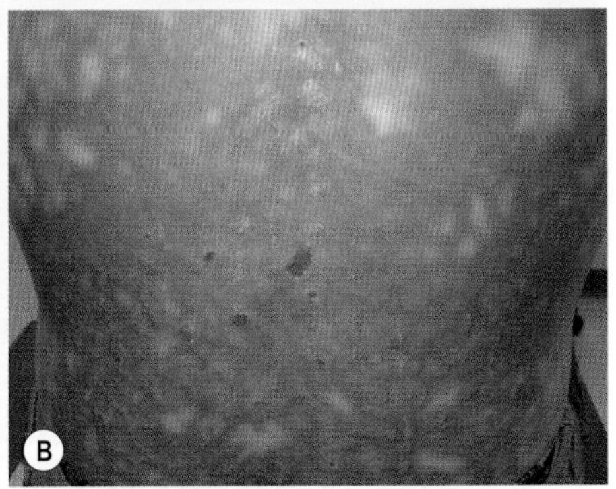

Fig. 74.3 Erythema ab igne. A Early phase with pink reticulated patches on the back, resulting from overuse of a heating blanket. **B** Later phase with large area of reticulated hyperpigmentation and superimposed pink keratotic plaques centrally. *A, Courtesy, Karynne O. Duncan, MD; B, Courtesy, Peter Klein, MD.*

- Classically presents with single or multiple erythematous to blue-violet macules, papules, or nodules distributed symmetrically on distal toes and fingers (Fig. 74.6), and less often on the remainder of the foot or hand, nose and ears.
- In severe cases, blistering and ulceration may be seen.
- Patients describe pruritus, burning, or pain; histopathology demonstrates a perivascular and perieccrine lymphohistiocytic infiltrate.
- Lesions typically resolve in 1–3 weeks but can take much longer or become chronic in elderly patients with venous insufficiency.

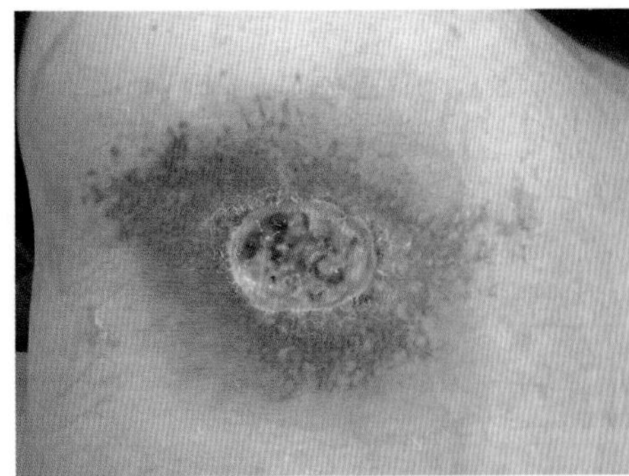

Fig. 74.4 Fluoroscopy-induced radiation dermatitis. The left upper back is a characteristic location for patients who have undergone attempts at coronary artery revascularization (e.g. angioplasty, stent placement). *Courtesy, Jeffrey P. Callen, MD.*

- **DDx:** chilblain lupus; frostbite; lupus pernio (a variant of sarcoidosis involving mainly the nose and ears) (Table 74.3).
- **Rx:** adequate clothing; avoidance of cold, damp conditions; keeping feet dry; avoidance of smoking; and use of nifedipine in recalcitrant cases.

Cutaneous Injury Due to Chemical Exposure

Chemical Hair Discoloration

- May be a voluntary cosmetic change or the result of chemical or metal exposure (Table 74.4).
- Most hair discoloration normalizes over time upon discontinuation of the offending exposure.
- Numerous anecdotal treatment remedies have been described, e.g. hot oil, hydrogen peroxide, and various shampoos (e.g. alkaline or EDTA-based).

Chronic Arsenical Dermatoses

- Chronic arsenic exposure most often occurs via contaminated drinking water or occupational exposure; long latency period (up to 40 years).
- Chronic arsenicism is characterized by mottled hyperpigmentation with areas of hypopigmentation; arsenical keratoses on the palms and soles (Fig. 74.7); multiple non-melanoma skin cancers (particularly Bowen disease); peripheral neuropathy and internal malignancies (e.g. bladder, lung, liver).

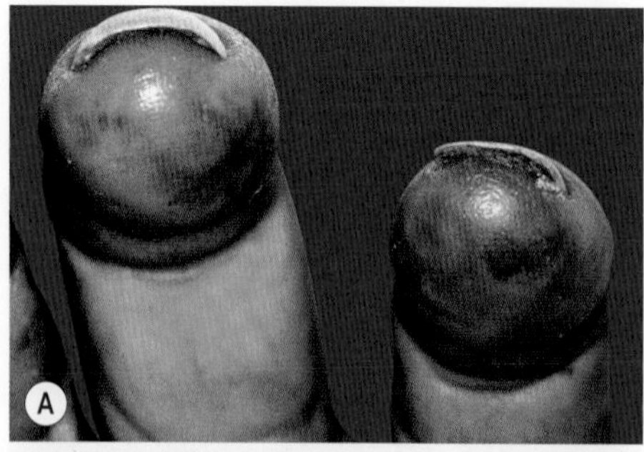

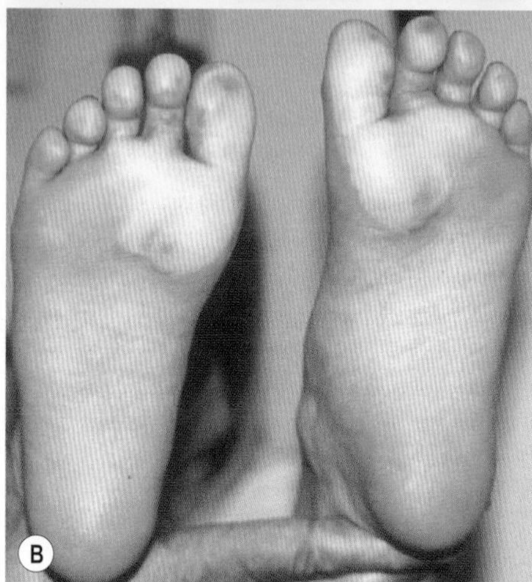

Fig. 74.5 Frostbite. A Erythema, edema, and hemorrhage are seen on the fingertips in a ***first-degree frostbite (frostnip)***; full recovery is expected, with only mild desquamation. **B** Bullae filled with clear fluid on the distal plantar surfaces in a ***second-degree frostbite***; many such patients develop long-term sensory neuropathies. In ***third-degree frostbite*** there is full-thickness dermal loss with hemorrhagic bullae or waxy, dry, mummified skin. In ***fourth-degree frostbite*** there is full-thickness loss of the entire part, with skin, muscle, tendon, and bone damage; amputation may occur. *A, Courtesy, Michael L. Smith, MD; B, Courtesy, Timothy Givens, MD.*

Cutaneous Findings Resulting from Toxic and Heavy Metal Exposure

- Various toxic and heavy metals are known to cause irritant and/or allergic contact dermatitis, including the following (Table 74.5):
  - ***Beryllium*** is a metal known to cause dermatitis and sarcoidosis-like granulomas of the skin and lung
  - ***Gold***, as an elemental salt, can cause a variety of cutaneous eruptions (Table 74.6)

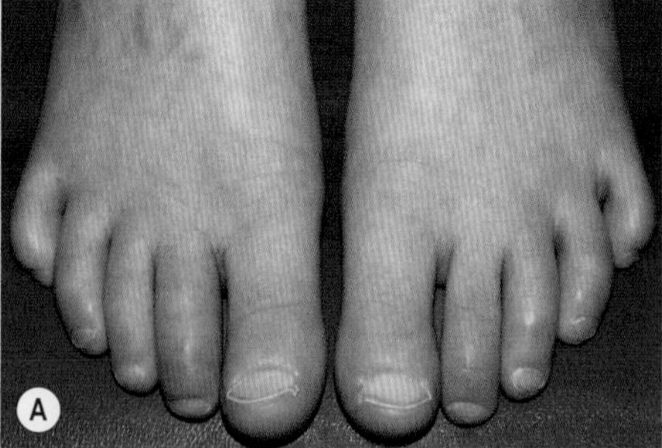

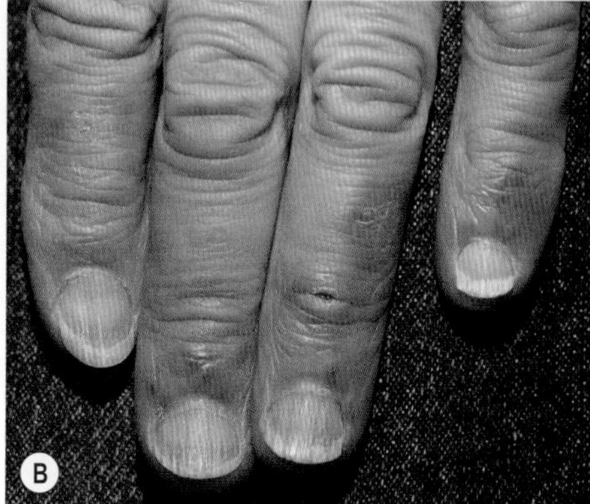

Fig. 74.6 Pernio. A Distal erythema of multiple toes with some edema in a symmetric pattern. **B** Erythematous papules and plaques of the distal fingers with scaling and an erosion. *Courtesy, Kalman Watsky, MD.*

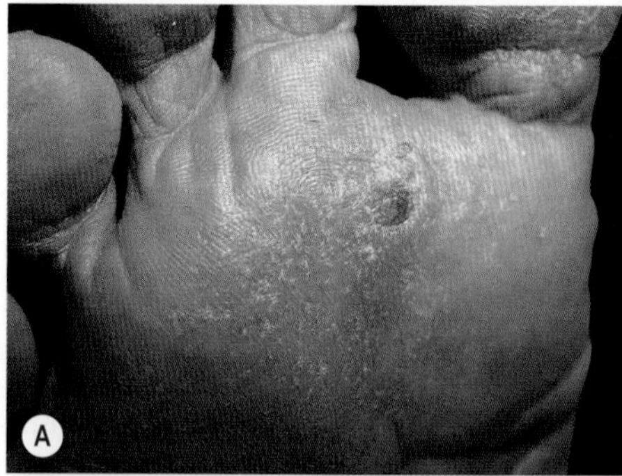

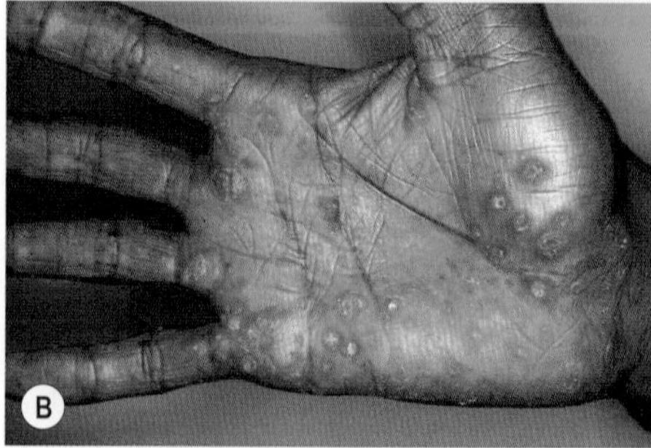

Fig. 74.7 Cutaneous manifestations of chronic arsenicism. A, B Arsenical keratoses on the plantar and palmar surface. *A, Courtesy, YDRSC; B, Courtesy, Jeffrey P. Callen, MD.*

DIFFERENTIAL DIAGNOSIS AND EVALUATION OF SKIN LESIONS INDUCED BY NON-FREEZING COLD EXPOSURE		
Disorder	**Features**	**Possible associated conditions**
Acrocyanosis	Red to purple discoloration Hands and feet Painless	Erythromelalgia Cryoproteins Anorexia nervosa
Pernio (chilblains) (see Fig. 74.6)	Erythrocyanotic Symmetric distribution of painful macules and papules, mostly on digits; scaling develops as lesions heal	Low body mass index SARS-CoV-2 infection Hematologic disorders (e.g. paraproteinemia) Viral hepatitis
Raynaud phenomenon (see Ch. 35)	Well-demarcated pallor, followed by blue, then red discoloration; painful Idiopathic form (common) – no nail-fold capillary changes; pulp ulcerations rare	AI-CTD (especially systemic sclerosis) Blood dyscrasias (e.g. polycythemia vera) Drugs (e.g. beta-blockers, bleomycin) Trauma
Livedo reticularis (see Ch. 87)	Bluish, broad reticulated patches corresponding to venous plexus May be idiopathic	Vascular occlusive diseases (e.g. severe atherosclerosis) AI-CTD (e.g. lupus erythematosus) Hematologic disorders (e.g. antiphospholipid syndrome) Infections (e.g. hepatitis C infection) Medications (e.g. amantadine)
Cold panniculitis (see Ch. 83)	Erythematous indurated plaques, most often on cheeks of children or thighs in equestrians	
Cold urticaria (see Ch. 14)	Cold-induced wheals	Cryoproteins Familial cold autoinflammatory syndrome
Chilblain lupus (see Ch. 33)	Cold-induced acral lesions, similar to pernio Histopathologic features of LE Coexistent LE	
Retiform purpura due to cryoproteins* • Cryoglobulins • Cryofibrinogen** • Cold agglutinins or hemolysins**	Favors acral sites (see Fig. 18.3) Cold serum protein precipitate Cold plasma protein precipitate RBCs agglutinate or lyse in cold Paroxysmal hemoglobinuria if RBC lysis	Type I (monoclonal) cryoglobulinemia due to plasma cell dyscrasias Lymphoproliferative disorders (e.g. Waldenström macroglobulinemia) Infections (e.g. hepatitis C infection) Malignancies (e.g. non-Hodgkin lymphoma) Infections (e.g. with *Mycoplasma*, EBV, CMV) Lymphoproliferative disorders

Table 74.3 Differential diagnosis and evaluation of skin lesions induced by non-freezing cold exposure. *Continued*

DIFFERENTIAL DIAGNOSIS AND EVALUATION OF SKIN LESIONS INDUCED BY NON-FREEZING COLD EXPOSURE
Evaluation considerations
• CBC with platelets and differential • ANA with profile • Hypercoagulable evaluation (see Table 18.5) • Cryoprotein analysis • Serum protein electrophoresis and immunofixation electrophoresis • Lesional biopsy

**Acrocyanosis, Raynaud phenomenon, livedo reticularis, and cold urticaria can also be observed in association with cryoproteins.*
***Rarely cause cold-related occlusion syndromes.*

Table 74.3 *Continued* **Differential diagnosis and evaluation of skin lesions induced by non-freezing cold exposure.** *Courtesy, Michael L. Smith, MD.*

CAUSES OF UNINTENTIONAL HAIR DISCOLORATION		
Green (chlorotrichosis)	**Yellow, orange, or golden**	**Purple**
Copper (swimming pools) Selenium sulfide Tar shampoo Cobalt Chromium Nickel Yellow mercuric oxide	Tar shampoo Anthralin Minoxidil Copper (cosmetic plant extracts, metallic eyeglass frames)	Alkalinized anthralin

Table 74.4 Causes of unintentional hair discoloration. *Courtesy, Michael L. Smith, MD.*

- ***Mercury***, in elemental, inorganic, or organic forms, may cause acrodynia, tattoo reaction (cinnabar), granulomas, exanthems, cutaneous hyperpigmentation, allergic and irritant contact dermatitis, baboon syndrome
- Cutaneous contact with ***silver*** may result in argyria, irritant contact dermatitis, or skin ulceration
- ***Thallium***, in its soluble form, may cause alopecia, acneiform papules, hyperkeratotic plaques on hands and feet, and Mees' lines in nails

• For most cutaneous exposures to these toxic and heavy metals, effective treatment requires prompt soap and/or water washing; an exception is lithium, in which washing is contraindicated and gentle brushing off is preferred.

Cutaneous Findings of Frictional and Traumatic Injury to the Skin

Corns and Calluses

• Keratotic lesions resulting from repeated trauma and the subsequent cycle of friction, pressure, and thickening (Fig. 74.8).

• Contributing factors include ill-fitting footwear, bony protuberances, abnormal biomechanical foot function, and specific activities that involve repetitive activity.

• *Hard corns* are usually located on the dorsal aspects of the toes, while *soft corns* are typically found in the interdigital web spaces.

• Corns and calluses can often be mistaken for verrucae; gentle paring of the lesions with a blade and noticing the lesion's effect on dermatoglyphics can help distinguish between these three entities (Table 74.7).

• Treatment involves both symptomatic relief and correction of the underlying biomechanical problem:

- Symptomatic relief:
  1. Paring of the callosity with removal of the corn's central core may bring immediate relief of discomfort, followed by periodic foot filing
  2. Application of keratolytic agents (e.g. 40% salicylic acid pads; 6% salicylic acid, 10–40% urea, or 12% ammonium lactate creams), from daily to twice weekly, depending on strength

SELECTED TOXIC AND HEAVY METALS KNOWN TO CAUSE CONTACT DERMATITIS	
Irritant contact dermatitis	**Allergic contact dermatitis**
• Cobalt salts • Copper salts • Lithium • Mercury, organic and inorganic • Selenium	• Chromium • Cobalt • Gold • Mercury, organic • Nickel

Table 74.5 Selected toxic and heavy metals known to cause contact dermatitis.

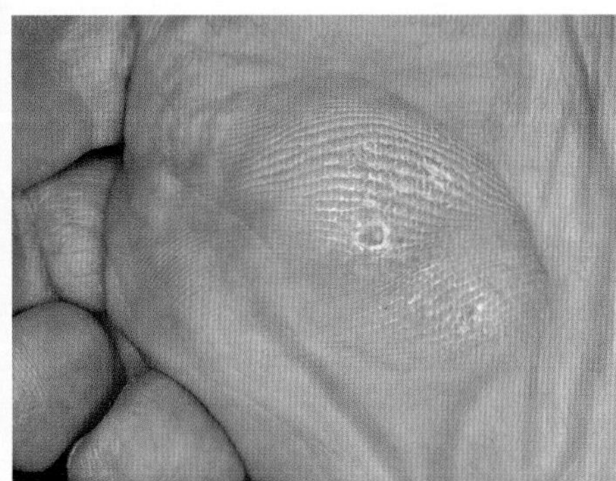

Fig. 74.8 Callus plus hard corns. Calluses are broad based and have increased skin markings while corns are round, more sharply defined papules with a central translucency and an interruption in dermatoglyphics. The skin overlying the second and third metatarsal heads is a common location for such lesions. *Courtesy, Jean L. Bolognia, MD.*

3. Soft cushions (e.g. silicone sheet, sheep skin) and donut-shaped corn pads

- *Biomechanical* correction – properly fitted footwear and use of appropriate orthotics
- *Recalcitrant* lesions – consider X-ray to look for exostoses and referral to orthopedic or podiatric surgeon

Black Heel (Talon Noir) and Black Palm

- Black macules on the palms or soles due to hemoglobin within the thickened stratum corneum (Fig. 74.9).

CUTANEOUS ERUPTIONS ASSOCIATED WITH GOLD EXPOSURE (AS AN ELEMENTAL SALT)	
Most common	**Less common**
• Lichen planus, lichenoid drug eruption • Allergic contact dermatitis • Pityriasis rosea-like eruptions • Erosive stomatitis	• Chrysiasis • Erythema nodosum • Erythema multiforme, toxic epidermal necrolysis • Exfoliative dermatitis

Table 74.6 Cutaneous eruptions associated with gold exposure (as an elemental salt).

- Secondary to impact trauma and resolves with paring or spontaneously with time.
- Harmless, but because of its dark color must be differentiated from acral cutaneous melanoma (does not resolve with gentle paring).

Chondrodermatitis Nodularis Helicis (CNH)

- A tender, inflammatory process of the ear that primarily affects patients older than 50 years of age; initiated by ischemia-related inflammation of the cartilage.
- Presents with a skin-colored to erythematous, dome-shaped papule or nodule with a central crust or keratin-filled crater; often exquisitely tender (Fig. 74.10).
- Most often a unilateral process affecting the most protuberant portion of the ear, primarily the upper helical rim or the middle to lower antihelical rim.
- **DDx:** SCC, KA, BCC, AK, cutaneous horn, weathering nodule, verruca, calcinosis cutis, gouty tophus; often distinguished via biopsy.
- **Rx:** mostly anecdotal and not standardized (e.g. intralesional CS, topical antibiotics, specially designed CNH pillows for sleeping, cryosurgery, electrodesiccation and curettage, CO_2 laser ablation); full-thickness excision is the most definitive and favored treatment for particularly bothersome lesions.

Acanthoma Fissuratum

- Results from ill-fitting eyeglass frames that create a frictional injury to the postauricular sulcus or the upper lateral nose (Fig. 74.11).

DISTINGUISHING FEATURES OF VERRUCAE, CORNS AND CALLUSES		
Lesion	**Paring revelations**	**Effect on dermatoglyphics**
Verruca	Thrombosed capillaries, multiple bleeding points	Interrupted
Corn	Central translucent, whitish-yellow core	Interrupted
Callus	Layers of yellowish keratin	Accentuated

Table 74.7 Distinguishing features of verrucae, corns, and calluses.

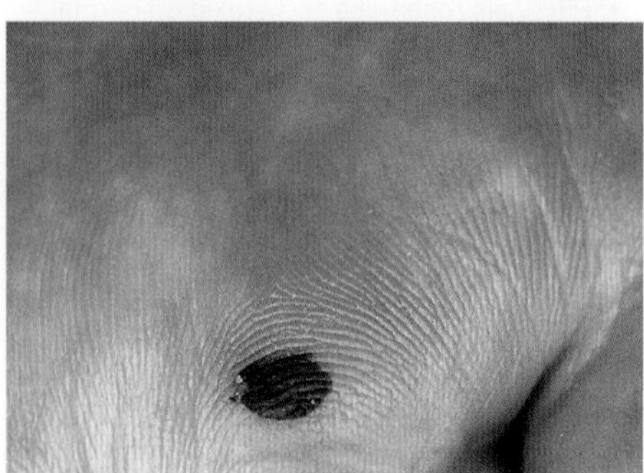

Fig. 74.9 Black heel (talon noir) and black palm. This black color is due to hemoglobin within the thickened stratum corneum of palmar skin. *Courtesy, Jean L. Bolognia, MD.*

- Presents as a firm or sometimes soft, skin-colored to erythematous nodule or plaque with a central vertical groove or fissure; occasionally tenderness, serous discharge, or slight hyperkeratosis.
- **DDx:** BCC, SCC, chronic dermatitis or benign acanthoma; biopsy is occasionally necessary to exclude a non-melanoma skin cancer.
- **Rx:** adjust or replace the offending eyeglasses.

Weathering Nodules of the Ears

- Multiple, bilateral, firm (feels like cartilage), asymptomatic, whitish, 2- to 3-mm papules located along the inner rim of the helices in older males >> females (Fig. 74.12).
- Associated consistently with a history of significant sun exposure and actinic damage.
- **DDx:** CNH, gouty tophi, calcinosis cutis, elastotic nodules, granuloma annulare.
- **Rx:** not necessary.

Sports-Related Dermatoses

- Participation in sports is often associated with a number of cutaneous injuries, dermatoses, or infections, related to acute and chronic mechanical trauma (Tables 74.8 and 74.9; Figs 74.13–74.16).

For further information see Ch. 88 from *Dermatology, Fourth Edition*.

For additional online figures and tables visit www.expertconsult.com 

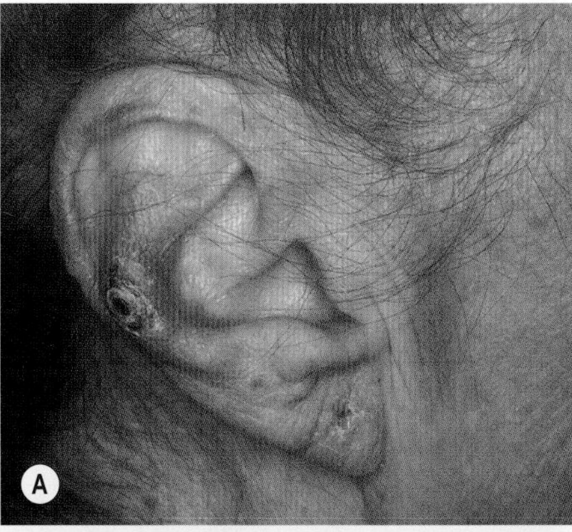

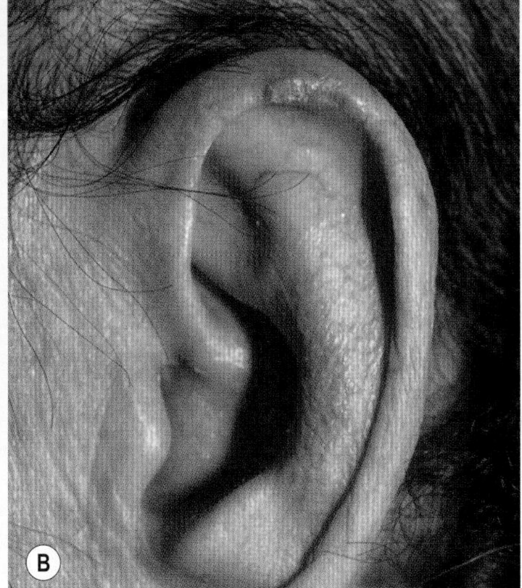

Fig. 74.10 Chondrodermatitis nodularis helicis (CNH). A Tender, erythematous papulonodule with central scale on the superior helix of an older woman. This represented the site most susceptible to pressure-induced ischemia. **B** Tender, erythematous papulonodule with central scale-crust on the mid antihelix of an older woman. *A, Courtesy, Kalman Watsky, MD; B, Courtesy, Harvey Lui, MD.*

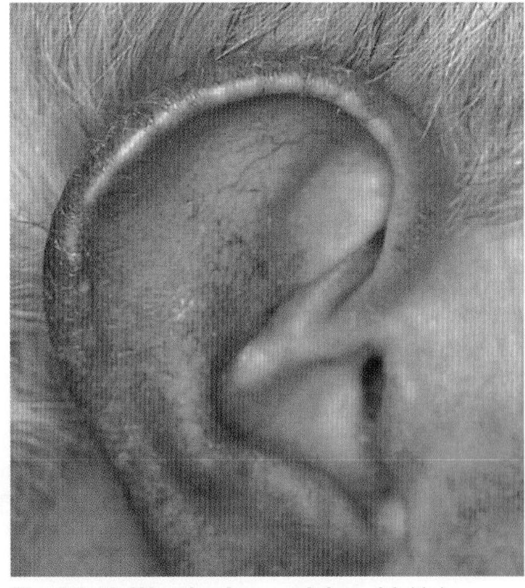

Fig. 74.12 Weathering nodules. Multiple asymptomatic, small, whitish papules along the helix of an older man with photodamage. *Courtesy, Jean L. Bolognia, MD.*

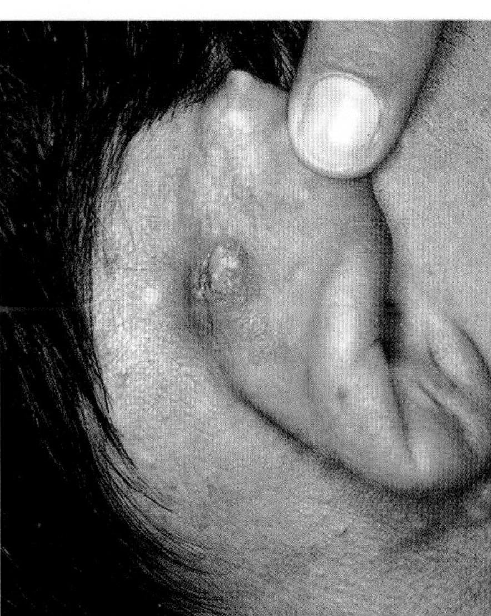

Fig. 74.11 Acanthoma fissuratum. Keratotic plaque of the postauricular sulcus; note the linear fissure. *Courtesy, Luis Requena, MD.*

SELECTED FRICTIONAL AND MECHANICAL DERMATOSES IN ATHLETES			
Condition	**Clinical features**	**Sports**	**Etiology/pathogenesis** **Prevention/treatment**
Subungual hematoma*	Red/maroon, purple or black discoloration beneath all or part of the nail (see Ch. 58 and Fig. 74.14)	Running Tennis	Sudden impact of toe tip with end of shoe Enlarged shoe toe box with proper arch and metatarsal support; drainage of hematoma may be necessary
Jogger's nipple	Pain, erythema, fissuring, occasional bleeding	Running	Repeated friction of rough shirt fabric Women: jogging bra Men: taping, lubrication, semisynthetic or silk shirt
Tennis toe	Toe tip callus, nail thickening, subungual hyperkeratosis (see Fig. 74.15)	Tennis Running	Repeated trauma of longest toe against inside of toe box Proper shoe fit, enlarged toe box, improved arch support
Fibrotic knots (e.g. surfer's nodules)	Thick fibrotic nodules on knees, knuckles, dorsal feet, and anterior lower ribs (surfers)	Surfing, boxing, football, marbles, yoga, video game playing	Chronic pressure over bony prominences Position change, padding

Table 74.8 Selected frictional and mechanical dermatoses in athletes. *Courtesy, Michael L. Smith, MD.*

CUTANEOUS INFECTIONS IN ATHLETES
Bacterial
• Impetigo (see Fig. 61.2) • Folliculitis (see Ch. 31) • Hot tub folliculitis (see Fig. 31.3) • *Pseudomonas* hot-foot syndrome (see Fig. 61.16) • Furuncles (boils) • Erythrasma (see Fig. 13.2 and/or Fig. 61.10) • Pitted keratolysis ("toxic sock syndrome") (see Fig. 61.11) • Otitis externa (swimmer's ear)
Mycobacterial
• Swimming pool granuloma (see Fig. 62.17)
Viral
• Verruca vulgaris (warts) (see Ch. 66) • Herpes simplex viral infection (herpes gladiatorum) (see Fig. 67.5) • Molluscum contagiosum (see Fig. 68.8)
Fungal (see Ch. 64)
• Tinea pedis (athlete's foot) • Tinea cruris (jock itch) • Tinea corporis (tinea gladiatorum) (see Fig. 74.16)
Other
• Seabather's eruption (sea lice) (see Fig. 72.9) • Swimmer's itch (see Fig. 70.14)

Table 74.9 Cutaneous infections in athletes. *Courtesy, Michael L. Smith, MD.*

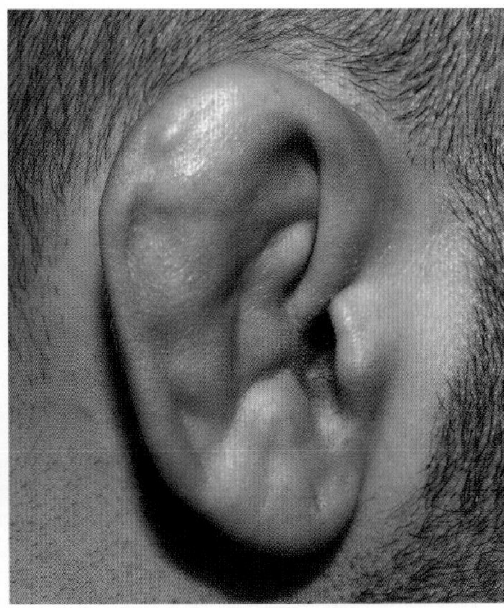

Fig. 74.13 Multinodular deformity of the external ear, often referred to as "cauliflower ear," in a jiu-jitsu fighter. It is the result of repeated auricular hematomas. *Courtesy, Kalman Watsky, MD.*

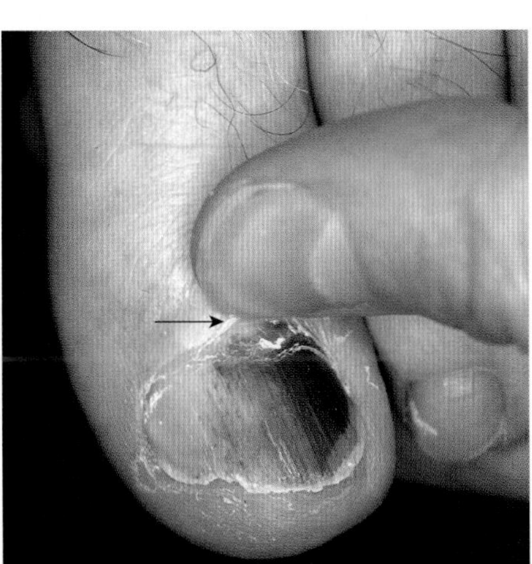

Fig. 74.14 Subungual hematoma. A common sports-related (e.g. tennis, running, basketball) injury due to the sudden impact of the toe tip with the end of the shoe. Note the subungual dark purplish discoloration, which may be misdiagnosed as melanoma. Clues to the diagnosis of subungual hematoma include: a normal-appearing proximal nail plate upon gentle retraction of the cuticle (arrow); characteristic dermoscopic features (e.g. red-brown to purplish-black round globules); and determination that the discoloration grows out distally. *Courtesy, Jean L. Bolognia, MD.*

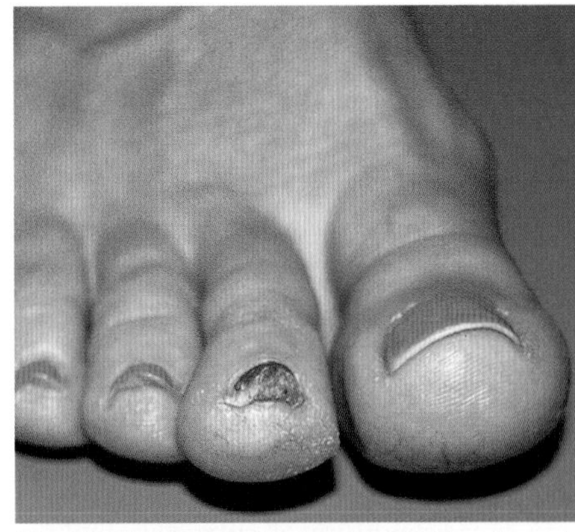

Fig. 74.15 Chronic "tennis toe." Chronic and repeated trauma of the longer second toe against the end of the tennis shoe toe box during sudden stops creates the distal callus formation and nail plate thickening known as "tennis toe." *Courtesy, Michael L. Smith, MD.*

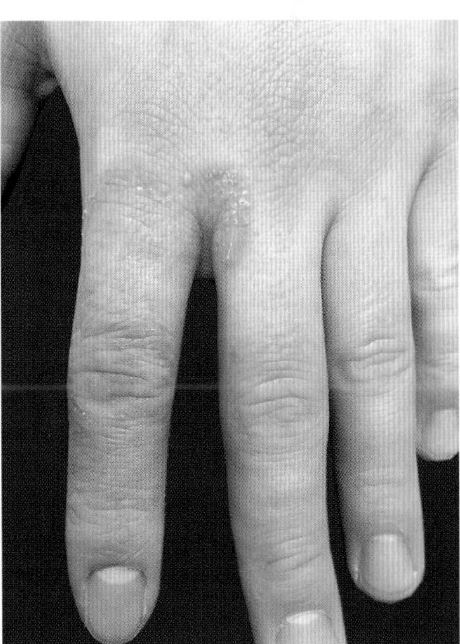

Fig. 74.16 Tinea gladiatorum. Erythematous, scaly, annular plaque with an active border on the dorsal hand of this high school wrestler. *Courtesy, Karynne O. Duncan, MD.*

75 Cutaneous Signs of Drug, Child, and Elder Abuse

Drug Abuse

- The skin often displays evidence of injection and inhalation drug abuse.
- A broad spectrum of cutaneous findings can result from local and systemic effects of the drug itself, adulterants, or associated infectious agents (Tables 75.1 and 75.2; Figs 75.1–75.10).
- Skin and soft tissue infections as well as thrombophlebitis are the most common conditions for which drug addicts seek medical care and are hospitalized.

Child Abuse

- Child abuse encompasses a broad spectrum of non-accidental maltreatment of children, including physical, emotional, and sexual abuse as well as neglect.
- Children with disabilities, behavioral problems, and stressful home situations (e.g. parental unemployment or substance use) are at increased risk of abuse, and serious injury is more frequent in boys.
- Cutaneous signs of physical abuse:
  - Unexplained bruises (Fig. 75.11), curvilinear or binding marks (e.g. produced by belts, ropes, or cords), buckle imprints, and burns (e.g. from cigarettes or scalding; Fig. 75.12)
  - Skin injuries in areas less prone to accidental trauma (e.g. ears, neck, trunk, buttocks, upper arms) or in infants who are not independently mobile
  - Delay between the injury and seeking medical care
- Physical signs are present in a small minority of sexually abused children; suggestive findings (in the absence of a plausible history of accidental injury) include acute laceration or bruising of genital/perianal tissues, complete transection of the posterior hymen, and scars of the perianal area or posterior fourchette.
- Anogenital warts in children may be perinatally acquired, transmitted during routine child care, autoinoculated from other sites, or acquired from sexual abuse; the latter is an uncommon etiology of anogenital warts in children <5 years of age.
- **DDx:** conditions that can mimic physical and sexual abuse in children are listed in Tables 75.3 and 75.4 (Fig. 75.13).
- **Rx:** guidelines for evaluation of suspected child abuse are available at http://pediatrics.aappublications.org/content/pediatrics/135/5/e1337.full.pdf (physical abuse) and http://pediatrics.aappublications.org/content/116/2/506.full.pdf (sexual abuse).

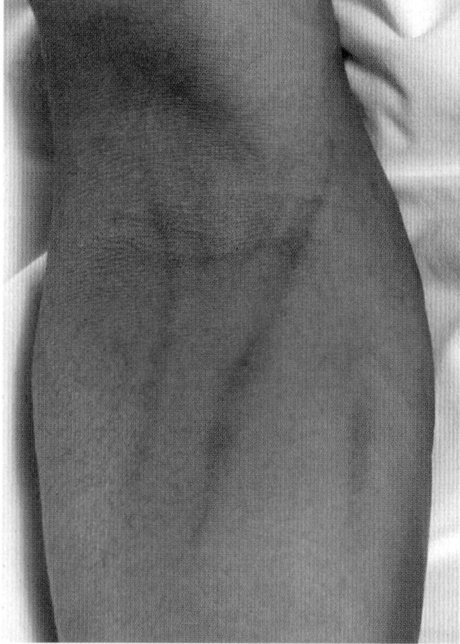

Fig. 75.1 Injection sites ("skin tracks") in an intravenous drug user. There is overlying hyperpigmentation and scarring of veins due to inflammation from repeated non-sterile injections as well as injections of irritating drugs and adulterants. *Courtesy, Mark Pittelkow, MD.*

MUCOCUTANEOUS SIGNS OF DRUG ABUSE	
Finding	**Route(s) and example drugs**
Sequelae of tissue injury	
Skin tracks (Fig. 75.1) and skin popping scars (Fig. 75.2)	IV and SC/intradermal, respectively
Lymphedema	IV, SC
Ulcers	IV – cocaine, propoxyphene* SC – barbiturates, pentazocine Intra-arterial injection leading to ischemia
Retiform purpura (Fig. 75.3) with ulceration (associated with neutropenia)	Snorting/IV cocaine or smoking crack cocaine adulterated with levamisole
Sclerosis	SC – pentazocine (Fig. 75.4), barbiturates, cocaine
Hyperkeratosis ± linear or circular black plaques on palms/fingers; erosions or blisters on lips; madarosis	Smoking crack cocaine
Circumferential pigmented bands due to tourniquet	IV
Pseudoaneurysm (tender pulsatile mass with bruit) associated with petechiae/purpura ± reduced pulses; distal purpuric papules/papulopustules due to embolization (Fig. 75.5)	Intra-arterial injection in groin or an extremity
Pressure erythema, bullae (Fig. 75.8), and ulcers	Overdose with barbiturates or other sedatives
Sequelae of CNS effects	
Pruritus ± excoriations	Methamphetamine (dry, leathery skin), heroin (associated with flushing), cocaine (with chronic use)
Formication/delusions of parasitosis leading to skin picking (Fig. 75.7) and self-induced ulcers	Cocaine, methamphetamine
Other skin findings	
Granulomas (Fig. 75.6; onset may be delayed)	Injection of talc (e.g. in narcotic tablets) or starch
Hyperhidrosis	Amphetamines, LSD
Acne vulgaris	Anabolic steroids†, methamphetamine (especially acne excoriée), marijuana
Perinasal or perioral irritant dermatitis	Sniffing volatile solvents/inhalants
Oral findings	
Xerostomia	Amphetamines, heroin
Dental caries, gingivitis, tooth loss	Methamphetamine, heroin

**Withdrawn from prescription drug market in 2010 in the United States and Europe.*
†May also be associated with androgenetic alopecia, hirsutism, clitoral enlargement, testicular atrophy, and gynecomastia.

Table 75.1 Mucocutaneous signs of drug abuse. Infections associated with drug abuse are presented in Table 75.2 A variety of cutaneous drug reactions can also develop, such as morbilliform or fixed drug eruptions, urticaria, small vessel vasculitis, and Stevens–Johnson syndrome/toxic epidermal necrolysis. LSD, lysergic acid diethylamide.

SKIN INFECTIONS RELATED TO DRUG ABUSE	
Finding	**Route(s) and example drugs**
Abscesses and cellulitis (Fig. 75.9): *Staphylococcus aureus* > *Streptococcus* spp. > GNRs, anaerobes; often polymicrobial and associated with lymphangitis*	IV, SC, intradermal • Adulterated (e.g. "black tar") heroin: *Clostridium* (including wound botulism from *C. botulinum*) • Heroin or pentazocine: *Pseudomonas* spp.
Necrotizing fasciitis (Fig. 75.10; severe, disproportionate pain): usually polymicrobial, may include anaerobes	IV, SC
Disseminated candidiasis with pustular folliculitis	Injection of heroin (e.g. brown heroin in 1980s)
Zygomycosis (necrotic cellulitic plaque or abscess)	IV
Nasal verrucae in setting of nasal irritation	Snorting cocaine or heroin
Hepatitis C > B viral infection leading to cryoglobulinemic vasculitis (e.g. palpable purpura)	Needle/syringe sharing

**May also be associated with osteomyelitis, septic arthritis, bacteremia, septic thrombophlebitis, and endocarditis (often tricuspid valve).*

Table 75.2 Skin infections related to drug abuse. GNRs, Gram-negative rods.

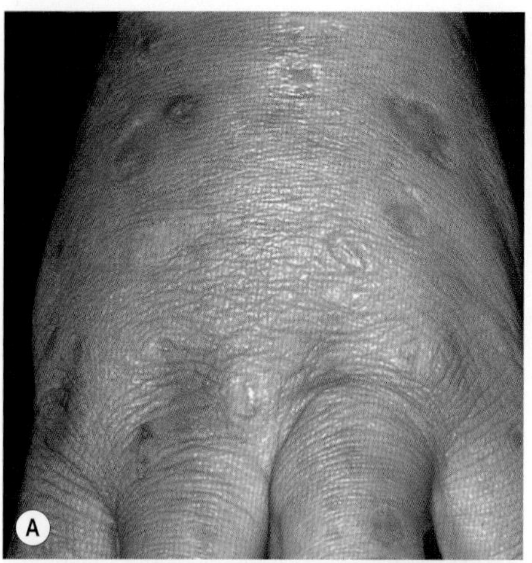

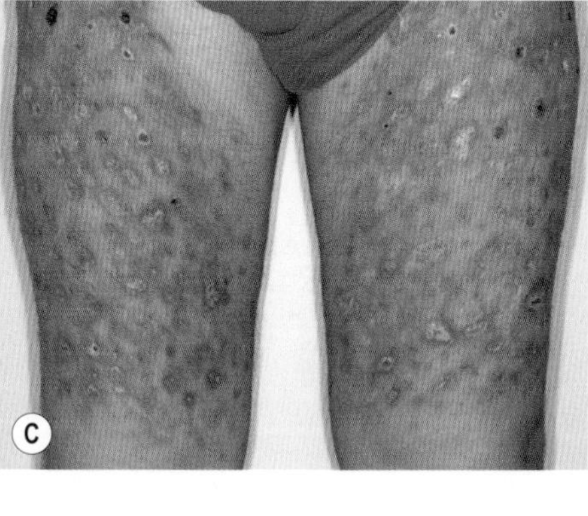

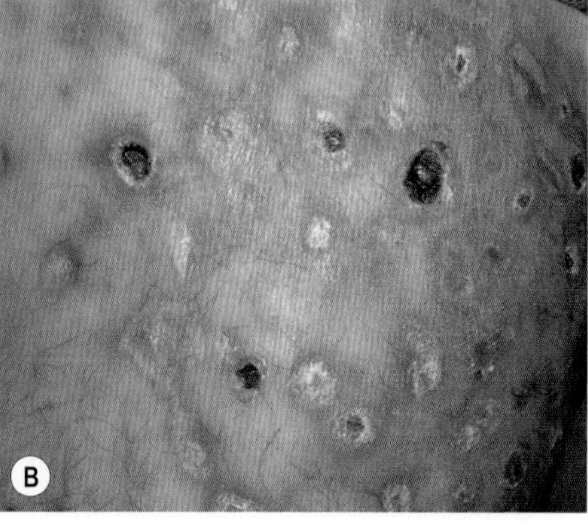

Fig. 75.2 "Skin popping" scars. A–C Multiple circular depressed scars, some with rims of postinflammatory hyperpigmentation, admixed with circular hemorrhagic crusts overlying ulcerations. Cocaine was injected into the thighs. *A, Courtesy Miguel Sanchez, MD; B, C, Courtesy, Mark Pittelkow, MD.*

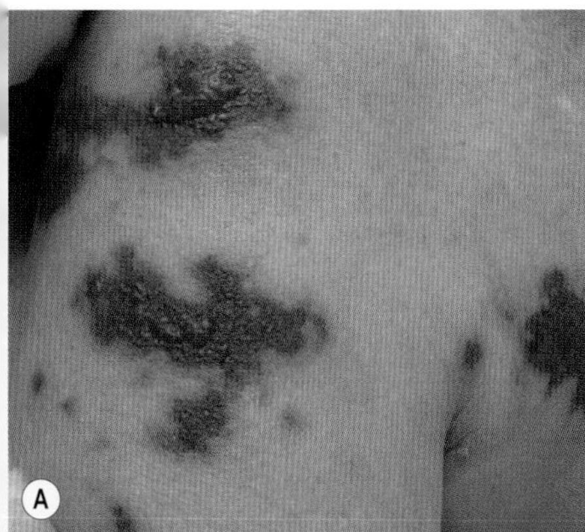

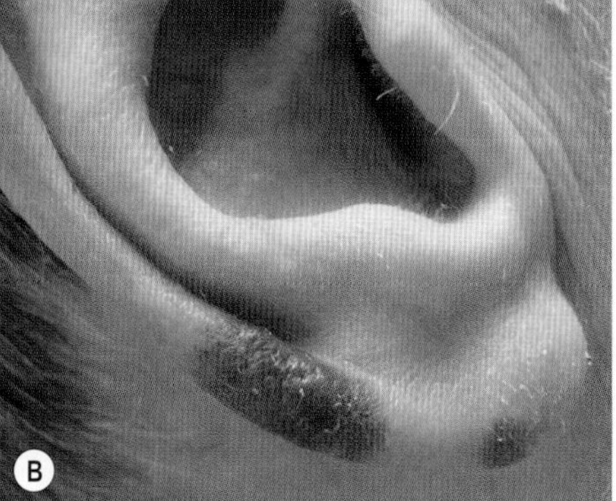

Fig. 75.3 Retiform purpura due to levamisole-adulterated cocaine. A, B The earlobe is a common site of involvement and purpuric lesions of the earlobe had been described previously as a side effect of levamisole. At the time of writing, up to 70% of the cocaine in the United States contained levamisole, compared to <3% of the heroin. *Courtesy, Jeffrey P. Callen, MD.*

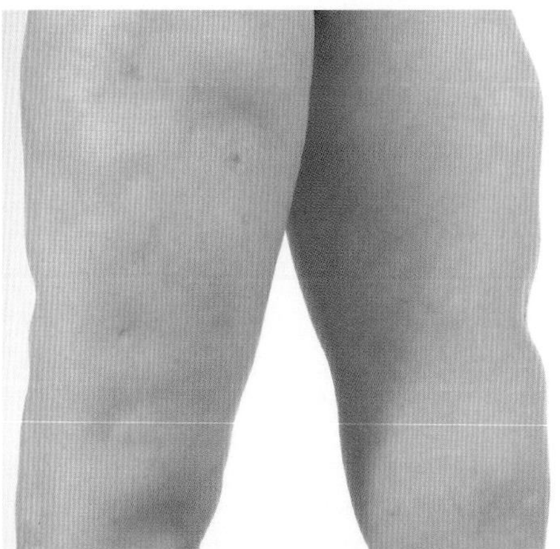

Fig. 75.4 Atrophic depressions on the thighs and extensive calcification from multiple pentazocine injections. The calcified areas are firm upon palpation. *Courtesy, Mark Pittelkow, MD.*

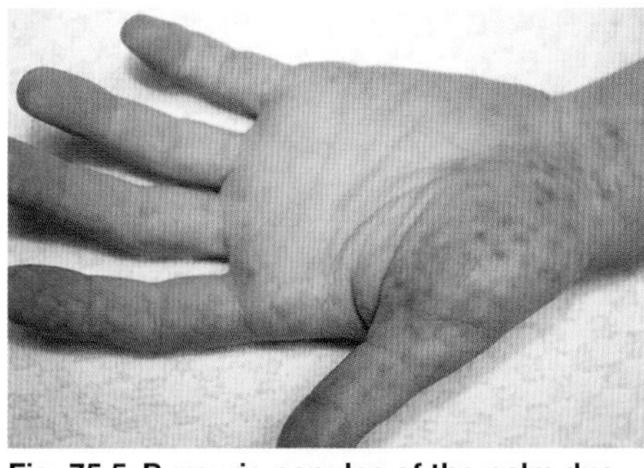

Fig. 75.5 Purpuric papules of the palm due to emboli of pill fragments following an intra-arterial injection. *Courtesy, Jean L. Bolognia, MD.*

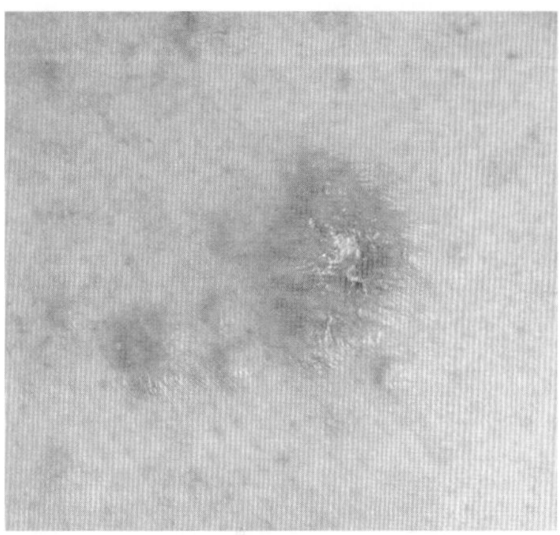

Fig. 75.6 Foreign body granuloma formation leading to papules at the sites of injection of adulterated heroin. *Courtesy, Mark Pittelkow, MD.*

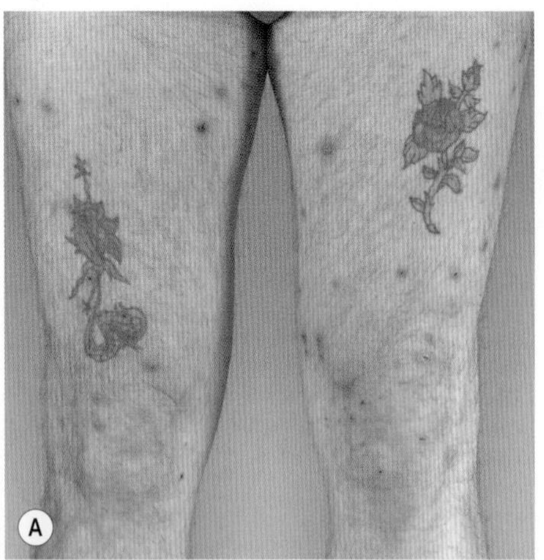

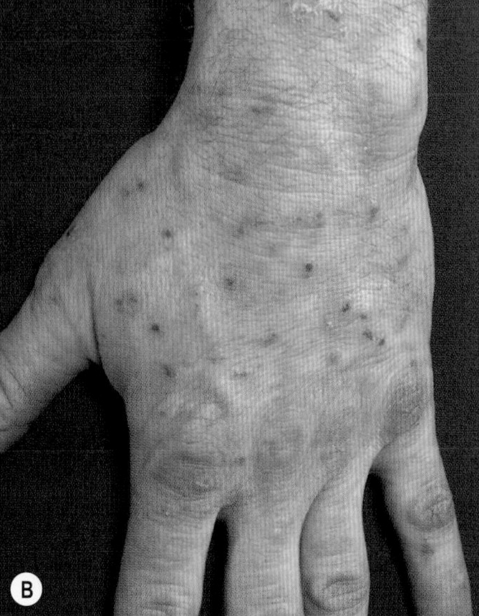

Fig. 75.7 Multiple excoriations in a cocaine addict. The patient felt "crawling" sensations in his skin. *Courtesy, Mark Pittelkow, MD.*

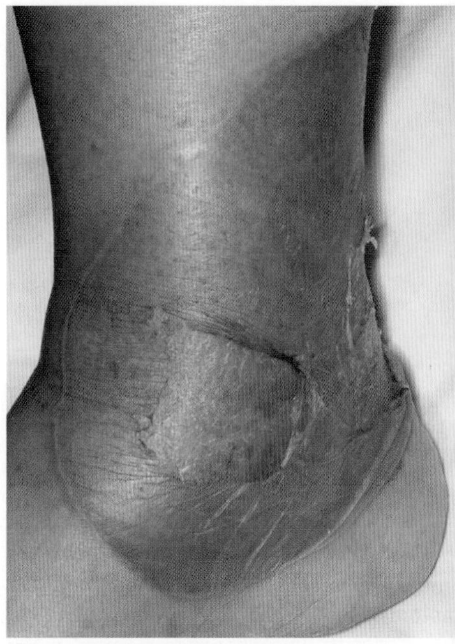

Fig. 75.8 Coma bulla. Large bulla with subsequent erosion on the medial ankle due to a prolonged coma from barbiturate overdose. *Courtesy, Mark Pittelkow, MD.*

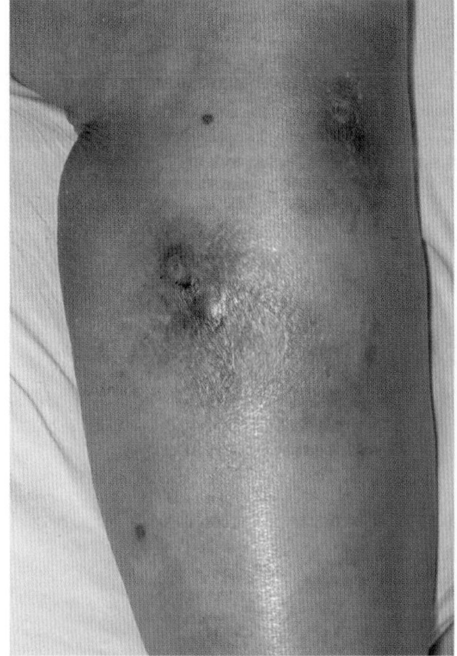

Fig. 75.9 Cellulitis of the lower extremity in an intravenous drug user. *Courtesy, Mark Pittelkow, MD.*

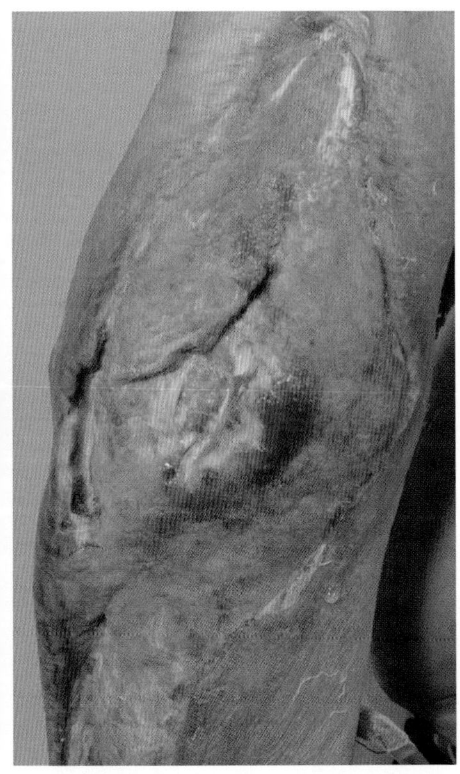

Fig. 75.10 Necrotizing fasciitis of the upper extremity with extensive tissue necrosis in an intravenous drug user. Surgical debridement has been performed. *Courtesy, Mark Pittelkow, MD.*

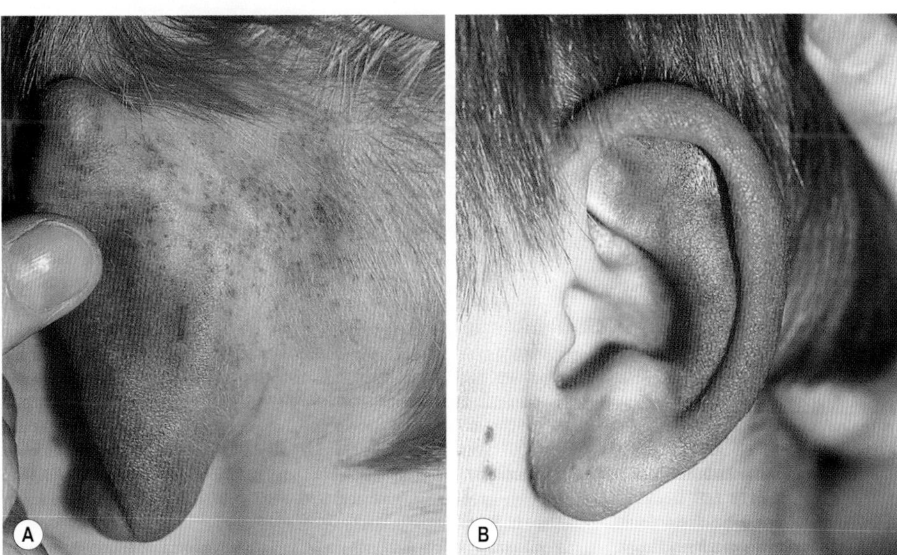

Fig. 75.11 Bruising and petechiae. A, B Bruising and petechiae of the pinna and post-auricular area in a 6-year-old boy, consistent with a hand slap by an adult. *From Hobbs CJ, Wynne JM. Physical Signs of Child Abuse. © 2001 WB Saunders. Continued*

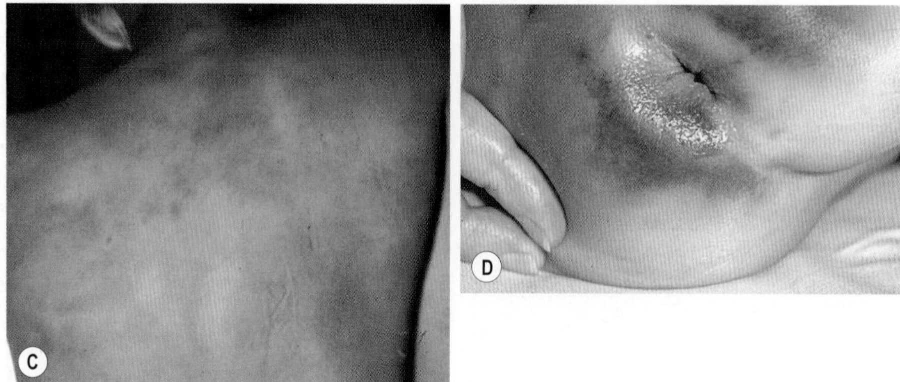

Fig. 75.11 *Continued* **Bruising and petechiae. C** Bruising from a belt and belt buckle on the back of an 8-year-old boy. **D** Bruising of the buttocks and perianal area of a sexually abused 2-year-old child. *Courtesy, Sharon Ann Raimer, MD.*

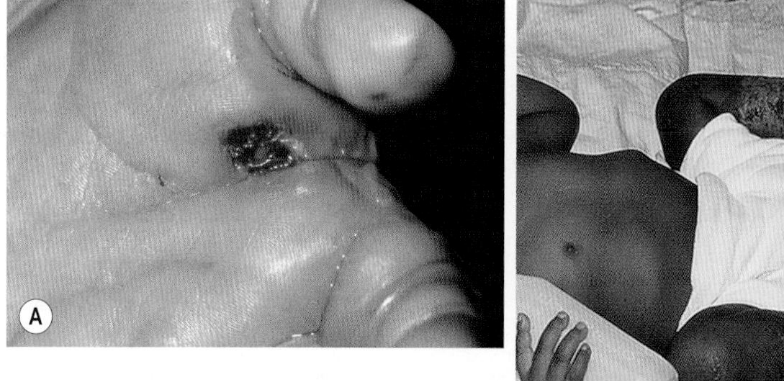

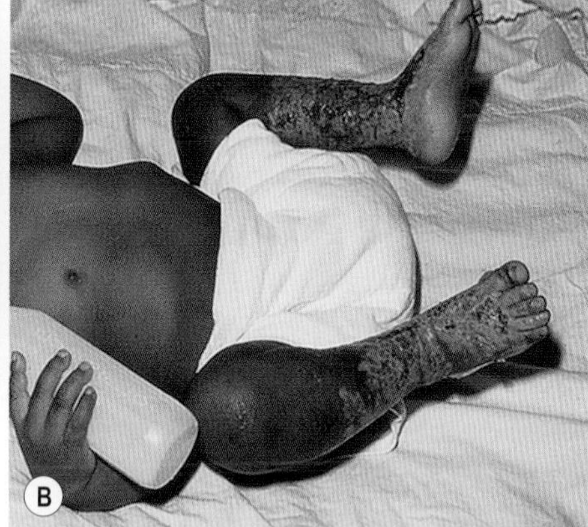

Fig. 75.12 Injuries produced by burns. A Cigarette burn. **B** Burn injury due to dunking in hot water, with a sharp line of demarcation on the lower legs. "Donut-type sparing" on the child's buttocks may be seen when the buttocks are held against the cooler tub while water scalds the surrounding immersed skin. *A, Courtesy, Sharon Ann Raimer, MD; B, Courtesy, Leo Litter, MD.*

Elder Abuse

- Elder abuse may involve intentional actions that cause harm (physical, psychological, sexual, or financial) as well as failure by a caretaker to satisfy the basic needs of an elder or to protect him or her from harm.
- Risk factors include dementia and social isolation.
- Elder self-neglect is a related entity where individuals fail or refuse to address their own basic needs in a way that threatens their health and safety.
- The National Center on Elder Abuse (https://ncea.acl.gov) provides resources to assist in the recognition and management of elder abuse.

For further information see Chs 89 and 90 from *Dermatology, Fourth Edition*.

For additional online figures visit www.expertconsult.com 

CONDITIONS THAT CAN MIMIC CHILD ABUSE
Bleeding into the skin (ecchymoses, purpura)
• Multiple bruises due to platelet/clotting disorders or Ehlers–Danlos syndrome (especially on shins, knees) • Bruising due to "cupping" or cao gio (coin rubbing) • Vasculitis, particularly Henoch–Schönlein purpura (HSP; favors lower extremities) and acute hemorrhagic edema of infancy (favors face)
Blue discoloration of skin mistaken as bruising
• Dermal melanocytosis (favors sacral area and back; color does not progress to green/yellow) • Infantile hemangioma (deep) or vascular malformation
Linear hyperpigmentation
• Phytophotodermatitis (Fig. 75.13A) • Sock-line or mitten-line hyperpigmentation
Vesicles, bullae, or erosions mistaken as non-accidental burns or other intentional injuries
• Impetigo, ecthyma, blistering distal dactylitis • Erythema multiforme, fixed drug eruption • Bullous mastocytosis • Irritant contact dermatitis (e.g. from laxative mimicking immersion burn, chemical burns from topical application of apple cider vinegar or garlic) (Fig. 75.13B) • Arthropod bite reaction • Moxibustion • Burn from a hot car seat or seat belt buckle • Genetic disorders of skin fragility, e.g. epidermolysis bullosa or porphyria
Other
• Osteogenesis imperfecta • Hair tourniquet • Self-inflicted injury

Table 75.3 Conditions that can mimic child abuse.

CONDITIONS OCCASIONALLY MISDIAGNOSED AS SEXUAL ABUSE IN CHILDREN

• Congenital anomalies or anatomic variants (e.g. white line in the posterior vestibule)
• Accidental injury
• Anal fissure due to constipation
• Perianal streptococcal infection
• Lichen sclerosus (Fig. 75.13C; may be associated with purpura or hemorrhagic bullae)
• Genital vitiligo
• Localized vulvar bullous pemphigoid or other bullous diseases
• Crohn disease (Fig. 75.13D)
• Infantile hemangioma (especially if ulcerated) or vascular malformation
• Entities misdiagnosed as genital or perianal warts
  – Perianal pyramidal protrusion (Fig. 75.13E)
  – Molluscum contagiosum
  – Pseudoverrucous papules and nodules due to encopresis or urinary incontinence

Table 75.4 Conditions occasionally misdiagnosed as sexual abuse in children.

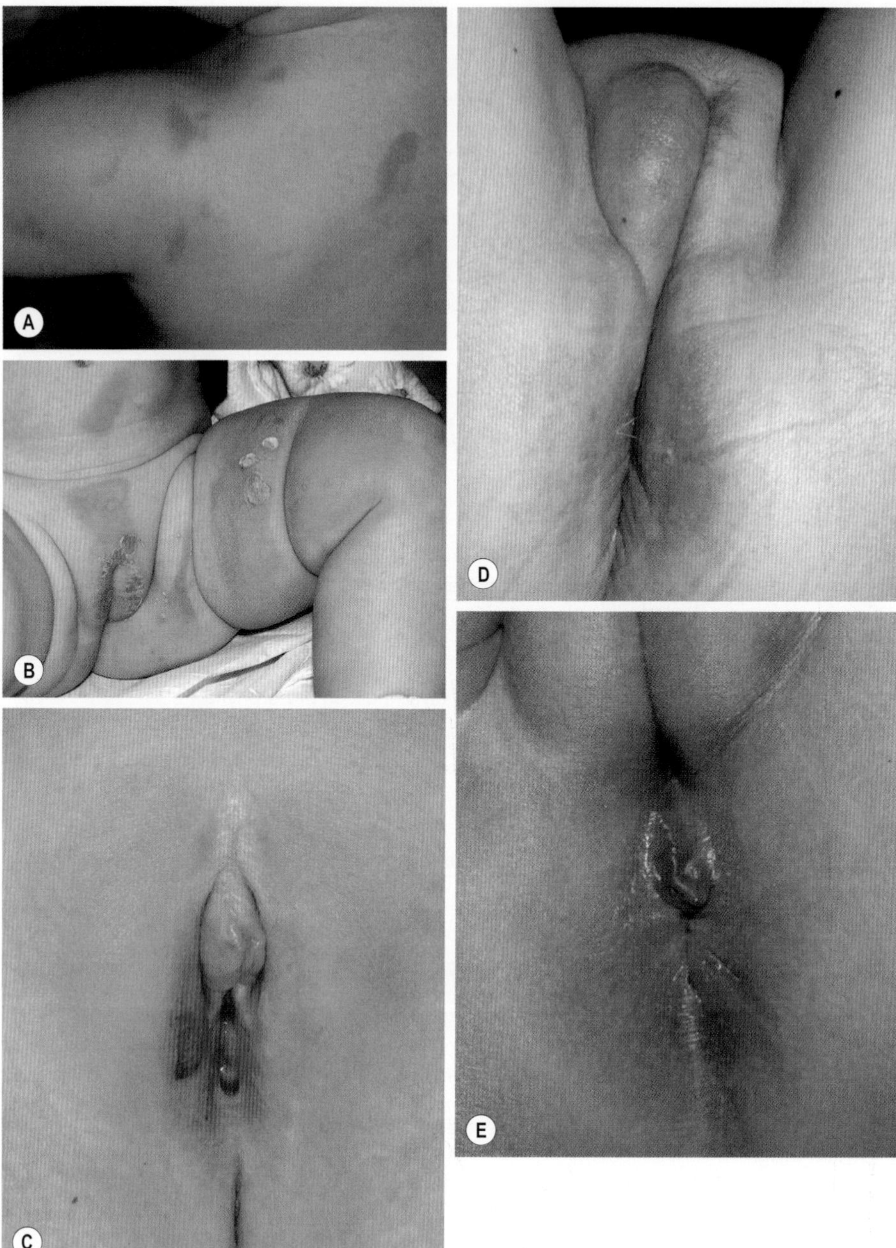

Fig. 75.13 Cutaneous disorders that may be misdiagnosed as physical or sexual abuse. **A** Linear hyperpigmented streaks due to phytophotodermatitis on the back of a 2-year-old girl; the mother had lime juice on her hand when she touched the child. **B** Chemical burn from topical application of apple cider vinegar in an infant. Note the sharply demarcated erythema with angular borders and sparing of the skin folds, as well as the superficial blistering and desquamation. **C** Genital lichen sclerosus may have associated purpura or hemorrhagic bullae. **D** Cutaneous Crohn disease can present with vulvar erythema and swelling as well as perianal ulcers. **E** A perianal pyramidal protrusion in the typical location, just anterior to the anus in the midline. This finding is most common in infant girls. *A, Courtesy, Anthony J. Mancini, MD; B, D, E, Courtesy, Julie V. Schaffer, MD; C, Courtesy, Sharon Ann Raimer, MD.*

Histiocytoses 76

- Group of disorders in which the predominant cell type is a Langerhans cell, a mononuclear cell/macrophage, or a dermal dendrocyte.
- Traditionally, there are two major groups: Langerhans cell histiocytoses and non-Langerhans cell histiocytoses. The V600E variant of BRAF has been detected in both groups.
- Within these two main groups, the disorders overlap and form a clinicopathologic spectrum.

Langerhans Cell Histiocytoses

- Langerhans cells, which represent the major antigen-presenting cells of the epidermis, are CD1a-positive, S-100 protein-positive, and langerin (CD207)-positive.
- Langerhans cells have Birbeck granules by electron microscopy.
- Common in children ages 1–3 years, but can occur at any age.

Multisystem Variant

- There is an acute, diffuse form (formerly termed Letterer–Siwe disease) that can have multisystem involvement (skin, lung, liver, lymph nodes, bone, bone marrow), classically in children <1–2 year(s) of age. Skin lesions are small, 1- to 3-mm, skin-colored to pink papules, which can coalesce; sometimes they are admixed with pustules or vesicles. Secondary changes include scale, crusts, and petechiae/purpura. These lesions favor the scalp, flexural neck, axilla, perineum, and trunk (Fig. 76.1).
- A triad (formerly termed Hand–Schüller–Christian disease) can occur, consisting of diabetes insipidus (in 30%), exophthalmos, and osteolytic bone lesions (especially in the cranium); the disease is usually chronic and progressive and classically affects children ages 2–6 years. Skin lesions (see Fig. 76.1) are present in ~30%. Due to the chronic course, older lesions are often more xanthomatous (i.e. yellow in color due to accumulations of lipid within macrophages) and occasionally they are ulcerated. Premature loss of teeth can occur.
- **DDx** includes seborrheic dermatitis (see Fig. 13.4), intertrigo (see Fig. 13.2), scabies, impetigo, atopic dermatitis, contact dermatitis. **DDx** of xanthomatous lesions includes juvenile xanthogranuloma.

Single System Variant

- Occasionally, there is localized bone involvement (formerly termed eosinophilic granuloma), classically in children (ages 7–12 years). It often presents as a single, asymptomatic bony lesion often favoring the cranium.
- A skin-limited, rapidly self-healing variant ("congenital self-healing reticulohistiocytosis" [Hashimoto–Pritzker disease]) presents at birth or during the first few days of life. Skin lesions are variable from a single nodule to widespread red-brown papules/nodules that crust and involute after several weeks (Fig. 76.2). Longitudinal follow-up is recommended because a small percentage of patients can develop systemic disease.

Non-Langerhans Cell Histiocytoses

Juvenile Xanthogranuloma

- Most common of the non-Langerhans cell histiocytoses.
- Appears primarily in infants and children (75% present during the first year of life).
- Usually a single papule or nodule (Fig. 76.3).

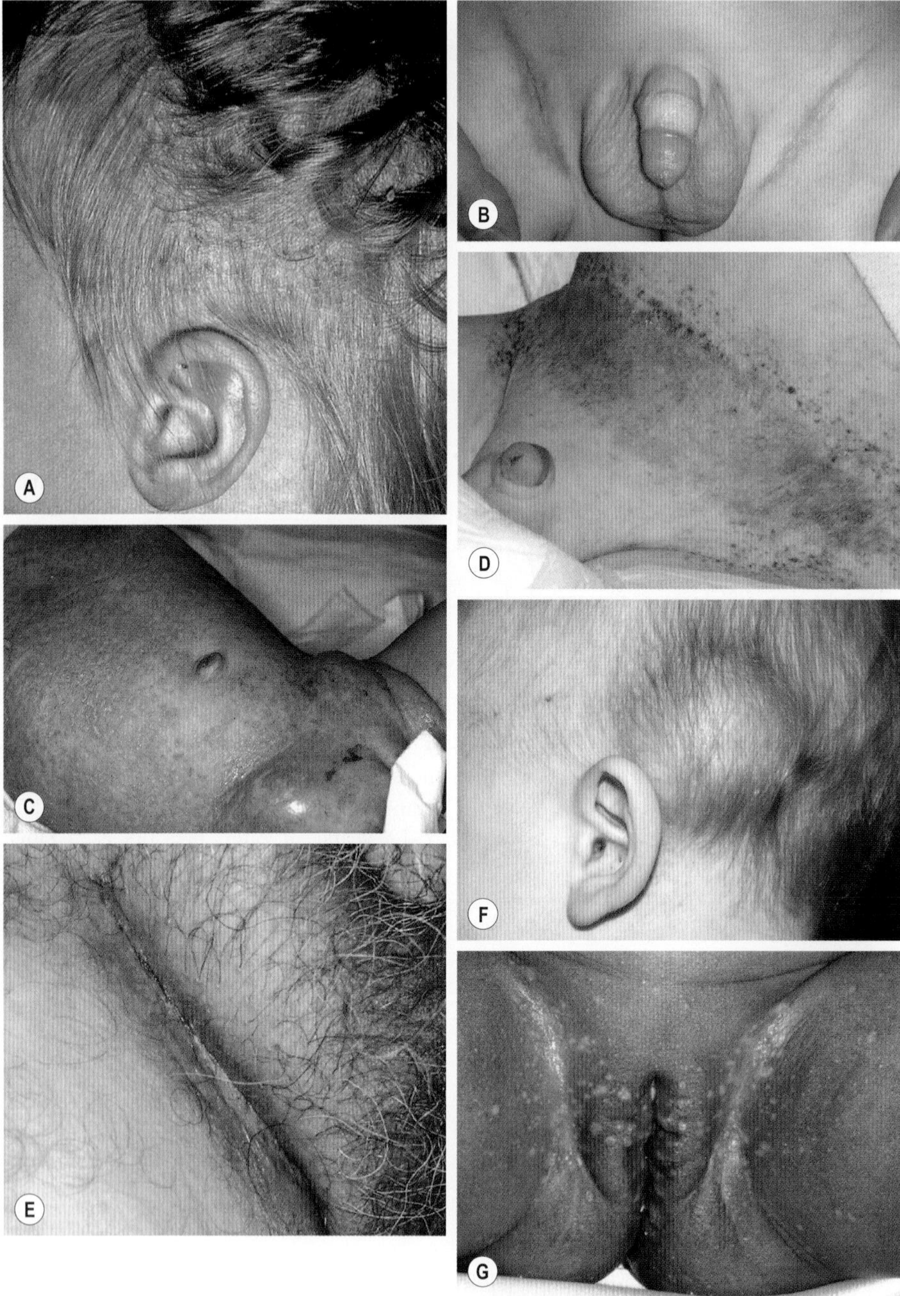

Fig. 76.1 Langerhans cell histiocytosis – clinical spectrum. **A** Scalp involvement may initially be diagnosed as seborrheic dermatitis; however, there are usually more discrete papules and crusting. **B** Pink, thin plaques with fissuring along the inguinal crease can also resemble seborrheic dermatitis. **C** Advanced disease with coalescence of papules into large plaques and prominent inguinal lymphadenopathy. **D** The presence of petechiae and purpuric papules is a clue to the diagnosis. **E** In an adult, the clinical presentation of inguinal involvement is similar to that of infants. **F** This subcutaneous nodule on the scalp involved the skull and represented the initial manifestation of multisystem Langerhans cell histiocytosis in an infant. **G** In patients with darkly pigmented skin, the papules can be hypopigmented. *A, C, E, Courtesy, YDRSC; B, Courtesy, Richard Antaya, MD; D, F, G, Courtesy, Julie V. Schaffer, MD.*

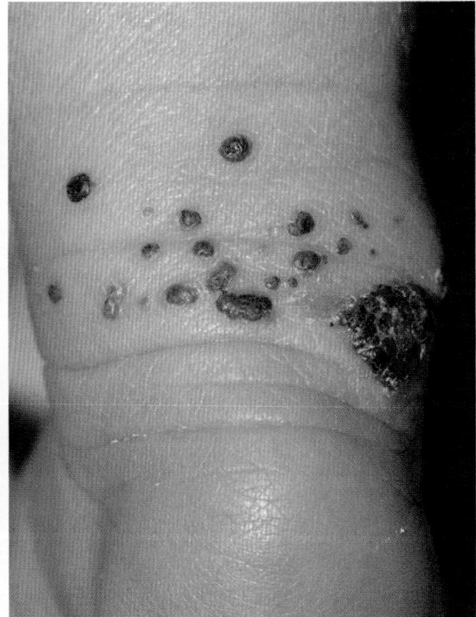

Fig. 76.2 Langerhans cell histiocytosis with spontaneous resolution in a neonate ("congenital self-healing reticulohistiocytosis"). Crusted papules and hemorrhagic crusts on the ankle. *Courtesy, Kristin Hook, MD.*

- The color is initially pink to red-brown, but over time a yellow hue develops due to accumulation of intracellular lipid.
- Head/neck > trunk > upper extremities > lower extremities.
- Self-limiting; no treatment necessary.
- If multiple lesions, consider ophthalmologic examination for ocular involvement.
- If multiple café-au-lait macules are present, then consider the rare triple association with neurofibromatosis type I and an increased risk of developing juvenile myelomonocytic leukemia (see Table 45.8).
- **DDx:** mollusca contagiosa; when solitary, Spitz nevus; in an adult with multiple lesions, Erdheim-Chester disease, a rare disorder with multi-system involvement frequently associated with BRAF V600E mutations.

Benign Cephalic Histiocytosis

- Rare, generally in infants <1 year old.
- 2- to 5-mm red-brown macules or papules on the face and neck, rarely elsewhere (Fig. 76.4).
- Self-limiting after months to years; no treatment necessary.

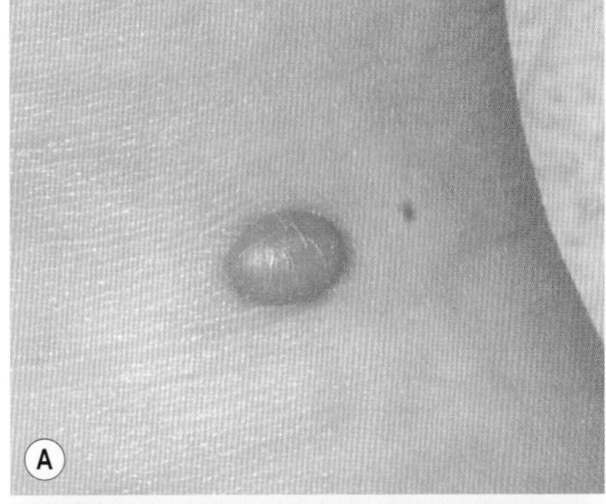

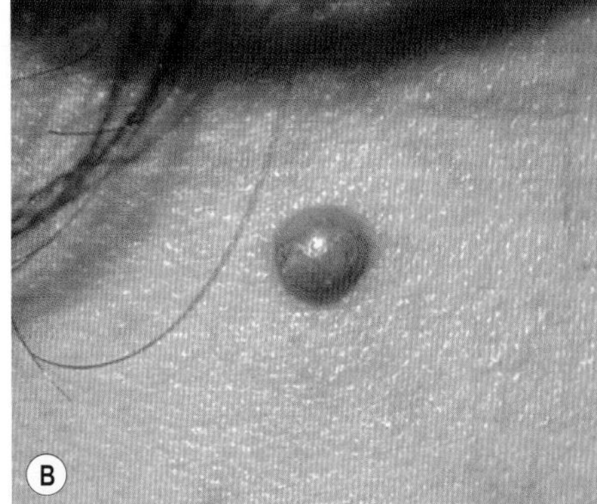

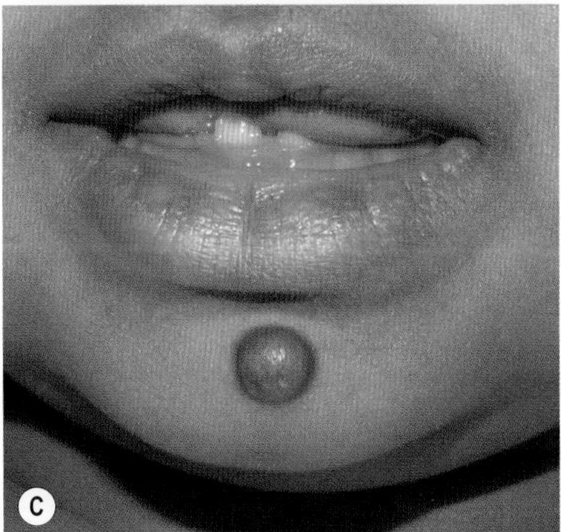

Fig. 76.3 Juvenile xanthogranuloma. Well-developed lesions that vary in color from pale yellow (**A**) to dark yellow/yellow-red (**B**) to yellow-brown (**C**), with the yellow hue reflecting the accumulation of lipid within histiocytes. *A, C, Courtesy, Julie V. Schaffer, MD; B, Courtesy, Luis Requena, MD.*

Generalized Eruptive Histiocytoma

- Rare, generally in adults.
- Recurrent crops of tens to hundreds of small red-brown, firm papules (Fig. 76.5).
- Widespread on trunk.
- Self-limiting; no treatment necessary.

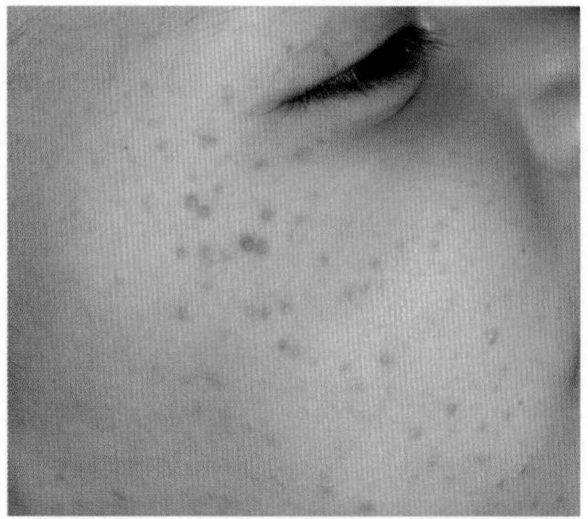

Fig. 76.4 Benign cephalic histiocytosis. Multiple light pink-brown papules on the face of a young child. *Courtesy, Julie V. Schaffer, MD.*

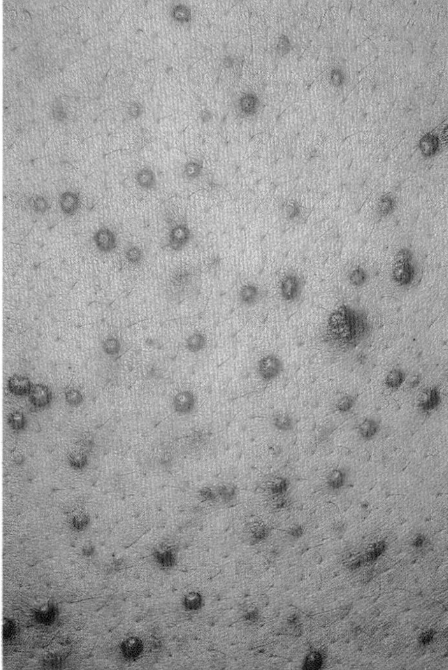

Fig. 76.5 Generalized eruptive histiocytoma. Multiple firm red papules on the trunk. *Courtesy, YDRSC.*

Indeterminate Cell Histiocytosis

- Rare, all ages affected.
- Clinically indistinguishable from generalized eruptive histiocytoma.
- Diagnosis made by evaluation of biopsy specimen, with cells expressing CD1a, S100 protein, and CD68 (a marker of macrophages); lack of Birbeck granules ultrastructurally.

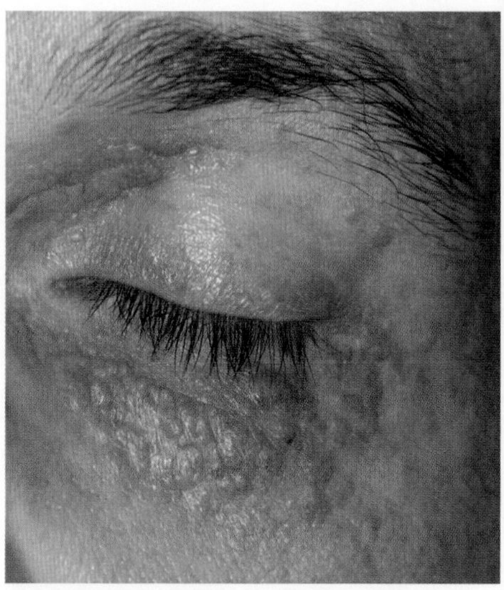

Fig. 76.6 Necrobiotic xanthogranuloma. Yellow-brown papules and plaques in a periorbital distribution in a patient with chronic lymphocytic leukemia. Such lesions may initially be mistaken for xanthelasma. *Courtesy, Kalman Watsky, MD.*

Necrobiotic Xanthogranuloma

- Rare, generally in adults >50 years of age.
- Firm, yellowish plaques or papulonodules; sometimes ulcerated.
- Classically periorbital (Fig. 76.6).
- IgG monoclonal gammopathy in at least 70% of patients (see Table 45.8); hepatosplenomegaly, increased ESR, leukopenia, hypocomplementemia.
- Underlying plasma cell dyscrasia common; also increased risk of lymphoproliferative disorders.

Multicentric Reticulohistiocytosis/ Giant Cell Reticulohistiocytoma

- Generally in adults.
- When single:
  - A skin-colored to pink papulonodule often on the head
  - Cutaneous disease only
- When multiple (Fig. 76.7):
  - Pink to red-brown papulonodules that favor the hands (especially periungual) and elbows; occasionally photodistributed
  - 50% with mucous membrane involvement

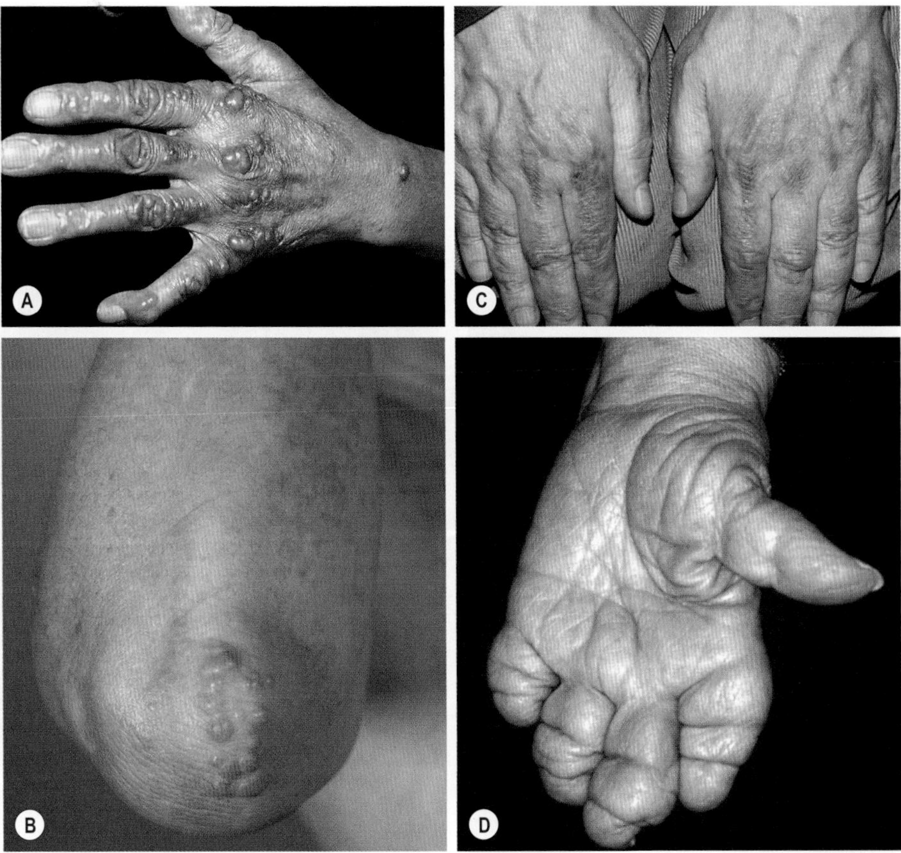

Fig. 76.7 Multicentric reticulohistiocytosis. A Grouped firm pink papules on the dorsal surface of the fingers, hand, and wrist of a 73-year-old African-American woman. **B** Grouped pink papulonodules on the elbow in a second patient. **C** A more subtle presentation in a third patient, with small pink papules and thin plaques that favor the skin overlying the small joints of the hands; this is the form that can initially be confused with dermatomyositis. **D** Telescoping of fingers due to arthritis mutilans.
A, Courtesy, Susan D. Laman, MD; B, Courtesy, Jean L. Bolognia, MD; C, D, Courtesy, Kalman Watsky, MD.

- Associated with destructive arthritis that can clinically resemble rheumatoid arthritis; in up to 50%, arthritis is preceded by skin disease
- Up to one third of affected patients can have an associated malignancy (see Table 45.8)

Rosai–Dorfman Disease (Sinus Histiocytosis with Massive Lymphadenopathy)

- Generally in children and young adults.
- Nonspecific red, red-brown, or yellow papulonodule(s) (Fig. 76.8).
- Favor eyelids and malar area.
- Skin-limited form being increasingly recognized.
- Often self-limited, but there may be a protracted course.
- Systemic disease presents as massive bilateral cervical lymphadenopathy; fever and IgG polyclonal hypergammaglobulinemia may be present.

Xanthoma Disseminatum

- Rare, generally before age 25 years.
- Triad of cutaneous xanthomas, mucous membrane xanthomas (in 40–60%), and diabetes insipidus (in 40%).
- Symmetric eruption of tens to hundreds of yellow, red, or brown papules and plaques.
- Favors face and flexural areas, including major folds (Fig. 76.9).
- Rarely sclerosis (Fig. 76.10).

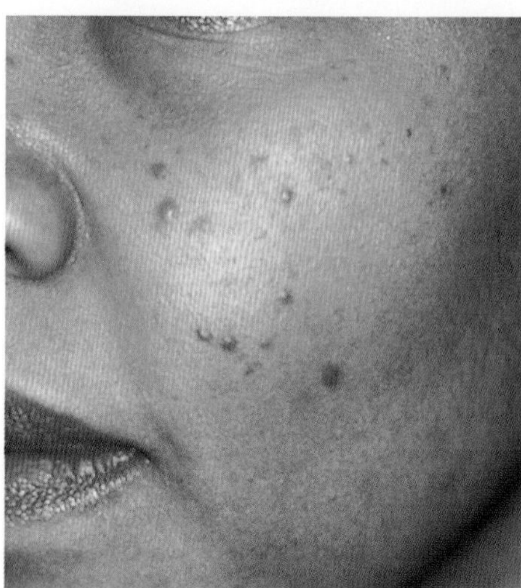
Fig. 76.8 Cutaneous Rosai–Dorfman disease. Discrete, dome-shaped, brown papules. *Courtesy, YDRSC.*

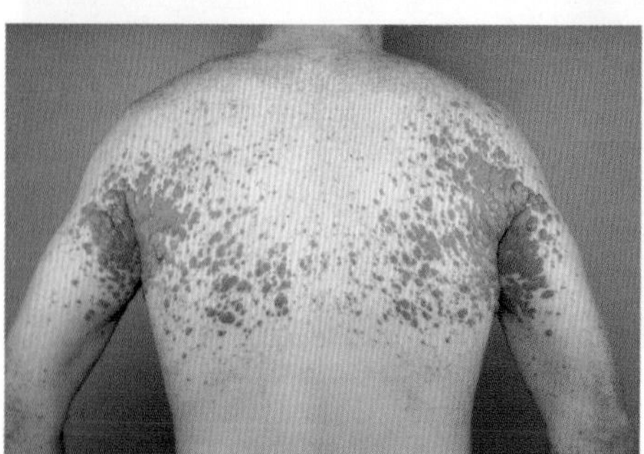
Fig. 76.9 Xanthoma disseminatum. Symmetric involvement of the major flexures is a characteristic finding. Note the yellow discoloration of some of the coalescing papulonodules. *Courtesy, David Wetter, MD.*

- Mucous membrane involvement: oral, upper airway, ocular (may threaten vision).
- Can be associated with a monoclonal gammopathy.
- May self-resolve, be persistent, or progressive.

Papular Xanthoma

- Any age.
- Generalized yellow papulonodules, sparing flexures.

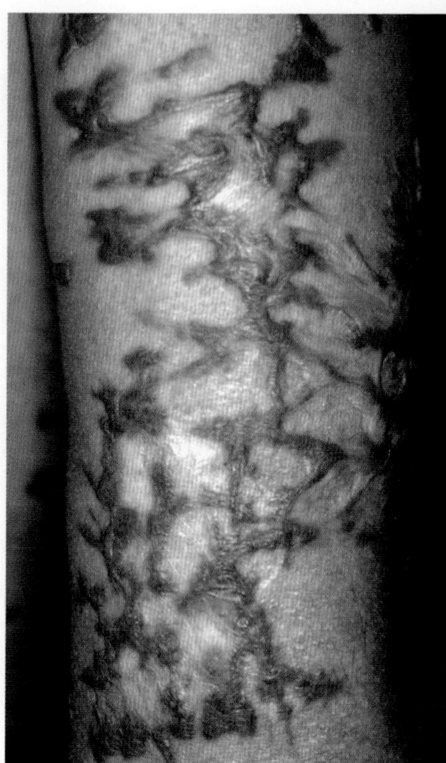
Fig. 76.10 Xanthoma disseminatum. Sclerotic form of xanthoma disseminatum in a patient who developed multiple myeloma. *Courtesy, YDRSC.*

Progressive Nodular Histiocytoma

- Any age.
- Generalized yellow papulonodules with prominent facial involvement.

Although we have made all these distinctions in the non-Langerhans cell histiocytoses, patients may have overlapping clinical and histopathologic features (including immunohistochemical staining). As a result, the evaluation of a patient with a non-Langerhans cell histiocytosis should include a total body skin examination and general physical examination, inclusive of eyes, mucosae, and lymph nodes. In addition, laboratory testing should include serum protein electrophoresis, immunofixation electrophoresis, and evaluation for diabetes insipidus.

For further information see Ch. 91 from *Dermatology, Fourth Edition*.

For additional online figures visit www.expertconsult.com 

Xanthomas 77

Key Points

- Cutaneous xanthomas are due to an accumulation of lipid, primarily within dermal macrophages (foam cells), and they have a characteristic yellow-orange hue.
- Four major types of xanthomas: eruptive, tuberous, tendinous, and plane.
- They may be a sign of hyperlipidemia, either primary or secondary, or an underlying monoclonal gammopathy.
- The type of xanthoma and its anatomic location are clues to the specific lipid abnormality or associated disorder (Tables 77.1 and 77.2; Fig. 77.1).
- **DDx** depends on the type of xanthoma (Table 77.3).
- In general, **Rx** is focused on correcting any underlying hyperlipidemia.

MAJOR TYPES OF HYPERLIPIDEMIA			
Type	**Laboratory findings**	**Clinical findings**	
		Skin (types of xanthoma)	**Systemic**
Type I (familial LPL deficiency, familial hyperchylomicronemia)	Slow chylomicron clearance Reduced LDL and HDL levels Hypertriglyceridemia	Eruptive	No increased risk of coronary artery disease
Type II (familial hypercholesterolemia or familial defective apo B-100)	Reduced LDL clearance Hypercholesterolemia	Tendinous, tuberoeruptive, tuberous, plane (xanthelasma, intertriginous areas, interdigital web spaces*)	Atherosclerosis of peripheral and coronary arteries
Type III (familial dysbetalipoproteinemia, remnant removal disease, broad beta disease, apo E deficiency)	Elevated levels of chylomicron remnants and IDLs Hypercholesterolemia Hypertriglyceridemia	Tuberoeruptive, tuberous Plane (palmar creases) – most characteristic Tendinous	Atherosclerosis of peripheral and coronary arteries
Type IV (endogenous familial hypertriglyceridemia)	Increased VLDLs Hypertriglyceridemia	Eruptive	Frequently associated with type 2 non-insulin-dependent diabetes mellitus, obesity, alcoholism
Type V	Decreased LDLs and HDLs Hypertriglyeridemia	Eruptive	Diabetes mellitus

Plane xanthomas in the interdigital web space are said to be pathognomonic for the homozygous state.

Table 77.1 Major types of hyperlipidemia. apo, apolipoprotein; HDL, high-density lipoprotein; IDL, intermediate-density lipoprotein; LDL, low-density lipoprotein; LPL, lipoprotein lipase; VLDL, very-low-density lipoprotein.

CAUSES OF HYPERTRIGLYCERIDEMIA	
Primary	
Genetic factors (see Table 77.1)	
Secondary	
Diabetes mellitus, especially when poorly controlled (see Table 45.10)	
Medications	Systemic retinoids (e.g. bexarotene, acitretin)
	Antiretrovirals (e.g. ritonavir, indinavir, stavudine)
	Azacitidine, cyclosporine, estrogen, olanzapine
Obesity	
Alcohol intake	
Other underlying systemic disorders (e.g. primary biliary cholangitis [see Table 45.6], hypothyroidism [see Table 45.12], nephrotic syndrome)	

Table 77.2 Causes of hypertriglyceridemia. Severe elevation is generally defined as triglycerides >500 mg/L, but eruptive xanthomas usually develop at much higher levels; more than one factor can be present in a patient. See Table 77.4 for recommended laboratory tests.

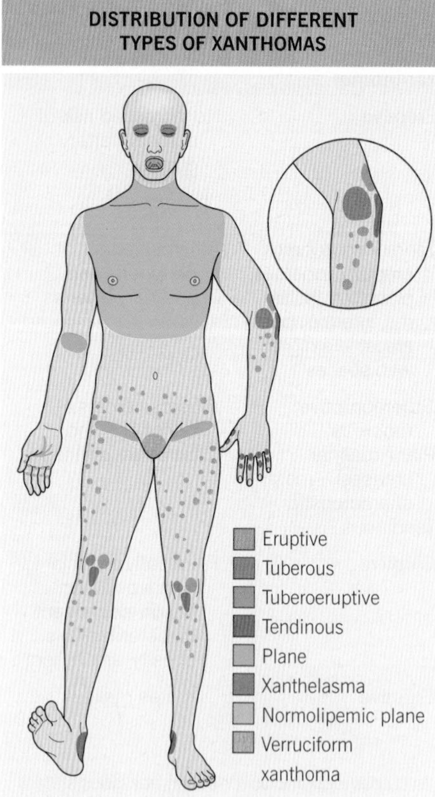

Fig. 77.1 Distribution of different types of xanthomas.

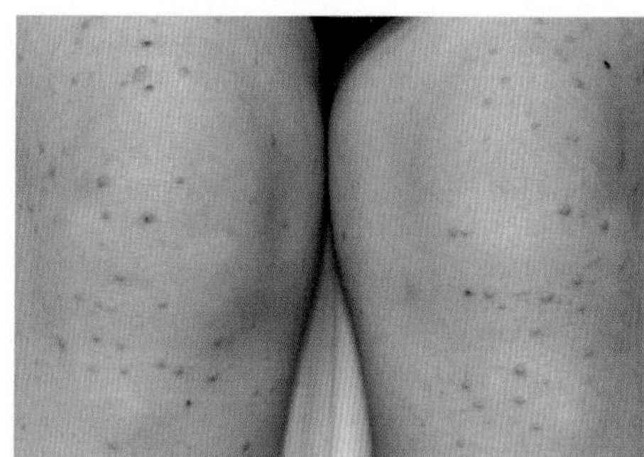

Fig. 77.2 Eruptive xanthomas due to hypertriglyceridemia. The lesions favored the extensor surface of the lower extremities, in particular the knees. *Courtesy, YDRSC.*

Xanthomas Associated with Hyperlipidemia

Eruptive Xanthomas

- Yellow-pink papules, 1–5 mm in diameter.
- May be widespread, but favor the extensor surfaces of the extremities and buttocks (Figs 77.2 and 77.3; see Fig. 45.10C).
- An inflammatory halo, tenderness, and/or pruritus may be present.
- Associated with hypertriglyceridemia (often >3000–4000 mg/dl) (see Table 77.2).
- Seen in the setting of type I, IV, or V hyperlipidemia and most commonly when associated

diabetes mellitus is under poor control (see Table 45.10).

- Lesions often resolve within weeks of aggressive **Rx:** insulin; triglyceride-lowering agents, e.g. fenofibrate.

Tuberous/Tuberoeruptive Xanthomas

- Pink-yellow to yellow-brown papules (tuberoeruptive) or nodules (tuberous) on extensor surfaces, especially the elbows and knees (Figs 77.4 and 77.5); tuberous xanthomas can be >3 cm in diameter.

DIFFERENTIAL DIAGNOSIS OF XANTHOMAS
Eruptive xanthomas
• Non-Langerhans cell histiocytosis – Xanthoma disseminatum – Papular xanthoma – Generalized eruptive histiocytoma – Indeterminate cell histiocytosis – Rosai–Dorfman disease – Juvenile xanthogranuloma (micronodular form) • Xanthomatous lesions of Langerhans cell histiocytosis • Disseminated granuloma annulare
Tuberous xanthomas
• Erythema elevatum diutinum • Multicentric reticulohistiocytosis
Tendinous xanthomas
• Giant cell tumor of the tendon sheath • Rheumatoid nodule • Subcutaneous granuloma annulare • Erythema elevatum diutinum
Xanthelasma
• Syringomas • Necrobiotic xanthogranuloma • Sebaceous hyperplasia • Palpebral sarcoidosis

Table 77.3 Differential diagnosis of xanthomas.

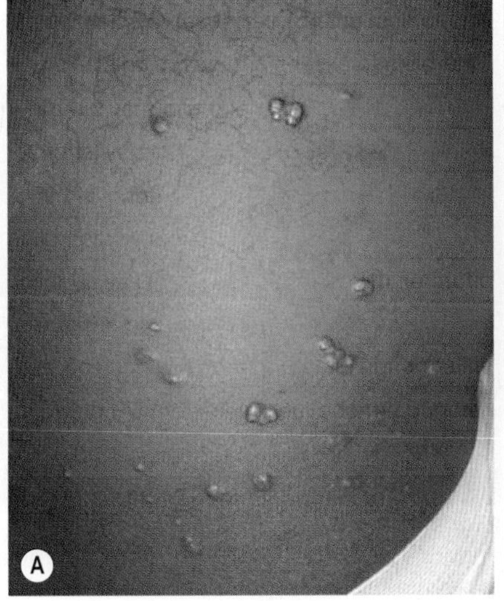

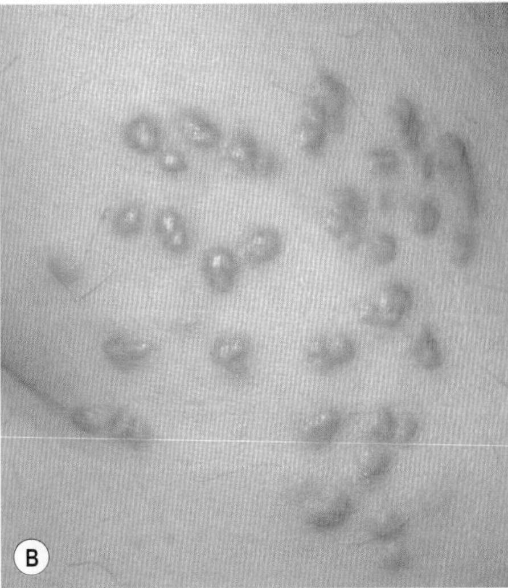

Fig. 77.3 Eruptive xanthomas. A, B The yellowish hue is influenced by the degree of pigmentation of the skin. Note the clustering of some of the lesions. *A, Courtesy, YDRSC; B, Courtesy, W. Trent Massengale, MD.*

• Associated with hypercholesterolemia (type II or III hyperlipidemia).

• May be slow to regress with cholesterol-lowering agents (e.g. "statins").

Tendinous Xanthomas

• Firm, smooth, skin-colored nodules due to lipid deposits within the Achilles tendons and the extensor tendons of the hands, knees, and/or elbows (Figs 77.6 and 77.7).

• Can serve as an early clue to the presence of type II hyperlipidemia.

• Rarely form as a consequence of accumulation of cholestanol (cerebrotendinous xanthomatosis) or plant sterols (β-sitosterolemia).

Plane Xanthomas and Xanthelasma

• Yellow to orange macules and patches or thin papules and plaques.

• Of the different types of xanthomas, xanthelasma is the most common; however, hyperlipidemia is detected in only 50% of patients.

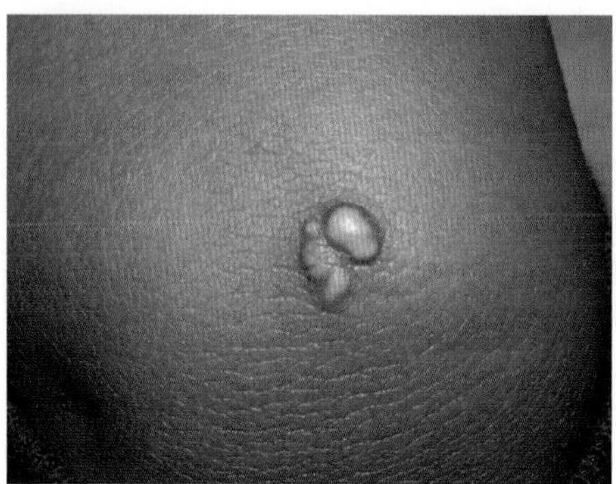

Fig. 77.4 Tuberoeruptive xanthomas on the elbow of a child with homozygous familial hypercholesterolemia. Note the yellowish hue. *Courtesy, Julie V. Schaffer, MD.*

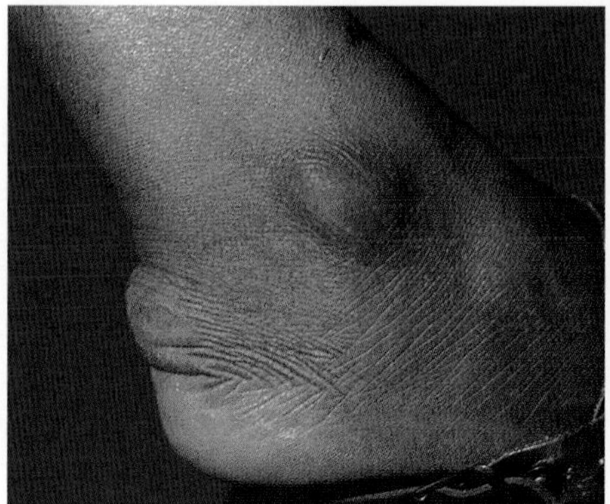

Fig. 77.6 Tendinous xanthoma. Linear swelling of the Achilles area, representing a tendinous xanthoma in a patient with dysbetalipoproteinemia. *Courtesy, W. Trent Massengale, MD, and Lee T. Nesbitt, Jr., MD.*

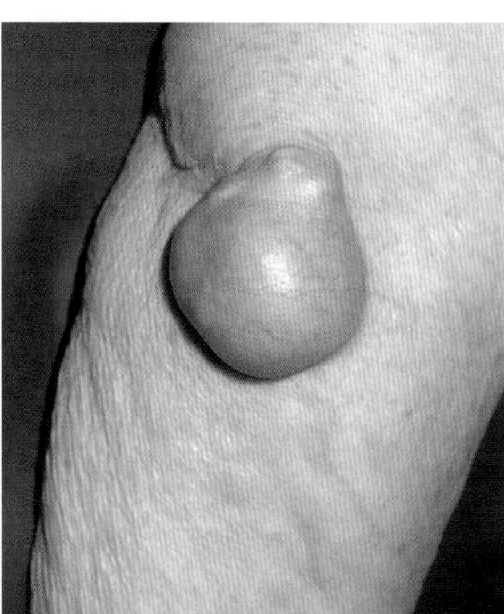

Fig. 77.5 Nodular tuberous xanthoma of the elbow. *Courtesy, Lorenzo Cerroni, MD.*

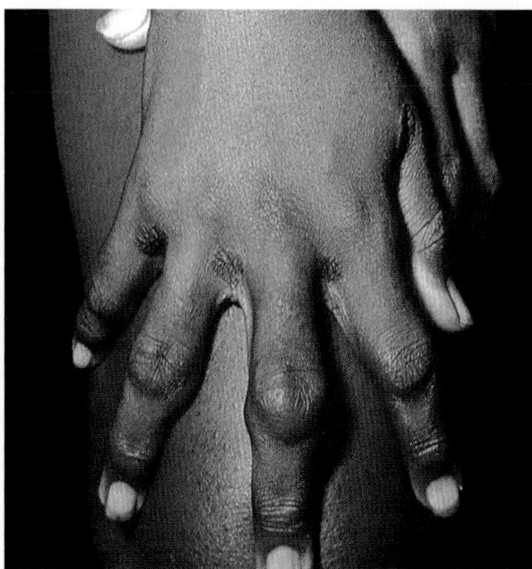

Fig. 77.7 Tendinous xanthomas of the fingers in a patient with homozygous familial hypercholesterolemia. Note interdigital plane xanthomas of the web spaces. *Courtesy, W. Trent Massengale, MD, and Lee T. Nesbitt, Jr., MD.*

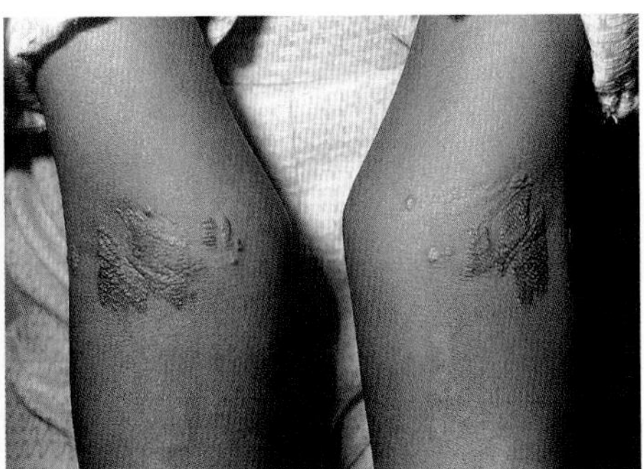

Fig. 77.8 Plane xanthomas of the antecubital fossae. This young patient had dysbetalipoproteinemia. *Courtesy, W. Trent Massengale, MD, and Lee T. Nesbitt, Jr., MD.*

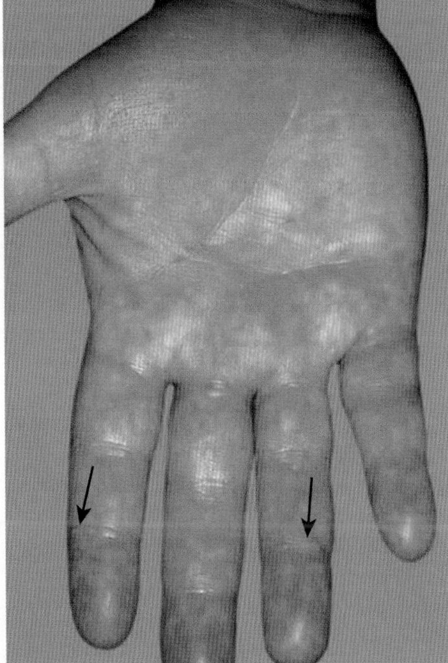

Fig. 77.9 Plane xanthomas of the palmar creases (arrows) in a patient with dysbetalipoproteinemia. They are seen in approximately two-thirds of patients with this disorder. Plane xanthomas are also seen in the setting of cholestasis, e.g. biliary atresia or primary biliary cholangitis. *Courtesy, W. Trent Massengale, MD, and Lee T. Nesbitt, Jr., MD.*

- Site:
  - Intertriginous – antecubital fossae, finger web spaces, and palmar creases (Figs 77.8 and 77.9)

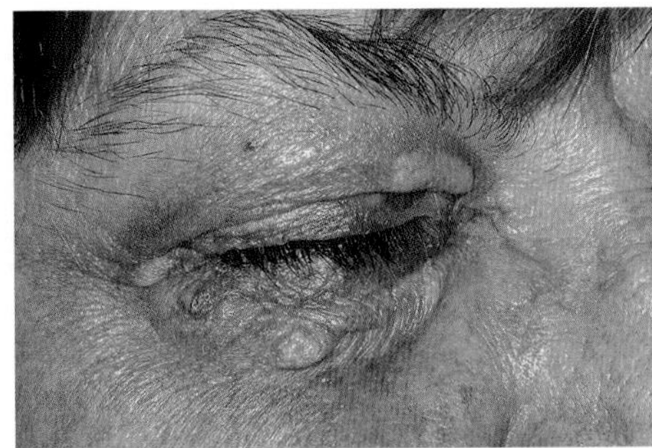

Fig. 77.10 Xanthelasma palpebrarum with typical yellowish hue. *Courtesy, YDRSC.*

  - Eyelids (xanthelasma), especially the medial aspect of the upper eyelid (Fig. 77.10)
- Intertriginous plane xanthomas can be seen in primary hyperlipidemia (type II or III) as well as secondary hyperlipidemia (e.g. biliary atresia, primary biliary cholangitis; see Table 45.6).
- **Rx** of xanthelasma: destructive methods (e.g. trichloroacetic acid application, laser ablation), surgical excision.

Laboratory evaluation for suspected hyperlipidemia is outlined in Table 77.4.

Normolipemic Xanthomas

Plane Xanthomas Associated with Monoclonal Gammopathy

- In contrast to plane xanthomas due to hyperlipidemia, these yellow-orange patches and thin plaques are usually larger in size and have a more extensive distribution pattern; the latter often includes the trunk (Fig. 77.11).
- In addition to the trunk, lesions may be seen on the neck, in flexural folds, and in the periorbital region.
- The monoclonal gammopathy is most commonly due to a plasma cell dyscrasia, and occasionally due to a lymphoproliferative disorder (see Table 45.8).

Verruciform Xanthoma

- Asymptomatic verrucous plaque, 1 to 2 cm in diameter (Fig. 77.12).
- Oral mucosa or anogenital region.
- May be seen in association with lymphedema, epidermolysis bullosa, and CHILD (congenital hemidysplasia with ichthyosiform erythroderma and limb defects) syndrome.

For further information see Ch. 92 from *Dermatology, Fourth Edition*.

For additional online figures and tables visit www.expertconsult.com 

LABORATORY EVALUATION OF SUSPECTED HYPERLIPIDEMIA
• Fasting lipid panel* • Fasting glucose level • Liver function tests** • Thyroid-stimulating hormone (TSH) level • Serum albumin
**Lipid panel: Total cholesterol, trigylcerides, HDL cholesterol, LDL cholesterol, calculated non-HDL cholesterol. If elevated serum lipids, evaluate for systemic disease (see Tables 77.1 and 77.2).* ***If elevated serum alkaline phosphatase and bilirubin, evaluate for biliary disease.*

Table 77.4 Laboratory evaluation of suspected hyperlipidemia.

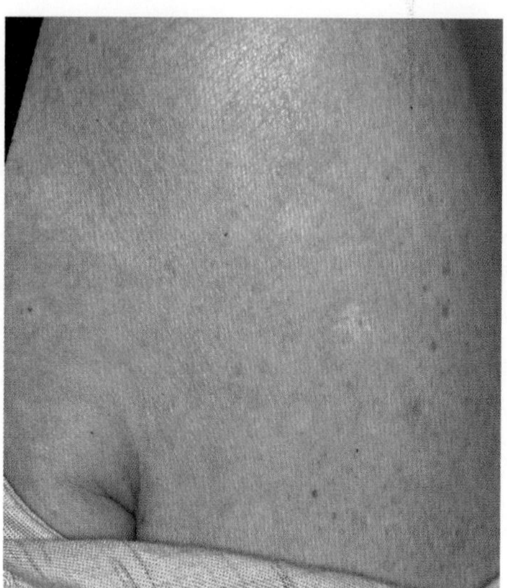

Fig. 77.11 Normolipemic plane xanthoma. The large thin plaques have a yellow-orange color. On longitudinal evaluation, the patient was found to have a monoclonal gammopathy. *Courtesy, Whitney High, MD, JD.*

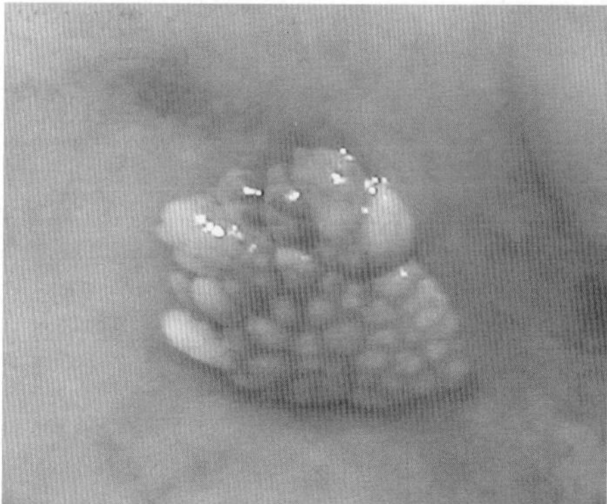

Fig. 77.12 Verruciform xanthoma of the oral mucosa. *Courtesy, Kishore Shetty, DDS.*

Non-infectious Granulomatous Disorders, Including Foreign Body Reactions

78

When histiocytes form granulomas within the skin, the cutaneous disorders are referred to as granulomatous. This group of disorders is further divided into infectious (e.g. mycobacterial infections, dimorphic fungal infections) and non-infectious (e.g. sarcoidosis, granuloma annulare). This chapter focuses on the latter category.

Sarcoidosis

- Disorder of unknown etiology in which granulomas develop in one or more organs, most commonly the lung, skin, liver, and spleen.
- Cutaneous manifestations occur in >30% of patients and may be the first and/or only sign of the disease (Table 78.1).
- The classic lesion is a red-brown papule or plaque with a yellowish color on compression (diascopy), most commonly on the face (Figs 78.1 and 78.2; see Fig. 45.1A).
- Variants:
  - Lupus pernio – purple to red-brown papules and plaques of the nose, ears, and cheeks; may be beaded along the nasal rim (Fig. 78.2C); associated with chronic pulmonary sarcoidosis (75% of patients), upper respiratory tract sarcoidosis (50%), and cysts within the distal phalanges
  - Darier–Roussy sarcoidosis (subcutaneous variant) – painless, firm, mobile nodules or plaques
  - Löfgren syndrome – hilar adenopathy, fever, migrating polyarthritis, and acute iritis; erythema nodosum is the primary skin finding (see Table 83.2); often spontaneously remits
  - Heerfordt syndrome – parotid gland enlargement, uveitis, fever, cranial nerve palsies
- Once the diagnosis of cutaneous sarcoidosis is established, evaluation for systemic involvement is necessary (Table 78.2)
- **DDx** of classic papule/plaque other entities in this chapter, granulomatous rosacea and perioral dermatitis, dimorphic fungal infections, cutaneous tuberculosis; in young children, consider Blau syndrome (see Ch. 37).
- **Rx** of cutaneous lesions: CS (topical, intralesional); oral medications include minocycline, antimalarials, methotrexate, tacrolimus, TNF inhibitors, thalidomide, and JAK inhibitors.

Granuloma Annulare

- May be a delayed-type hypersensitivity reaction to an unknown antigen; by history can follow an arthropod bite, trauma.
- Common clinical variants (see Table 78.1) – localized, often acral (Fig. 78.3); subcutaneous on hands, shins, and scalp in children; generalized (Fig. 78.4).
- Less common variants are perforating, often on the hands (Fig. 78.5), patch type on the trunk, and micropapular (Fig. 78.6).
- Generalized granuloma annulare, also referred to as disseminated, is more likely to be associated with diabetes mellitus (see Table 45.10) or lipid abnormalities (e.g. hypercholesterolemia) compared to other variants; atypical presentations seen in HIV-infected patients.
- **DDx:** other entities in this chapter (see Table 78.1), tinea, interstitial granulomatous dermatitis, inflammatory morphea.
- **Rx:** spontaneous resolution may occur; first-line – CS (topical including under occlusion, intralesional); second-line – cryosurgery, niacinamide +/– tetracycline, antimalarials, retinoids, PUVA/UVA1/excimer laser and apremilast.

Necrobiosis Lipoidica

- Formerly referred to as "necrobiosis lipoidica diabeticorum," a term abandoned given that not all patients with this disorder have diabetes mellitus (see Table 45.10).

CLINICAL FEATURES OF THE MAJOR GRANULOMATOUS DERMATITIDES						
	Sarcoidosis*	**Classic granuloma annulare^**	**Necrobiosis lipoidica**	**IGD/PNGD**	**Cutaneous Crohn disease**	**Rheumatoid nodule (see Fig. 37.2)**
Average age (years)	25–35, 45–65	<30	30	40–70	35	40–50
Sex predilection	Female	Female	Female	IGD: Female	Female	Male†
Racial/ethnic predilection in United States	African-American	None	None	Caucasian	Ashkenazi Jews	None
Sites	Symmetric on face, neck, upper trunk, extremities	Hands, feet, extensor aspects of extremities	Anterior and lateral aspects of shins	IGD: lateral trunk, medial arms/thighs; PNGD: elbows, fingers	Anogenital region, buttocks, lower > upper extremities	Juxta-articular areas, especially elbows, hands, ankles, feet
Appearance	Protean; most commonly red-brown or violaceous papules and plaques; occasionally violaceous or annular	Papules coalescing into annular plaques	Plaques with elevated borders, telangiectasias centrally	IGD: erythematous papules and plaques, sometimes annular; PNGD: umbilicated papules	Dusky erythema, lymphedema, ulceration, vegetating plaques	Skin-colored, firm, mobile subcutaneous nodules
Size of lesions	0.2 to >5 cm	1- to 3-mm papules, annular plaques usually <6 cm	3 to >10 cm	IGD: 5 mm to > 2 cm; PNGD: 1–4 mm	Variable	1–3 cm
No. of lesions	Variable	1–10	1–10	1 to >20	1–5	1–10
Associations	Systemic manifestations of sarcoidosis; can be drug-induced (e.g. IFN, TNF inhibitors) or reaction pattern to underlying lymphoma	Possible diabetes mellitus, thyroid disease, or hyperlipidemia; rare reports of HIV infection, malignancy	Diabetes mellitus	Medications, e.g. statins, TNF inhibitors; autoimmune disease, e.g. rheumatoid arthritis	Intestinal Crohn disease	Rheumatoid arthritis
Special clinical characteristics	Occasional central atrophy and hypopigmentation; develop within scars and tattoos	Central hyperpigmentation	Yellow-brown atrophic centers, ulceration	"Rope sign" (linear cords)	Draining sinuses and fistulas	Occasional ulceration, especially at sites of trauma

**Clinical variants include lupus pernio and subcutaneous (Darier–Roussy), psoriasiform, ichthyosiform, angiolupoid, and ulcerative sarcoidosis .*
^Clinical variants include generalized/disseminated, micropapular, nodular, perforating, subcutaneous, and patch granuloma annulare.
†Although rheumatoid arthritis has a female:male ratio of 2–3:1.

Table 78.1 Clinical features of the major granulomatous dermatitides. [illegible]

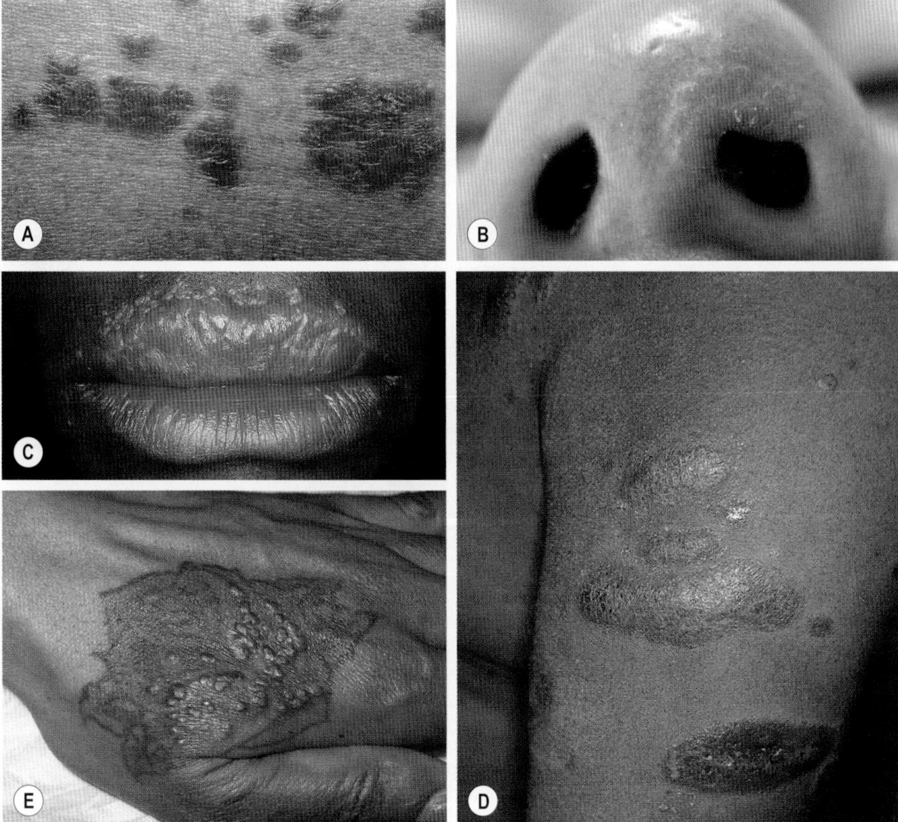

Fig. 78.1 Sarcoidosis. A Cutaneous sarcoidosis usually consists of papules and plaques with a typical reddish-brown color. **B, C** Lesions often favor the nose, lips, and perioral region. **D** Hyperpigmented plaques, some of which have scale. **E** Papules of cutaneous sarcoidosis arising within a tattoo; the differential diagnosis includes foreign body reaction. *A, C–E, Courtesy, YDRSC; B, Courtesy, Misha Rosenbach, MD.*

- Typically red-brown plaques on the shins with central clearing that may become yellow and atrophic over time; occasionally, lesions involve the upper extremities, face, and scalp (Fig. 78.7; see Table 78.1; see Fig. 45.10D).
- **DDx:** granuloma annulare, sarcoidosis, and non-Langerhans cell histiocytoses, in particular necrobiotic xanthogranuloma.
- **Rx:** CS (topical, intralesional, rarely systemic) are the mainstay; for intralesional CS, test sites are recommended.

Annular Elastolytic Giant Cell Granuloma

- Clinically most closely resembles granuloma annulare but lesions have an atrophic, hypopigmented center and sites of predilection are sun-exposed sites including the face, neck, and forearms (Fig. 78.8; see Table 78.1).
- Biopsy needs to be elliptical and involve the center, the border, and uninvolved skin with longitudinal sectioning.
- **Rx:** often ineffective, can try topical and intralesional CS.

Interstitial Granulomatous Dermatitis (IGD) and Palisaded Neutrophilic and Granulomatous Dermatitis (PNGD) (Reactive Granulomatous Dermatitis)

- Two clinicopathologic patterns of granulomatous dermatitis that occur in patients (women > men) with rheumatoid arthritis (RA) and other autoimmune disorders.

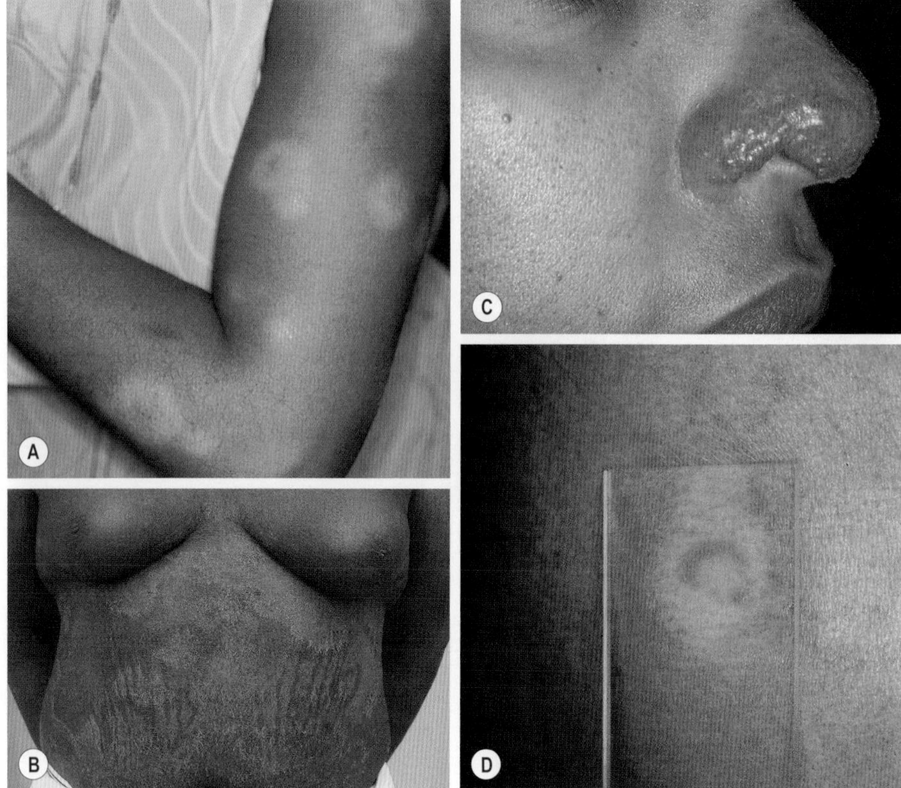

Fig. 78.2 Sarcoidosis – clinical variants and appearance with diascopy. A The hypopigmented variant is more noticeable in individuals with dark skin. **B** Ichthyosiform presentation with obvious scale. **C** Coalescing violaceous papules on the nose in lupus pernio; note the notching of the nasal rim. **D** Diascopy: pressure applied to a lesion creates a yellow-brown, "apple-jelly", color. *A, Courtesy, Louis A. Fragola, Jr., MD; B, Courtesy, Jean L. Bolognia, MD; C, D, Courtesy, YDRSC.*

SUGGESTED INITIAL SYSTEMIC EVALUATION OF A PATIENT WITH CUTANEOUS SARCOIDOSIS
In ALL patients: • **CXR (PA and lateral)*** • **PFTs with DLCO** • **Ophthalmologic examination** • **CBC, LFTs, BUN/Cr, TSH, serum calcium, serum 25-hydroxy- and 1,25-dihydroxy-vitamin D levels, ACE level** • TST or IFN-gamma release assay (e.g. QFT-GIT)** • ECG*** *Based upon findings from thorough history, review of systems, physical examination:* • Heart palpitations, syncopal or pre-syncopal episodes, abnormal ECG: refer to cardiology (further cardiac imaging will be performed, e.g. cardiac MRI or PET) • Extensive facial involvement (e.g. lupus pernio, multiple nasal/perinasal lesions): refer to otolaryngology (evaluation for sinus and/or upper airway involvement) • Cough, chest pain, dyspnea, velcro rales in lung base, abnormal CXR or PFTs: refer to pulmonology • Neuropathy (e.g. peripheral, cranial, small fiber): refer to neurology

*Items in **bold** should be repeated annually.*
**High resolution chest CT scan is more sensitive than CXR and should be ordered if any suspicious findings on CXR or if normal CXR but high clinical suspicion for pulmonary involvement.*
***To exclude tuberculosis, which can present with similar radiographic signs.*
****Any abnormalities should prompt referral to cardiology.*

Table 78.2 Initial systemic evaluation of a patient with cutaneous sarcoidosis. ACE, angiotensin converting enzyme; DLCO, diffusing capacity for carbon monoxide; PET, positron emission tomography; PFTs, pulmonary function tests; QFT-GIT, Quantiferon-gold TB In-Tube test.

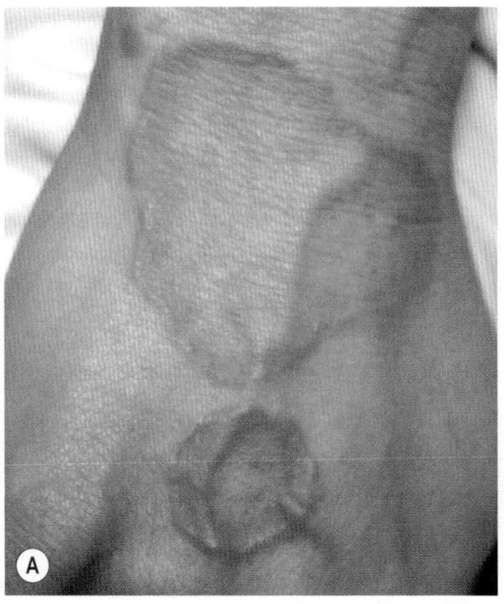

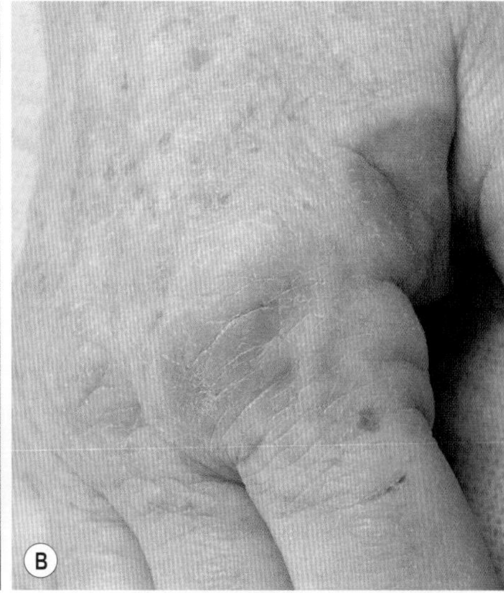

Fig. 78.3 Granuloma annulare. A,B Annular pink to pink-brown plaques; discrete papules may be seen. The dorsal aspect of the hand is a common location. *A, Courtesy YDRSC; B, Courtesy, Misha A. Rosenbach, MD.*

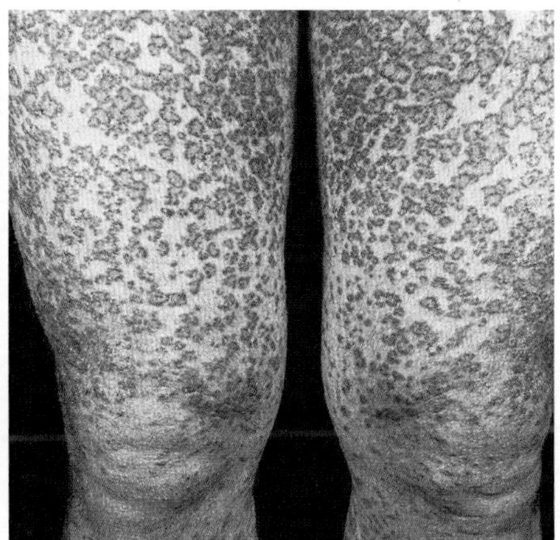

Fig. 78.4 Generalized granuloma annulare. Numerous papules and small annular plaques. *Courtesy, YDRSC.*

- *IGD* presents as annular erythematous plaques or linear cords ("rope sign") that favor the lateral and upper trunk, axillae, medial thighs, and buttocks (Fig. 78.9); patients often have RA or seronegative arthritis.
- *PNGD* presents as skin-colored to erythematous, umbilicated papulonodules that are often crusted and favor the elbows (see Fig. 19.11B) and extensor hands/fingers; associated with RA, SLE, and ANCA-positive systemic vasculitides (e.g. eosinophilic granulomatosis with polyangiitis); see Table 45.1.

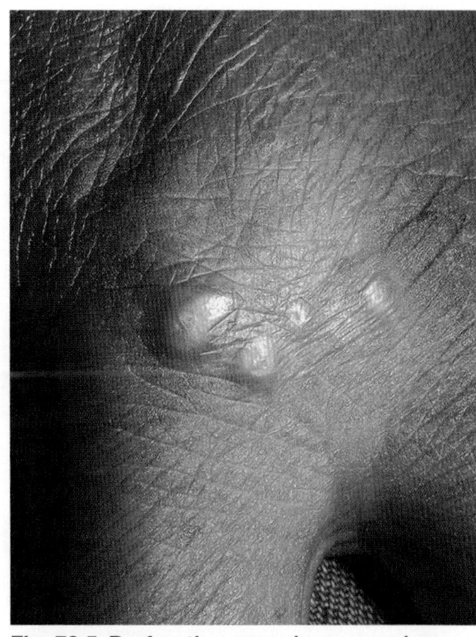

Fig. 78.5 Perforating granuloma annulare. Papules can have a central keratotic plug or umbilication. *Courtesy, Ronald P. Rapini, MD.*

- Because interstitial granulomatous drug reactions can have clinical and histologic features similar to those of IGD and PNGD, a review of all medications should be performed; culprit drugs include calcium channel blockers, angiotensin-converting enzyme inhibitors, statins, and TNF inhibitors.

• Histologically, a dense pandermal infiltrate is seen in both entities; IGD features rosettes of palisading histiocytes surrounding tiny foci of degenerated collagen, while findings in PNGD range from a predominance of neutrophils with foci of leukocytoclastic vasculitis to well-developed palisaded granulomas surrounding basophilic degenerated collagen.

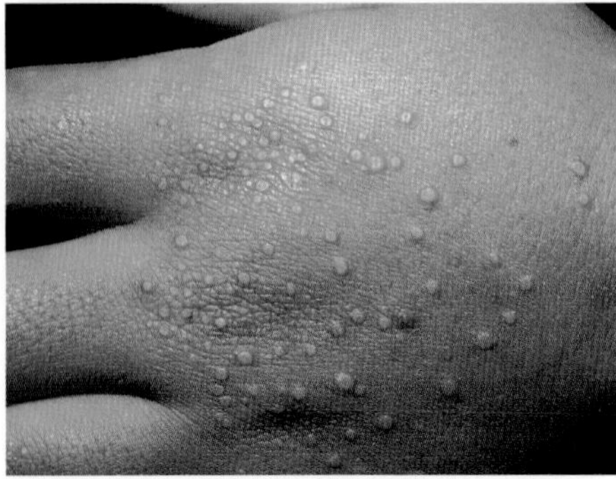

Fig. 78.6 Papular granuloma annulare of the dorsal hand. Several of the lesions have a central dell. *Courtesy, Joyce Rico, MD.*

• **DDx:** interstitial granulomatous drug reaction (see above); *for IGD* – patch-type granuloma annulare (GA), morphea (inflammatory stage), mycosis fungoides and leprosy; *for PNGD* – papular GA, rheumatoid nodules/nodulosis, perforating disorders.

• **Rx:** high-potency topical or intralesional CS, dapsone (if prominent neutrophils); may improve with treatment of the underlying disorder.

Cutaneous Crohn Disease

• Skin lesions may be the presenting sign of Crohn disease in up to 20% of patients and they may be specific or nonspecific; examples of the latter include pyoderma gangrenosum and erythema nodosum (see Table 45.4).

• Specific lesions can be contiguous or noncontiguous (metastatic), and both show granulomas on biopsy:

  – Contiguous lesions are seen in the mouth, perioral or anogenital region, and

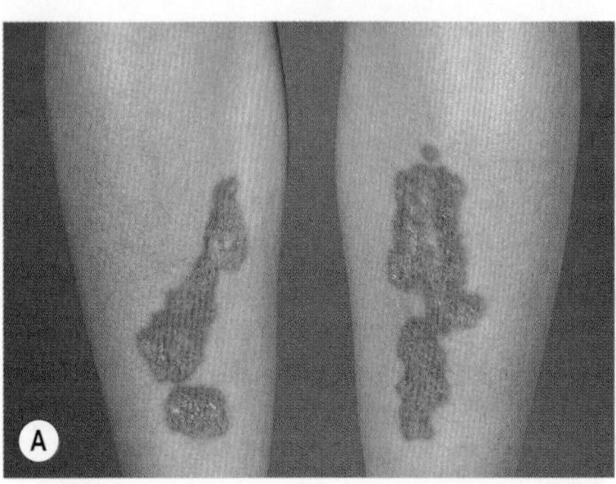

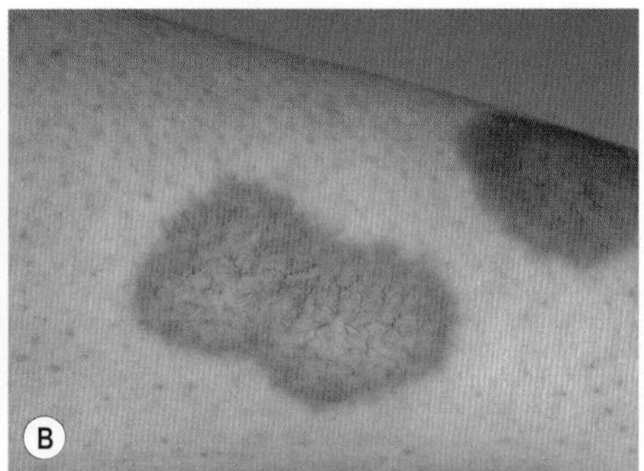

Fig. 78.7 Necrobiosis lipoidica. A Pink-brown atrophic plaques on the shins. **B** Annular plaques with central telangiectasias. *A, B, Courtesy, NYUDSC.*

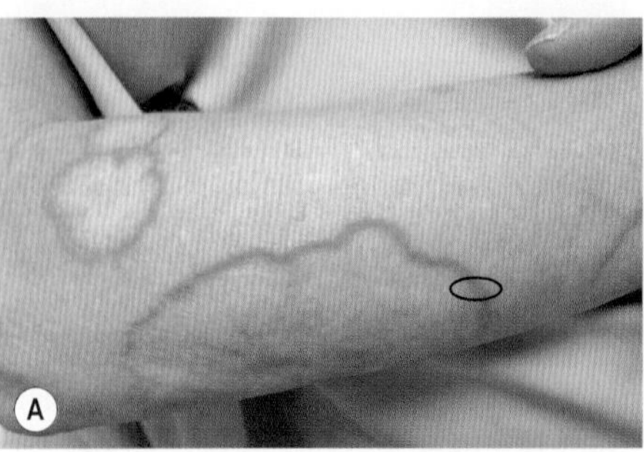

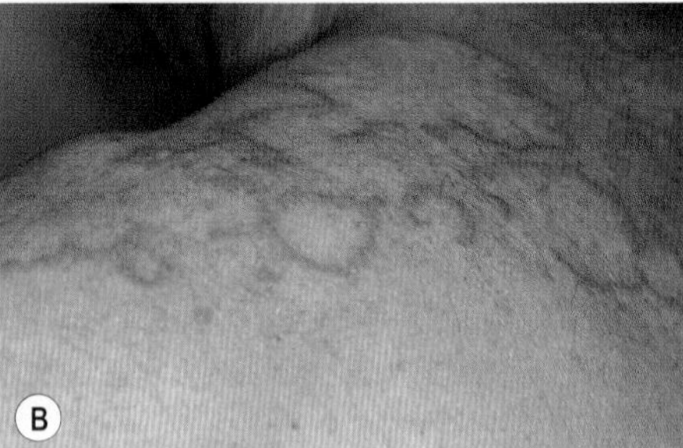

Fig. 78.8 Annular elastolytic giant cell granuloma. The border resembles granuloma annulare but the central portion is hypopigmented and/or atrophic **(A, B)**. A biopsy specimen that includes the area outlined in **A** would contain the three characteristic histologic zones: absence of elastic fibers, granulomatous inflammation, and normal skin. Longitudinal sectioning of the surgical specimen is preferred. *A, Courtesy, Misha A. Rosenbach, MD; B, Courtesy, Kalman Watsky, MD.*

peristomal areas with clinical presentations varying from fissures to cobblestoning to swelling (Figs 78.10 and 78.11; see Fig. 45.4A)
  - Metastatic lesions present as vegetating plaques or nodules, most commonly on the lower extremities (see Table 78.1)
  - Sinuses from GI disease may extend to the skin, particularly in the anogenital region or surgical sites on the abdomen
- **Rx of skin lesions**: often improve with systemic Rx of GI disease; oral metronidazole (250 mg three times daily); topical, intralesional, and oral CS; other systemic agents (e.g. sulfasalazine, TNF inhibitors).

Foreign Body Granulomas

- An inflammatory reaction to inorganic (e.g. suture) or organic (e.g. keratin) materials implanted into the skin.
- The most common foreign body is keratin due to ruptured cysts or hair follicles (Table 78.3; Figs 78.12–78.18).
- The clinical presentation is usually a red to red-brown papule, nodule, or plaque that may be ulcerated or extruding the foreign material.
- History and histologic findings including polarization can aid in identifying the foreign material; occasionally other procedures (e.g. energy dispersive X-ray analysis) are necessary.

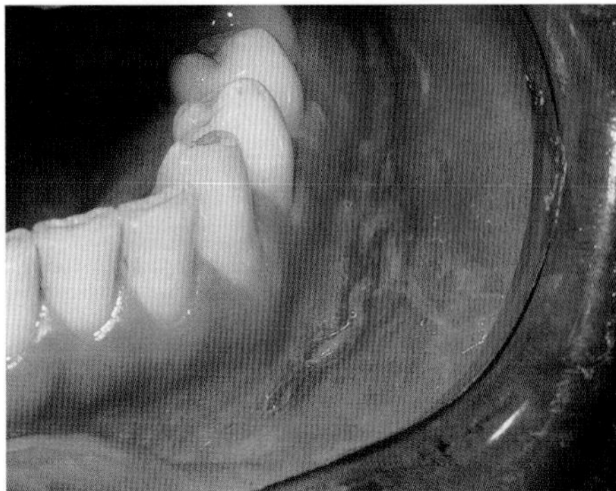

Fig. 78.10 Crohn disease. Linear ulceration of the mandibular vestibule: the classic oral manifestation of this disease. *Courtesy, Charles Camisa, MD.*

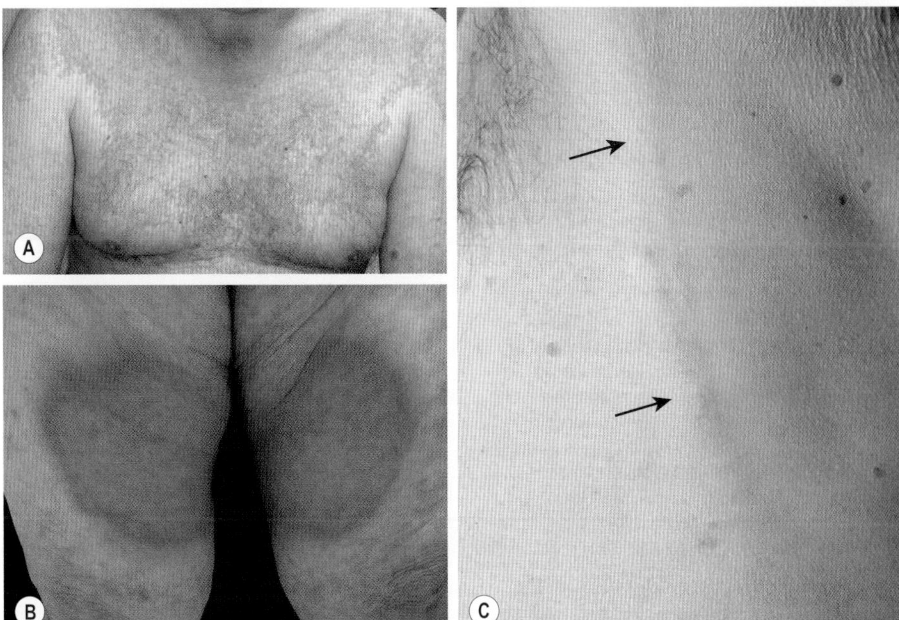

Fig. 78.9 Interstitial granulomatous dermatitis (IGD). A Large, symmetric pink patches and thin plaques that often resemble patch-type granuloma annulare. **B** Annular lesions on the medial thighs. **C** Firm linear cord along the axillary line in a patient with rheumatoid arthritis. *A, YDRSC; B, Courtesy, Jeffrey P. Callen, MD; C, Courtesy Kathryn Schwarzenberger, MD.*

For further information see Chs 93 and 94 from *Dermatology, Fourth Edition*.

For additional online figures and tables visit www.expertconsult.com 

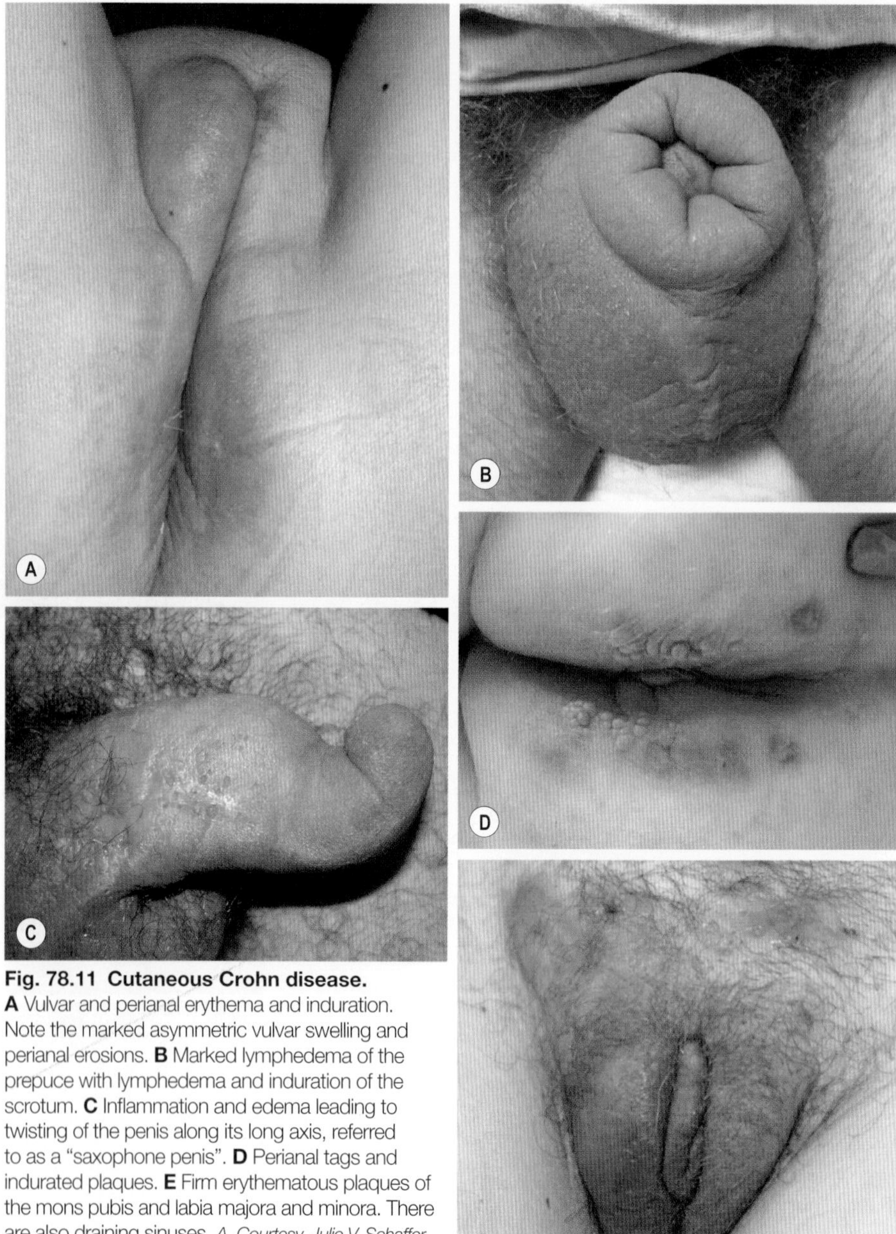

Fig. 78.11 Cutaneous Crohn disease. **A** Vulvar and perianal erythema and induration. Note the marked asymmetric vulvar swelling and perianal erosions. **B** Marked lymphedema of the prepuce with lymphedema and induration of the scrotum. **C** Inflammation and edema leading to twisting of the penis along its long axis, referred to as a "saxophone penis". **D** Perianal tags and indurated plaques. **E** Firm erythematous plaques of the mons pubis and labia majora and minora. There are also draining sinuses. *A, Courtesy, Julie V. Schaffer, MD; B,D, Courtesy, Misha Rosenbach, MD; C, E, Courtesy, Luis Requena, MD; D, Courtesy, Mary Stone, MD.*

FEATURES OF SELECTED FOREIGN BODY REACTIONS		
Foreign body	**Clinical presentations**	**Cause/common site(s)**
Endogenous material		
Keratin	• Erythema, induration, papules, nodules • Pseudofolliculitis/acne keloidalis nuchae • Pyogenic granuloma-like lesions • Pilonidal disease	• Ruptured follicle/cyst • Ingrown hair/nail • Beard area • Neck • Sacral area
Generally exogenous material		
Tattoo pigment	• Erythema, induration, papules, nodules (Fig. 78.12) • Lichenoid papules and plaques • Eczematous dermatitis (including photoallergic reactions)	• Decorative/cosmetic • Accidental (Fig. 78.13) • Iatrogenic
Silica (silicon dioxide)	• Nodules, indurated plaques within scar (Fig. 78.14) • Disseminated papules (blast injury) • Prolonged incubation period (sometimes decades)	• Wound contamination • Blast injury
Zirconium	• Persistent, brown, soft papules • Involvement of axillary skin	• Topical application of deodorants, antipruritic medications
Beryllium	• Nodule, ulcer • Widely scattered papules (systemic reaction)	• Laceration by broken fluorescent lamps • Inhalation
Cactus	• Dome-shaped, skin-colored papules with a central black dot	• Accidental • Occupational
Jellyfish, corals, sea urchin spines	• Pruritic lichenoid papules and plaques (onset 2–3 weeks after exposure) • Linear, zigzag, and whip-like (flagellate) patterns of erythema/edema (early), hyperpigmentation or lichenoid papules (late) (Fig. 78.15)	• Accidental • Swimming or diving
Implanted/injected material during procedures (Fig. 78.16)		
Suture	• Wound/scar appears inflamed and edematous (or develops papules or nodules) and opens to form a fistula	
Intralesional corticosteroids	• Skin-colored to yellow-white papules or nodules develop at the site of a previous intralesional injection of corticosteroid • Incubation period varies from weeks to months	
Talc	• Sarcoidosis-like papules • Thickening and erythema of an old scar • Involvement of intertriginous zones, IV injection sites (e.g. self-prepared drugs) • Pyogenic granuloma-like papulonodules of the umbilicus in infants (following talc application to umbilical stump)	
Starch	• Papules and nodules	
Aluminum	• Persistent subcutaneous nodule at vaccine injection site	
Zinc	• Furuncles at insulin injection sites	

Table 78.3 Features of selected foreign body reactions. *Continued*

FEATURES OF SELECTED FOREIGN BODY REACTIONS		
Foreign body	**Clinical presentations**	**Cause/common site(s)**
Injected material for tissue augmentation		
Paraffin	• Firm nodules, indurated plaques on genitalia or breasts • Ulceration or abscess formation (Fig. 78.17) • Occasionally periorbital (due to topical paraffin-containing preparations)	
Silicone	• Erythema, induration, nodules, ulcers on breasts • Often appears after years • Sometimes injected into the buttocks or face for cosmetic purposes, including for HIV-associated lipodystrophy (Fig. 78.18; see Ch. 84)	
Bovine collagen,* hyaluronic acid,* fillers containing synthetic particles	• Generally injected into the face • Induration and erythema • Papules and nodules (Fig. 78.19) • Abscesses	

*Often resorbable.

Table 78.3 *Continued* **Features of selected foreign body reactions.**

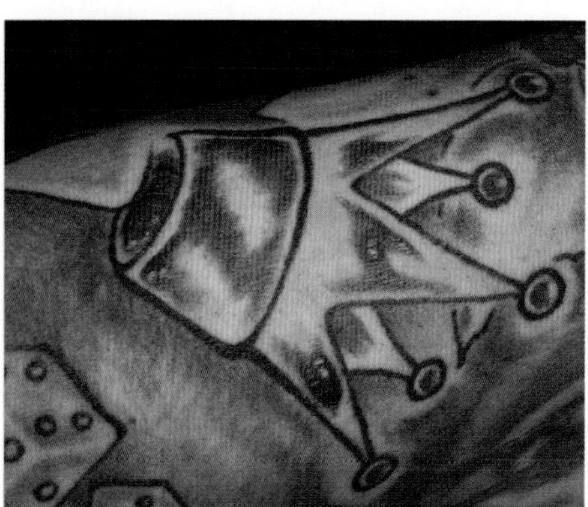

Fig. 78.12 Granulomatous reaction within the red portions of a tattoo. Over the past several years, cinnabar (mercuric sulfide) has been gradually replaced by cadmium selenide (cadmium red), ferric hydrate (sienna), and organic compounds. *Courtesy, Lorenzo Cerroni, MD.*

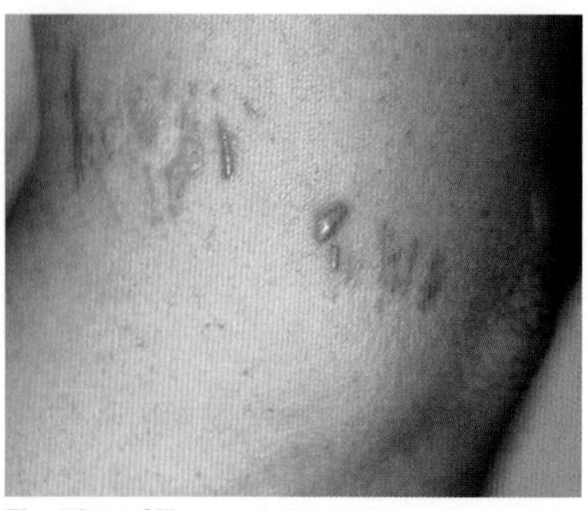

Fig. 78.14 Silica granulomas. *Courtesy, Kenneth Greer, MD.*

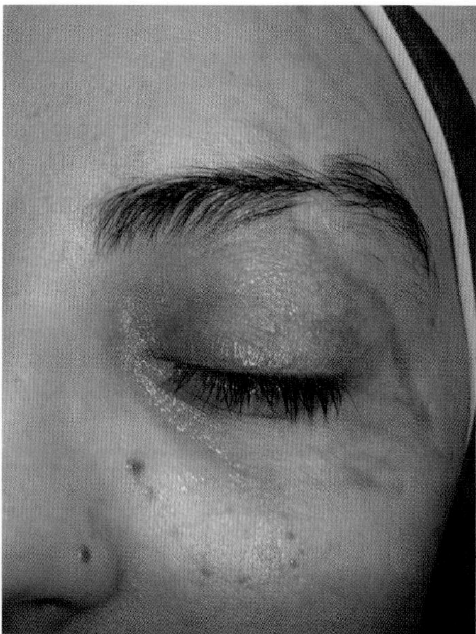

Fig. 78.13 Traumatic tattoo of the eyelid due to asphalt following a motor vehicle accident. This type of tattoo responds favorably to Q-switched laser therapy. *Courtesy, M. Abdel Rahim Abdallah, MD.*

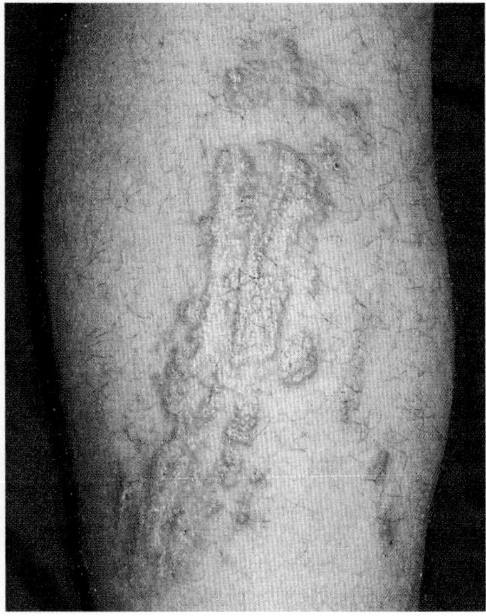

Fig. 78.15 Coral envenomation. Delayed lichenoid reaction on the calf. The patient accidentally came into contact with a coral reef and developed acute dermatitis that resolved, to be followed 3 weeks later by this severely itchy eruption that responded favorably to intralesional triamcinolone injection. *Courtesy, M. A. Abdallah, MD.*

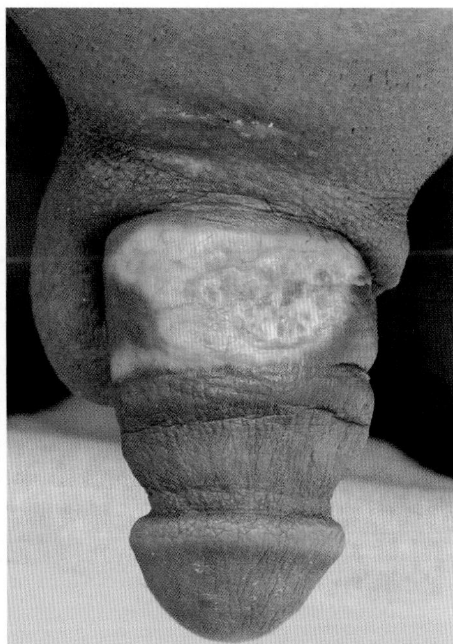

Fig. 78.17 Sclerosing lipogranuloma of the penis. The penis was injected in order to relieve urinary retention following a motorbike accident, and an ulcerated, indurated yellow plaque with telangiectasias developed at the site. *Courtesy, Glen Foxton, MD, and Clare Tait, MD.*

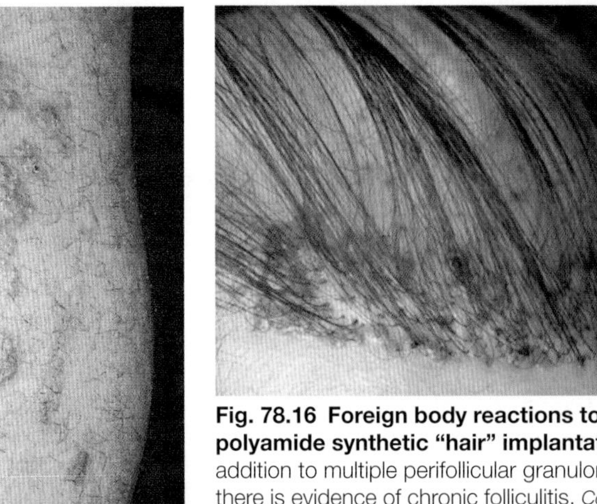

Fig. 78.16 Foreign body reactions to polyamide synthetic "hair" implantation. In addition to multiple perifollicular granulomas, there is evidence of chronic folliculitis. *Courtesy, Marwa Abdallah, MD.*

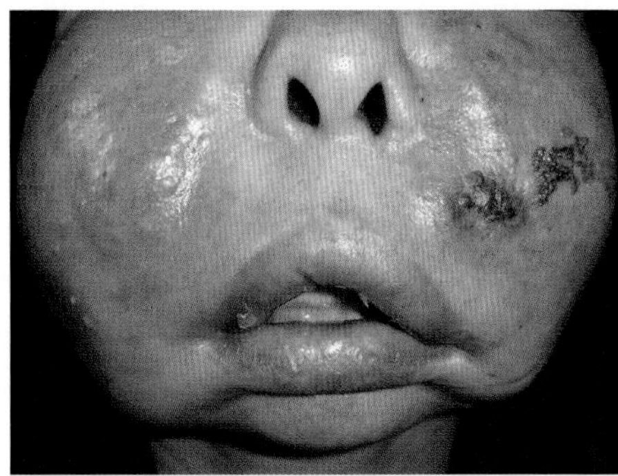

Fig. 78.18 Granulomatous reaction due to silicone injections. The procedure was performed in a beauty salon for cosmetic purposes. *Courtesy, M. Abdel Rahim Abdallah, MD.*

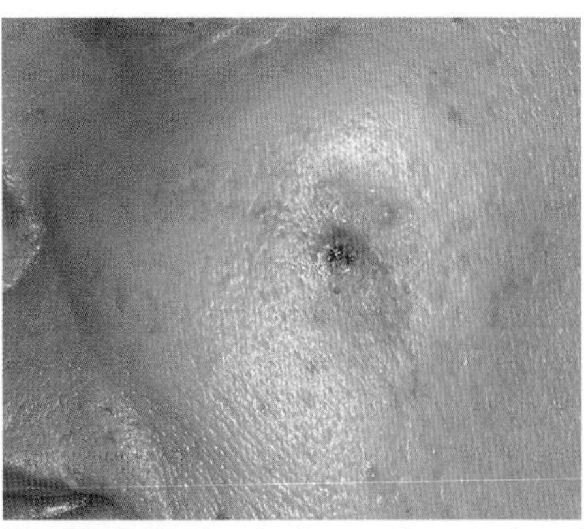

Fig. 78.19 Foreign body reaction at site of bovine collagen injection. Formation of granulomas at bovine collagen injection sites occurs in ~1% of patients who have had two negative skin tests. *Courtesy, YDRSC.*

79 Perforating Disorders

Classically, a group of disorders in which there is transepidermal elimination ("perforation") of components of the dermis, in particular collagen and/or elastic fibers (Table 79.1). Etiologies are multiple and include inherited as an isolated cutaneous disease or inherited in association with genetic disorders that affect connective tissue (e.g. Ehlers–Danlos syndrome). Most commonly, however, the perforating disorder is acquired and is related to the cutaneous trauma that results from scratching pruritic skin, especially in the setting of chronic kidney disease. A number of other cutaneous diseases occasionally undergo perforation, e.g. granuloma annulare, calcinosis cutis, chondrodermatitis nodularis helicis.

Acquired Perforating Dermatosis (APD)

- The most commonly observed perforating disorder (see Table 79.1); it is an acquired disease that affects primarily adults; the term APD encompasses several overlapping entities including *acquired* reactive perforating collagenosis (RPC), Kyrle disease, and perforating folliculitis.
- In general, affected individuals have pruritic skin that has been scratched; the vast majority of patients have chronic kidney disease and/or diabetes mellitus, with most of the latter individuals having diabetic nephropathy; it affects up to 10% of patients receiving chronic hemodialysis.
- Occurs less often in patients with pruritus due to other causes, e.g. insect bites, scabies, primary biliary cholangitis, Hodgkin disease.
- Erythematous, skin-colored or hyperpigmented papules and papulonodules with a central keratotic core that favor the extensor surfaces of the extremities (Figs 79.1–79.3); the central core is a reflection of the transepidermal elimination of collagen and/or elastic fibers as well as hyperkeratosis associated with epidermal hyperplasia.
- **DDx:** see Table 79.2.
- **Rx:** difficult; topical antipruritics (e.g. pramoxine), sedating antihistamines, CS-impregnated tape, intralesional CS, cryotherapy, tangential excision, Unna boot (impregnated gauze wrapping that serves as a physical barrier against scratching), NB- or BB-UVB, topical or oral retinoids.

Elastosis Perforans Serpiginosa (EPS)

- Annular or serpiginous plaques composed of keratotic papules that are usually skin-colored (Fig. 79.4); lesions favor flexural sites, in particular the neck and antecubital fossae, and can be several centimeters in diameter.
- Occurs in patients with inherited disorders that affect connective tissue (~40% of cases of EPS; Fig. 79.5) or as a consequence of medications that disrupt elastin formation, e.g. penicillamine; in the first group, the onset is during childhood or early adulthood; there is also a skin-limited childhood form that may be inherited.
- Elastic fibers are surrounded by a hyperplastic epidermis and then eliminated transepidermally.
- **DDx:** see Table 79.2.
- **Rx:** lesions may spontaneously resolve over a period of years; cryotherapy, tangential excision, nonaggressive electrosurgical or laser therapy (to avoid scarring).

Familial Reactive Perforating Collagenosis (RPC)

- Rare inherited disorder with an onset during childhood; affects sites of trauma, especially the arms and hands (Fig. 79.6).

MAJOR PERFORATING DISORDERS					
Disease	**Incidence**	**Time of onset**	**Most common location**	**Perforating substance**	**Associations**
Acquired perforating dermatosis (APD)	Common	Adulthood	Extensor extremities (legs > arms); occasionally generalized	Necrotic material +/or collagen >> elastic fibers	Pruritus, usually in the setting of chronic kidney disease +/or diabetes mellitus* affects 10% of patients on chronic hemodialysis
Elastosis perforans serpiginosa (EPS)	Rare	Childhood, early adulthood; variable if drug-induced	Flexures, especially neck, antecubital fossae; face	Elastic fibers	Genetic disorders (see Fig. 79.5); penicillamine
Familial reactive perforating collagenosis (RPC)	Rare	Childhood	Arms, hands, sites of trauma	Collagen	None
Perforating calcific elastosis	Rare, but more common in African-American women	Adulthood	Periumbilical, abdomen > breast	Calcified elastic tissue	Primarily multiparity, obesity; occasionally chronic kidney disease
Perforating folliculitis (in the absence of pruritus)	Uncommon	Early adulthood	Extremities, trunk	Necrotic tissue	May represent rupture of ordinary folliculitis

**Occasionally affects patients with pruritus due to other disorders, e.g. scabies, Hodgkin disease, primary biliary cholangitis; can also be induced by several medications (see Fig. 79.5).*

Table 79.1 Major perforating disorders. *Courtesy, Ronald Rapini, MD.*

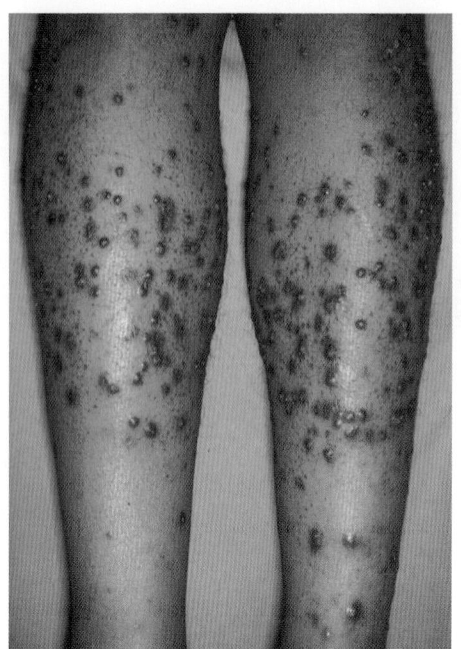

Fig. 79.1 Acquired perforating dermatosis. Numerous papules and papulonodules on the legs in a patient with diabetes mellitus and chronic kidney disease. Note the central keratotic core. *Courtesy, Ronald Rapini, MD.*

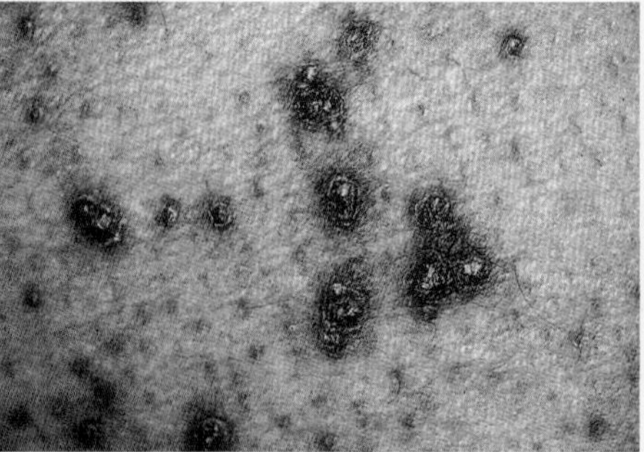

Fig. 79.2 Acquired perforating dermatosis. Keratotic papules on the arm of a diabetic woman on hemodialysis. Note the central keratotic core which is sometimes dislodged by the patient. *Courtesy, YDRSC.*

DIFFERENTIAL DIAGNOSIS OF PERFORATING DISEASES
Acquired perforating dermatosis and reactive perforating collagenosis
• Excoriations from a variety of causes (prurigo simplex) • Prurigo nodularis • Folliculitis • Arthropod bites • Perforation of exogenous foreign material • Perforation of endogenous substances (e.g. calcium) • Multiple keratoacanthomas • Dermatofibromas • If Koebner phenomenon, psoriasis, lichen planus, verrucae (autoinoculation)
Elastosis perforans serpiginosa (see Ch. 15 for DDx of annular lesions)
• Granuloma annulare } Common annular diseases • Tinea } • Sarcoidosis • Annular elastolytic giant cell granuloma (actinic granuloma) • Perforating pseudoxanthoma elasticum • Porokeratosis • Discoid lupus erythematosus

Table 79.2 Differential diagnosis of perforating diseases. This is in addition to other perforating disorders discussed in this chapter.

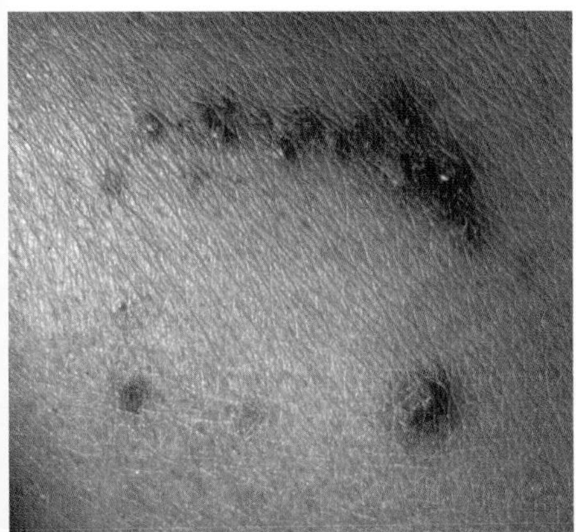

Fig. 79.3 Acquired perforating dermatosis. Note the linear arrangement of the keratotic papules (Koebner phenomenon). *Courtesy, Ronald Rapini, MD.*

- Skin-colored papules with a central core composed of "perforating" collagen fibers; a linear array due to Koebner phenomenon may be seen.
- **DDx:** other perforating disorders, perforating GA.
- **Rx:** lesions spontaneously resolve over a period of a few months.

Perforating Calcific Elastosis

- Most common site of involvement is periumbilical (Fig. 79.7); may be seen on the breast in the setting of chronic kidney disease.
- The periumbilical form favors obese, middle-aged, multiparous black women.

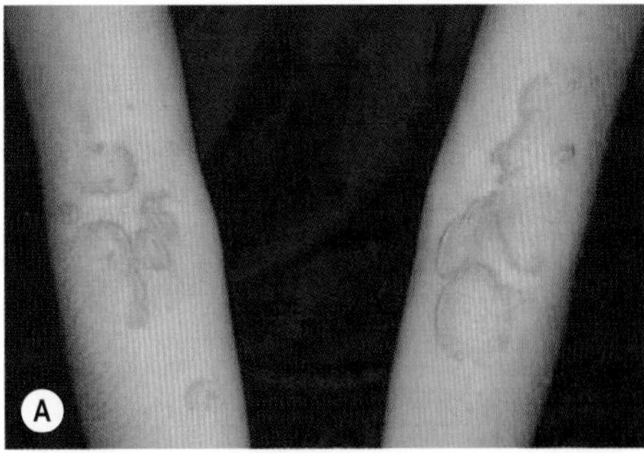

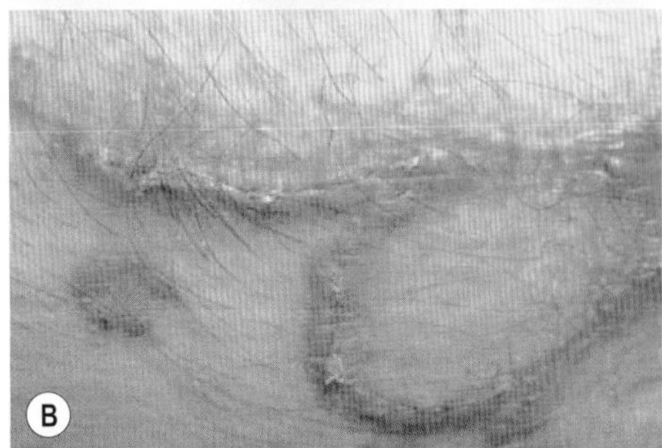

Fig. 79.4 Elastosis perforans serpiginosa. **A** Multiple annular plaques favoring the antecubital fossae, a flexural site. **B** Closer view with foci of hyperkeratosis at sites of transepidermal elimination. The patient had received penicillamine. *Courtesy, YDRSC.*

- Plaques usually have a keratotic or verrucous rim and may have a yellowish hue; histologically, calcified elastic fibers (with an appearance similar to the elastic fibers of pseudoxanthoma elasticum [PXE]) are undergoing transepidermal elimination.
- Although this entity has been referred to as perforating PXE, these patients do not have the genetic disorder PXE.

For further information see Ch. 96 from *Dermatology, Fourth Edition*.

For additional online figures visit www.expertconsult.com 

APPROACH TO THE PATIENT WITH A PRIMARY PERFORATING DISEASE

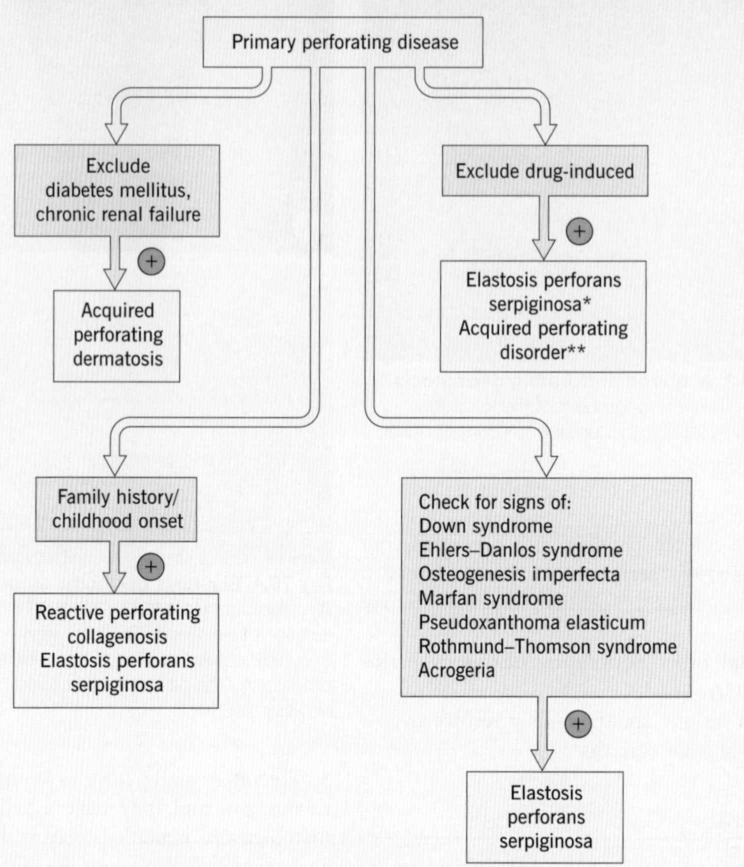

Fig. 79.5 Approach to the patient with a primary perforating disease. *Penicillamine. **Tumor necrosis factor inhibitors, epidermal growth factor receptor inhibitors (e.g. gefitinib) and other kinase inhibitors (e.g. nilotinib), antivirals (e.g. telaprevir, indinavir), sirolimus, several monoclonal antibodies (e.g. natalizumab, bevacizumab).

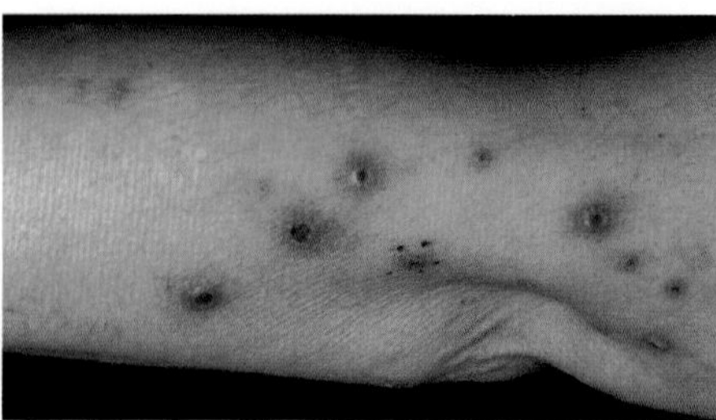

Fig. 79.6 Reactive perforating collagenosis of the arm. Several erythematous papules with a central scale-crust core. *Courtesy, Lorenzo Cerroni, MD.*

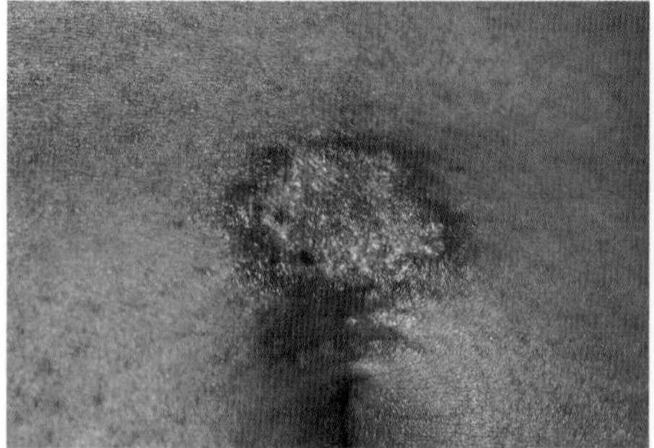

Fig. 79.7 Perforating calcific elastosis. When a biopsy was performed from the elevated edge of this supraumbilical plaque in a multiparous African-American woman, resistance was felt, as well as a grinding sound. *Courtesy, YDRSC.*

Heritable Connective Tissue Disorders

80

Heritable connective tissue disorders present with a broad range of cutaneous and extracutaneous manifestations. Recognition of characteristic skin findings is often critical to establishing the diagnosis and identifying associated internal involvement, which may include life-threatening cardiovascular disease, e.g. in the vascular type of Ehlers–Danlos syndrome (EDS) and pseudoxanthoma elasticum (PXE).

Ehlers–Danlos Syndrome

- Clinically and genetically heterogeneous group of connective tissue disorders caused by defective function of various collagens, extracellular matrix-processing enzymes, and associated proteins.
- The cardinal physical findings of hyperextensible, fragile skin and hypermobile joints (Fig. 80.1) are present to varying degrees in different subtypes of EDS (Table 80.1).
- Manifestations of cutaneous fragility include easy bruising (sometimes leading to suspicion of a bleeding disorder; see Fig. 80.1D) and gaping, "fish-mouth" wounds from minor trauma that heal with widened, atrophic scars (see Fig. 80.1C); additional findings may include smooth velvety skin, molluscoid pseudotumors (fleshy nodules in sites of repetitive trauma), subcutaneous spheroids over bony prominences (small, hard nodules that represent calcified fat lobules), piezogenic papules (see Ch. 82), and elastosis perforans serpiginosa (see Ch. 79).
- **Rx:** prevention of trauma; patients with the vascular type of EDS require close monitoring (especially during pregnancy) to avoid serious complications.

Pseudoxanthoma Elasticum

- Uncommon autosomal recessive disorder characterized by distorted and calcified elastic fibers in the skin, eyes, and cardiovascular system; typically caused by mutations in the *ABCC6* gene, which encodes an ABC-cassette transporter (expressed primarily in the liver) that facilitates the export of anti-mineralization factors into the circulation.
- Skin changes and asymptomatic ocular findings usually appear during the first two decades of life, with ocular and cardiovascular complications typically developing in the third and fourth decades.
- Thin yellowish papules coalesce to form cobblestoned plaques (resembling "plucked chicken skin") on the lateral neck and in other flexural sites (e.g. antecubital and popliteal fossae, axillae, groin) (Fig. 80.2); decreased elasticity leads to sagging skin in affected areas (see Fig. 80.2D), and yellow papules on the oral mucosa may be evident (see Fig. 80.2E).
- Early ocular findings include angioid streaks, which reflect breaks in the calcified elastic lamina of Bruch's membrane (also seen in other metabolic/genetic disorders, e.g. sickle cell anemia), and mottling of the retinal pigment epithelium; choroidal neovascularization and hemorrhage can result in progressive loss of vision.
- Calcification of elastic fibers in the walls of medium-sized arteries leads to luminal narrowing and clinical sequelae such as intermittent claudication, renovascular hypertension, angina, myocardial infarction, and stroke; GI hemorrhage may also occur.
- **DDx:** PXE-like cutaneous and extracutaneous findings can be seen in generalized arterial calcification of infancy (*ENPP1* mutations), PXE-like disorder with coagulation factor deficiency (*GGCX* mutations), β-thalassemia, and sickle cell anemia; other conditions featuring PXE-like skin lesions are outlined in Table 80.2.
- **Rx:** an approach to management of PXE is presented in Table 80.3.

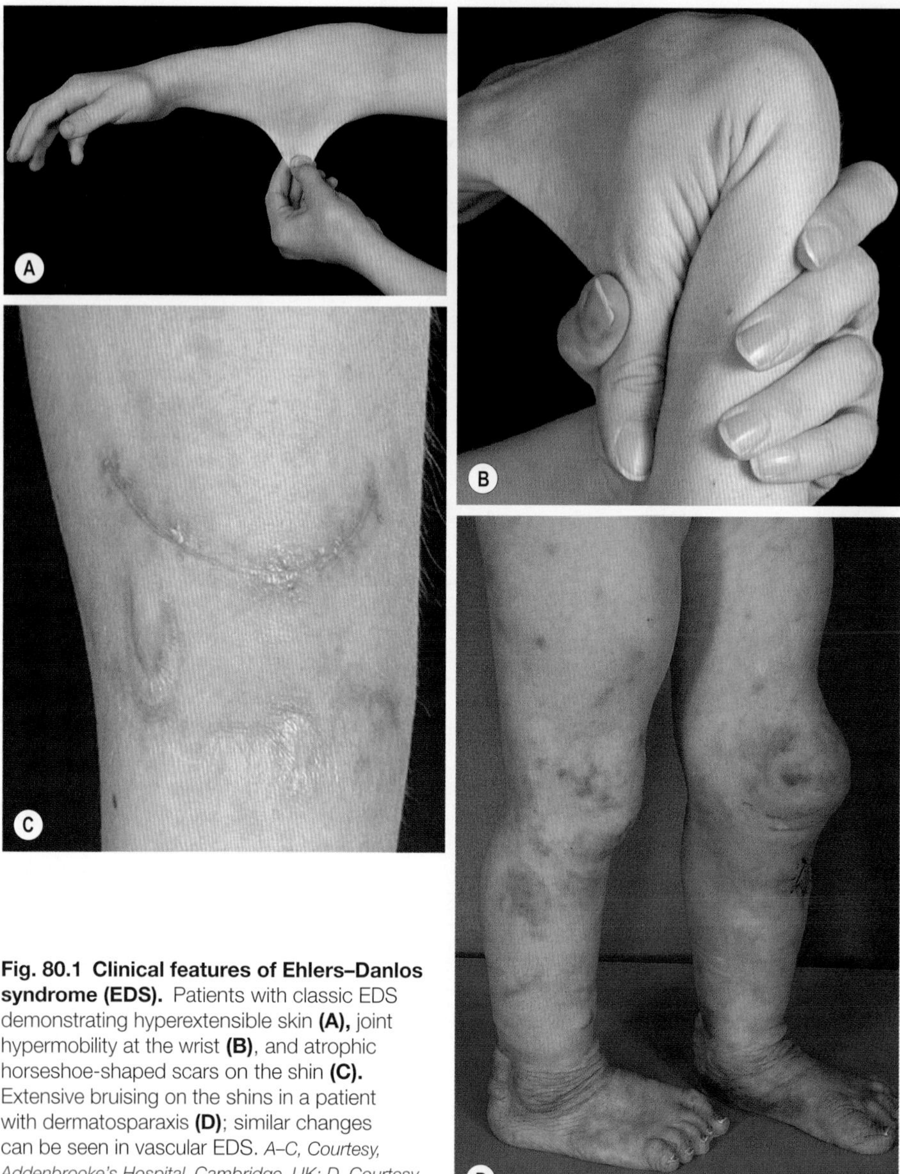

Fig. 80.1 Clinical features of Ehlers–Danlos syndrome (EDS). Patients with classic EDS demonstrating hyperextensible skin **(A),** joint hypermobility at the wrist **(B)**, and atrophic horseshoe-shaped scars on the shin **(C).** Extensive bruising on the shins in a patient with dermatosparaxis **(D)**; similar changes can be seen in vascular EDS. *A–C, Courtesy, Addenbrooke's Hospital, Cambridge, UK; D, Courtesy, Julie V. Schaffer, MD.*

Cutis Laxa

- Heterogeneous group of heritable and acquired disorders (Table 80.4) characterized by loose, sagging skin due to sparse and fragmented elastic fibers.
- Skin involvement is often generalized, giving patients a prematurely aged appearance (Fig. 80.3), but it may be localized to acral or periorbital sites; cutaneous findings are present at birth in most heritable forms of cutis laxa, developing later in acquired cutis laxa and some autosomal dominant variants.
- Extracutaneous manifestations can include emphysema, hernias (e.g. umbilical, inguinal), diverticula (e.g. GI, genitourinary),

MAJOR TYPES OF EHLERS–DANLOS SYNDROME			
EDS type	**Cutaneous findings**	**Extracutaneous manifestations**	**Inheritance, mutated protein**
Classic (I/II)*	Hyperextensible and fragile skin, with easy bruising and atrophic scars	Joint hypermobility, absence of inferior labial and lingual frenula, ability to touch nose with tongue (Gorlin sign)	AD, type V collagen
Hypermobility (III)	Hyperextensible skin	Joint hypermobility, pain and dislocations	AD, tenascin-X (F > M)
Vascular (IV)†	Thin, translucent skin with excessive bruising; decreased facial fat	Distal joint hypermobility; arterial, gastrointestinal, and uterine rupture	AD, type III collagen
Kyphoscoliosis (VIA)	Hyperextensible and fragile skin	Joint hypermobility, congenital scoliosis, osteopenia; neonatal hypotonia; ocular fragility	AR, lysyl hydroxylase
Musculocontractural (VIB)	Hyperextensible and fragile skin; wrinkled palms	Joint hypermobility, contractures, scoliosis, craniofacial anomalies; ocular fragility	AR, dermatan-4-sulfotransferase 1 or dermatan sulfate epimerase
Arthrochalasia (VIIA/B)	Hyperextensible and fragile skin	Severe joint hypermobility with congenital bilateral hip dislocation	AD, type I collagen
Dermatosparaxis (VIIC)	Sagging, doughy and extremely fragile skin, with easy bruising and tearing	Hernias; PROM; delayed closure of fontanelles, puffy eyelids, micrognathia	AR, procollagen I N-peptidase

**Most common form of Ehlers–Danlos syndrome. Tenascin-X deficiency is an AR condition with similar findings except for normal scarring, and it may be associated with congenital adrenal hyperplasia due to a contiguous gene syndrome.*
†Loeys–Dietz syndrome (see Table 80.5) can have a similar clinical presentation.

Table 80.1 Major types of Ehlers–Danlos syndrome. AD, autosomal dominant; AR, autosomal recessive; PROM, premature rupture of fetal membranes.

cardiovascular defects, musculoskeletal or craniofacial anomalies, and developmental delay; these findings are most common in autosomal recessive variants and occasionally occur in acquired forms.

- **DDx:** PXE and related conditions, mid-dermal elastolysis (see Ch. 82), anetoderma (see Ch. 82; smaller, circumscribed lesions), hereditary gelsolin amyloidosis.
- **Rx:** reconstructive surgery for cutaneous disease; multidisciplinary approach for internal involvement.

Other Disorders

- Additional heritable connective tissue disorders with cutaneous manifestations are summarized in Table 80.5.

For further information see Chs 95 and 97 from *Dermatology, Fourth Edition*.

For additional online figures visit www.expertconsult.com 

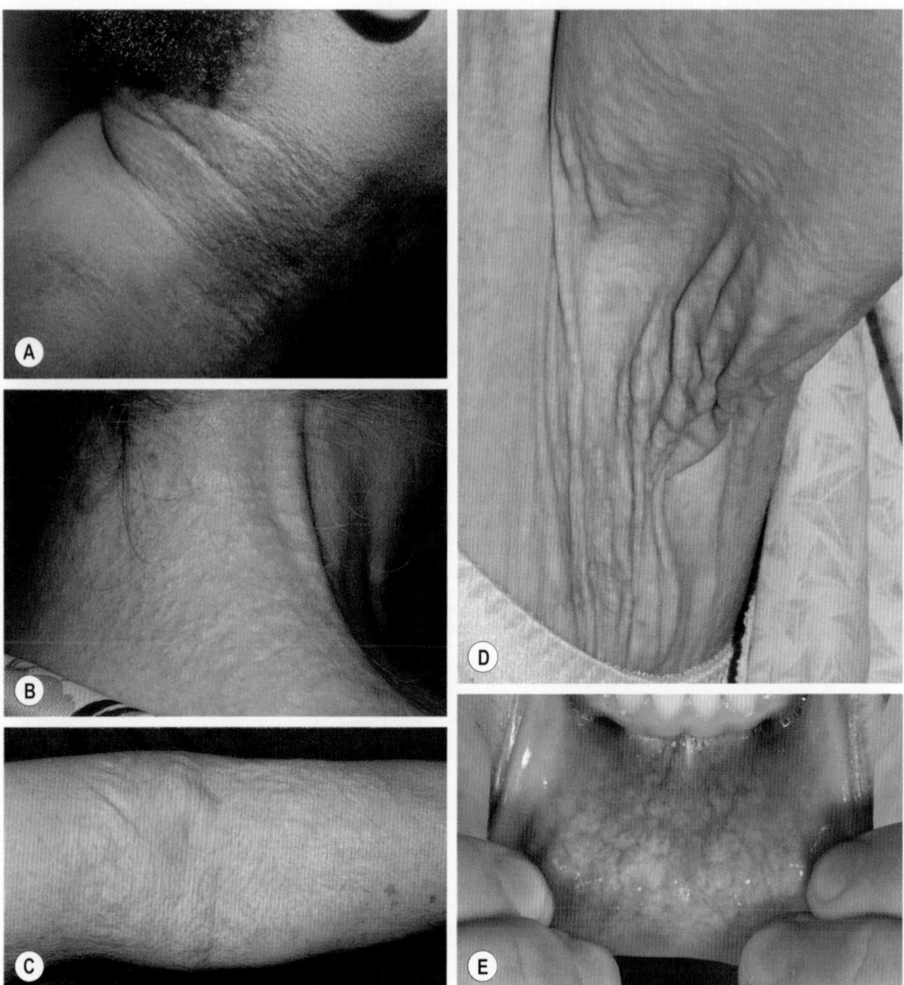

Fig. 80.2 Mucocutaneous findings in pseudoxanthoma elasticum. Yellowish papules and "cobblestoned" plaques on the neck **(A, B)** and in the antecubital fossa **(C).** Thickened, yellowish, sagging skin in the axilla **(D)**. Yellow papules on the inner aspect of the lower lip **(E)**. *A, B, Courtesy, YDRSC; C, D, Courtesy, Julie V. Schaffer, MD; E, Courtesy, Addenbrooke's Hospital, Cambridge, UK.*

DIFFERENTIAL DIAGNOSIS OF PSEUDOXANTHOMA ELASTICUM (PXE)-LIKE SKIN FINDINGS		
Disorder	**Patient characteristics**	**Clinical features**
Actinic elastosis	Middle-aged and older adults with lightly pigmented skin and a history of chronic sun exposure	Yellow to gray, thickened, lax, finely to coarsely wrinkled skin; photodistribution on the lateral forehead, neck, dorsal aspect of the forearms
Perforating calcific elastosis*	5th–8th decades; primarily multiparous black women**	Plaque composed of coalescing keratotic papules (most apparent at the periphery); periumbilical area >> breasts
PXE-like papillary dermal elastolysis (PPDE)† and white fibrous papulosis of the neck (WFPN)†	5th–9th decades; primarily Caucasian women and (for WFPN) Japanese men	Multiple 2- to 3-mm yellow, skin-colored, or (in WFPN) whitish papules; in PPDE, coalesce to form plaques with a cobblestone appearance; neck > upper trunk, axillae, flexor forearms, lower abdomen

**Also referred to as periumbilical perforating PXE.*
***Occasionally associated with an increased calcium-phosphate product in chronic kidney disease.*
†Related conditions within the spectrum of fibroelastolytic papulosis; late-onset focal dermal elastosis has a similar clinical presentation.

Table 80.2 Differential diagnosis of pseudoxanthoma elasticum (PXE)-like skin findings. Additional considerations may include PXE-like skin lesions in patients receiving D-penicillamine, exposed to saltpeter, or with chronic kidney disease, β-thalassemia, or sickle cell anemia.

A MULTIDISCIPLINARY APPROACH TO THE MANAGEMENT OF PSEUDOXANTHOMA ELASTICUM
General
• Antioxidant and magnesium supplementation, moderate calcium intake • Regular exercise, weight control, avoidance of smoking or excessive alcohol intake
Skin
• Surgical intervention for excessive skin folds
Eyes
• Biannual funduscopic examination, use of Amsler grid to assess for central visual field defects • Use of sunglasses; avoidance of head trauma or heavy straining • Laser photocoagulation or photodynamic therapy for choroidal neovascularization if visual symptoms • Intravitreal injections of VEGF antagonists
Cardiovascular system
• Baseline electrocardiogram and echocardiogram, annual cardiac examination • Low-dose acetylsalicylic acid (if not contraindicated), correction of hyperlipidemia and hypertension • Pentoxyfylline, cilostazol or clopidogrel for intermittent claudication

Table 80.3 A multidisciplinary approach to the management of pseudoxanthoma elasticum. VEGF, vascular endothelial growth factor.

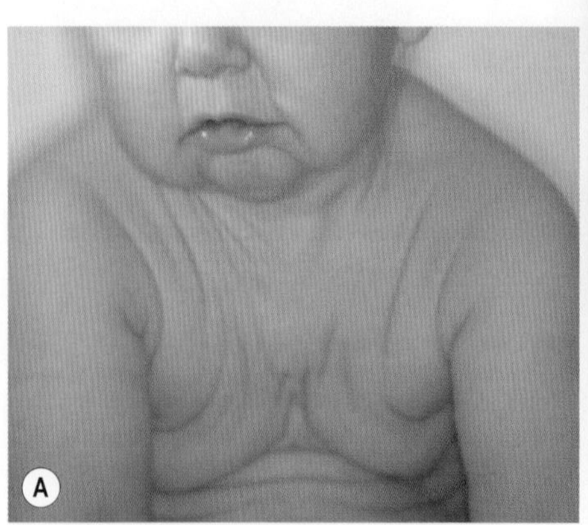

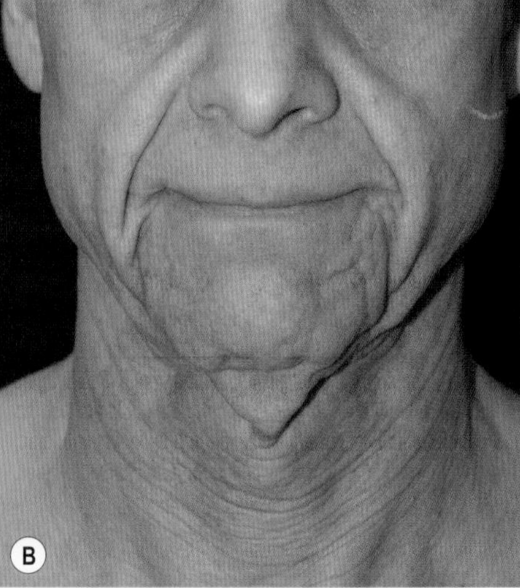

Fig. 80.3 Clinical features in cutis laxa. A Loose skin and drooping jowls in an infant with heritable cutis laxa. **B** Sagging folds of skin giving a prematurely aged appearance to a man with acquired cutis laxa associated with multiple myeloma. *A, Courtesy, Thomas Schwarz, MD; B, Courtesy, Jeffrey P Callen, MD.*

ETIOLOGIES OF CUTIS LAXA
Hereditary cutis laxa
Defects in elastic fiber components, e.g. elastin, fibulin-4/5 or latent TGF-β binding protein-4 Defective glycosylation and vesicular trafficking of elastic fiber components Defective mitochondrial proline biosynthetic enzymes
Acquired cutis laxa*
Skin disorders, e.g. Sweet syndrome-like eruptions (Marshall syndrome),* urticaria/angioedema, drug eruptions, cutaneous lymphoma **Monoclonal gammopathies** with various underlying plasma cell dyscrasias; cutis laxa may be acral or (especially with heavy chain disease) generalized **Direct effects of drug intake**, particularly penicillamine
**Sometimes in the setting of α_1-antitrypsin deficiency.*

Table 80.4 Etiologies of cutis laxa. TGF-β, transforming growth factor-β.

ADDITIONAL HERITABLE CONNECTIVE TISSUE DISORDERS WITH CUTANEOUS FINDINGS			
Disease	**Cutaneous findings**	**Extracutaneous manifestations**	**Inheritance, mutated protein**
Marfan syndrome	Striae, elastosis perforans serpiginosa, decreased fat in extremities	Tall stature with long limbs, arachnodactyly, scoliosis; lens subluxations (upward), myopia; dilation/dissection of ascending aorta*	AD, fibrillin-1
Loeys–Dietz syndrome	Translucent skin, easy bruising, atrophic scarring, ± multiple facial milia	Marfanoid habitus, joint hypermobility; aortic aneurysms, arterial tortuosity; hypertelorism, bifid uvula	AD, TGF-β receptors 1 & 2, TGF-β2 & 3, SMAD family member 3
Homocystinuria	Malar flush, livedo reticularis, diffuse pigmentary dilution, tissue paper-like scars	Marfanoid habitus, lens subluxations (downward), thrombosis, intellectual disability	AR, cystathionine synthase > other enzymes
Buschke–Ollendorff syndrome	Connective tissue nevi with increased elastin or collagen (dermatofibrosis lenticularis disseminata); occasionally cutaneous sclerosis associated with melorheostosis	Osteopoikilosis ("spotted" bones); occasionally melorheostosis (sclerotic bone resembling "dripping candle wax" on radiographs)	AD, LEM domain-containing 3 (antagonist of TGF-β signaling)

**Rx:* *β-blockers and angiotensin II receptor blockers, which antagonize pathogenic TGF-β signaling.*

Table 80.5 Additional heritable connective tissue disorders with cutaneous findings. AD, autosomal dominant; AR, autosomal recessive; TGF-β, transforming growth factor-β.

81 Dermal Hypertrophies

Hypertrophic Scar

- Firm, initially pink to purple in color then becomes skin-colored to hypopigmented, occasionally hyperpigmented; papule or plaque limited to an excision site or wound (Figs 81.1 and 81.2).
- Most commonly seen on the trunk and shoulders.
- Sometimes pruritic.
- With treatment, can reduce pruritus and height but not width of scar.
- **Rx** options include silicone gel sheets, intralesional triamcinolone (initially 5–10 mg/ml), re-excision (but may recur), laser (e.g. pulsed dye laser to improve color), massage/pressure, postoperative radiotherapy.

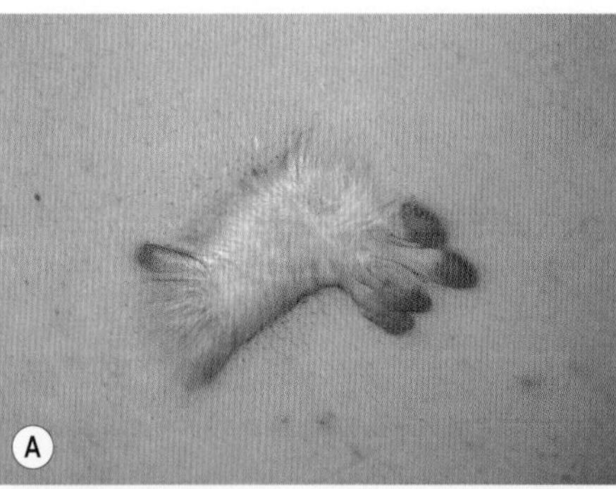

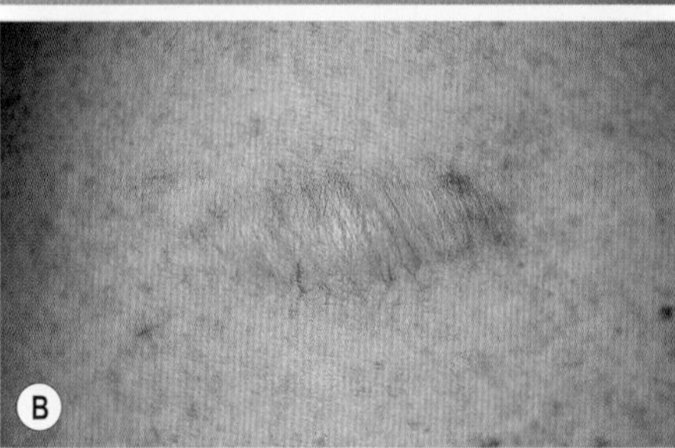

Fig. 81.1 Comparison of a keloid and a hypertrophic scar. A The keloid has claw-like extensions that extend beyond the original wound margin into adjacent normal skin. **B** The hypertrophic scar remains confined to the site of the original surgical wound. *A, Courtesy, Edward Cowen, MD; B, Courtesy, Jean L. Bolognia, MD.*

Keloid

- More common in patients with darkly pigmented skin who have a familial predisposition.
- Rarely associated with syndromes (e.g. Rubinstein–Taybi or Goeminne syndromes).
- Raised, often skin-colored firm plaque(s) that, in contrast to hypertrophic scars, extend beyond the wound margin (Fig. 81.3; Table 81.1); color may vary as in hypertrophic scars.
- Follow trauma from surgical procedures (including ear piercing) and inflammatory disorders, especially acne, but can occur spontaneously (Fig. 81.4).
- Poor response to treatment.
- **Rx** options include silicone gel sheets; intralesional injections of triamcinolone (initially 10–20 mg/ml), interferon-α-2b, or 5-fluorouracil; pressure; laser (e.g. pulsed dye laser to improve color); excision followed by other modalities such as low-dose radiation or topical imiquimod.

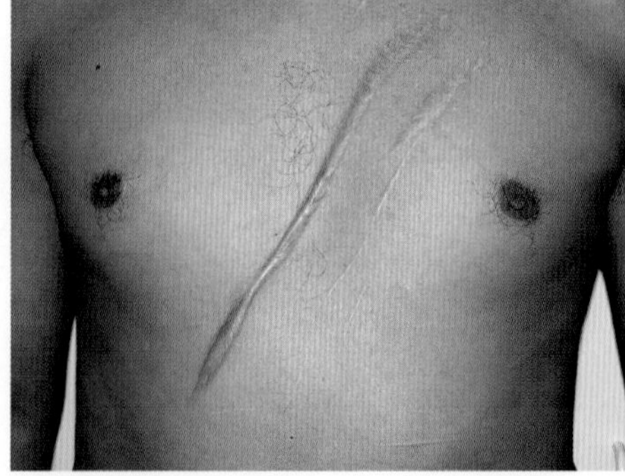

Fig. 81.2 Hypertrophic scar at the site of a knife injury. *Courtesy, Luis Requena, MD.*

CLINICAL FEATURES OF CONVENTIONAL SCARS, HYPERTROPHIC SCARS, AND KELOIDS			
	Conventional scar	**Hypertrophic scar**	**Keloid scar**
Preceded by injury	Yes	Yes	Not always
Onset	Immediate	Immediate	Delayed
Erythema	Temporary	Prominent	Varies
Profile	Flat	Raised	Raised
Symptomatic	No	Yes	Yes
Confined to wound margin	Yes	Yes	No
Increased mast cells	No	Yes	Yes
Spontaneous resolution	N/A	Possible, gradual	Rare
Treatment response	N/A	Good	Poor

Table 81.1 Clinical features of conventional scars, hypertrophic scars, and keloids. N/A, not applicable.

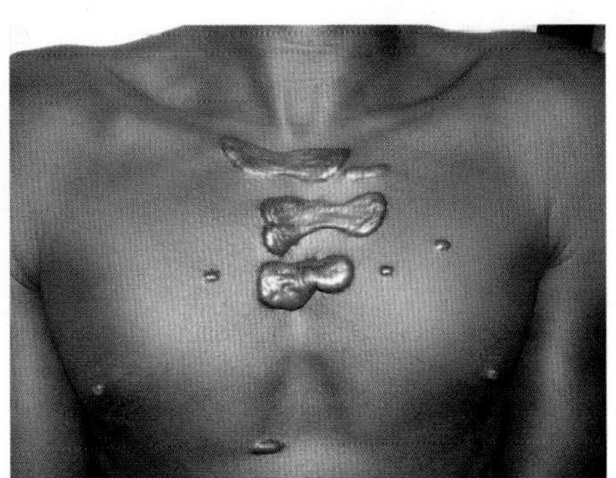

Fig. 81.3 Keloid of the chest, a common site. Note the extension of the keloid into the normal surrounding skin and the central flattening in larger lesions. *Courtesy, Luis Requena, MD.*

Dupuytren Disease

- Fibromatosis of the fascia of the ventral aspect of the digit and the palm.
- Starts as a linear thickening proximal to the fourth > fifth finger that is most apparent with extension of the digits.
- May gradually progress to flexion contractures (Fig. 81.5).
- Associated with other fibromatoses (e.g. plantar, penile), alcoholism, and diabetes mellitus; vemurafenib may cause new onset or worsening of existing disease.
- Surgical correction usually helpful; injection of collagenase also sometimes effective.

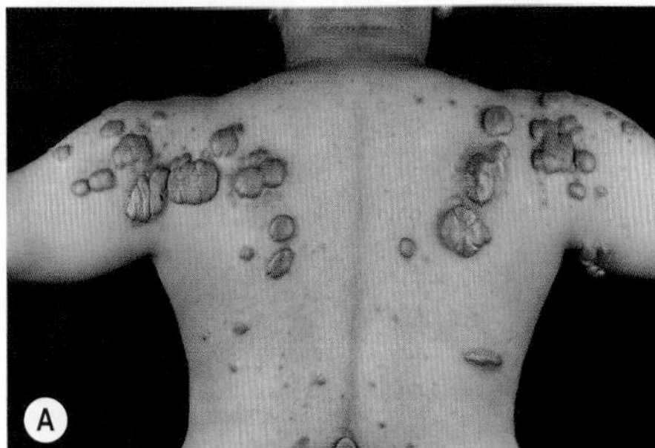

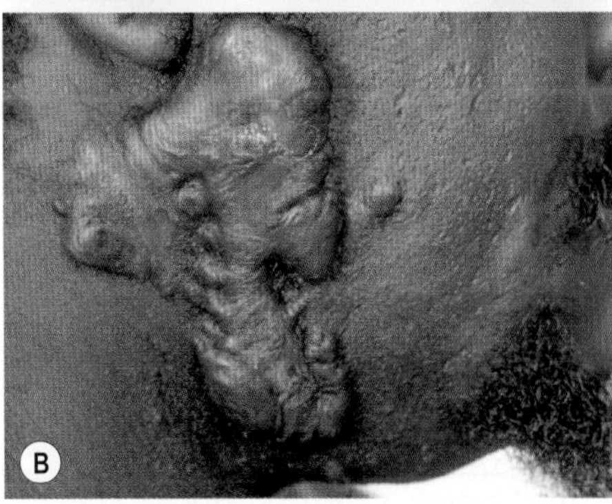

Fig. 81.4 Keloids. The upper trunk **(A)** and neck **(B)** are common sites. There is a higher prevalence of keloids in patients with darkly pigmented skin, but they can occur in individuals with any skin phototype. Note the extension of keloids into the normal surrounding skin in a claw-like manner. *A, Courtesy, Lorenzo Cerroni, MD; B, Courtesy, YDRSC.*

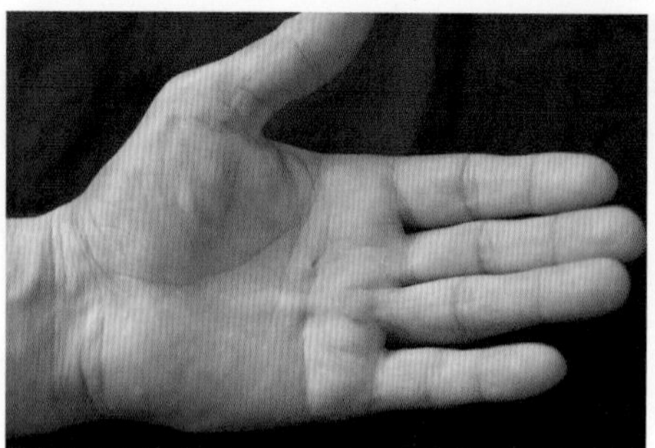

Fig. 81.5 Dupuytren disease. Fibrotic nodule at the base of the fourth finger with an obvious cord extending proximally. In addition to palpation, fibrotic cords can be accentuated by extension of the digit. Eventually, flexion contractures develop. *Courtesy, Luis Requena, MD.*

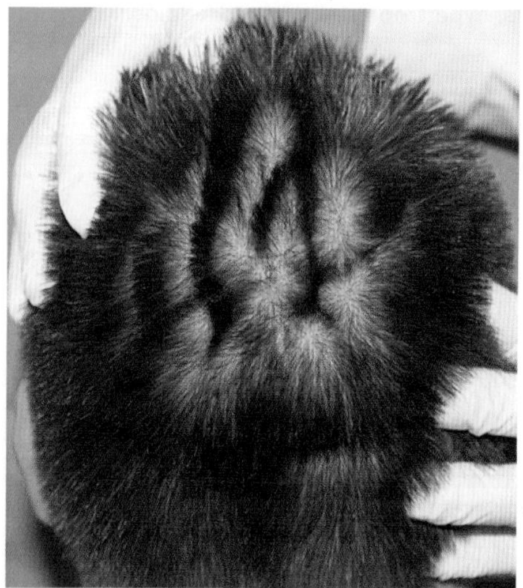

Fig. 81.6 Cutis verticis gyrata. Cerebriform folding of the skin of the scalp. *Courtesy, Luis Requena, MD.*

Elastic Tissue-Related Disorders

- See Figs 73.2A–C and E, 79.4, 79.7; Tables 80.2, 80.5.

Cutis Verticis Gyrata

- Hypertrophy and linear folding of the scalp only (Fig. 81.6); male predominance with onset during puberty in idiopathic cases.
- Primary (idiopathic) form is more common and may be associated with systemic findings (neurologic, ophthalmologic).

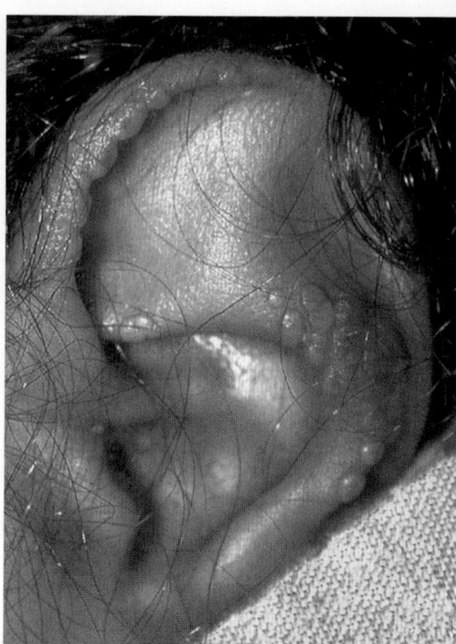

Fig. 81.7 Juvenile hyaline fibromatosis. Firm pearly papules favor the ears. *Courtesy, YDRSC.*

- Secondary form associated with endocrinopathies (e.g. acromegaly, myxedema), insulin resistance, and genetic disorders (e.g. Turner syndrome).
- **DDx** includes several disorders, including benign tumors or hamartomas (e.g. cerebriform congenital melanocytic nevus of the scalp, plexiform neurofibroma), pachydermoperiostitis (involves the face and acral sites as well as the scalp), and dissecting cellulitis (scalp is boggy and painful).

Hyaline Fibromatosis Syndrome (Juvenile Hyaline Fibromatosis and Infantile Systemic Hyalinosis)

- Autosomal recessive spectrum of disorders due to *ANTXR2* mutations.
- Presents during infancy or early childhood with papulonodules on the ears, hands, and periorificial areas (Fig. 81.7), in addition to gingival hypertrophy and flexion contractures.
- Severe form (infantile systemic hyalinosis) has internal organ involvement.

For further information see Ch. 98 from *Dermatology, Fourth Edition*.

For additional online figures and table on treatment options visit www.expertconsult.com

Atrophies of Connective Tissue 82

This chapter focuses primarily on entities in which there is a reduction in collagen and/or elastic tissue within the dermis. They vary from very common skin disorders such as striae to cutaneous manifestations of rare genetic syndromes. Loss of subcutaneous fat, i.e. lipoatrophy, is covered in Chapter 84, while acrodermatitis chronica atrophicans is covered in Chapter 97 and Ehlers–Danlos syndrome and cutis laxa are covered in Chapter 80.

Striae (Distensae)

- Linear atrophic lesions that reflect dermal damage ("breaks") at sites of mechanical stress due to stretching of the skin, hence the popular term "stretch marks"; most commonly observed in adolescents undergoing growth spurts or weight gain and on the abdomen in up to 75% of pregnant women.
- Striae are multiple, symmetric, and arranged along the lines of cleavage, with the typical sites of involvement and characteristic patterns shown in Fig. 82.1; early lesions may be red-purple in color (striae rubra) but with time, most striae become skin-colored to white with fine wrinkling (striae alba) (Fig. 82.2).
- Additional causes include hypercortisolism (e.g. Cushing syndrome), application of potent topical CS (especially in areas of occlusion such as major body folds), and heredity; in weightlifters, mechanical stress and muscle enlargement can lead to striae.
- **DDx:** linear focal elastosis, in particular when lesions are present on the lower mid-back.
- **Rx:** difficult, but striae often become less noticeable over a period of years; possible modest improvement with topical tretinoin 0.1% cream; lasers (e.g. pulsed dye for striae rubra, 308 nm excimer for striae alba) have reportedly led to improvement.

Pizogenic Pedal Papules (Piezogenic Papules)

- Herniations of fat in the heel region where there is reduced dermal connective tissue; the skin-colored papules appear with the pressure of weight-bearing and disappear when the leg is raised (Fig. 82.3A); occasionally they occur on the wrist.
- In an infantile variant, larger nodules occur on the medial aspect of the heel and their appearance does not require weight-bearing (Fig. 82.3B).

Anetoderma

- Well-circumscribed, skin-colored, flaccid lesions that result from a marked focal decrease in elastic tissue within the dermis (Fig. 82.4).
- Often arises *de novo* (primary form), with lesions usually measuring 1–2 cm in diameter; there are also secondary forms of anetoderma that can follow inflammation or infection of the skin (e.g. varicella, lepromatous leprosy, acute cutaneous lupus) or are seen in association with cutaneous tumors (e.g. involuted infantile hemangiomas) or the antiphospholipid antibody syndrome.
- Anetoderma of prematurity presents as atrophic lesions resulting from minor iatrogenic trauma to immature skin in the setting of neonatal intensive care.
- Although the individual lesions of the primary form are often elevated, they can be even with the skin surface or depressed (Fig. 82.4C); however, all lesions are soft to palpation and the focal reduction in elastic tissue results in a feel similar to that of an abdominal hernia (referred to as a "buttonhole" sign, which is also seen in neurofibromas).

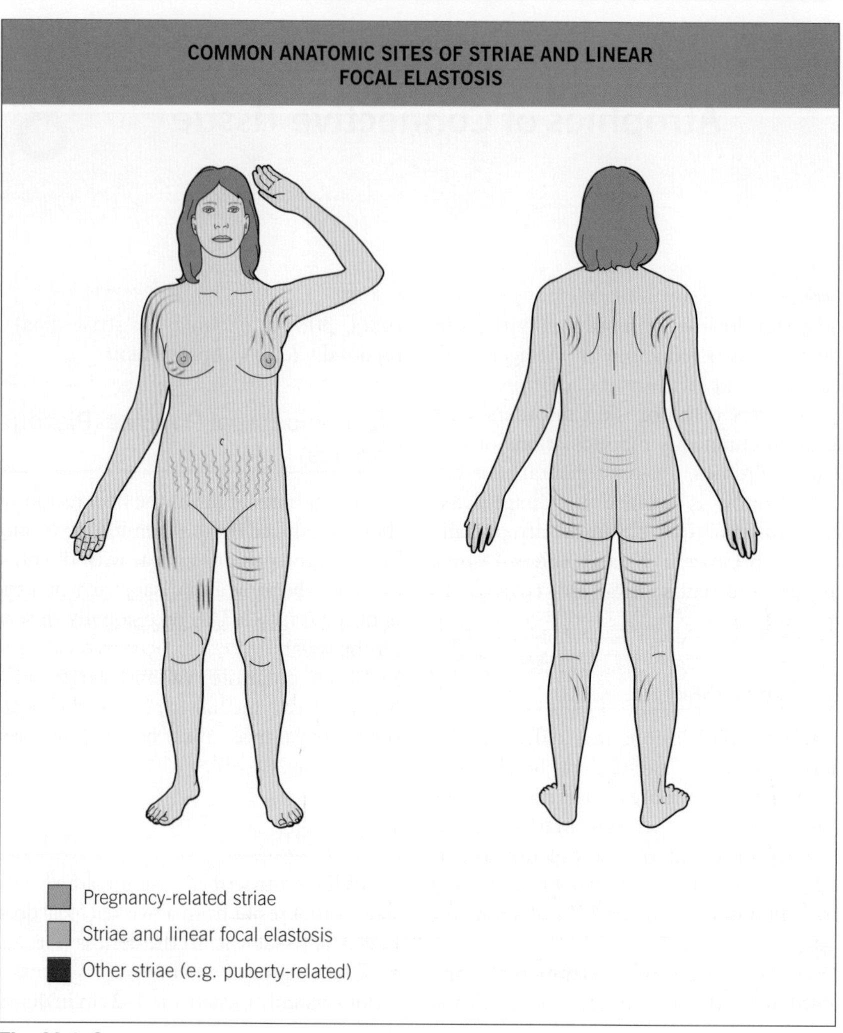

Fig. 82.1 Common anatomic sites of striae and linear focal elastosis. In teenage boys, striae are commonly seen in the same site and in the same orientation as focal elastosis.

- The primary form favors the neck, upper trunk, and upper extremities of young adults, with lesions appearing over a period of years, while the distribution pattern of the secondary form reflects that of the preceding inflammatory disorder.
- **DDx:** post-traumatic scars, papular elastorrhexis (similar clinical appearance but firm to palpation), anetoderma-like scars (perifollicular elastolysis) due to acne vulgaris, pseudoxanthoma elasticum-like papillary dermal elastolysis (flexural areas; see Table 80.2).
- **Rx:** difficult; for secondary form, treatment of underlying disease may prevent new lesions; surgical excision can lead to scars.

Atrophoderma of Pasini and Pierini

- Minimally depressed hyperpigmented patches, primarily of the posterior trunk (Fig. 82.5); the characteristic "cliff-drop" sign at the peripheral edge may be subtle; significant overlap with "burnt-out" plaque-type morphea, and notably a minority of patients have both disorders.

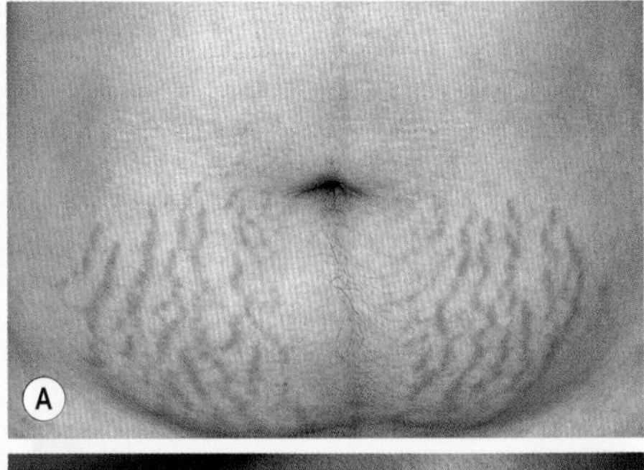

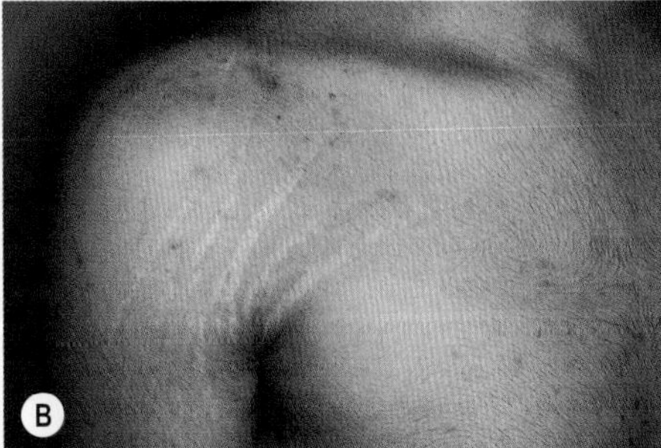

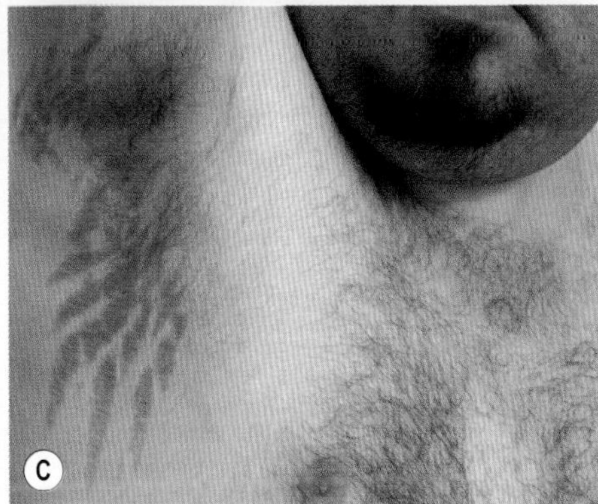

Fig. 82.2 Striae. A Linear erythematous lesions on the abdomen (striae rubra). **B** Multiple linear atrophic streaks of striae alba in a teenager. **C** Large axillary striae in a patient receiving chronic, high-dose systemic corticosteroids. *A, Courtesy, USCDRSC; B, Courtesy, Kalman Watsky, MD; C, Courtesy, YDRSC.*

- Onset typically during adolescence or young adulthood; the patches are often oval in shape, 2–8 cm in diameter, number from one to several, and persist for decades; rarely, lesions are present at birth or arise along the lines of Blaschko (atrophoderma of Moulin; Fig. 82.6; see Ch. 51).
- Because the reduction in the thickness of the dermis is subtle, an elliptical biopsy that includes both involved and uninvolved skin and is sectioned longitudinally is usually required for diagnosis.
- **DDx:** morphea, but in contrast to atrophoderma, induration and/or an inflammatory rim is observed; postinflammatory hyperpigmentation; if a limited number of lesions, dermatofibrosarcoma protuberans (primarily in children).
- **Rx:** difficult; modest improvement in hyperpigmentation reported with pigment-specific laser therapy.

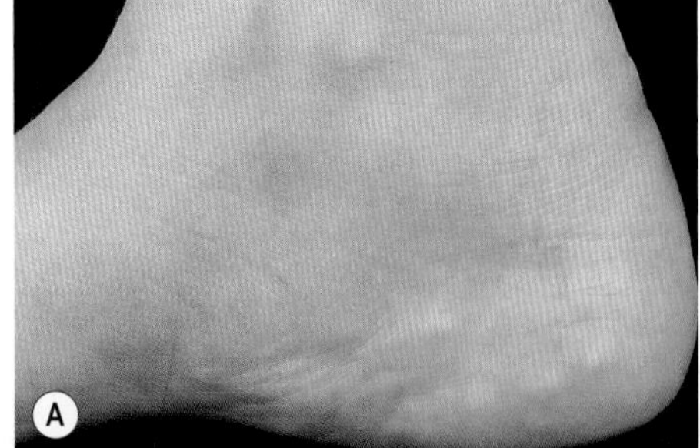

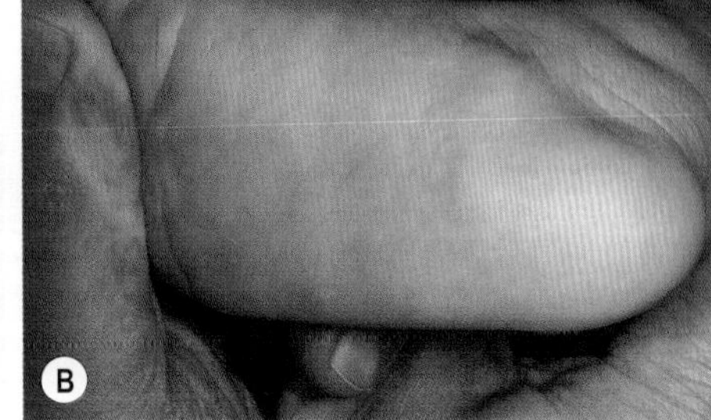

Fig. 82.3 Pizogenic pedal papules. A Skin-colored to yellowish outpouchings on the heel represent herniation of subcutaneous fat through the plantar fascia and they are sometimes painful. **B** Soft nodules on the medial and plantar surface of the foot in an infant. *B, Courtesy, Julie V. Schaffer, MD.*

Mid-Dermal Elastolysis

- Idiopathic disorder characterized by large, skin-colored patches with fine wrinkling and occasionally follicular papules with central delling; the lesions are often clinically subtle (Fig. 82.7) and histologically, there is a selective loss of elastic tissue in the mid dermis best demonstrated by special elastic stains.
- Most commonly affects the trunk, neck, and arms of middle-aged Caucasian women.
- **DDx:** the major entity is generalized acquired cutis laxa.
- **Rx:** none currently available.

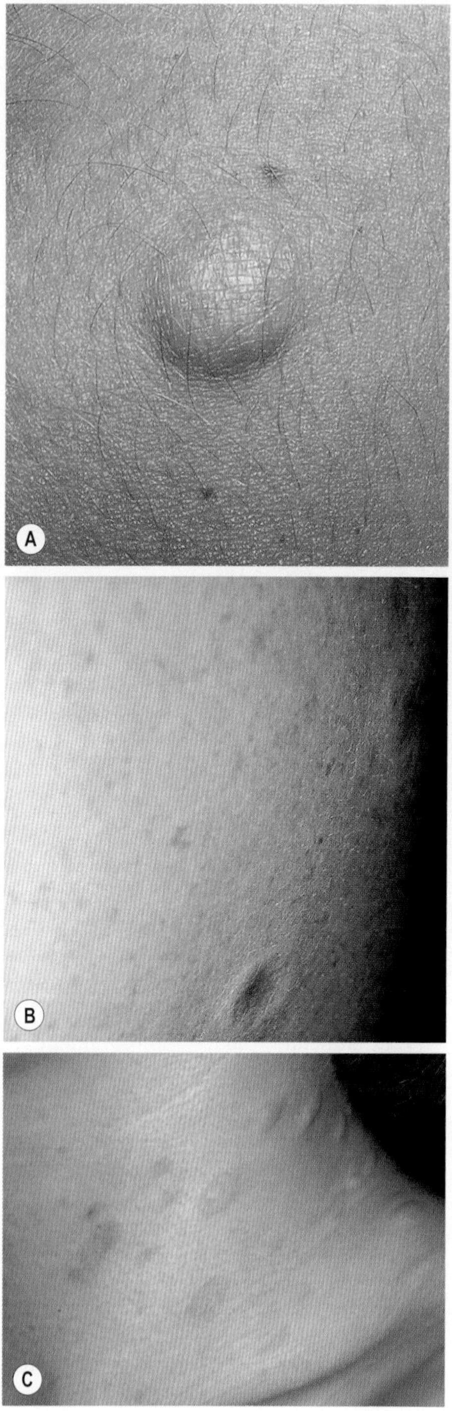

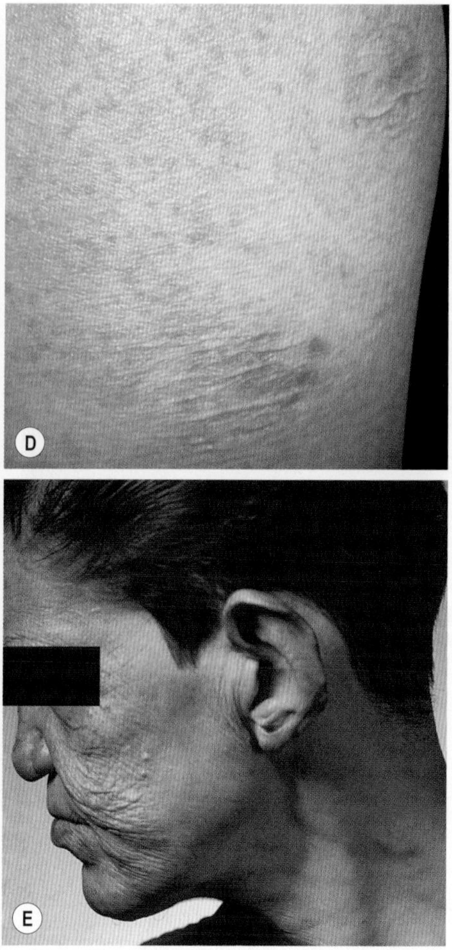

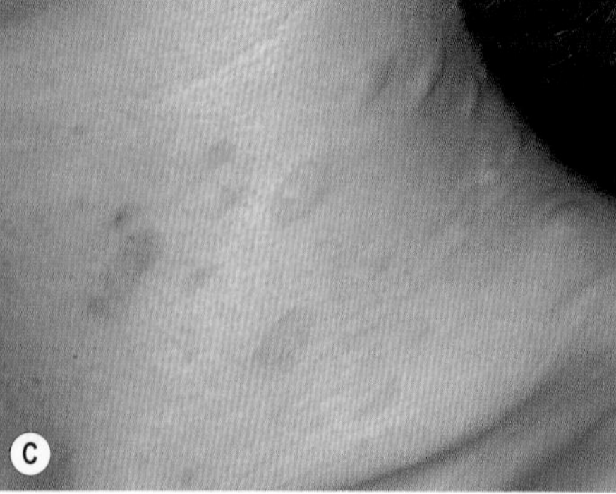

Fig. 82.4 Anetoderma – primary and secondary. Lesions can range from soft, skin-colored papules that herniate upon palpation **(A)** to flaccid papules that have a central depression **(B)**. The upper trunk and neck is a common location for primary anetoderma; an admixture of elevated, macular and depressed lesions is seen **(C)**. Wrinkling of the skin from secondary anetoderma due to sarcoidosis **(D)** and lepromatous leprosy **(E).** *A, Courtesy, Ronald Rapini, MD; B, Courtesy, Catherine Maari, MD, and Julie Powell, MD; C, Courtesy, Thomas Schwarz, MD; D, Courtesy, Catherine Maari, MD, and Julie Powell, MD; E, Courtesy, Louis A. Fragola, Jr., MD.*

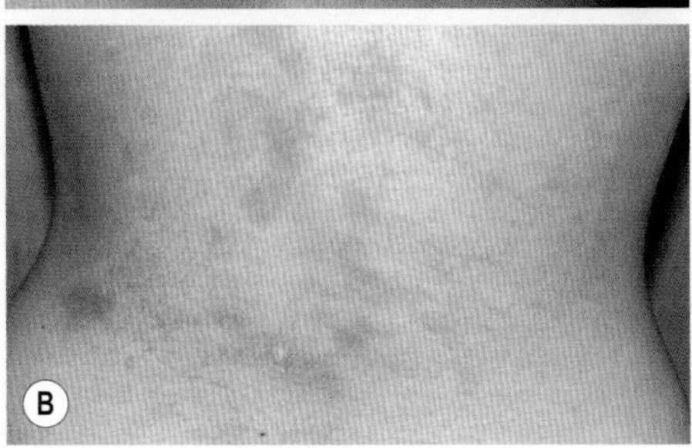

Fig. 82.5 Atrophoderma of Pasini and Pierini. **A, B** Multiple light brown patches on the back; note the subtle depression of the lesions with a "cliff-drop" edge. In **(B)**, dermal blood vessels are seen within a few patches; the white papule is a healed biopsy site. *A, Courtesy, Catherine C. McCuaig, MD; B, Courtesy, Julie V. Schaffer, MD.*

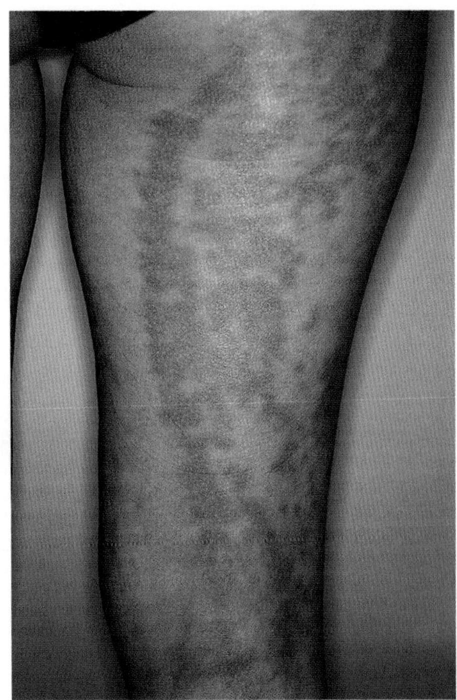

Fig. 82.6 Atrophoderma of Moulin. Linear hyperpigmented streaks along the lines of Blaschko. Note the subtle depression of the lesions on the upper lateral thigh. *Courtesy, Jean L. Bolognia, MD.*

Follicular Atrophoderma

- Small depressions at the sites of hair follicles.
- Clinical presentations include:
  - As atrophoderma vermiculatum of the cheeks (Fig. 82.8), which can be sporadic, inherited in an autosomal dominant manner, or be a component of the keratosis pilaris atrophicans spectrum in which there is also follicular hyperkeratosis (Table 82.1; Fig. 82.9)
  - As patulous follicles on the dorsal aspect of the hands and feet in the X-linked dominant Bazex–Dupré–Christol syndrome in which patients also develop BCCs and alopecia
  - As follicular pits within streaks along the lines of Blaschko in the X-linked dominant disorder Conradi–Hünermann–Happle syndrome (form of chondrodysplasia punctata)

Atrophia Macularis Varicelliformis Cutis (AMVC)

- Acquired thin linear depressions on the face that measure 2–10 mm in length and can be admixed with small circular depressions; there is no history of preceding inflammation, acne, or trauma (Fig. 82.10).

For further information see Ch. 99 from *Dermatology, Fourth Edition*.

For additional online figures and table visit www.expertconsult.com 

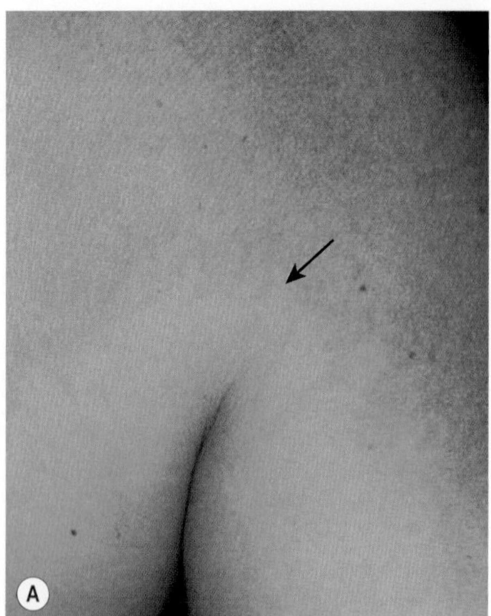

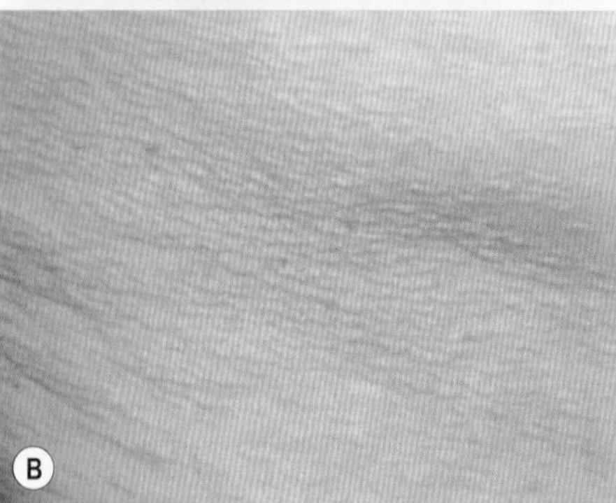

Fig. 82.7 Mid-dermal elastolysis. A Large patch with fine wrinkling and a slightly reticulated border on the upper back and shoulder. The junction of involved and uninvolved skin is marked with an arrow. **B** Both circumscribed areas of wrinkling and follicular papules are present. *A, Courtesy, Judit Stenn, MD; B, Courtesy, Lorenzo Cerroni, MD.*

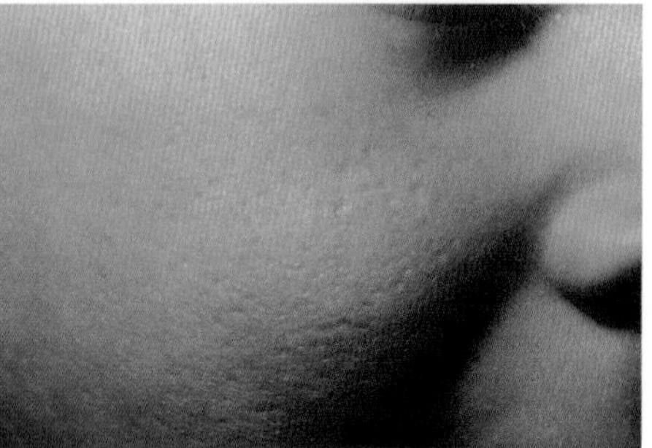

Fig. 82.8 Atrophoderma vermiculatum. Multiple small pitted scars on the cheek of a young girl. Note the honeycomb pattern on the lower inner cheek; the skin is said to appear "worm-eaten." The atrophic lesions may be preceded by inflammatory papules. *Courtesy, Robert Hartmann, MD.*

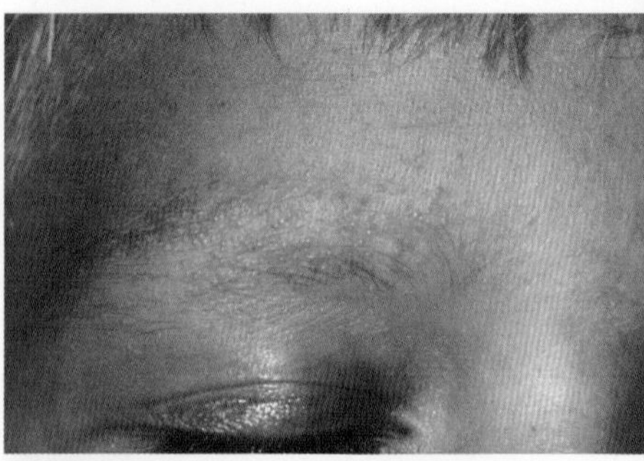

Fig. 82.9 Ulerythema ophryogenes. Alopecia of the eyebrows admixed with tiny follicular papules with a thin erythematous rim. *Courtesy, Jean L. Bolognia, MD.*

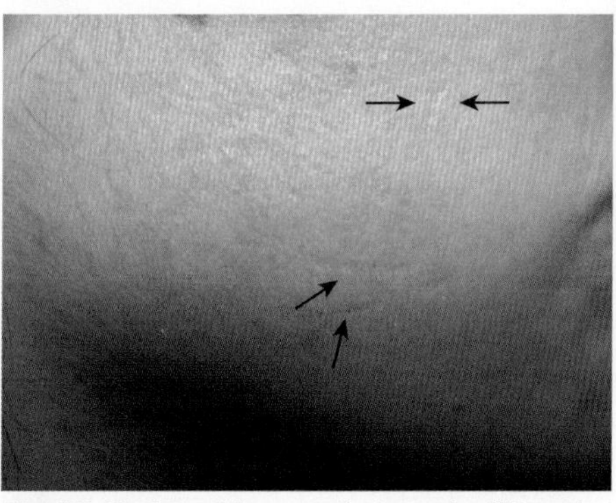

Fig. 82.10 Atrophia macularis varicelliformis cutis. Multiple linear scar-like depressions (between and above arrows) with no history of trauma. *Courtesy, Jean L. Bolognia, MD.*

THE SPECTRUM OF KERATOSIS PILARIS ATROPHICANS						
Disorder	**Mode of inheritance**	**Age of onset**	**Distribution**	**Cutaneous features**	**KP***	**Other findings and associations**
Keratosis pilaris atrophicans faciei (ulerythema ophryogenes)	AD AR (*LRP1* mutations)	Infancy	Eyebrows, particularly the lateral third (Fig. 82.9) > temples, cheeks, forehead	• Erythematous follicular papules with central keratotic plugs, eventuating in follicular atrophy • Scarring alopecia of the lateral eyebrows distinguishes it from KP rubra	+	Associated with Noonan syndrome and other RASopathies
Atrophoderma vermiculata	See text and Fig. 82.8				–	
Keratosis follicularis spinulosa decalvans (KFSD)	XR (*MBTPS2* mutations)	Childhood	Face, scalp, limbs, trunk	• Erythematous follicular papules with central keratotic plugs, eventuating in follicular atrophy • Scarring alopecia of the scalp, eyebrows, and eyelashes	++	• Palmoplantar keratoderma, facial erythema • Keratitis, photophobia

**Associated keratosis pilaris (KP) on the extremities and trunk, which does not typically eventuate in atrophy.*

Table 82.1 The spectrum of keratosis pilaris atrophicans. There is also an autosomal dominant form of KFSD with scalp involvement. AD, autosomal dominant; MBTPS2, membrane-bound transcription factor peptidase, site 2 (involved in sterol regulation); XR, X-linked recessive; +, mild to moderate; ++, severe.

83 Panniculitis

Introduction

- Adipose tissue plays many active roles in the body beyond insulation, e.g. storing and releasing lipids, mediating inflammation, and modulating endocrine and reproductive systems.
- Panniculitis = inflammation of adipose tissue.
- Clinically and histopathologically, the adipose tissue has a limited repertoire of responses to insults and inflammation.
- Most often clinically presents as tender, inflamed, subcutaneous nodules or plaques; with the exception of erythema nodosum, ulceration with drainage may develop.
- There are various etiologies, and a clinical classification system is presented in Table 83.1.
- Diagnosis is challenging and involves consideration of (1) patient characteristics such as age, immune status, underlying dis-

CLINICAL CLASSIFICATION OF THE PANNICULITIDES
Reactive panniculitis
• Erythema nodosum (EN) • Subacute nodular migratory panniculitis • Erythema induratum (EI)
Predominantly childhood panniculitis (see Table 83.3)
Metabolic panniculitis
• α_1-Antitrypsin deficiency panniculitis • Pancreatic panniculitis
Connective tissue disease panniculitis
• Lupus erythematosus panniculitis • Dermatomyositis-associated panniculitis • Morphea/systemic sclerosis (see Chs 35 and 36)
Physical/traumatic panniculitis
• Cold panniculitis • Factitial panniculitis • Blunt trauma panniculitis • Injection-related panniculitis (e.g. abatacept, glatiramer acetate) • Sclerosing lipogranuloma
Infection-induced panniculitis (see Table 83.2)
Panniculitis-like T-cell lymphomas (see Table 83.4 and Ch. 98)
Other
• Lipodermatosclerosis (LDS) • Idiopathic neutrophilic lobular panniculitis (overlapping with subcutaneous Sweet syndrome) • Cytophagic hemophagocytic panniculitis (CHP)*

**The majority represent an underlying subcutaneous lymphoma.*

Table 83.1 Clinical classification of the panniculitides.

eases; (2) location of the lesions (Fig. 83.1); (3) the presence or absence of ulceration and/or drainage; and (4) histopathologic findings.

- A biopsy is usually necessary to establish the diagnosis, and it is critical that the specimen include a generous portion of the subcutaneous (SC) fat.
- Excisional biopsies or narrow incisional biopsies that incorporate a broad expanse of SC fat are preferable to punch biopsies.
- Once the diagnosis of panniculitis is made, further evaluation for an underlying etiology or associated conditions is necessary (Tables 83.2–83.4).
- **DDx:** primarily differentiating among the various forms of panniculitis, superficial thrombophlebitis.
- **Rx:** involves specific treatment of the panniculitis and often treatment of an underlying disorder (see Tables 83.2–83.4).

MOST COMMON LOCATIONS FOR SEVERAL FORMS OF PANNICULITIS

Erythema nodosum
Erythema induratum
Lipodermatosclerosis
Lupus panniculitis
α_1-Antitrypsin deficiency panniculitis

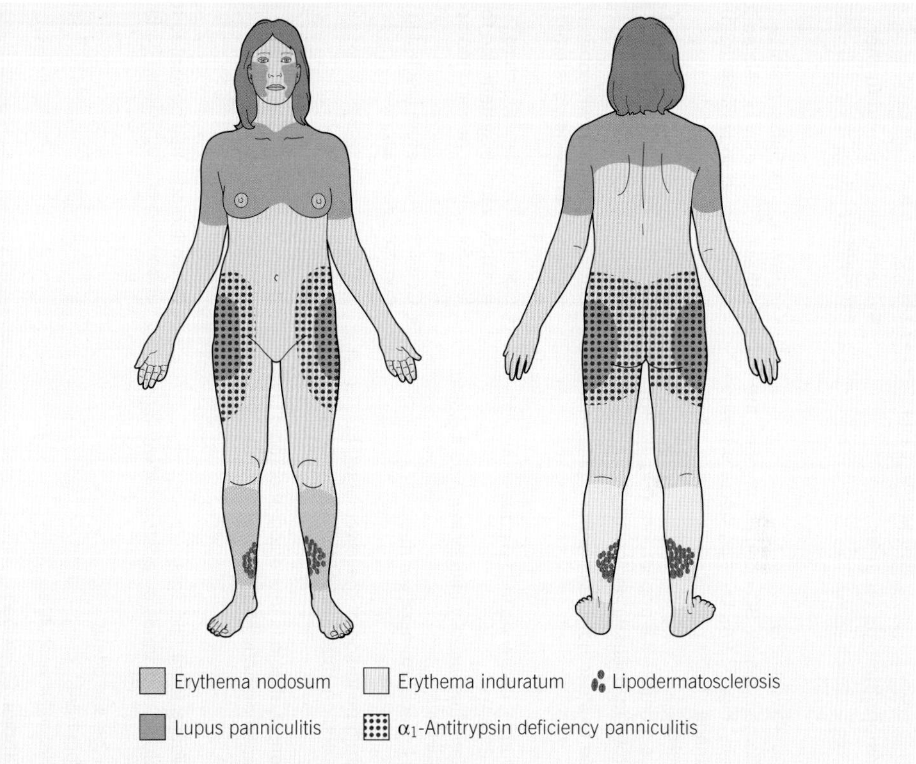

Fig. 83.1 Most common locations for several forms of panniculitis.

For further information see Ch. 100 from *Dermatology, Fourth Edition*.

For additional online figures and tables visit www.expertconsult.com 

THE MORE COMMON PANNICULITIDES			
Panniculitis	**Classic clinical and histopathologic features**	**Systemic findings and further evaluation**	**Treatment**
Most common			
Erythema nodosum (EN)	• Females > males; 2nd–4th decade • Acute eruption of inflamed, tender SC nodules, favoring the pretibial area bilaterally (Fig. 83.2A), but may occur elsewhere • No ulceration or drainage • May last days to weeks • Late lesions can have a bruise-like appearance (Fig. 83.2B) • Histopathology: prototypical septal panniculitis	• ± Fevers, arthralgias, malaise • Other findings may be related to underlying etiology (Table 83.5)	• Address and treat underlying etiology (Table 83.6)
Lipodermatosclerosis (LDS)	• Typically middle-aged to older individuals with chronic venous disorders (CVD) **ACUTE** • Painful, warm, red-purple, poorly defined plaques with variable induration (Fig. 83.3A) • Favors the lower extremities, usually initially involves the skin above the medial malleolus • Sometimes involves lower abdominal pannus **CHRONIC** • Induration and hyperpigmentation of the lower legs (Fig. 83.3B), with an "inverted champagne bottle" appearance **ACUTE on CHRONIC** • Occasionally acute onset of pain in the region of chronic LDS • Histopathology: lipomembranous change	• Strong association with obesity, venous insufficiency, systemic hypertension • Consider Doppler studies to evaluate venous system and to look for valvular or vein incompetence • Consider ABI before instituting compression therapy	**ACUTE** • Compression therapy (consider the Velcro strip variant) • If too painful for compression therapy alone, add fibrinolytic agent (e.g., anabolic steroids such as oxandrolone 10 mg BID) plus pentoxifylline (400–800 mg TID) **CHRONIC** • Compression stockings (≥20–30 mmHg) • Consider endovenous laser or radiofrequency ablation of incompetent veins
Less common			
Erythema induratum (nodular vasculitis)	• Females >> males; young to middle-aged • Tender, inflamed nodules or plaques on posterior lower legs (Fig. 83.4) • Ulceration and drainage can occur • Heal with scarring; recurrent • Histopathology: neutrophilic vasculitis	• Other findings may be related to underlying etiology (Table 83.5)	• Address and treat underlying etiology (Table 83.6)

Table 83.2 The more common panniculitides. *Continued*

Panniculitis	Classic clinical and histopathologic features	Systemic findings and further evaluation	Treatment
α_1-Antitrypsin deficiency panniculitis	• Inherited in an autosomal co-dominant pattern • Panniculitis may be initial presentation of disease or develop well into its course • Painful red or purpuric SC nodules or plaques favoring the lower trunk or proximal extremities (Fig. 83.5) • May spontaneously ulcerate and drain an oily material • Histopathology: liquefactive necrosis of dermis and SC septa	• COPD • Chronic liver disease • Dx made by demonstrating low plasma concentrations of α_1-antitrypsin (AAT) and either observation of a deficient variant of the protein AAT by protease inhibitor typing (PI ZZ variant most common) or by molecular genetic testing for *SERPINA1* gene mutations	• **MILD disease** – Doxycycline, dapsone • **SEVERE disease** – Intravenous α_1-antitrypsin replacement • **REFRACTORY disease** – Plasma exchange, liver transplant
Lupus erythematosus panniculitis	• Uncommon form of chronic cutaneous LE • Associated with SLE in at least 10% of cases • Associated with discoid LE (DLE) in at least one-third of cases, but may be an isolated finding • Painful SC nodules or plaques in a characteristic pattern – on face, shoulders, upper arms, breasts, hips, and buttocks (Fig. 83.6), notably sparing lower extremities • Chronic remitting course; can be elicited by trauma • Overlying skin may be normal, depressed, bound down, or have changes of DLE ("lupus profundus") • Histopathology: hyaline necrosis and lymphoplasmacytic infiltrate	• May have other findings of SLE (see Ch. 33) • If associated with SLE often portends a good prognosis • ANA often (+) but in low titers • Hematologic abnormalities may be the only other abnormality • Needs to be distinguished from subcutaneous panniculitis-like T-cell lymphoma (see Ch. 98)	• Intralesional CS • Systemic medications most effective • **First-line** – Antimalarials • **Second-line** – Methotrexate, dapsone, mycophenolate mofetil, azathioprine, thalidomide
Infection-induced panniculitis • Bacterial • Mycobacterial • Fungal • Viral • Parasitic	• Most often seen in immunocompromised patients, but not exclusively • Three typical clinical scenarios: – Direct inoculation of infectious organisms into the SC fat (may see sporotrichoid pattern) – Hematogenous spread to SC fat, as in septicemia (disseminated lesions) – Extension to the SC fat from underlying infection • Typically presents with ≥1 fluctuant nodules that ulcerate and drain • Favors lower extremities • Histopathology: necrosis and neutrophils; special stains can highlight organisms, but tissue culture ± PCR also recommended	• May be profoundly ill (e.g. septicemia) or appear well (e.g. normal host with isolated lesion) • Dx requires a high index of suspicion, *pre*-biopsy, so that a sterile, deep biopsy specimen can be sent to microbiology for tissue culture ± PCR, in addition to pathology	• Empirical, broad-spectrum coverage in severely ill host • Otherwise tailored to identified organism

Table 83.2 *Continued* **The more common panniculitides.**

PREDOMINANTLY CHILDHOOD PANNICULITIDES			
Panniculitis	**Classic features***	**Systemic findings and further evaluation**	**Treatment**
Subcutaneous fat necrosis of the newborn†	• Usually seen in full-term neonates • Onset during the first 2–3 weeks of life • Mobile, firm SC nodules or plaques, favoring the cheeks, shoulders, back, buttocks, and thighs (Fig. 83.7)	• Hypercalcemia (usually within 2 months of onset), thrombocytopenia, hypertriglyceridemia • May be precipitated by hypothermia, hypoglycemia, perinatal distress/hypoxia	• Spontaneous resolution common • Favorable prognosis • Supportive care
Post-steroid panniculitis†	• Onset usually within 10 days after the rapid withdrawal of systemic CS • Firm red plaques on the cheeks, arms, trunk	• May be related to the condition that required the systemic CS	• May resolve spontaneously • Consider readministration and slower tapering of systemic CS
Cold panniculitis	• Favors the cheeks of infants and children due to popsicles or ice cubes and the medial thighs of equestrians due to riding in cold temperatures plus tight-fitting clothing (Fig. 83.8)	• Possibly other signs of hypothermia	• Remove cold exposure and rewarm
Sclerema neonatorum†	• Seen in premature, extremely ill neonates • Onset during the first week of life • Diffusely cold, rigid, board-like skin	• Death common due to septicemia • May be precipitated by hypothermia, dehydration, perinatal asphyxia	• No good treatment • Supportive care

**All entities, except for cold panniculitis, will demonstrate needle-shaped clefts on histopathology.*
†Seen exclusively in infants or children.

Table 83.3 Predominantly childhood panniculitides.

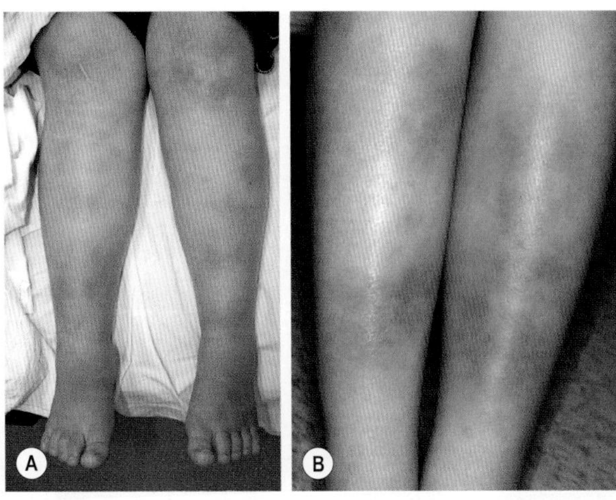

Fig. 83.2 Erythema nodosum. **A** Erythematous, tender nodules bilaterally on the shins and dorsal feet; the patient is pregnant. **B** The nodules and plaques may develop a bruise-like appearance. *A, Courtesy, Ian Odell, MD, PhD; B, Courtesy, Kalman Watsky, MD.*

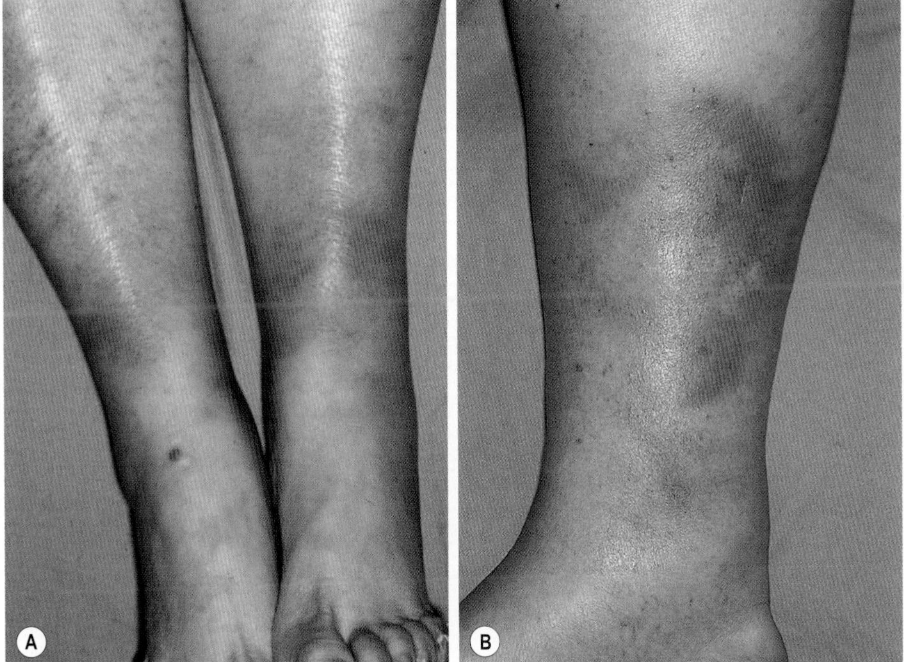

Fig. 83.3 Lipodermatosclerosis. **A** Acute phase with tender erythematous plaques on both lower extremities. This condition is often misdiagnosed as "bilateral recurrent cellulitis." **B** Chronic phase with sclerotic red-brown plaque on the lower medial leg. *A, Courtesy, James Patterson, MD; B, Courtesy, Kenneth E. Greer, MD.*

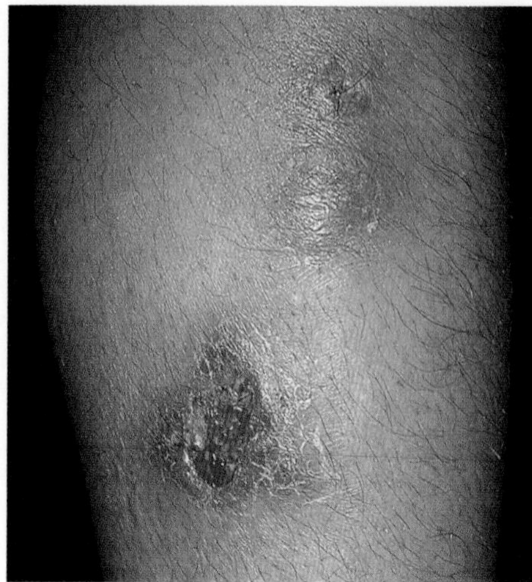

Fig. 83.4 Erythema induratum. Nodular lesions on the lower leg, with evidence of ulceration. *Courtesy, Kenneth E. Greer, MD.*

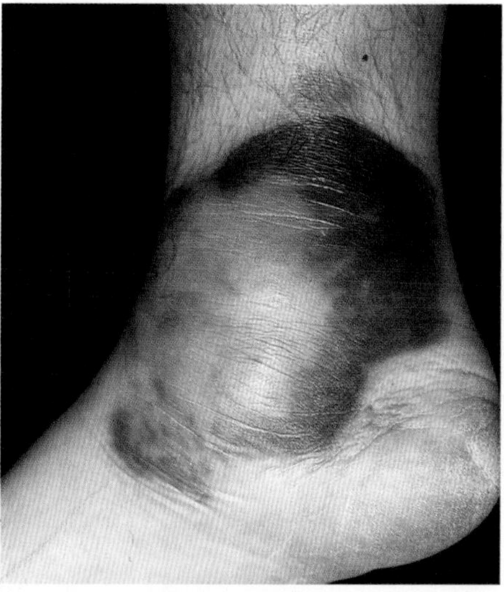

Fig. 83.5 α_1-Antitrypsin deficiency panniculitis. Purpuric nodules on the ankles. *Courtesy, Kenneth E. Greer, MD.*

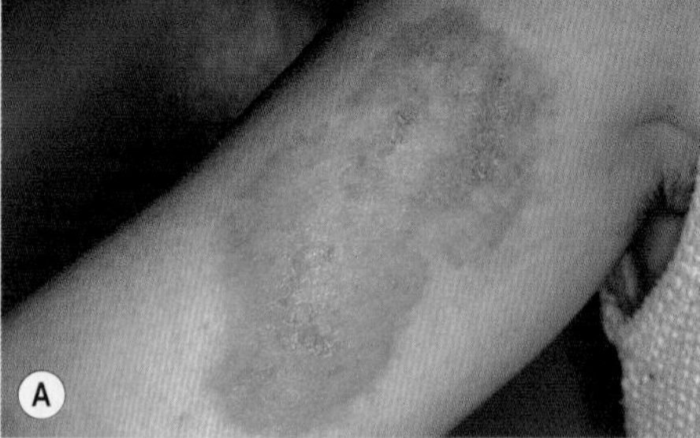

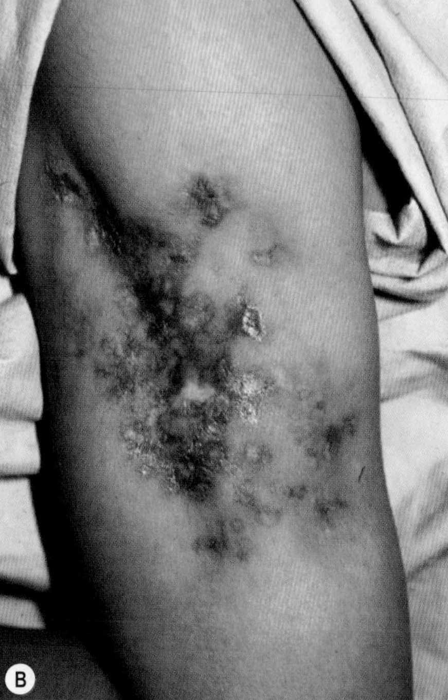

Fig. 83.6 Lupus panniculitis. A Erythematous plaque on the upper arm. The lesions may resolve with lipoatrophy. **B** Red-brown plaques on the upper outer arm. Note the significant subcutaneous atrophy and overlying lesions of discoid lupus erythematosus. *A, Courtesy, YDRSC; B, Courtesy, Kenneth E. Greer, MD.*

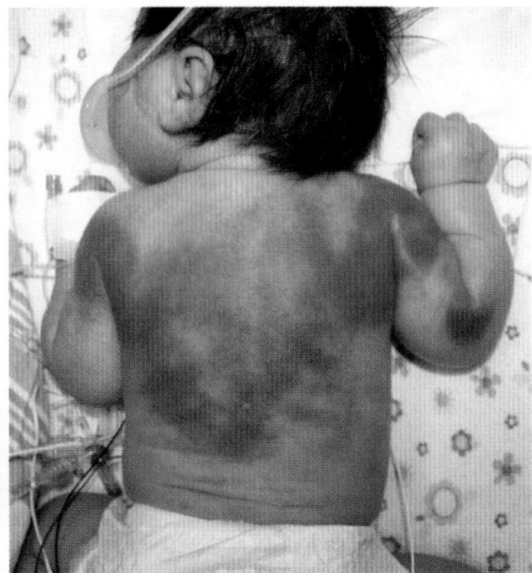

Fig. 83.7 Subcutaneous fat necrosis of the newborn. Red-violet indurated plaques, primarily on the back and shoulders. *Courtesy, Lorenzo Cerroni, MD.*

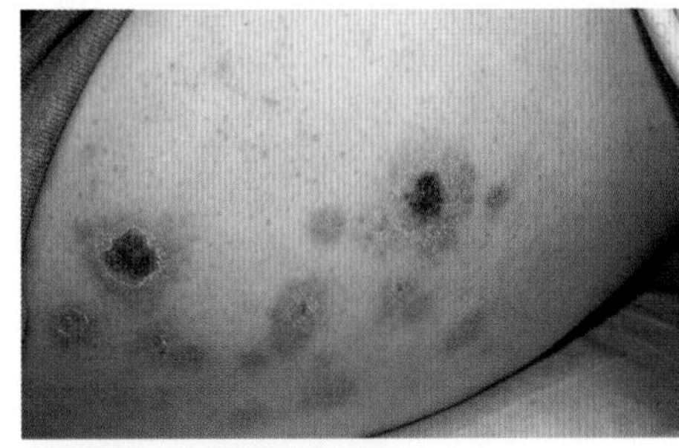

Fig. 83.8 Cold panniculitis. Violaceous nodules and plaques, some with central crusting, on the thigh of a young woman. *Courtesy, Kendra Lesiak, MD.*

THE LESS COMMON PANNICULITIDES	
Panniculitis	**Classic features**
Subacute nodular migratory panniculitis (chronic EN)	• Resembles EN but is typically chronic, unilateral, and tends to migrate and/or form annular lesions • May be associated with streptococcal infections or thyroid disease
Pancreatic panniculitis	• May be the initial presentation of pancreatic disease (pancreatitis > cancer) or develop during its course • Favors lower legs (Fig. 83.9), but also arms, chest, abdomen • May become fluctuant, ulcerate, and drain an oily substance • Eosinophilia and polyarthritis are associated findings
Dermatomyositis-associated panniculitis	• More common in juvenile dermatomyositis • Tender SC nodules or plaques on thighs, arms, buttocks, and abdomen; calcify with time
Panniculitis-like T-cell lymphomas (see Ch. 98)	• Dx is often suggested after a biopsy is performed in a patient whose lesions fail to improve or worsen, e.g. in a patient with a clinical Dx of EN • Two major types, requiring histopathologic differentiation: subcutaneous panniculitis-like T-cell lymphoma ($\alpha\beta$ type) and $\gamma\delta$ T-cell lymphoma • Evaluation for systemic involvement is necessary • DDx includes lupus panniculitis
Cytophagic histiocytic panniculitis (CHP)	• Dx is usually made after histopathologic examination of SC nodules or plaques (Fig. 83.10) when the finding of hematophagocytosis is identified • The majority of patients have subcutaneous involvement with an aggressive lymphoma, e.g. $\gamma\delta$ T-cell lymphoma; may have a fatal course due to a hemophagocytic syndrome

Table 83.4 The less common panniculitides. EN, erythema nodosum.

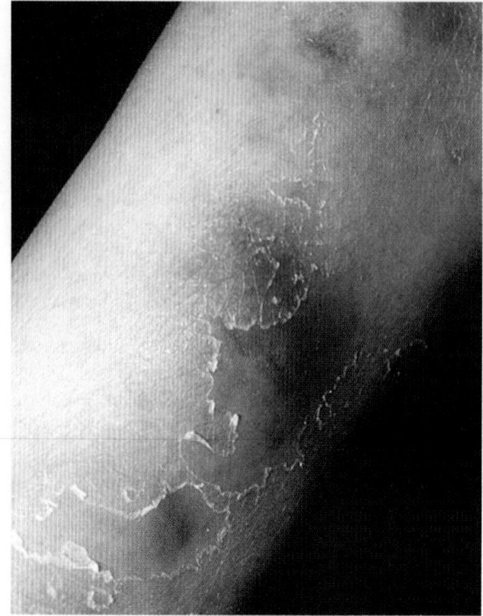

Fig. 83.9 Pancreatic panniculitis. Multiple red to violet-brown nodules on the arm. There is also postinflammatory desquamation. *Courtesy, Lorenzo Cerroni, MD.*

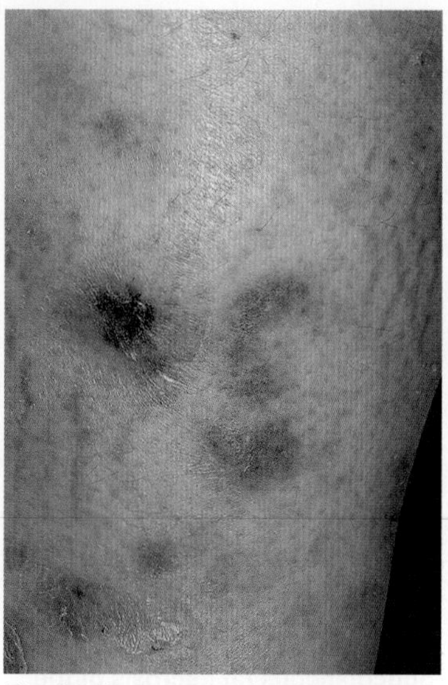

Fig. 83.10 Cytophagic histiocytic panniculitis. Subcutaneous nodules with purpura. The majority of these patients have an underlying subcutaneous lymphoma. *Courtesy, Kenneth E. Greer, MD.*

TRIGGERS OF ERYTHEMA NODOSUM AND ERYTHEMA INDURATUM AND SUGGESTED EVALUATIONS		
	Erythema nodosum	**Erythema induratum**
Most common causes	• Idiopathic • Streptococcal infections, especially of the upper respiratory tract • Other infectious associations: – Bacterial gastroenteritis – *Yersinia* > *Salmonella*, *Campylobacter* – Viral upper respiratory tract infections – Coccidioidomycosis • Sarcoidosis* • Inflammatory bowel disease • Drugs: – Estrogens/oral contraceptives – Antibiotics (e.g. sulfonamides, penicillins)	• Tuberculosis • Idiopathic
Less common causes	• Other infections (e.g. brucellosis, tuberculosis, hepatitis B†) • Neutrophilic dermatoses (e.g. Sweet syndrome, Behçet disease) • Pregnancy • Drugs: – TNF inhibitors (e.g. etanercept, infliximab, adalimumab)** – Immune checkpoint inhibitors (e.g. ipilimumab, nivolumab)*** – BRAF inhibitors (e.g. vemurafenib, dabrafenib)‡ – Bromides, iodides • Malignancy (e.g. acute myelogenous leukemia)	• Other infections (e.g. *Nocardia*, *Pseudomonas*, viral hepatitis) • Non-infectious associations (e.g. superficial thrombophlebitis, hypothyroidism, RA, Crohn disease) • Drugs (e.g. propylthiouracil)

Table 83.5 Triggers of erythema nodosum and erythema induratum and suggested evaluations. *Continued.*

TRIGGERS OF ERYTHEMA NODOSUM AND ERYTHEMA INDURATUM AND SUGGESTED EVALUATIONS		
	Erythema nodosum	**Erythema induratum**
Suggested workup[§]	• Anti-streptolysin O and/or anti-DNase B titers • Chest X-ray • Tuberculin skin test or IGRA • Viral hepatitis panel • If diarrhea, check fecal WBC and stool culture for bacteria, ova and parasites • Consider GI referral if bloody diarrhea, fecal WBC, and negative cultures • β-HCG in women • Malignancy workup as indicated by history and physical exam	• Chest X-ray • Tuberculin skin test or IGRA • Consider PCR of skin biopsy for *M. tuberculosis* • Viral hepatitis panel • TSH • CBC, ESR • Rheumatoid factor • Consider GI referral if diarrhea

**Löfgren syndrome is an acute, spontaneously resolving form of sarcoidosis characterized by erythema nodosum, fever, hilar lymphadenopathy, polyarthritis, and uveitis.*
***Also lupus-like.*
****Also sarcoid-like.*
†Erythema nodosum secondary to hepatitis B vaccine has also been reported.
‡Also neutrophilic lobular as with other tyrosine kinase inhibitors (e.g. imatinib, dasatinib, ibrutinib).
§Basic workup in patients with erythema nodosum and erythema induratum with no obvious etiology.

Table 83.5 *Continued* **Triggers of erythema nodosum and erythema induratum and suggested evaluations.** HCG, human chorionic gonadotropin; IGRA, interferon-γ release assay; RA, rheumatoid arthritis.

TREATMENT RECOMMENDATIONS FOR ERYTHEMA NODOSUM AND ERYTHEMA INDURATUM		
Treatment	**Erythema nodosum**	**Erythema induratum**
In all patients	• Discontinue possible causative medications • Diagnose and treat underlying cause/infection • Bed rest and leg elevation • Compression	
First-line	• Nonsteroidal anti-inflammatory medications • Salicylates • Potassium iodide (see Appendix)	
Second-line, *once infection excluded or treated*	• Colchicine* • Infliximab** • Hydroxychloroquine*** • Adalimumab*** • Etanercept • Mycophenolate mofetil	• Systemic CS • Tetracyclines • Mycophenolate mofetil
Third-line, *once infection excluded or treated*	• Systemic CS • Thalidomide** • Cyclosporine* • Dapsone	

**Helpful for erythema nodosum occurring in the setting of Behçet disease.*
***Helpful for erythema nodosum occurring in the setting of inflammatory bowel disease.*
****Helpful for chronic erythema nodosum.*

Table 83.6 Treatment recommendations for erythema nodosum and erythema induratum.

84 Lipodystrophies

• Lipodystrophy is characterized by areas of fat loss/absence (lipoatrophy), and/or fat accumulation (lipohypertrophy), with both often coexisting in the same patient; lipoatrophy can lead to the appearance of muscular hypertrophy (Fig. 84.1).

• Lipoatrophy may be classified as:
  - Generalized, partial, or localized (Fig. 84.2)
  - Inherited (often appears during childhood) or acquired
  - Stable or progressive

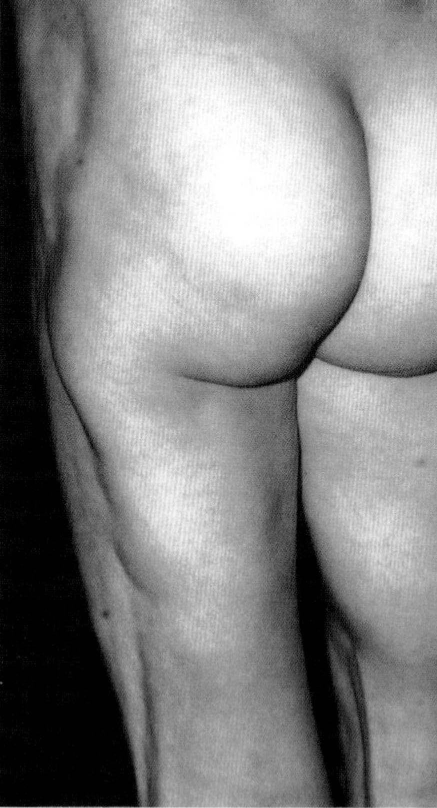

Fig. 84.1 Lipoatrophy of the lower extremities, leading to the appearance of muscular hypertrophy. *Courtesy, William D. James, MD.*

• Localized lipo*atrophy* may be idiopathic (Fig. 84.3) or secondary to various causes, e.g. injection of medications (in particular CS), pressure (Figs 84.4 and 84.5), trauma, autoimmune connective tissue disease (e.g. lupus panniculitis; Figs 84.6 and 84.7), and other panniculitides due to inflammation or lymphoma.

• Localized lipo*hypertrophy* is most commonly seen in the setting of multiple insulin injections.

• HIV/antiretroviral therapy (HIV/ART) causes a distinct syndrome of central lipohypertrophy and peripheral lipoatrophy (Fig. 84.8).

• Extensive lipodystrophy syndromes have characteristic distributions of fat atrophy and hypertrophy (Figs 84.2 and 84.9–84.11).

• Fat is a metabolically active tissue with important endocrine functions; therefore, non-localized lipodystrophy is often seen in conjunction with the metabolic syndrome (insulin resistance, diabetes mellitus, hyperinsulinemia, dyslipidemia, cardiovascular disease, and fatty hepatic steatosis).

• Other associations include hormonal abnormalities, anabolic syndrome, glomerulonephritis, and autoinflammatory syndromes (e.g. CANDLE syndrome, see Table 37.3).

• **Rx:** depends in part on underlying etiology (see Fig. 84.2); (1) remove inciting cause (e.g. relieve pressure or rotate sites of injections); (2) address the metabolic syndrome if present; (3) consider metreleptin for inherited or acquired generalized lipoatrophy; (4) improve cosmetic appearance (e.g. injection of poly-L-lactic acid or autologous fat transfer into the cheeks).

For further information see Ch. 101 from *Dermatology, Fourth Edition*.

For additional online figures visit www.expertconsult.com 

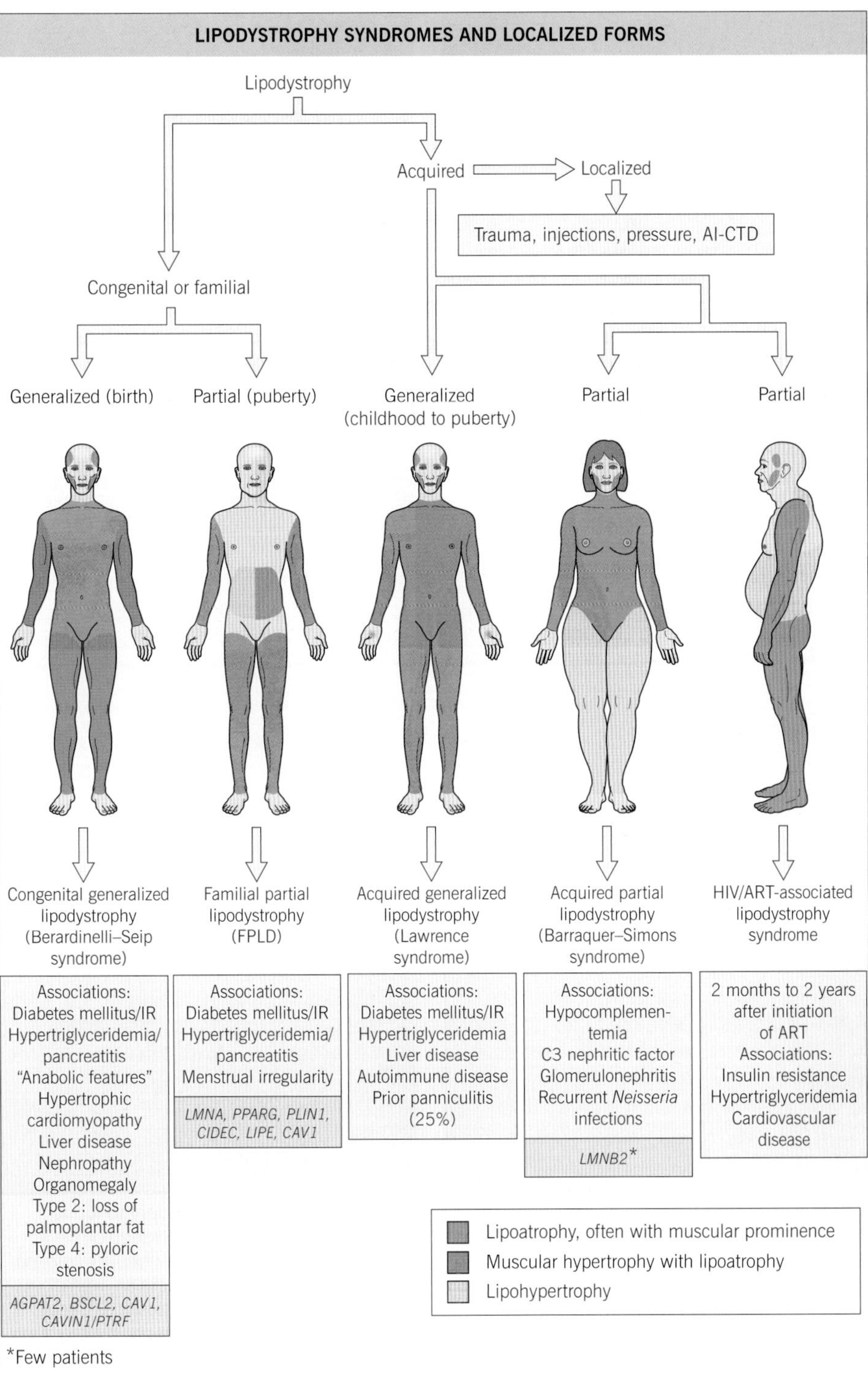

Fig. 84.2 Lipodystrophy syndromes and localized forms. Schematic representation of the predominant sites of lipoatrophy and lipohypertrophy. Shaded boxes include best-described underlying genetic mutations. In familial partial lipodystrophy, *LMNA* mutations are associated with facial lipohypertrophy and abdominal lipoatrophy while *PPARG* mutations are associated with abdominal lipohypertrophy. IR, insulin resistance.

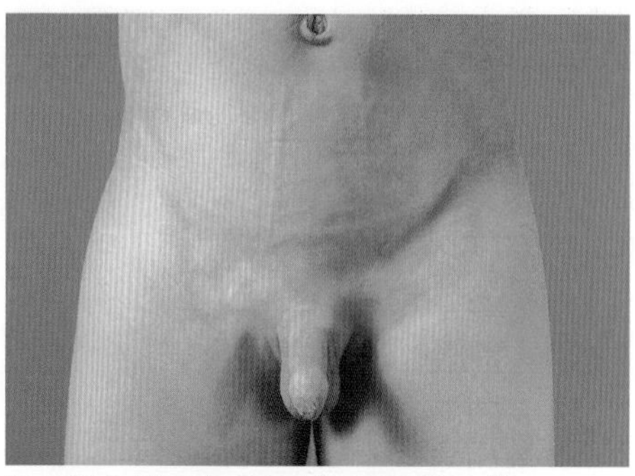

Fig. 84.3 Lipodystrophia centrifugalis abdominalis infantilis (centrifugal lipodystrophy). A 5-year-old Malay boy with a two-year history of progressive lipoatrophy involving the groin bilaterally and the lower abdomen. The veins in the involved area are readily visible. *Courtesy, National Skin Centre, Singapore.*

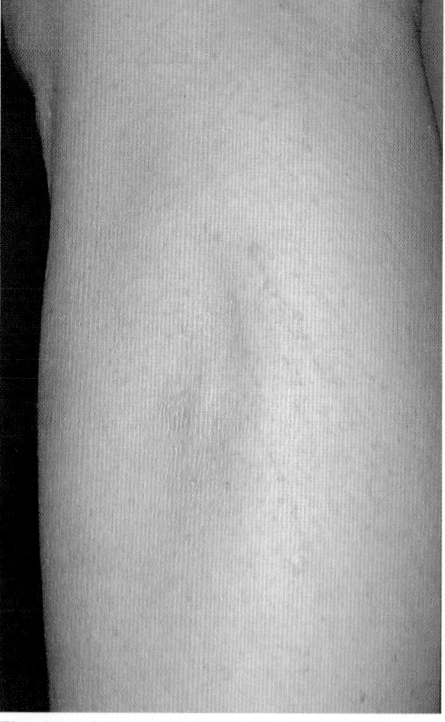

Fig. 84.4 Localized lipoatrophy of the upper lateral calf due to pressure. A fairly common finding in women who cross their legs while seated. *Courtesy, Jean L. Bolognia, MD.*

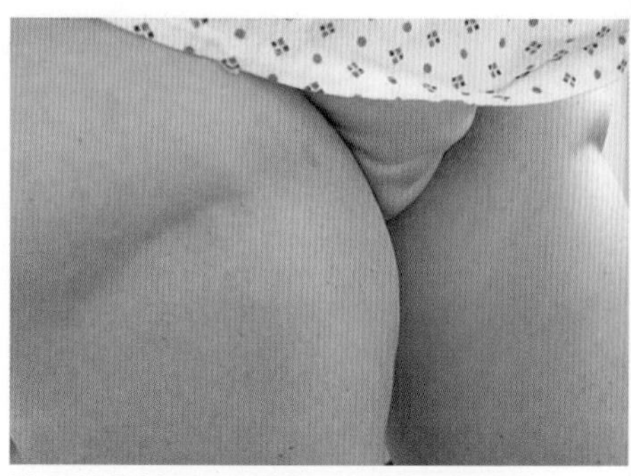

Fig. 84.5 Lipoatrophia semicircularis (semicircular lipoatrophy). Bilateral slightly curved depressions on the anterolateral thighs. *Courtesy, Diane Thaler, MD.*

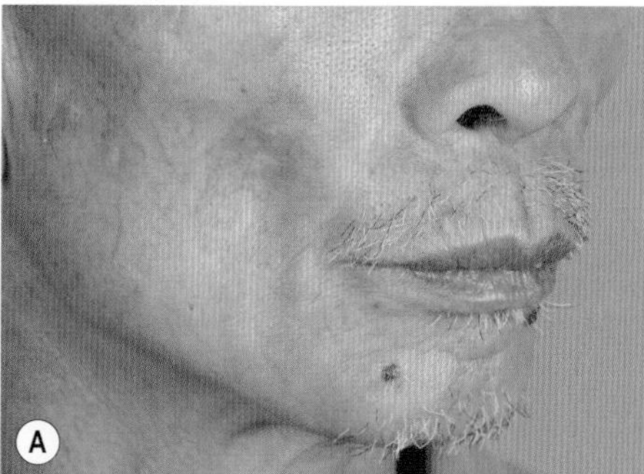

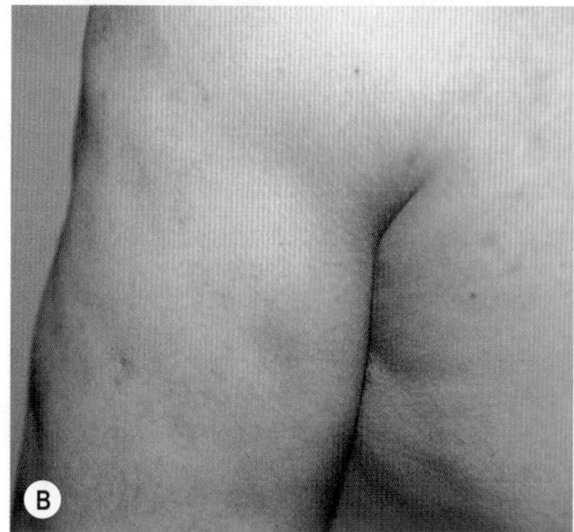

Fig. 84.6 Lipoatrophy secondary to lupus panniculitis. A An area of depression on the cheek due to burnt-out lupus panniculitis; note the dyspigmentation and scarring from an overlapping lesion of discoid lupus erythematosus. **B** Circular depressions on the upper arm, a common location for lupus panniculitis. Lipoatrophy can be seen with other connective tissue disorders, including dermatomyositis in children. *A, Courtesy National Skin Centre, Singapore; B, Courtesy, YDRSC.*

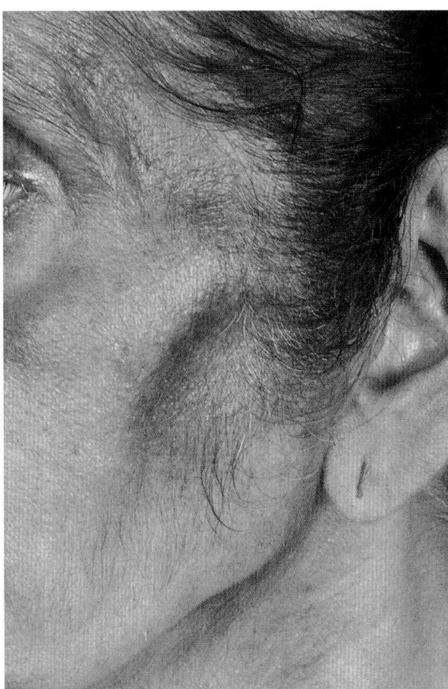

Fig. 84.7 Acquired partial lipodystrophy syndrome in a patient with Sjögren syndrome. Lipoatrophy of the face with sunken eyes and loss of temporal and buccal fat pads. The facial pigmentation is related to lichen planus. *Courtesy, Priya Sen, MD.*

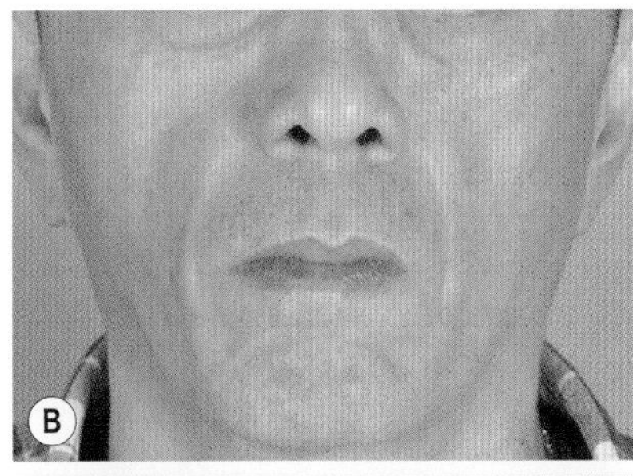

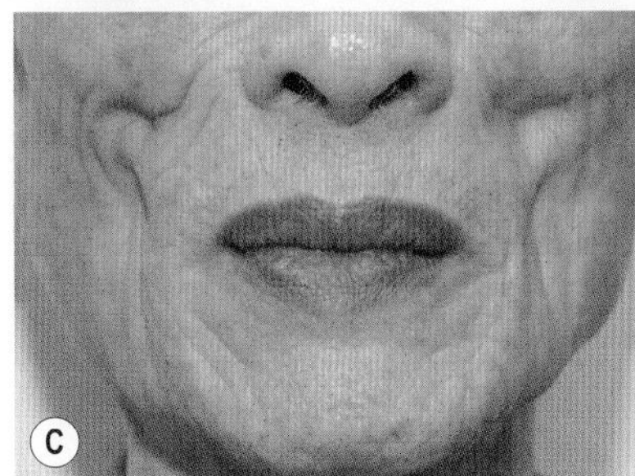

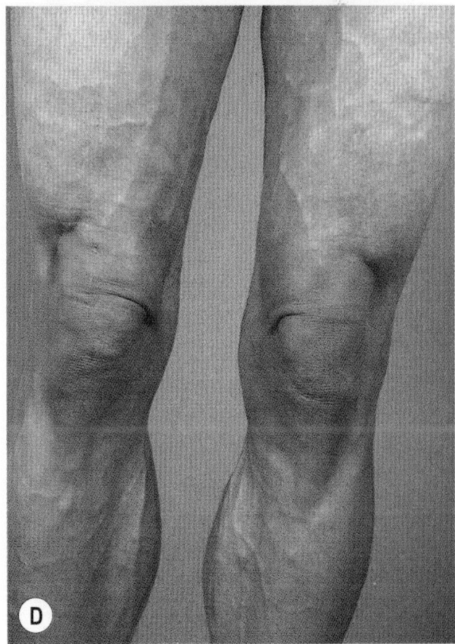

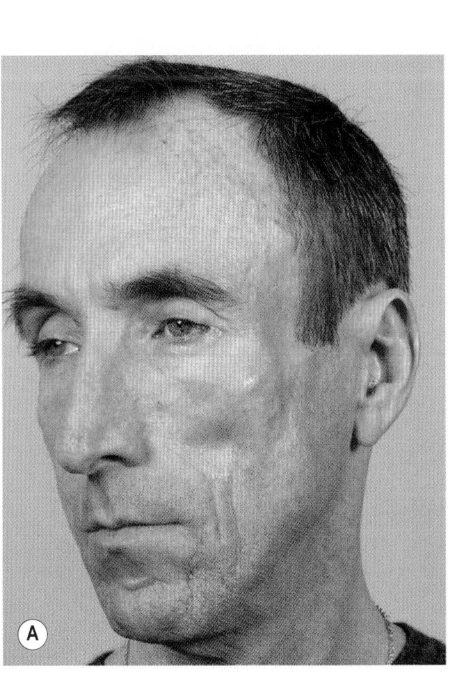

Fig. 84.8 HIV/ART-associated lipodystrophy. A The side view highlights the loss of temporal fat. **B** There is symmetric loss of buccal and parotid fat, resulting in prominent zygomata and a cachectic appearance. **C** Marked indentation of the medial cheeks in an older patient with redundancy of the melolabial folds. In particular, stavudine and protease inhibitors are most strongly associated with lipoatrophy. **D** Lower extremities with defined veins and prominent musculature. *A, Courtesy, Ken Katz, MD; B, Courtesy, National Skin Centre, Singapore; C, Courtesy, Priya Sen, MD; D, Courtesy, Alison Sharpe Avram, MD and Matthew Avram, MD.*

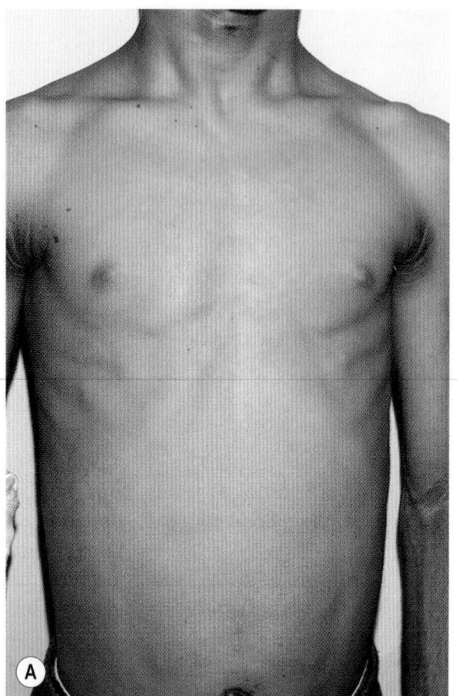

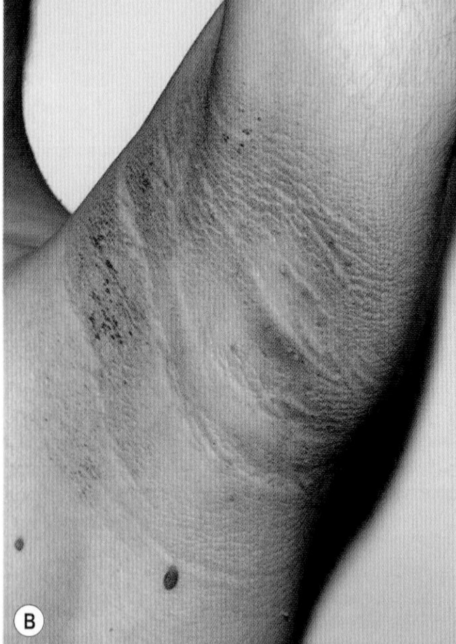

Fig. 84.9 Congenital generalized lipodystrophy syndrome (Berardinelli–Seip syndrome). A Lipoatrophy of the trunk leading to muscle definition. **B** Extensive acanthosis nigricans. *A, B, Courtesy, Edward Cowen, MD.*

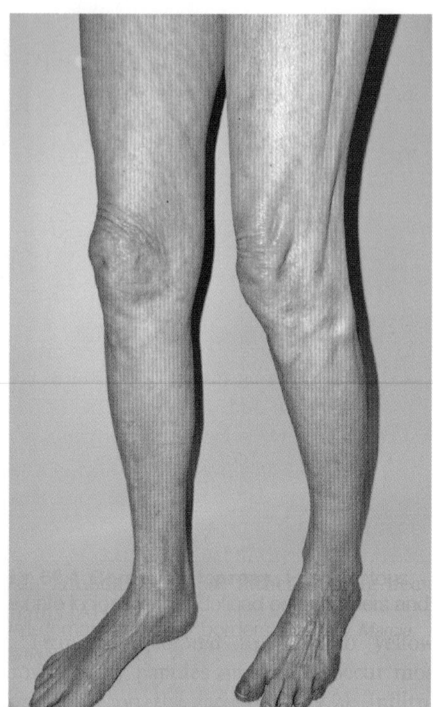

Fig. 84.10 Acquired generalized lipodystrophy. There is loss of subcutaneous fat, resulting in a muscular appearance of the legs and accentuation of the tendons. *Courtesy, Jacqueline Junkins-Hopkins, MD.*

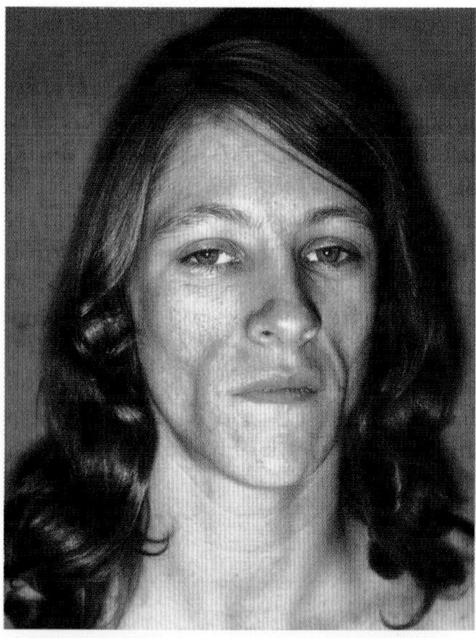

Fig. 84.11 Acquired partial lipodystrophy in a patient with nephritic factor and renal disease. Lipoatrophic features are most prominent on the face, with a marked loss of buccal fat. Axillary acanthosis nigricans was present. *Courtesy, Kenneth E. Greer, MD.*

Infantile Hemangiomas and Vascular Malformations

85

- Vascular anomalies, which often present at birth or during early infancy, are classified into two groups based on their biologic and clinical behavior:
  - *Vascular tumors*, most commonly the infantile hemangioma (IH), that are characterized by endothelial cell proliferation
  - *Vascular malformations* that result from abnormal vascular morphogenesis
- Features that distinguish IHs from vascular malformations are presented in Table 85.1, and differences in their natural histories are depicted in Fig. 85.1.
- Additional vascular neoplasms are discussed in Chapter 94; other vascular ectasias,

COMPARISON OF INFANTILE HEMANGIOMAS WITH VASCULAR MALFORMATIONS		
Characteristic	**Infantile hemangiomas**	**Vascular malformations**
Epidemiology	More common in: • Girls (female:male ratio 3–5:1) • Premature and/or low-birth-weight infants • Infants whose mothers are older or underwent CVS	• Equal sex ratio • No predilection based on gestational history • Certain variants have autosomal dominant inheritance (see text)
Appearance at birth	• Often absent • ~50% with a subtle precursor lesion, e.g. telangiectatic, vasoconstricted, pink or bluish bruise-like macules or patches (Fig. 85.2)	• Typically present and already demonstrate characteristic clinical findings
Natural history	• *Postnatal proliferation* for 6–9 months, followed by *slow involution* over several years	• *Lifelong persistence*, with commensurate growth during childhood and often *gradual worsening* (e.g. thickening of capillary malformations) over time
Radiology	• Well-defined mass with high-flow vessels	• Varies depending on the type (see text)
Pathology	In the proliferative phase: • Dense lobules of hyperplastic endothelial cells forming capillaries with tiny lumens • Increased cellular turnover demonstrated by markers of proliferation (e.g. Ki-67)	• Ectatic or distorted vascular channels • Typically no increase in cellular turnover
Immunophenotype	• GLUT1-positive	• GLUT1-negative

Table 85.1 Comparison of infantile hemangiomas with vascular malformations. CVS, chorionic villus sampling; GLUT1, glucose transporter protein-1 (expressed by the placenta as well as infantile hemangiomas, but no diffuse expression in other vascular tumors).

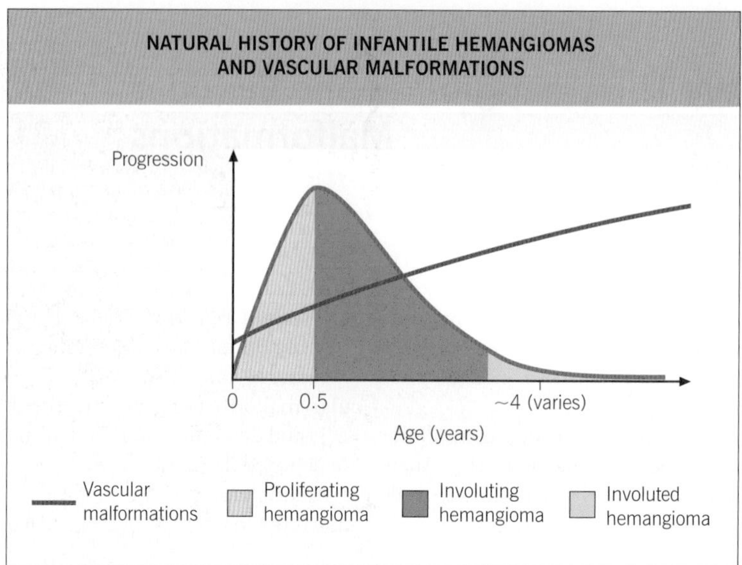

Fig. 85.1 Natural history of infantile hemangiomas and vascular malformations.

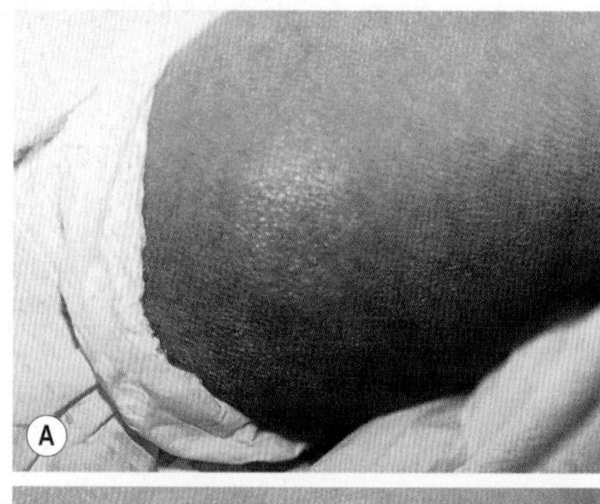

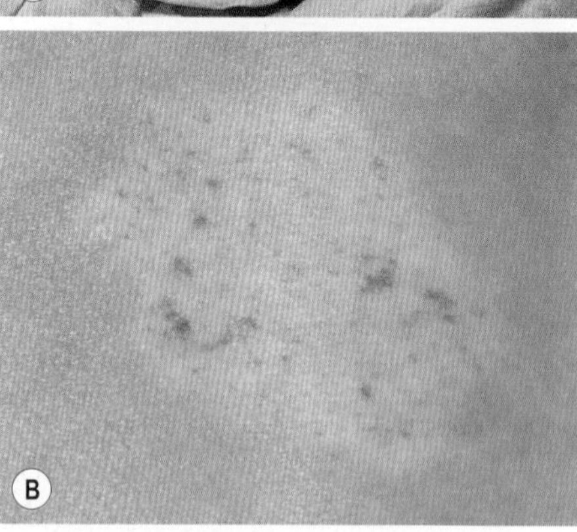

Fig. 85.2 Hemangioma precursors. These initial lesions can have a "bruised" **(A)** or blanched **(B)** appearance. *A, Courtesy, Maria Garzon, MD; B, Courtesy, Julie V. Schaffer, MD.*

such as telangiectasias and angiokeratomas, are covered in Chapter 87.

Infantile Hemangioma (IH)

- Benign vascular neoplasm that represents the most common tumor of infancy.
  - Affects ~5% of infants, with a predilection for girls and premature neonates (see Table 85.1)
- IHs appear during the first few weeks of life, with a characteristic course:
  - *Proliferation* for 5–9 months, tending to "mark out their territory" early on and then grow primarily in volume; overall, ~80% of growth is in the first 5 months of life, with the most rapid growth in the first 2–3 months
  - Subsequent *involution* gradually over several years (completed at a median age of 3 years), with development of a duller, lighter red to gray color and softening followed by flattening (Fig. 85.3)
  - Some IHs involute with little or no visible sequelae, whereas others (especially pedunculated or exophytic lesions) leave atrophic, fibrofatty, or telangiectatic residua in addition to scars at sites of previous ulceration (discussed later; Fig. 85.4)

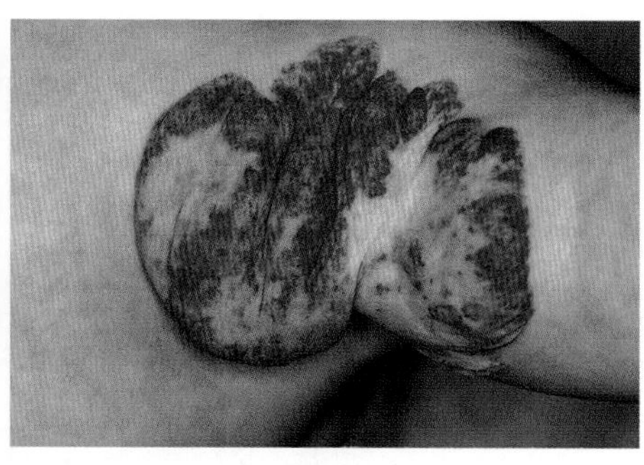

Fig. 85.3 Involuting infantile hemangioma. Note the duller red to grayish color with areas of complete fading. These color changes were accompanied by gradual softening and flattening. *Courtesy, YDRSC.*

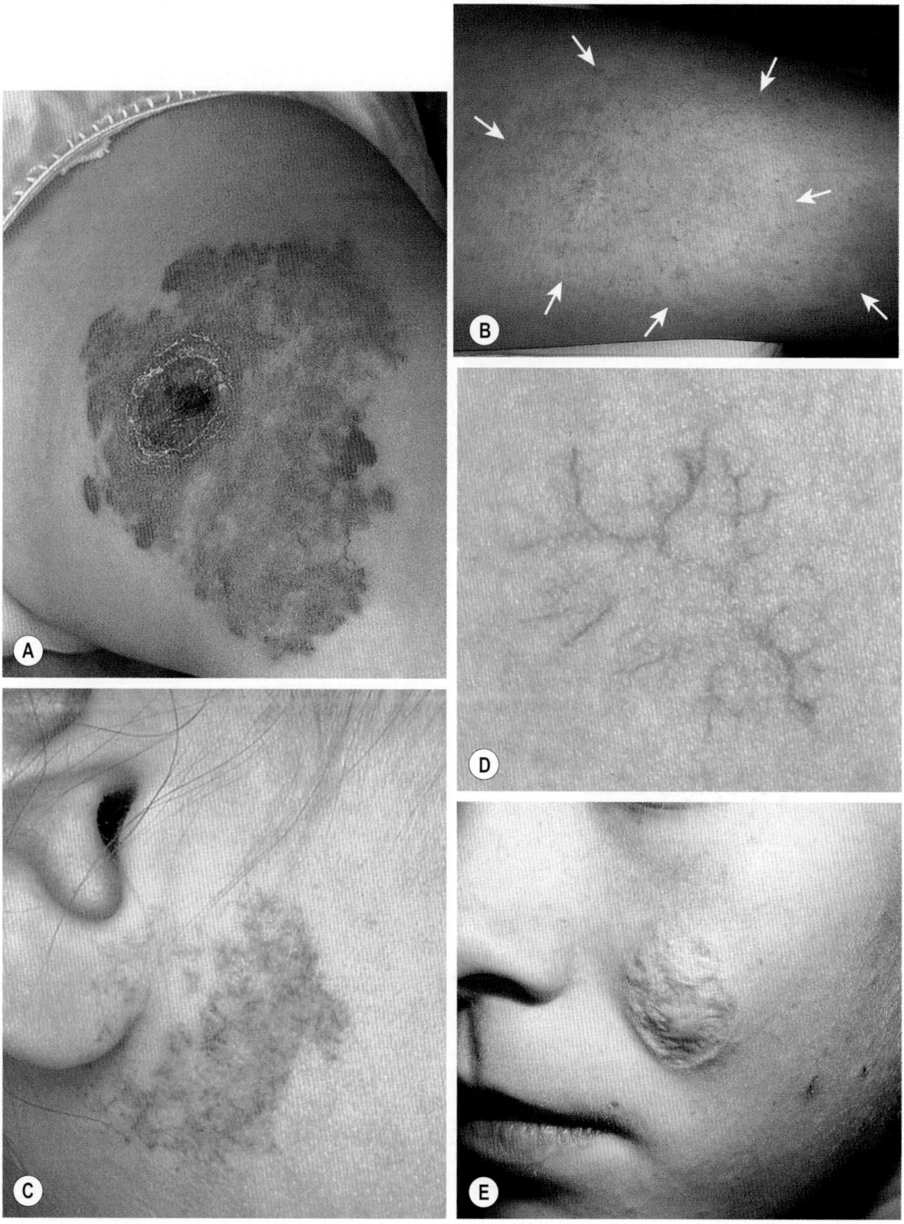

A B C D E

Fig. 85.4 Residua of infantile hemangiomas. A Superficial hemangioma with a healing ulcer in an infant. **B** Hypopigmentation (arrows) and a circular scar at the site of the previous ulcer in the same patient 20 years later. **C, D** Residual telangiectasias. **E** Atrophy and fibrofatty changes. *A, B, E, Courtesy, Ronald P. Rapini, MD; C, Courtesy, YDRSC; D, Courtesy, Jean L. Bolognia, MD.*

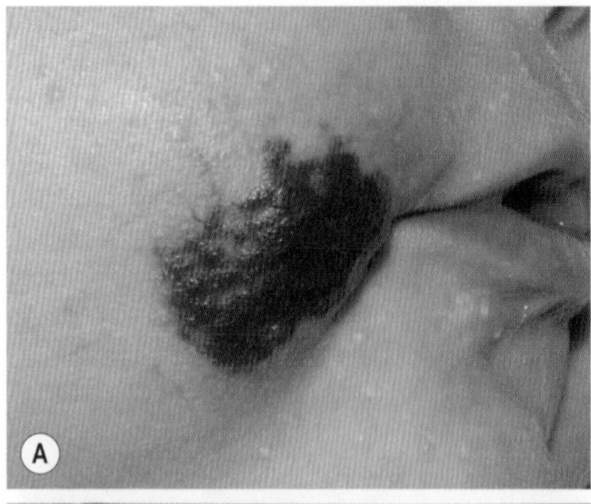

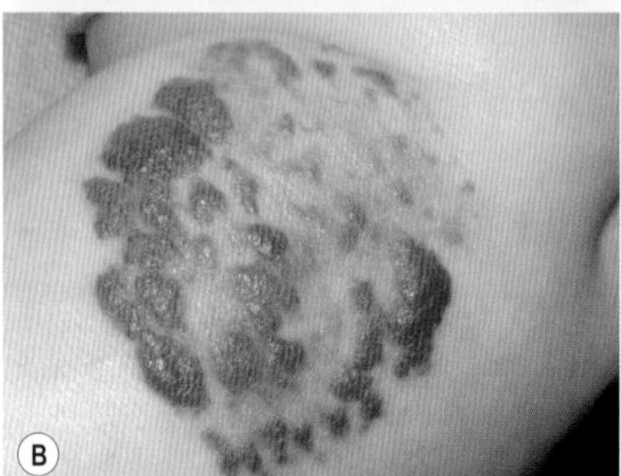

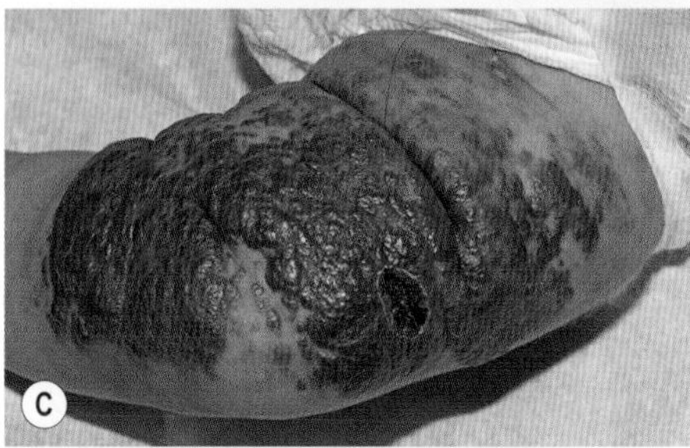

Fig. 85.5 Superficial infantile hemangiomas. Note the bright red color and finely lobulated surface. Involvement may be diffuse or broken up, and lesions can be focal (**A**, **B**) or have a broader, segmental distribution (**C**). *Courtesy, Julie V. Schaffer, MD.*

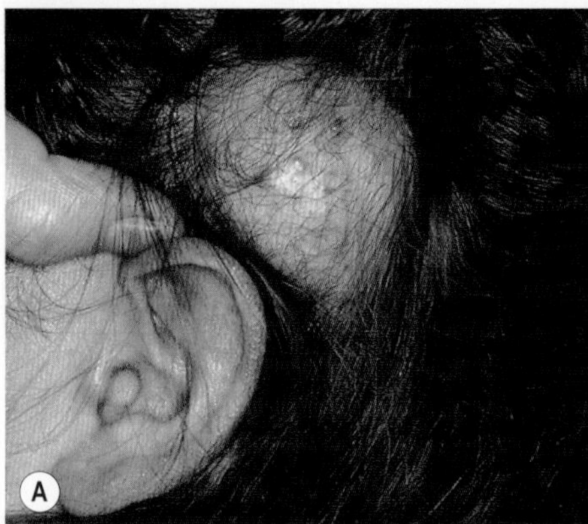

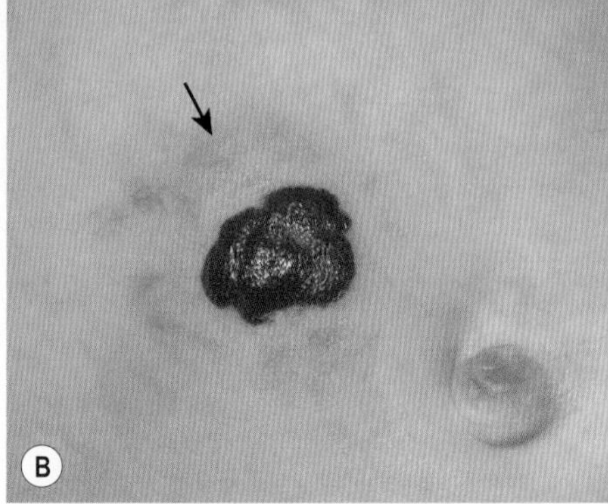

Fig. 85.6 Deep and mixed infantile hemangiomas. A Skin-colored deep hemangioma with overlying telangiectasias and alopecia on the scalp. **B** Mixed hemangioma composed of a well-demarcated, bright red superficial plaque plus a broader, ill-defined underlying deep nodule with a subtle light bluish hue (arrow) and scattered telangiectasias. *A, Courtesy, YDRSC; B, Courtesy, Julie V. Schaffer, MD.*

- Divided into three clinical subtypes based on the depth of cutaneous involvement:
  - *Superficial* lesions (~50%; upper dermis) are bright red with a finely lobulated surface ("strawberry" hemangiomas) during proliferation, changing to a mixture of purple-red and gray during involution (Fig. 85.5)
  - *Deep* lesions (~15%; lower dermis and subcutis) present as warm, ill-defined, light blue-purple, rubbery nodules or masses (Fig. 85.6A); often become evident later and proliferate ~1 month longer than superficial lesions
  - *Mixed* lesions (~35%) have superficial and deep components – e.g. a well-defined red plaque overlying a poorly circumscribed bluish nodule (Fig. 85.6B)
- IHs have two major distribution patterns:
  - *Focal* lesions arise from a localized nidus (see Fig. 85.5A,B)
  - *Segmental* lesions cover a broader area or developmental unit and are more likely to be associated with regional extracutaneous abnormalities – e.g. PHACE(S) and LUMBAR syndromes (discussed later) (Fig. 85.7; see Fig. 85.5C)

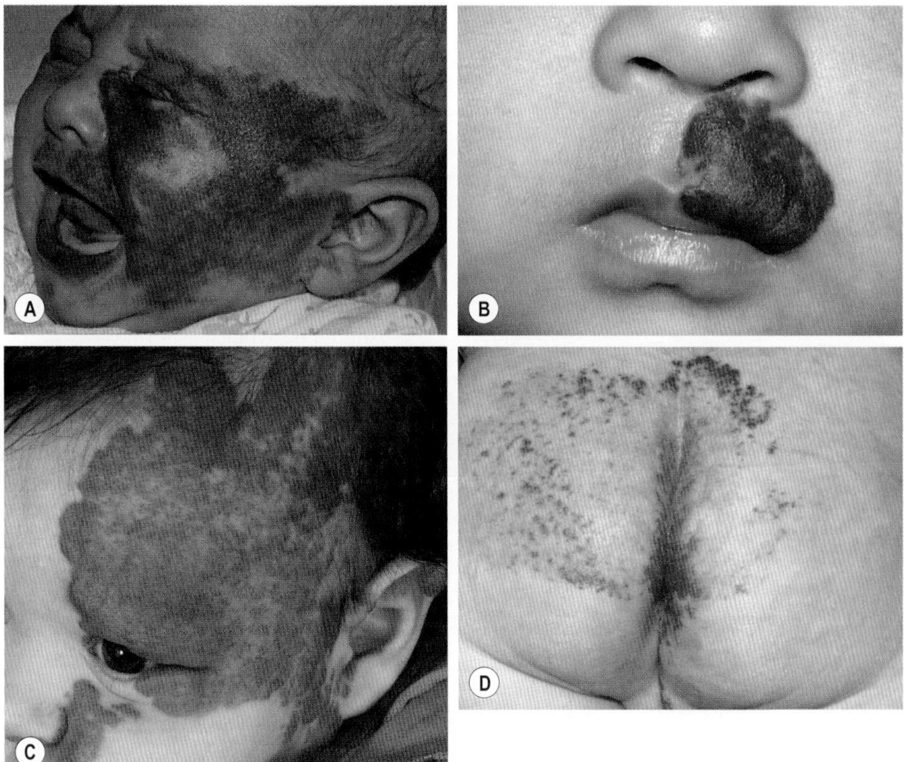

Fig. 85.7 Segmental infantile hemangiomas. A Segmental facial hemangioma mimicking a capillary malformation. **B** Smaller segmental hemangioma on the lip. This is a cosmetically sensitive site, especially when lesions cross the vermilion border. Hemangiomas on the vermilion lip are prone to ulceration. **C** Thicker segmental facial hemangioma partially obstructing the visual axis. This patient and the one depicted in **A** had PHACE(S) syndrome. **D** Segmental lumbosacral hemangioma. This child is at risk for LUMBAR syndrome. *Courtesy, Julie V. Schaffer, MD.*

• Some superficial IHs have *minimal or arrested growth (IH-MAG)*, presenting as patches of reticulated erythema with telangiectasias, often on a vasoconstricted background, and variable development of small red papules involving <25% of the surface area (Fig. 85.8).

• **DDx:** *precursors and early lesions*: capillary malformation, telangiectasias; *well-developed lesions*: pyogenic granuloma, other vascular tumors (e.g. kaposiform hemangioendothelioma, which can lead to Kasabach–Merritt phenomenon, see Ch. 94 and Fig. 85.15D), venous/lymphatic malformation, and rare entities such as nasal glioma and soft tissue sarcomas (see Table 53.1); *multiple lesions:* glomuvenous malformations, blue rubber bleb nevus syndrome, multifocal lymphangioendotheliomatosis with thrombocytopenia, "blueberry muffin baby" (see Ch. 99).

• When an atypical clinical appearance or natural history leads to consideration of entities in the DDx of an IH, additional evaluation may include ultrasonography, other imaging, and biopsy.

Complications of IHs

• *Ulceration*: occurs in ~10% of lesions, especially those on the lip and in the anogenital region or other skin folds, at a median age of 4 months (Fig. 85.9); whitish discoloration of an IH in an infant <3 months of age may signal impending ulceration; results in pain, a risk of infection (relatively uncommon), and eventual scarring (see Fig. 85.4A,B).

• *Disfigurement and interference with function due to the IH's location and/or large size.*

  – *Periocular IH* – risk of astigmatism if puts pressure on globe, amblyopia if

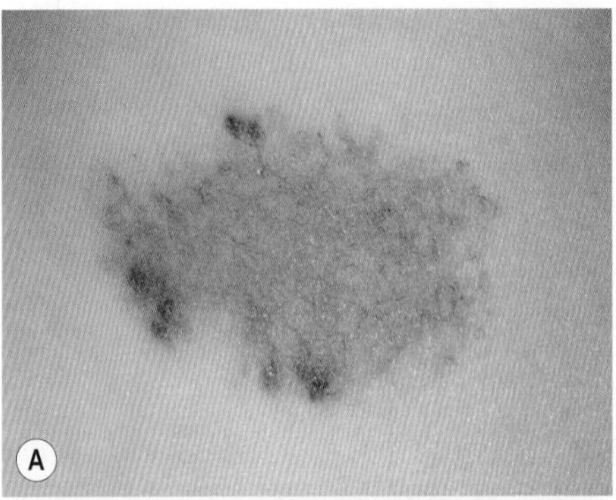

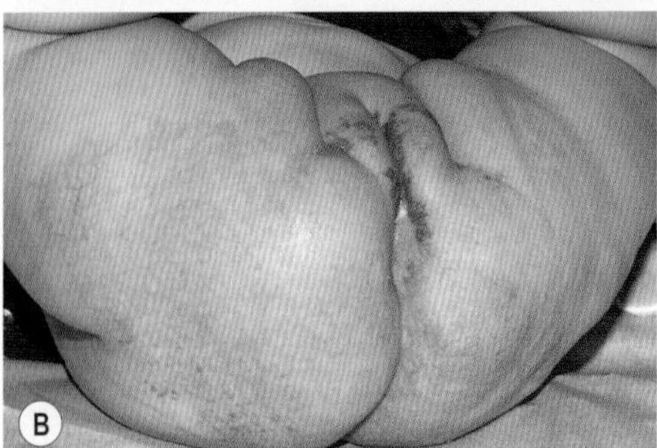

Fig. 85.8 Infantile hemangiomas with minimal or arrested growth (IH-MAG). Focal small bright red papules cover <25% of the surface area and are evident at the periphery (**A**) and on the vulva and upper buttock (**B**). Presence of these papules (which may be subtle or absent), reticulated erythema, and characteristic fine to coarse telangiectasias help to distinguish these lesions from capillary–venous malformations. *Courtesy, Julie V. Schaffer, MD.*

obstructs the visual axis, and strabismus if affects orbital musculature (see Fig. 85.7A,C); requires ophthalmologic evaluation

- *IH on nasal tip, columella, or lip (especially if crosses the vermilion border)* – high risk of distortion of facial structures (as well as ulceration if on the lip) (see Fig. 85.7B)
- *IH on breast* (in girls) – may affect underlying breast bud, so early surgery should be avoided

- *Associated extracutaneous abnormalities.*
  - *IHs in "beard" area of the lower face* – often associated with *airway IHs*, which may present with noisy breathing or biphasic stridor; otolaryngologic evaluation is needed for infants with symptoms or when the IH is likely to be actively proliferating (i.e. <5 months of age) (Fig. 85.10)
  - *Large facial IHs, particularly segmental lesions* – risk of *PHACE(S)* syndrome: *P*, *p*osterior fossa malformations; *H*, *h*emangioma; *A*, *a*rterial abnormalities (cervical, cerebral); *C*, *c*ardiac defects, especially *c*oarctation of the aorta; *E*, *e*ye anomalies; *S*, *s*ternal defects and *s*upraumbilical raphe (Table 85.2; Figs 85.11 and 85.12; see Fig. 85.7A,C)

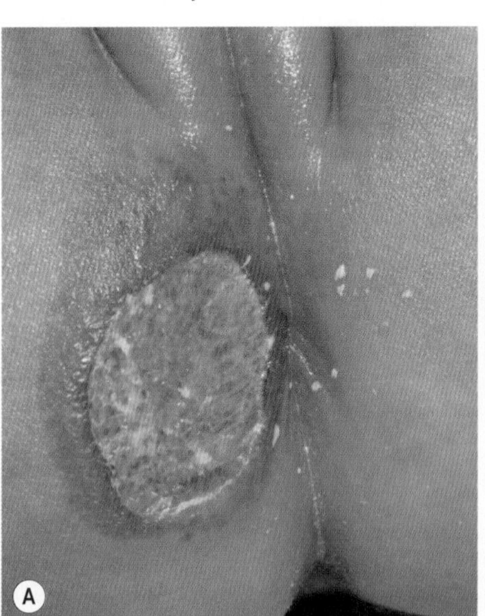

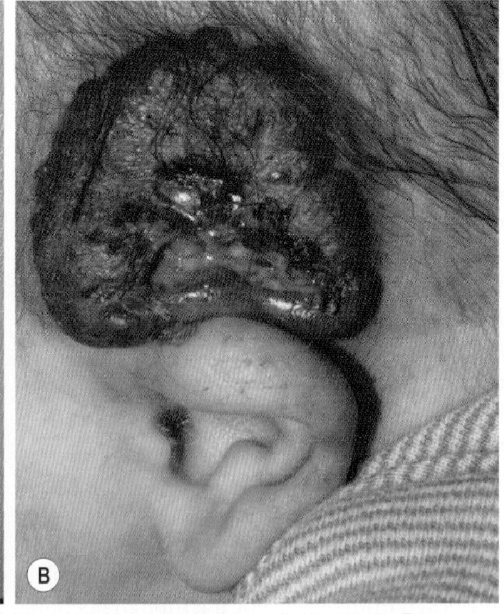

Fig. 85.9 Ulcerated infantile hemangiomas. A Ulcerated hemangioma on the buttock. Because the hemangioma component may not be obvious, this diagnosis should be considered when an infant presents with an ulcer in the diaper area. **B** Ulcerated superficial hemangioma above the ear. Note the distortion of the pinna. *Courtesy, Julie V. Schaffer, MD.*

HEMANGIOMAS IN A "BEARD" DISTRIBUTION

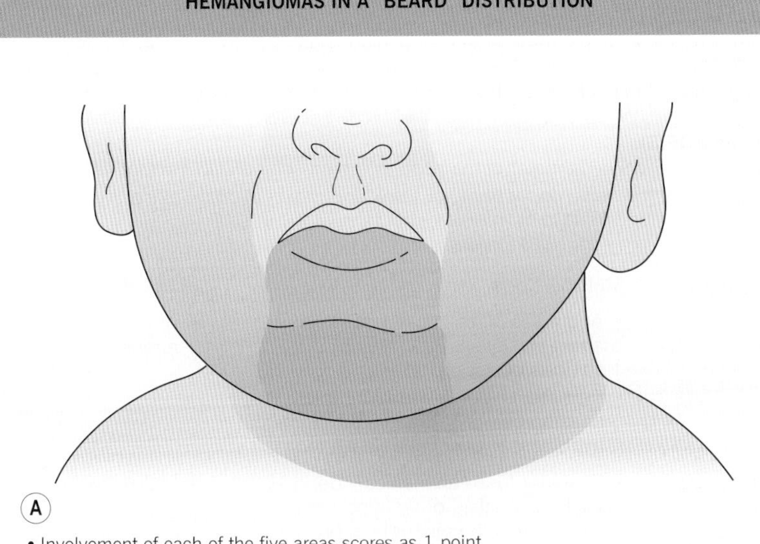

A

- Involvement of each of the five areas scores as 1 point
- In one study of 16 children with a score ≥ 4, 63% had some degree of symptomatic airway involvement

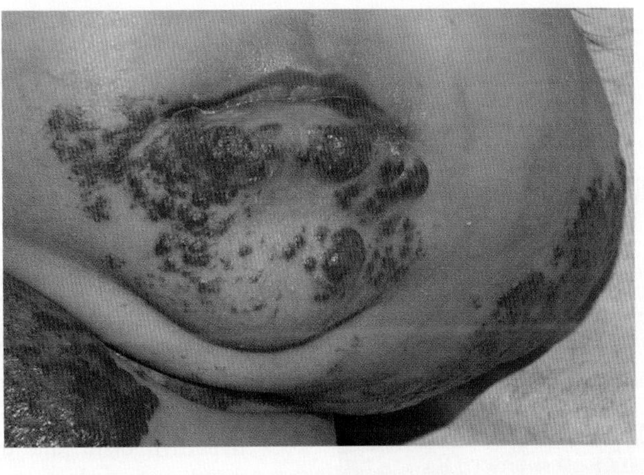

B

Fig. 85.10 Infantile hemangiomas in a "beard" distribution. A Anatomic sites associated with risk of an airway hemangioma. **B** Infant with a laryngeal hemangioma in addition to cutaneous lesions in a "beard" distribution. *A, Adapted with permission from Orlow SJ, Isakoff MS, Blei F. Increased risk of symptomatic hemangiomas of the airway in association with cutaneous hemangiomas in a 'beard' distribution. J Pediatr 1997;131:643–6; B, Courtesy, Julie V. Schaffer, MD.*

- *Large IHs on the lower body, particularly segmental lesions (often IH-MAG)* – risk of *LUMBAR* syndrome: *L*, *l*ower body/*l*umbosacral IH and *l*ipomas; *U*, *u*rogenital anomalies and *u*lceration; *M*, *m*yelopathy (spinal dysraphism); *B*, *b*ony deformities; *A*, *a*norectal and *a*rterial anomalies; *R*, *r*enal anomalies (Fig. 85.13; see Figs 85.7D and 85.12)
- *Midline lumbosacral IHs* – risk of *spinal dysraphism* (see Ch. 53)
- *Multifocal IHs (≥5)* – may be associated with *extracutaneous hemangiomas*, most often hepatic; the cutaneous IHs are usually relatively small and superficial, but hepatic involvement can be associated with complications such as high-output cardiac failure and

DIAGNOSTIC CRITERIA FOR PHACE(S) SYNDROME		
Definite PHACE(S): • Hemangioma >5 cm in diameter of the head including scalp PLUS 1 major criterion or 2 minor criteria • Hemangioma of the neck, upper trunk, or trunk and proximal upper extremity PLUS 2 major criteria **Possible PHACE(S):** • Hemangioma >5 cm in diameter of the head including scalp PLUS 1 minor criterion • Hemangioma of the neck, upper trunk, or trunk and proximal upper extremity PLUS 1 major criterion or 2 minor criteria • No hemangioma PLUS 2 major criteria		
Organ system	**Major criteria**	**Minor criteria**
Arterial	• Anomalies of major cerebral or cervical arteries* – dysplasia**, hypoplasia, stenosis/occlusion, aberrant origin/course • Persistent carotid–vertebrobasilar anastomosis (e.g. proatlantal segmental, hypoglossal, otic, trigeminal arteries)	• Aneurysm of cerebral arteries
Structural brain	• Posterior fossa anomalies – Dandy–Walker complex, other hypoplasia/dysplasia of the mid or hind brain	• Midline anomalies • Malformation of cortical development
Cardiovascular	• Aortic arch anomalies • Aberrant origin of subclavian artery ± vascular ring	• Ventricular septal defect • Right/double aortic arch • Systemic venous anomalies
Ocular	• Posterior segment anomalies – persistent hyperplastic primary vitreous/persistent fetal vasculature, retinal vascular anomalies, optic nerve hypoplasia, morning glory disc anomaly	• Anterior segment anomalies, e.g. sclerocornea, cataract, coloboma, microphthalmia
Ventral or midline	• Sternal defect/pit/cleft • Supraumbilical raphe	• Hypopituitarism • Ectopic thyroid • Midline sternal papule/hamartoma

**Includes internal carotid artery; middle, anterior, or posterior cerebral artery; and vertebrobasilar system.*
***Includes kinking, looping, tortuosity, and/or dolichoectasia.*

Table 85.2 Diagnostic criteria for PHACE(S) syndrome.

REASONS TO CONSIDER SYSTEMIC THERAPY FOR INFANTILE HEMANGIOMAS
Threatened vital functions
• Vision • Airway
Potential for disfigurement
• Nasal tip or columella • Lip, especially if crosses the vermilion border • Large or rapidly growing lesion, especially if on the face
Severe/recalcitrant ulceration
High-output cardiac failure

Table 85.3 Reasons to consider systemic therapy for infantile hemangiomas.

hypothyroidism (due to iodothyronine deiodinase production by the IH) (Fig. 85.14; see Fig. 85.12)

Treatment of IHs

• "Active non-intervention," including education of parents and observation with periodic photography, is sufficient for most small IHs expected to have a good cosmetic outcome.

• Patients with a potentially problematic IH should be referred for systemic therapy by 4–6 weeks of age.

• **Local Rx:** topical timolol, e.g. one drop (0.25 mg) of 0.5% gel-forming ophthalmic solution applied BID (systemic absorption

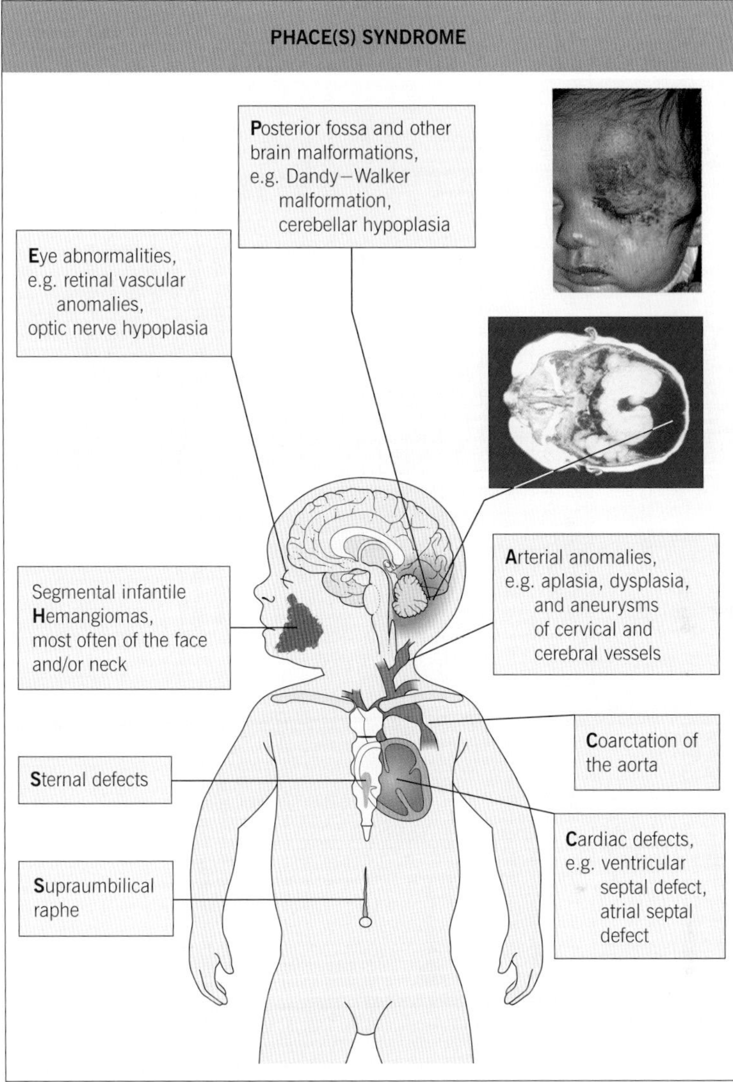

Fig. 85.11 PHACE(S) syndrome. Major clinical features are illustrated. Additional possible associated features include hearing impairment and endocrine abnormalities such as hypothyroidism.

possible, especially if ulcerated or involving mucous membranes; limit to <0.25 mg/kg/day), or superpotent CS for thin superficial lesions; intralesional CS for thicker lesions (avoiding the periocular area); pulsed dye laser for residual telangiectasias and possibly for thin superficial lesions.

- **Systemic Rx:** indications are listed in Table 85.3; oral propranolol (Table 85.4) has replaced prednisolone as the first-line systemic therapy.
- Management of an ulcerated IH includes wound care (e.g. hydrocolloid dressings), pain management, monitoring for infection, and specific therapies directed at the ulcer (e.g. pulsed-dye laser) or IH (e.g. β-blockers; faster healing with propranolol dose ≤1 mg/kg/d).
- Surgical excision is useful to remove fibrofatty tissue and redundant skin in involuted or partially involuted IHs; often done in preschool-aged children with cosmetically significant lesions (e.g. on the lip), and earlier resection may be considered when eventual surgery is inevitable (e.g. for some pedunculated lesions).

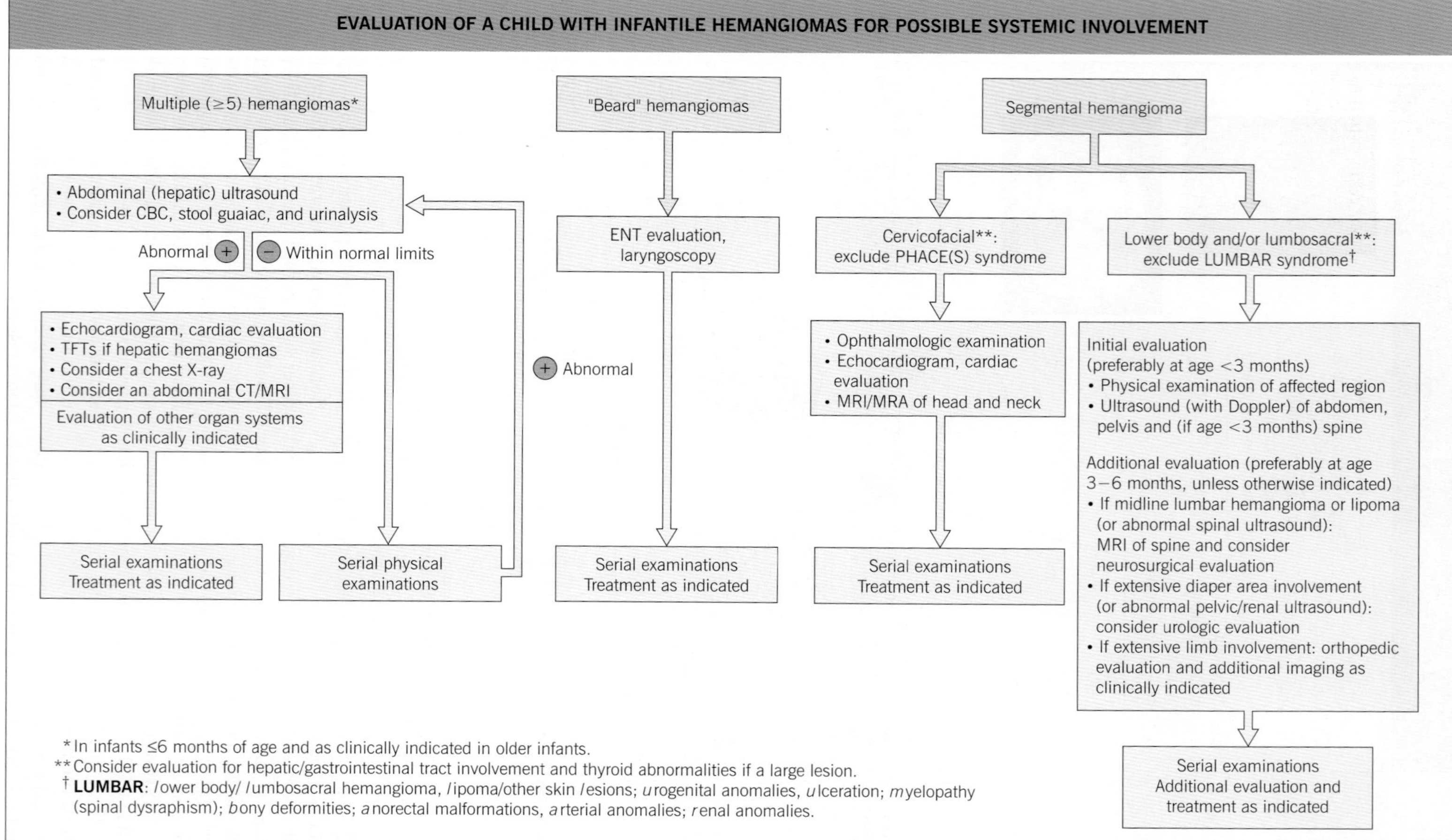

Fig. 85.12 Evaluation of a child with infantile hemangiomas for

ADMINISTRATION OF PROPRANOLOL FOR INFANTILE HEMANGIOMAS (IHS): PRETREATMENT EVALUATION, DOSING, AND MONITORING
Pretreatment evaluation
• *If history of bronchospasm/reactive airway disease* (a relative contraindication to propranolol therapy): consult with a pulmonologist or consider alternate therapy • *If at risk for PHACE(S) syndrome**: MRI/MRA of head/neck and echocardiogram to exclude arterial and cardiovascular anomalies (see Fig. 85.12); if abnormal, consult with a neuroradiologist, neurologist, and/or cardiologist as indicated • Cardiac examination, heart rate, and manual blood pressure; also consider an electrocardiogram (ECG); bradycardia (<80 beats per minute), greater than first degree heart block, blood pressure <50/30 mmHg, and decompensated heart failure are considered to be contraindications
Dosing and course
• Initial: usually ~1 mg/kg/day divided into 2 (or 3) doses** • Goal: 2–3 mg/kg/day divided into 2 (or 3) doses**; the target dose for the FDA-approved formulation (Hemangeol™) is as high as 3.4 mg/kg/day, whereas doses ≤1 mg/kg/day may lead to shorter healing times for ulcerated hemangiomas • For a proliferating IH, treatment is typically continued for 6–12 months, depending on the clinical setting and course¶   – The dose should be adjusted to account for weight gain and maintain the goal dose/kg, especially during the proliferative phase • Taper over 2–4+ weeks before discontinuing, primarily to assess for rebound growth
Monitoring

• Risks of propranolol include bradycardia, hypotension, hypoglycemia, sleep disturbances, and bronchospasm
• Consider a brief inpatient stay (e.g. 1–2 days) with telemetry for initiation of treatment if <5 weeks of age (using corrected age for premature infants) and/or complications such as cardiovascular or cerebrovascular anomalies
• Outpatient initiation of therapy
  – Monitor heart rate and blood pressure for 2 hours after the initial dose or a significant dose increase
  – Measure heart rate and blood pressure every 4–8 weeks while on a stable dose
  – Normal ranges for pediatric vital signs are available at: www.emedicinehealth.com/pediatric_vital_signs/article_em.htm
• Educate parents about signs of hypoglycemia – *early* (may be masked by β-blockade): sweating, rapid heart rate, shakiness, fussiness; *late*: lethargy, poor feeding, hypothermia, seizures
• Administer during or immediately after a feeding; twice daily doses should be ≥9 hours apart
  – Dose should be lowered or therapy suspended during intercurrent illnesses with decreased oral intake or vomiting

**Segmental hemangioma ≥5 cm in diameter on the head or upper body (see Table 85.2).*
***The dose is typically increased in increments of 1 mg/kg/day weekly in an outpatient setting or after 1–3 doses in an inpatient setting, until reaching the goal dose. A lower starting dose and slower escalation may be required for patients at higher risk of complications or when treatment is initiated without in-office monitoring (e.g. starting with 0.5 mg/kg/d and increasing by 0.5 mg/kg/d every 3-4 days). The FDA-approved Hemangeol™ 4.28 mg/ml solution has a dosing chart in the package insert; the concentration differs slightly from generic propranolol 20 mg/5 ml (4 mg/ml) solution.*
¶A longer duration of treatment may be required for IHs with prolonged growth or rebound growth after reduction/discontinuation of propranolol.

Table 85.4 Administration of propranolol for infantile hemangiomas (IHs): pretreatment evaluation, dosing, and monitoring. Propranolol, a nonselective β-blocker, binds to β_2-adrenergic receptors on hemangioma endothelial cells, with effects including vasoconstriction (leading to softening and dulling of color within 24 hours), decreased expression of pro-angiogenic growth factors, and induction of apoptosis. Practices vary, and the patient's age, hemangioma-related issues, and medical comorbidities also affect management.

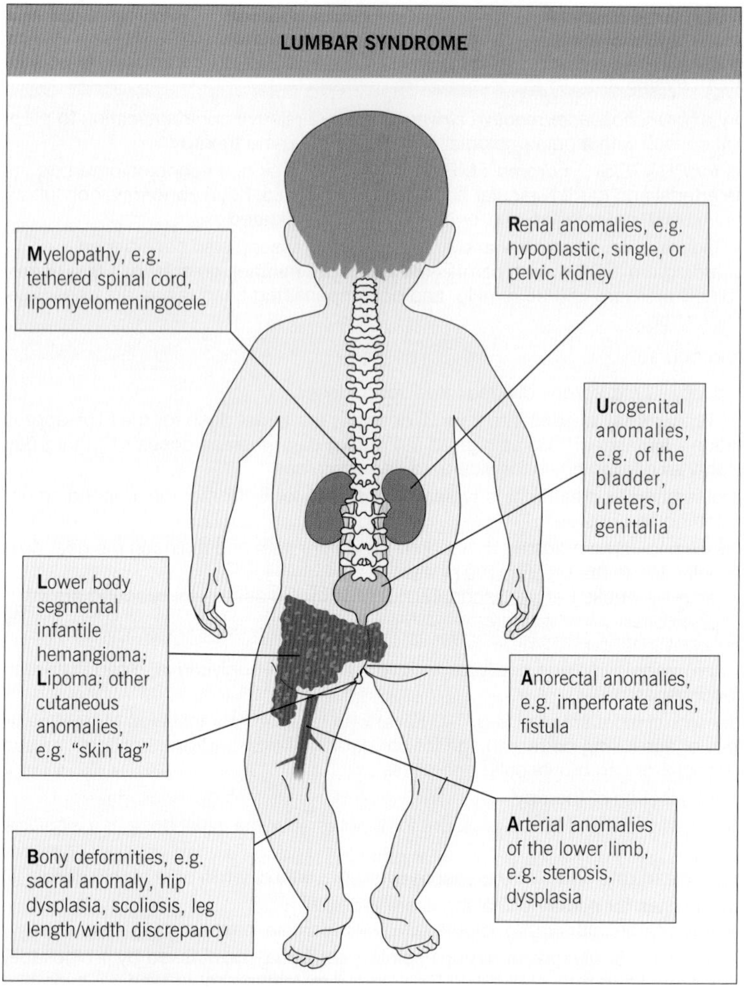

LUMBAR SYNDROME

Myelopathy, e.g. tethered spinal cord, lipomyelomeningocele

Renal anomalies, e.g. hypoplastic, single, or pelvic kidney

Urogenital anomalies, e.g. of the bladder, ureters, or genitalia

Lower body segmental infantile hemangioma; **L**ipoma; other cutaneous anomalies, e.g. "skin tag"

Anorectal anomalies, e.g. imperforate anus, fistula

Arterial anomalies of the lower limb, e.g. stenosis, dysplasia

Bony deformities, e.g. sacral anomaly, hip dysplasia, scoliosis, leg length/width discrepancy

Fig. 85.13 LUMBAR syndrome. Major clinical features are illustrated. The segmental hemangioma is often ulcerated.

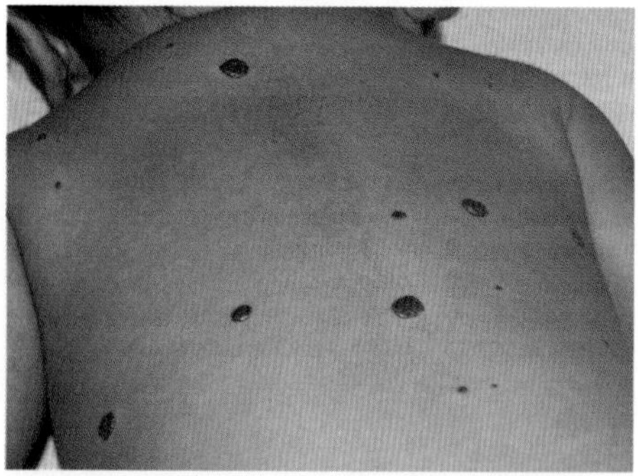

Fig. 85.14 Multifocal infantile hemangiomas with extracutaneous hemangiomas. This infant had many small, superficial skin lesions in a miliary pattern plus hemangiomas in the liver. Historically, this was referred to as "diffuse neonatal hemangiomatosis." *Courtesy, Julie V. Schaffer, MD.*

Hemangioma Variants

- *Congenital hemangiomas* are fully developed at birth, typically presenting as a warm, pink to blue-violet mass or plaque with overlying coarse telangiectasias, surrounded by a vasoconstricted rim and/or radiating veins; unlike IHs, congenital hemangiomas are GLUT1-negative and often have an underlying somatic mutation in *GNAQ* or *GNA11* that activates G protein α-subunits.
  - *Rapidly involuting congenital hemangioma (RICH)* – rapid involution during the first year of life (Fig. 85.15A,B)
  - *Partially involuting congenital hemangioma (PICH)* – incomplete involution early in life

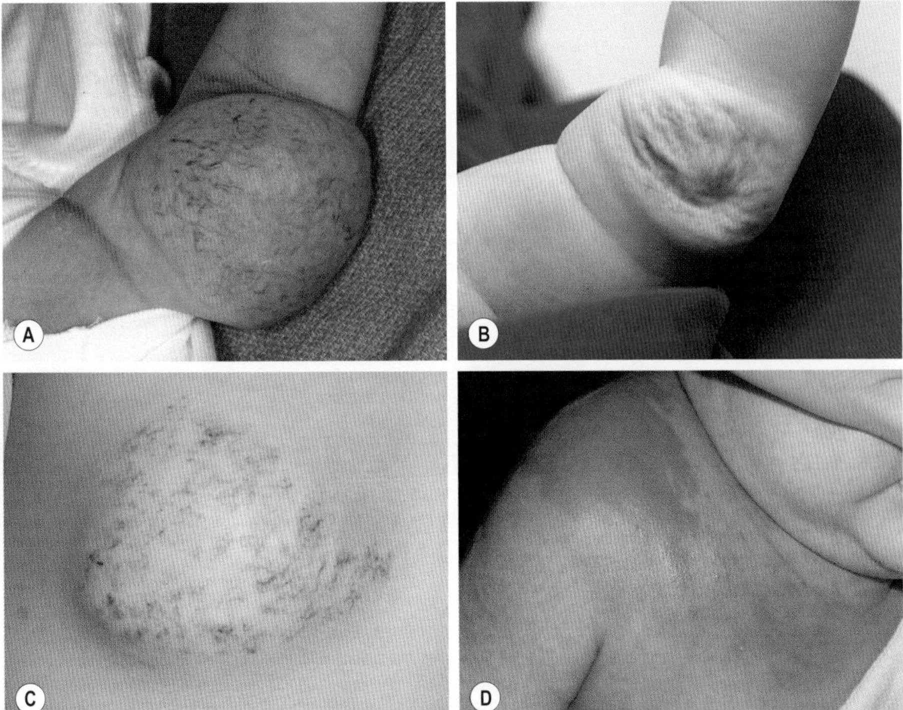

Fig. 85.15 Congenital hemangiomas and other vascular tumors. A Rapidly involuting congenital hemangioma (RICH) presenting as a violaceous tumor on the upper extremity with surface telangiectasias in a neonate. **B** Spontaneous involution of the RICH at 5 months of age, with fibrofatty residua. **C** Non-involuting congenital hemangioma (NICH) in a school-aged child. This lesion was fully formed at birth and is still warm and firm to palpation. Note the coarse telangiectasias and pallor. **D** Kaposiform hemangioendothelioma associated with Kasabach–Merritt phenomenon in a 5-week-old boy. Progressive induration and ecchymosis developed rapidly over a 24-hour period. An eczematous eruption is also evident. *A, B, Courtesy, Annette Wagner, MD; C, D, Courtesy, Julie V. Schaffer, MD.*

  - *Non-involuting congenital hemangioma (NICH)* – postnatal growth in proportion to the child, without involution (Fig. 85.15C); tardive expansion occasionally occurs during childhood

Vascular Malformations

- Categorized based on the predominant type(s) of vascular channels, which are divided into slow- and fast-flow groups:
  - *Slow-flow*: capillary (port-wine stain), venous, microcystic lymphatic ("lymphangioma"), and macrocystic lymphatic ("cystic hygroma")
  - *Fast-flow*: arteriovenous (arterial anomalies + arteriovenous shunting)
- Vascular malformations may contain only one type of vessel or an arteriovenous malformation (*simple*) or ≥2 types of vessels (*combined*; e.g. capillary–lymphatic–venous malformation).
- Although they can affect any organ, vascular malformations are most easily identified in the skin and mucous membranes, where they may extend into deeper structures or be associated with other extracutaneous abnormalities.

Capillary Malformations (CMs) and Related Conditions

NEVUS SIMPLEX (SALMON PATCH)

- Common congenital capillary stain (*not* a true CM) on the mid face (forehead, glabella, nasal tip, and philtrum), eyelids, occiput, and nape ("stork bite") (Fig. 85.16A,B); multiple lesions may be present (*nevus simplex complex*) and can occur in the lumbar area.
- Facial lesions often fade by early childhood.

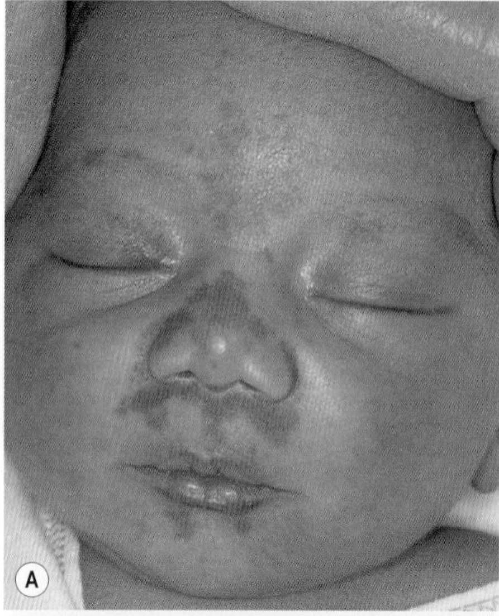

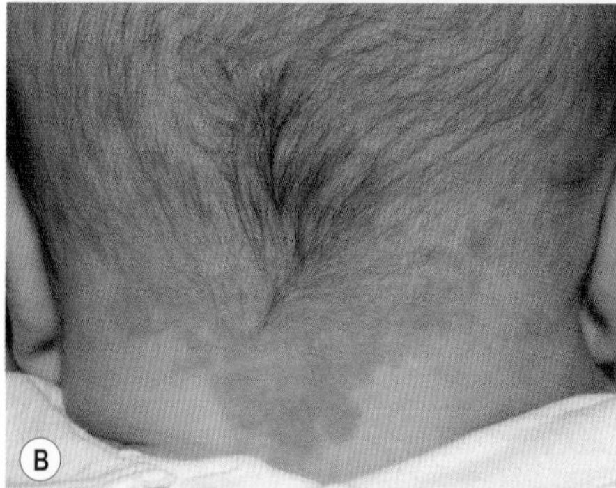

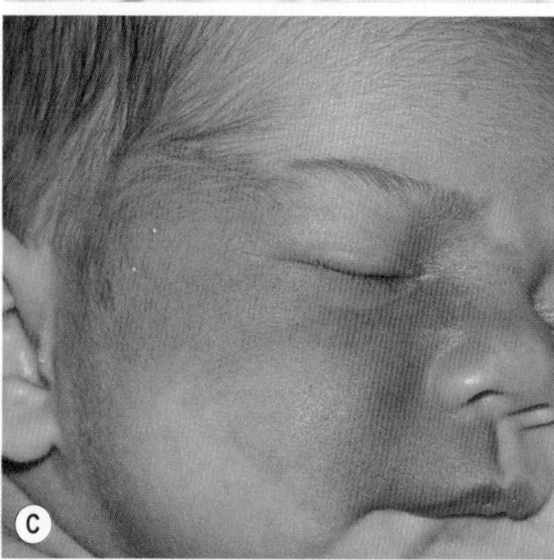

Fig. 85.16 Nevus simplex versus port-wine stain (PWS). **A** Involvement of the central face in a symmetric pattern is common with a nevus simplex (salmon patch); such lesions fade over the first few years of life but are sometimes misdiagnosed as a PWS. **B** Nevus simplex in the nape area ("stork bites") tends to be more persistent. **C** In this young infant with a PWS in the maxillary region, the affected skin is smooth. This lesion will persist. *A, Courtesy, YDRSC; B, C, Courtesy, Julie V. Schaffer, MD.*

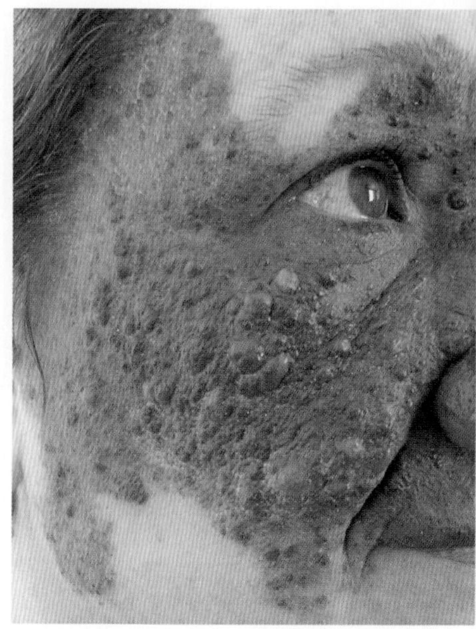

Fig. 85.17 Facial port-wine stains in the maxillary region with hypertrophic changes in an adult. Note the prominent skin thickening and nodularity. *Courtesy, Pablo Boixeda, MD.*

PORT-WINE STAIN (PWS)

- Mosaic activating mutations in the *GNAQ* gene, which encodes a G protein α-subunit, underlie both nonsyndromic PWSs and Sturge–Weber syndrome.
- PWSs present at birth as pinkish-red macules and patches, often in a segmental pattern (Fig. 85.16C).
- Over time, may develop a deeper purplish-red color, and affected skin (especially on the face) often thickens and becomes nodular; overgrowth of underlying soft tissues and bones can also occur (Figs 85.17 and 85.18).
- **DDx:** *in infant*: nevus simplex, early or arrested-growth IH; CMTC (especially if on an extremity), stage 1 arteriovenous malformation, *verrucous venocapillary malformation* ("verrucous hemangioma"; congenital red-purple hyperkeratotic plaques, often in a segmental pattern favoring the extremities, with growth proportional to the child).
- **Rx:** pulsed dye laser therapy, preferably initiated during infancy for facial lesions to avoid psychosocial distress and lesional thickening.
- *Sturge–Weber syndrome:* ocular and/or leptomeningeal vascular malformations may accompany a facial PWS involving the "forehead area," which also includes the upper

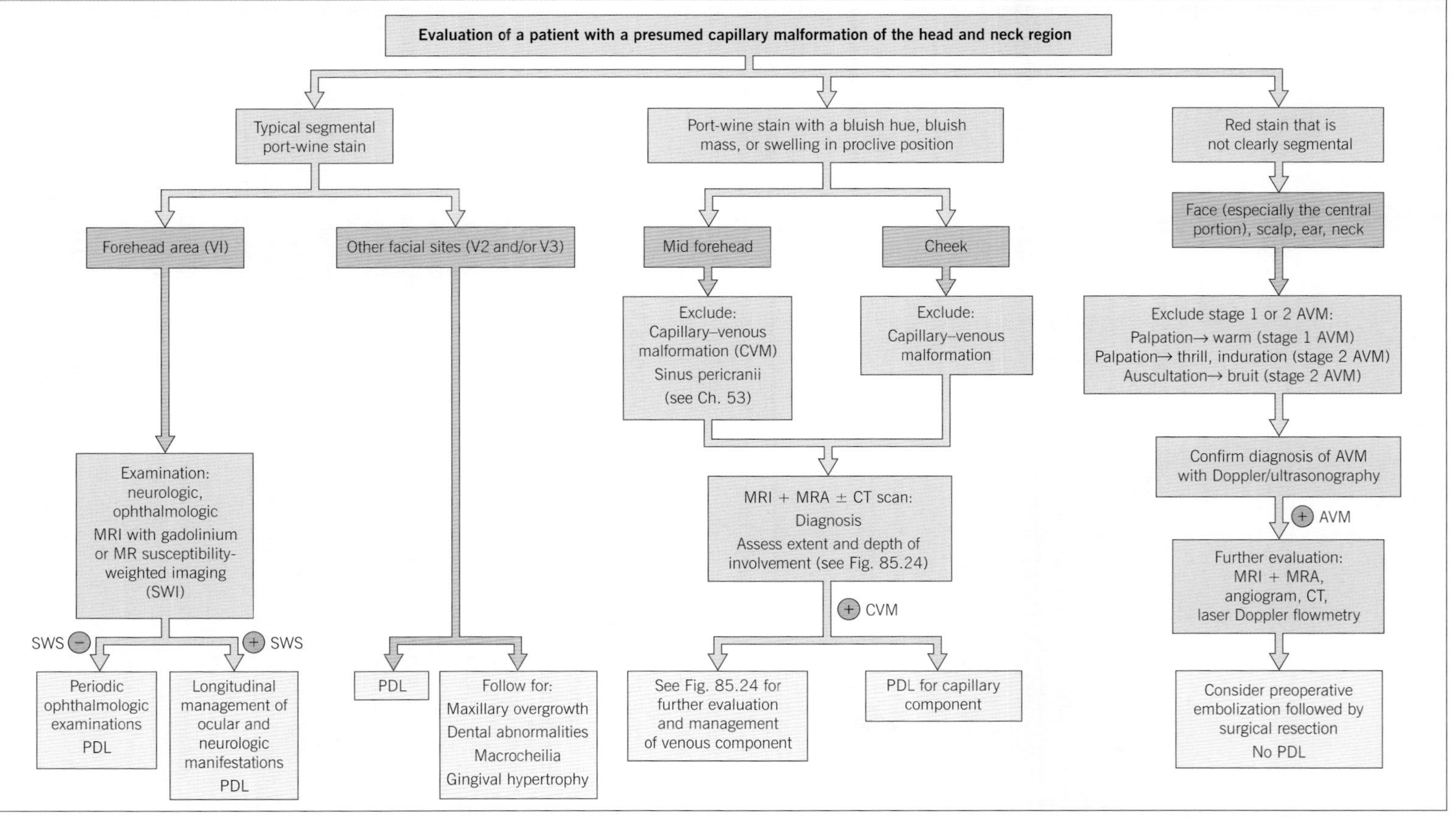

Fig. 85.18 Evaluation of a patient with a presumed capillary malformation of the head and neck region. AVM, arteriovenous malformation; CVM, capillary venous malformation; PDL, pulsed dye laser; PET, positron emission tomography; SPECT, single photon emission computed tomography; SWS, Sturge–Weber syndrome.

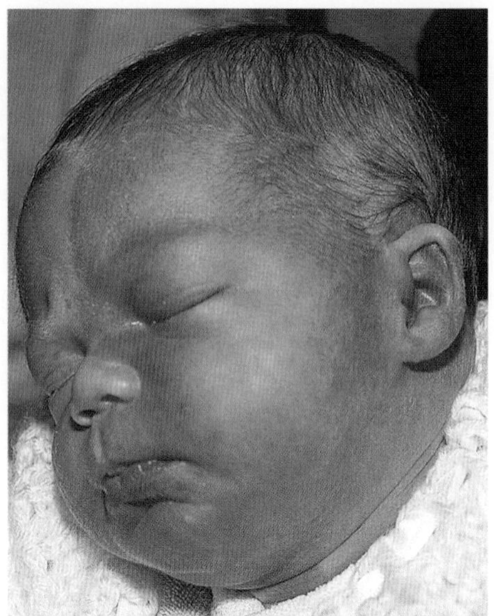

Fig. 85.19 Infant at risk for Sturge–Weber syndrome (SWS). The port-wine stain covers most of the left side of the face, with involvement of the "forehead area" conferring risk of SWS. *Courtesy, Odile Enjolras, MD.*

eyelid and is delineated inferiorly by a line drawn from the outer canthus to the top of the ear; this area encompasses most of the trigeminal V1 and small portions of the V2/V3 dermatomes (Fig. 85.19). Affected individuals can develop glaucoma and neurologic sequelae such as developmental delay and contralateral seizures or hemiparesis. Neuroimaging (e.g. susceptibility-weighted MRI) can reliably exclude leptomeningeal involvement by 1 year of age, and prophylactic aspirin administration may reduce the likelihood of neurologic symptoms in SWS patients.

- *Phakomatosis pigmentovascularis (PPV)*: PWS coexisting with aberrant Mongolian spots (dermal melanocytosis; both caused by mosaic *GNAQ/11* mutations) (Fig. 85.20) or a nevus spilus; a nevus anemicus may also be present.
- *Diffuse capillary malformation with overgrowth*: widespread reticulated CM associated with soft tissue hypertrophy that does not necessarily correlate with the CM location and is not progressive (Fig. 85.21A); may be due to a *GNA11* mutation.
- *Megalencephaly–capillary malformation* (previously *macrocephaly–CMTC*): reticulated PWS and persistent nevus simplex associated with asymmetric overgrowth, macrocephaly, and developmental delay; due to mosaic *PIK3CA* mutations (Fig. 85.21B).

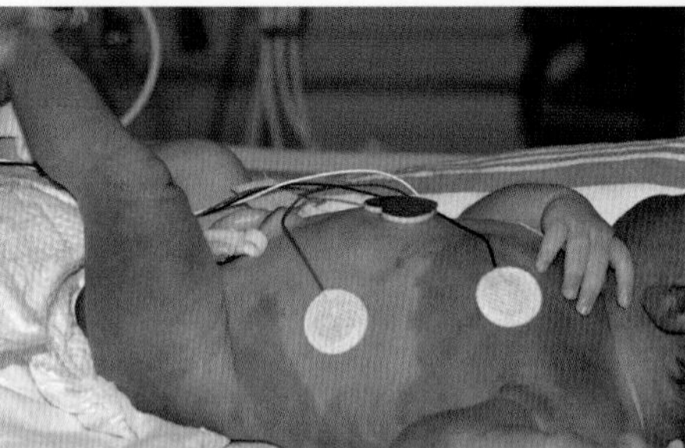

Fig. 85.20 Phakomatosis pigmentovascularis type 2. A large port-wine stain and extensive dermal melanocytosis are seen. *Courtesy, Julie V. Schaffer, MD.*

CUTIS MARMORATA TELANGIECTATICA CONGENITA (CMTC)

- Red-purple, broad reticulated vascular pattern intermingled with telangiectasias, ± prominent veins and atrophy; most often affects a limb, which may be hypoplastic; occasionally generalized (Fig. 85.22).
- *Adams–Oliver syndrome* features CMTC together with aplasia cutis congenita and limb defects (see Table 53.3).

Venous Malformations (VMs; Former Misnomer of "Cavernous Hemangioma")

CLASSIC VMs

- Soft, compressible bluish nodules that fill with dependency; may be focal, segmental, or widespread, and often extend into underlying muscles and bones (Fig. 85.23).
- Both *multiple cutaneous and mucosal VMs* with autosomal dominant inheritance and sporadic VMs can result from mutations in the *TEK* gene, which encodes an endothelial cell-specific tyrosine kinase, or *PIK3CA*.
- *Blue rubber bleb nevus (Bean) syndrome* also presents with multiple cutaneous and mucosal (e.g. GI) VMs.
- An approach to the evaluation and management of VMs at different sites is presented in Fig. 85.24.

GLOMUVENOUS MALFORMATIONS (GVMs; PREVIOUSLY KNOWN AS GLOMANGIOMATOSIS)

- Pink to blue-purple nodules and cobblestoned plaques that resist full compression

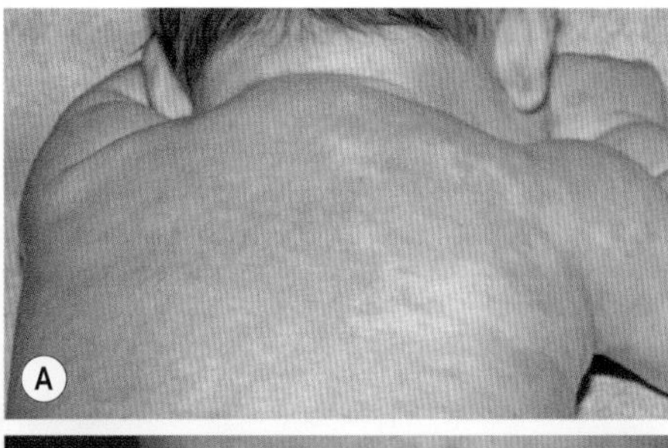

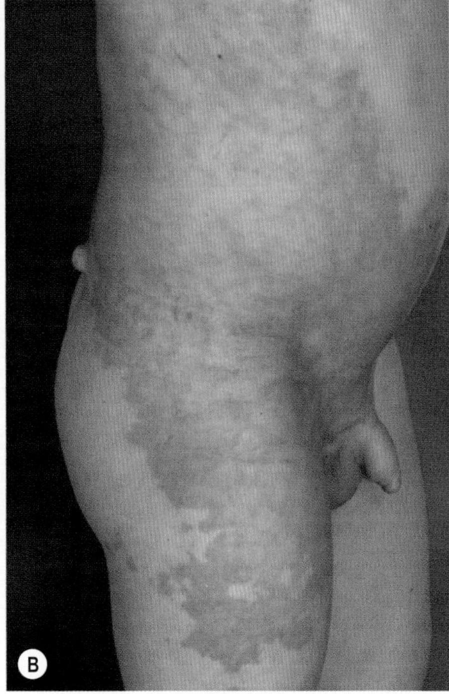

Fig. 85.21 Reticulated capillary malformations. A Diffuse capillary malformation with overgrowth. This normocephalic infant has an extensive reticulated capillary malformation involving the trunk, one arm, and both legs. **B** Megalencephaly–capillary malformation syndrome. This boy has hemihypertrophy of the side of the body *opposite* to the PWS. *Courtesy, Julie V. Schaffer, MD.*

and are painful upon palpation; may be focal, segmental, or widespread and (unlike classic VMs) are typically limited to the skin and subcutis (Fig. 85.25).

• Autosomal dominant inheritance due to mutations in the glomulin gene (*GLMN*).

MAFFUCCI SYNDROME

• Association of VMs with enchondromas, most often of the extremities; skin lesions may also have features of a spindle cell hemangioma.

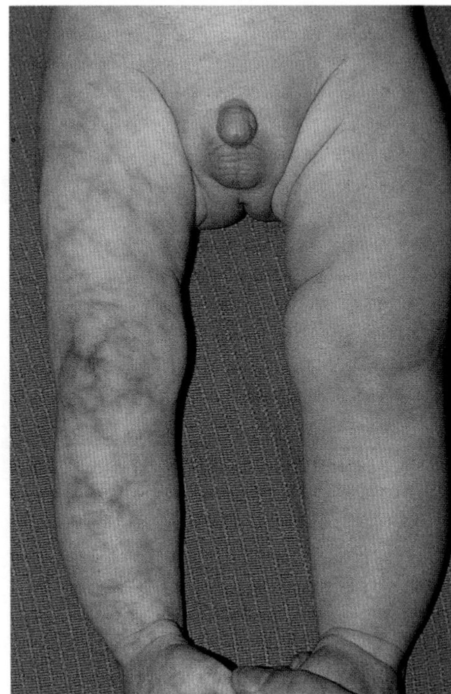

Fig. 85.22 Cutis marmorata telangiectatica congenita (CMTC) with atrophy of the affected limb. The color of the broad vascular network can be red-purple (as in this infant) to brownish-purple. *Courtesy, YDRSC.*

Lymphatic Anomalies

• *Lymphatic malformations (LMs)* are due to excessive aberrant lymphatic channels, often due to an underlying mosaic *PIK3CA* mutation, whereas *lymphedema* results from hypoplasia or disruption of the lymphatics.

LYMPHATIC MALFORMATIONS

• *Microcystic LM ("lymphangioma circumscriptum")*: clusters of clear or hemorrhagic, vesicle-like papules favoring the proximal limbs and chest; intermittent hemorrhage and leakage of lymph can occur (Fig. 85.26A–D). A subset of superficial LM presents as red-purple, geographic patches with a finely reticulated, net-like pattern of vascular structures.

• *Macrocystic LM ("cystic hygroma")*: ballotable subcutaneous masses representing

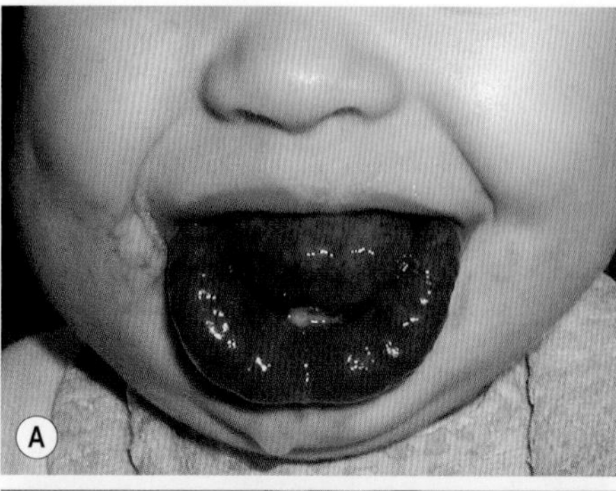

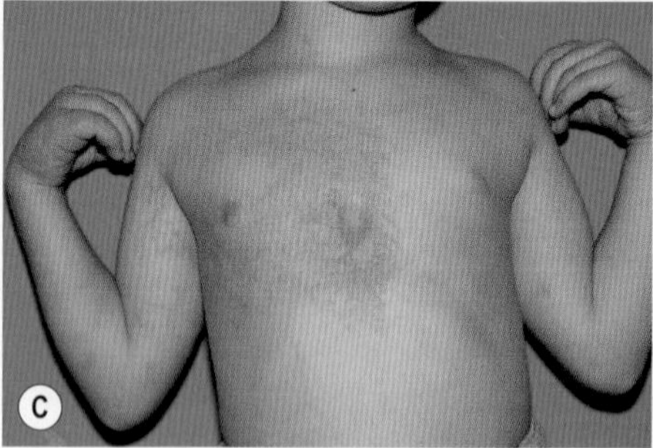

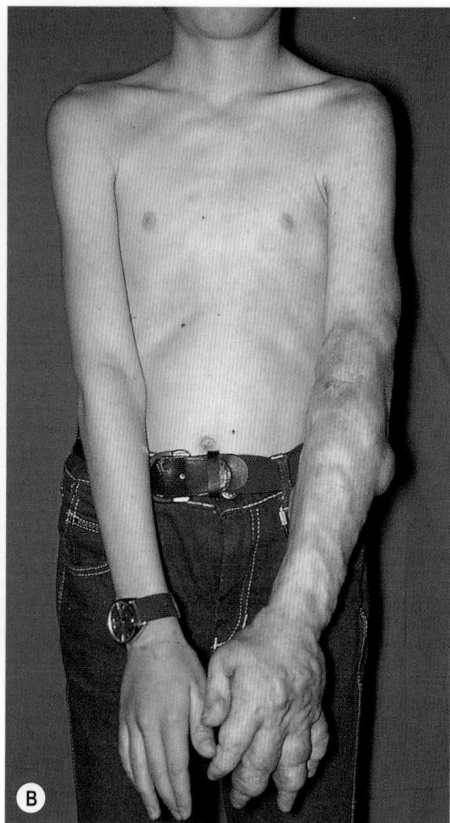

Fig. 85.23 Venous malformations (VMs). A Distortion of the tongue and lower lip has led to an open bite. **B** The skin and muscles of the entire arm are affected, with soft bluish nodules and obvious swelling in the dependent position. **C** This VM has a segmental distribution on the right trunk and involvement of the ipsilateral arm. *Courtesy, Odile Enjolras, MD.*

larger lymphatic cysts; favor the neck, axilla, and lateral chest wall (Fig. 85.26E).

• Cellulitis-like inflammatory reactions can be triggered by trauma or infection and may result in expansion and worsening over time.

• Cervicofacial lesions often distort underlying bony structures, and oropharyngeal involvement can lead to airway compromise; rare complications include visceral "lymphangiomatosis" and massive osteolysis (*Gorham–Stout [disappearing bone] disease*).

• **DDx:** acquired cutaneous lymphangiectasia (e.g. due to Crohn disease, recurrent cellulitis, or intralymphatic metastases).

• Radiologic evaluation: ultrasonography, MRI with gadolinium (lack enhancement).

• **Rx:** topical or oral sirolimus, sclerotherapy, laser therapy (for microcystic lesions), surgical excision (but recurrences are common).

PRIMARY LYMPHEDEMA

• Most often affects the extremities (lower > upper), with occasional genital, cephalic, or generalized involvement; may be associated with pulmonary or GI lymphangiectasia.

• *Congenital lymphedema* is present at birth or develops during infancy; etiologies include *Milroy disease* (mutations in the gene encoding vascular endothelial growth factor receptor 3) and *Turner* and *Noonan syndromes.*

• *Lymphedema praecox* presents around puberty; etiologies include *Meige disease* and *lymphedema–distichiasis syndrome.*

• Secondary lymphedema is discussed in Chapter 86.

Arteriovenous Malformations (AVMs)

• Fast-flow malformations with potential for serious complications (e.g. amputation, deformity); frequently due to a mosaic mutation

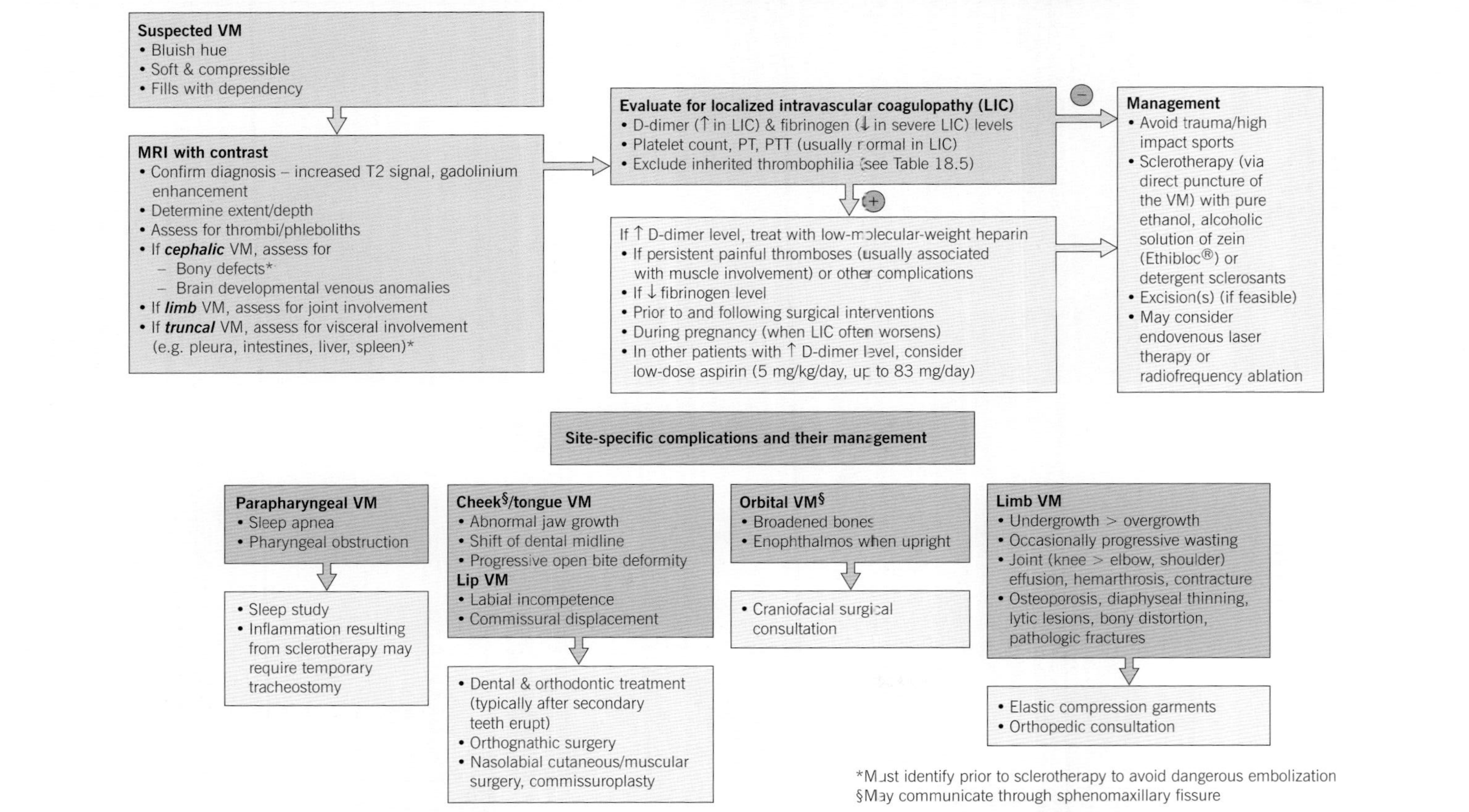

Fig. 85.24 An approach to the evaluation and management of venous malformations (VMs).

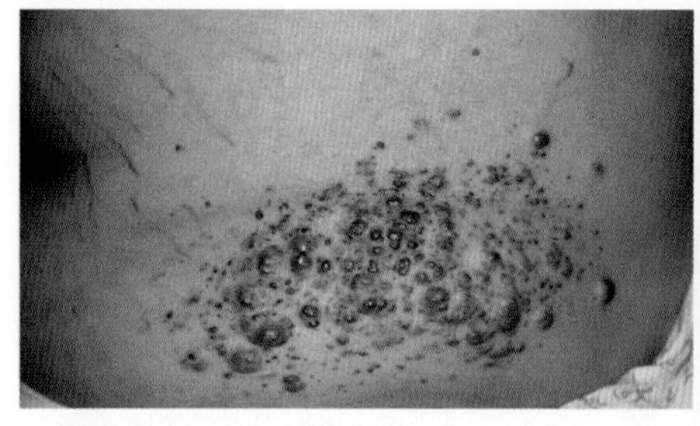

Fig. 85.25 Segmental glomuvenous malformation on the abdomen. Coalescing blue-purple papulonodules. *Courtesy, Paula North, MD.*

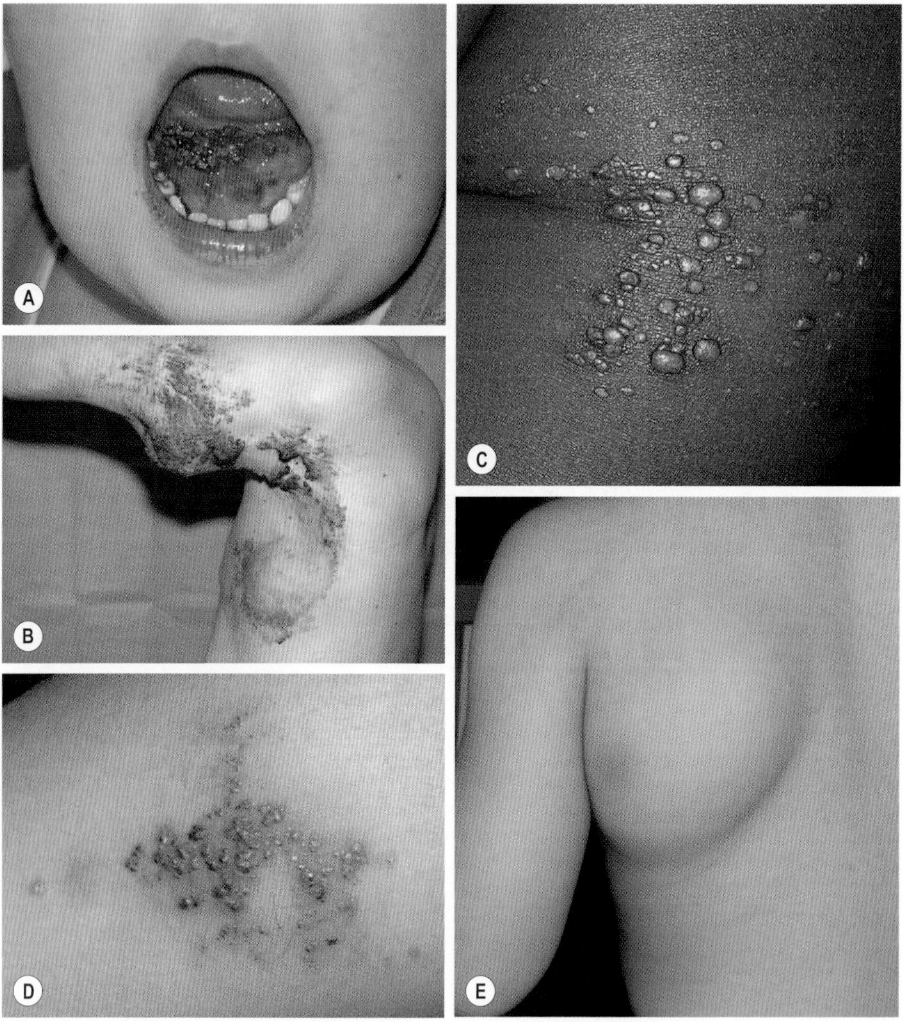

Fig. 85.26 Lymphatic malformations (LMs). A–D Microcystic LMs presenting as clusters of clear or hemorrhagic vesicles, with active bleeding from lesions in the mouth **(A)**. The crops of vesicles in **(B)** recurred years after surgical resection (utilizing grafting and linear closure) of a large microcystic LM affecting the skin and deeper structures of the arm and thorax. **E** Macrocystic LM on the lateral trunk. The mass was soft except for a focal firm area of hemorrhage associated with bruise-like discoloration of the overlying skin. *A, B, Courtesy, Odile Enjolras, MD; C, Courtesy, YDRSC; D, E, Courtesy, Julie V. Schaffer, MD.*

affecting the mitogen-activated protein kinase (MAPK) pathway (e.g. *KRAS, MAP2K1*).

- Often involve the cephalic region, especially the central face, with approximately half of lesions evident at birth; may worsen with puberty, pregnancy, trauma, partial excision, or proximal embolization.
- Divided into four stages based on clinical severity:
  - *Stage 1 – dormant*: red, warm and macular (mimicking a PWS) or slightly infiltrated (Fig. 85.27A,B)
  - *Stage 2 – expansion*: warm mass with thrill/throbbing and dilated draining veins
  - *Stage 3 – destruction*: pain, necrosis, and ulceration; ± lytic bone lesions (Fig. 85.27C)
  - *Stage 4 – cardiac decompensation*: high-output cardiac failure
- Radiologic evaluation: ultrasonography, MRI/MRA, arteriography.
- **Rx:** complete excision after judicious preoperative embolization.
- *Acroangiodermatitis* (pseudo-Kaposi sarcoma; see Ch. 86) can occur in association with a lower extremity AVM.
- *Metameric AVMs*.
  - *Cobb syndrome*: cutaneous (may mimic a CM or angiokeratomas) in dermatomal distribution + intraspinal/vertebral
  - *Bonnet–Dechaume–Blanc (Wyburn–Mason) syndrome*: cutaneous facial + orbit/eye and/or brain

PIK3CA-Related Overgrowth Spectrum and Other Syndromes Associated with Combined Vascular Malformations

- *Klippel–Trenaunay syndrome*: CM + VM ± LM due to a mosaic *PIK3CA* mutation, associated with progressive overgrowth of the affected extremity; well-demarcated geographic stains usually have a lymphatic component, which increases the likelihood of massive overgrowth and cellulitis; risk of deep venous thrombosis/pulmonary embolism (Fig. 85.28).
- *Proteus syndrome* (see Table 51.3): mosaic disorder due to *AKT1* mutations; can feature CM, VM, and/or LM.
- *CLOVES syndrome: c*ongenital *l*ipomatous *o*vergrowth, *v*ascular malformations (slow- or

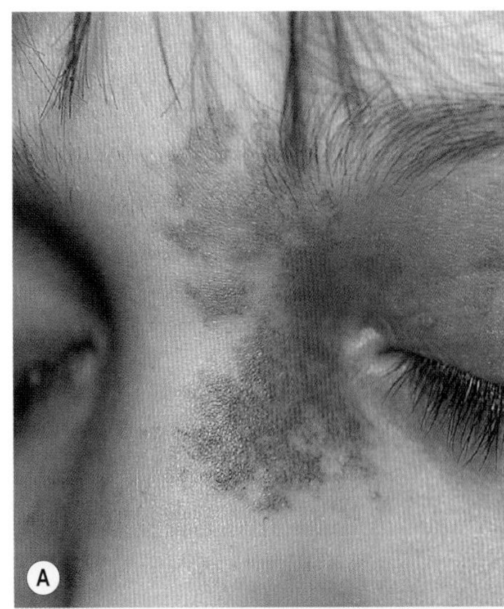

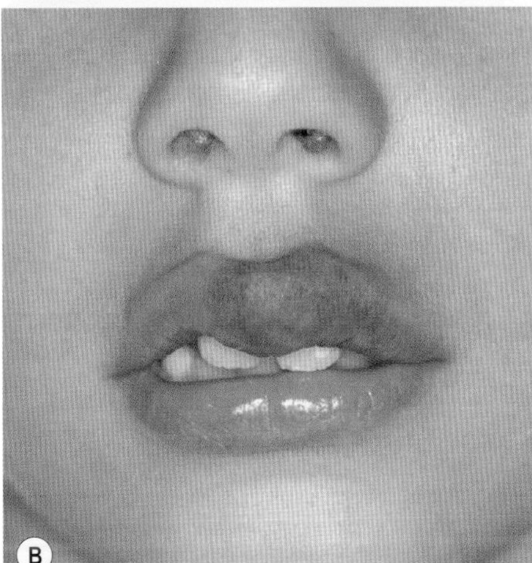

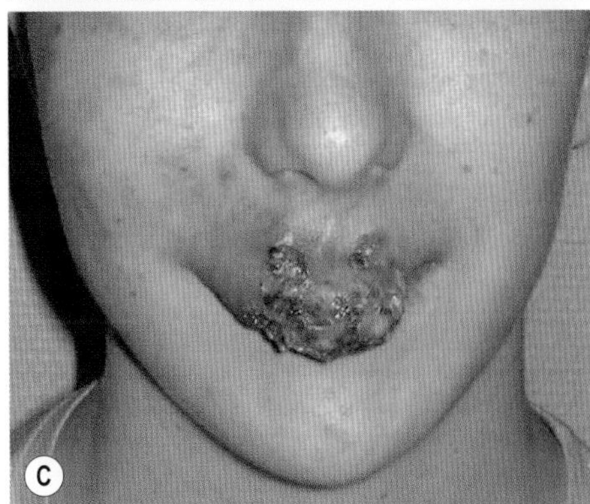

Fig. 85.27 Arteriovenous malformations (AVMs). A, B Dormant (stage 1) AVMs mimicking a port-wine stain **(A)** and infantile hemangioma **(B)**. **C** Destructive (stage 3) AVM that has led to cutaneous necrosis. *A, B, Courtesy, Odile Enjolras, MD; C, Courtesy, Juan Carlos Lopez, MD.*

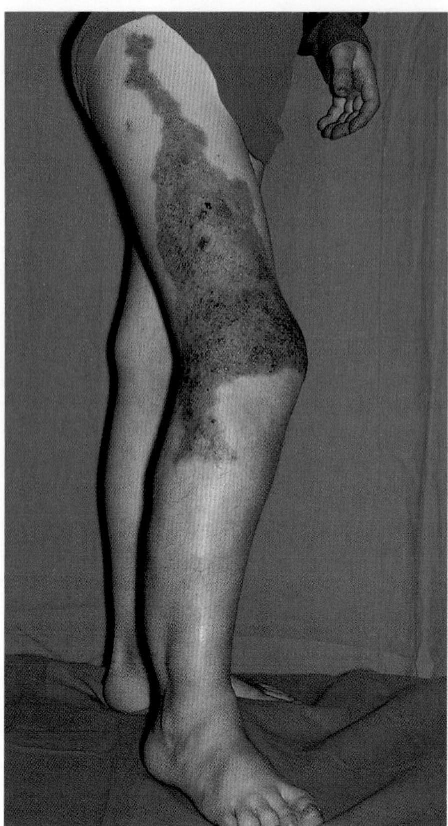

Fig. 85.28 Klippel–Trenaunay syndrome (KTS). Dilated incompetent veins and an enlarged lower limb are evident. The sharply demarcated *geographic* borders of this capillary stain and the superimposed purple papulovesicles (representing lymphangiectasias) are clues to the presence of a lymphatic malformation. In contrast, KTS without a lymphatic component often presents with an ill-defined *patchy* capillary stain in a segmental or haphazard distribution. *Courtesy, USCDRSC.*

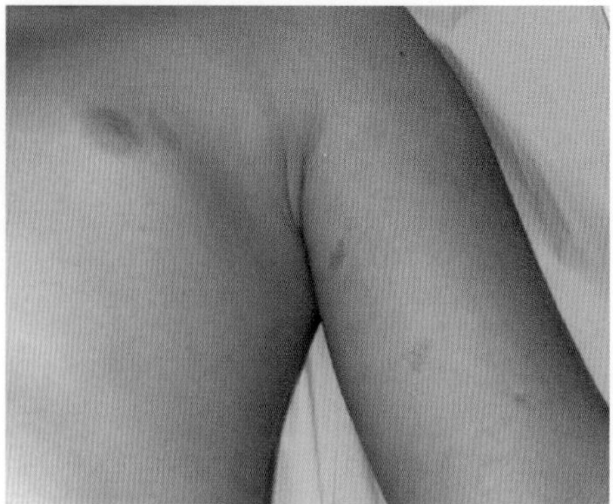

Fig. 85.29 Capillary malformation–arteriovenous malformation due to a *RASA1* mutation. Multiple pink-red macules. A blanched halo is often evident at the periphery of lesions. *Courtesy, Eulalia Baselga, MD.*

fast-flow), *e*pidermal nevi, and *s*keletal anomalies (e.g. scoliosis, splayed feet) due to mosaic *PIK3CA* mutations.

- *PTEN hamartoma tumor syndrome* (see Ch. 52): often intramuscular fast-flow anomalies associated with ectopic fat and dilated draining veins; ± CM and LM components.
- *Cerebral CM and hyperkeratotic cutaneous CM-VM:* autosomal dominant disorder, usually due to *KRIT1* mutations; congenital red-purple plaques and red-brown macules with peripheral telangiectatic puncta.
- *CM-AVM syndrome*: autosomal dominant disorder due to *RASA1* or *EPHB4* mutations; presents with multiple small CMs ± AVM(s) (Fig. 85.29) and sometimes *Parkes–Weber syndrome* (limb overgrowth associated with an AVM).

For further information see Chs 103 and 104 from *Dermatology, Fourth Edition*.

For additional online figures and tables visit www.expertconsult.com 

Ulcers 86

• An ulcer is defined as a wound with loss of the entire epidermis plus dermal tissue, sometimes extending as deep as the subcutis.
• The most common types of leg ulcers – venous, arterial, and neuropathic – as well as pressure ulcers, lymphedema, and an approach to wound healing are reviewed (see below); additional physical, inflammatory, infectious, metabolic, and neoplastic causes of leg ulcers are outlined in Fig. 86.1.
• Features to consider in the history and physical examination of patients with a leg ulcer are presented in Table 86.1, and routine laboratory testing often includes a CBC, ESR, and blood glucose and serum albumin levels; microbial cultures, evaluation for thrombophilia (previously referred to as hypercoagulability; see Table 18.5), and additional studies depend on the clinical setting.
• Ulcers with atypical features or a lack of response to appropriate therapy should be re-evaluated, with expansion of the DDx and consideration of a skin biopsy (preferably including the ulcer margin and bed) to exclude less common etiologies, such as SCC, vasculitis, and fungal or mycobacterial infections (via tissue culture).

Venous Ulcers

• Venous hypertension and insufficiency represent the most common causes of chronic leg ulcers.
• Prevalence increases with age, and risk factors include female sex, obesity, pregnancy, prolonged standing, and family history of venous insufficiency; thrombophilia can be a contributing factor, especially in patients with a history of deep vein thrombosis or livedoid vasculopathy (Fig. 86.3; see Ch. 18).
• Ulcers tend to have irregular borders and a yellow fibrinous base, with a predilection for the area above the medial malleolus (Fig. 86.4); the ulcers can become large but are often fairly shallow, with granulation tissue evident upon debridement.
• Surrounding skin has signs of venous hypertension such as yellow-brown discoloration due to hemosiderin deposits, pinpoint petechiae, stasis dermatitis, lipodermatosclerosis, and, occasionally, acroangiodermatitis (Fig. 86.5; see Table 11.1).
• Other findings include varicosities and edema > lymphedema of the lower extremities (Fig. 86.6); swelling and aching of the legs is worsened by dependency (e.g. prolonged standing) and improved by leg elevation and the use of compression therapy; other dependent sites, such as a large pannus, can develop similar clinical changes (Fig. 86.7).
• **DDx:** see Fig. 86.1; coexistent arterial insufficiency (see below) or uncompensated congestive heart failure should be excluded before initiating compression therapy.
• Evaluation and **Rx:** an approach to the patient with a chronic venous ulcer is presented in Fig. 86.8.
• Compression represents a mainstay of therapy.
  – *Graduated compression stockings*: pressures of 30–40 mmHg at the ankle are required for moderate edema and to promote healing of venous ulcers, although lower pressures (20–30 mmHg) can be used for mild edema and as an initial step; stockings should be applied immediately upon arising from bed in the morning, and lifelong use is recommended
  – *Compression bandages*: the *Unna boot*, a zinc oxide-impregnated bandage that is covered by a self-adherent elastic wrap such as Coban™, provides semi-rigid compression and is usually changed weekly; four-layer bandages represent another option for highly exudative wounds

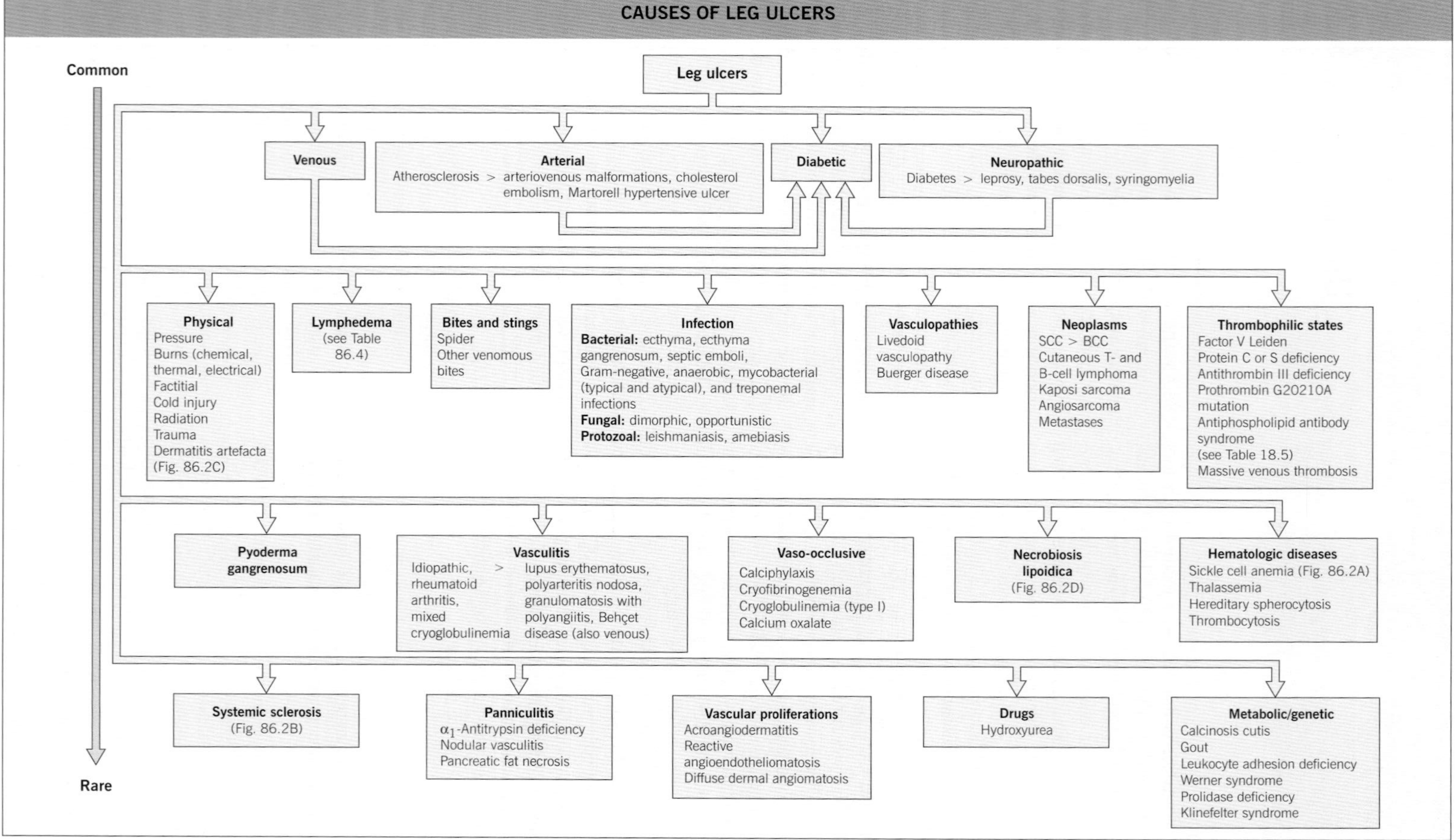

Fig. 86.1 Causes of leg ulcers. Patients with Behçet disease can also develop leg ulcers due to vasculitis and/or venous insufficiency related to deep vein thromboses. Erosive pustular dermatosis is another occasional cause of leg ulcers.

POINTS TO INCLUDE IN THE HISTORY AND PHYSICAL EXAMINATION OF PATIENTS WITH A LEG ULCER	
History	**Physical examination**
• Onset and clinical course of ulcer • Symptoms, including those of vascular disease or neuropathy • Alleviating and exacerbating factors • Past medical history, e.g. diabetes mellitus, atherosclerotic cardiovascular disease, AI-CTD • Family history • Medications, topical and systemic • Personal habits (e.g. smoking, alcohol intake)	General, emphasizing the following: • Ulcer characteristics – Location and size – Morphology, including depth, shape, border, and base – Surrounding skin, e.g. edema, dermatitis, fibrosis, cellulitis, necrosis • Peripheral pulses • Capillary refill time • Evidence of peripheral neuropathy • Deep tendon reflexes

Table 86.1 Points to include in the history and physical examination of patients with a leg ulcer. *Courtesy, Tania Phillips, MD.*

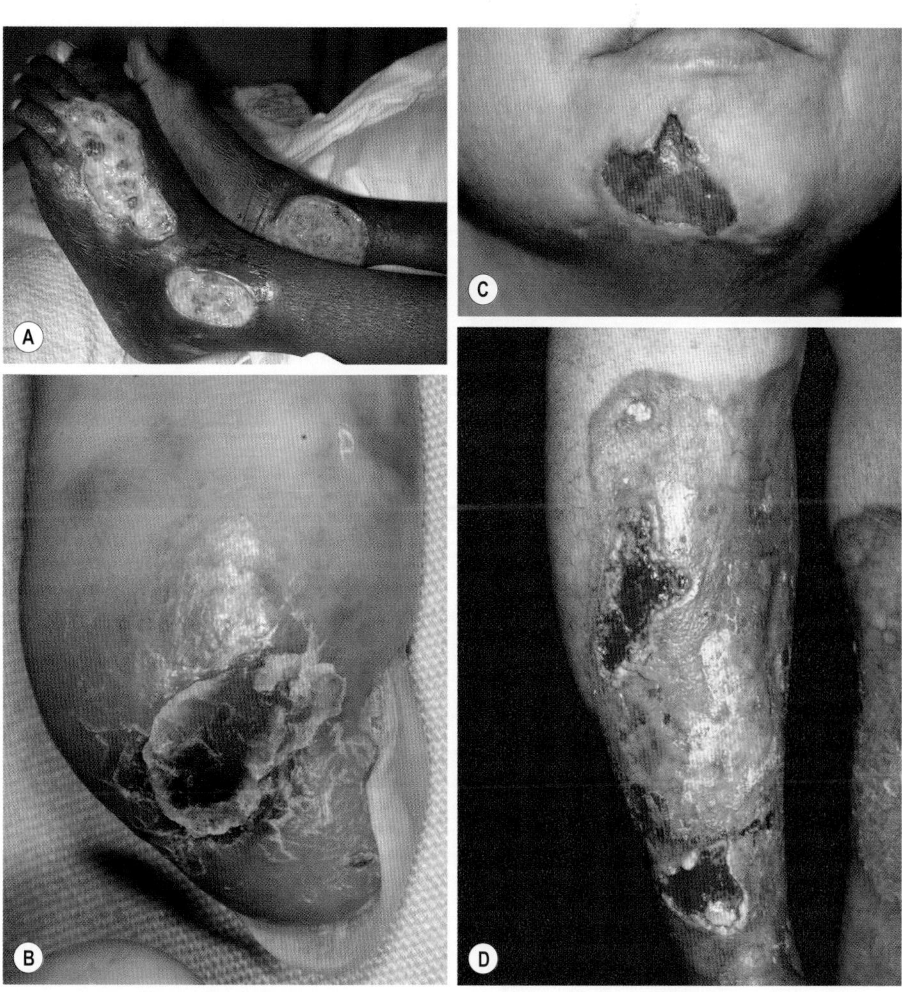

Fig. 86.2 Diverse causes of ulcers. A Multiple ulcers in a patient with sickle cell anemia. **B** Ulcer of the fingertip in a patient with systemic sclerosis. **C** Ulcer with a “bizarre” shape and angulated borders due to dermatitis artefacta. **D** Ulcerated necrobiosis lipoidica, which is associated with diabetes mellitus in a subset of affected individuals. *A, B, Courtesy, YDRSC; C, Courtesy, Kalman Watsky, MD; D, Courtesy, Jeffrey Callen, MD.*

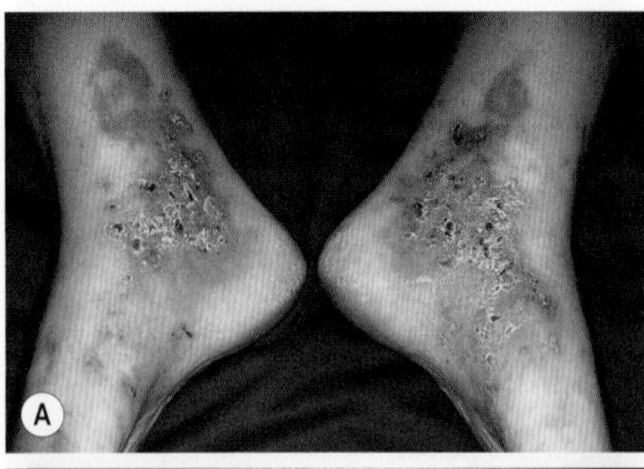

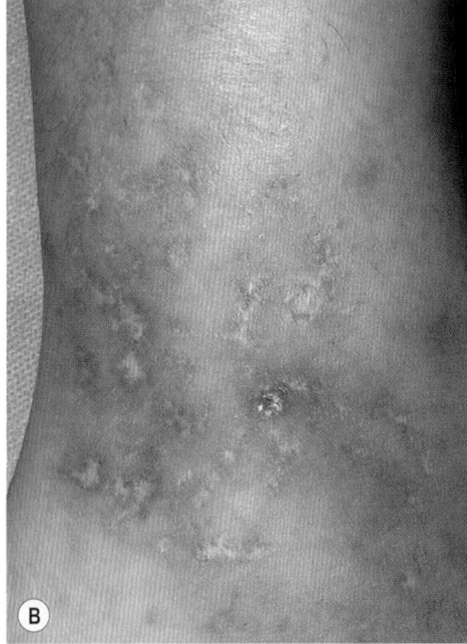

Fig. 86.3 Livedoid vasculopathy. A Multiple hemorrhagic crusts and small, very painful ulcers associated with brown discoloration due to hemosiderin deposits. **B** Stellate, porcelain-white atrophic scars with peripheral telangiectatic papules, referred to as atrophie blanche. *A, Courtesy, YDRSC; B, Courtesy, Julie V. Schaffer, MD.*

Arterial Ulcers

- Peripheral arterial disease (PAD), a manifestation of atherosclerosis, is present in up to 25% of patients with leg ulcers; risk factors include cigarette smoking, diabetes mellitus, dyslipidemia, and hypertension; ulceration is often precipitated by trauma.
- Well-demarcated, round, "punched out" ulcers with a dry necrotic base; occur primarily on the distal lower extremities, favoring the toes and sites of pressure.
- Surrounding skin is typically hairless, shiny, and atrophic (Fig. 86.9).
- Other findings include cool feet, weak or absent peripheral pulses, prolonged capillary refill time (>3–4 seconds), pallor ± pain upon leg elevation (45° for 1 minute), and dependent rubor; patients may report pain induced by ambulation and relieved by rest.
- **DDx:** other causes of ulcers in patients with PAD include cholesterol emboli (Fig. 86.10), diffuse dermal angiomatosis (painful violaceous plaques with central ulceration), and Buerger disease (thrombangiitis obliterans; inflammatory and vaso-occlusive disorder in smokers affecting upper and lower extremities); patients with co-existing diabetes mellitus may have overlapping features (see below).
- Evaluation: the ankle–brachial index (ABI) is used to screen for PAD (Table 86.2); additional assessment may include duplex ultrasonography, CT angiography, and magnetic resonance angiography.
- **Rx:** surgical or endovascular restoration of blood flow; wound care (see below), but with avoidance of sharp debridement.

Neuropathic (Mal Perforans) and Diabetic Ulcers

- Diabetes mellitus confers a 15–25% lifetime risk of foot ulcers, ~15% of which eventuate in an amputation; diabetic neuropathy is the major cause of these ulcers, although ischemia, venous hypertension, and infection often contribute to pathogenesis.
- *Sensory* neuropathy leads to unrecognized foot trauma, *motor* neuropathy leads to altered biomechanics and structural deformities that increase mechanical stress, and *autonomic* neuropathy leads to both arteriovenous shunting that decreases perfusion and reduced sweating that predisposes to dryness and fissuring.
- Neuropathic ulcers are typically "punched out" with a hyperkeratotic rim, arising in a background of callused skin; they are usually located on pressure points and over bony prominences (e.g. metatarsal heads, heels, great toes) (Fig. 86.11).
- Other findings include decreased sensation due to peripheral neuropathy and sometimes foot deformities (e.g. hammer toes, Charcot foot).
- Evaluation: neurologic examination using nylon monofilament to test sensation ± nerve

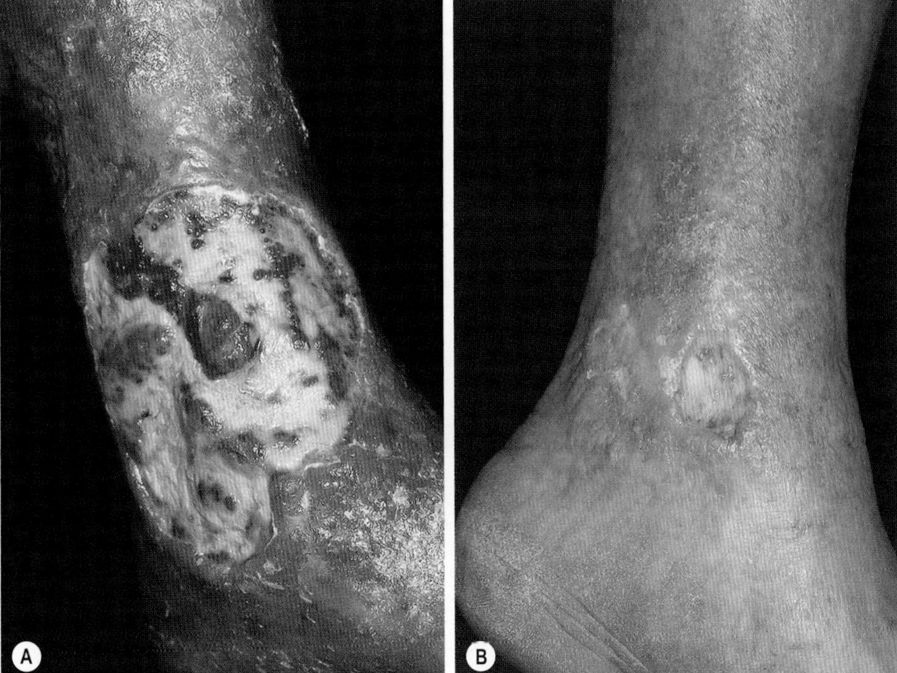

Fig. 86.4 Venous ulcers over the medial malleolus. A Note the yellowish fibrinous base over most of the ulcer and focal areas of granulation tissue. There is surrounding stasis dermatitis with erythema, crusting, and scaling as well as scarring. **B** Induration due to lipodermatosclerosis, hemosiderin deposition, and atrophie blanche scars are present in the surrounding skin. *A, Courtesy, YDRSC; B, Courtesy, Jean L. Bolognia, MD.*

conduction studies/electromyography and determination of the ABI (see Table 86.2); assessment for infection utilizing laboratory studies (e.g. CBC, ESR/C-reactive protein), wound cultures (tissue from biopsy is higher yield than swabs), and imaging to exclude osteomyelitis (e.g. radiographs [low sensitivity], MRI) as indicated by clinical suspicion.

• **Rx:** wound care with debridement of necrotic material and the hyperkeratotic rim, eradication of infection, and mechanical offloading (e.g. bed rest, wheelchair, crutches, total contact casting, felted foam, orthotic shoes); additional options include hyperbaric oxygen and becaplermin gel (recombinant platelet-derived growth factor [PDGF]); patient instructions are provided in Table 86.3.

Pressure (Decubitis) Ulcers (Bed Sores)

• Occur as a consequence of prolonged immobility, affecting ~10% of hospitalized patients and ~25% of nursing home residents; other risk factors include sensory deficits, older age, and poor nutrition.

• Soft tissues are compressed between a bony prominence (e.g. sacrum, ischial tuberosity; Figs 86.12 and 86.13) and an external surface; pathogenic factors include continuous pressure, shearing forces/friction, and moisture (e.g. perspiration, urine, feces).

• Classified according to a four-stage system (Fig. 86.14); ulcers do not necessarily progress sequentially through these stages, and extensive deep tissue damage may initially have few superficial manifestations.

• Prevention: frequent position changes together with use of softer surfaces (e.g. containing foam, air, or liquid) and devices (e.g. pillows, foam wedges) to relieve pressure; optimize nutrition.

• **Rx:** relief of pressure and wound care – for example, utilizing an occlusive dressing (see below); stage IV ulcers may require surgical intervention.

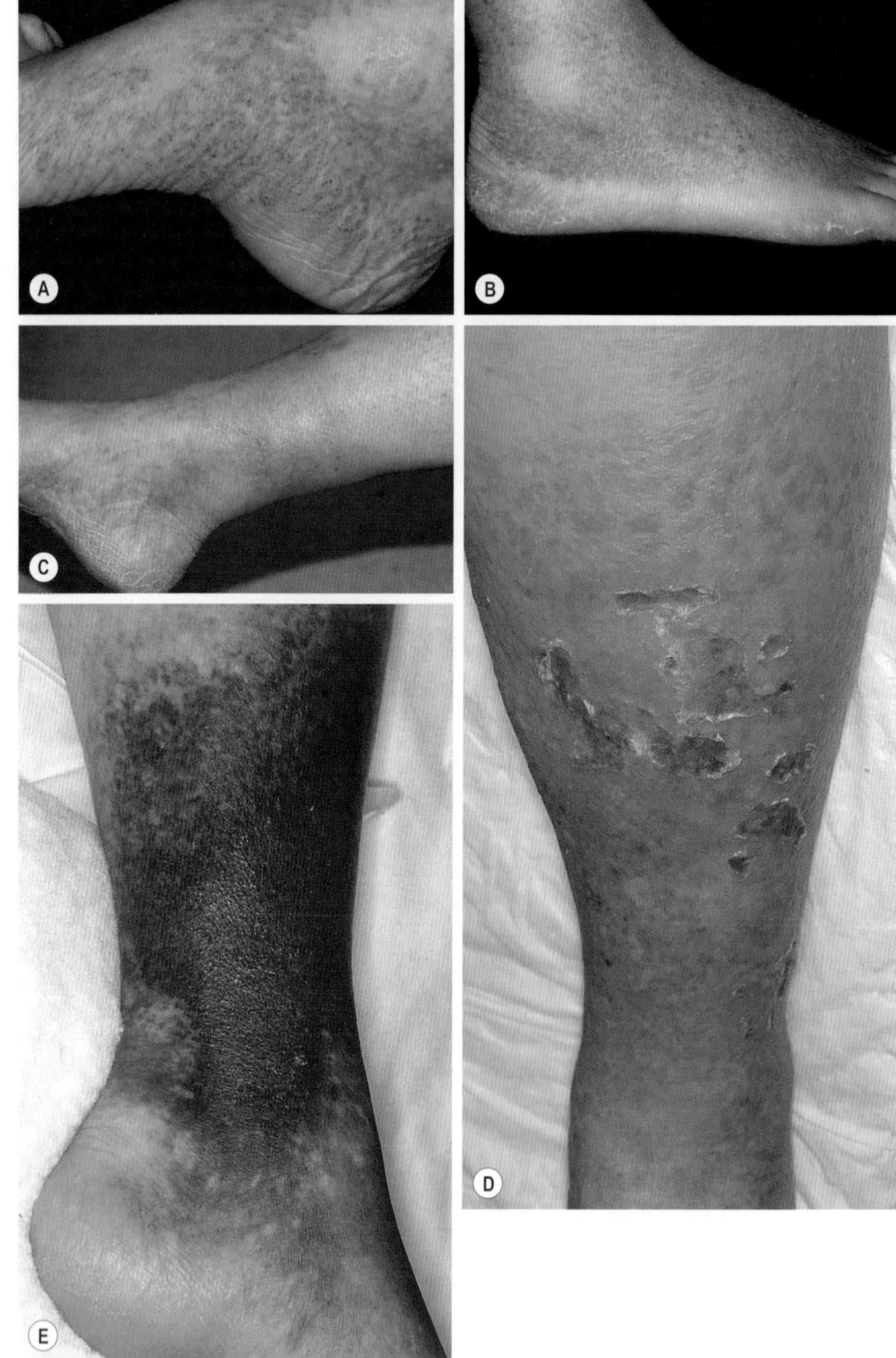

Fig. 86.5 Associated findings in patients with venous hypertension and insufficiency. **A** Venulectasias of the instep referred to as corona phlebectasia. **B** Brown discoloration of the foot and ankle due to hemosiderin deposits within dermal macrophages in addition to hyperpigmentation. Note the cutoff at Wallace's line. **C** Lipodermatosclerosis with violet-brown discoloration, tenderness, and induration that typically begins above the medial malleolus. **D** Stasis dermatitis and chronic lipodermatosclerosis with serous crusts and the "inverted champagne bottle" or "bowling pin" configuration. **E** Acroangiodermatitis (pseudo-Kaposi sarcoma). Violaceous plaque in a patient with venous hypertension. Histologically, these lesions can resemble Kaposi sarcoma. *A, B, Courtesy, Jean L. Bolognia, MD; C, Courtesy, Kalman Watsky, MD; D, Courtesy, Ariela Hafner, MD, and Eli Sprecher, MD; E, Courtesy, YDRSC.*

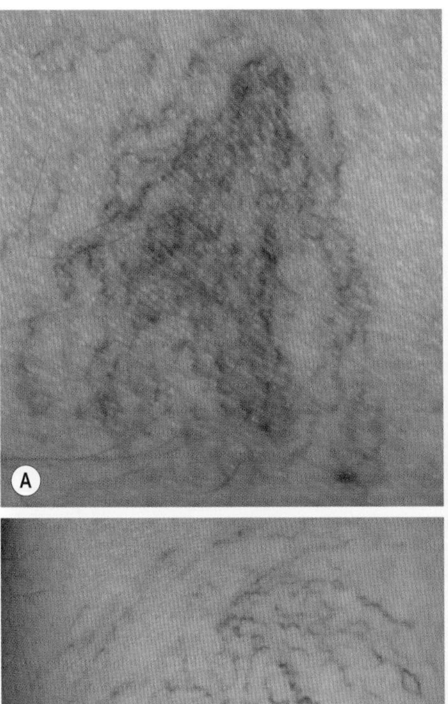

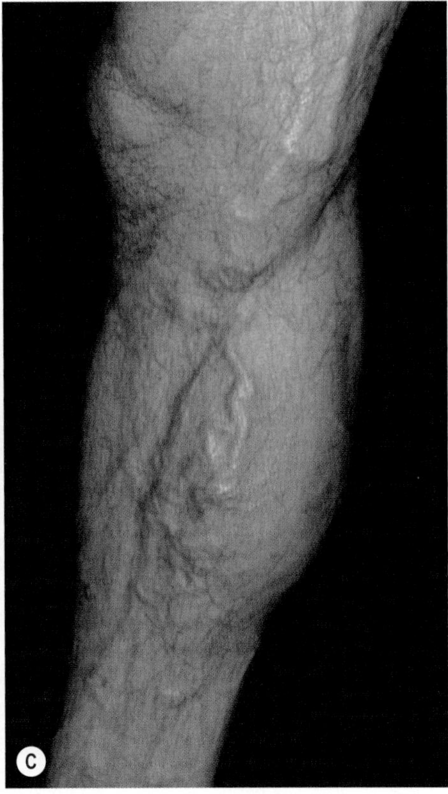

Fig. 86.6 Venous abnormalities of the lower extremity. A Venulectasias and a few reticular varicosities at the site of a perforator vein. **B** Reticular varicosities; note the blue-green color. **C** Larger saphenous varicosities may also be evident. *Courtesy, Jean L. Bolognia, MD.*

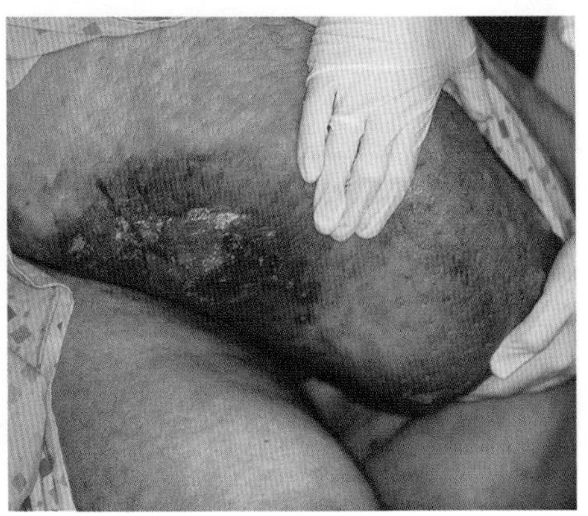

Fig. 86.7 Lymphedema, lipodermatosclerosis, and chronic ulceration of the dependent portion of the pannus. The changes are similar to those that can be seen on the distal lower extremities. *Courtesy, Jean L. Bolognia, MD.*

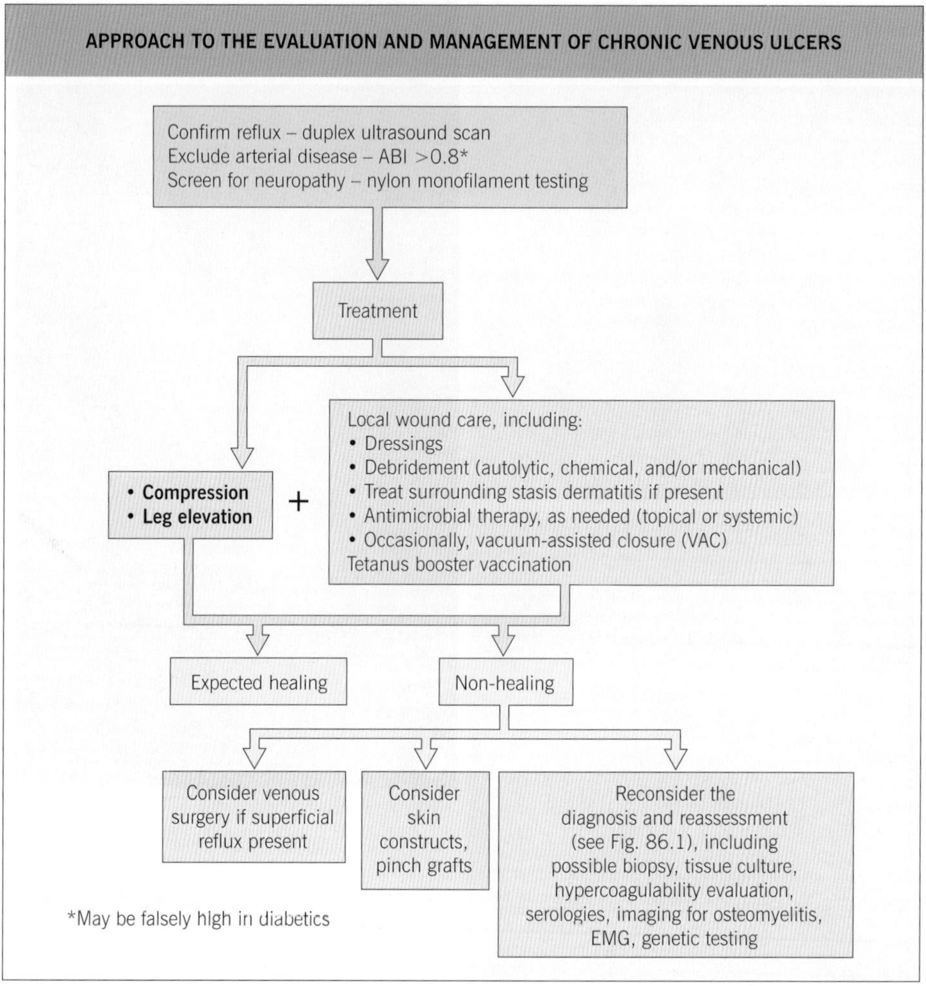

APPROACH TO THE EVALUATION AND MANAGEMENT OF CHRONIC VENOUS ULCERS

Confirm reflux – duplex ultrasound scan
Exclude arterial disease – ABI >0.8*
Screen for neuropathy – nylon monofilament testing

↓

Treatment

↓

- **Compression**
- **Leg elevation**

\+

Local wound care, including:
- Dressings
- Debridement (autolytic, chemical, and/or mechanical)
- Treat surrounding stasis dermatitis if present
- Antimicrobial therapy, as needed (topical or systemic)
- Occasionally, vacuum-assisted closure (VAC)

Tetanus booster vaccination

↓

Expected healing | Non-healing

Non-healing ↓

- Consider venous surgery if superficial reflux present
- Consider skin constructs, pinch grafts
- Reconsider the diagnosis and reassessment (see Fig. 86.1), including possible biopsy, tissue culture, hypercoagulability evaluation, serologies, imaging for osteomyelitis, EMG, genetic testing

*May be falsely high in diabetics

Fig. 86.8 Approach to the evaluation and management of chronic venous ulcers. *Courtesy, Tania Phillips, MD.*

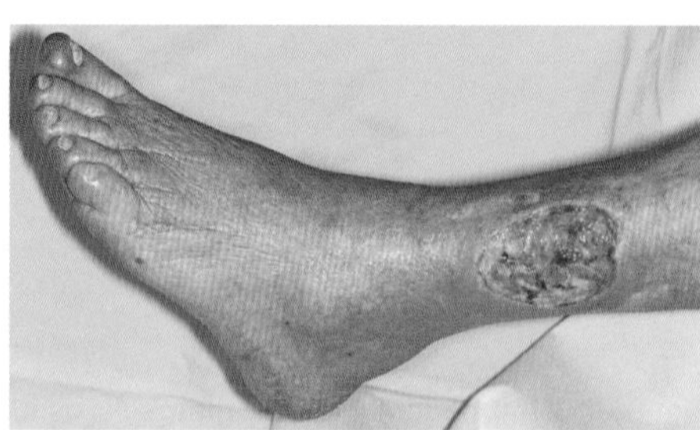

Fig. 86.9 Arterial ulcer. The punched-out appearance and surrounding smooth shiny skin are common features. *Courtesy, Ariela Hafner, MD, and Eli Sprecher, MD.*

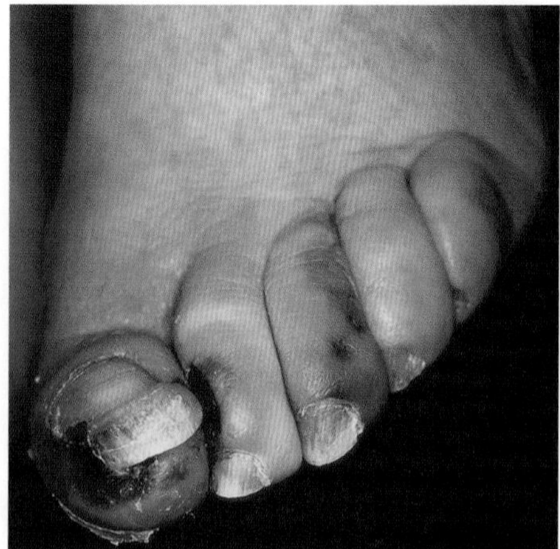

Fig. 86.10 Cholesterol emboli. Ischemia of the toes and necrosis with early ulcer formation. *Courtesy, YDRSC.*

DETERMINATION AND INTERPRETATION OF THE ANKLE–BRACHIAL INDEX (ABI)
• With the patient in a supine position, the systolic blood pressure is measured in the: – Brachial arteries (right and left) – Dorsalis pedis and posterior tibial arteries (right and left) • The ABI is determined by: $\frac{\text{the highest of the systolic pressures from the dorsalis pedis or posterior tibial arteries}}{\text{the higher of the brachial artery systolic pressures}}$ • Interpretation of the ABI: 0.91–1.30 = normal range >1.30 = suggests incompressible tibial arteries due to medial calcification (diabetes mellitus, chronic renal insufficiency) <0.9 = indicative of peripheral artery disease (PAD) 0.41–0.90 = mild to moderate PAD 0.00–0.40 = severe PAD

Table 86.2 Determination and interpretation of the ankle–brachial index (ABI).

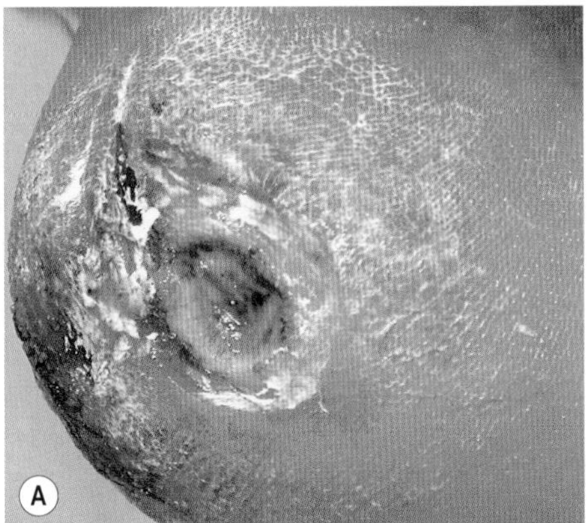

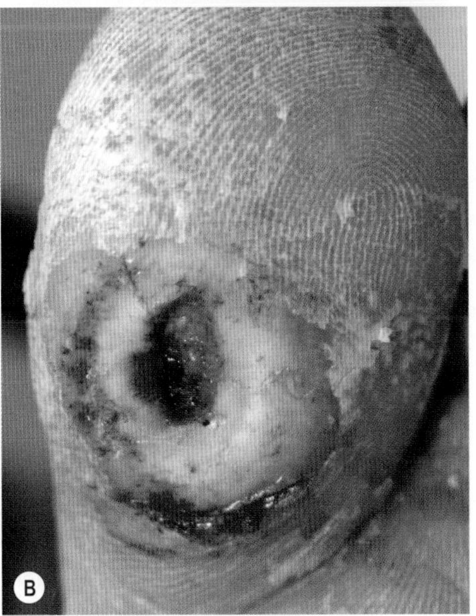

Fig. 86.11 Neuropathic ulcers in patients with diabetes mellitus and peripheral neuropathy. Common locations are the plantar surface of the heel **(A)** and the great toe **(B)**. Note the thick rim of callus. *A, Courtesy, Ariela Hafner, MD, and Eli Sprecher, MD; B, Courtesy, YDRSC.*

INSTRUCTIONS FOR THE PATIENT WITH A DIABETIC OR NEUROPATHIC ULCER
Foot care • Inspect feet daily for blisters, scratches, and red areas. If your vision is impaired, get someone to do this for you. • Wash your feet daily in warm water. Dry carefully between the toes. • Apply petroleum jelly to dry areas of skin but not between the toes. • Do not remove corns or apply strong chemicals to your feet. • Cut nails straight across. • If you develop any breaks in the skin or blisters, inform your doctor. • See your podiatrist regularly.
Shoe choice and use • Wear properly fitting shoes. New shoes should be worn for 1–2 hours daily only. Check your feet for red spots afterwards. • Inspect the insides of your shoes before putting them on. • Avoid open-toed sandals and shoes with pointed toes. • Never walk barefoot.
General medical care and safety • Stop smoking, control blood sugar levels, and lose weight if overweight. • Always test water temperature before bathing. • See your doctor regularly.

Table 86.3 Instructions for the patient with a diabetic or neuropathic ulcer. *Adapted with permission from Levin M, O'Neal ME. The Diabetic Foot. St. Louis: Mosby, 1988.*

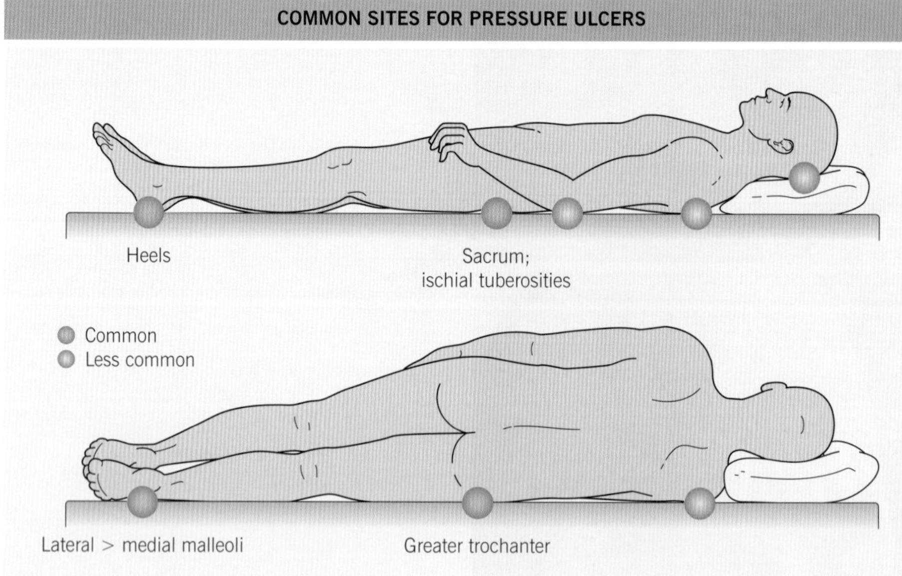

Fig. 86.12 Common sites for pressure ulcers.

Lymphedema

• Lymphedema is the interstitial accumulation of lymphatic fluid due to reduced drainage by lymphatic vessels.

• Divided into *primary* forms due to abnormal lymphatic development (see Ch. 85) and *secondary* forms due to lymphatic damage or obstruction (Table 86.4).

• Usually presents as chronic, painless swelling and heaviness of an extremity (leg > arm), typically beginning distally (e.g. on the dorsal foot) and progressing proximally (Fig. 86.15); initially pitting, but becomes indurated

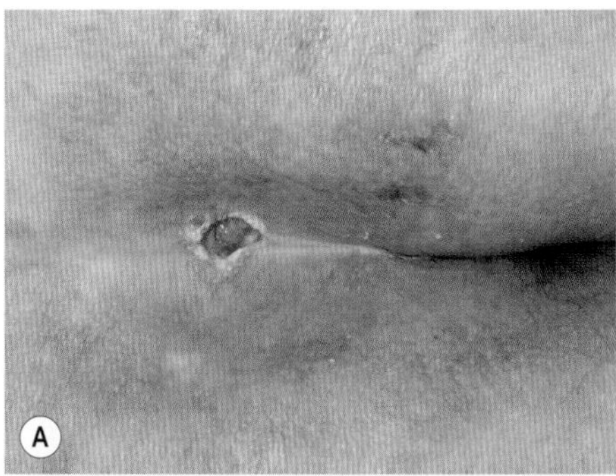

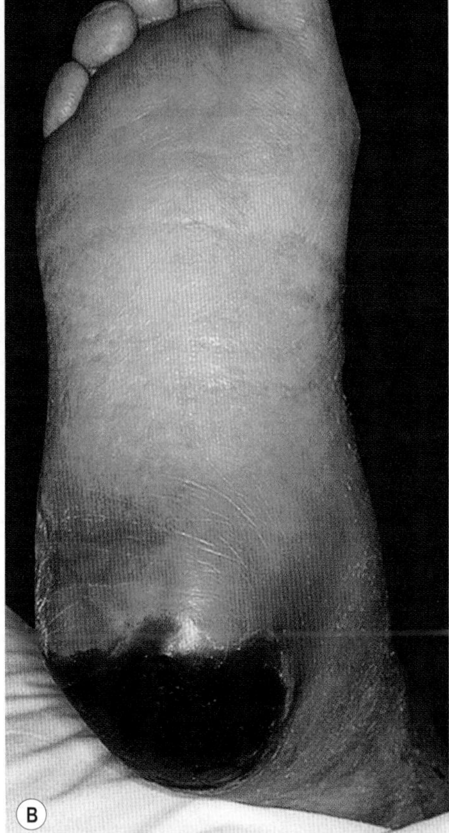

Fig. 86.13 Pressure ulcers. A Stage III ulcer over the sacrum. **B** Black eschar on the heel due to pressure necrosis. *A, Courtesy, Ariela Hafner, MD, and Eli Sprecher, MD; B, Courtesy, YDRSC.*

and non-pitting as fibrosis develops; prone to ulceration and often worsens following secondary infections.

- *Elephantiasis nostras verrucosa* is a complication of severe lymphedema characterized by massive enlargement of the affected area, marked fibrosis, and verrucous epidermal changes with a mossy, cobblestoned appearance (Fig. 86.16).
- **DDx:** edema secondary to venous insufficiency, lipedema (bilateral lower extremity swelling that spares the feet, almost exclusively affecting women; Fig. 86.17), obesity-associated lymphedematous mucinosis.
- **Rx:** difficult; compression (e.g. garments, wrapping), pneumatic pumps and massage to decrease accumulation of lymph; treatment of secondary infections.

General Approach to Wound Healing

- In a patient with an ulcer, modifiable local and systemic factors that may impair wound healing should be addressed, including deleterious mechanical forces, inadequate perfusion, and poor nutritional or immune status.
- A moist wound environment such as that provided by a semipermeable "occlusive" dressing enhances healing by stimulating collagen synthesis, promoting angiogenesis, encouraging re-epithelialization, and providing autolytic debridement.
- The choice of dressing depends on the wound type and amount of exudate (Tables 86.5 and 86.6), and it may be helpful to protect the skin around the wound with a thin coat of ointment to prevent maceration; the frequency of dressing changes is based on their absorbency as well as the amount of exudate.
- Debridement of non-viable tissue from the wound bed also promotes healing.
  - *Autolytic debridement* utilizing the body's own proteolytic enzymes is provided by moist retentive dressings; it is best suited for non-infected wounds with minimal debris
  - *Mechanical debridement* (e.g. "sharp" with surgical instruments, wet-to-dry [can disrupt viable tissue]) may be helpful for wounds with large amounts of necrotic and/or infected tissue
  - *Enzymatic debridement* utilizes topical proteolytic enzyme preparations such as collagenase and papain-urea
  - *Maggot debridement* can be considered for recalcitrant ulcers with excessive necrotic tissue
- Bacterial colonization occurs in all chronic wounds and must be distinguished from true

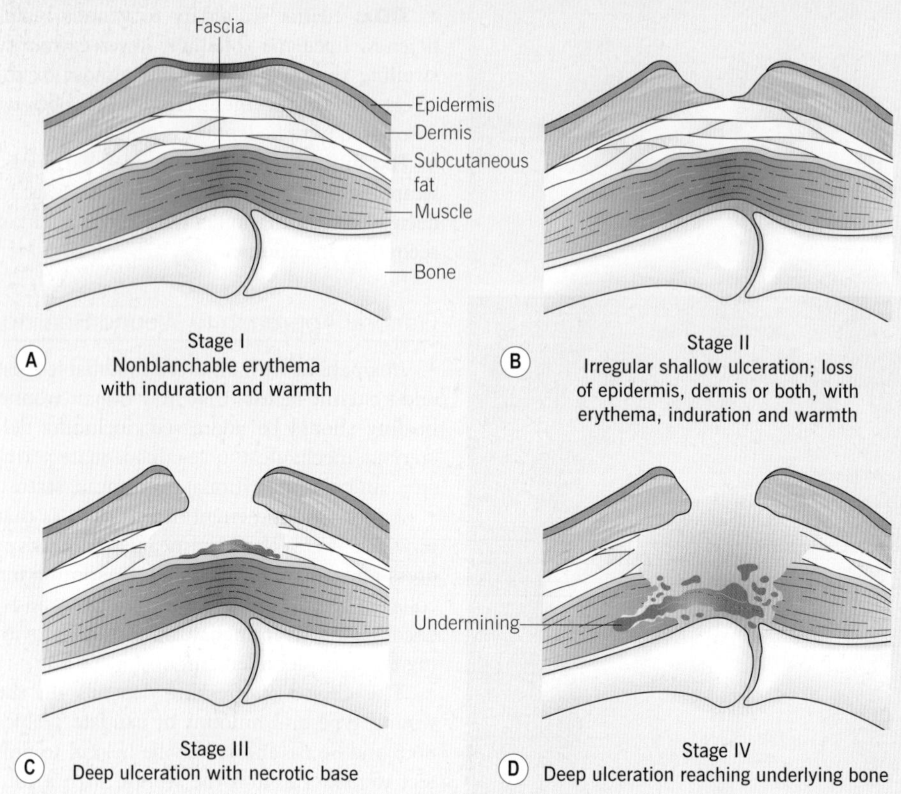

Fig. 86.14 National Pressure Ulcer Advisory Panel classification of pressure ulcers. A Stage I: nonblanchable erythema of intact skin. This lesion is the heralding sign of impending skin ulceration. For darker-skinned individuals, other signs may be indicators and include warmth, edema, discoloration of the skin, and induration. **B** Stage II: partial-thickness skin loss involving the epidermis, dermis, or both. This superficial lesion presents as an abrasion, blister, or shallow crater. **C** Stage III: full-thickness skin loss, in which subcutaneous tissue is damaged or necrotic and may extend down into, but not including, the underlying fascia. This deep lesion presents as a crater and sometimes involves adjacent tissue. **D** Stage IV: full-thickness skin loss and extensive tissue necrosis, destruction to muscle, bone, or supporting structures such as a tendon or joint capsule. Undermining or sinus tracts can be present.

soft tissue infection; wounds with clinical evidence of infection (e.g. purulent discharge, surrounding cellulitis) should be cultured and treated with systemic antibiotics (initially broad-spectrum and then adjusted based on sensitivities); topical antimicrobial agents (e.g. dressings containing silver or cadexomer-iodine) can be considered for non-healing wounds with "critical colonization" ($>10^6$ colony-forming units of bacteria per gram of tissue).

- In addition to wound care, treatment of ulcers should be directed at the underlying cause (see above).
- Other adjuncts to wound care may include topical growth factors (e.g. PDGF), topical negative pressure therapy, and tissue-engineered skin equivalents.

For further information see Ch. 105 from *Dermatology, Fourth Edition*.

For additional online figures and tables visit www.expertconsult.com

CAUSES OF SECONDARY LYMPHEDEMA
Infections
• Recurrent cellulitis and lymphangitis • Parasitic infections (e.g. filariasis)
Cancer-related, including iatrogenic
• Lymph node dissection (e.g. for melanoma or breast cancer) or other surgical excisions (e.g. mastectomy) • Radiation injury • Malignant obstruction (e.g. by lymphoma or Kaposi sarcoma)
Inflammatory
• Acne vulgaris and rosacea (midfacial) • Granulomatous disorders (e.g. anogenital in Crohn disease)
Other
• Obesity • Podoconiosis (exposure to mineral microparticles in volcanic soils)

Table 86.4 Causes of secondary lymphedema.

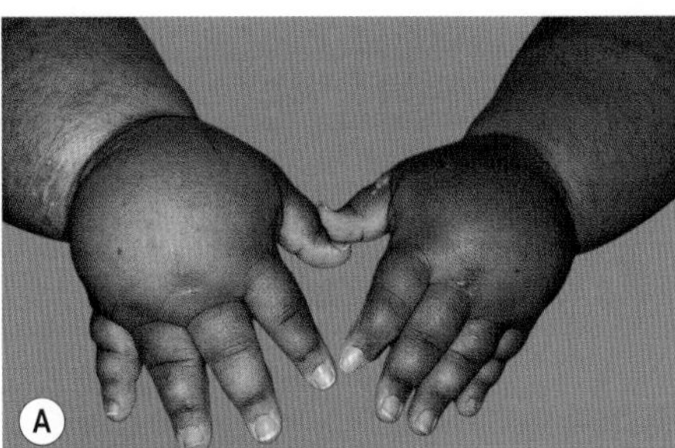

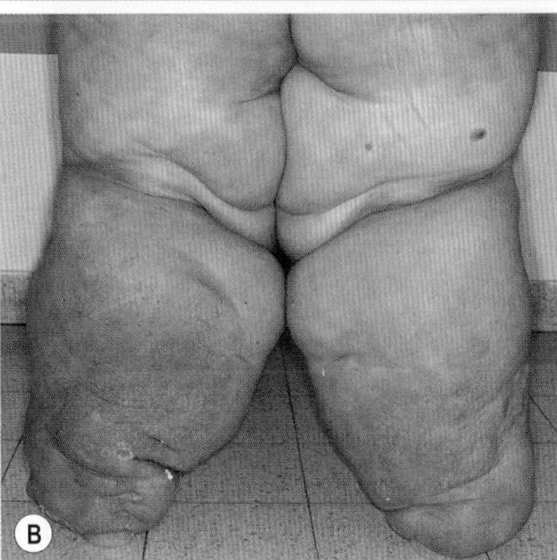

Fig. 86.15 Lymphedema. A Primary lymphedema of the upper extremities due to Milroy disease (see Ch. 85). **B** Lymphedema of the lower extremities secondary to morbid obesity and associated with myxedema. *A, Courtesy, YDRSC; B, Courtesy, Ariela Hafner, MD, and Eli Sprecher, MD.*

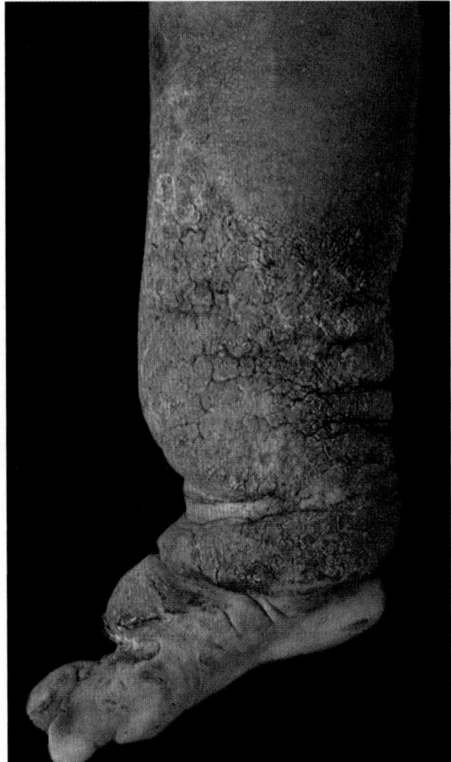

Fig. 86.16 Elephantiasis nostras verrucosa. The patient had both lymphedema and venous insufficiency. Note the involvement of the foot. *Courtesy, Ariela Hafner, MD, and Eli Sprecher, MD.*

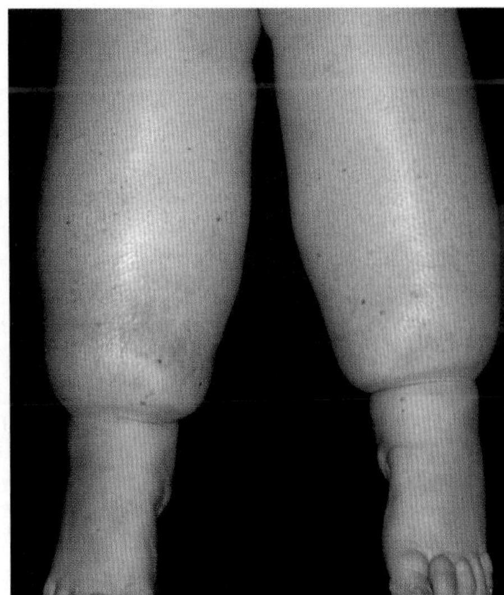

Fig. 86.17 Lipedema. This middle-aged woman has bilateral "stovepipe" enlargement of the legs and minimal involvement of the feet. Note the sharp demarcation between normal and abnormal tissue at the ankle, referred to as the "cuff sign." *Courtesy, Jean L. Bolognia, MD.*

TYPES OF WOUND DRESSINGS		
Dressing type	**Properties**	**Disadvantages**
Gauzes	• Good absorption • Can be impregnated with: – NaCl to become highly absorbent, discourage bacterial overgrowth, and prevent formation of excess granulation tissue – Petrolatum so less drying and adherent, but then less absorbent – Iodine or silver as an antiseptic	• Adhere to wound bed and promote desiccation • Can cause pain and trauma, including disruption of epithelium, upon removal
Films	• Thin polyurethane membranes • Maintain a moist environment • Semipermeable (only to vapors, not to liquids) • Transparency enables wound visualization	• Non-absorbent • Can cause maceration of surrounding skin if applied to wounds with heavy exudate
Hydrogels	• Maintain a moist environment • Promote autolytic debridement • Non-adhesive • Relieve pain	• Can cause maceration of surrounding skin if applied to wounds with heavy exudate
Hydrocolloids	• Adhesive, occlusive dressings that absorb exudates with the formation of hydrophilic gel • Provide a moist environment	• Not suitable for wounds with heavy exudate or infected wounds • May produce a brown, malodorous gel • May lead to maceration of surrounding skin, and removal can be traumatic
Alginates	• Fibrous dressings derived from brown seaweed • Highly absorbent and require moisture to function • Ion exchange between calcium in the alginate and sodium in the wound fluid leads to the formation of a moist retentive gel • Hemostatic	• May adhere to dry wounds • May leave fibrous debris in the wound • Can lead to maceration around the wound unless cut to the size of the wound bed
Foams (polyurethane)	• Good absorbance capacity • Non-traumatic upon removal • Provide thermal and shear protection	• Not suitable for dry wounds • Maceration around wound possible
Collagens	• Collagen matrix that physically entraps MMPs and facilitates growth factor activity	• Nonspecific inhibition of MMPs

Table 86.5 Types of wound dressings. A conventional layered dressing usually has three components: (1) a nonadherent, fluid-permeable material that directly contacts the wound; (2) an absorbent layer (e.g. cotton pad or gauze); and (3) an outer wrap. However, some dressings (e.g. hydrocolloids) that are waterproof and adhere directly do not require secondary layers. MMPs, matrix metalloproteinases. *Courtesy, Ariela Hafner, MD, and Eli Sprecher, MD.*

DRESSING CHOICES FOR DIFFERENT WOUND TYPES						
	Gauze	Film	Hydrogel	Hydrocolloid	Alginate*	Foam
Wound exudate:						
Minimal		✓	✓			
Mild				✓		
Moderate				✓	✓	✓
Heavy	✓				✓	✓
Use as a secondary dressing	✓	✓				

**Helpful for undermined or tunneling wounds.*

Table 86.6 Dressing choices for different wound types. Collagens may also be useful for recalcitrant chronic wounds that are clean and non-infected.

87 Other Vascular Disorders

This chapter covers a range of vascular disorders from livedo reticularis to common vascular ectasias such as venous lakes and telangiectasias. Additional disorders characterized by a proliferation of blood vessels are covered in Chapters 85 (infantile hemangiomas and vascular malformations) and 94 (vascular neoplasms).

Livedo Reticularis

- Blue-violet netlike pattern that reflects an increase in deoxygenated blood within the venous plexus of the skin (Fig. 87.1); this increase can be due to a number of causes, including vasospasm of arterioles supplying the skin and sluggish flow due to hypercoagulability or luminal pathology.
- A common physiologic vasospastic response to cold that resolves with rewarming, as well as a sign of a number of systemic diseases, from severe atherosclerosis to SLE (Table 87.1; Fig. 87.2).
- Most commonly observed on the legs but may be more widespread, especially in the setting of systemic diseases. When the pattern is larger and more branching and irregular ("broken up"), as well as more widespread, it is often described as *livedo racemosa* (Fig. 87.3).
- **DDx:** early phase of erythema ab igne; viral exanthems (e.g. erythema infectiosum),

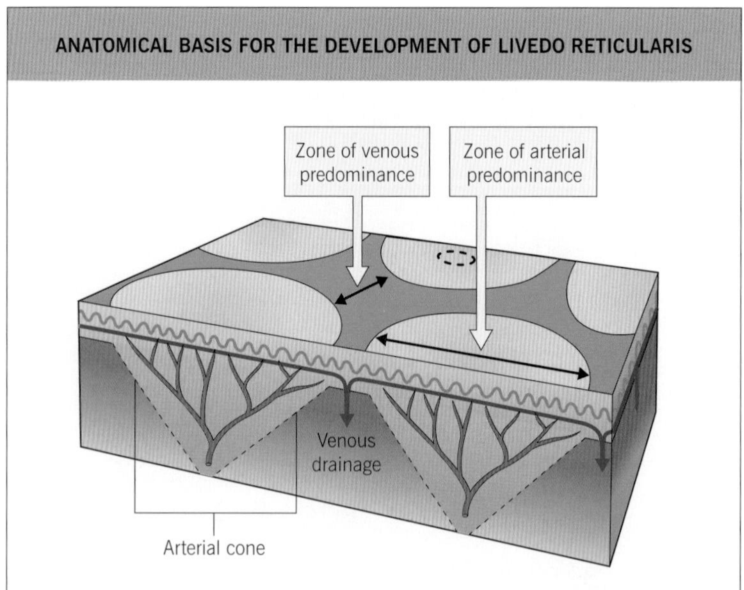

Fig. 87.1 Anatomic basis for the development of livedo reticularis. At the edges of arterial cones, the venous plexus is prominent. An increase in deoxygenated blood within this plexus (due to a decrease in blood flow into or through the skin or impeded drainage of blood) leads to livedo reticularis. If disease of the feeding arteriole is suspected, a wedge biopsy of the central paler cone (dashed oval) can be performed.

CAUSES OF LIVEDO RETICULARIS
Congenital livedo reticularis
Cutis marmorata telangiectatica congenita
Acquired livedo reticularis
Vasospasm
• Cutis marmorata/physiologic livedo reticularis (more common in young children) • Primary (idiopathic) livedo reticularis • Autoimmune connective tissue diseases (e.g. SLE) • Raynaud phenomenon/disease
Vessel wall pathology
• Vasculitis (medium-sized arterioles) – Cutaneous polyarteritis nodosa (nearly all patients) – Systemic polyarteritis nodosa – Cryoglobulinemic vasculitis* – Autoimmune connective tissue-associated vasculitis (e.g. rheumatoid arthritis, SLE, Sjögren syndrome)* • Calciphylaxis • Sneddon syndrome • Livedoid vasculopathy (also intraluminal obstruction) • Adenosine deaminase 2 deficiency (can present as Sneddon syndrome or PAN)
Intraluminal pathology
• Increased normal blood components (e.g. thrombocythemia, polycythemia vera) • Abnormal proteins (e.g. cryoglobulinemia, paraproteinemia; see Ch. 18) • Hypercoagulability (e.g. antiphospholipid antibody syndrome, protein C or S deficiency, antithrombin III deficiency, factor V Leiden mutation, DIC; see Table 18.5) • Thrombotic thrombocytopenic purpura • Emboli (e.g. cholesterol, septic) • Hyperoxaluria • Intralymphatic histiocytosis
Other
• Medications (e.g. amantadine, norepinephrine, interferon) • Infections (e.g. hepatitis C [vasculitis], *Mycoplasma* spp. [cold agglutinins], syphilis) • Neoplasms (e.g. pheochromocytomas, multiple myeloma) • Neurologic disorders (e.g. complex regional pain syndrome [reflex sympathetic dystrophy], paralysis) • Moyamoya disease

**Can also present with cutaneous small vessel vasculitis.*

Table 87.1 Causes of livedo reticularis. DIC, disseminated intravascular coagulation; PAN, polyarteritis nodosa.

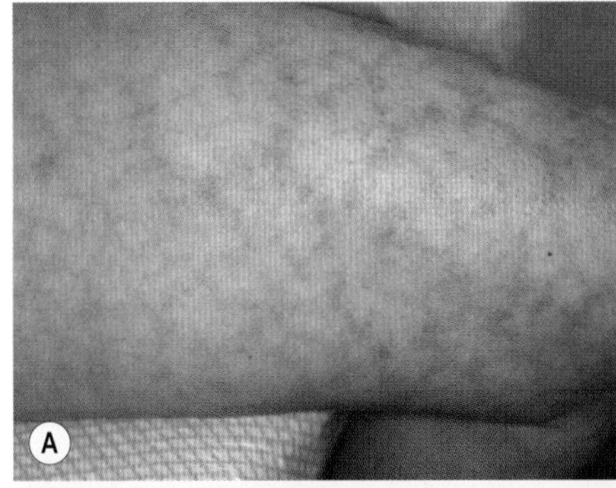

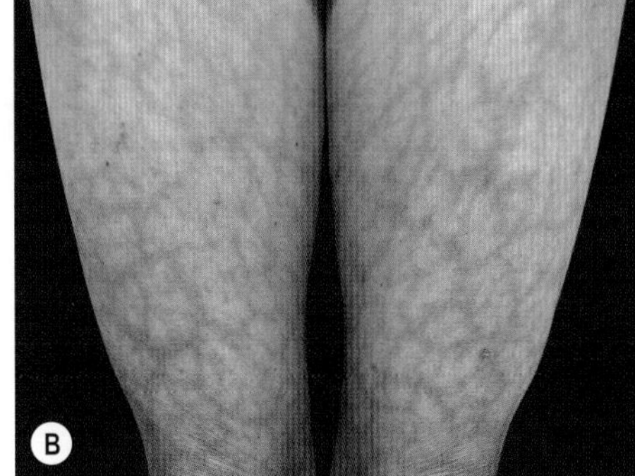

Fig. 87.2 Livedo reticularis. A An even, netlike pattern is seen on the thigh in physiologic livedo reticularis; in primary (idiopathic) livedo reticularis, the pattern persists with rewarming. **B** Livedo reticularis in a patient with SLE. *A, Courtesy, Christopher Baker, MD, and Robert Kelly, MD; B, Courtesy, Jeffrey P. Callen, MD.*

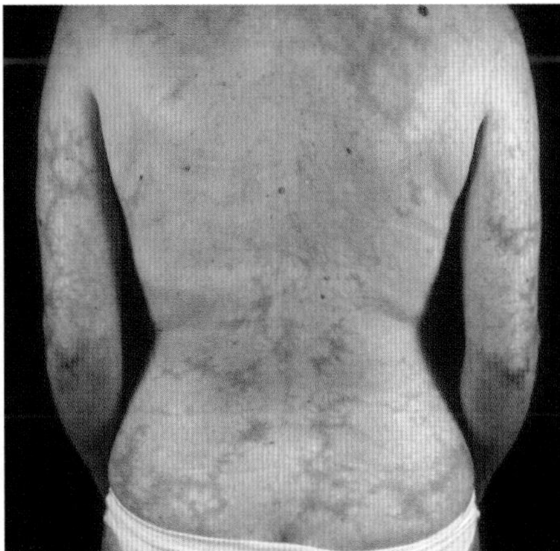

Fig. 87.3 Sneddon syndrome. The characteristic irregular, broken, branching pattern of livedo racemosa is seen on the back and arms. Pediatric-onset livedo racemosa and stroke with or without polyarteritis nodosa should prompt consideration of adenosine deaminase 2 deficiency. *Courtesy, Christopher Baker, MD, and Robert Kelly, MD.*

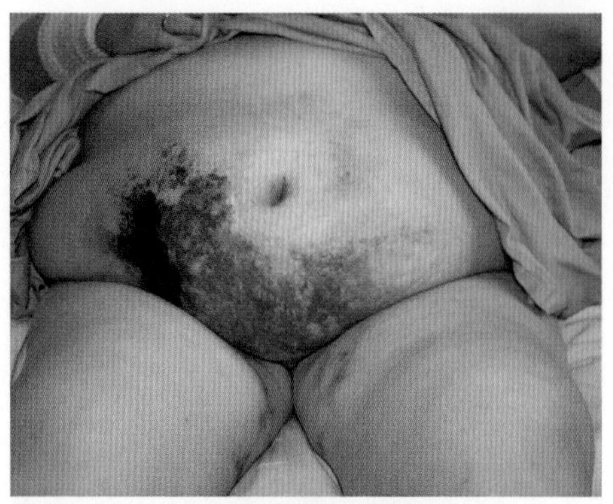

Fig. 87.4 Calciphylaxis in a patient with end-stage chronic renal disease. There is retiform purpura and a large black eschar overlying cutaneous necrosis. Note the violaceous reticulated pattern on the inner thighs. Because the patient was also receiving warfarin, the differential diagnosis included warfarin necrosis. *Courtesy, Alicia Little, MD.*

retiform purpura and necrosis due to more complete disruption of blood flow (Fig. 87.4; see Ch. 18); underlying etiologies are outlined in Table 87.1.

- **Rx:** can improve with treatment of an underlying systemic disorder; no treatment currently available for the idiopathic form.

Flushing

- Exaggerated physiologic dilatation of superficial cutaneous blood vessels that can be triggered by a number of factors, including heat, spicy foods, hot drinks, and anxiety; the resultant erythema of the skin is episodic and transient and may be accompanied by sweating.
- Common etiologies are menopause, other causes of estrogen deficiency (e.g. tamoxifen), rosacea, and medications (e.g. nicotinic acid, nitrates); uncommon causes are carcinoid syndrome, mastocytosis, and pheochromocytoma (Table 87.2).
- Sites of involvement, primarily the face > ears, neck, and chest, are both visible and characterized by greater vasculature capacitance; an approach to the evaluation of a patient with flushing is outlined in Table 87.3.
- **Rx:** avoidance of exacerbating factors; addressing any underlying systemic disorder; for physiologic flushing – propranolol, nadolol, or clonidine; for menopausal "hot flashes" – hormone replacement therapy, SSRIs, or clonidine; laser therapy can address telangiectasias that may result from repeated episodes of flushing.

CAUSES OF FLUSHING
• Physiologic • Estrogen deficiency (e.g. menopause, tamoxifen, raloxifene*) • Rosacea (also triggered by exogenous agents) • Exogenous agents – Alcohol, especially poor metabolizers – Drugs (e.g. nicotinic acid, nitrates, PDE5 inhibitors [e.g. sildenafil], prostaglandins, disulfiram**, chlorpropamide**, methylphenidate, calcium channel blockers, calcitonin) • Foods (e.g. spoiled scombroid fish) • Food additives (e.g. monosodium glutamate, sodium nitrite, sulfites) • Neurologic disorders – Anxiety – Autonomic dysfunction – Tumors (e.g. hypogonadal pituitary tumors) – Migraine – Frey syndrome (auriculotemporal syndrome) • Systemic disease – Carcinoid syndrome (also vascular rosacea-like changes, pellagra, facial edema)*** – Mastocytosis (also red-brown papules, plaques, or nodules) – Pheochromocytoma (also macular amyloidosis if MEN 2a) – Medullary carcinoma of the thyroid (also macular amyloidosis if MEN 2a) – Thyrotoxicosis (also hyperhidrosis) – POEMS syndrome – Pancreatic tumors (e.g. VIPomas)

**Agonist effects on bone and cholesterol.*
***With alcohol intake.*
****Midgut tumors with liver metastases, type III gastric tumors, and bronchial tumors.*

Table 87.2 Causes of flushing. PDE5, phosphodiesterase type 5; POEMS, polyneuropathy, organomegaly, endocrinopathy, M-protein (monoclonal gammopathy), skin changes; VIP, vasoactive intestinal polypeptide.

Erythromelalgia

- Erythema, warmth, and painful burning sensation of the distal extremities (lower > upper) that is usually episodic but may be constant (Fig. 87.5); relieved by cooling and

CLINICAL APPROACH TO THE EVALUATION OF FLUSHING
1. Identify provocative factors • Direct questioning (e.g. menopause, perimenopause) • Patient diary (food, medications, supplements, activities)
2. Check for associated symptoms • Sweating • Urticaria • Diarrhea • Bronchospasm
3. Investigation (not required in all cases) Indicated if flushing: • Of sudden or recent onset • Severe • Associated with systemic symptoms Investigations to consider: • Serum estradiol, FSH, LH (in women) • Complete blood count with differential and platelets • Thyroid function tests • Serum tryptase [M] and/or chromogranin A levels [C]; plasma free metanephrines [P] • 24-hour urine collection for: – Serotonin metabolites such as 5-hydroxyindole acetic acid (5-HIAA) [C] – Fractionated metanephrines [P] – Histamine metabolites such as methylimidazole acetic acid (MIAA) [M] • CT/MRI scans; somatostatin receptor scintigraphy (using radiolabeled analogue of somatostatin)
4. Elimination • Exclude suspected drugs and food additives

Table 87.3 Clinical approach to the evaluation of flushing. C, carcinoid; FSH, follicle stimulating hormone; LH, luteinizing hormone; M, mastocytosis; P, pheochromocytoma.

precipitated by warming, with attacks often beginning in the evening.

• Three major forms: (1) associated with thrombocythemia, (2) primary or "idiopathic" that can be familial, and (3) associated with underlying disorders other than thrombocythemia (e.g. myelodysplasia, SLE); in some families, gain-of-function mutations in *SCN9A*, which encodes a subunit of a voltage-gated sodium channel, have been identified and are thought to lead to "overexcitability" of pain-signaling sensory neurons.

• **DDx:** complex regional pain syndrome (reflex sympathetic dystrophy), peripheral neuropathy, autonomic dysfunction, acrodynia, thromboangiitis obliterans, administration of calcium channel blockers.

• **Rx:** cooling techniques, leg elevation, oral analgesics, topical anesthetics, SSRIs, tricyclic antidepressants, gabapentin, carbamazepine, magnesium; for those with thrombocythemia, aspirin; for those with *SCN9A* mutations, sodium channel blocking agents (e.g. mexiletine, flecainide).

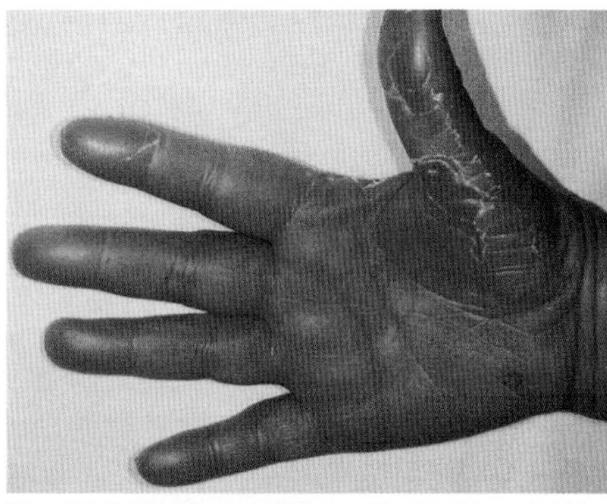

Fig. 87.5 Erythromelalgia. Red hot hand with painful burning sensation. *Courtesy, Agustin Aloma, MD.*

Telangiectasias

• Permanently dilated superficial cutaneous blood vessels; fine (diameter 0.1–1 mm), red to blue-violet in color, and usually fade with pressure (Fig. 87.6).

• Although most commonly seen on the face and on the lower extremities in the settings of photodamage and venous hypertension, respectively, telangiectasias are associated with a number of conditions (Table 87.4) and have several variants (see later).

• **Rx:** fine wire diathermy, injection sclerotherapy (legs), laser or intense pulsed light therapy.

Spider Telangiectasia (Spider Angioma)

• Characterized by a red papule with multiple radiating fine vessels ("legs"); the papular component is the site of the feeding arteriole; usually present as isolated lesions in children but are often multiple when associated with hyperestrogenemia, e.g. in the setting of pregnancy or hepatic cirrhosis in men.

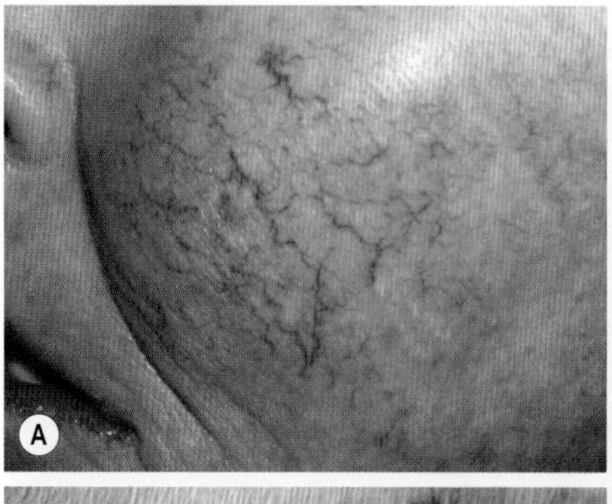

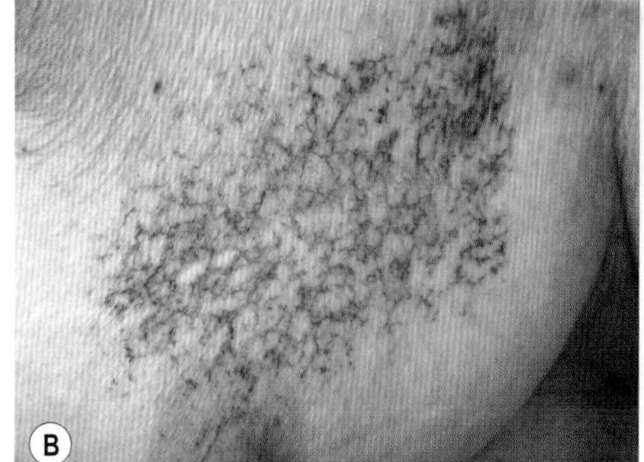

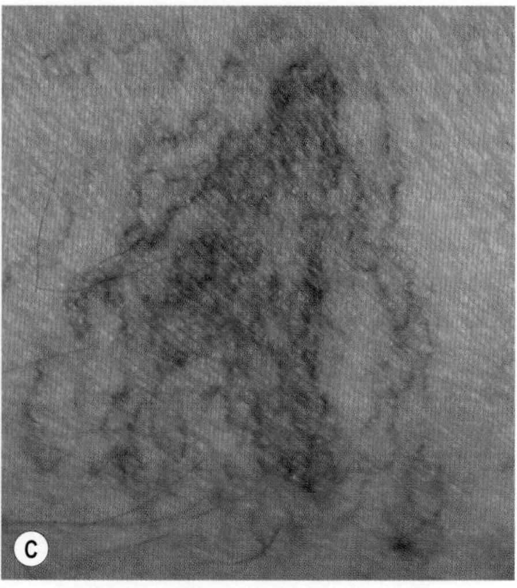

Fig. 87.6 Telangiectasias. A Sun-induced linear and branching telangiectasias on the cheek. **B** Prominent telangiectasias on the breast following radiation therapy. Note the overall rectangular configuration. **C** Venulectasias of the leg, which have a larger diameter (1–2 mm). The latter are a reflection of venous hypertension. *A, B, Courtesy, Christopher Baker, MD, and Robert Kelly, MD; C, Courtesy, Jean L. Bolognia, MD.*

CAUSES OF TELANGIECTASIAS
Primary
• Spider telangiectasias (also associated with estrogen excess) (Fig. 87.8) • Hereditary benign telangiectasia (Fig. 87.7) • Costal fringe • Angioma serpiginosum (Fig. 87.9) • Unilateral nevoid telangiectasia (Fig. 87.10) • Generalized essential telangiectasia (Fig. 87.11) • Cutaneous collagenous vasculopathy
Secondary to physical changes or damage
• Photodamage (Fig. 87.6A) • Post radiation therapy (Fig. 87.6B) • Traumatic • Venous hypertension (Fig. 87.6C)
Skin disease
• Telangiectatic rosacea (see Ch. 30) • Incipient, minimally progressive, or involuted infantile hemangiomas (see Figs 85.2 and 85.3) • Basal cell carcinoma
Hormonal/metabolic

• Estrogen-related
  – Liver disease
  – Pregnancy
  – Exogenous estrogens
• Corticosteroids

Table 87.4 Causes of telangiectasias. *Continued*

CAUSES OF TELANGIECTASIAS
Systemic conditions
• Carcinoid syndrome • Mastocytosis (telangiectasia macularis eruptiva perstans) (see Fig. 96.5) • Autoimmune connective tissue diseases – Lupus erythematosus – Dermatomyositis (see Fig. 34.3) – Systemic sclerosis (see Fig. 35.6) • Mycosis fungoides, including poikilodermatous • B-cell lymphomas • Angiolupoid sarcoidosis • GVHD (in the context of poikiloderma) • HIV infection (anterior chest)
Congenital malformations and genodermatoses*
• Cutis marmorata telangiectatica congenita • Hereditary hemorrhagic telangiectasia (Fig. 87.12) • Ataxia–telangiectasia (see Fig. 49.1) • Bloom syndrome (see Ch. 73) • Goltz syndrome (in lines of Blaschko)

**Not exhaustive list.*

Table 87.4 *Continued* **Causes of telangiectasias.**

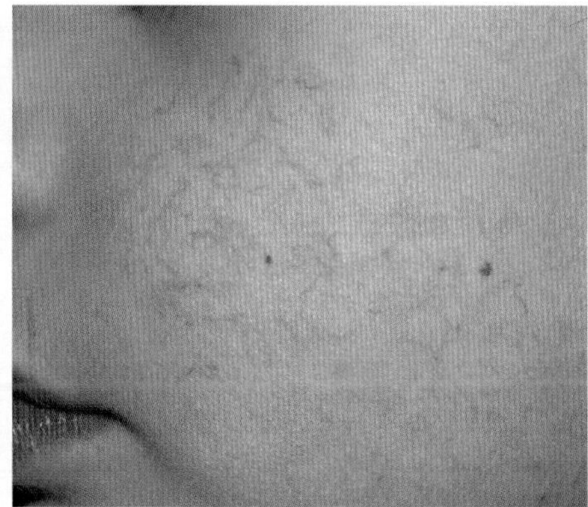

Fig. 87.7 Hereditary benign telangiectasia. Multiple linear and arborizing telangiectasias appear during childhood and favor the sun-exposed areas of the face and upper extremities; the vermilion lips and palate are occasionally affected, but there is no visceral involvement. *Courtesy, Julie V. Schaffer, MD.*

• Usually develop in otherwise healthy women and children, with the most common locations being the face, neck, chest, and hands (Fig. 87.8).

Generalized Essential Telangiectasia

• Broad areas composed of multiple linear telangiectasias that vary in color from red to purple; involvement is often symmetrical and usually begins on the ankles, primarily of adult women (Fig. 87.11); over time, there is typically proximal spread.

• Although these linear telangiectasias can become quite extensive, the disorder remains a cosmetic one, i.e. there are no associated systemic manifestations.

• **DDx:** cutaneous collagenous vasculopathy (similar clinical appearance but central distribution and perivascular deposits of type IV collagen histologically); initially, telangiectasias due to venous hypertension.

Hereditary Hemorrhagic Telangiectasia (Osler–Weber–Rendu Disease)

• Autosomal dominant disorder due to mutations in several genes, particularly the two that encode endoglin and ALK-1, both of which are TGF-β receptors expressed in the vascular endothelium.

• The vascular lesions are actually arteriovenous malformations (AVMs) and are found in the skin, mucous membranes, GI tract, CNS, and other visceral organs (e.g. lung, liver); the disorder most often initially presents as recurrent epistaxis due to involvement of the nasal mucosa, with hemorrhage at other sites usually occurring later in life.

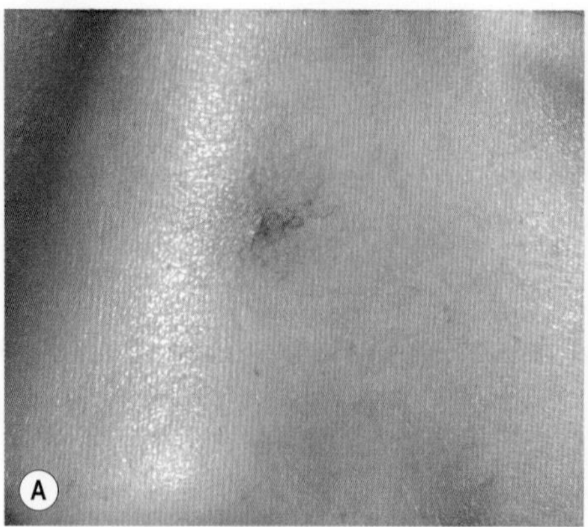

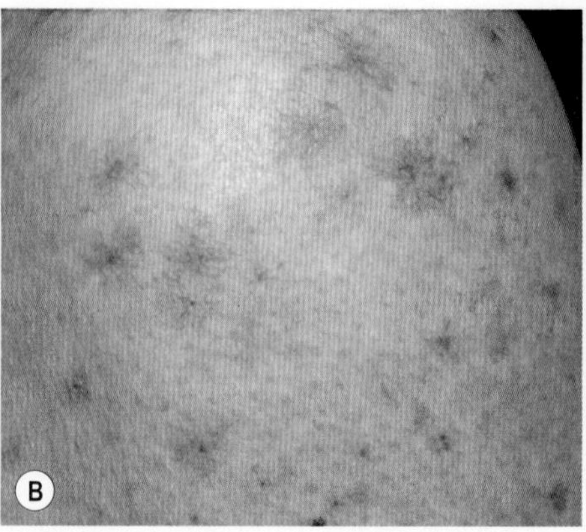

Fig. 87.8 Spider telangiectasias. They are characterized by a central arteriole with radiating telangiectatic "legs". **A** Single lesion on the nose of a young child. **B** Multiple lesions on the shoulder of an adult with liver disease. *A, Courtesy, Julie V. Schaffer, MD; B, Courtesy, Jeffrey P. Callen, MD.*

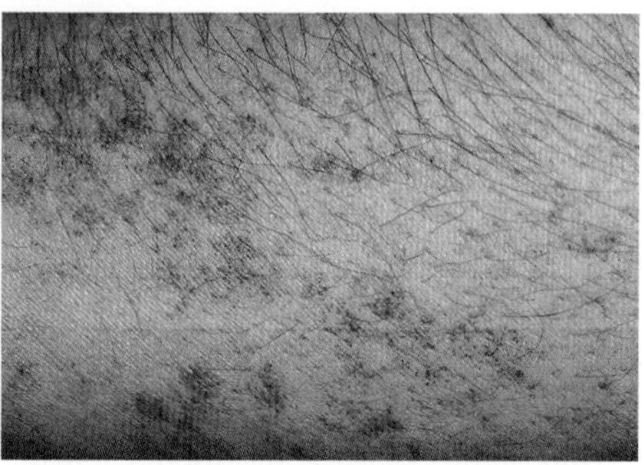

Fig. 87.9 Angioma serpiginosum. Clusters of dark red puncta on the arm in a serpiginous pattern. This disorder initially favors a single extremity, usually in a girl, and may be confused with a pigmented purpuric eruption. *Courtesy, YDRSC.*

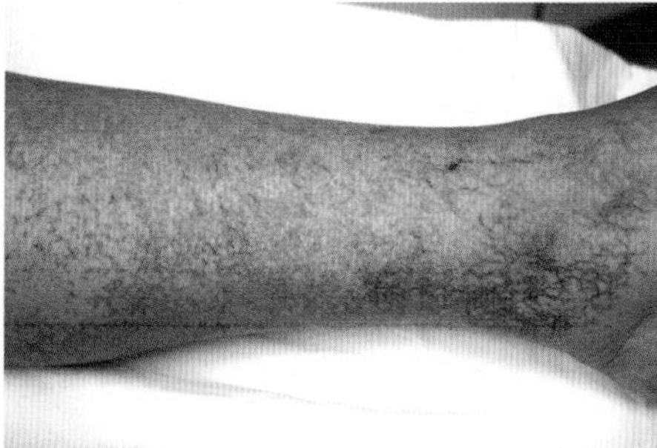

Fig. 87.11 Generalized essential telangiectasia. The site of initial involvement is usually the distal lower extremities. Sheets of asymptomatic blanchable telangiectasias appear bilaterally and over time can become widespread. *Courtesy, Jean L. Bolognia, MD.*

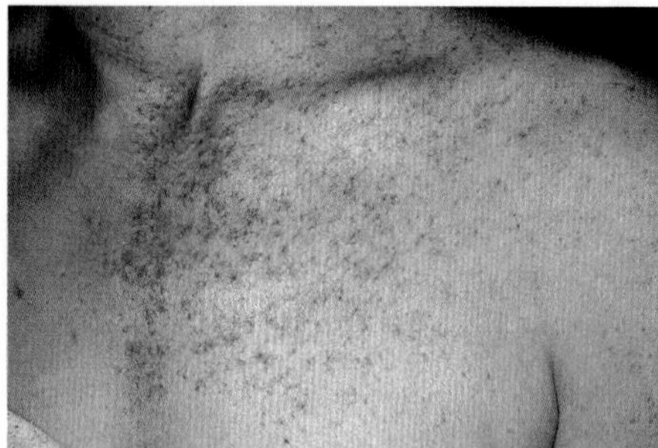

Fig. 87.10 Unilateral nevoid telangiectasia. Discrete telangiectasias in a unilateral, segmental distribution pattern. This is a common location. *Courtesy, Robert Hartman, MD.*

- The oral mucosal lesions (tongue, lips) usually appear during adolescence and predate the cutaneous "telangiectasias" (face, hands); there is an increase in the overall number of lesions with time (Fig. 87.12).
- Clinical criteria: (1) spontaneous recurrent epistaxis, (2) characteristic mucocutaneous telangiectasias/AVMs, (3) visceral telangiectasias/AVMs, and (4) HHT in a first-degree relative; definite diagnosis if ≥3 criteria and possible/suspected diagnosis if 1 or 2 criteria (especially in children and young adults).
- Evaluation is outlined in Table 87.5.

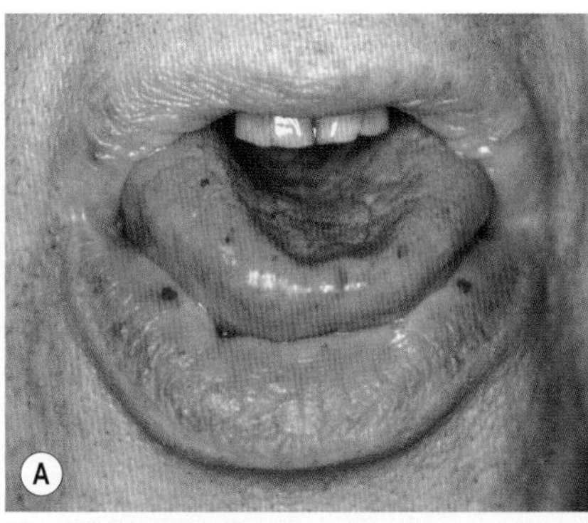

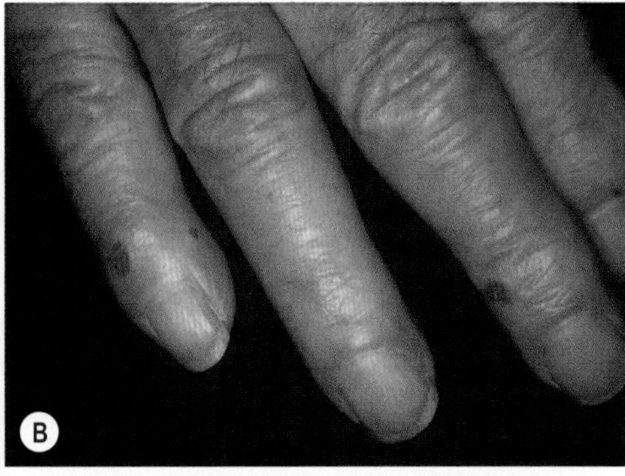

Fig. 87.12 Hereditary hemorrhagic telangiectasia (Osler–Weber–Rendu disease). The majority of lesions are papular, but occasionally they resemble the mat telangiectasias observed in systemic sclerosis. **A, B** Common locations include the tongue and lips as well as the fingers, with the former predating the latter. *A, Courtesy, YDRSC; B, Courtesy, Irwin Braverman, MD.*

STUDIES RECOMMENDED TO SCREEN FOR SYSTEMIC INVOLVEMENT AND ASSIST IN THE DIAGNOSIS OF HEREDITARY HEMORRHAGIC TELANGIECTASIA (HHT)			
Study and purpose	**Frequency**	**Indication(s)**	**% of HHT patients**
Transthoracic contrast echocardiography (bubble study) to detect **pulmonary** AVMs	If initial screening negative, repeat every 5–10 years as well as prior to and following pregnancies	Suspected or confirmed HHT	15–50
Brain MRI with and without gadolinium to detect **cerebral** AVMs and other vascular malformations	If initial screening negative, repeat at age 18 years	Suspected or confirmed HHT	~25
Hemoglobin and hematocrit levels to detect GI bleeding due to **GI** AVMs	Yearly after age 35 years	HHT patients	~25
Doppler ultrasonography or triphasic spiral CT of liver to detect **hepatic** AVMs	If signs or symptoms of heart failure or hepatobiliary disease	HHT patients	30–80
	As a clinical criterion (see text)	Suspected or confirmed HHT	
Genetic analysis of *ENG* and/or *ACVRL1* (then *SMAD4* or *GDF2* if negative) of index case	Once unless additional genes identified or improved methodology	Also performed in first-degree relatives of HHT patients or suspected HHT	~75 for *ENG* or *ACVRL1*; 1–3 for *SMAD4*

Table 87.5 Studies recommended to screen for systemic involvement and assist in the diagnosis of hereditary hemorrhagic telangiectasia (HHT).

- **Rx:** laser therapy, diathermy, transcatheter embolotherapy (e.g. for lung AVMs so as to avoid right-to-left shunting and risk of paradoxical embolization), surgical intervention.

Ataxia–Telangiectasia (see Ch. 49)

- Primary immunodeficiency syndrome inherited in an autosomal recessive manner in which telangiectasias appear on the bulbar conjunctivae during childhood as

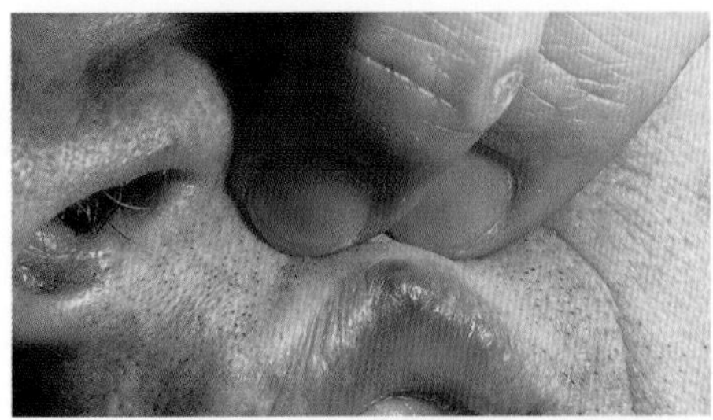

Fig. 87.13 Venous lake on the vermilion lip. This dark blue papule is soft and, with compression, can be emptied of most of its blood content. *Courtesy, Ronald Rapini, MD.*

well as in the head and neck region (eyelids, malar, ears) and antecubital and popliteal fossae.

Venous Lake

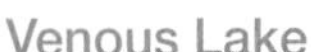

- A blue, soft papule that is compressible and, with pressure, both its color and elevation are diminished (Fig. 87.13); represents dilation of superficial blood vessels.
- Most common sites are vermilion lip > face, ears.
- **Rx:** electrosurgery, vascular laser therapy.

Angiokeratomas

- See Chapter 94

Nevus Anemicus

- Congenital circumscribed area of pale vasoconstriction, often 5–10 cm in diameter and occurs most commonly on the trunk (Fig. 87.14).
- The edges are irregular and disappear via diascopy (pressure), allowing distinction from nevus depigmentosus or vitiligo; application of heat or an ice cube accentuates the border as a result of hyperemia of surrounding uninvolved skin.

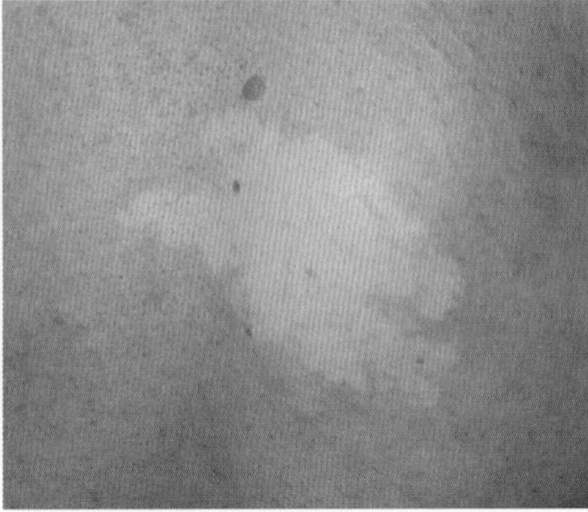

Fig. 87.14 Nevus anemicus. Pale area of vasoconstriction with irregular borders on the back. *Courtesy, YDRSC.*

Angiospastic Macules (Bier Spots)

- Pale macules due to relative vasoconstriction within areas of subtle vascular mottling (Fig. 87.15); as with nevus anemicus, the border disappears with diascopy (pressure); dependency leads to accentuation of lesions due to venous congestion.
- Most commonly observed in young healthy adults with lightly pigmented skin; no effective **Rx.**

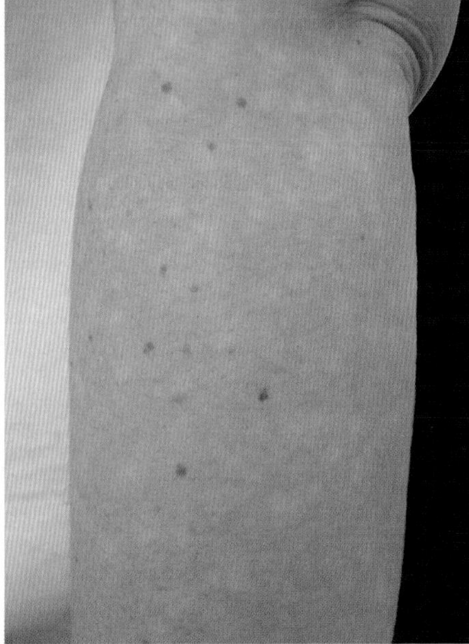

Fig. 87.15 Angiospastic macules (Bier spots). Multiple pale macules due to vasoconstriction within a background of erythema on the forearm.

For further information see Ch. 106 from *Dermatology, Fourth Edition*.

For additional online figures visit www.expertconsult.com 

Actinic Keratosis, Basal Cell Carcinoma, and Squamous Cell Carcinoma

Introduction

- Keratinocyte carcinoma (KC), also referred to as non-melanoma skin cancer (NMSC), is the most frequently observed malignancy in Caucasians.
- KC typically refers to basal cell carcinoma (BCC) and squamous cell carcinoma (SCC).
- In individuals with fair skin, ~75–80% of KCs are BCCs, and up to 25% are SCCs.
- The two most important risk factors for developing KC are skin phototype (see Appendix) and exposure to UVR (Table 88.1).
- The presence of actinic keratoses (AKs) and/or KCs increases the likelihood of future KCs and cutaneous melanoma, particularly lentigo maligna; such persons require lifelong surveillance via total body skin examination (TBSE).
- Based upon epidemiologic studies, KCs have been associated with an increased risk of internal malignancies; the risk is greatest in persons with numerous KCs and in those with younger age of onset of KCs.

Actinic Keratoses (AKs)

- Also referred to as solar keratoses, AKs are considered "precancerous" lesions that have the potential to progress into invasive SCC; estimates of progression vary from a rate of 0.075–0.1% per lesion per year to ~10% over 10 years.
- The atypical keratinocytes are confined to the lower portion of the epidermis (Fig. 88.1).
- AKs are one of the most frequently encountered lesions in clinical practice.
- Occur primarily in sites that have received the greatest amount of cumulative sun exposure (e.g. scalp in bald individuals, face, ears, neck, dorsal forearms and hands, shins); seen primarily in middle-aged to older, fair-skinned individuals.
- Classic presentation is a gritty papule with an erythematous base; the associated scale is usually white to yellow in color and feels rough (Fig. 88.2).
- Common clinical variants: pigmented (Fig. 88.2C), hypertrophic (referred to as HAK [Fig. 88.2D, E]), lichenoid, and atrophic (Fig. 88.2B); in actinic cheilitis, there is scaling and roughness of the lower vermilion lip (Fig. 88.2F).
- Dx: usually made by visual inspection and palpation; because of the rough texture, it is sometimes easier to detect lesions via touch.
- AKs have the potential to persist, spontaneously regress, or progress to SCC, but clinically it is difficult to predict which course a given AK will take.
- Clinical clues of progression to invasive SCC and need for biopsy: tenderness, volume (particularly thickness), inflammation, and failure to respond to appropriate therapy.
- **DDx:** SCC *in situ*, BCC, lichen planus-like keratosis (LPLK; see Ch. 89), irritated seborrheic keratosis (SK) or verruca vulgaris, and amelanotic melanoma; for thicker lesions (e.g. HAK), invasive SCC; for lesions on extensor extremities, actinic porokeratosis; occasionally, isolated lesions of psoriasis or seborrheic dermatitis may resemble an AK.
- **Rx:** localized or lesion-targeted treatments are best for an isolated or limited number of lesions; field treatments are best for more numerous or larger lesions (Table 88.2).
- Prevention is possible with broad-spectrum sunscreens and sun avoidance measures; in patients with a history of KCs, use of oral nicotinamide may reduce the development of additional AKs and KCs.

RISK FACTORS FOR THE DEVELOPMENT OF BASAL CELL CARCINOMAS (BCC) AND SQUAMOUS CELL CARCINOMAS (SCC)		
	SCC	**BCC**
Environmental exposures		
UV exposure	+	+
Other exposures to UV light (PUVA, tanning beds)	+	+
Ionizing radiation	+	+
Chemicals, including arsenic, mineral oil, coal tar, soot, mechlorethamine (nitrogen mustard), polychlorinated biphenyls, 4,4′ bipyridyl, psoralen (plus UVA)	+	+
Medications (e.g. HCTZ, voriconazole, BRAF inhibitors [especially when used alone], hydroxyurea)	+	(+)
Human papillomavirus (HPV)	+	(+)
Cigarette smoking	+	
Pigmentary phenotype		
Fair skin, always burns, never tans	+	+
Freckling	+	+
Red hair	+	+
Genetic syndromes		
Xeroderma pigmentosum	+	+
Oculocutaneous albinism	+	+
Epidermodysplasia verruciformis	+	(+)
Dystrophic epidermolysis bullosa (primarily recessive)	+	
Ferguson–Smith syndrome	+	
Muir–Torre syndrome	+*	+*
Basal cell nevus syndrome		+
Bazex–Dupré–Christol and Rombo syndromes		+
Predisposing clinical settings		
Chronic non-healing wounds	+	
Longstanding discoid lupus erythematosus, lichen planus (erosive), or lichen sclerosus	+	
Porokeratosis (especially linear)	+	
Nevus sebaceus	+	+†
Immunosuppression		
Organ transplantation	+	+
Immunosuppressive medications (e.g. azathioprine, cyclosporine, tacrolimus, biologics, prednisone)	+	+
Other (e.g. chronic lymphocytic leukemia treated with fludarabine, AIDS patients with HPV infection, childhood cancer survivors)	+	(+)

**Both SCCs (keratoacanthoma type) and BCCs typically have sebaceous differentiation.*
†More often trichoblastomas.

Table 88.1 Risk factors for the development of basal cell carcinomas (BCC) and squamous cell carcinomas (SCC).

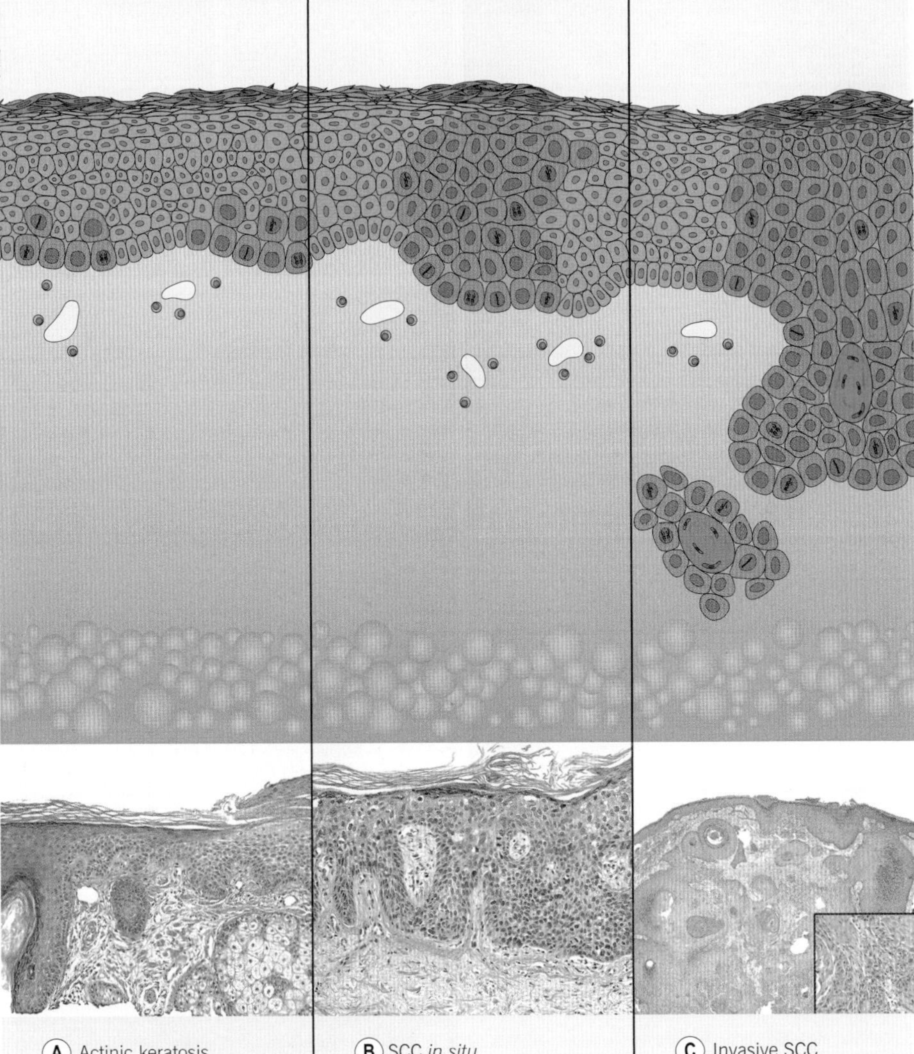

Fig. 88.1 The histopathologic features of actinic keratosis (AK), SCC *in situ*, and invasive SCC. **A** An AK consists of a lower epidermal proliferation of cytologically abnormal keratinocytes; the adnexal epithelium is notably spared. **B** In SCC *in situ*, the atypical keratinocytes occupy the entire epidermis and intraepidermal portion of adnexal structures, without invasion into the dermis. **C** Invasive SCC is distinguished by the extension of the malignant keratinocytes into the dermis. If an invasive SCC is clinically suspected, the biopsy specimen should be deep enough to determine the extent of dermal invasion.

SCC *In Situ* (Bowen Disease)

- May arise *de novo* or from a pre-existing AK; sometimes caused by oncogenic strains of human papillomavirus (HPV, e.g. periungual [see Ch. 66]).
- Keratinocyte atypia is seen throughout the entire epidermis (full-thickness) (see Fig. 88.1) and has the potential to progress to invasive SCC, with an estimated risk of ~3–5% if untreated.
- With the exception of HPV- or arsenic-related SCC *in situ*, the risk factors for and the locations of SCC *in situ* are similar to those for AKs (see above and Table 88.1).

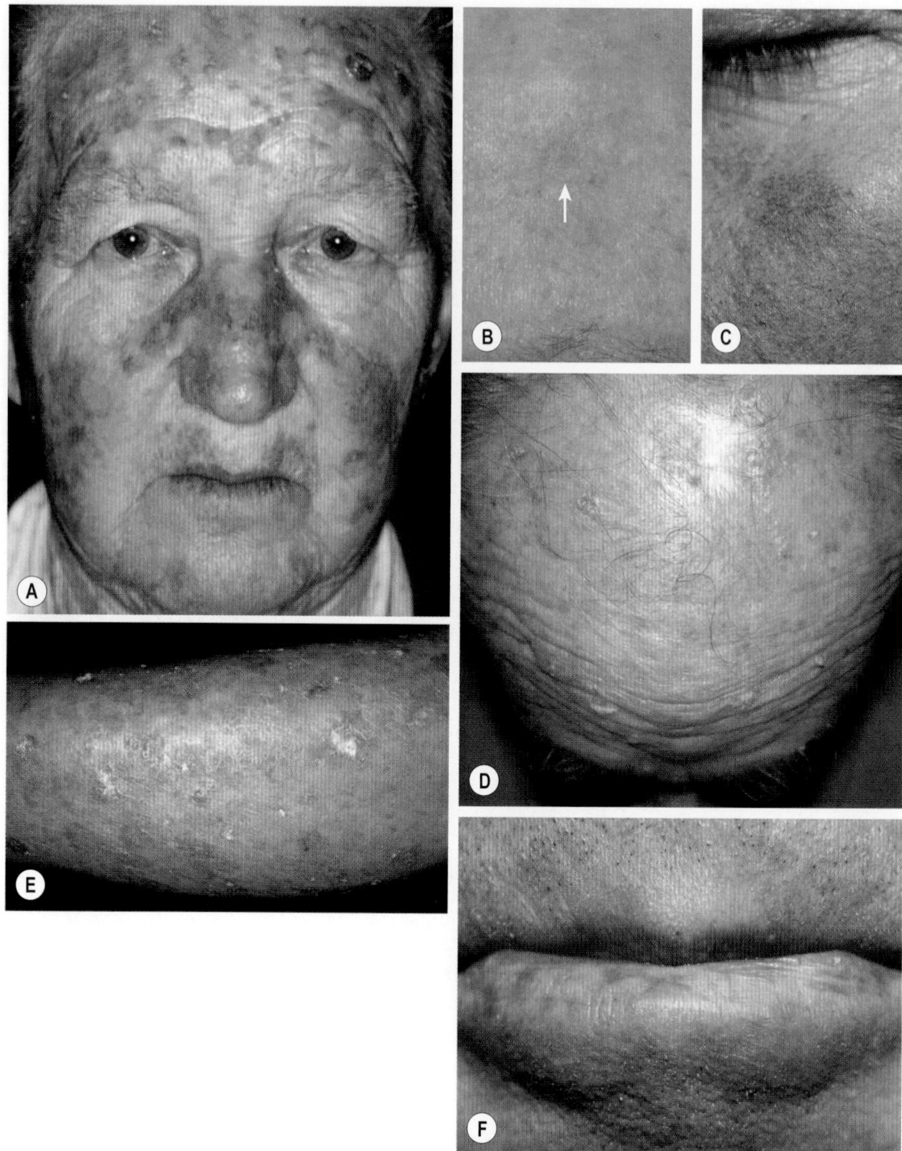

Fig. 88.2 Actinic keratoses (AKs). A Multiple AKs on the face of an elderly woman with fair complexion, blue eyes, and moderate to severe photodamage; the AKs vary in size from a few millimeters to more than 1 cm. On the left forehead, the red nodule with slight scale-crust represents a well-differentiated SCC. **B** Pink-colored atrophic AK with minimal scale on the forehead. **C** Pigmented AK presenting as a subtle hyperpigmented, reticulated macule on the cheek; there may be associated scale but an absence of erythema. **D** Multiple AKs on the bald scalp, some of which are hypertrophic; the area of hypopigmentation represents a site of previous treatment and due to the field defect, recurrence at the edge is commonly seen. **E** Multiple, large hypertrophic AKs on the shin of an elderly woman; note the thick scale. **F** Actinic cheilitis presenting with erythema and scale of the entire lower vermilion lip; note the erosions and areas of leukoplakia. *A, Courtesy, H. Peter Sawyer, MD; B, Courtesy, Iris Zalaudek, MD; C, F, Courtesy Kalman Watsky, MD; D, Courtesy, Luis Requena, MD; E, Courtesy, Jean L. Bolognia, MD.*

COMMON TREATMENT OPTIONS FOR ACTINIC KERATOSES (AKS)	
Localized/lesion-targeted treatments*	
Lesion-targeted treatment	**Helpful hints**
Liquid nitrogen cryosurgery	• No cutting or anesthesia necessary • 10- to 14-day healing period • Risk of hypopigmentation
Curettage (> curettage + electrodesiccation)	• Requires local anesthesia • Risk of hypopigmentation and scarring (less so if curettage alone)
Shave excision	• Requires local anesthesia • Risk of hypopigmentation and scarring

Topical field treatments,†**		
Although these are the recommended FDA dosing schedules, if the patient develops significant burning with application or significant erosive erythema, the treatment should be held or discontinued.		
Topical agent	**Dosing**	**Helpful hints**
5-Fluorouracil	• 1.0% or 5.0% cream – apply twice a day for 2–4 weeks • 2.0% and 5.0% solutions – apply twice a day for 2–4 weeks • 0.5% cream – apply at bedtime × 4 weeks • When treating extensor extremities, pretreatment with a topical retinoid for 1–2 weeks may be required • For severe leg involvement, occluded "chemowraps" may be used • 5.0% cream can be combined with topical 0.005% calcipotriene (calcipotriol) ointment twice a day for 4 days	• Warn of photosensitivity, which can be severe • Optimal results occur if treatment continues until there is significant inflammation or mild superficial erosions • Healing usually occurs within 2 weeks of stopping treatment • Solution is best for hair-bearing areas, such as the scalp
Imiquimod	• 2.5% or 3.75% cream – apply at bedtime for 2 weeks; take a 2-week break, and then repeat 2-week application cycle • 5% cream – apply twice a week for 16 consecutive weeks • Recommended treatment area is 25 cm^2	• May cause systemic flu-like symptoms • Not recommended if patient has an underlying autoimmune condition • May cause hypopigmentation at the treated site
Diclofenac	• 3% gel – apply twice a day for 90 days • A maximum amount of 8 gm daily should not be exceeded	• Do not use if patient is allergic to NSAIDs • Although it may have a less severe cutaneous reaction, compliance is an issue given a longer application period
Ingenol mebutate[$]	• 0.015% gel – apply at bedtime for 3 consecutive nights (face and scalp) • 0.05% gel – apply at bedtime for 2 consecutive nights (trunk and extremities)	• Rapid onset of action; typically within 24 hours of application, patient will experience erythema and burning • Healing occurs within 10–14 days • Supposedly does not cause hypopigmentation

Table 88.2 Common treatment options for actinic keratoses (AKs). *Continued*

COMMON TREATMENT OPTIONS FOR ACTINIC KERATOSES (AKS)	
Procedural field treatments**,†	
Procedure	Helpful hints
Photodynamic therapy (e.g. 5-ALA + blue light)	• Can be painful • Requires 48 hours of no outdoor exposure post-treatment • Relatively quick recovery over 1–2 weeks
Chemical peels (e.g. trichloroacetic acid)	• May require local anesthesia • May cause significant irritation and temporary discoloration • Healing typically over 7 days
Ablative laser techniques (e.g. ablative fractional lasers, erbium:YAG laser)	• Requires local anesthesia • Depending on the technique, recovery period varies • Hypopigmentation a potential complication

**Most appropriate for an isolated or limited number of AKs.*

***Most appropriate for numerous or larger AK lesions; a recent study favored 5-fluorouracil over other topical therapies.*

†In practice, combination or sequential therapy is sometimes used (e.g. liquid nitrogen to several thicker lesions followed by 5-fluorouracil or imiquimod).

$Ingenol mebutate has been withdrawn from the EU, UK, and Canadian markets because of concern over an associated increase in cutaneous malignancy.

Table 88.2 *Continued* **Common treatment options for actinic keratoses (AKs).** ALA, aminolevulinic acid.

- Clinically presents as an erythematous patch or thin plaque with scale (Fig. 88.3); occasionally, the lesions are pigmented.
- Less common sites (may be related to HPV infection): beard area, periungual (see Figs 88.3C and 58.8) and subungual, anogenital (now referred to as intraepithelial neoplasia, further qualified by anatomic site [see Ch. 60 and Fig. 88.4]); SCC *in situ* in non-sun-exposed sites may also be related to arsenic exposure.
- Dx: biopsy; dermoscopy may assist in diagnosis (Fig. 88.3B).
- **DDx:** AK, invasive SCC, BCC, LPLK, irritated SK, amelanotic melanoma; occasionally may be misdiagnosed as an isolated lesion of psoriasis or nummular eczema, but a clue is its lack of response to appropriate therapy.
- **Rx:** tangential excision with curettage or electrodesiccation and curettage (especially for smaller lesions), excision, Mohs micrographic surgery (e.g. head and neck, acrogenital); imiquimod cream and topical 5% fluorouracil (twice daily for a longer period, e.g. 8 weeks) may be used when a surgical approach would prove difficult to perform because of location or extent.

Squamous Cell Carcinoma (SCC)

- An invasive mucocutaneous malignancy arising from keratinocytes; may develop *de novo* or from precursor AK or SCC *in situ* (see Fig. 88.1).
- More common in males than females, and incidence increases with age.
- In fair-skinned individuals, the risk factors for and the locations of invasive SCC are similar to those for AKs and SCC *in situ* (see above and Table 88.1).
- In all phototypes, invasive SCC may develop in sites of HPV infection, scars, chronic injury or inflammation, previous radiation therapy, or chemical exposure (e.g. polycyclic aromatic hydrocarbons; see Table 88.1).
- Common clinical presentation is an erythematous, keratotic papule or nodule that arises within a background of sun-damaged skin; tenderness is common; often a history of rapid enlargement (Fig. 88.5) and sometimes a history of antecedent trauma (see Fig. 88.5B).
- Clinical variants: keratoacanthoma (KA) (Fig. 88.6), verrucous carcinoma (Fig. 88.7), mucosal (Fig. 88.8), periungual and subungual.
- Dx: biopsy (should be deep enough to determine extent of dermal invasion); palpate regional lymph node basin.
- **DDx:**
  - *Most common*: AK, HAK, SCC *in situ*, BCC, verruca vulgaris, irritated SK
  - *Less common*: amelanotic melanoma, atypical fibroxanthoma (AFX), Merkel cell carcinoma, adnexal tumors, prurigo nodularis

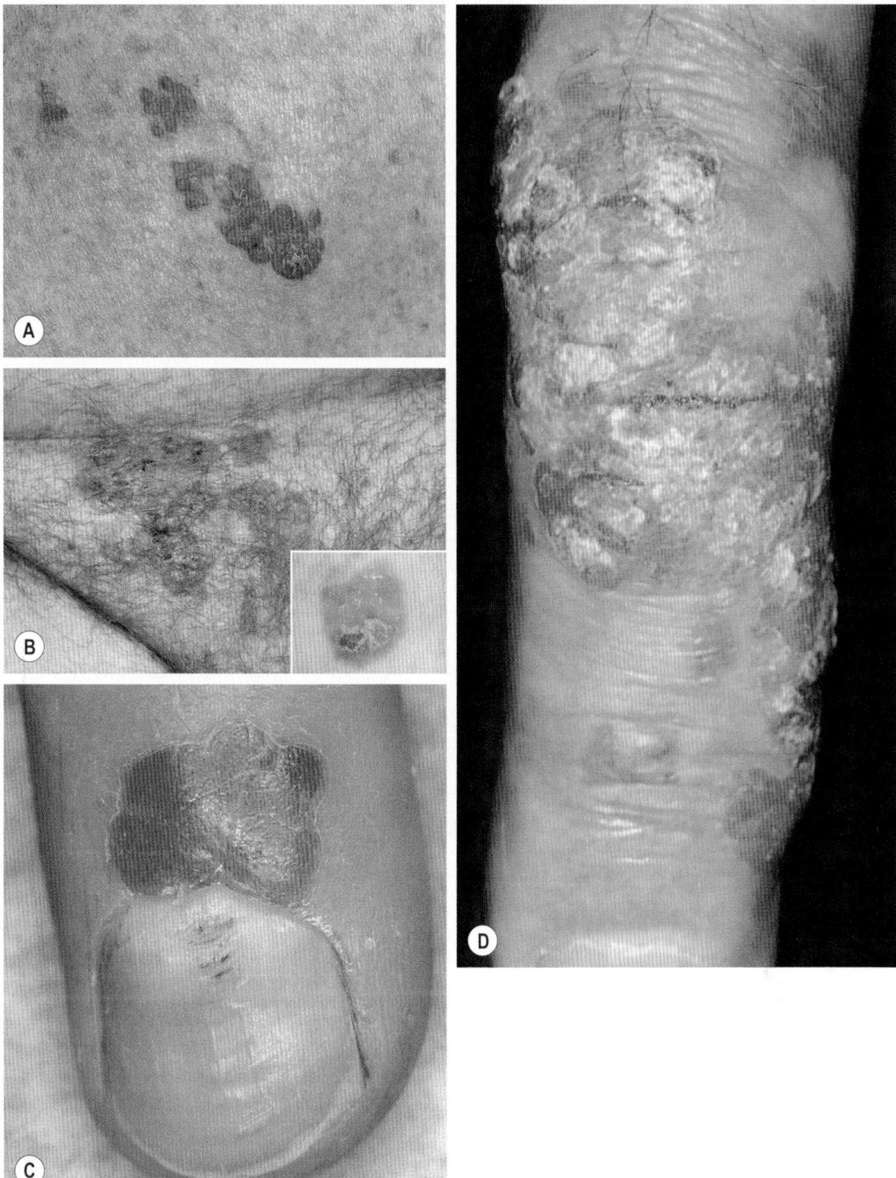

Fig. 88.3 Squamous cell carcinomas *in situ*, Bowen disease type. A Scaly red plaque on the chest with skip areas and background photodamage. **B** Larger broken up pink plaque with scale-crust in the pubic region, a sun protected site. This type of lesion is often misdiagnosed as dermatitis or psoriasis and treated with topical CS; (inset) dermoscopic examination of a pink scaly plaque of SCC *in situ* with tiny dotted vessels in the upper half of the lesion combined with superficial scales. **C** Bright-red, well-demarcated plaque on the proximal nail fold with associated horizontal nail ridging; the possibility of HPV infection needs to be considered. **D** Extensive involvement of the finger, which was misdiagnosed clinically as an inflammatory dermatosis and treated for years with topical CS. *A, C, Courtesy, YDRSC; B, Courtesy, Kalman Watsky, MD; inset, Courtesy, Iris Zalaudek, MD; D, Courtesy, H. Peter Sawyer, MD.*

• A cutaneous SCC staging format has been proposed by the American Joint Commission on Cancer, incorporating the TNM criteria, prognostic factors (tumor thickness, ± perineural invasion, high-risk locations, ± lymph node involvement), histologic grade, and the presence or absence of lymphatic/vascular invasion on histology (Table 88.3).

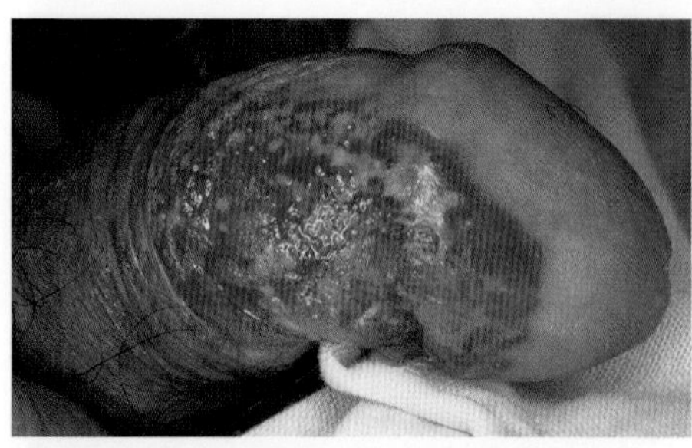

Fig. 88.4 Squamous cell carcinoma, *in situ*, of the penis, also known as penile intraepithelial neoplasia (PIN). Formerly called SCC *in situ*, erythroplasia of Queyrat type. Large eroded erythematous plaque with well-demarcated borders. The lesion began on the shaft of the penis. *Courtesy, YDRSC.*

- Long-term prognosis for adequately treated SCC is excellent.
- Overall, the risk of nodal metastases from invasive SCC has been estimated at 2–4%; ~20% of all skin cancer deaths are due to SCC.
- There are several risk factors for metastasis: lesions on the lips, ear, and mucosae (e.g. tongue, vulva, penis); development within a scar; host immunosuppression; tumor thickness >2 mm; tumor diameter ≥2 cm; poorly differentiated histopathology; development within Bowen disease; perineural invasion.
- Significant cause of morbidity and mortality in solid organ transplant recipients, who are more likely to experience local and regional recurrences, as well as metastases.
- **Rx:** primarily excision, but based on risk factors (Table 88.4), ranges from electrodesiccation and curettage (e.g. smaller, minimally invasive lesion in an elderly patient) to Mohs micrographic surgery (Table 88.5).
- Prophylaxis in high-risk patients: acitretin, low-dose oral capecitabine in solid organ transplant recipients.

Basal Cell Carcinoma (BCC)

- Most common KC in humans; arises *de novo*, with no known precursor lesion.
- More common in males than females; primarily seen in middle-aged to older adults who are fair-skinned; however, the incidence is rising, especially in young women.
- UVR exposure is the greatest risk factor, but in contrast to AK/SCC, intense episodes of burning are more important than chronic long-term exposure; in addition, BCCs can also arise in relatively non-sun-exposed areas, e.g. retroauricular crease and inner canthus (Fig. 88.9C).
- Usually slow-growing; without adequate treatment, BCCs will gradually increase in size and they may ulcerate and cause local destruction of surrounding tissue; metastases are exceedingly rare (regional lymph nodes > lung).
- Multiple clinical variants and varied presentations exist:
  - *Most common*: nodular (pearly papule with telangiectasias and/or umbilication; Fig. 88.9), superficial (typically an erythematous thin plaque on trunk > extremities; Fig. 88.10), pigmented (Fig. 88.11)
  - *Less common*: morpheaform (scar-like; Fig. 88.12), micronodular, cystic, basosquamous, and fibroepithelial (fibroepithelioma of Pinkus) (Fig. 88.13)
- Dx: biopsy; dermoscopy can assist in diagnosis (see Figs 88.9B and 88.11C).
- **DDx:** *nodular*: intradermal melanocytic nevus, fibrous papule, sebaceous hyperplasia, invasive SCC, amelanotic melanoma; *superficial*: LPLK, AK, SCC *in situ*, isolated lesion of psoriasis, seborrheic dermatitis or nummular eczema, amelanotic melanoma; *morpheaform*: scar, adnexal tumors (e.g. desmoplastic trichoepithelioma, microcystic adnexal carcinoma [see Ch. 91]); *pigmented*: melanocytic nevus, seborrheic keratosis, pigmented SCC *in situ*, nodular melanoma.
- Categorize tumor into histologic subtype and whether or not meets criteria for high-risk BCC (e.g. morpheaform, micronodular, or infiltrative; see Table 88.4) or indications for Mohs micrographic surgery to determine best treatment (see Table 88.5); basosquamous lesions are treated as invasive SCCs (see above).
- Nevoid BCC syndrome (NBCS): rare, autosomal dominant, caused by mutations in human *PTCH* gene; characterized by multiple BCCs, palmoplantar pits, odontogenic keratocysts of jaw, skeletal abnormalities, macrocephaly, and calcification of the falx cerebri; patients may develop medulloblastomas during childhood or ovarian fibromas.

For further information see Chs 107–108 from *Dermatology, Fourth Edition*.

For additional online figures and tables visit www.expertconsult.com 

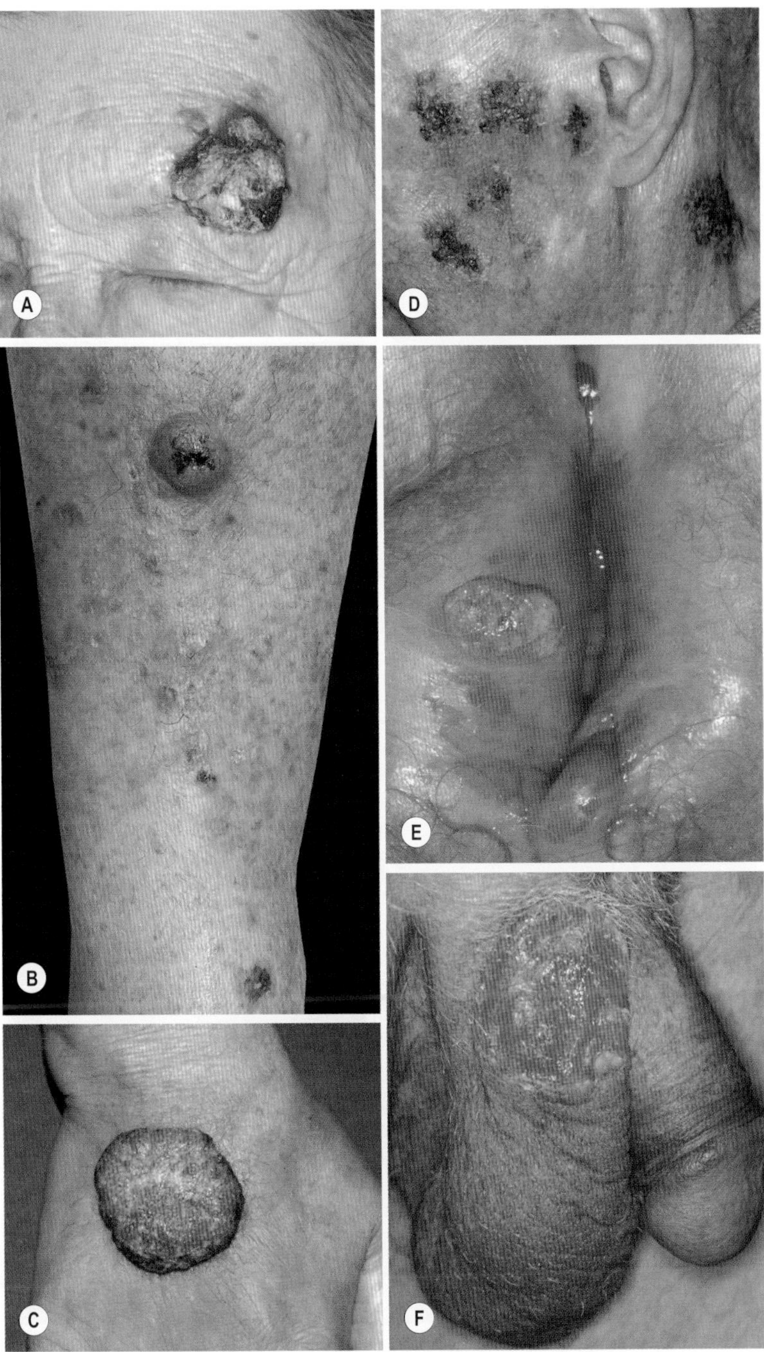

Fig. 88.5 Squamous cell carcinomas (SCCs). A A large keratotic nodule on the supraorbital region in an elderly woman; note the coarse wrinkling and solar elastosis of the face. **B** Eroded and keratotic nodule that developed rapidly at the site of trauma on the shin in a patient with severe photodamage; this has also been described as a reactive process, termed "atypical squamous proliferation". **C** Large, fungating nodule on the dorsum of the hand. **D** Multiple eroded superficial SCCs in association with hypertrophic AKs on the cheek and neck of an elderly man. **E** Erosive, slightly vegetating, thick plaque arising within lichen sclerosus of the vulva. **F** Firm, eroded red plaque on the scrotum; histopathologically, the SCC was moderately differentiated. *A, C–F, Courtesy, H. Peter Sawyer, MD; B, Courtesy, Jean L. Bolognia, MD.*

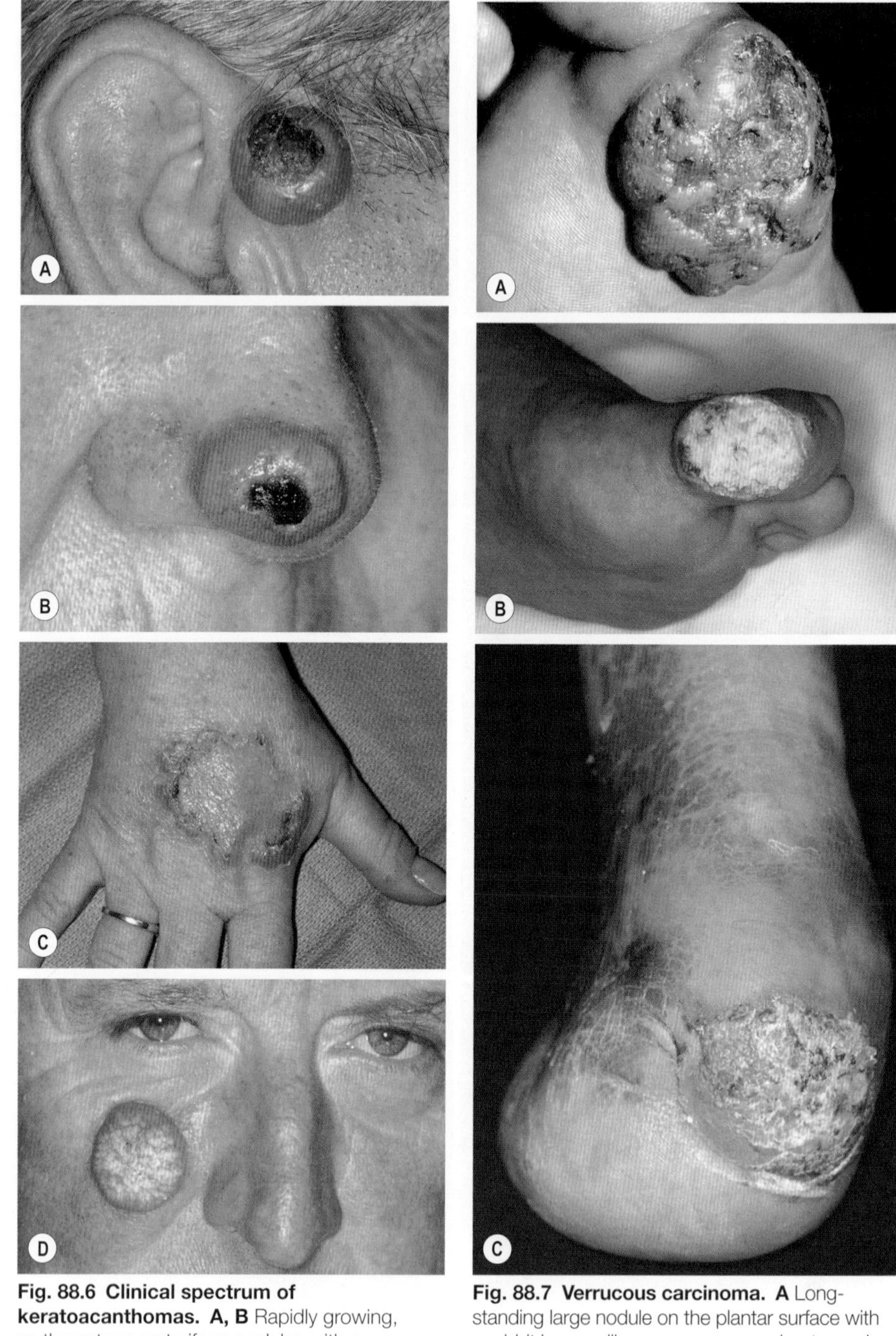

Fig. 88.6 Clinical spectrum of keratoacanthomas. A, B Rapidly growing, erythematous crateriform nodules with a rolled border and central keratotic core. **C** Progressive peripheral expansion and central involution with residual atrophy characterize keratoacanthoma centrifugum marginatum. **D** Giant keratoacanthoma with a yellow-red color and a history of rapid growth. *A, D, Courtesy, H. Peter Sawyer, MD; B, C, Courtesy, YDRSC.*

Fig. 88.7 Verrucous carcinoma. A Long-standing large nodule on the plantar surface with a rabbit burrow-like appearance; such a tumor is also referred to as an epithelioma cuniculatum. **B** Keratotic and ulcerated plaque on the ventromedial aspect of the great toe. The lesion was originally misdiagnosed as a plantar wart. **C** A classic location in an amputation stump. In general, these well-differentiated SCCs enlarge slowly. *A, C, Courtesy, H. Peter Sawyer, MD; B, Courtesy, YDRSC.*

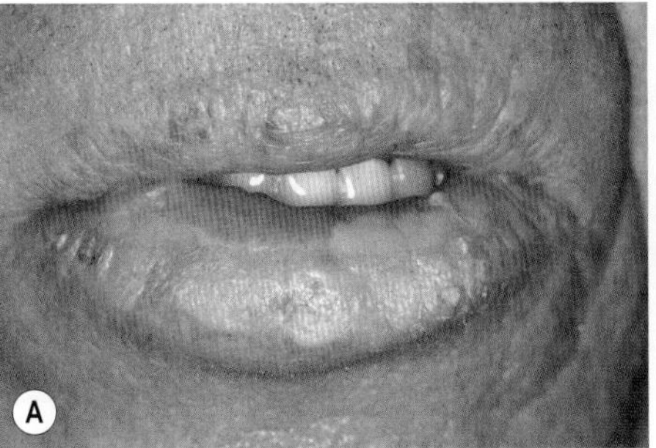

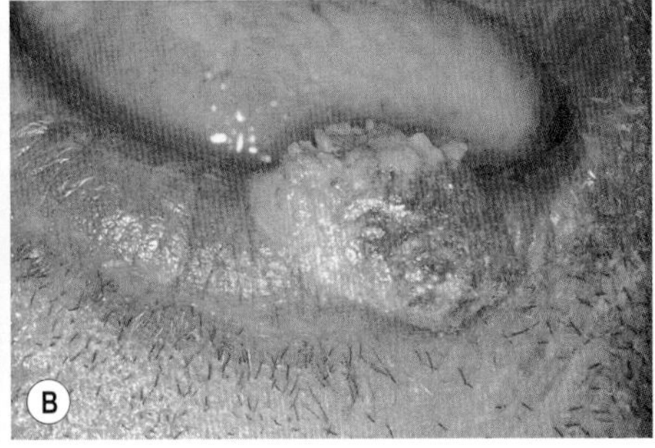

Fig. 88.8 Squamous cell carcinoma (SCC) of the lower lip. A Extensive hyperkeratosis and leukoplakia of the lower vermilion lip; histopathologically, the SCC was superficially invasive and well-differentiated. **B** Verrucous and eroded nodule on the lower vermilion lip in a heavy smoker. *Courtesy, H. Peter Sawyer, MD.*

STAGING OF CUTANEOUS SQUAMOUS CELL CARCINOMA (SCC) OF THE HEAD AND NECK	
T, N, M	
Primary tumor (T)	
TX	Primary tumor cannot be identified
Tis	Carcinoma *in situ*
T1	Tumor <2 cm in greatest dimension
T2	Tumor 2 cm or larger, but smaller than 4 cm in greatest dimension
T3	Tumor 4 cm or larger in maximum dimension or minor bone erosion or perineural invasion or deep invasion*
T4	Tumor with gross cortical bone/marrow invasion (4a); skull base invasion and/or skull base foramen involvement (4b)
Regional lymph nodes (clinical) (cN)	
NX	Regional lymph nodes cannot be assessed
N0	No regional lymph node metastasis
N1	Metastasis in a single ipsilateral lymph node, ≤3 cm in greatest dimension and ENE(–)
N2	Metastasis in a single ipsilateral lymph node, >3 cm but <6 cm in greatest dimension and ENE(–) (2a); or in multiple ipsilateral lymph nodes, none >6 cm in greatest dimension and ENE(–) (2b); or in bilateral or contralateral lymph nodes, none >6 cm in greatest dimension and ENE(–) (2c)
N3	Metastasis in a lymph node, >6 cm in greatest dimension and ENE(–) (3a); or metastasis in any node(s) and ENE(+) (3b)
Distant metastasis (M)	
M0	No distant metastasis
M1	Distant metastasis

Table 88.3 Staging of cutaneous squamous cell carcinoma (SCC) of the head and neck. *Continued*

STAGING OF CUTANEOUS SQUAMOUS CELL CARCINOMA (SCC) OF THE HEAD AND NECK			
Stage			
	T	**N**	**M**
0	Tis	N0	M0
I	T1	N0	M0
II	T2	N0	M0
III	T3	N0	M0
	T1	N1	M0
	T2	N1	M0
	T3	N1	M0
IV	T1	N2	M0
	T2	N2	M0
	T3	N2	M0
	T Any	N3	M0
	T4	N Any	M0
	T Any	N Any	M1

**Deep invasion is defined as invasion beyond the subcutaneous fat or >6mm (as measured from the granular layer of adjacent normal epidermis to the base of the tumor); perineural invasion for T3 classification is defined as tumor cells within the nerve sheath of a nerve lying deeper than the dermis or measuring 0.1mm or larger in caliber, or presenting with clinical or radiographic involvement of named nerves without skull base invasion or transgression.*

Table 88.3 *Continued* **Staging of cutaneous squamous cell carcinoma (SCC) of the head and neck.** The Brigham and Women's Hospital (BWH) T staging system divides T2 into a and b and considers T1 = 0 high-risk factors (HRF), T2a = 1 HRF, T2b = 2–3 HRF, and 3 = ≥4 HRF or bone invasion; the HRF are diameter ≥2cm, poorly differentiated, perineural invasion ≥0.1mm, or invasion beyond fat. ENE, extranodal extension. *Adapted from American Joint Committee on Cancer, 2017.*

CHARACTERISTICS OF HIGH-RISK BCC AND SCC	
Clinical characteristics	**Histopathologic characteristics**
• Area L ≥20 mm Area M ≥10 mm Area H (any size) • Poorly defined borders • Recurrent tumor • Immunosuppressed host • Tumor at site of previous XRT • Tumor at site of chronic inflammatory process or ulceration • Rapidly growing tumor (SCC only) • Neurologic symptoms: pain, paresthesia, paralysis	• Morpheaform (sclerosing), infiltrative, micronodular or basosquamous subtypes (BCC only) • Adenoid, adenosquamous, desmoplastic or metaplastic subtypes (SCC only) • Poorly differentiated (SCC only) • Arising within Bowen disease (SCC only) • Depth ≥2 mm or Clark level IV or V (SCC only) • Perineural involvement (BCC and SCC) • Lymphatic or vascular involvement (SCC)

Table 88.4 Characteristics of high-risk basal cell carcinoma (BCC) and squamous cell carcinoma (SCC). The presence of these high-risk characteristics increases the likelihood of recurrence of BCC and SCC, as well as the possibility of metastasis (primarily SCC). In addition, these high-risk features are used to determine indication for Mohs micrographic surgery. Area L – low-risk anatomic sites: trunk, extremities (excluding hands, feet, nail units, pretibia, ankles). Area M – middle-risk anatomic sites: cheeks, forehead, neck, jawline, scalp, pretibia. Area H – high-risk anatomic sites: central face, eyelids, eyebrows, periorbital skin, nose, lips, chin, mandible, pre- and post-auricular skin/sulci, temple, ear, genitalia, hands, feet, ankles, nipple/areola.

COMMON TREATMENT OPTIONS FOR BCC AND SCC	
Squamous cell carcinoma	**Basal cell carcinoma**
Low-risk lesions	**Low-risk lesions**
Surgical: • Tangential excision with curettage • Electrodesiccation and curettage • Standard excision with 4- to 6-mm margins Nonsurgical**: • XRT† for nonsurgical candidates • Topical therapies (e.g. imiquimod, 5-FU) and PDT are typically *not* recommended for treatment of *invasive* SCC; occasionally they are used for treatment of *in situ* SCC when a patient declines or is not a candidate for surgical therapy.	Surgical: • Tangential excision with curettage • Electrodesiccation and curettage • Standard excision with 4-mm margins Nonsurgical (primarily for superficial variant)**: • Topical imiquimod (e.g. 5 days/week × 6 weeks)*** • Topical 5% 5-FU (e.g. BID × 3-6 weeks)*** • MAL- or ALA-PDT • XRT† for nonsurgical candidates
High-risk* lesions	**High-risk* lesions**
• Mohs micrographic surgery • Standard excision with 10+ mm margins$ • XRT† for nonsurgical candidates • Adjuvant XRT (if perineural involvement)	
Inoperable or metastatic#	**Inoperable or metastatic#**
• Immune checkpoint inhibitors (e.g. cemiplimab)	• Hedgehog pathway inhibitors (e.g. vismodegib, sonidegib)
Indications for Mohs micrographic surgery	
• Lesions noted as "high-risk" (see Table 88.4) • Site of positive margin on prior excision • Underlying genetic syndrome (e.g. xeroderma pigmentosum, nevoid BCC syndrome)	

**See characteristics of such lesions in Table 88.4.*
***The cure rate with topical therapies is lower than with surgical therapies.*
****Dosing regimen should be adjusted based upon tolerance of side effects (e.g. crusting, erosive erythema).*
†Excluding genitalia, hands, and feet.
$May be considered for select high-risk tumors, but the concern is the inability of complete margin assessment.
#Referral to an oncologist is also necessary.

Table 88.5 Common treatment options for basal cell carcinoma (BCC) and squamous cell carcinoma (SCC). 5-FU, 5-fluorouracil; ALA, aminolevulinic acid; MAL, methylaminolevulinate; PDT, photodynamic therapy.

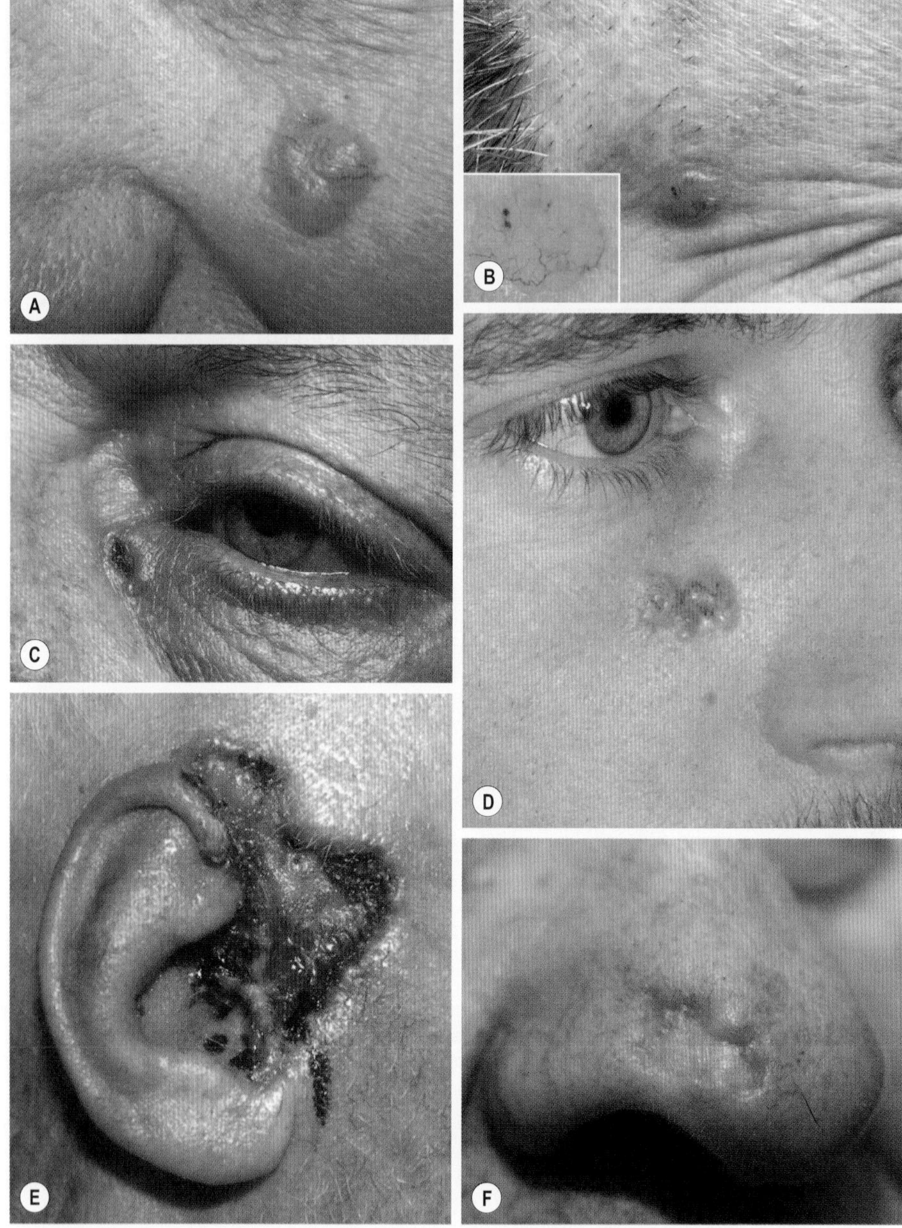

Fig. 88.9 Clinical spectrum of nodular basal cell carcinoma (BCC). A, B Translucent papulonodules with prominent telangiectasias on the infraorbital cheek (**A**) and forehead (**B**); on dermoscopy (**B**, inset) the arborizing telangiectasias are in sharp focus. **C** Classic presentation with a pearly rolled border and central hemorrhagic crust. **D** Larger plaque with rolled borders and multiple telangiectasias. **E** Nodulo-ulcerative tumor of the preauricular region with translucent rolled borders, most obvious at "noon." **F** Depressed scar on the nose. *A, Courtesy, Stanley J. Miller, MD; B, D, E, Courtesy, H. Peter Sawyer, MD; C, Courtesy, YDRSC; F, Courtesy, Kalman Watsky, MD.*

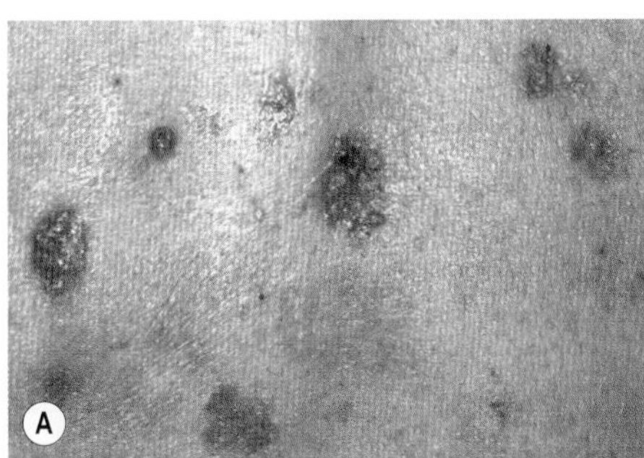

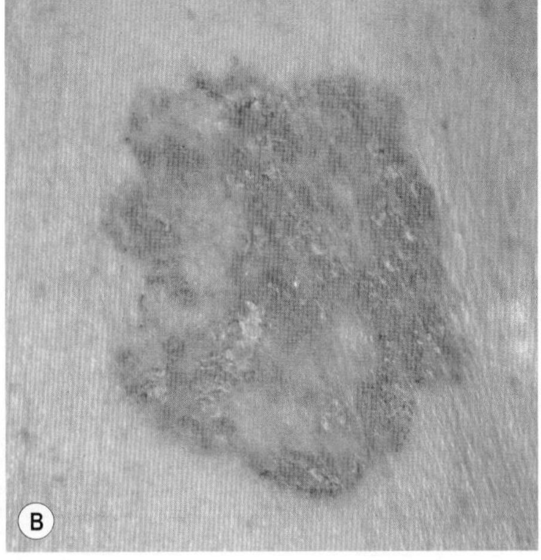

Fig. 88.10 Superficial basal cell carcinoma (BCC). A Numerous erythematous patches and thin plaques on the back of a man with a history of arsenic exposure decades previously. **B** A solitary large, thin, dark pink plaque. There are scattered areas of fine scaling and small foci of brown pigment within the rolled border. As a rule, these lesions are neither pruritic nor tender. *Courtesy, H. Peter Sawyer, MD.*

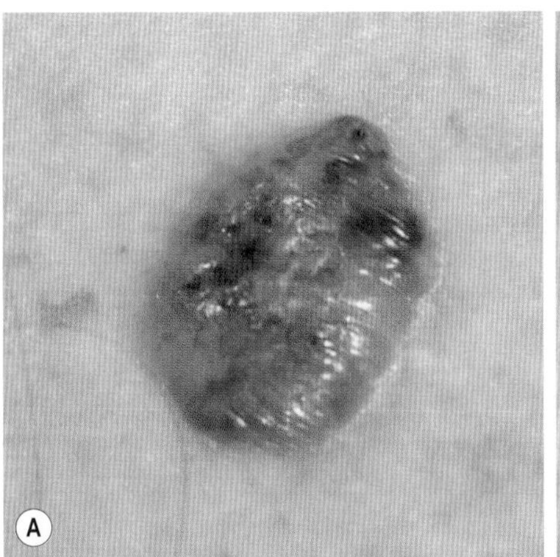

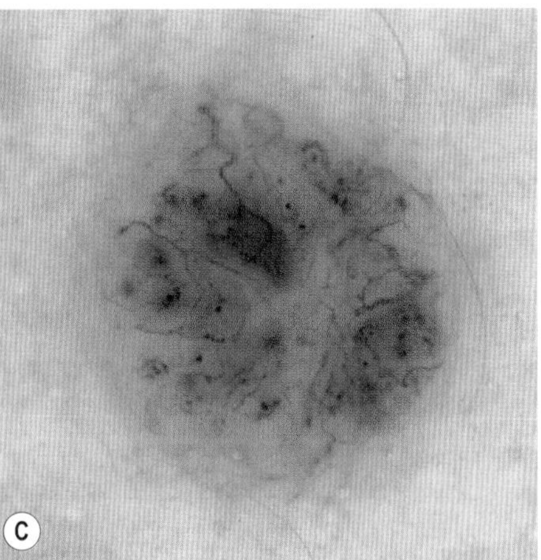

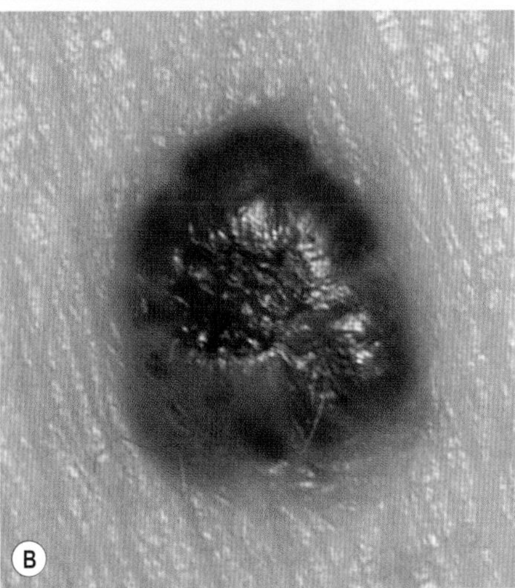

Fig. 88.11 Pigmented basal cell carcinoma (BCC). A, B Pigmented nodular BCCs with varying degrees of melanin pigmentation that may clinically resemble cutaneous melanoma. However, the glassy translucency, in concert with characteristic dermoscopic features such as arborizing telangiectasias and multiple blue-gray ovoid globules (**C**), point to the diagnosis of pigmented BCC. *A, Courtesy, Kalman Watsky, MD; B, Courtesy, H. Peter Sawyer, MD; C, Courtesy, Giuseppe Argenziano, MD.*

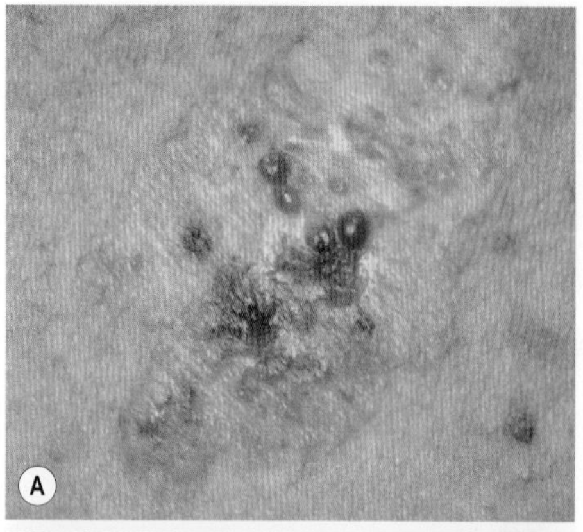

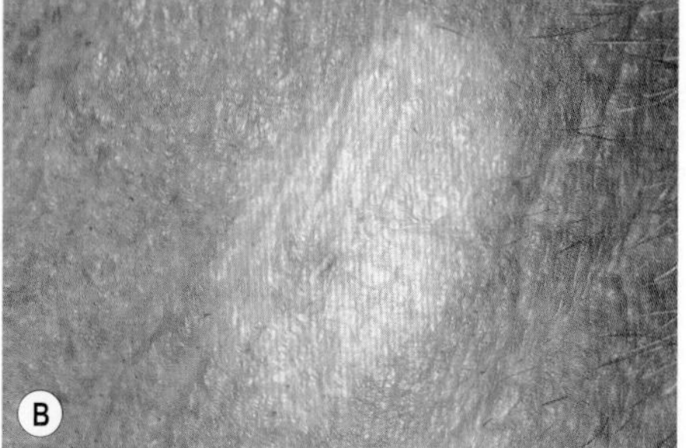

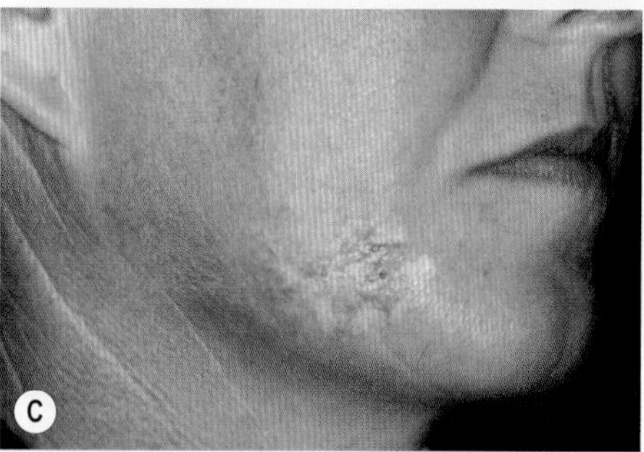

Fig. 88.12 Morpheaform basal cell carcinoma (BCC). A Recurrent tumor two years after microscopically controlled surgery; note the scar-like appearance with superimposed glassy pink and brown papules. **B** Oval hypopigmented firm plaque that resembles a scar (e.g. post electrodesiccation and curettage). While there is a light pink color between 6 and 9 o'clock, no translucency or rolled border is present. **C** A classic example with indistinct borders and scar-like appearance. *A, Courtesy, Darrell S. Rigel, MD; B, C Courtesy, H. Peter Sawyer, MD.*

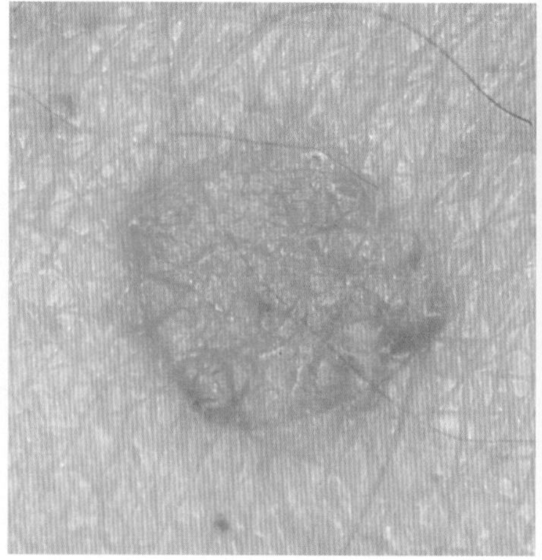

Fig. 88.13 Fibroepithelial basal cell carcinoma (fibroepithelioma of Pinkus). A soft, skin-colored to light pink, broad, sessile plaque on the lower back is a classic presentation for a fibroepithelial BCC. *Courtesy, Oscar R. Colegio, MD, PhD.*

Benign Epithelial Tumors and Proliferations

89

The entities in this chapter can be further classified according to the algorithm in Fig. 89.1.

COMMON

Seborrheic Keratosis

- Begin to appear during the 4th decade of life and then gradually increase in number.
- Macular, papular, or verrucous; colors vary from white to black but most commonly brown.
- Typically has a "stuck-on" appearance with a smooth to verrucous surface (Fig. 89.2).
- Spares the palms, soles, and mucosal surfaces.
- May resemble a melanoma clinically but has no pigment network (by dermoscopy) and has horn pseudocysts.
- Sudden appearance of multiple lesions may be associated with internal malignancy (*sign of Leser–Trélat*) or erythroderma; the former may also be associated with skin tags, irritated seborrheic keratoses, tripe palms, and acanthosis nigricans.
- Histopathology: a spectrum of different architectures, most commonly acanthotic, papillomatous and hyperkeratotic, or irritated (Fig. 89.3).
- Variants:
  - **Dermatosis papulosa nigra** (Fig. 89.4): common in dark-skinned individuals; 1- to 5-mm hyperpigmented papules on the face
  - **Stucco keratosis** (Fig. 89.5): 1- to 4-mm gray-white papules on the lower extremities (especially dorsal feet and ankles) of older adults

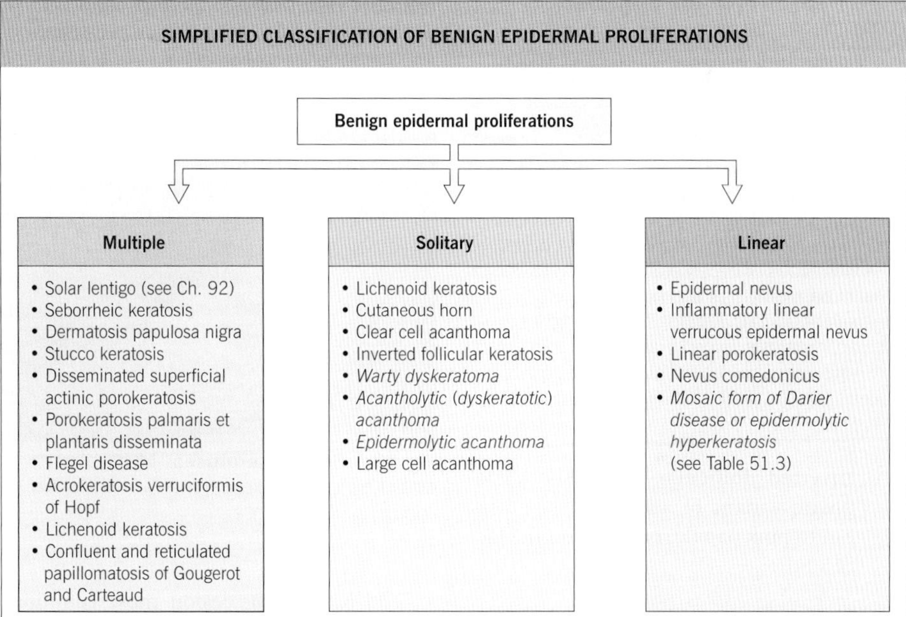

Fig. 89.1 Simplified classification of benign epidermal proliferations. Although the term solitary lichenoid keratosis is sometimes used, patients may develop multiple lesions, especially those with skin phototypes I or II and significant actinic damage. Entities in *italics* are not covered. *Courtesy, Luis Requena, MD.*

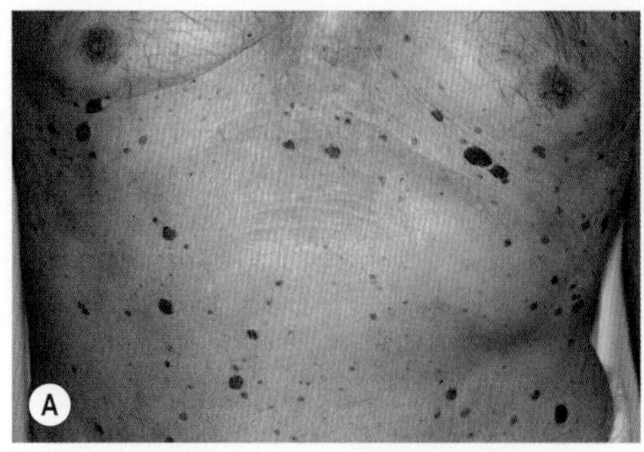

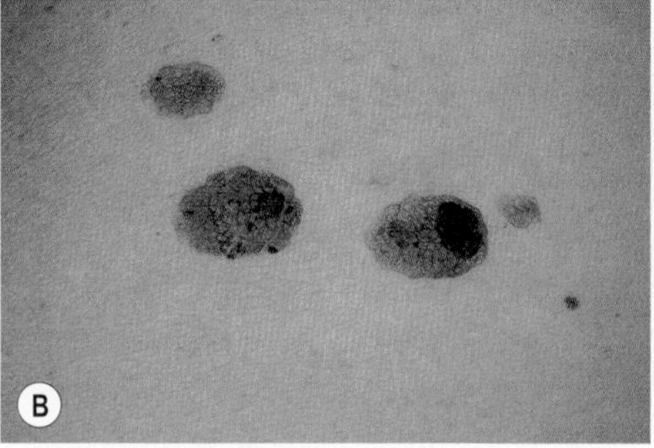

Fig. 89.2 Seborrheic keratoses. A Multiple seborrheic keratoses of the anterior trunk that vary in size and color. **B** Sharply demarcated pigmented papules and plaques with a papillomatous surface and horn pseudocysts. Note the "stuck-on" appearance. *B, Courtesy, YDRSC.*

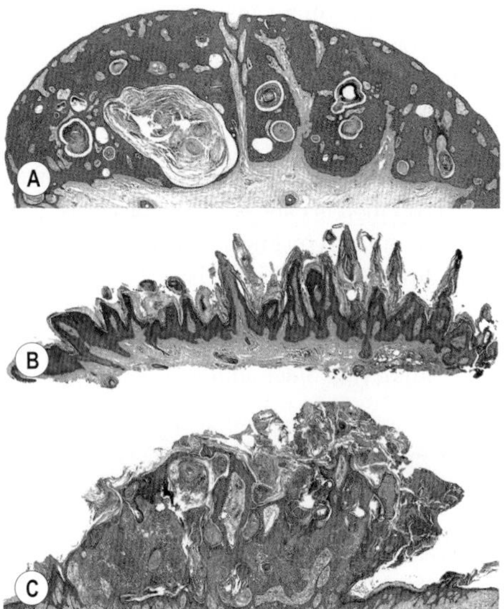

Fig. 89.3 Seborrheic keratoses – spectrum of histologic subtypes. A Acanthotic type with lobular hyperplasia with prominent horn cysts. **B** Papillomatous or hyperkeratotic type with church spires of papillomatosis and hyperkeratosis. **C** Irritated seborrheic keratosis. Exophytic lesion with papillomatosis, hyperkeratosis, hemorrhagic crust, and dermal inflammation. *A, B, Courtesy, Luis Requena, MD; C, Courtesy, Lorenzo Cerroni, MD.*

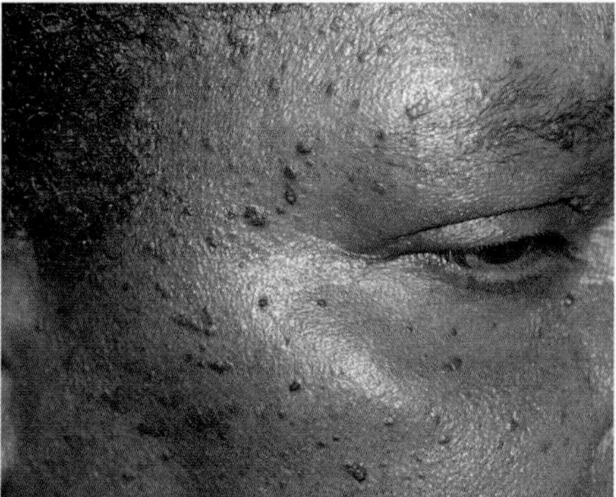

Fig. 89.4 Dermatosis papulosa nigra. Multiple hyperpigmented papules with typical location on the cheeks. *Courtesy, Luis Requena, MD.*

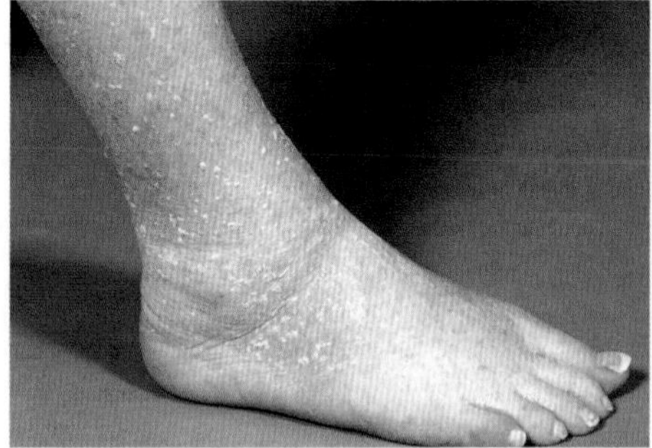

Fig. 89.5 Stucco keratoses. Multiple gray-white keratotic papules, primarily on the ankle and dorsal foot.

- **Inverted follicular keratosis**: endophytic variant of seborrheic keratosis; tan to pink papule, typically on the face of adults

Cutaneous Horn

- Clinical term for marked hyperkeratosis arising from a papule or nodule (Fig. 89.6).
- The base of the lesion most commonly represents an actinic keratosis or wart, but of the entities in this chapter, a seborrheic keratosis is most common; sometimes the base is a squamous cell carcinoma.

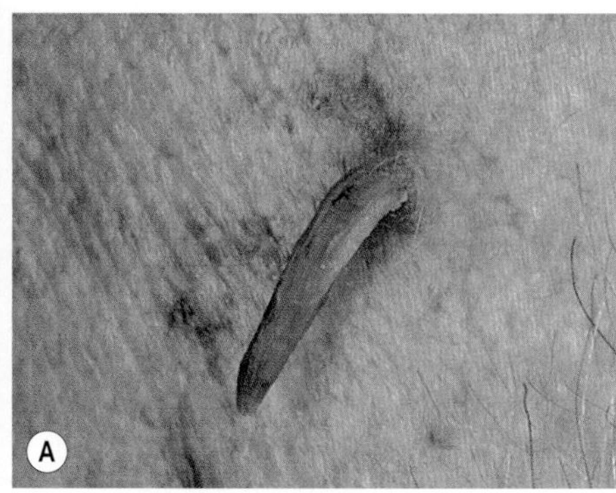

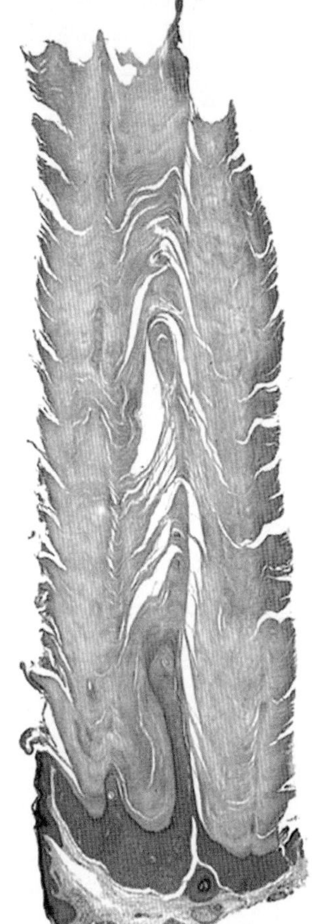

Fig. 89.6 Cutaneous horn. A This cutaneous horn arose from an actinic keratosis. **B** Striking column of hyperkeratosis with hyperplasia of the underlying epidermis. *A, Courtesy, YDRSC; B, Courtesy, Luis Requena, MD.*

Solitary Lichenoid Keratosis/Lichen Planus-Like Keratosis

- Pink to pink-brown papule or plaque (Fig. 89.7); arises in chronically sun-damaged skin, most commonly on the chest, arms, and shins.

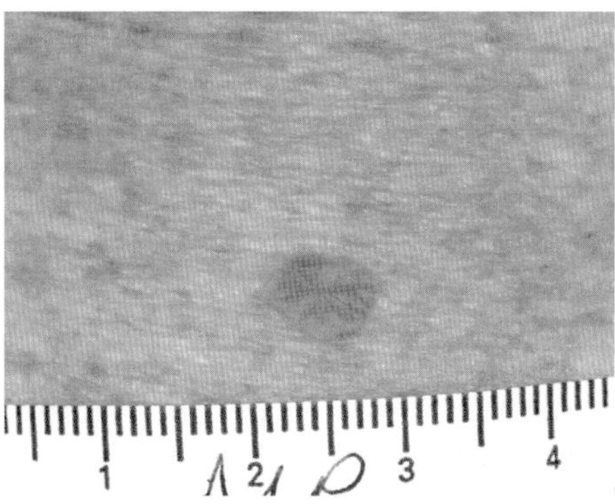

Fig. 89.7 Lichenoid keratosis. Pink, flat-topped papule in a fair-skinned individual. *Courtesy, Jean L. Bolognia, MD.*

- Occasionally multiple.
- Clinically mimics basal cell carcinoma or Bowen disease.

Porokeratosis

- Several different types (Table 89.1; Fig. 89.8).
- All have a distinctive thread-like border of scale that corresponds histopathologically to the cornoid lamella (column of parakeratosis histologically).
- The most common form, disseminated superficial actinic porokeratosis (DSAP), is sometimes misdiagnosed as multiple actinic keratoses.

Confluent and Reticulated Papillomatosis (of Gougerot and Carteaud)

- Onset during puberty.
- Scaly to verrucous hyperpigmented plaques.
- Centrally confluent and reticulated at periphery (Fig. 89.9).
- Favors neck, central chest, submammary regions.
- **Rx:** oral tetracyclines (e.g. minocycline).

LESS COMMON

Clear Cell Acanthoma

- Red, shiny papule or plaque, sometimes with a peripheral collarette of scale (Fig. 89.10).
- Favors the leg.
- Histopathology: acanthosis of characteristically well-demarcated pale or clear keratinocytes with overlying parakeratosis.

CLINICAL VARIANTS OF POROKERATOSIS	
Type	**Clinical features**
Porokeratosis of Mibelli	Plaque that arises during infancy or childhood, usually on a distal extremity; usually several cm in diameter
Disseminated superficial actinic porokeratosis	Pink to brown papules and plaques with peripheral scale; arise in sun-exposed sites, especially the forearms and shins; usually measure from a few mm to 1.5 cm; in some patients, autosomal dominant inheritance
Large-sized lesions	Usually in immunocompromised patients, especially solid organ transplant recipients; in sun-exposed areas
Linear porokeratosis	Streaks along the lines of Blaschko; arise during infancy or childhood Risk of development of squamous cell carcinoma
Punctate porokeratosis	Palmoplantar papules that measure 1 to 2 mm in diameter; arise during adolescence or adulthood
Porokeratosis palmaris et plantaris et disseminata	Palmoplantar papules in addition to involvement of the trunk, extremities, and even mucous membranes; onset during childhood or adolescence
Porokeratosis ptychotropica	Red to brown papules or plaques in the intergluteal cleft and on the buttocks; there may be coalescence of lesions centrally with scattered papules peripherally

Table 89.1 Clinical variants of porokeratosis. There have been scattered case reports of eruptive disseminated porokeratosis in which numerous, inflamed keratoses were thought to be a sign of associated malignancy.

Large Cell Acanthoma

- Variably colored papule or plaque in sun-exposed sites in older individuals (Fig. 89.11).
- A variant of actinic keratosis and seborrheic keratosis.
- Histopathology: orthokeratosis overlying a thin epidermis composed of enlarged keratinocytes.

Flegel Disease (Hyperkeratosis Lenticularis Perstans)

- Rare; may have an autosomal dominant inheritance.
- Onset usually during adulthood.
- Lentil-like keratotic papules on the distal lower extremities (Fig. 89.12).

Acrokeratosis Verruciformis

- Autosomal dominant disorder; sometimes associated with Darier disease.
- Multiple, skin-colored, flat-wart-like papules on dorsal aspect of hands and feet (see Fig. 48.10).
- Benign neoplasm of keratinocytes showing papillomatosis with overlying hyperkeratosis in "church spires".
- May have *ATP2A2* gene mutation.

LINEAR

Epidermal Nevus (See Ch. 51)

- Hyperpigmented (rarely hypopigmented) papules and plaques (Fig. 89.13) along lines of Blaschko.
- Verrucous, keratotic, velvety or barely elevated.
- May have a sebaceous or other adnexal component (i.e. nevus sebaceus), especially if on the scalp or face.
- Can be caused by mosaicism for mutations in *FGFR3* (fibroblast growth factor receptor-3), *PIK3CA*, *HRAS* (also in nevus sebaceus), keratin 1 or 10 (if histologic finding of epidermolytic hyperkeratosis), and other genes.
- May be associated with extracutaneous manifestations (see Ch. 51).

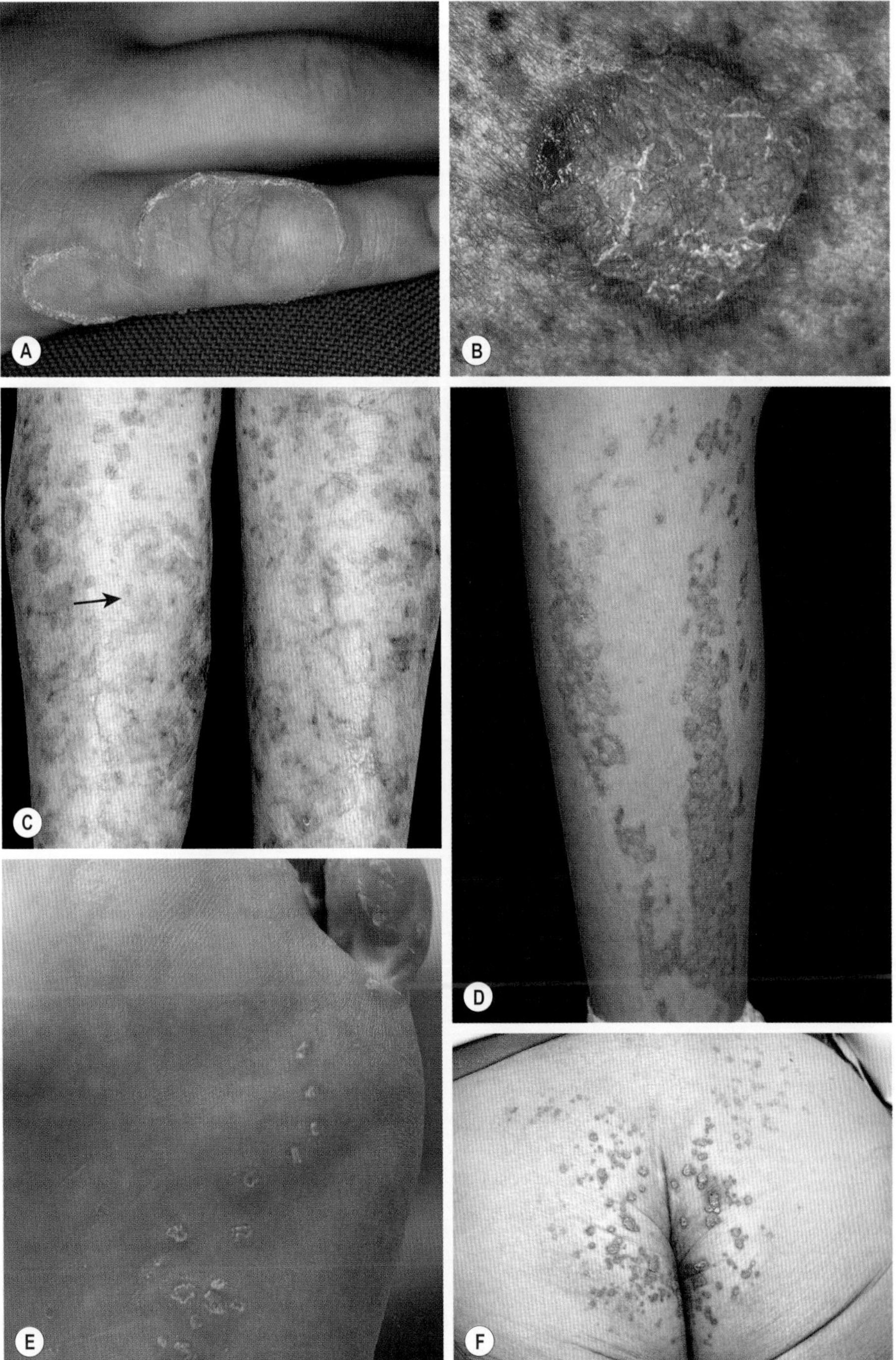

Fig. 89.8 Porokeratoses. A Porokeratosis of Mibelli on the hand of a child. **B** Actinic porokeratosis in a renal transplant patient with significant solar damage. Note the narrow, elevated rim. **C** Multiple lesions of disseminated superficial actinic porokeratosis (DSAP). Note the hyperpigmented, peripheral keratotic edge (black arrow) which is where the biopsy should be obtained in order to see the cornoid lamellae; lesions can range in color from light brown to pink. **D** Several streaks of linear porokeratosis on the lower extremity. **E** Multiple keratotic papules on the plantar surface due to punctate porokeratosis. **F** Porokeratosis ptychotropica with pink to brown papules localized to the intergluteal cleft and buttocks. *A, Courtesy, YDRSC; B, D, Courtesy, Jean L. Bolognia, MD; C, Courtesy, Karynne O. Duncan, MD; E, Courtesy, Kalman Watsky, MD; F, Courtesy, César Cosme Álvarez Cuesta, MD.*

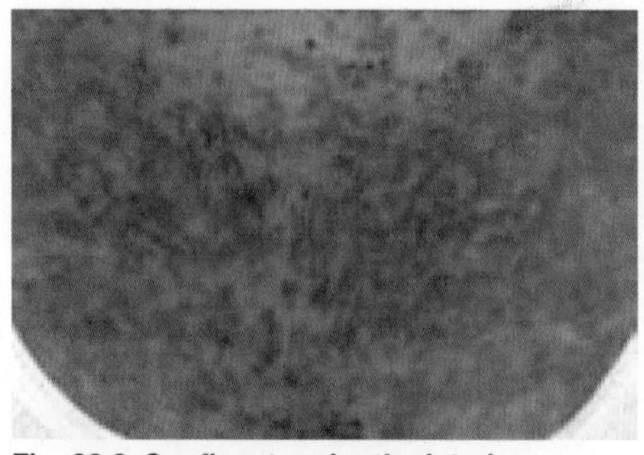

Fig. 89.9 Confluent and reticulated papillomatosis (CARP). Multiple hyperpigmented papules that are confluent centrally and assume a reticulated pattern laterally. *Courtesy, Julie V. Schaffer, MD.*

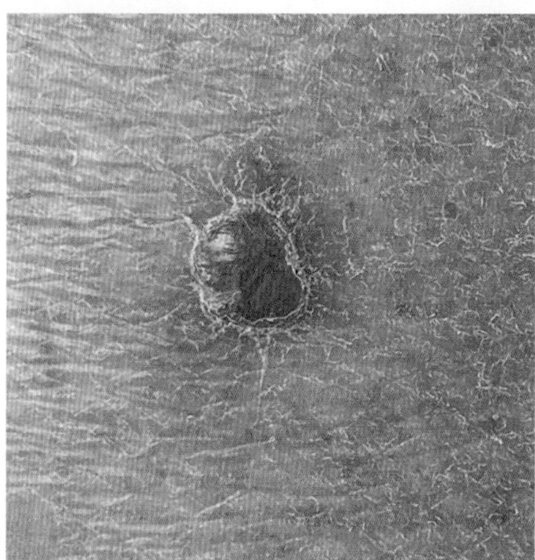

Fig. 89.10 Clear cell acanthoma. Well-demarcated, dark, red, shiny papule with a wafer-like collarette of scale. *Courtesy, Karynne O. Duncan, MD.*

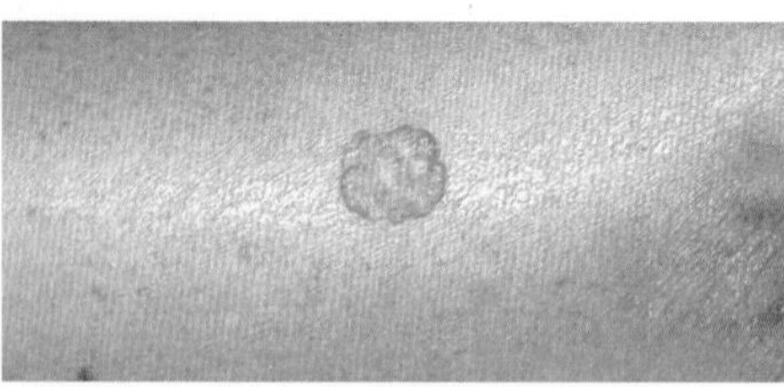

Fig. 89.11 Large cell acanthoma. Well-demarcated, thin, pink-brown plaque. *Courtesy, Luis Requena, MD.*

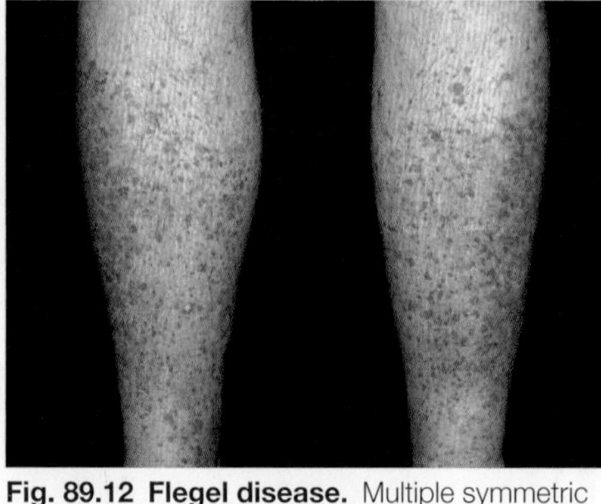

Fig. 89.12 Flegel disease. Multiple symmetric hyperpigmented keratotic papules are present on the shins. *Courtesy, Luis Requena, MD.*

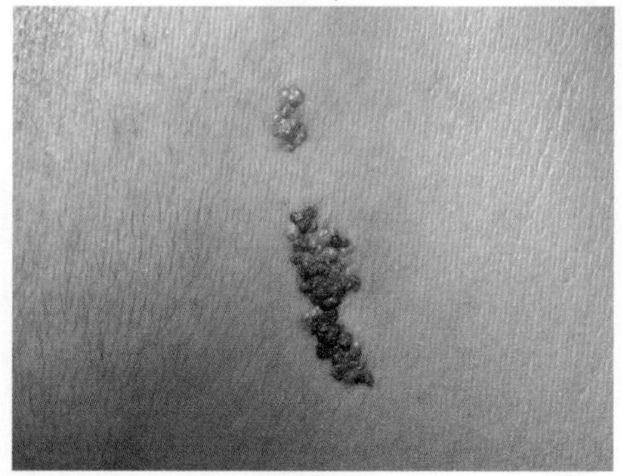

Fig. 89.13 Epidermal nevus. Obvious papillomatosis in a single thin linear plaque; this is the most common clinical presentation. *Courtesy, Julie V. Schaffer, MD.*

Inflammatory Linear Verrucous Epidermal Nevus

- Linear, pruritic, psoriasiform (erythematous with scale) plaques, usually on an extremity (see Fig. 51.2C).
- 75% appear before age 5 years.
- **DDx:** primarily linear psoriasis (see Ch. 6).

Nevus Comedonicus

- Linear plaques composed of grouped comedones; may develop inflammatory acneiform lesions (see Fig. 51.3G).
- 50% present at birth; otherwise, generally appear before age 10 years.
- May be due to mosaicism for a mutation in *FGFR2*.

For further information see Ch. 109 from *Dermatology, Fourth Edition*.

Cysts 90

Introduction

- Variably sized papules or nodules.
- Cysts can be divided into true cysts with an epithelial lining (histologically and sometimes visible clinically) and false cysts without such a lining.
- Appreciation of the actual size of the cyst often requires palpation.
- Different types of cysts often have characteristic anatomic locations and histologic features.
- Treatment of true cysts (if symptomatic) is primarily surgical.
- Congenital cysts (e.g. dermoid, branchial cleft, omphalomesenteric duct) are covered in Ch. 53.

True Cysts – Common

Epidermoid Cyst (Epidermoid Inclusion Cyst [EIC], "Sebaceous Cyst", Epidermal Cyst)

- Most commonly on the face and the upper trunk; skin-colored to yellow-white unless inflamed; size varies from a few millimeters to several centimeters.
- A visible comedonal-like opening or pore (resembles a blackhead) may be seen on the surface of the papule or nodule (Fig. 90.1A).
- A soft cheese-like, sometimes malodorous, material composed primarily of keratin can usually be expressed from the opening.
- Cyst contents may rupture into the dermis, eliciting an acute and chronic inflammatory reaction, leading to significant redness and pain; this inflammation is often confused with a bacterial infection (Fig. 90.1B).
- Most commonly sporadic; multiple lesions rarely associated with Gardner syndrome or Gorlin syndrome. Facial cysts may also develop in patients receiving targeted oncologic drugs, e.g. selective BRAF inhibitors.
- **DDx:** see Fig. 95.18.
- **Rx:** *inflamed* lesions: if fluctuant, can be incised and drained ± packed with gauze (a wick); if non-fluctuant, can be injected with intralesional CS; *non-inflamed* ("cold") lesions can be excised surgically but may result in a significant scar.

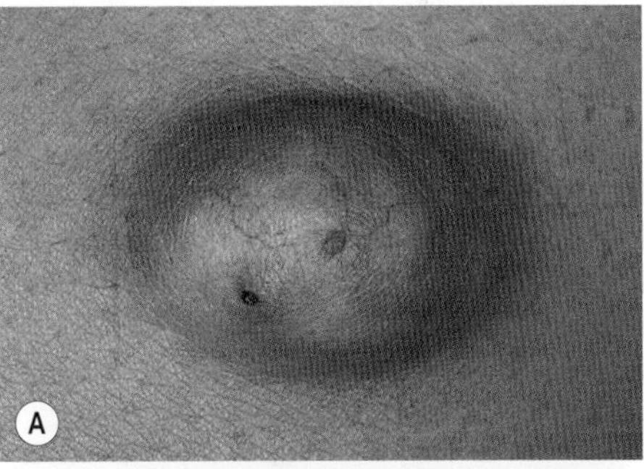

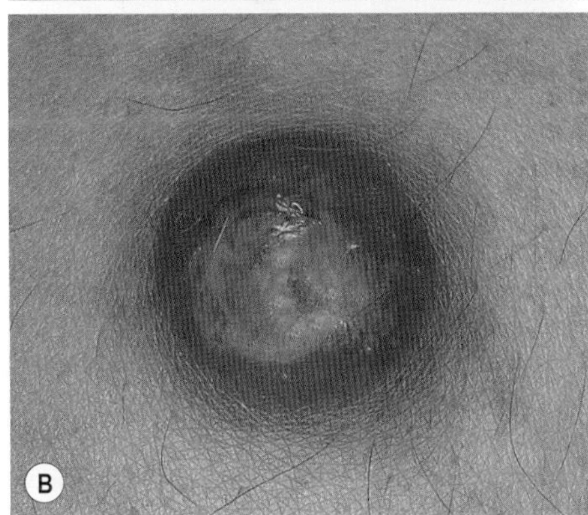

Fig. 90.1 Epidermoid inclusion cysts. **A** Typical clinical appearance of an epidermoid inclusion cyst with a yellowish hue. Two pores are present in this example. **B** Painful inflammatory reactions to cyst rupture are a frequent cause for presentation to a physician. Culture will often prove these lesions to be sterile, even if draining pus. Antibiotic treatment can be helpful due to their anti-inflammatory effects. *A, Courtesy, YDRSC; B, Courtesy, Mary S. Stone, MD.*

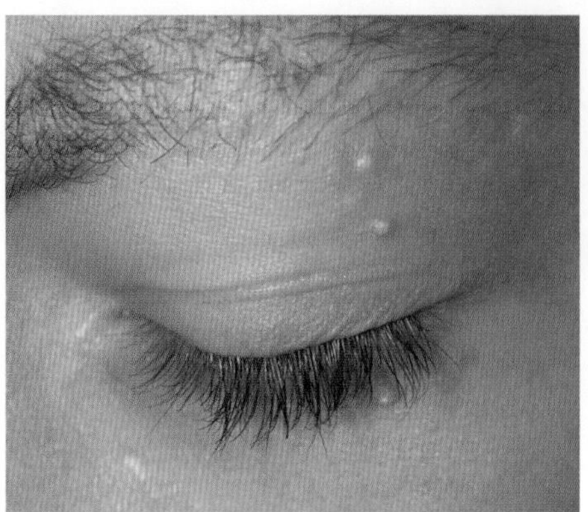

Fig. 90.2 Milia. Tiny (1–2 mm), white, dome-shaped papules on the face. *Courtesy, YDRSC.*

CONDITIONS ASSOCIATED WITH MULTIPLE MILIA
• Trauma, e.g. burn • Bullous diseases – Metabolic (e.g. porphyria cutanea tarda) – Autoimmune (e.g. epidermolysis bullosa acquisita >> bullous pemphigoid) – Inherited (e.g. epidermolysis bullosa) – Exposures (e.g. poison ivy) • Other genodermatoses (e.g. Bazex–Dupré–Christol syndrome) • Follicular mycosis fungoides

Table 90.1 Conditions associated with multiple milia.

Milium (Milia – Plural)

- A small, superficial (1–2 mm) epidermoid cyst that is white in color and is sometimes confused with a whitehead (Fig. 90.2); occasionally they are grouped.
- Occurs most frequently on the central face, especially the periorbital region; seen in both children and adults.
- Commonly observed on the face in newborns; in this setting, they often resolve spontaneously.
- The majority of patients with multiple facial milia have no underlying condition; however, there may be a secondary cause (Table 90.1).
- **DDx:** whitehead (closed comedone), syringoma.
- **Rx:** because a milium lies beneath intact epidermis, the lesion must be punctured with a needle or sharp blade (e.g. #11) in order to express the keratin contents.

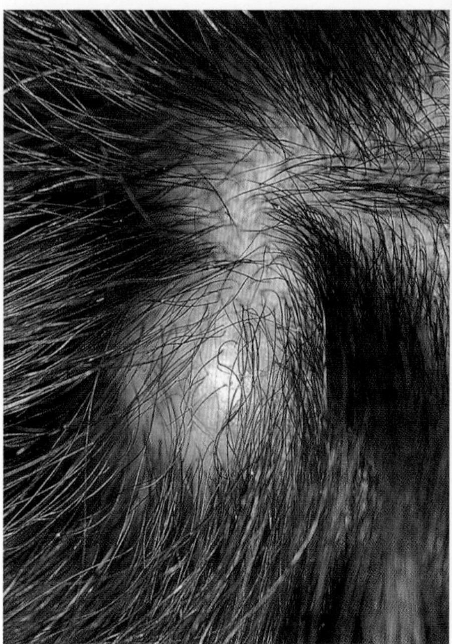

Fig. 90.3 Pilar cyst. A non-inflamed pilar cyst is skin-colored, mobile, and has a smooth surface. *Courtesy, Mary S. Stone, MD.*

Pilar Cyst (Tricholemmal Cyst, Wen)

- Most common location is the scalp; sometimes there is associated overlying alopecia (Fig. 90.3).
- Solitary or multiple relatively firm nodules.
- May be inherited (autosomal dominant).
- Surgical removal is easier than for an EIC because less dissection from surrounding normal tissue is required; a small incision with lateral pressure may be all that is necessary.

Pilonidal Cyst (Pilonidal Sinus, Pilonidal Disease)

- Most common location is the upper gluteal cleft in association with a sinus tract ± fragments of hairs (Fig. 90.4).
- May have a history of draining malodorous material.
- More common in men.
- May be associated with acne conglobata, hidradenitis suppurativa, and dissecting cellulitis (follicular occlusion tetrad).

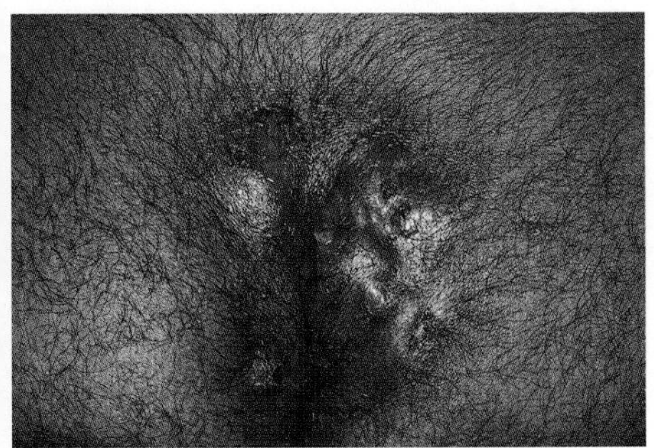

Fig. 90.4 Pilonidal sinus and abscess formation at the superior portion of the intergluteal cleft. *Courtesy, Kalman Watsky, MD.*

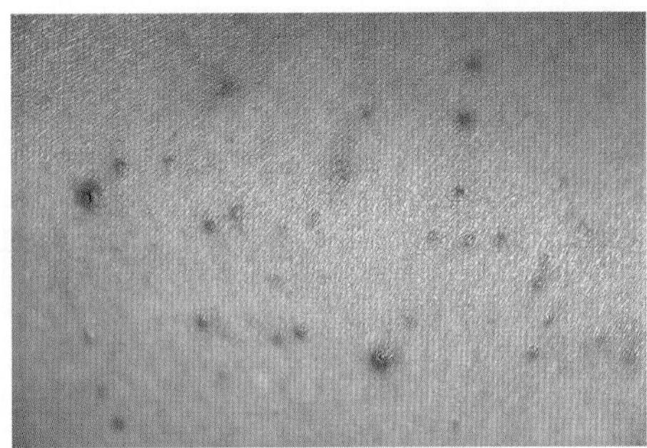

Fig. 90.5 Eruptive vellus hair cysts. Pigmented small papules on the thigh of a young woman. *Courtesy, Mary S. Stone, MD.*

True Cysts – Less Common

Vellus Hair Cyst

- 1- to 3-mm, skin-colored to brown-blue papule(s), commonly on the trunk (Fig. 90.5).
- Occasionally inflamed.
- When multiple, may be inherited (autosomal dominant); can occasionally be associated with pachyonychia congenita 6b/17 > 6a/16.
- Bedside diagnostic test: nick the cyst and examine expressed contents for vellus hairs.
- **DDx:** acne, steatocystomas (may have overlap).

Steatocystoma

- 2- to 10-mm, skin-colored to pigmented papule or nodule, usually multiple and grouped (steatocystoma multiplex); commonly develop on the trunk or in the axillae and groin (Fig. 90.6). May be solitary (steatocystoma simplex).
- Can drain oily fluid.
- Multiple lesions may be inherited as an isolated finding (autosomal dominant, *KRT17* mutation) or represent a clinical feature of pachyonychia congenita 6b/17 > 6a/16.

Hidrocystoma

APOCRINE

- Often a solitary, translucent to bluish papule on the eyelid margin (Fig. 90.7).
- Histology: the lining resembles that of an apocrine gland (decapitation secretion).
- **Rx:** if bothersome or symptomatic, excision by an experienced surgeon.

ECCRINE

- Multiple or solitary bluish, translucent papule(s) on the face (Fig. 90.8).
- Can become more prominent with sweating.
- Bedside diagnostic test: nicking the surface results in drainage of clear liquid.

"False" Cysts (No True Epithelial Lining)

Mucocele

- Compressible mucosal-colored to bluish papule or nodule, most commonly seen on the lower, inner mucosal lip (Fig. 90.9).
- Secondary to disruption of the minor salivary ducts.
- May resolve spontaneously.
- **Rx:** if persistent, excision or other destructive procedure, intralesional CS.

Digital Mucous Cyst (Digital Myxoid Cyst)

- Skin-colored to translucent papule or nodule most commonly on digits, in particular the dorsal, distal finger near the distal interphalangeal joint (Fig. 90.10).
- There may be a connection to the joint space.
- Occurs in the setting of osteoarthritis.
- Longitudinal nail deformity, usually a depression, may be present when the lesion compresses the nail matrix.
- Puncture can result in drainage of a gelatinous material.
- **Rx:** observation, intralesional CS, excision, repeated incision and drainage.

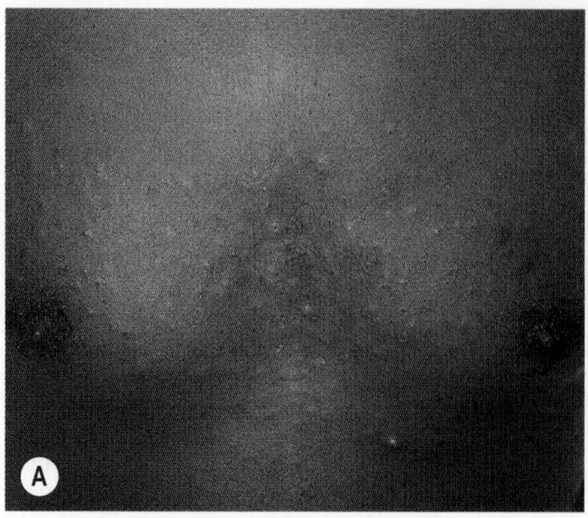

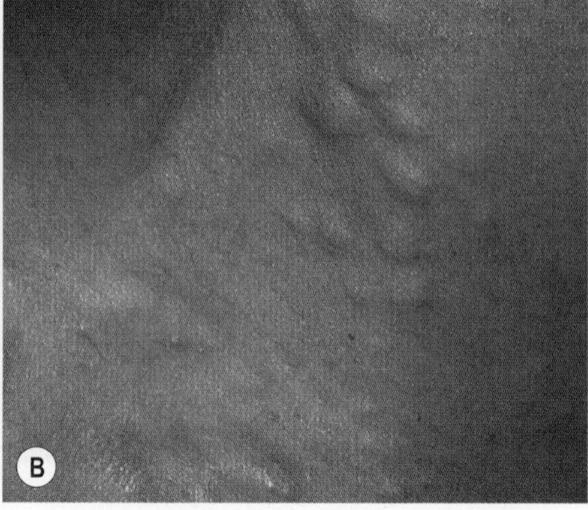

Fig. 90.6 Steatocystoma multiplex. A, B Numerous cystic papules on the trunk and multiple cystic nodules on the neck. *A, Courtesy, Mary S. Stone, MD; B, Courtesy, YDRSC.*

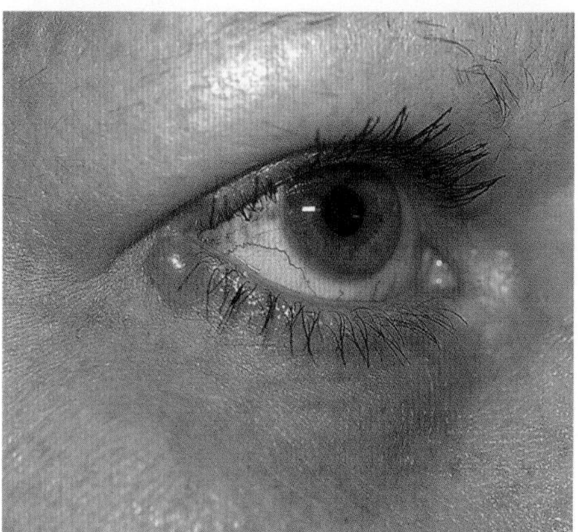

Fig. 90.7 Apocrine hidrocystoma. A single, slightly bluish, translucent papule on the lower eyelid near the lateral canthus. *Courtesy, Mary S. Stone, MD.*

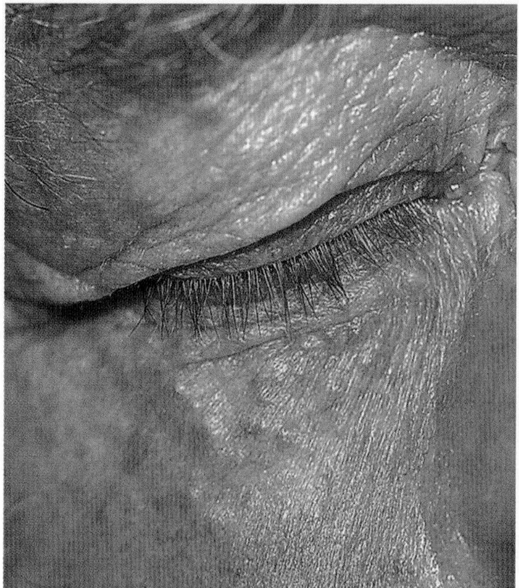

Fig. 90.8 Eccrine hidrocystomas. Numerous, tiny translucent or bluish papules on the lower eyelid.

Ganglion Cyst (Synovial Cyst)

- Soft, cystic nodule up to 4 cm in diameter, most commonly on the wrist > ankle (Fig. 90.11).
- **Rx:** may spontaneously resolve but recurrence common; treatment modalities include compression, aspiration and intralesional CS, excision.

Pseudocyst of the Auricle

- Painless swelling, generally unilateral, of the scaphoid fossa of the ear (Fig. 90.12).
- More common in men than in women.
- **Rx:** aspiration ± intralesional CS, incision and drainage; any treatment should be followed by pressure dressings.

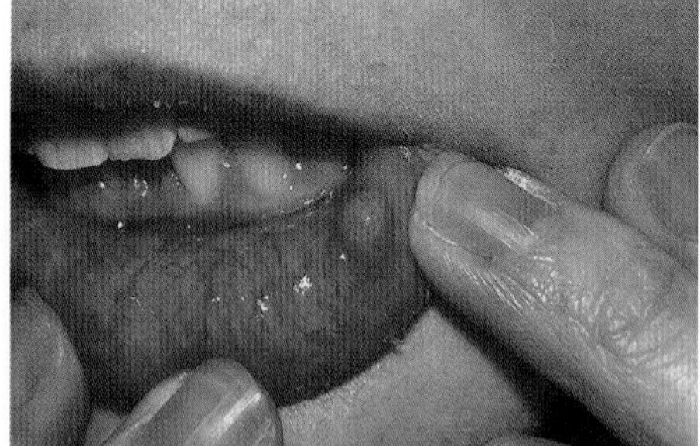

Fig. 90.9 Mucocele. A bluish translucent papule on the lower mucosal lip. *Courtesy, Mary S. Stone, MD.*

For further information see Ch. 110 from *Dermatology, Fourth Edition*.

For additional online figures visit www.expertconsult.com 

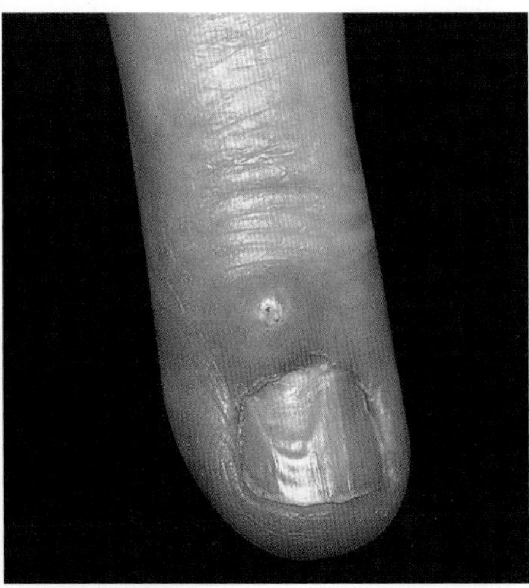

Fig. 90.10 Digital mucous cyst. A translucent papule on the dorsal distal phalanx of the finger causing a depression in the nail plate. *Courtesy, Mary S. Stone, MD.*

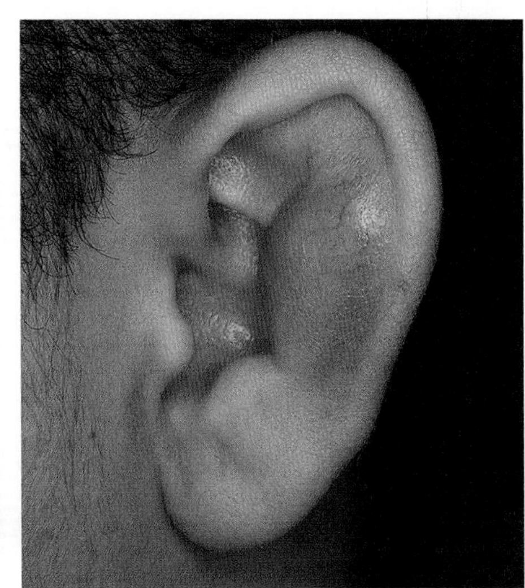

Fig. 90.12 Pseudocyst of the auricle. Erythematous firm nodule on the ear. *Courtesy, YDRSC.*

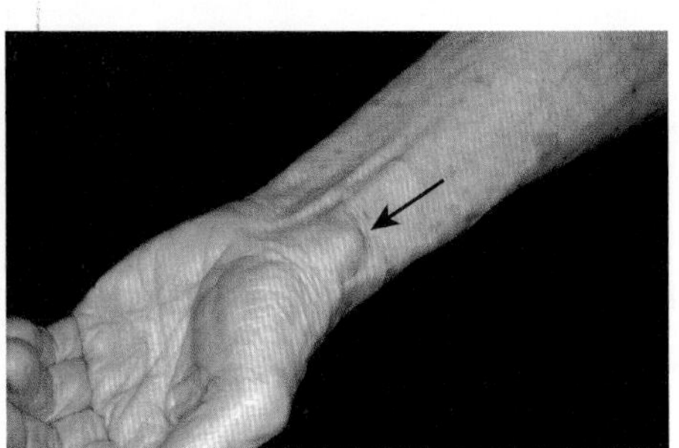

Fig. 90.11 Ganglion (cyst). A skin-colored, compressible, subcutaneous nodule is present on the wrist (arrow), the most common location. *Courtesy, Jean L. Bolognia, MD.*

91 Adnexal Neoplasms

- Adnexal neoplasms are tumors, more commonly benign, that show features of cutaneous adnexal structures (Fig. 91.1), e.g. hair (Table 91.1), sebaceous glands (Table 91.2), apocrine glands and eccrine glands (Table 91.3).

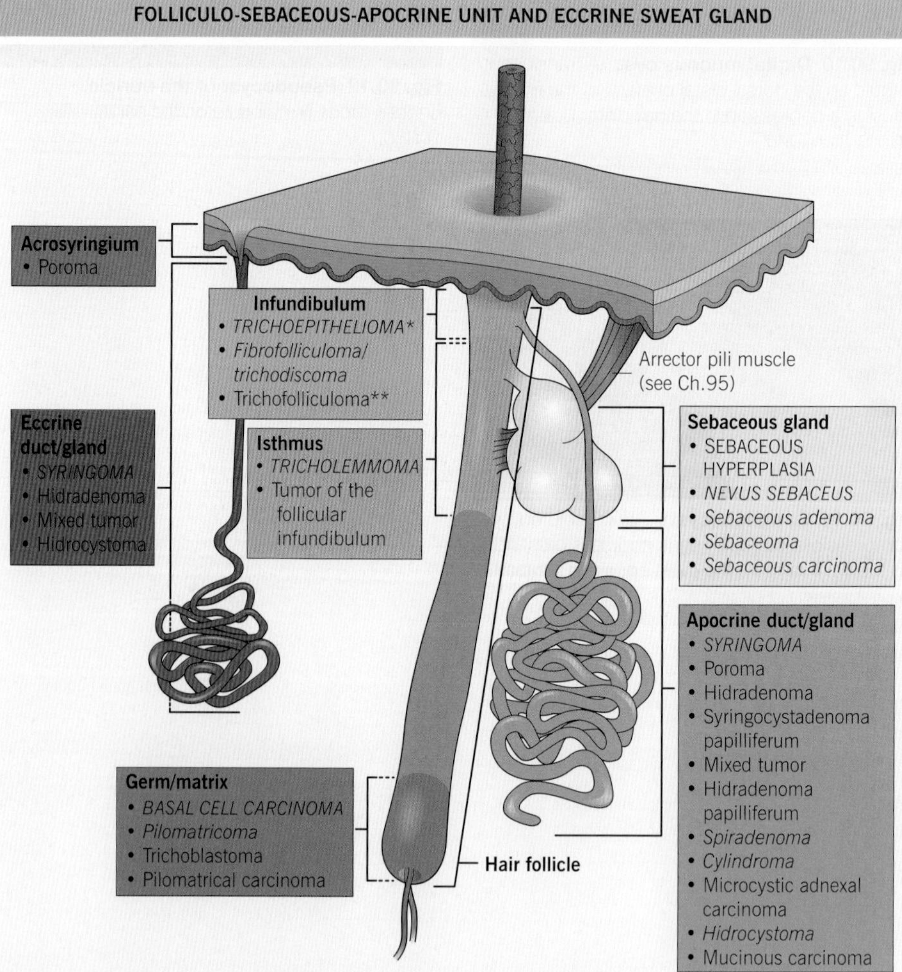

Fig. 91.1 Folliculo-sebaceous-apocrine unit and eccrine sweat gland. Adnexal tumors showing differentiation toward the hair follicle, sebaceous gland, apocrine gland, and eccrine gland are listed in correspondingly colored boxes. Important entities are in capital letters; entities associated with syndromes are in italics (see Tables 91.1–91.3). *Can show germinal differentiation; **differentiation toward entire follicle.

BENIGN AND MALIGNANT TUMORS WITH FOLLICULAR DIFFERENTIATION

	Morphology	Common site(s)	Distinctive characteristic(s)	Association(s)*
Benign				
Pilomatricoma	Firm to hard (calcified) papule, nodule, or dermal plaque	Head > upper trunk (Fig. 91.2)	Common in children; may have a characteristic "shelf-like" feel, possibly due to calcification; sometimes has associated anetoderma	Tumor has *CTNNB1* mutation (encodes β-catenin) Occasionally associated with myotonic dystrophy, Gardner syndrome (when cystic; *APC* mutation), Rubinstein–Taybi syndrome
Tricholemmoma	Skin-colored papule > nodule	Central face, especially nose or upper lip	May be wart-like (verrucous)	Cowden disease (PTEN hamartoma tumor syndrome) (*PTEN* mutation) (Fig. 91.16)
Desmoplastic trichoepithelioma	Skin-colored to erythematous plaque	Cheek or upper lip	Annular; more common in women	
Trichofolliculoma	Papule or nodule	Face > scalp > upper trunk	Occasionally has a tuft of white, wispy hairs protruding from center (Fig. 91.3)	
Fibrofolliculoma/ trichodiscoma	Subtle skin-colored to hypopigmented papule	Face, ears (Fig. 91.4), neck > scalp > upper trunk		Birt–Hogg–Dubé syndrome (*BHD* mutation) (Fig. 91.16)
Tumor of the follicular infundibulum	Hypopigmented, subtle macule or papule or plaque	Face (Fig. 91.5)	Sometimes atrophic	Rarely, Cowden disease (PTEN hamartoma tumor syndrome) (Fig. 91.16)
Trichoepithelioma	Pink-red to skin-colored papule or nodule	Face (especially medial cheeks, nose) > upper trunk (Fig. 91.6)		Brooke–Spiegler syndrome (*CYLD* mutation), multiple familial trichoepitheliomas
Trichoblastoma	Nodule			Most common tumor to develop in nevus sebaceus
Proliferating pilar tumor	Skin-colored to pink-red nodule	90% of cases on scalp		
Malignant†				
Basal cell carcinoma	See Ch. 88			

**Patients generally have multiple tumors when associated with a syndrome.*
†Rare tumors include pilomatrical carcinoma and trichilemmal carcinoma.

Table 91.1 Benign and malignant tumors with follicular differentiation. Cysts (e.g. epidermoid and pilar) are discussed in Chapter 90. *BHD* encodes folliculin, a tumor suppressor; *CYLD* encodes a deubiquinating enzyme; *APC* encodes a protein that regulates cell adhesion/migration.

BENIGN AND MALIGNANT TUMORS WITH SEBACEOUS DIFFERENTIATION				
	Morphology	**Site(s)**	**Distinctive characteristic(s)**	**Association(s)**
Benign				
Nevus sebaceus (see Ch. 51)	Yellow-orange, hairless linear plaque (Fig. 91.7)	Scalp > face/neck	Along lines of Blaschko, minimally raised and waxy during childhood, becoming thicker and verrucous at puberty; can develop secondary tumors, most commonly trichoblastoma	Mosaic *HRAS* > *KRAS* mutation; more extensive lesions may be associated with Schimmelpenning syndrome (see Ch. 51)
Sebaceous hyperplasia	Yellowish papule (Fig. 91.8)	Face (rarely other sites)	Sometimes telangiectatic, with central dell	
Sebaceous adenoma	Papule or nodule	Head and neck > upper trunk		Muir–Torre syndrome (especially in patients <50 years of age; *MSH2* or *MLH1* >> *MSH6* mutation) (Fig. 91.16)*
Sebaceoma	Deep nodule or "cyst"	Face (especially nose) > upper trunk		Muir–Torre syndrome (Fig. 91.16)
Malignant				
Sebaceous carcinoma	Occasionally yellowish nodule or plaque, sometimes ulcerated or crusted	Eyelid or other sites	Early lesions may resemble blepharitis or ocular rosacea	Muir–Torre syndrome (Fig. 91.16)

**MSH2, MLH1, and MSH6 encode mismatch repair proteins.*

Table 91.2 Benign and malignant tumors with sebaceous differentiation.

BENIGN AND MALIGNANT TUMORS WITH APOCRINE/ECCRINE (GLANDULAR) DIFFERENTIATION				
	Morphology	Site(s)	Distinctive characteristic(s)	Associated syndrome(s)*
Benign				
Syringoma	2–4 mm firm, skin-colored to yellow or pink papule	Most commonly eyelids > vulva > disseminated on trunk and upper extremities (Fig. 91.9)	More discrete than xanthelasma	Down syndrome, rarely metabolic syndrome (diabetes) with clear cell syringomas (Fig. 91.16)
Mixed tumor	Nodule	Head and neck (Fig. 91.10)		
Poroma	Red-blue papule, plaque, or nodule	Head and neck or palmoplantar	May have a vascular appearance (Fig. 91.11)	
Hidradenoma	Dermal or subcutaneous nodule (Fig. 91.12)			
Syringocystadenoma papilliferum	Papule or plaque, often crusted	Scalp (Fig. 91.13)	May arise within nevus sebaceous (see Fig. 91.7B)	
Hidradenoma papilliferum	Smooth dermal or subcutaneous nodule	Vulva		
Spiradenoma	Dermal or subcutaneous papule or nodule, may have bluish hue		Sometimes painful	Brooke–Spiegler syndrome (Fig. 91.16)
Cylindroma	Pink, single or multiple papule(s) or nodule(s)	Head and neck, especially scalp (Fig. 91.14)	May become confluent/extensive on head ("turban" tumor)	Cylindromatosis, Brooke–Spiegler syndrome (Fig. 91.16)
Malignant†				
Microcystic adnexal carcinoma	Nodule or plaque	Face (Fig. 91.15)	Young or middle-aged adults, female > male; more aggressive than basal cell carcinoma	

Patients generally have multiple tumors when associated with a syndrome.
†Other rare tumors include porocarcinoma and adenoid cystic carcinoma.

Table 91.3 Benign and malignant tumors with apocrine/eccrine (glandular) differentiation. Cysts (e.g. hidrocystoma) are discussed in Chapter 90.

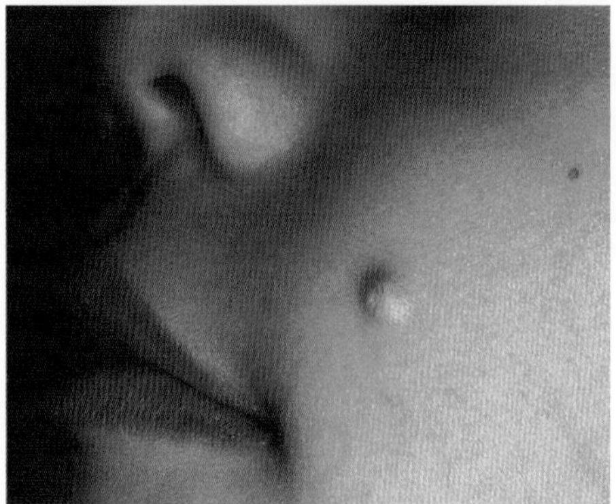

Fig. 91.2 Pilomatricoma. A nodule on the cheek of a child. *Courtesy, YDRSC.*

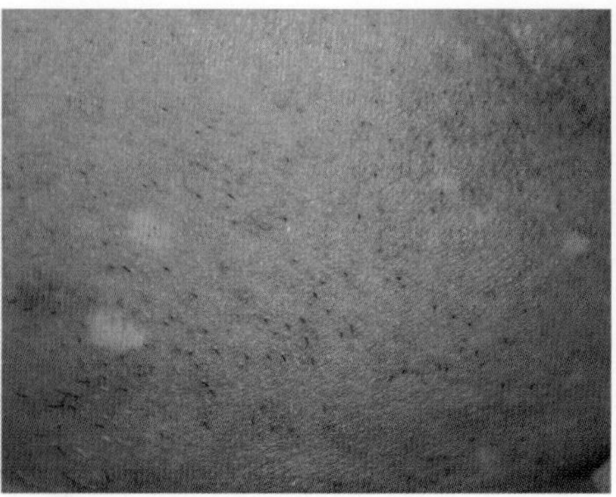

Fig. 91.5 Tumor of the follicular infundibulum. Multiple hypopigmented thin papules on the cheek. *Courtesy, YDRSC.*

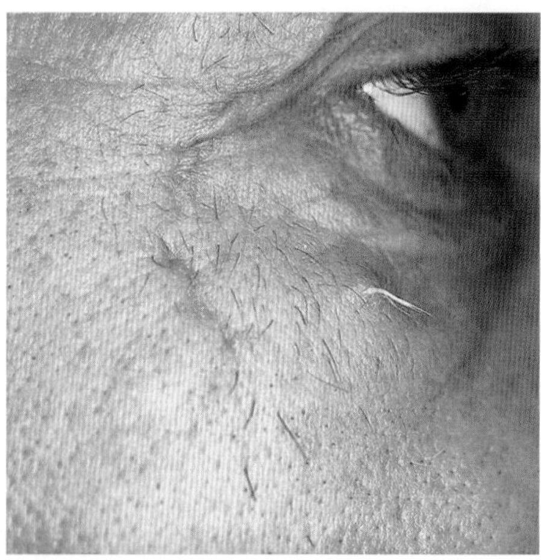

Fig. 91.3 Trichofolliculoma. Wispy vellus hairs emerge from a skin-colored papule with a dilated central pore. *Courtesy, YDRSC.*

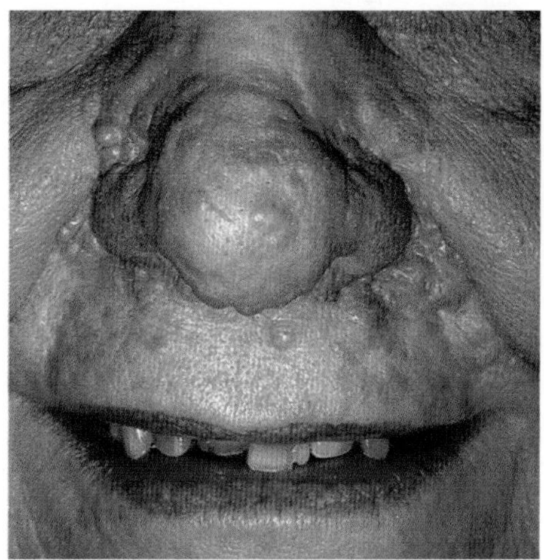

Fig. 91.6 Multiple familial trichoepitheliomas. Numerous skin-colored papules and nodules on the mid-face. *Courtesy, YDRSC.*

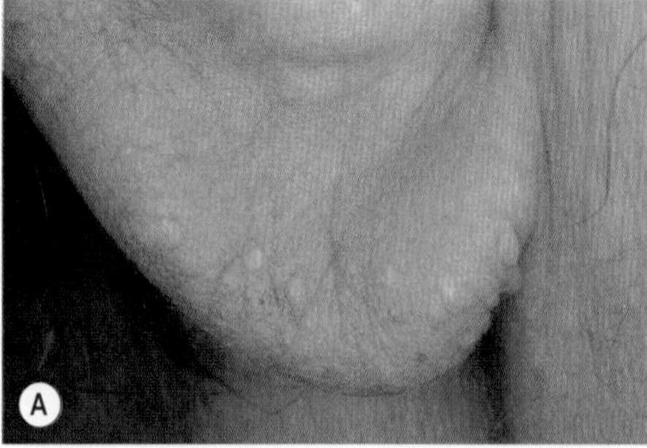

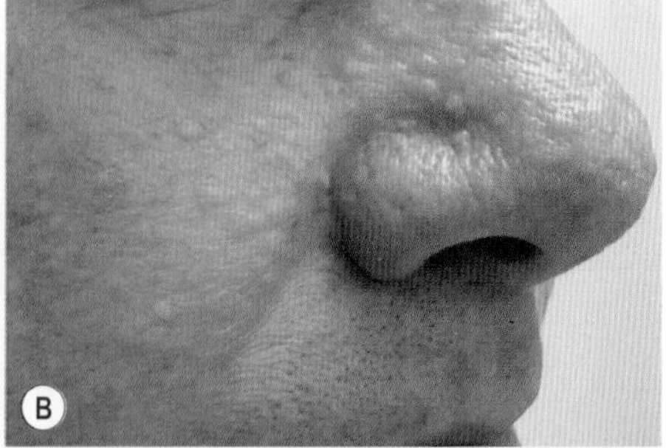

Fig. 91.4 Fibrofolliculomas in association with Birt–Hogg–Dubé syndrome. A Several skin-colored papules are present on the ear. **B** Multiple smooth papules of the cheek that are skin-colored to relatively hypopigmented; they lack the telangiectasias of the background skin. *A, Courtesy, YDRSC; B, Courtesy, Barry Goldberg, MD.*

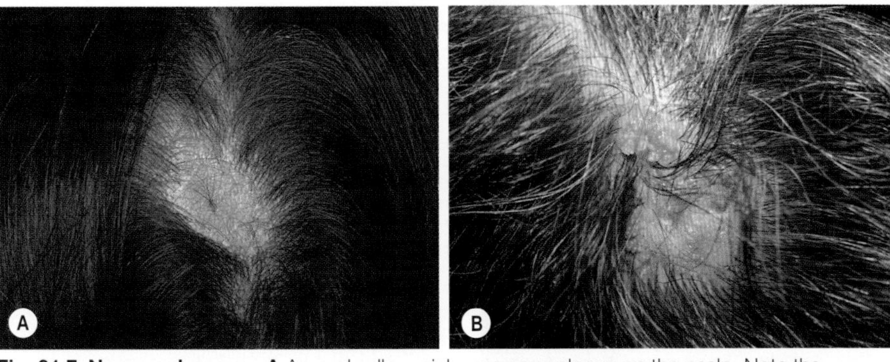

Fig. 91.7 Nevus sebaceus. A An oval yellow-pink verrucous plaque on the scalp. Note the alopecia. **B** Syringocystadenoma papilliferum arising within a nevus sebaceous. Yellow-brown verrucous plaque in which an eroded, pink, lobulated papulonodule developed. *A, Courtesy, YDRSC; B, Courtesy, Kalman Watsky, MD.*

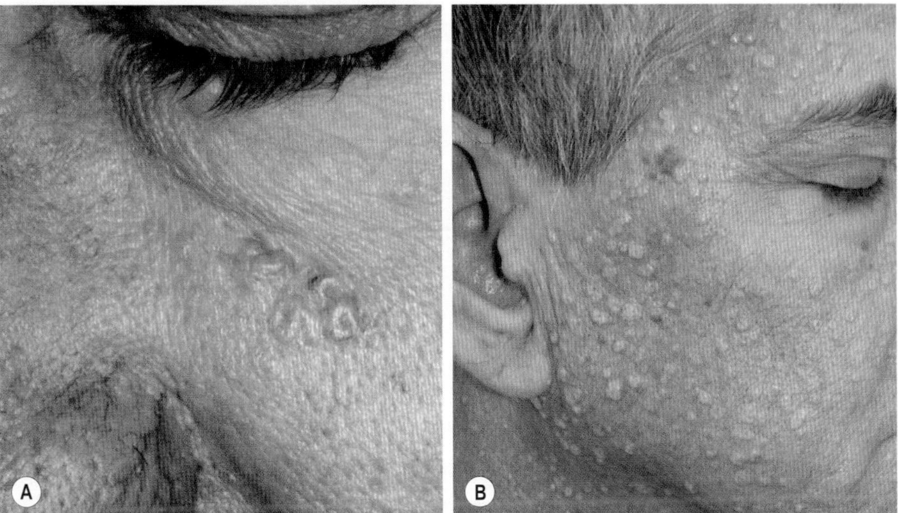

Fig. 91.8 Sebaceous hyperplasia. A Skin-colored to yellowish papules with a central dell. **B** Numerous lesions of sebaceous hyperplasia in a solid organ transplant recipient receiving long-term cyclosporine. *A, Courtesy, YDRSC; B, Courtesy, Oscar Colegio, MD, PhD.*

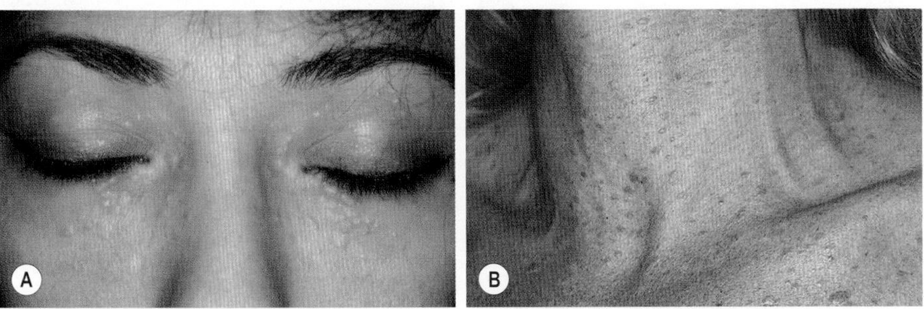

Fig. 91.9 Syringomas. A Aggregated skin-colored papules on the eyelids. **B** Multiple skin-colored to pink, smooth papules on the neck and upper chest. The lesions favor the ventral surface of the trunk, a distribution pattern referred to as *"en demicuirasse"*. *A, Courtesy, YDRSC; B, Courtesy, Jean L. Bolognia, MD.*

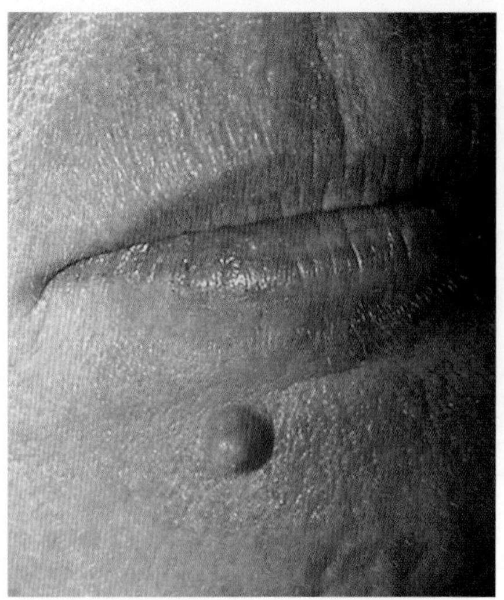

Fig. 91.10 Mixed tumor (chondroid syringoma). Nodule on the chin. *Courtesy, Ronald P. Rapini, MD.*

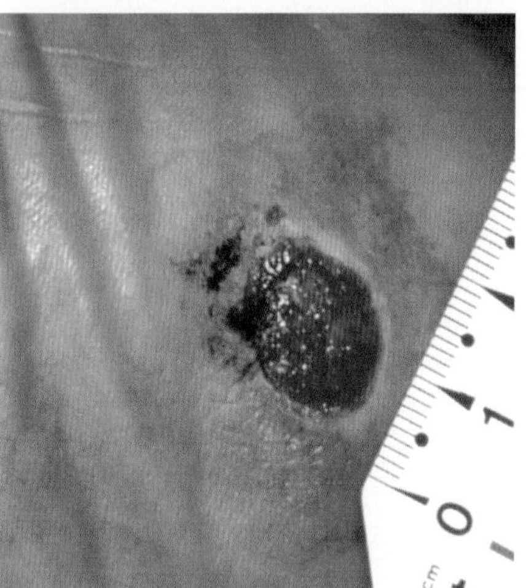

Fig. 91.11 Poroma. A solitary eroded red plaque on the plantar surface. The differential diagnosis often includes amelanotic melanoma and pyogenic granuloma. *Courtesy, YDRSC.*

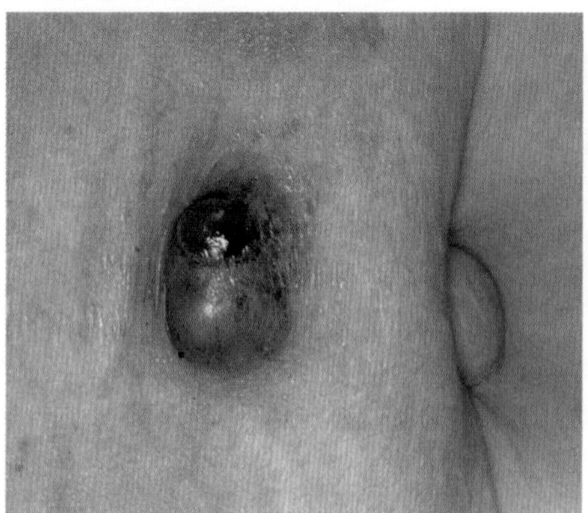

Fig. 91.12 Hidradenoma. A solitary violaceous nodule on the abdomen with serous drainage. *Courtesy, USCDRSC.*

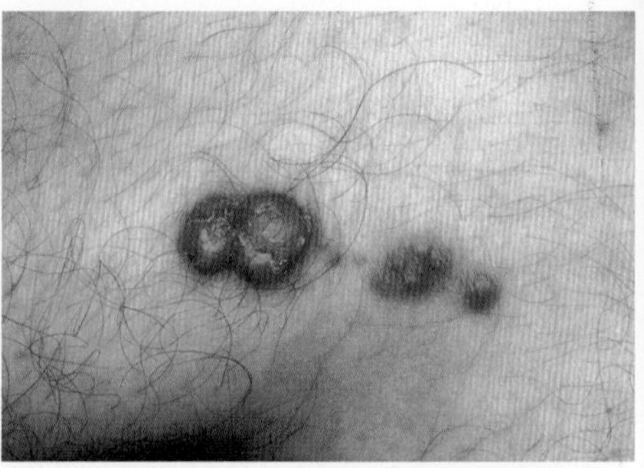

Fig. 91.13 Syringocystadenoma papilliferum. Grouped papules and nodules. The possibility of an associated nevus sebaceus needs to be considered. *Courtesy, YDRSC.*

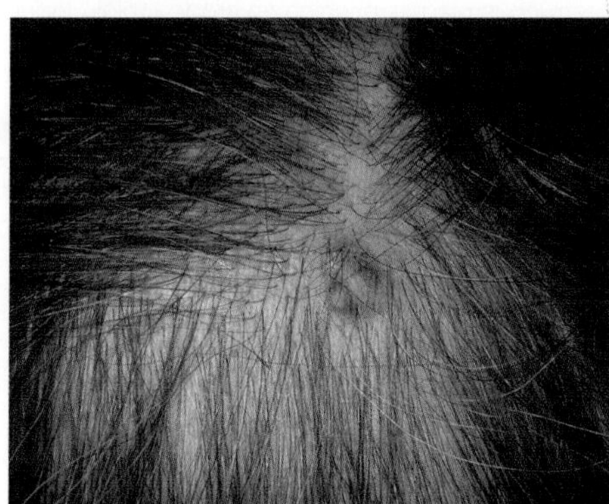

Fig. 91.14 Cylindroma. Whereas numerous tumors aggregated on the scalp are called turban tumors, solitary lesions usually present as smooth erythematous nodules. *Courtesy, YDRSC.*

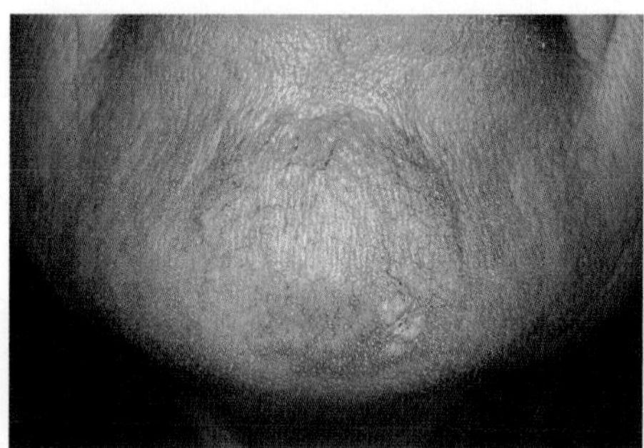

Fig. 91.15 Microcystic adnexal carcinoma. This tumor presents as a slowly expanding, firm plaque. *Courtesy, YDRSC.*

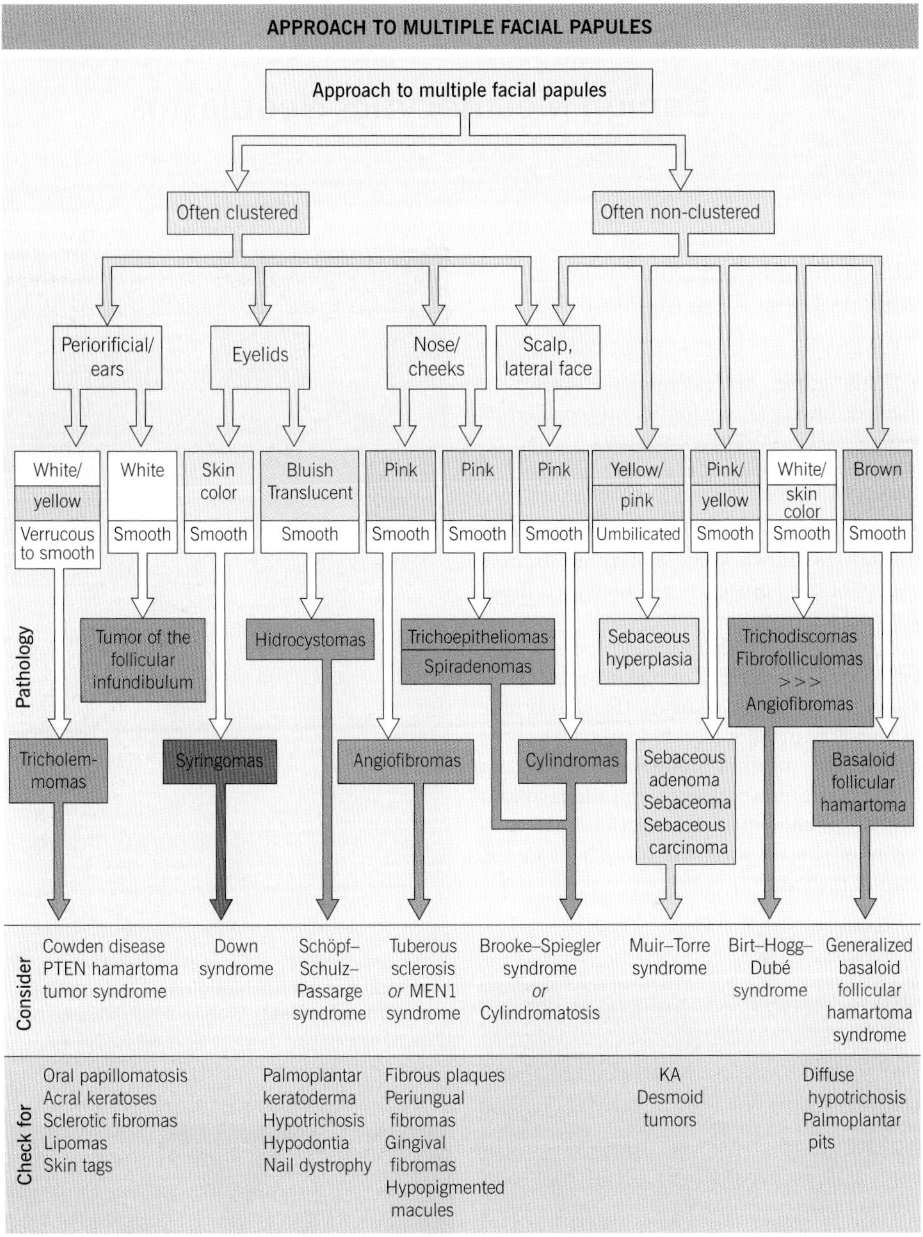

APPROACH TO MULTIPLE FACIAL PAPULES

Approach to multiple facial papules

Distribution	Location	Color	Surface	Pathology	Consider	Check for
Often clustered	Periorificial/ ears	White/ yellow	Verrucous to smooth	Tricholemmomas	Cowden disease PTEN hamartoma tumor syndrome	Oral papillomatosis Acral keratoses Sclerotic fibromas Lipomas Skin tags
Often clustered	Periorificial/ ears	White	Smooth	Tumor of the follicular infundibulum		
Often clustered	Eyelids	Skin color	Smooth	Syringomas	Down syndrome	
Often clustered	Eyelids	Bluish Translucent	Smooth	Hidrocystomas	Schöpf–Schulz–Passarge syndrome	Palmoplantar keratoderma Hypotrichosis Hypodontia Nail dystrophy
Often clustered	Nose/ cheeks	Pink	Smooth	Angiofibromas	Tuberous sclerosis *or* MEN1 syndrome	Fibrous plaques Periungual fibromas Gingival fibromas Hypopigmented macules
Often clustered	Nose/ cheeks	Pink	Smooth	Trichoepitheliomas Spiradenomas	Brooke–Spiegler syndrome *or* Cylindromatosis	
Often clustered / Often non-clustered	Scalp, lateral face	Pink	Smooth	Cylindromas	Brooke–Spiegler syndrome *or* Cylindromatosis	
Often non-clustered		Yellow/ pink	Umbilicated	Sebaceous hyperplasia		
Often non-clustered		Pink/ yellow	Smooth	Sebaceous adenoma Sebaceoma Sebaceous carcinoma	Muir–Torre syndrome	KA Desmoid tumors
Often non-clustered		White/ skin color	Smooth	Trichodiscomas Fibrofolliculomas >>> Angiofibromas	Birt–Hogg–Dubé syndrome	
Often non-clustered		Brown	Smooth	Basaloid follicular hamartoma	Generalized basaloid follicular hamartoma syndrome	Diffuse hypotrichosis Palmoplantar pits

Fig. 91.16 Approach to multiple facial papules. As a general rule, multiple lesions are suggestive of a syndrome, but exceptions are syringoma and tumor of the follicular infundibulum (rarely syndromic). Other causes of multiple facial papules include BCCs (acquired and inherited in nevoid basal cell carcinoma syndrome), miliary osteomas, milia, verrucae, and acne. KA, keratoacanthoma

For further information see Ch. 111 from *Dermatology, Fourth Edition*.

For additional online figures visit www.expertconsult.com 

92 Benign Melanocytics Neoplasms

Benign Pigmented Cutaneous Lesions Other Than Melanocytic Nevi

- This group of lesions can further be divided into: (1) predominantly epidermal lesions (Table 92.1; Figs 92.1–92.5); and (2) dermal melanocytoses (Table 92.2; Figs 92.6 and 92.7).
- In the predominantly epidermal lesions, the tan to brown color can result from a variety of mechanisms – e.g. increased melanocyte activity (melanogenesis), increased melanin content in keratinocytes, and a mild increase in the number of melanocytes.
- In dermal melanocytoses, the skin is blue to blue-gray in color (ceruloderma) due to the presence of melanin-producing melanocytes in the mid to lower dermis and the resultant Tyndall phenomenon (the preferential scattering of shorter wavelengths of light by the dermal melanin).

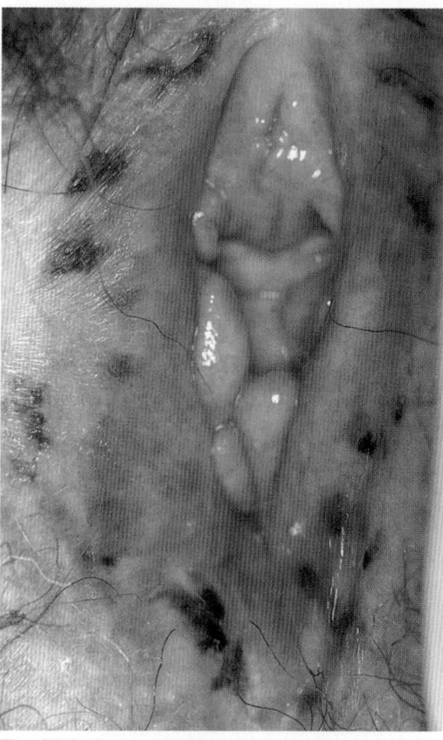

Fig. 92.2 Anogenital lentiginosis (anogenital melanotic macules). Biopsy of the clinically most atypical lesion (at 7 o'clock) showed no cellular atypia. Over a period of 10 years, several of the macules faded. *Courtesy, Jean L. Bolognia, MD.*

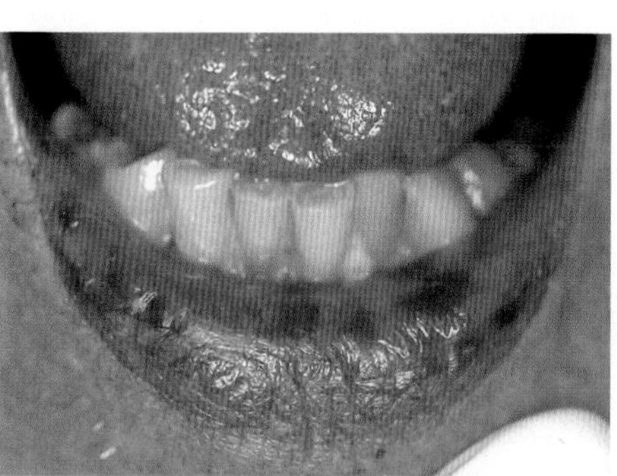

Fig. 92.1 Labial lentigines in a patient with Laugier–Hunziker syndrome. Multiple hyperpigmented macules on the lower lip (labial melanotic macules) and a few on the tongue; Peutz–Jeghers syndrome can have a similar clinical appearance. *Courtesy, YDRSC.*

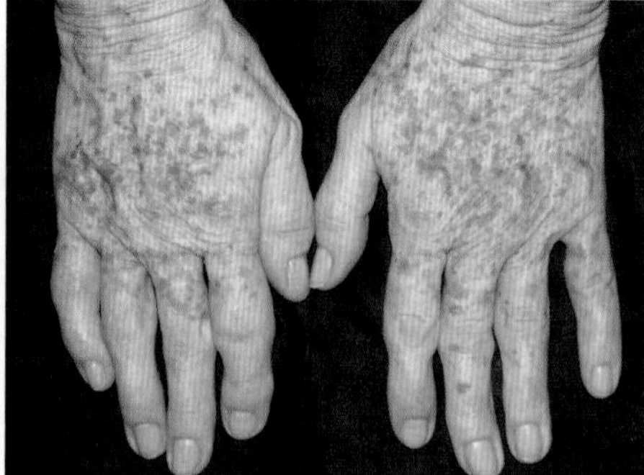

Fig. 92.3 Solar lentigines. Multiple, round to irregularly shaped, brown macules on the dorsal aspect of the hands in an older woman. *Courtesy, Luis Requena, MD.*

BENIGN PIGMENTED LESIONS OTHER THAN MELANOCYTIC NEVI (PREDOMINANTLY EPIDERMAL LESIONS)	
Lesion	**Major clinical features**
Ephelid (freckle)	• Onset in childhood (UVR-induced) and tends to fade with age and in the absence of sun exposure (e.g. winter months) • Small, well-circumscribed, usually multiple, tan to brown macules on sun-exposed areas in fair-skinned individuals
Lentigo simplex and mucosal melanotic lesions	• Onset usually in childhood; not related to sun exposure • Small, sharply circumscribed, brown to black macule that can occur at any site, including mucosae; typically a few lesions • Multiple or generalized lentigines may be an isolated phenomenon or a marker of an underlying disorder (Table 92.3)
• **Oral melanotic macules** (Fig. 92.1)	• Onset in adulthood • Typically, an isolated to a few, brown to brown-black macule(s) on the vermilion portion of the lower lip (labial melanotic macules); occasionally on the gingiva, buccal mucosa, tongue, or palate (Fig. 92.1) • Multiple lesions (lentiginosis) may be a marker of Peutz–Jeghers or Laugier–Hunziker syndromes
• **Anogenital lentiginosis** (anogenital melanotic macules) (Fig. 92.2)	• Onset typically in adulthood; females > males • One or more brown to black macules, sometimes with irregular or jagged borders, mottled pigmentation, and occasionally of large size (>1 cm) • In *females* favors the labia minora > labia majora, vaginal introitus, perineum; in *males* favors the glans penis and penile shaft • Multiple lesions are a feature of lichen sclerosis, Laugier–Hunziker syndrome, and Bannayan–Riley–Ruvalcaba syndrome (see Table 52.1)
• **Conjunctival melanosis** (conjunctival melanotic macules)	• Conjunctival brown to black pigmented macules, streaks, or patches • While congenital form is typically benign, primary acquired ocular melanosis is considered a precursor lesion of conjunctival melanoma
Solar lentigo (lentigo senilis, "liver spot") (Fig. 92.3)	• Onset in adulthood (UVR-induced); persists throughout life and may darken with sun exposure, but does not fade • Typically, multiple tan to dark brown macules, often with irregular borders, ranging from a few millimeters to >1 cm in diameter • Distribution limited to sun-exposed sites, favoring those areas of greatest cumulative exposure (e.g. face, dorsal hands and forearms, upper trunk) • Clinical variants: ink spot lentigo, PUVA lentigo, tanning bed lentigo, sunburn lentigo • If present or widespread in young children, consider: xeroderma pigmentosum, type 2 oculocutaneous albinism (lesions are unusually large and jagged)
Café-au-lait macule (CALM) (Fig. 92.4)	• Onset at birth or in early childhood; not UVR-induced, but may first become noticeable following sun exposure • Uniformly colored, tan to brown macule or patch, varying in size from a few millimeters to >15 cm; grows proportionately with the child • Usually isolated but occasionally multiple; single CALM seen in ~25–35% of children; <1% of children have ≥3 CALMs • Multiple CALMs may be associated with a variety of disorders (see Table 50.3)

Table 92.1 Benign pigmented lesions other than melanocytic nevi (predominantly epidermal lesions). *Continued*

BENIGN PIGMENTED LESIONS OTHER THAN MELANOCYTIC NEVI (PREDOMINANTLY EPIDERMAL LESIONS)	
Lesion	**Major clinical features**
Becker melanosis (nevus) (Fig. 92.5; see Fig. 57.3 and Table 57.1)	• May be present at birth, but the majority appear around puberty; male:female ratio ~5:1; stimulated by androgens • Classically, unilateral, tan to brown patch or thin plaque on the shoulder and/or upper trunk, but can occur elsewhere; margins typically irregular and break up into "islands" at the periphery; hypertrichosis in ~50% • Associated smooth muscle hamartoma often present and is clinically apparent by the presence of perifollicular papules that are accentuated with rubbing • Infrequently associated with ipsilateral developmental anomalies (e.g. supernumerary nipples, breast hypoplasia, hypoplasia of the pectoralis major muscle, bony abnormalities)

Table 92.1 *Continued* **Benign pigmented lesions other than melanocytic nevi (predominantly epidermal lesions).**

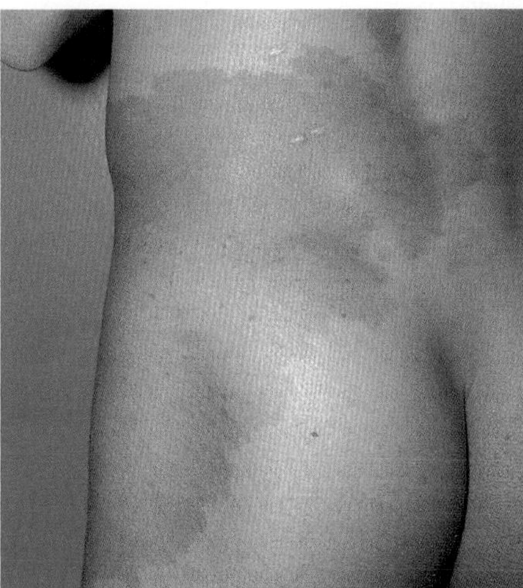

Fig. 92.4 Café-au-lait macule (CALM). Large tan patch in a geographic pattern on the lateral trunk. The patient did not have McCune–Albright syndrome (see Ch. 50). *Courtesy, YDRSC.*

Acquired Melanocytic Nevi (Moles)

• Benign proliferations of a type of melanocyte called a "nevus cell".
• Nevus cells differ from "ordinary" melanocytes, which typically reside as single units in the basal layer of the epidermis, in that they: (1) usually cluster as nests in the lower epidermis and/or dermis; and (2) do not have dendritic processes (except when found in a blue nevus).
• Both "ordinary" melanocytes and nevus cells can produce melanin.
• Acquired melanocytic nevi can be categorized as **common** (banal) or **atypical** (dysplastic), and they are further named based on the histopathologic location of the collections of nevus cells (Fig. 92.8):
  – ***Junctional*** *melanocytic nevus*: dermal–epidermal junction
  – ***Compound*** *melanocytic nevus:* dermal–epidermal junction plus dermis
  – ***Intradermal*** *melanocytic nevus:* dermis
• Variants include halo, blue, Spitz, and "special site" nevi (Figs 92.9A–F and 92.10).
• Risk factors for developing acquired melanocytic nevi: (1) a family history of numerous nevi; (2) a greater degree of sun exposure during childhood, especially intermittent and intense; and (3) lightly pigmented skin (individuals with phototype II have the greatest number of nevi).
• The vast majority of acquired melanocytic nevi remain as benign neoplasms throughout one's life and do not require treatment.
• Having numerous melanocytic nevi (>50–100) or multiple atypical nevi are phenotypic markers for an entire skin surface at risk for developing cutaneous melanoma; such persons should have lifelong surveillance with periodic total body skin examinations (beginning around puberty) and counseling regarding home self-skin examinations and sun protective measures.
• Cutaneous melanoma may arise within a pre-existing nevus, but more than half of cutaneous melanomas arise *de novo* – i.e. in previously normal-appearing skin.

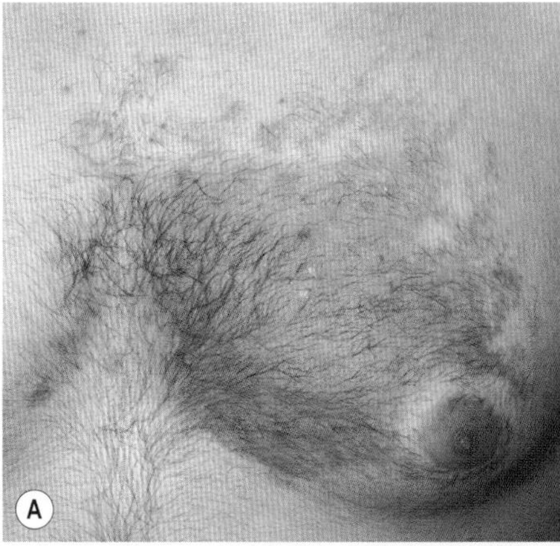

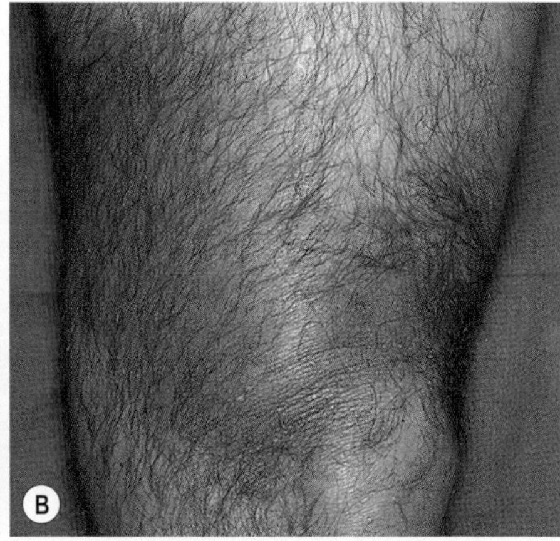

Fig. 92.5 Becker melanosis (nevus). A Unilateral, block-like configuration with hyperpigmentation and hypertrichosis; the patient had an underlying smooth muscle hamartoma. **B** Large patch of hyperpigmentation on the leg, which is medium brown in color. Such lesions may be misdiagnosed as café-au-lait macules or congenital melanocytic nevi, especially when they do not occur on the upper trunk. *A, Courtesy, Edward Cowen, MD; B, Courtesy, Jean L. Bolognia, MD.*

THE SPECTRUM AND CLINICAL FEATURES OF DERMAL MELANOCYTOSES	
Lesion	**Major clinical features**
Congenital dermal melanocytosis (Mongolian spots) (Fig. 92.6)	• Typically apparent at birth or within the first few weeks of life • Regresses in >95% of patients by age 18 years; more likely to persist in extensive or extra-sacral variants; most common in Asians and Blacks • Presents as a single or multiple, uniform, blue-gray patch(es) with indefinite borders; favors the lumbosacral area and buttocks > back; varies in size from a few centimeters to >20 cm • CALM and melanocytic nevi that reside within these areas often have a "halo" that lacks dermal melanocytes (Fig. 92.6) • **DDx:** ecchymosis, child abuse, patch blue nevus, venous malformation • Extensive lesions may be associated with a port-wine stain (phakomatosis pigmentovascularis; see Ch. 85), developmental abnormalities (e.g. cleft lip), or inborn errors of metabolism (e.g. Hurler syndrome)
Nevus of Ota*,** (oculodermal melanocytosis, nevus fuscocaeruleus ophthalmomaxillaris) (Fig. 92.7)	• Bimodal age of onset, with the majority (50–60%) present at birth or in infancy (before 1 year of age), and the remainder (40–50%) appearing at or around puberty; lifelong persistence • More common in Asians and Blacks; females > males • Involves those areas innervated by the first and second divisions of the trigeminal nerve, including the skin, conjunctiva, sclera, tympanic membrane, and/or oral and nasal mucosa; 10% of cases are bilateral • Lesions are characterized by speckled or mottled, grayish-brown to blue-black patches; may extend in size over time but usually stable by adulthood • Occasionally associated with neurocutaneous melanosis, glaucoma, ipsilateral sensorineural hearing loss, ocular melanoma (yearly ophthalmologic exams recommended)

Table 92.2 The spectrum and clinical features of dermal melanocytoses. *Continued*

THE SPECTRUM AND CLINICAL FEATURES OF DERMAL MELANOCYTOSES	
Lesion	**Major clinical features**
Nevus of Ito* (nevus fuscocaeruleus acromiodeltoideus)	• Favored populations and clinical appearance are similar to nevus of Ota (see above) • Involves areas of skin innervated by the posterior supraclavicular and lateral brachiocutaneous nerves, namely the supraclavicular, scapular, or deltoid regions; typically unilateral
Nevus of Ota-like macules** (acquired dermal melanocytosis, acquired bilateral nevus of Ota-like macules, Hori's nevus)	• Most often seen in middle-aged Asian females • Multiple grayish-brown macules arising in a symmetric, bilateral distribution on the malar cheeks and forehead and sometimes the eyelids, temple, and nose; does not involve mucosa • Important to distinguish from melasma, as laser therapy improves nevus of Ota-like macules

**DDx* *for nevus of Ota or Ito: patch or plaque blue nevus, ecchymosis, venous malformation; for nevus of Ito: extra-sacral Mongolian spot.*
***Rx* *(if desired): pulsed Q-switched lasers (e.g. Q-switched ruby, alexandrite, or Nd:YAG lasers) beneficial but often requires multiple sessions.*

Table 92.2 *Continued* **The spectrum and clinical features of dermal melanocytoses.** CALM, café-au-lait macule.

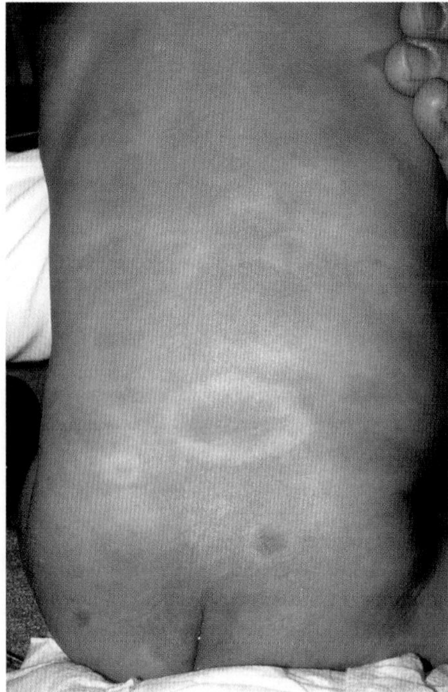

Fig. 92.6 Dermal melanocytosis (Mongolian spots) in a child with neurofibromatosis 1. Surrounding each café-au-lait macule, there is an absence of the characteristic blue discoloration. *Courtesy, YDRSC.*

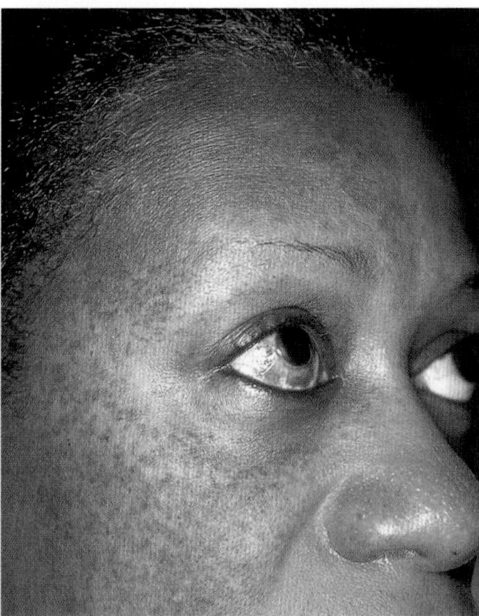

Fig. 92.7 Nevus of Ota (oculodermal melanocytosis). Unilateral blue-gray discoloration of the face, which is either mottled or confluent. There is also involvement of the sclera. *Courtesy, YDRSC.*

• Most patients with numerous nevi and atypical nevi will have a prominent morphologic type of nevus ("signature nevus"); by recognizing signature nevi, the "ugly duckling" can be identified and closely examined.

• Persons with more darkly pigmented skin will typically have darker colored nevi.

DISORDERS ASSOCIATED WITH MULTIPLE LENTIGINES	
Disorder, inheritance, gene mutation	**Comments**
Generalized	
LEOPARD syndrome (now referred to as Noonan syndrome with multiple lentigines) AD *PTPN11* > *RAF1* > *BRAF*	• *L*entigines present in infancy/early childhood • Café-noir macules • *E*CG changes (conduction defects, hypertrophic cardiomyopathy), *o*cular hypertelorism, *p*ulmonary stenosis, *a*bnormal genitalia, growth *r*etardation and *d*eafness
Generalized lentigines AD	• Café-au-lait macules
Carney complex (NAME/LAMB syndrome) AD *PRKAR1A*	• Lentigines, mucocutaneous myxomas, blue nevi (including epithelioid) • Psammomatous melanotic schwannomas • Atrial myxoma • Myxoid mammary fibroadenomas • Pigmented nodular adrenocortical disease; testicular (calcifying Sertoli cell), thyroid, and pituitary tumors
Arterial dissection plus lentiginosis	• Cutaneous lentigines with onset in childhood • Dissection of aortic, internal carotid, and vertebral arteries
Localized	
Head and neck (including oral mucosa) ± acral	
Peutz–Jeghers syndrome AD *STK11*	• Lentigines favor perioral region†, oral mucosa‡, and hands; longitudinal melanonychia • Multiple hamartomatous GI polyps • Pancreatic carcinoma; ovarian (adenoma malignum)/testicular tumors
Laugier–Hunziker syndrome	• Similar distribution of lentigines as in Peutz–Jeghers, including lips, oral mucosa, and digits • Longitudinal melanonychia and genital melanosis
Hyperkeratosis–hyperpigmentation (Cantú) syndrome AD	• Punctate palmoplantar keratoderma • Multiple small (1 mm) macules on the face, forearms, hands/feet
Cowden disease AD *PTEN* (See Ch. 52 and Table 52.1)	• Periorificial and acral pigmented macules

Table 92.3 Disorders associated with multiple lentigines. *Continued*

DISORDERS ASSOCIATED WITH MULTIPLE LENTIGINES	
Disorder, inheritance, gene mutation	**Comments**
Centrofacial lentiginosis (neurodysraphic) AD	• Lentigines in a butterfly distribution on the nose, cheeks > forehead, eyelids, upper lip • Onset in infancy; increase in number in childhood • Possibly associated with neuropsychiatric illness and osseous anomalies
Inherited patterned lentiginosis AD	• Blacks with more lightly pigmented skin • Pigmented macules appear in early childhood • Present on central face and lips > buttocks, elbows, hands/feet • Rare oral mucosal involvement
Cronkhite–Canada syndrome	• Typically affects older men • Lentigines of buccal mucosa, face, hands/feet • Alopecia (diffuse, non-scarring), nail dystrophy, intestinal polyposis, diarrhea, malabsorption
Genital	
Bannayan–Riley–Ruvalcaba syndrome AD *PTEN* (see Table 52.1)	• Penile > vulvar pigmented macules
"Photodistribution"	
Xeroderma pigmentosum AR Mutations in genes encoding DNA repair proteins	• Lentigines favor, but are not limited to, chronically sun-exposed sites • Multiple skin cancers
Segmental	
Partial unilateral lentiginosis	• Multiple lentigines in a segmental distribution • Café-au-lait macules in same distribution

†*May fade.*
‡*Persists.*

Table 92.3 *Continued* **Disorders associated with multiple lentigines.** AD, autosomal dominant; AR, autosomal recessive; LAMB, lentigines/atrial myxoma/mucocutaneous myxoma/blue nevi syndrome; LEOPARD, lentigines/ECG abnormalities/ocular hypertelorism/pulmonary stenosis/abnormalities of genitalia/retardation of growth/deafness syndrome; NAME, nevi/atrial myxoma/myxoid neurofibroma/ephelides syndrome. *Adapted from Bolognia JL. Disorders of hypopigmentation and hyperpigmentation. In Harper J, Oranje A, Prose N (eds.), Textbook of Pediatric Dermatology, 2nd edn. Oxford: Blackwell, 2006;997–1040.*

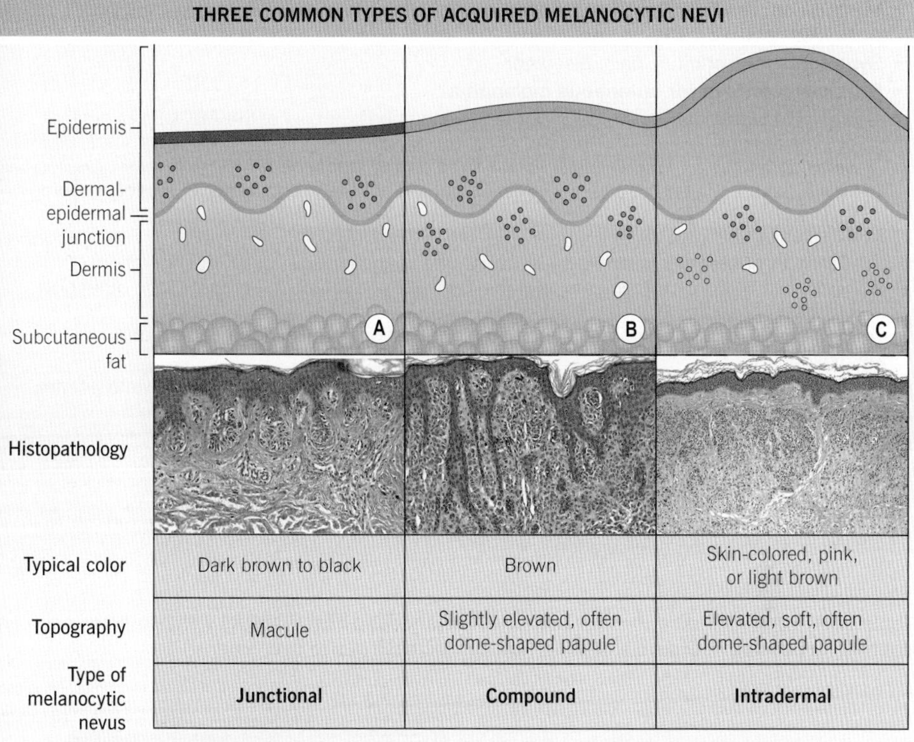

Fig. 92.8 Three common types of acquired melanocytic nevi. (A) Junctional, **(B)** compound, and **(C)** intradermal. The latter may also be pedunculated or papillomatous (see Ch. 1).

- **Rx:** it is not necessary to remove clinically atypical nevi prophylactically in order to confirm the presence of histopathological atypia; biopsies of nevi are indicated primarily when a severely atypical nevus or cutaneous melanoma is in the **DDx** (Table 92.4); if banal nevi become irritated (e.g. by clothing or jewelry), shave removal can be done.
- When cutaneous melanoma is in the **DDx**, complete removal of the nevus is recommended as well as submission to a dermatopathologist; removal can be accomplished by several methods (see Fig. 1.6); providing additional information (e.g. eccentric hyperpigmented area) is also helpful.

Common (Banal) Acquired Melanocytic Nevi

- Benign lesions with varied clinical appearance, but typically ≤6 mm in diameter, symmetric, well-circumscribed, evenly pigmented, and round or oval in shape; perifollicular hypopigmentation or stippled pigmentation is often present upon closer inspection.
- Distribution favors intermittently sun-exposed areas of the trunk and extremities and, less frequently, acral sites (palms, soles, nail matrix); in patients who eventually develop many nevi, the scalp may be one of the first sites of involvement.
- Classically appear after the first 6 months of life, increase in number during childhood and adolescence, peak by the third decade, and then slowly regress with age.
- As nevi "age" over time, they often become more elevated, softer, and less pigmented.

Atypical (Dysplastic or Clark) Acquired Melanocytic Nevi

- Benign lesions that share, to a lesser extent, many clinical features of cutaneous melanoma (e.g. asymmetry, border irregularity, color variegation, and diameter >6 mm) but usually they "age" in a manner similar

POTENTIAL INDICATIONS FOR BIOPSY OF MELANOCYTIC NEVI
• **Patient concern for cutaneous melanoma** (e.g. new nevus, changing nevus, anxiety-provoking nevus) • **Symptoms** (e.g. pruritus, pain, bleeding) • **Physician concern for cutaneous melanoma** – Marked *a*symmetry (e.g. irregular *b*orders, variegated *c*olor) – i.e. the ABCDEs of cutaneous melanoma* – Areas of regression (often seen as white or blue-gray areas) – Development of areas of pink or red color that are not easily explained by a benign etiology (e.g. acne or trauma) – Surrounding cloak of erythema ("little red riding hood sign") – History or photographic evidence of worrisome change in size, color, configuration – "Ugly duckling" nevus (i.e. a nevus with a different phenotype than most of the other nevi in a given patient) • **Acral nevus –** marked asymmetry, mottled pigmentation, parallel ridge pattern on dermoscopy • **Nail matrix-derived nevus –** single band that is dark or has an irregular color, width ≥4 mm, progressive darkening with time, or extension of pigmentation beyond the nail fold • **Halo nevus –** the central nevus is markedly atypical or has worrisome features • **Cellular blue nevus –** has undergone change (e.g. a new papule or nodule) • **Spitz nevus with clinically atypical features** – see text • **Congenital melanocytic nevus –** new papulonodule whose color can vary from red to black, new area of induration or ulceration

**D and E represent large diameter and evolution.*

Table 92.4 Potential indications for biopsy of melanocytic nevi. Patients with numerous nevi can continue to develop new nevi, and banal nevi can increase in size over time.

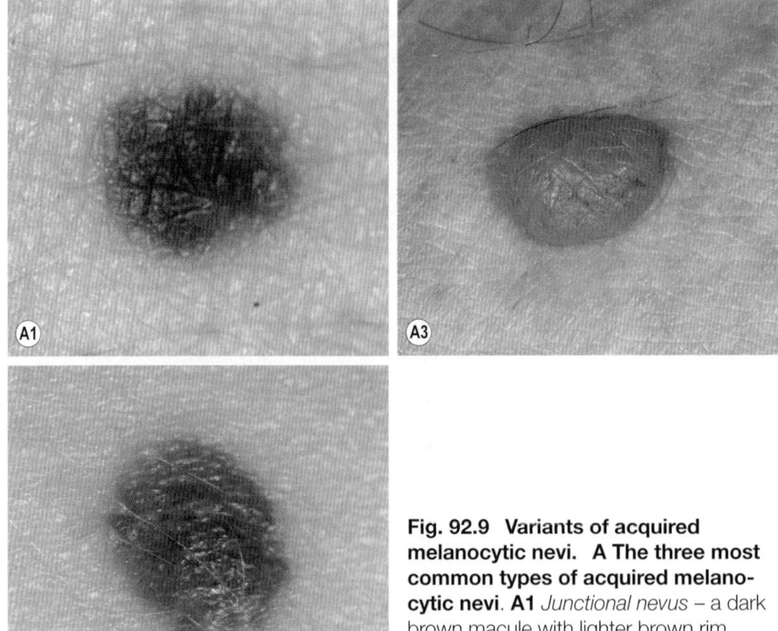

Fig. 92.9 Variants of acquired melanocytic nevi. A The three most common types of acquired melanocytic nevi. **A1** *Junctional nevus* – a dark brown macule with lighter brown rim. **A2** *Compound nevus* – clinically, a light to medium brown papule. **A3** *Intradermal nevus* – a soft, light pink papule. *Continued*

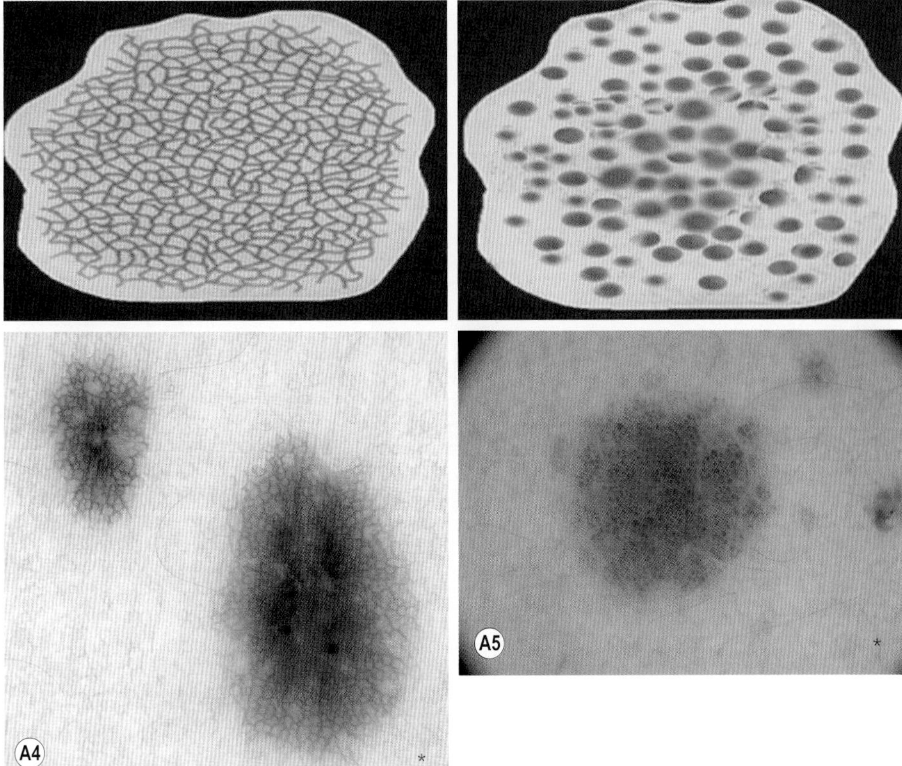

Fig. 92.9 *Continued* **A4** A reticular pattern on dermoscopy* is commonly seen in typical acquired nevi. **A5** The globular pattern is another common dermoscopic* finding in acquired melanocytic nevi.

to banal nevi and only a tiny proportion may develop melanoma within them.

- Histopathologically, architectural disorder is seen and cytologic atypia may be present; sometimes the latter is categorized as mild, moderate, or severe.
- The major risk factor for developing atypical nevi is genetic predisposition.
- The *"atypical mole syndrome"* has been variably described in the literature, ranging from individuals with atypical nevi but no personal or family history of melanoma to the *f*amilial *a*typical *m*ultiple *m*ole and *m*elanoma syndrome (FAMMM syndrome), in which an individual with numerous nevi (>50), multiple atypical nevi, and ≥1 first- or second-degree relative with cutaneous melanoma has a very high risk of developing melanoma (see Ch. 93).
- Atypical nevi often appear around puberty and are thought to develop throughout life.
- Although the majority of atypical nevi are located in intermittently sun-exposed sites (e.g. trunk and extremities [lower > upper in females]), often they can be seen on the breasts and buttocks.
- *Clinically*, atypical nevi are recognized by various features – e.g. varied colors (pink, brown, tan), a "fried-egg" appearance with a papular component and a macular rim, a larger size than banal nevi, and borders that are ill-defined, "fuzzy," and sometimes notched or irregular (see Fig. 92.9B).
- Adjuncts to monitoring these patients include baseline and follow-up nevus and total body photography; dermoscopy; patient/partner education on skin self-examination and

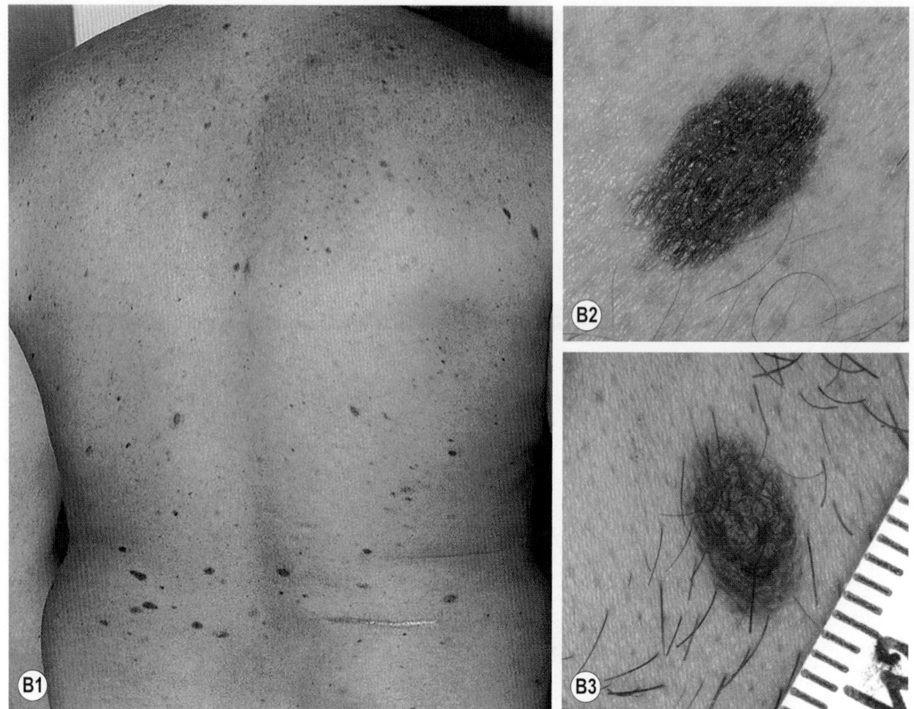

Fig. 92.9 *Continued* **B Clinically atypical melanocytic nevi. B1** In addition to multiple atypical nevi, patients can have numerous banal nevi. **B2** There is asymmetry as well as several shades of brown, simulating the clinical features seen in cutaneous melanoma. **B3** Although this "fried egg" nevus is at least 7 mm in size, it is symmetric and does not need to be excised.

signs of melanoma; and possibly alternating examinations between two dermatologists.

- Nevi with mild cytologic atypia histopathologically and most with moderate cytologic atypia do not require re-excision, especially when the biopsy attempted to remove the entire nevus; it is generally recommended, however, that severely atypical nevi be completely excised or re-excised with conservative margins (e.g. 3–5 mm).

Blue Nevi

- Benign lesions due to a proliferation of dendritic melanocytes within the dermis; blue in color because of the Tyndall effect (see above).
- Sites of predilection are those areas in which active dermal melanocytes are still present at the time of birth (e.g. head, neck, dorsal hands and feet, sacral region).
- Most blue nevi have a somatic activating mutation in *GNAQ* (more often than *GNA11*), both of which encode Q-class G-protein α subunits.
- The ***common blue nevus*** typically presents as a solitary, blue to blue-black, dome-shaped papule, usually <1 cm in diameter and most often occurring on the dorsal hands or feet (see Fig. 92.9C); frequently arises in adolescence; no malignant potential.

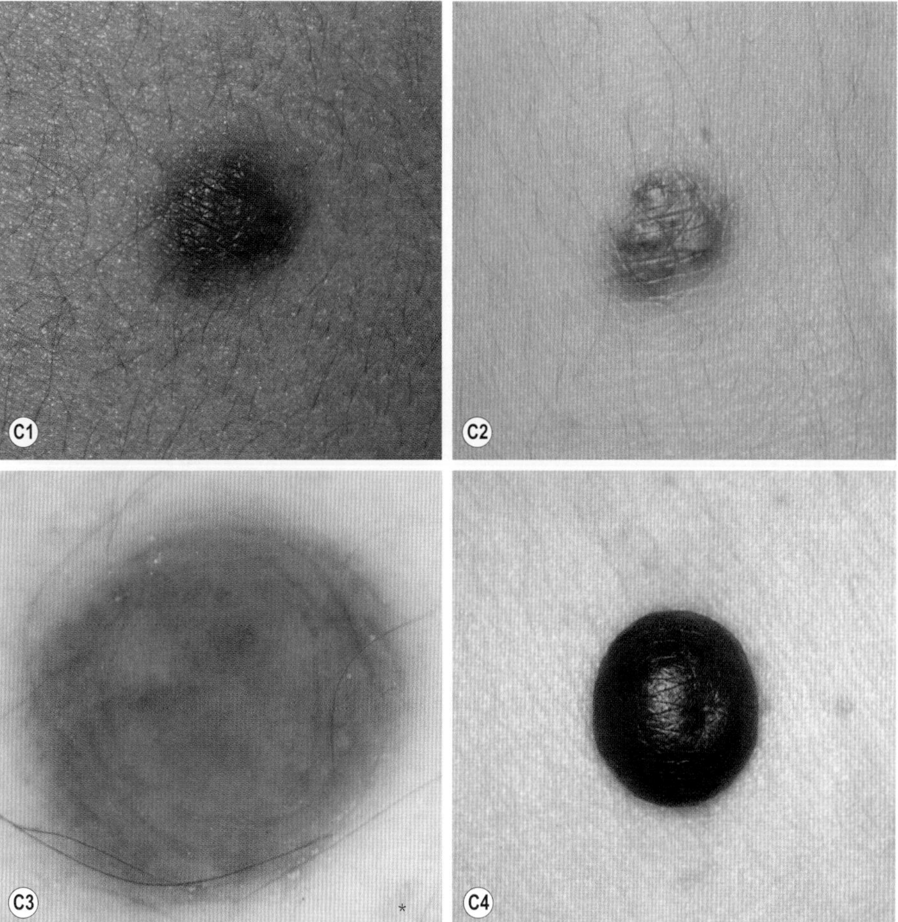

Fig. 92.9 *Continued* **C Blue nevi**. **C1–C3** *Common blue nevus* – clinically a dark blue-black papule in a patient with more darkly pigmented skin (**C1**). Blue papule with an irregular, micropapular surface (**C2**). Dermoscopically* – blue homogeneous color (**C3**). **C4** *Cellular blue nevus* – a black nodule is seen.

- The ***cellular blue nevus*** tends to be larger in size (i.e. more plaque-like), and it can be congenital or acquired (see Fig. 92.9C4); favors the head, sacral region, and buttocks; melanoma (malignant blue nevus) can develop within cellular blue nevi (see Ch. 93); if location (e.g. scalp) or patient awareness prevents satisfactory observation, then complete excision can be performed.
- The ***combined blue nevus*** typically presents as a blue to gray-brown macule or papule with a subtle brown rim; it usually represents a combination of a blue nevus with a banal nevus, but in theory can be a combination of any two types of nevi.
- **DDx:** traumatic tattoo (e.g. carbon from a pencil), which typically can be distinguished by history, or a venous lake (compressible) > melanoma metastasis, primary cutaneous melanoma.
- **Rx:** none for common blue nevi and as noted above for cellular blue nevi; lesions with a history of recent growth or change should be biopsied.
- Multiple blue nevi (normal in Asians) may signify an underlying syndrome, e.g. Carney complex (see Table 92.3).

Spitz Nevus (Spindle and Epithelioid Cell Nevus)

- Benign proliferation of epithelioid and/or spindled melanocytes.

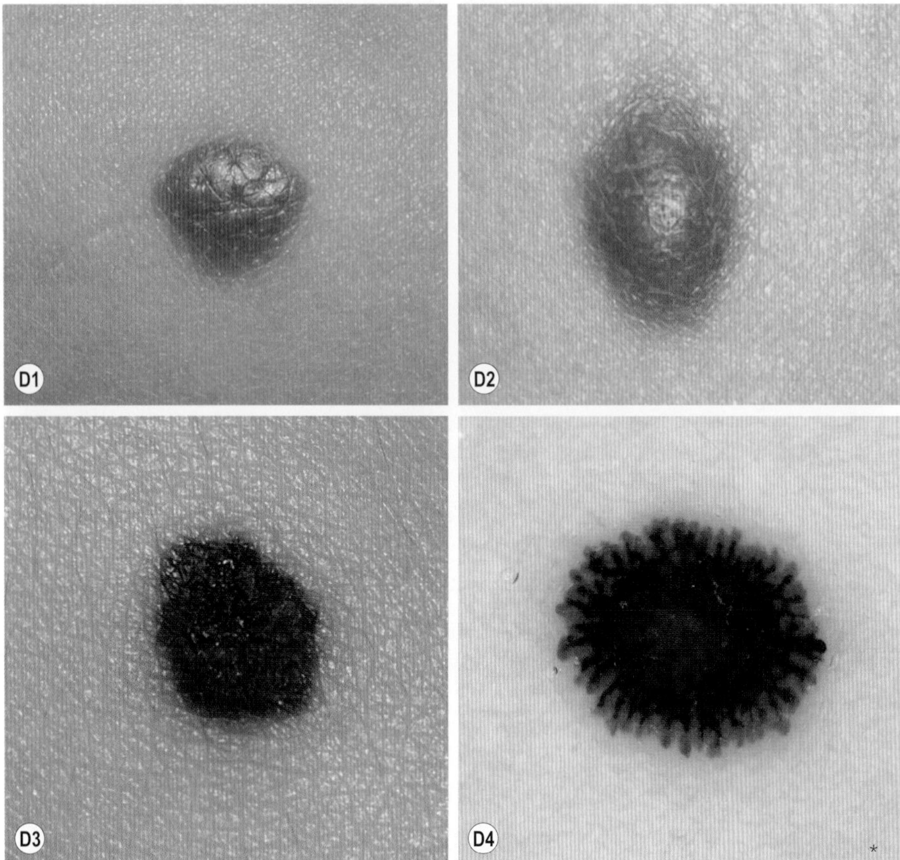

Fig. 92.9 *Continued* **D Spitz nevi. D1** Red, symmetric, dome-shaped papule on the thigh of a child. **D2** Medium-brown, symmetric, dome-shaped papule with a thinner rim in an adolescent. **D3** Darkly pigmented Spitz nevus in a child with a flatter surface. **D4** *Reed nevus*, typified dermoscopically* by the classic starburst pattern (irregular streaks at the periphery of a heavily pigmented and symmetric small macule).

- Majority appear during childhood or young adulthood and most commonly occur on the face and lower extremities.
- Classically, a Spitz nevus is symmetric, well-circumscribed, <1 cm in diameter, uniformly pink, tan, red, or red-brown, smooth, and dome-shaped (see Fig. 92.9D); occasionally, lesions are verrucous or darkly pigmented.
- ***Pigmented spindle cell nevus of Reed*** is a variant that typically presents in young women as a very dark brown to black minimally elevated papule, most often on the thigh; characteristic "starburst pattern" on dermoscopy (see Fig. 92.9D4).
- **DDx:** *clinical:* pyogenic granuloma, juvenile xanthogranuloma, molluscum contagiosum, verruca vulgaris, intradermal melanocytic nevus (in adults), cutaneous melanoma, dermatofibroma, solitary mastocytoma; *histopathologic:* when atypical features, cutaneous melanoma.
- The **DDx** also includes "BAP-omas," which in general are amelanotic (pink) and occur in patients with germline *BAP1* mutations (see Ch. 93).
- Molecular techniques (e.g. FISH or CGH analysis, *BRAF* V600E and *H-RAS* mutational status) are sometimes used to differentiate atypical Spitz nevi from melanoma.
- Spitz nevi have a tendency to involute over time, and monitoring is an option for a presumed Spitz nevus that develops during childhood and has classic clinical and dermoscopic features.

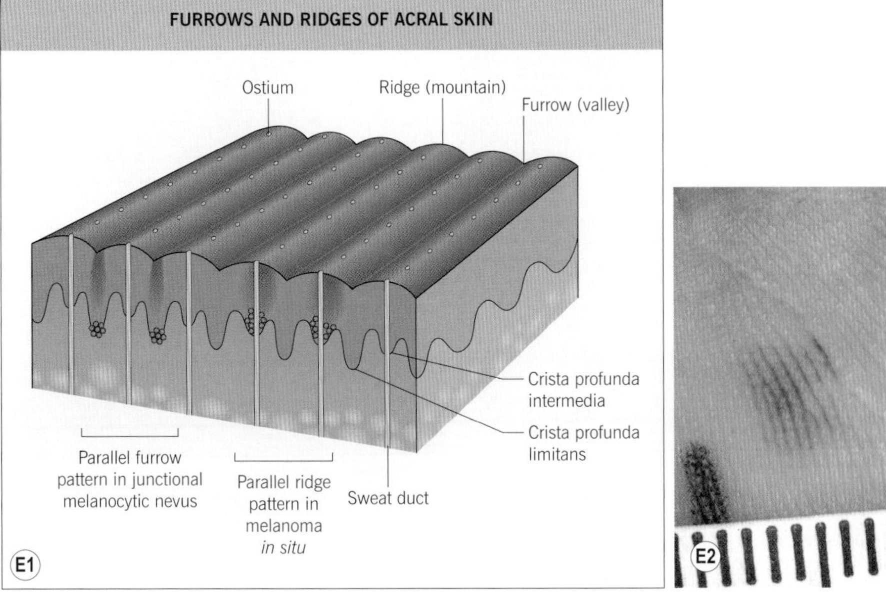

Fig. 92.9 *Continued* **E Nevi of "special sites" (e.g. scalp, acral, genital, milk-line). E1** *Acral melanocytic nevus* – furrows and ridges of acral skin. **E2** The parallel furrow pattern is evident with a small focus of the lattice pattern. The ostia of the eccrine ducts within the epidermal ridges can also be seen, especially at the site of blue ink.

- Any presumed Spitz nevus with *clinically* atypical features (e.g. size >1 cm, ulceration, asymmetry) should be biopsied.
- Any Spitz nevus with unusual features *histopathologically* should be completely excised.

Nevi of Special Sites

- Nevi in certain anatomic locations (e.g. scalp) may exhibit *atypical clinical* features, whereas those in several specific sites (e.g. acral, genital, auricular, milk line, flexural, and scalp nevi) may have *atypical histopathologic* features that simulate cutaneous melanoma (see Fig. 92.9E).
- Recognition of this phenomenon prevents overdiagnosis of cutaneous melanoma.

Other "Specially Named" Nevi

- ***Meyerson or eczematous nevus***: a melanocytic nevus with an eczematous halo; eczematous reaction typically resolves spontaneously or with the application of a topical CS.
- ***Eclipse nevus***: benign melanocytic nevus most often found on the scalp of children; presents as a tan, occasionally pink, central macule or papule with a brown, often stellate rim (see Fig. 92.9F1); ages into an intradermal nevus; when present on the scalp, may be a marker for developing numerous nevi elsewhere over time.
- ***Cockade nevus***: a benign melanocytic nevus with a target configuration, namely a central pigmented papule surrounded by a concentric tan rim, which is then surrounded by another pigmented annulus (see Fig. 92.9F2); occurs in patients with eclipse nevi.
- ***Recurrent nevus***: the reappearance of pigment within the scar of a previously biopsied or excised nevus (see Fig. 92.9F4); if symmetric, re-evaluation of the original histopathology and observation is generally all that is required; if asymmetric or continues to enlarge after its initial appearance, then biopsy is prudent.
- ***Agminated nevus***: a clustering of melanocytic nevi within normal-appearing skin.

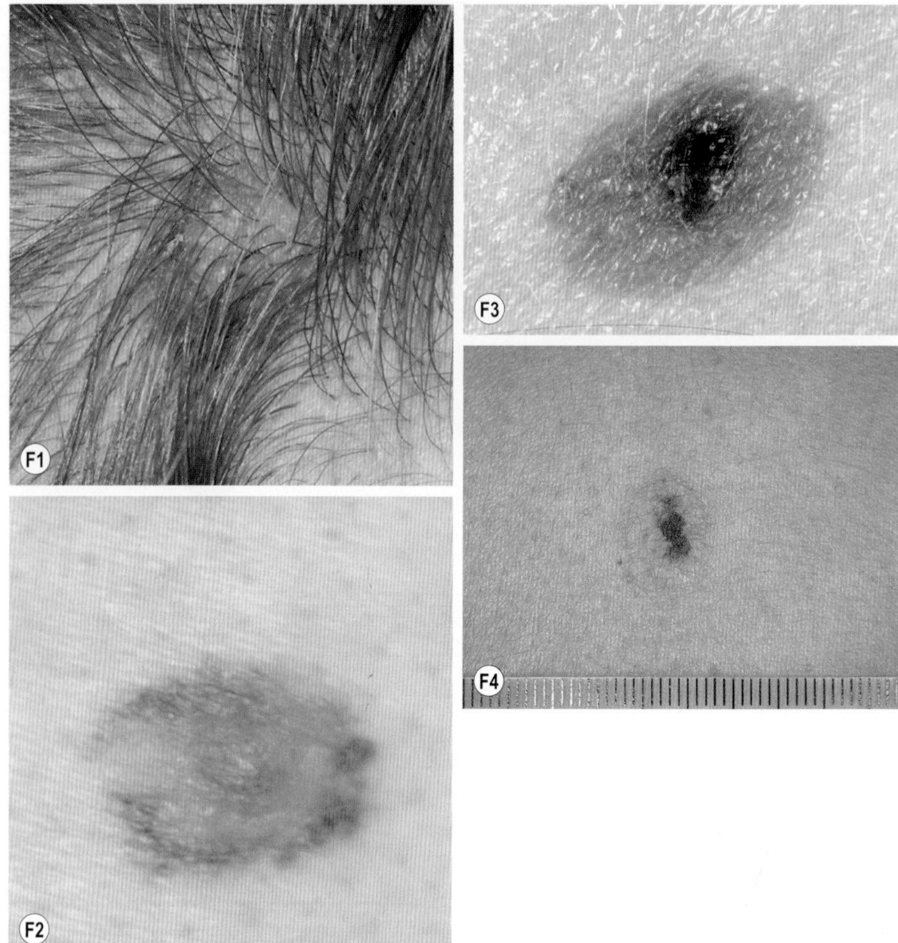

Fig. 92.9 *Continued* **F Other "specially named" nevi. F1** *Eclipse nevus,* characterized by a tan center and brown rim, is commonly found on the scalp of children who go on to develop numerous melanocytic nevi. The associated dermoscopic patterns are those seen in benign melanocytic nevi. **F2** *Cockade or target nevus*, characterized by a central lightly pigmented papule surrounded by a tan annulus then a brown ring. **F3** One variant of *combined melanocytic nevus* – dark brown to black papule within an otherwise uniformly pigmented light brown nevus. The differential diagnosis includes the possibility of a melanoma developing in a nevus. **F4** *Recurrent melanocytic nevus*. Irregular dark brown pigmentation within the center of a circular scar; the pigmentation reflects the proliferation of melanocytes within the epidermis. Note that there is no extension of the recurrence beyond the scar itself, one of the signs that favors observation rather than repeat biopsy. *A1–A3, Courtesy, Raymond L. Barnhill, MD; A4, Courtesy, AAD Dermoscopy Group and Iris Zalaudek, MD & Giuseppe Argenziano, MD; A5, Courtesy, AAD Dermoscopy Group and Iris Zalaudek, MD & Giuseppe Argenziano, MD; B1, B2, Courtesy, Raymond L. Barnhill, MD; B3, C5, E2, F4, Courtesy, Jean L. Bolognia, MD; C1, C2, D1, D3, F1, Courtesy, Julie V. Schaffer, MD; C3, D4, Courtesy, Iris Zalaudek, MD & Giuseppe Argenziano, MD; C4, D2, F3, Courtesy, Lorenzo Cerroni, MD; E1, Courtesy, Jean L. Bolognia, MD and Julie V. Schaffer, MD; F2, Courtesy, Jean L. Bolognia, MD.*

Halo Nevus

- A melanocytic nevus that is surrounded by a round or oval, usually symmetric, halo of complete depigmentation (i.e. white color).
- The central nevus is most often a common acquired melanocytic nevus, but it can also be other nevus subtypes.
- The halo of depigmentation is believed to represent a T-cell-mediated immune response against nevus antigens, analogous to vitiligo (see Ch. 54).
- Halo nevi are seen in up to 5% of Caucasian children aged 6–15 years; they are more common in patients with an increased number of nevi and a personal or family history of vitiligo.
- The most common location is the back; multiple halo nevi are seen in ~50% of cases.
- There are four clinical stages in the life of a halo nevus, and the evolution usually occurs over years to decades (Fig. 92.10).
- The central nevus should be assessed for suspicious or clinically atypical features; if none are present, then no treatment is necessary (vast majority of lesions); if present, then biopsy of just the central nevus should be performed.
- A new onset of multiple halo nevi is unusual in middle-aged and older adults; this clinical scenario should raise the possibility of the halo nevi representing an autoimmune reaction against a cutaneous or ocular melanoma.
- **DDx:** other pigmented lesions that can have halos (e.g. solar lentigo, seborrheic keratosis), halo primary cutaneous melanoma, halo melanoma metastasis.

Congenital Melanocytic Nevus (CMN)

- Classically defined as a melanocytic nevus present at birth; may be subtle at birth and not readily apparent for a few months.
- Melanocytic nevi that become apparent after 3 months of age, but before 2 years of age, have been termed "tardive CMN," "congenital nevus-like nevi," or "early onset nevi."
- CMN are due to a proliferation of melanocytes that arise during embryogenesis; melanocytes extend deep into the dermis and subcutaneous tissues and often follow follicular and neurovascular structures; in classic large/giant CMN, the most commonly observed mutations are in *NRAS*.
- Incidence of small CMN is estimated at 1–2%, with large CMN having an incidence of ~1 in 20,000 individuals.
- CMN are classified into four groups, based on their **final adult size**:
  - ***Small CMN***: <1.5 cm (Fig. 92.11A)
  - ***Medium CMN***: 1.5–20 cm (Fig. 92.11B–E)
  - ***Large CMN***: >20–40 cm (in a neonate, large CMN are ≥9 cm on the head or ≥6 cm on the body)
  - ***Giant CMN***: >40 cm (Fig. 92.11F)
- ***Small*** or ***medium-sized CMN*** are usually solitary, can occur anywhere on the body, range in color from tan to black, and may have increased terminal hair growth (hypertrichosis).
- ***Giant CMN*** are sometimes referred to as "bathing suit" or "garment" nevi because of their distribution pattern; multiple smaller, widely disseminated "satellite" nevi are also commonly associated with these giant CMN.
- CMN grow proportionately with the child and over time can change from initially flat, evenly pigmented patches to elevated, mottled, pebbly or verrucous plaques; scalp CMN may lighten in color and gradually regress; papules or nodules can develop within the CMN, but signs of rapid growth, induration, or ulceration should raise suspicion for the development of melanoma and prompt a biopsy.
- CMN are a known risk factor for melanoma and neurocutaneous melanosis (NCM), with the absolute risk being associated with the severity of the cutaneous phenotype.
- The risk of developing melanoma within a small or medium-sized CMN is thought to be <1% over a lifetime; the risk for giant CMN is ~5%, with greater risk being a function of nevus size and number of satellite lesions; in giant CMN, the majority of melanomas develop in childhood (~50% in the first 5 years of life).
- Cutaneous melanomas can arise within the dermis or subcutaneous tissues of a CMN, making clinical diagnosis difficult.

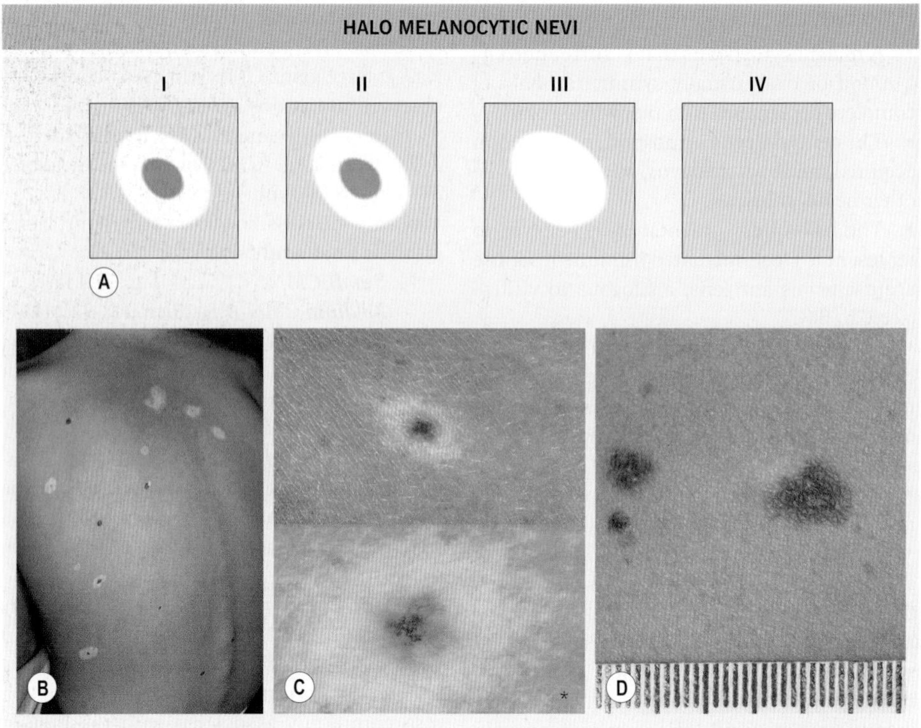

HALO MELANOCYTIC NEVI

I II III IV

Fig. 92.10 Halo melanocytic nevi. A Four potential clinical stages in the life of a halo nevus. *Stage I*: central pigmented melanocytic nevus with a halo of depigmentation; *Stage II*: central nevus is pink with a halo of depigmentation; *Stage III*: no central nevus, just a depigmented macule; *Stage IV*: repigmentation (partial or complete). **B** Multiple halo nevi (seen here in all four of the various stages) are seen most commonly in children and young adults with numerous nevi. **C** Close-up of a halo nevus with a depigmented macular halo surrounding a central dark brown papule. Dermoscopically*, a symmetric white structureless area surrounding the remaining network of the nevus. **D** Asymmetric halos can also be seen, as in this photo surrounding a benign compound melanocytic nevus. *B, Courtesy, YDRSC; C, Courtesy, Harold Rabinovitz, MD; D, Courtesy, Jean L. Bolognia, MD.*

- Patients with a giant CMN in a posterior axial location that is associated with multiple satellite nevi (≥20) have the greatest risk of developing melanoma; although the melanoma can develop within the CMN itself (not the satellite lesions), the CNS, or the retroperitoneum, the primary site may remain unknown.
- In **neurocutaneous melanosis (NCM)**, also referred to as leptomeningeal melanocytosis, there is a proliferation of melanocytes in the CNS (as well as the skin); individuals with multiple (≥3, but usually 10–20+), disseminated medium-sized CMN are at greatest risk of NCM, followed by those with a giant CMN in a posterior axial location with multiple satellites.
- NCM-associated signs – e.g. hydrocephalus, seizures, developmental delay, increased intracranial pressure, cranial nerve palsies, sensorimotor defects, and hypotonia – tend to manifest by 2–3 years of age.
- An approach to the management of CMN is presented in Table 92.5 and Fig. 92.12.

Nevus Spilus (Speckled Lentiginous Nevus [SLN])

- A subtype of congenital melanocytic nevus with a prevalence of ~2% in the general population.

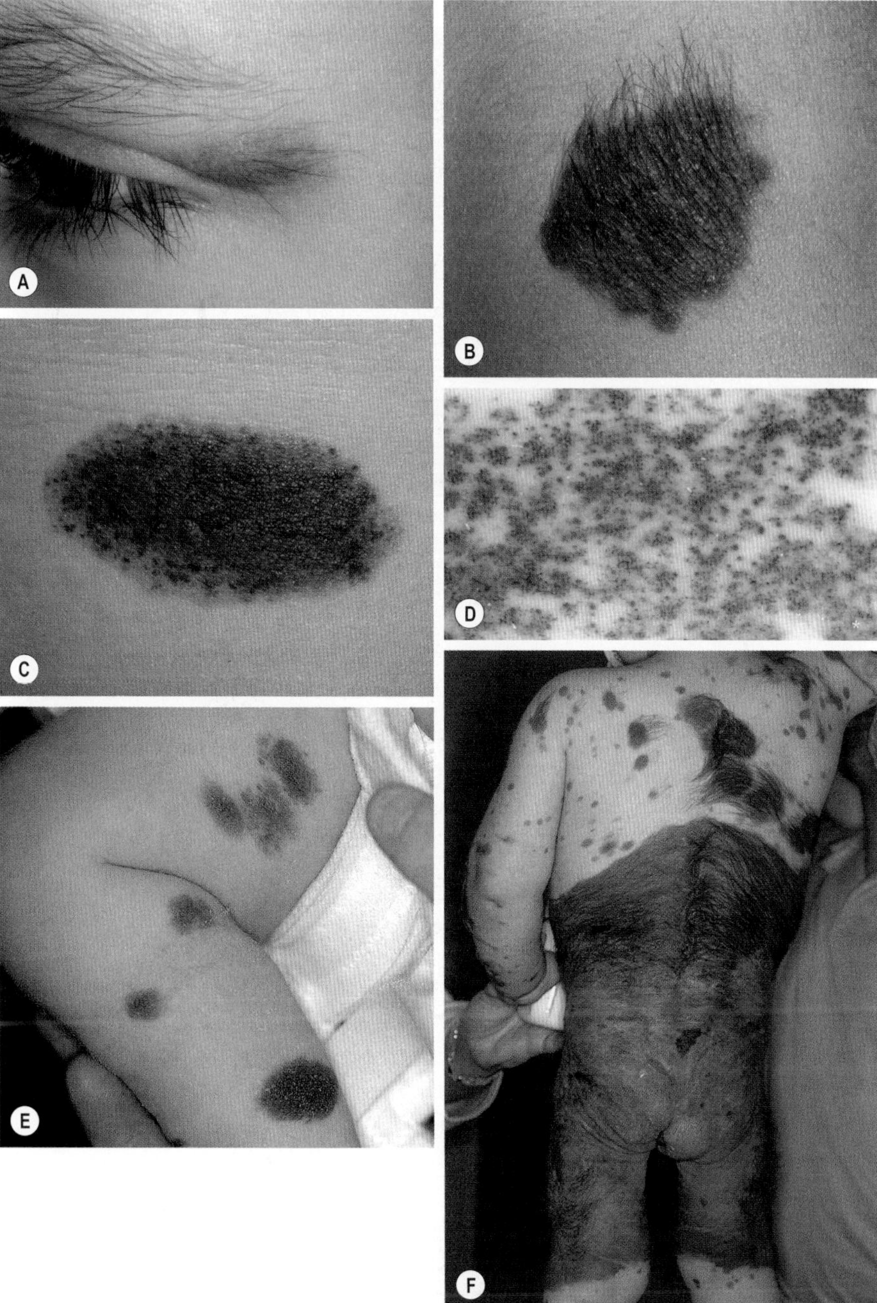

Fig. 92.11 Congenital melanocytic nevi (CMN). A Small CMN. Note the hypertrichosis and slight heterogeneity in pigmentation, reflecting its hamartomatous nature. **B, C** Medium-sized CMN, also with hypertrichosis and slight heterogeneity in pigmentation (**B**). Note the pebbly appearance on clinical examination (**C**) and the globular pattern with hyphae-like structures on dermoscopy* (**D**). **E** Multiple medium-sized CMN. This patient had 25–30 such lesions. This presentation can be associated with neurocutaneous melanosis (NCM). **F** Giant CMN, also called a "bathing suit" nevus. It is situated in a posterior axial location with numerous satellite nevi, some of which have hypertrichosis. This patient died of intractable ascites due to the migration of benign melanocytes from the brain to the peritoneal cavity via his VP shunt. In the perianal region, the nevus was softer and somewhat "boggy" due to neurotization. *A, Courtesy, Lorenzo Cerroni, MD; B, C, Courtesy, Julie V. Schaffer, MD; D, Courtesy, Raymond L. Barnhill, MD, and Harold S. Rabinovitz, MD; E, F, Courtesy, Jean L. Bolognia, MD.*

APPROACH TO THE PATIENT WITH A SMALL OR MEDIUM-SIZED CONGENITAL MELANOCYTIC NEVUS (CMN)	
Longitudinal evaluation*	**Excision**
• No worrisome features	• Worrisome clinical or histopathologic features
• Observation is easy because of: – Location – Color – Smooth surface and uniform texture	• Observation is difficult because of: – Location (e.g. scalp) – Color (e.g. black) – Irregular or multinodular surface – Dense hypertrichosis
• Parents/patient are: – Motivated and knowledgeable – Not anxious regarding the small chance (<1%) of melanoma – Not concerned regarding cosmetic appearance	• Parents/patient are: – Reluctant to observe – Anxious regarding small chance (<1%) of melanoma – Concerned regarding cosmetic appearance

Includes baseline photography, measurements, and periodic skin examinations.

Table 92.5 Approach to the patient with a small or medium-sized congenital melanocytic nevus (CMN).

- Often presents at or around birth as a tan patch; over time numerous macules and papules develop within the tan patch, ranging from lentigines to junctional, compound and intradermal nevi to Spitz and blue nevi (Fig. 92.13).
- The risk of developing melanoma within the nevus spilus is thought to be similar to classic congenital melanocytic nevi of the same size range, but may be related to the type of nevi that develop within it.
- **DDx:** agminated nevus (see above); partial unilateral lentiginosis.
- Nevus spilus should be followed with periodic examinations, photography, and biopsies as clinically indicated.

For further information see Ch. 112 from *Dermatology, Fourth Edition*.

For additional online figures and tables visit www.expertconsult.com 

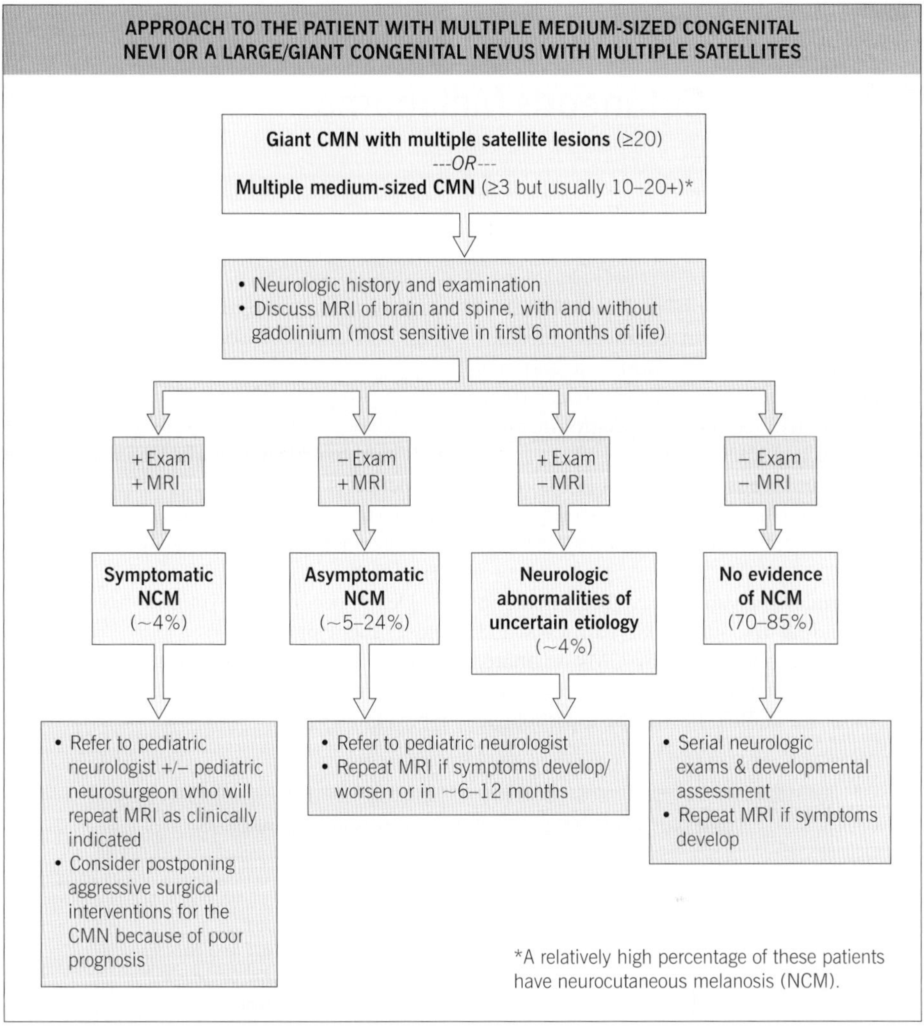

APPROACH TO THE PATIENT WITH MULTIPLE MEDIUM-SIZED CONGENITAL NEVI OR A LARGE/GIANT CONGENITAL NEVUS WITH MULTIPLE SATELLITES

Giant CMN with multiple satellite lesions (≥20)
---*OR*---
Multiple medium-sized CMN (≥3 but usually 10–20+)*

↓

- Neurologic history and examination
- Discuss MRI of brain and spine, with and without gadolinium (most sensitive in first 6 months of life)

↓

+Exam +MRI	−Exam +MRI	+Exam −MRI	− Exam − MRI
Symptomatic NCM (~4%)	**Asymptomatic NCM** (~5–24%)	**Neurologic abnormalities of uncertain etiology** (~4%)	**No evidence of NCM** (70–85%)
• Refer to pediatric neurologist +/– pediatric neurosurgeon who will repeat MRI as clinically indicated • Consider postponing aggressive surgical interventions for the CMN because of poor prognosis	• Refer to pediatric neurologist • Repeat MRI if symptoms develop/ worsen or in ~6–12 months	• Refer to pediatric neurologist • Repeat MRI if symptoms develop/ worsen or in ~6–12 months	• Serial neurologic exams & developmental assessment • Repeat MRI if symptoms develop

*A relatively high percentage of these patients have neurocutaneous melanosis (NCM).

Fig. 92.12 Approach to the patient with multiple medium-sized congenital nevi or a large/ giant congenital nevus with multiple satellites. CMN, congenital melanocytic nevus.

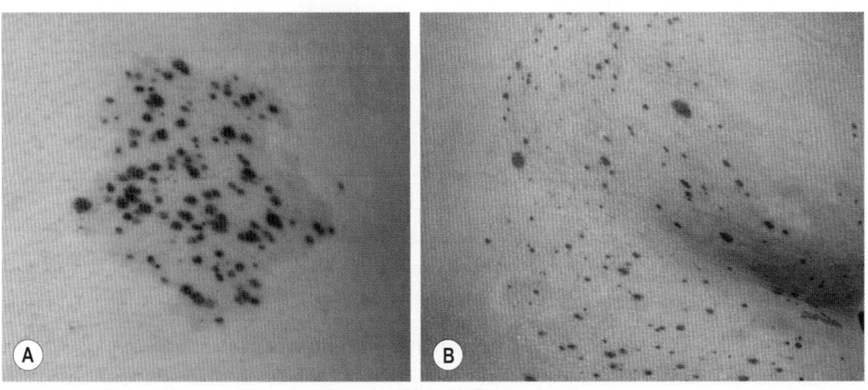

Fig. 92.13 Nevus spilus (speckled lentiginous nevus). A Multiple medium to dark brown macules and papules superimposed upon a tan patch. **B** Larger lesion of the lateral trunk with dark brown to black nevi of varying sizes; sometimes the tan background is subtle and not initially recognized. *Courtesy, Jean L. Bolognia, MD.*

93 Cutaneous Melanoma

- A malignant tumor of melanocytes, most commonly arising from cutaneous melanocytes; can also develop from melanocytes residing elsewhere – e.g. in the uveal tract, retinal pigment epithelium, gastrointestinal mucosa, or leptomeninges.
- Some cutaneous melanomas (CMs) arise *de novo*, whereas others arise within precursor lesions (e.g. melanocytic nevi; see Ch. 92).
- Tremendous advances have been made in understanding the molecular pathways and mutations from which many CMs originate, resulting in identification of genetic markers, tools for aiding in the histopathologic diagnosis, and targeted treatments for CM (Figs 93.1 and 93.2; see Table 93.14).

Epidemiology

- There has been a marked increase in the incidence of CM, especially thinner lesions, during the past 40–50 years, with a modest increase in mortality, primarily in older men (Fig. 93.3).
- Death occurs at a younger age than for most other cancers.
- Risk factors are divided into three major groups: genetic, environmental, and phenotypic (Table 93.1).

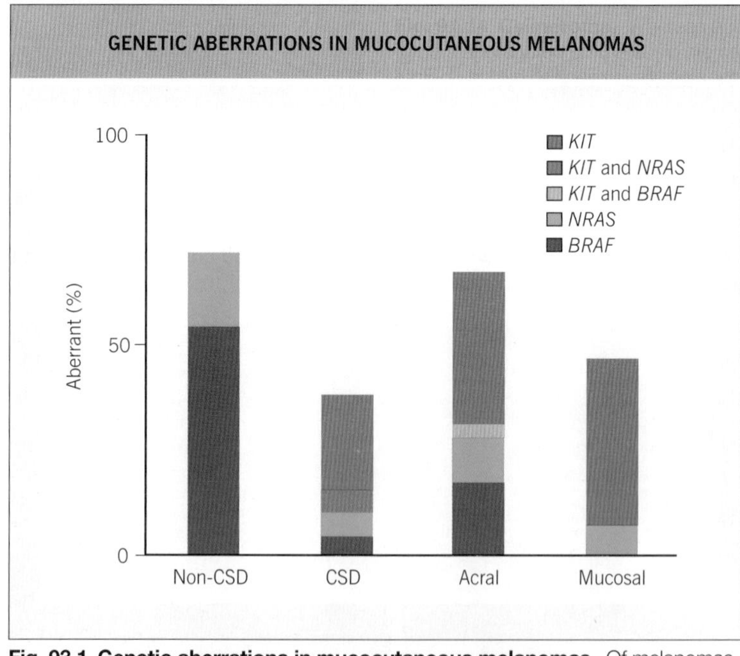

Fig. 93.1 Genetic aberrations in mucocutaneous melanomas. Of melanomas with somatic mutations in *BRAF*, at least 80% lead to substitution of glutamic acid (E) for Valine (V) at codon 600, i.e. V600E. CSD, skin with chronic sun-induced damage such as marked solar elastosis; non-CSD, skin without chronic sun-induced damage. *From Curtin JA, Busam K, Pinkel D, Bastian BC. J Clin Oncol 2006;24:4340–6.*

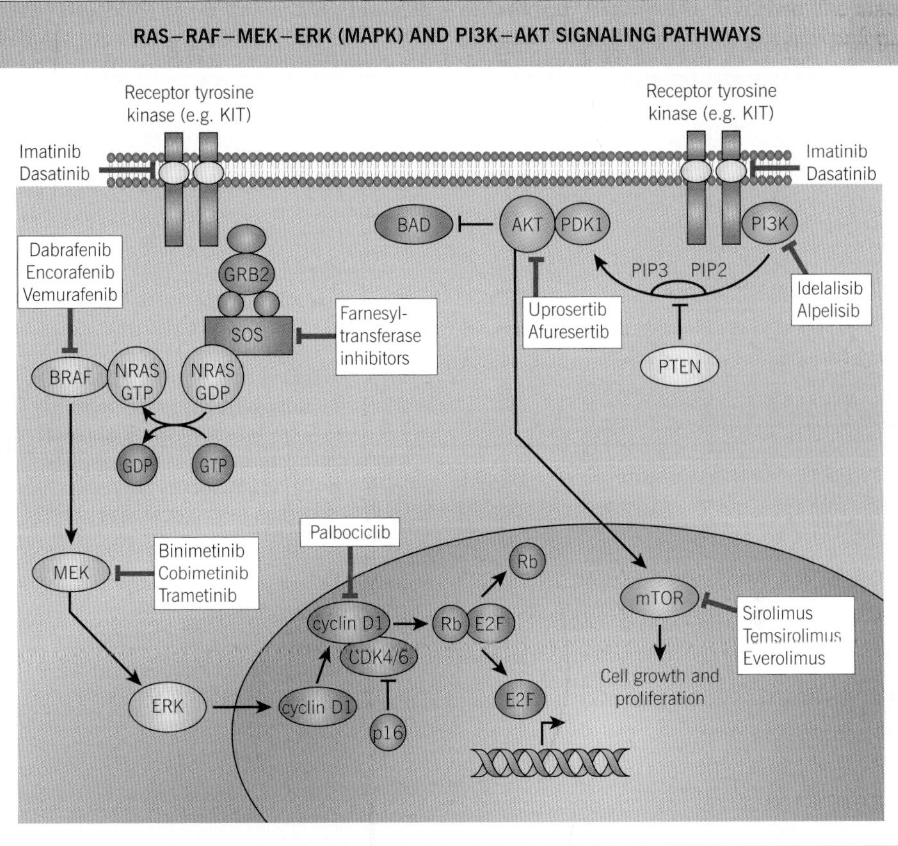

Fig. 93.2 RAS–RAF-MEK–ERK (MAPK) and PI3K–AKT signaling pathways. The *m*itogen-activated *p*rotein *k*inase (MAPK) pathway (orange color), also referred to as the MAP kinase pathway, is physiologically activated by growth factor binding to receptor tyrosine kinases. The stimulus is relayed to the nucleus via the GTPase activity of NRAS and the kinase activity of BRAF, MEK, and ERK. Within the nucleus, this results in increased transcription of genes involved in cell growth, proliferation and migration. The central role of this pathway in melanocytic neoplasia is highlighted by the fact that either *NRAS* or *BRAF* is mutated in ~80% of all cutaneous melanomas and melanocytic nevi. The PI3K–AKT pathway is another important regulator of cell survival, growth, and apoptosis (green color). A key inhibitor of this pathway is PTEN, and inactivation of the gene that encodes PTEN via mutations, deletions, or promoter methylation also occurs in cutaneous melanomas. As a result, there is increased activity of the PI3K–AKT signaling pathway. Examples of farnesyltransferase inhibitors are tipifamib and ionafamib. BAD, BCL-2 associated agonist of cell death; CDK, cyclin-dependent kinase; E2F, transcription factor that controls transcription of cyclins; ERK, extracellular signal-regulated kinase; GDP, guanosine-5′-diphosphate; GRB2, growth factor receptor-bound protein 2, an adaptor protein that contains one Src homology 2 (SH2) domain and two SH3 domains; GTP, guanosine-5′-triphosphate; MEK, MAPK kinase; mTOR, mammalian target of rapamycin (aka sirolimus); p16, protein product of *CDKN2A*; PDK1, phosphoinositide-dependent kinase-1; PI3K, phosphoinositide 3-kinase; PIP2, phosphatidylinositol 4,5-bisphosphate; PIP3, phosphatidylinositol 3,4,5-triphosphate; PTEN, phosphatase and tensin homolog; Rb, retinoblastoma protein; SOS, son of sevenless.

- Approximately 10% of melanomas are familial, and germline mutations have been detected in several melanoma-dominant genes (e.g. *CDKN2A, CDK4*) as well as genes responsible for a more general predisposition to malignancies ("mixed cancer syndromes" such as Lynch and Li–Fraumeni; Tables 93.2 and 93.3).
- Primary prevention: sun protective measures, avoidance of tanning beds.

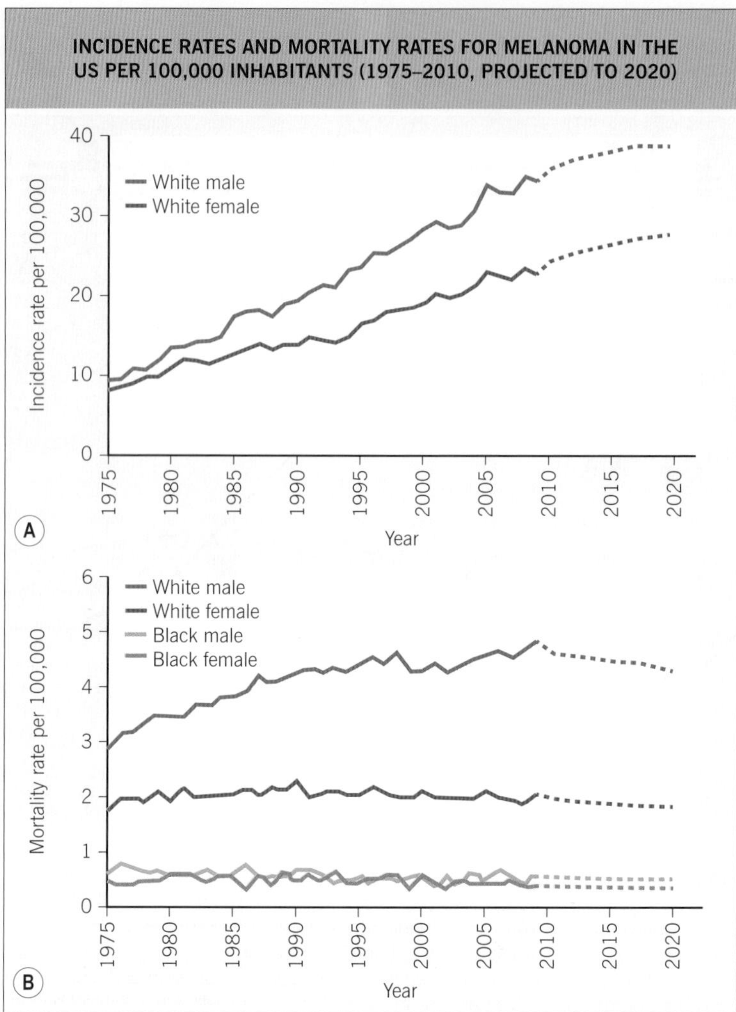

Fig. 93.3 Incidence rates and mortality rates for melanoma in the US per 100,000 inhabitants (1975–2010, projected to 2020). A,B While the incidence has increased significantly in white men and women over the past four decades, there has been a modest increase in mortality in white men. *Data from* www.cdc.gov/cancer/dcpc/research/articles/cancer_2020_incidence.htm.

- Secondary prevention: early detection, screening of higher-risk individuals.

Clinical

- The clinical presentation of CM varies greatly; although the **ABCDE**s (**A**symmetry, **B**order irregularity, **C**olor variegation, **D**iameter >6 mm, **E**volution) are often used in public awareness campaigns to help promote the clinical recognition of CM, they have their shortcomings; to rectify this, the **EFG** rule (**E**levated, **F**irm, **G**rowing) has been added for nodular and amelanotic CMs.
- As banal nevi age, they also become more elevated, but in contrast to nodular CMs, they are soft to palpation.
- In CM *in situ* (MIS), the malignancy is confined to the epidermis and/or the hair follicle epithelium (Fig. 93.4); all types of CM (except for nodular melanoma) can have an *in situ* phase; *lentigo maligna* (Fig. 93.5) is a type of MIS that arises within chronically sun-damaged skin and can remain *in situ* for years to decades.

RISK FACTORS FOR THE DEVELOPMENT OF CUTANEOUS MELANOMA
Genetic factors
• Family history of cutaneous melanoma (see Table 93.2) • Family history of "mixed cancer syndrome" (see Table 93.2) • Lightly pigmented skin • Tendency to burn, inability to tan • Red hair color • DNA repair defects (e.g. xeroderma pigmentosum)
Environmental factors
• Intense intermittent sun exposure • Chronic sun exposure • Residence in equatorial latitudes • PUVA (possible) • Tanning bed use, especially under the age of 35 years • Iatrogenic or acquired immunosuppression
Phenotypic expressions of gene/environment interactions
• Melanocytic nevi and solar lentigines: – Increased total number of acquired melanocytic nevi (MN) >100 MN, relative risk ~8- to 10-fold increased – Atypical melanocytic nevi (AMN) >5 AMN, relative risk ~4- to 6-fold increased • Multiple solar lentigines (SL): – Multiple SL, relative risk ~3- to 4-fold increased – Relative risks (RR) are multiplicative: e.g. a person with >100 MN + >5 AMN + multiple SL has a relative risk ~10 × 5 × 3 = 150-fold • Personal history of cutaneous melanoma

Table 93.1 Risk factors for the development of cutaneous melanoma.

FAMILIAL MELANOMA – DOMINANT AND SUBORDINATE SYNDROMES		
Susceptibility gene	**Syndrome**	**Characteristic features (in addition to cutaneous melanoma)**
Melanoma dominant syndromes – multiple & early-onset melanomas + strong family history of melanoma		
*CDKN2A/ p16**	Familial atypical multiple mole–melanoma syndrome (FAMMM) Melanoma–astrocytoma syndrome (MAS)	• Numerous nevi (>50), atypical nevi**, ≥1 first- or second-degree relative with melanoma • Increased risk for pancreatic cancer • CNS tumors (e.g. astrocytoma)
CDK4	Rare cases of FAMMM syndrome	• Similar presentation as patients with *CDKN2A* mutations
BAP1	BAP1 tumor syndrome	• Multiple "BAP-omas" – atypical melanocytic proliferations which appear clinically benign (e.g. dome-shaped, often pink papules) with histopathologically spitzoid features • Uveal melanoma • Mesothelioma, renal cell carcinoma, other internal malignancies
MITF (E318K) variant	MITF-related melanoma and renal cell carcinoma predisposition syndrome	• Often high atypical nevus count • Early-onset melanoma • Renal cell carcinoma, pancreatic carcinoma

Table 93.2 Familial melanoma – dominant and subordinate syndromes. *Continued*

FAMILIAL MELANOMA – DOMINANT AND SUBORDINATE SYNDROMES		
Susceptibility gene	**Syndrome**	**Characteristic features (in addition to cutaneous melanoma)**
Shelterin complex genes (e.g. *POT1*, *ACD*, *TERF2IP*)		• Early-onset and multiple primary melanomas • Many different internal malignancies (e.g. breast, prostate, lung)
TERT		• Numerous atypical nevi (possible) • Hematologic malignancies and multiple types of internal malignancies
Melanoma subordinate syndromes – in the context of a "mixed cancer syndrome"		
BRCA1 and *BRCA2*	Hereditary breast and ovarian carcinoma syndrome (HBOC)	• Breast, ovarian, pancreatic, prostate cancers
TP53	Li–Fraumeni syndrome	• Childhood (e.g. sarcomas, leukemias, CNS) and multiple primary lifetime cancers (e.g. breast, others)
PTEN	Cowden syndrome/PTEN hamartoma tumor syndrome (see Table 52.1)	• Tricholemmomas, papillomatous papules, mucosal lesions, palmar–plantar keratosis • Breast, thyroid, endometrial, and colorectal carcinomas
RB	Hereditary retinoblastoma	• Early onset, often bilateral, ocular retinoblastoma • Pineoblastoma, osteosarcoma, soft tissue sarcomas
MLH1, MSH2, MSH6, PMS2, EPCAM	Lynch syndrome	• Colorectal, endometrial, stomach, breast and other cancers
Other possible hereditary factors		
MC1R		• Red hair, freckling, fair skin • Childhood/adolescent melanomas

*The major high-penetrance susceptibility gene locus associated with familial melanoma; MAS may be more linked to the functional loss of the *CDKN2A* gene product p14^{ARF}.
**Not all patients/families with *CDKN2A* mutation have numerous/atypical nevi.

Table 93.2 *Continued* **Familial melanoma – dominant and subordinate syndromes.** About 45% of familial melanomas are due to an inherited mutation in a highly penetrant predisposition gene.

- There are four **major subtypes** of primary invasive CM, based on clinicopathologic features:
  - *Superficial spreading melanoma* (SSM; ~60% of melanomas) (Fig. 93.6)
  - *Nodular melanoma* (NM; ~20%) (Fig. 93.7)
  - *Lentigo maligna melanoma* (LMM; ~9%) (Fig. 93.8)
  - *Acral lentiginous melanoma* (ALM; ~4%) (Fig. 93.9)
- **Less common variants of CM:**
  - *Amelanotic melanoma*: color ranges from pink to red and any type of CM may be amelanotic (Fig. 93.10); children can develop amelanotic nodular CM, and the lesion may resemble a pyogenic granuloma or wart
  - *Nail matrix melanoma*: see Table 58.3 and Fig. 93.11

SUGGESTED CRITERIA FOR REFERRAL TO A GENETICS COUNSELOR FOR A SUSPECTED FAMILIAL MELANOMA SYNDROME
Suspected melanoma dominant syndrome*
• Family history, defined as ≥3 affected members on 1 side of the family, of invasive melanoma or pancreatic cancer or CNS tumor (e.g. astrocytoma) or renal cell carcinoma
• ≥3 primary invasive melanomas, including 1 early-onset melanoma (≤45 years of age)
• ≥2 *BAP1*-mutated atypical melanocytic proliferations ("BAP-omas")
• ≥1 *BAP1*-mutated atypical melanocytic proliferations ("BAP-omas") + a family history of mesothelioma, meningioma, renal cell carcinoma, and/or uveal melanoma
Suspected melanoma subordinate syndrome**
• Personal history of melanoma + personal/family history of other malignancies that suggest a mixed cancer syndrome (e.g. breast, ovarian, prostate, pancreatic, colon; see Table 93.2)

**Familial cancer syndrome in which melanoma is the predominant cancer type, although other cancers may also be observed (see Table 93.2).*

***Familial cancer syndrome in which there is a lower risk of melanoma than that of other malignancies seen in the syndrome (see Table 93.2).*

Table 93.3 Suggested criteria for referral to a genetics counselor for a suspected familial melanoma syndrome. Melanoma predisposition genes can be associated with other malignancies and other cancer predisposition genes can increase the risk of melanoma. A discussion regarding genetic counseling should be held with melanoma patients who have any of the proposed criteria in this table. HBOC, hereditary breast and ovarian cancer.

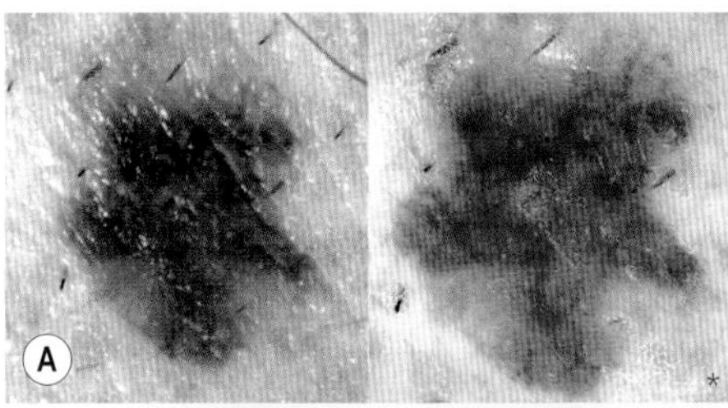

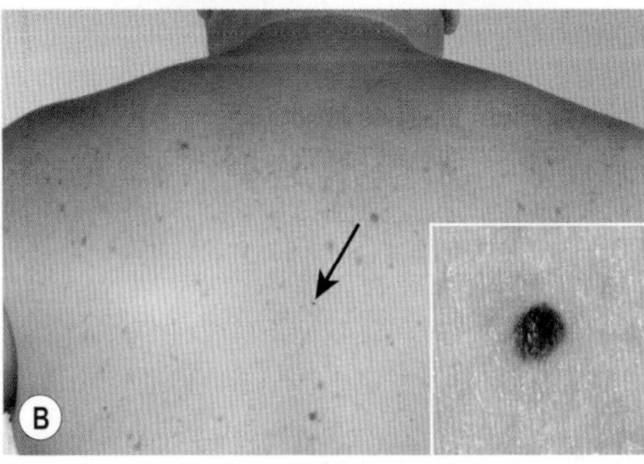

Fig. 93.4 Melanoma *in situ*. A Clinically, note the asymmetry, border irregularity, color variation, and erythema ("little red riding hood" sign); by dermoscopy*, findings include a broadened network, dots, and some globules. **B** This melanoma *in situ* measured less than 3 mm in diameter. Small melanomas can be easily overlooked, especially if they are less heavily pigmented. This lesion was the "ugly duckling" of all of this patient's nevi. Dermoscopy assists in making an earlier diagnosis. *Courtesy, Claus Garbe, MD.*

- *Mucosal melanoma*: mouth (e.g. palate, gingiva), anus > nasopharynx, larynx, vagina; ~35% are amelanotic
- *Desmoplastic* and *neurotropic melanomas*: skin-colored or pink > brown to black, firm nodule, usually in sun-exposed sites; may arise *de novo* or within a lentigo maligna; a deeper biopsy is necessary for diagnosis; local recurrence is a common problem
- *Ocular melanoma:* divided into conjunctival or uveal melanomas, with a majority of the latter harboring *GNA11* or *GNAQ* mutations; partial or total loss of chromosome 3 portends a poor prognosis (*BAP1* is on its short arm)

• Childhood CM is rare; prepubertal patients tend to have amelanotic (pink or red), thicker lesions that can be difficult to distinguish from atypical Spitz nevi histopathologically.

• Controlling for Breslow depth of invasion (in sites where the Breslow depth can be measured), all CMs have the same prognosis, including pregnancy-associated CM; however, some types of CM tend to have a deeper Breslow depth at presentation due to delayed diagnosis (e.g. amelanotic, ALM).

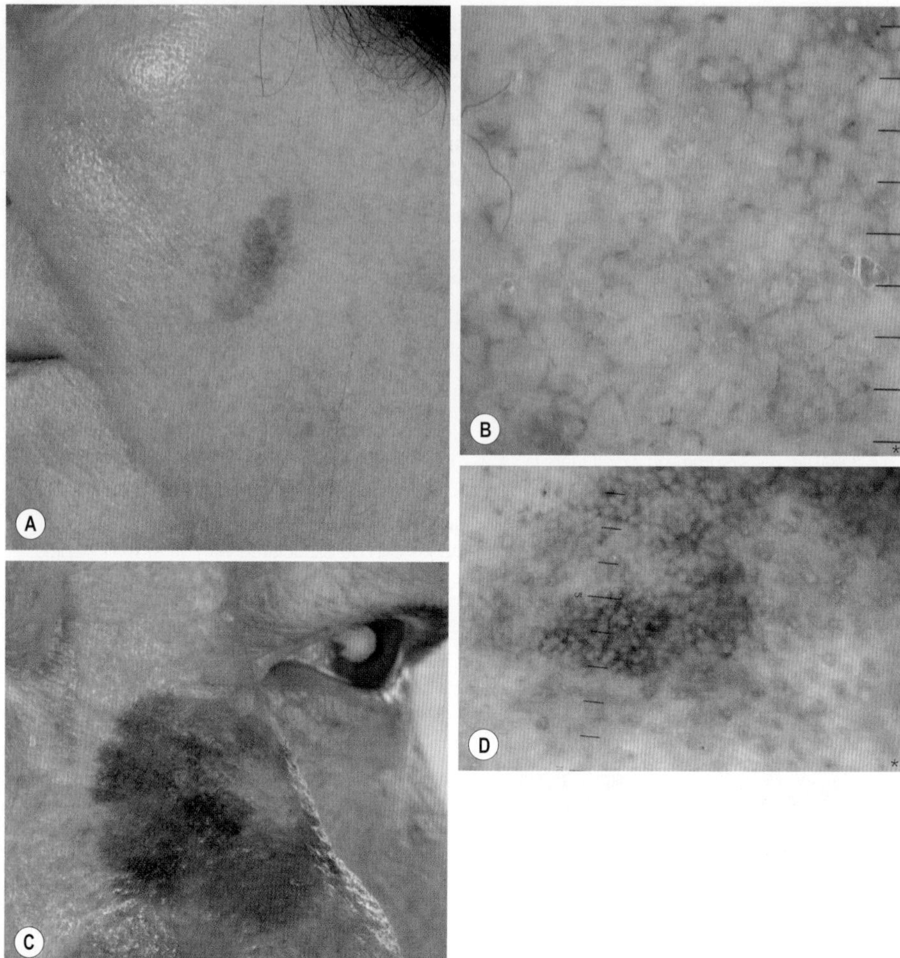

Fig. 93.5 Lentigo maligna (LM). A, C An early LM presenting as a light brown patch with subtle asymmetric pigmentation (**A**) is compared to a more advanced lesion with readily apparent variation in pigmentation (**C**). **B, D** By dermoscopy*, follicular openings surrounded by annular pigmentation are seen, referred to as a "circle in a circle". Findings are more subtle in **B** and a few rhomboidal structures are seen in **D**. *Courtesy, Claus Garbe, MD and Jürgen Bauer, MD.*

Diagnosis

- Early detection is key to improved survival; diagnosis is based upon clinical suspicion (e.g. visual inspection, dermoscopy), followed by histopathologic confirmation.
- The biopsy should attempt to remove the entire lesion, including a depth adequate to determine an accurate Breslow depth (Fig. 93.12); if limited by large size, representative samples should be obtained; histopathologic evaluation is then performed by a dermatopathologist.
- When doing a total body skin examination (TBSE), signs such as the "ugly duckling sign" (a pigmented lesion that stands out as atypical within the context of surrounding nevi; see Fig. 93.4B and Ch. 92) and the "little red riding hood sign" can prove useful (see Fig. 93.4A).
- In addition to dermoscopy, photography can aid in diagnosis; for the former, the first step is to determine if the lesion is melanocytic (Table 93.4) and then assess for worrisome features (Tables 93.5 and 93.6).

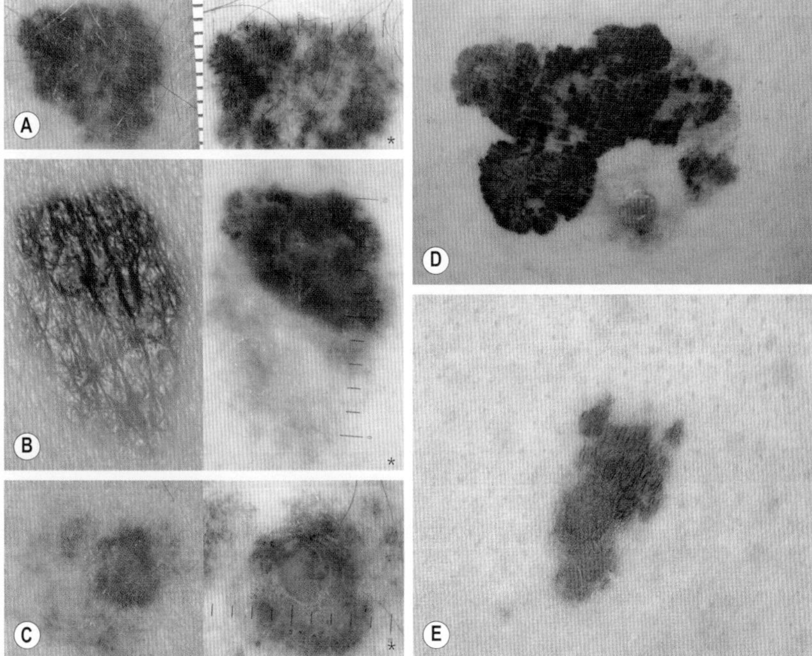

Fig. 93.6 Superficial spreading melanomas. A–C Clinically, all of these lesions demonstrate asymmetry due to variation in color and irregularity in outline. Breslow depths for **A–C** were <0.5 mm, 0.58 mm, and 1.60 mm, respectively. By dermoscopy*, there is asymmetry, atypical pigment networks, irregular blotches, and multiple colors; in **B** and **C** a blue-white veil is present. **D** In this more advanced lesion, note the asymmetry, irregular borders, variation in colors, scar-like regression zones, and an inferior pink papule, indicating vertical growth phase. **E** Superficial spreading melanoma arising within a compound melanocytic nevus. Note the irregular outline and variable pigmentation. *A–C, Courtesy, Claus Garbe, MD and Jürgen Bauer, MD; D, Courtesy, Claus Garbe, MD; E, Courtesy, YDRSC.*

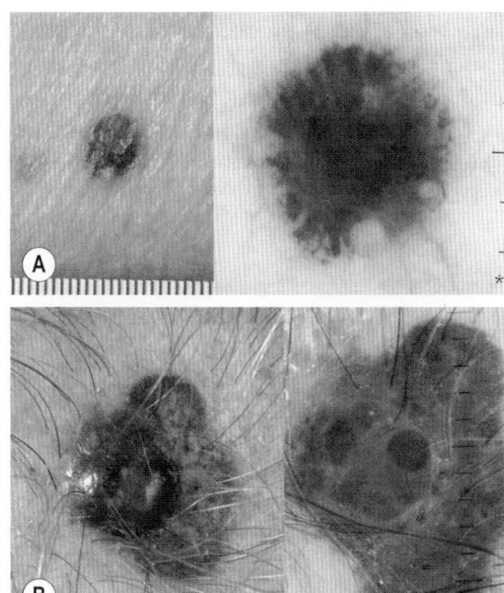

Fig. 93.7 Nodular melanomas. A Clinically, a darkly pigmented papule measuring ~3 mm in diameter with a Breslow depth of 0.95 mm; by dermoscopy*, a blue color, atypical pigment network, and streaks are seen. **B** Darkly pigmented plaque on the scalp with an eccentric nodule and a Breslow depth of 2.75 mm; by dermoscopy*, multiple colors including blue-gray are seen. *Courtesy, Claus Garbe, MD and Jürgen Bauer, MD.*

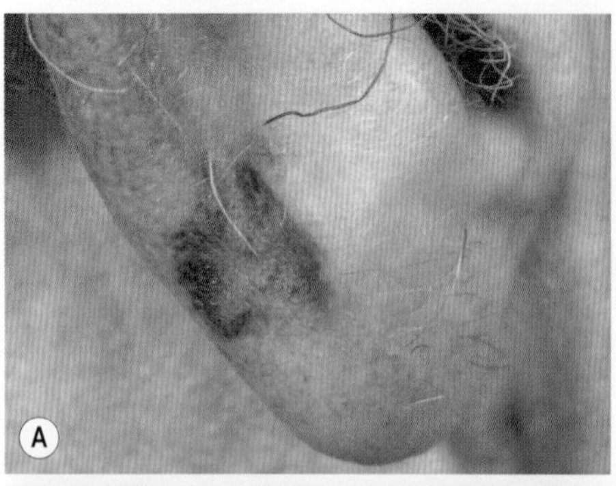

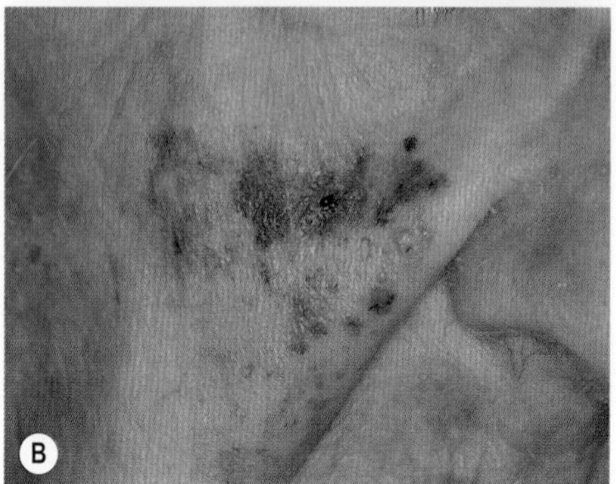

Fig. 93.8 Lentigo maligna melanoma (LMM). A Asymmetric pigmented lesion on the earlobe, with irregular borders and significant variation in pigmentation; the Breslow depth was 0.45 mm. **B** Larger triangular brown patch in which there are multiple dark brown, black, and blue-gray papules and plaques; Breslow depth was 1.1 mm. *A, Courtesy, Claus Garbe, MD and Jürgen Bauer, MD; B, Courtesy, Kalman Watsky, MD.*

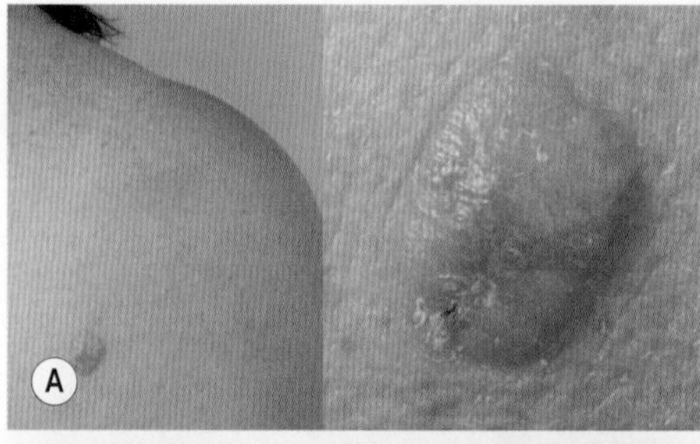

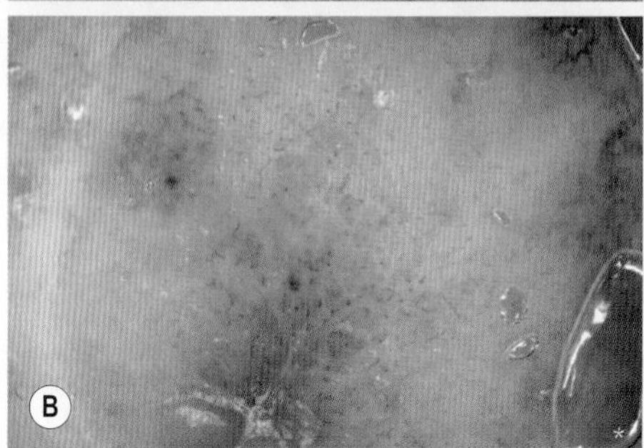

Fig. 93.10 Amelanotic melanoma. A Skin-colored to light pink nodule on the right scapula of a female patient; Breslow depth was 4 mm. **B** By dermoscopy*, some pigmented globules allow one to identify the tumor as a melanocytic lesion. Dotted, point and linear-irregular vessels are suggestive of melanoma. *Courtesy, Claus Garbe, MD.*

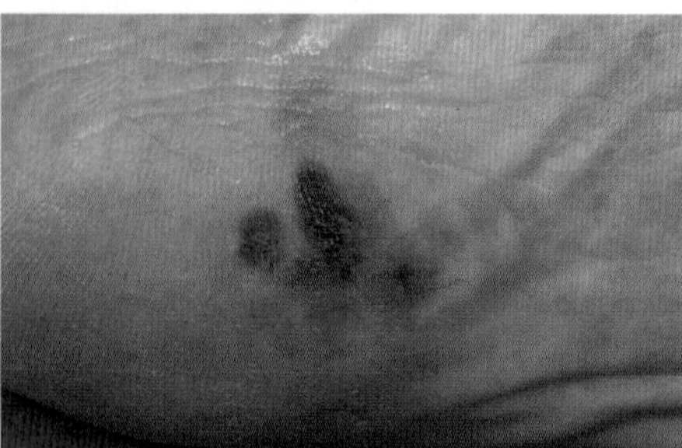

Fig. 93.9 Acral lentiginous melanoma. Irregularly pigmented lesion on the plantar surface of the foot. These tumors may become amelanotic and are then easily overlooked or misdiagnosed as verrucae or other benign lesions, often resulting in a significantly delayed diagnosis. Dermoscopic findings include irregular diffuse pigmentation and a parallel ridge pattern. *Courtesy, Claus Garbe, MD.*

- Not all cutaneous melanomas present with typical features and in early lesions, clinical findings can be subtle; therefore, concern by a patient for one particular lesion needs to be factored into the evaluation.
- **DDx:** outlined in Table 93.7.

Prognosis and Staging

- Of the histopathologic features of a primary invasive CM, the Breslow depth (measured in millimeters) is the strongest predictor of survival (see Fig. 93.12); the presence or absence of lymph node involvement is an even stronger predictor of survival.
- The American Joint Committee on Cancer's (AJCC) TNM classification and staging system for CM are outlined in Tables 93.8 and 93.9.

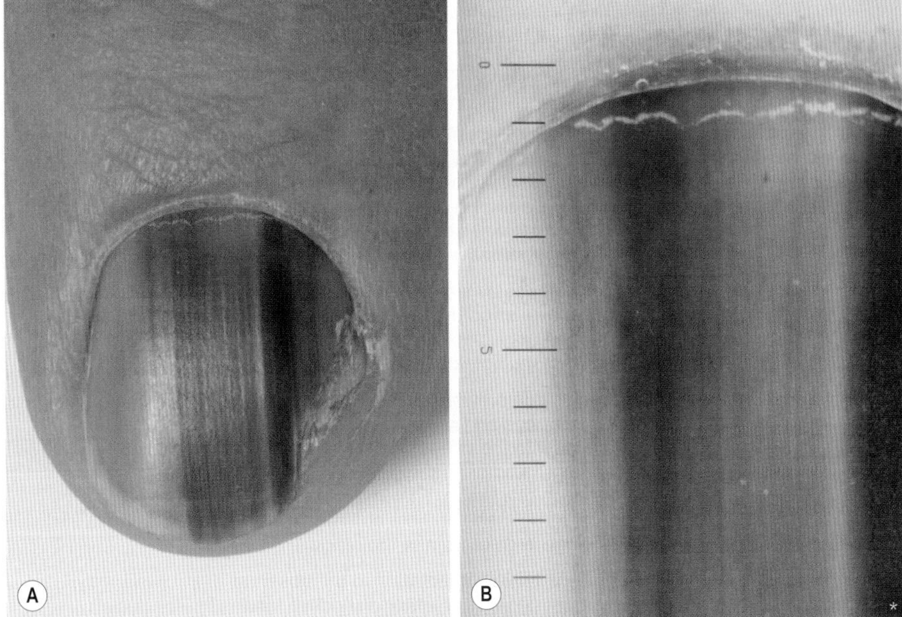

Fig. 93.11 Melanoma of the nail matrix. A, B The longitudinal pigmentation of the nail plate is non-homogeneous, both clinically (**A**) and dermoscopically* (**B**); the Breslow depth was 0.7 mm. *Courtesy, Claus Garbe, MD and Jürgen Bauer, MD.*

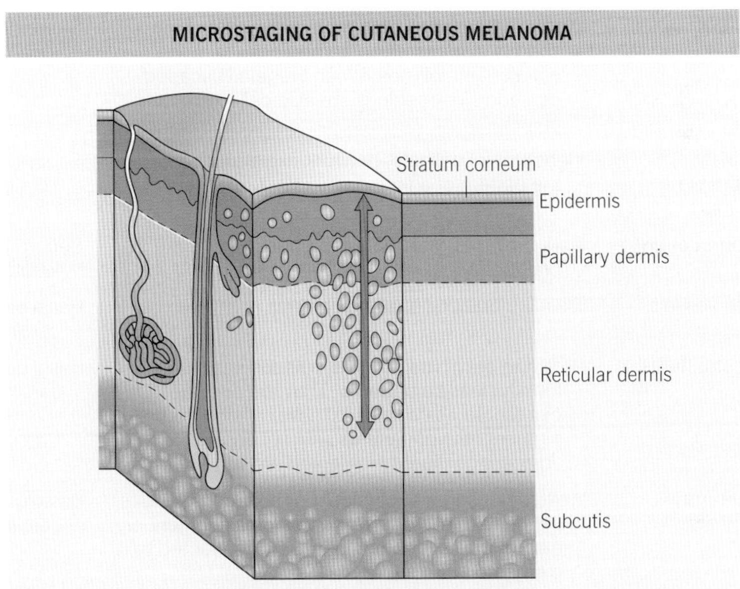

Fig. 93.12 Microstaging of cutaneous melanoma: Breslow tumor thickness (blue vertical arrow). Breslow method: measure in millimeters from the top of the granular layer of the epidermis (or the base of an ulcer) to the deepest part of the tumor.

DERMOSCOPIC PATTERN ANALYSIS: FIRST-STEP ALGORITHM FOR DIFFERENTIATION BETWEEN MELANOCYTIC AND NON-MELANOCYTIC LESIONS		
Dermoscopic criterion	**Definition**	**Diagnostic significance**
Pigment network – pseudo-network†	Network of brownish interconnected lines over a background of tan diffuse pigmentation. In facial skin, a peculiar pigment network, also called a pseudo-network, is typified by round, equally sized network holes corresponding to the pre-existing follicular ostia.	Melanocytic lesion
Aggregated globules	Numerous, variously sized, more or less clustered, round to oval structures with various shades of brown and gray-black. They should be differentiated from multiple blue-gray globules.	Melanocytic lesion
Streaks	These have been previously described separately as pseudopods and radial streaming, but are now combined into the one term. They are bulbous and often kinked or finger-like projections seen at the edge of a lesion. They may arise from network structures but more commonly do not. They range in color from tan to black.	Melanocytic lesion
Homogeneous blue pigmentation‡	Structureless blue pigmentation in the absence of pigment network or other distinctive local features	Melanocytic lesion
Parallel pattern	Seen in melanocytic lesions of palms/soles and mucosal areas. On palms/soles, the pigmentation may follow the sulci or the cristae (i.e. furrows or ridges) of the dermatoglyphics. Rarely arranged at right angles to these structures.	Melanocytic lesion
Multiple milia-like cysts	Numerous, variously sized, white or yellowish, roundish structures	Seborrheic keratosis
Comedo-like openings	Brown-yellowish to brown-black, round to oval, sharply circumscribed keratotic plugs in the ostia of hair follicles. When irregularly shaped, comedo-like openings are also called irregular crypts.	Seborrheic keratosis
Light brown fingerprint-like structures	Light brown, delicate, network-like structures with the pattern of a fingerprint	Seborrheic keratosis
Cerebriform pattern	Dark brown furrows between ridges typifying a brainlike appearance	Seborrheic keratosis
Arborizing vessels	Tree-like branching telangiectasias	Basal cell carcinoma*
Leaf-like structures	Brown to gray/blue discrete bulbous structures forming leaflike patterns. They are discrete pigmented nests (islands) never arising from a pigment network and usually not arising from adjacent confluent pigmented areas.	Basal cell carcinoma*
Large blue-gray ovoid nests	Well-circumscribed, confluent or near confluent, pigmented, ovoid or elongated areas, larger than globules, and not intimately connected to a pigmented tumor body	Basal cell carcinoma*
Multiple blue-gray globules	Multiple globules (not dots) that should be differentiated from multiple blue-gray dots (melanophages)	Basal cell carcinoma*

Table 93.4 Dermoscopic pattern analysis: first-step algorithm for differentiation between melanocytic and non-melanocytic lesions. *Continued*

DERMOSCOPIC PATTERN ANALYSIS: FIRST-STEP ALGORITHM FOR DIFFERENTIATION BETWEEN MELANOCYTIC AND NON-MELANOCYTIC LESIONS		
Dermoscopic criterion	**Definition**	**Diagnostic significance**
Spoke-wheel areas	Well-circumscribed radial projections, usually tan in color but sometimes blue or gray, meeting at an often darker (dark brown, black or blue) central axis	Basal cell carcinoma*
Ulceration§	Absence of the epidermis, often associated with congealed blood, not due to a well-described recent history of trauma	Basal cell carcinoma*
Red-blue lacunae	More or less sharply demarcated, roundish or oval areas with a reddish, red-bluish, or dark red to black coloration	Vascular lesion
Red-bluish to reddish-black homogeneous areas	Structureless homogeneous areas of red-bluish to red-black coloration	Vascular lesion
None of the listed criteria	Absence of the above-mentioned criteria	Melanocytic lesion

**To diagnose a basal cell carcinoma, the negative feature of pigment network must be absent and one or more of the positive features listed here must be present.*

†Exception 1: Pigment network or pseudo-network is also present in solar lentigo and rarely in seborrheic keratosis and pigmented actinic keratosis. A delicate, annular pigment network is also commonly seen in dermatofibroma and accessory nipple (clue for diagnosis of dermatofibroma and accessory nipple: central white patch).

‡Exception 2: Homogeneous blue pigmentation (dermoscopic hallmark of blue nevus) is also seen (uncommonly) in some hemangiomas and basal cell carcinomas and (commonly) in intradermal melanoma metastases.

§Exception 3: Ulceration is also seen less commonly in invasive melanoma.

Table 93.4 *Continued* **Dermoscopic pattern analysis: first-step algorithm for differentiation between melanocytic and non-melanocytic lesions.** *Adapted from Argenziano G, Soyer HP, Chimenti S, et al. Dermoscopy of pigmented skin lesions: Results of a consensus meeting via the Internet. J Am Acad Dermatol 2003;48:679–93.*

DERMOSCOPIC PATTERN ANALYSIS: SECOND-STEP ALGORITHM FOR DIFFERENTIATION BETWEEN MELANOCYTIC NEVI AND MELANOMA		
Dermoscopic criterion	**Definition**	**Diagnostic significance**
Global features		
Reticular pattern	Pigment network covering most parts of the lesion	Melanocytic nevus
Globular pattern	Numerous, variously sized, round to oval structures with various shades of brown and gray-black	Melanocytic nevus
Cobblestone pattern	Large, closely aggregated, somehow angulated globule-like structures resembling a cobblestone	Dermal nevus
Homogeneous pattern	Diffuse, brown, gray-blue to gray-black pigmentation in the absence of other distinctive local features	Melanocytic (blue) nevus
Starburst pattern	Pigmented streaks in a radial arrangement at the edge of the lesion	Spitz/Reed nevus

Table 93.5 Dermoscopic pattern analysis: second-step algorithm for differentiation between melanocytic nevi and melanoma. *Continued*

DERMOSCOPIC PATTERN ANALYSIS: SECOND-STEP ALGORITHM FOR DIFFERENTIATION BETWEEN MELANOCYTIC NEVI AND MELANOMA		
Dermoscopic criterion	**Definition**	**Diagnostic significance**
Parallel pattern	Pigmentation on palms/soles that follows the sulci or the cristae (furrows or ridges), rarely arranged at right angles to these structures	Acral nevus/ melanoma (see below)
Multicomponent pattern	Combination of three or more of the above patterns	Melanoma
Nonspecific pattern	Pigmented lesion lacking above patterns	Possible melanoma
Local features		
Pigment network	Typical pigment network: light to dark brown network with small, uniformly spaced network holes and thin network lines distributed more or less regularly throughout the lesion and usually thinning out at the periphery	Benign melanocytic lesion
	Atypical pigment network: black, brown, or gray network with irregular holes and thick lines	Melanoma
Dots/globules	Black, brown, round to oval, variously sized structures regularly or irregularly distributed within the lesion	If regular, benign melanocytic lesion If irregular, melanoma
Streaks	These have been previously described separately as pseudopods and radial streaming. Streaks are bulbous and often kinked or finger-like projections seen at the edge of a lesion. They may arise from network structures but more commonly do not. They range in color from tan to black.	If regular, benign melanocytic lesion (Spitz/Reed nevus) If irregular, melanoma
Blue-whitish veil	Irregular, structureless area of confluent blue pigmentation with an overlying white “ground-glass” film. The pigmentation cannot occupy the entire lesion and usually corresponds to a clinically elevated part of the lesion.	Melanoma
Regression structures	White scarlike depigmentation and/or blue pepper-like granules usually corresponding to a clinically flat part of the lesion	Melanoma
Hypopigmentation	Areas with less pigmentation than the overall pigmentation of the lesion	Nonspecific
Blotches	Black, brown, and/or gray structureless areas with symmetrical or asymmetrical distribution within the lesion	If symmetrical, benign melanocytic lesion If asymmetrical, melanoma

Table 93.5 Dermoscopic pattern analysis: second-step algorithm for differentiation between melanocytic nevi and melanoma. *Continued*

DERMOSCOPIC PATTERN ANALYSIS: SECOND-STEP ALGORITHM FOR DIFFERENTIATION BETWEEN MELANOCYTIC NEVI AND MELANOMA		
Dermoscopic criterion	**Definition**	**Diagnostic significance**
Site-related features		
Face	Typical pseudo-network (round, equally sized network holes corresponding to the pre-existing follicular ostia)	Benign melanocytic lesion
	Annular–granular structures (multiple blue-gray dots surrounding the follicular ostia with an annular–granular appearance)	Melanoma
	Gray pseudo-network (gray pigmentation surrounding the follicular ostia, formed by the confluence of annular–granular structures)	Melanoma
	Rhomboidal structures (gray-brown pigmentation surrounding the follicular ostia with a rhomboidal appearance)	Melanoma
	Asymmetric pigmented follicles (eccentric annular pigmentation around follicular ostia)	Melanoma
Palms/soles	Parallel-furrow pattern (pigmentation following the sulci)	Acral nevus
	Lattice-like pattern (pigmentation following and crossing the furrows)	Acral nevus
	Fibrillar pattern (numerous, finely pigmented filaments perpendicular to the furrows and ridges)	Acral nevus
	Parallel-ridge pattern (pigmentation aligned along the cristae)	Melanoma

Table 93.5 *Continued* **Dermoscopic pattern analysis: second-step algorithm for differentiation between melanocytic nevi and melanoma.** *Adapted from Argenziano G, Soyer HP, Chimenti S, et al. Dermoscopy of pigmented skin lesions: Results of a consensus meeting via the Internet. J Am Acad Dermatol 2003;48:679–93.*

DEFINITIONS OF DERMOSCOPIC CRITERIA FOR THE 3-POINT CHECKLIST	
Criterion	**Definition**
Asymmetry	Asymmetrical distribution of colors and dermoscopic structures
Atypical network*	More than one type of network (in terms of color and thickness of the meshes) irregularly distributed within the lesion
Blue-white structures†	Presence of any type of blue and/or white color

**Usually found in early melanoma.*
†Usually found in both melanoma and pigmented basal cell carcinoma.

Table 93.6 Definitions of dermoscopic criteria for the 3-point checklist. The presence of more than one criterion suggests a suspicious lesion. *Adapted from Argenziano G, Puig S, Zalaudek I, et al. Dermoscopy improves accuracy of primary care physicians to triage lesions suggestive of skin cancer. J Clin Oncol. 2006;24:1877–82.*

DIFFERENTIAL DIAGNOSIS OF CUTANEOUS MELANOMA	
General	**Location-based**
If pigmented • Atypical (dysplastic) nevus • Other nevi (e.g. black [hypermelanotic], blue, genital, acral, Spitz, recurrent) • Seborrheic keratosis • Pigmented BCC • Pigmented Bowen disease • Thrombosed hemangioma • Dermatofibroma **If amelanotic (pink, red)** • Pyogenic granuloma (nodular) • BCC; SCC, *in situ* or invasive • Merkel cell carcinoma • Pink intradermal nevus • Spitz nevus • Dermatofibroma • Wart • Lichen planus-like keratosis (LPLK) • Isolated patch of psoriasis or eczema	**Lentigo maligna melanoma** • Pigmented actinic keratosis • Solar lentigo • Macular seborrheic keratosis **Nail matrix melanoma** • Longitudinal melanonychia (see Table 58.2) • Drug-induced nail pigmentation (see Table 58.4) • SCC, *in situ* or invasive • Subungual hematoma • Wart **Mucosal melanoma** • Melanosis of mucosal regions • Venous lake (vermilion lip) • Amalgam tattoo • Angiokeratoma (genital) • SCC, *in situ* or invasive **Acral lentiginous melanoma** • Black heel or palm (see Fig. 74.9) • Plantar wart • Tinea nigra • Plantar callosity • Trophic ulcers

Table 93.7 Differential diagnosis of cutaneous melanoma.

AJCC MELANOMA TNM CLASSIFICATION – 2017		
T category	**Thickness**	**Ulceration status**
Tis (melanoma *in situ*)	NA	NA
T1	<0.8 mm	a. –
	<0.8 mm 0.8–1.0 mm	b. + b. +/–
T2	>1.0–2.0 mm	a. –
		b. +
T3	>2.0–4.0 mm	a. –
		b. +
T4	>4.0 mm	a. –
		b. +

N category	Number of tumor-involved regional lymph nodes	Presence of in-transit, satellite, and/or microsatellite metastases*
N0	No regional metastases detected	No
N1	One tumor-involved node –*or*– in-transit, satellite, and/or microsatellite metastases with no tumor-involved nodes	
N1a	One clinically occult (i.e. detected by SLN biopsy)	No

Table 93.8 AJCC melanoma TNM classification – 2017. *Continued.*

AJCC MELANOMA TNM CLASSIFICATION – 2017		
N category	**Number of tumor-involved regional lymph nodes**	**Presence of in-transit, satellite, and/or micro-satellite metastases***
N1b	One clinically detected	No
N1c	No regional lymph node disease	Yes
N2	Two or three tumor-involved nodes *–or–* in-transit, satellite, and/or microsatellite metastases with one tumor-involved node	
N2a	Two or three clinically occult	No
N2b	Two or three, at least one of which was clinically detected	No
N2c	One clinically occult or clinically detected	Yes
N3	Four or more tumor-involved nodes *–or–* in-transit, satellite, and/or microsatellite metastases with two or more tumor-involved nodes *–or–* any number of matted nodes without or with in-transit, satellite, and/or microsatellite metastases	
N3a	Four or more clinically occult	No
N3b	Four or more, at least one of which was clinically detected, or presence of any number of matted nodes	No
N3c	Two or more clinically occult or clinically detected and/or presence of any number of matted nodes	Yes
M category	**Anatomic site**	**LDH level**
M0	No evidence of distant metastasis	NA
M1a	Distant metastasis to skin, soft tissue including muscle, and/or non-regional lymph node	Not recorded or unspecified
		(0) Not elevated
		(1) Elevated
M1b	Distant metastasis to lung with or without M1a sites of disease	Not recorded or unspecified
		(0) Not elevated
		(1) Elevated
M1c	Distant metastasis to non-CNS visceral sites with or without M1a or M1b sites of disease	Not recorded or unspecified
		(0) Not elevated
		(1) Elevated
M1d	Distant metastasis to CNS with or without M1a, M1b or M1c sites of disease	Not recorded or unspecified
		(0) Not elevated
		(1) Elevated

**In-transit metastases are >2 cm from the primary tumor but not beyond the regional lymph nodes, while satellite lesions are within 2 cm of the primary. Satellite lesions can be detected clinically or microscopically; the latter are referred to as microsatellite metastases.*

Table 93.8 *Continued* **AJCC melanoma TNM classification – 2017.** Histologic evaluation of lymph nodes must include at least one immunohistochemical marker (e.g. HMB45, MART-1/Melan-A). NA, not applicable; SLN, sentinel lymph node. *Adapted from: AJCC Cancer Staging Manual. American Joint Committee on Cancer, 8th edn. Springer, 2017:563–85.*

AJCC STAGE GROUPINGS FOR CUTANEOUS MELANOMA – 2017							
	Survival (%)*	Clinical staging†			Pathologic staging‡		
		T	N	M	T	N	M
0		Tis	N0	M0	Tis	N0	M0
IA	97	T1a	N0	M0	T1a	N0	M0
					T1b		
IB	93	T1b	N0	M0	T2a	N0	M0
		T2a					
IIA	82	T2b	N0	M0	T2b	N0	M0
	79	T3a			T3a		
IIB	68	T3b	N0	M0	T3b	N0	M0
	71	T4a			T4a		
IIC	53	T4b	N0	M0	T4b	N0	M0
III§		Any T, Tis	≥N1	M0			
IIIB					T0	N1b, N1c	M0
IIIC					T0	N2b, N2c, N3b or N3c	M0
IIIA	78				T1a/b–T2a	N1a or N2a	M0
IIIB	59				T1a/b–T2a	N1b/c or N2b	M0
					T2b/T3a	N1a–N2b	
IIIC	40				T1a–T3a	N2c or N3a/b/c	M0
					T3b/T4a	Any N ≥ N1	
					T4b	N1a–N2c	
IIID					T4b	N3a/b/c	M0
IV	9–27¶	Any T	Any N	M1	Any T, Tis	Any N	M1

**Approximate 5-year survival (%), adapted from Balch et al. 2009 AJCC melanoma staging and classification. J Clin Oncol. 2009;27:6199–206; based upon 2009 AJCC melanoma TNM classification and prior to advent of targeted therapy and immunotherapy.*
†Clinical staging includes microstaging of the primary melanoma and clinical/radiologic evaluation for metastases. By convention, it should be used after complete excision of the primary melanoma with clinical assessment for regional and distant metastases.
‡Pathologic staging includes microstaging of the primary melanoma and pathologic information about the regional lymph nodes after partial or complete lymphadenectomy. Pathologic stage 0 or stage IA patients are the exception.
§There are no stage III subgroups for clinical staging.
¶Higher survival rate associated with normal serum LDH levels and lower rate with elevated LDH levels.

Table 93.9 AJCC stage groupings for cutaneous melanoma – 2017. *Adapted from Balch CM, Gershenwald JE, Soong SJ, et al. Final version of 2009 AJCC melanoma staging and classification. J Clin Oncol 2009;27:6199–6206. Reprinted with permission from the American Society of Clinical Oncology.*

- As with other cancers, prognosis is dependent on the stage at the time of diagnosis (Fig. 93.13); other independent prognostic factors for survival have also been identified (Table 93.10).
- Molecular testing of the primary CM (e.g. gene expression profiling) for prognostication is still considered investigational.

Management

- Once the histopathologic diagnosis of CM is confirmed and prior to re-excision (Table 93.11), evaluation should include a thorough history, TBSE, palpation of the surrounding skin and lymph node basins, and

COMPARISON OF SURVIVAL CURVES IN FOUR STAGES OF MELANOMA

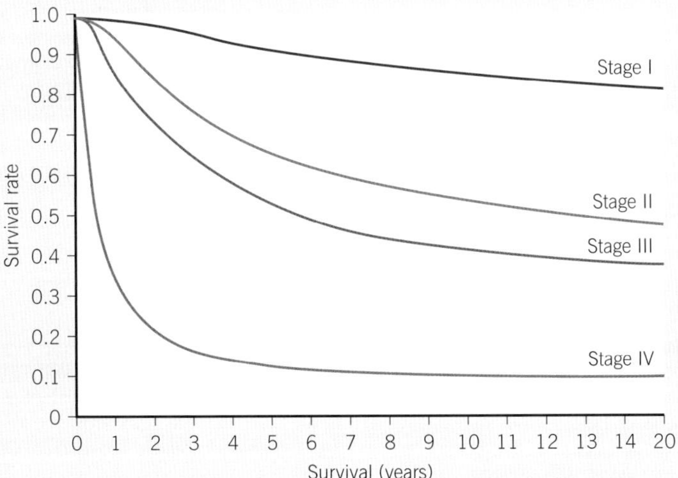

Fig. 93.13 Comparison of survival curves in four stages of melanoma. *Redrawn from Balch CM. Melanoma of the skin. In Edge SB, Byrd DR, Compton CC, et al., eds. AJCC Cancer Staging Manual, 7th edn. New York: Springer, 2009.*

MELANOMA – MAJOR INDEPENDENT PROGNOSTIC FACTORS FOR SURVIVAL IN MULTIVARIATE ANALYSES	
Prognostic factor	**Commentary**
Tumor thickness	≤1 mm, low risk; >1 mm, higher risk
Ulceration	Worse prognosis with ulceration
Mitotic rate	Worse prognosis with ≥1 mitoses/mm^2
Age	Worse prognosis with older age
Sex	Men have poorer prognosis (only for localized disease)
Anatomic site	Trunk, head, and neck associated with poorer prognosis than extremities
Number of involved lymph nodes	Cutoff points: 1, 2–3, 4 or more lymph nodes (see Table 93.8)
Regional lymph node tumor burden	Clinically detectable (palpable) nodal metastases with poorer prognosis than clinically occult (non-palpable) nodal metastases
Site of distant metastases	Visceral metastases associated with poorer prognosis than non-visceral metastases (skin, subcutaneous, distant lymph nodes)

Table 93.10 Melanoma – major independent prognostic factors for survival in multivariate analyses.

determination of whether or not a sentinel lymph node biopsy (SLNB) should be considered (Table 93.12).

- **Sentinel lymph node biopsy (SLNB):**
  - SLNB is useful as a staging and prognostic tool, but to date its usefulness as a therapeutic modality has not been established
  - SLN status is also an important determinant for consideration of adjuvant therapy (e.g. immune checkpoint inhibitors) for patients with stage III disease
  - Typically, SLNB is performed at the time of re-excision
  - If the SLNB is positive for *micro*-metastases, complete lymph node

SURGICAL TREATMENT OF PRIMARY CUTANEOUS MELANOMA		
Tumor thickness	**Excision margins* (cm)**	**Comments**
In situ	0.5	Lentigo maligna of the face may be excised with 1-cm margins (especially when lesions are >1.5–2 cm in diameter) or treated by Mohs micrographic surgery or radiotherapy; postoperative topical imiquimod is often used
≤1 mm	1.0	Mohs micrographic surgery may be employed in acral and facial melanomas
1.01–2 mm	1.0–2.0	
>2 mm	2.0	

**Measurement of the excision margins should begin at the outermost edge of the biopsy site or the clinical lesion, whichever is furthest out.*

Table 93.11 Surgical treatment of primary cutaneous melanoma. Evidence from available randomized trials is insufficient to address the optimal margins for the excision of primary cutaneous melanoma, but multiple expert international committees have produced fairly consistent guidelines, as summarized here. Of note, further investigative efforts will likely alter the standards of care over time. *Adapted from Sladden MJ, et al. Surgical excision margins for primary cutaneous melanoma. Cochrane Database Syst Rev 2009;(4):CD004855.*

CRITERIA FOR CONSIDERATION OF SENTINEL LYMPH NODE BIOPSY (SLNB)
Discuss SLNB • Stage T1a: <0.8 mm without ulceration but with any adverse features* • Stage T1b: <0.8 mm with ulceration • Stage T1b: 0.8–1.0 mm with or without ulceration
Discuss and offer SLNB • Stage >T2a: >1.0 mm

**Young age (<40 years), presence of lymphovascular invasion, positive deep biopsy margin (especially if diffuse), high mitotic rate.*

Table 93.12 Criteria for consideration of sentinel lymph node biopsy (SLNB). The patient should also be informed of the FDA-approved therapies for stage III disease.

dissection used to be the standard procedure, but nowadays clinical surveillance (including ultrasound of the regional basin) is often chosen instead

  – *Disadvantages*: can cause lymphedema; expensive; usually requires general anesthesia

• Regional nodal ultrasound surveillance may also be used to monitor the regional lymph node basin in patients who are eligible for SLNB but elect not to undergo the procedure.

• Imaging studies for identification of metastases include: ultrasound of lymph node basins; CT scan of the chest, abdomen, and pelvis or PET scan in high-risk patients; and if symptoms, cranial MRI; serum LDH is measured serially in stage IV patients, as it influences prognosis (see Table 93.8).

• Additional **Rx**, in particular immunotherapy and targeted therapies, is outlined in Tables 93.13 and 93.14.

• A melanoma patient worksheet can help organize all of this information for both the patient and the clinician (see Appendix).

Follow-Up

• Primary objectives include identification of potentially curable local recurrences (~4% of patients; Fig. 93.14) or regional metastases (e.g. in transit, lymph node; Fig. 93.15) and to identify second primary CMs (up to 10% of patients).

GENERAL GUIDELINES FOR TREATMENT OF CUTANEOUS MELANOMA (CM) BASED ON STAGE AT DIAGNOSIS, IN ADDITION TO RE-EXCISION OF THE PRIMARY CM	
Stage	**Recommended treatment**
Stage 0 (melanoma *in situ)*	
• Tis	• Re-excision (see Table 93.11)
Stages I and II	
• T1a <0.8 mm (no ulceration and no other adverse features*)	• Re-excision (see Table 93.11)
• T1a <0.8 mm (no ulceration but (+) adverse features*) • T1b <0.8 mm (+) ulceration or 0.8–1.0 mm +/– ulceration	• Re-excision (see Table 93.11) • Discussion of SLNB**
• ≥T2a (>1.0 mm +/– ulceration)	• Re-excision (see Table 93.11) • Discussion and offering of SLNB**
Stage III	
• Lymph node metastases, including clinically occult disease noted by SLNB	• Offer adjuvant therapy (see Table 93.14) • Consider clinical trial enrollment
• In-transit or satellite metastases†	*Depending on number of lesions, local, regional or systemic therapy is chosen or may be combined:* • *Systemic therapy* (see Table 93.14) • *Local therapy*: – Complete surgical excision to clear margins if possible – T-VEC¶, BCG, interferon alpha, or IL-2 injection in tumor – Topical imiquimod cream – Consider radiotherapy if can't be removed by surgery • *Regional therapy:* – Isolated limb infusion/perfusion with melphalan
Stage IV	
• Skin or subcutaneous metastases	• Depends upon size and number of lesions (see above, in-transit metastases)
• Solid organ metastases	• Systemic therapy (see Table 93.14) +/– surgery or radiotherapy (including stereotactic)

**Adverse features include young age (<40 years), presence of lymphovascular invasion, positive deep biopsy margin (especially if diffuse), high mitotic rate.*
***SLNB should be performed before or at the time of re-excision.*
†The distinction between in-transit and satellite metastases is not clinically necessary as both are considered manifestations of intralymphatic disease and are grouped together in the new AJCC staging system.
¶An oncolytic virus therapy that uses a genetically modified herpes virus to infect and kill cancer cells.

Table 93.13 General guidelines for treatment of cutaneous melanoma (CM) based on stage at diagnosis, in addition to re-excision of the primary CM. BCG, Bacillus Calmette–Guérin; SLNB, sentinel lymph node biopsy; T-VEC, talimogene laherparepvec.

• Visits should include: (1) review of systems that focuses on signs or symptoms of metastases to soft tissue, liver, lung, GI tract, and CNS; (2) TBSE; (3) examination and palpation of the melanoma scar/excision site and surrounding area for local recurrences or in-transit metastases; (4) lymph node examination; and (5) laboratory and radiologic tests as indicated by signs and symptoms.

• Follow-up intervals during the first 3–5 years after diagnosis vary from 3 to 6 months, depending on stage, in addition to the number of primary melanomas, melanocytic nevi, and atypical nevi as well as family history of melanoma; lifelong follow-up is recommended.

• Patients should be counseled to adhere to sun protective measures; perform skin self-examinations at home; stay up-to-date on

TARGETED THERAPIES AND CHECKPOINT INHIBITORS		
Targeting the MAPK pathway (see Fig. 93.2)		**FDA approved as of June 2021**
BRAF inhibitors (selective*,**)	Dab*rafe*nib***	√
	Enco*rafe*nib	√
	Vemu*rafe*nib	√
MEK inhibitors**	Bini*meti*nib	√
	Cobi*meti*nib	√
	Tra*meti*nib***	√
Immune checkpoint inhibitors		
Anti-CTLA-4 antibody	Ipilimumab***	√
	Tremelimumab	
Anti-PD-1 antibody	Nivolumab***	√
	Pembrolizumab***	√
	Pidilizumab	
	Cemiplimab	Approved for advanced cutaneous SCC and BCC
Anti-PD-L1 antibodies	Atezolizumab	√
	Avelumab	Approved for metastatic Merkel cell carcinoma and urothelial carcinoma
	Durvalumab	Approved for bladder cancer (PD-L1-positive) and extensive-stage small cell lung cancer

**Target melanomas that have specific amino acid substitutions at position 600 in BRAF, most commonly V600E and less often V600D or V600K.*
***For melanomas with activating BRAF mutations, the combination of a selected BRAF inhibitor with a MEK inhibitor is recommended to minimize the development of drug resistance and cutaneous toxic effects (see Table 17.9), most notably eruptive SCCs and KAs.*
****Dabrafenib + trametinib, ipilimumab, nivolumab, and pembrolizumab have been approved for* ***adjuvant therapy*** *of melanoma; peginterferon alpha 2b is also approved but is rarely used.*

Table 93.14 Major systemic treatments for metastatic melanoma – targeted therapies and checkpoint inhibitors. MAPK, mitogen-activated protein kinase.

their other health maintenance and recommended cancer screenings; and take an oral vitamin D supplement if needed.

- Family members can be screened by a dermatologist, who can then determine frequency of subsequent screenings.
- Genetic counseling/testing for germline mutations should be considered in patients suspected of having a familial melanoma syndrome (see Tables 93.2 and 93.3).

For further information see Ch. 113 from *Dermatology, Fourth Edition*.

For additional online figures and tables visit www.expertconsult.com 

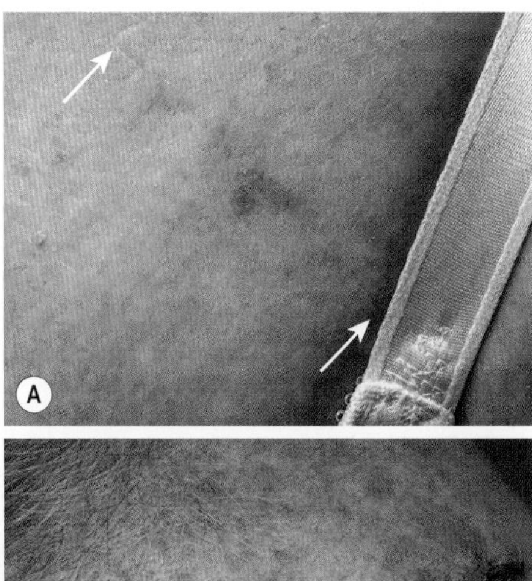

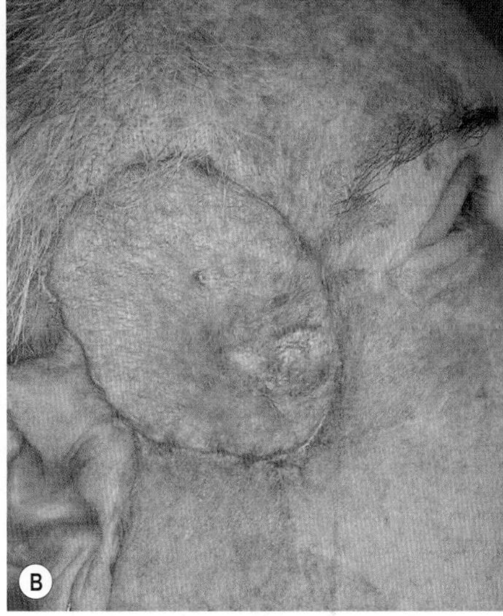

Fig. 93.14 Local recurrences of cutaneous melanoma. A Recurrent melanoma *in situ* occurring midway along the excision scar (demarcated by arrows) on the right upper back in a female with Lynch syndrome (*PMS2* mutation). **B** Amelanotic nodular recurrence of a desmoplastic melanoma within the skin graft. *A, Courtesy, Karynne O Duncan, MD; B, Courtesy, Jean L. Bolognia, MD.*

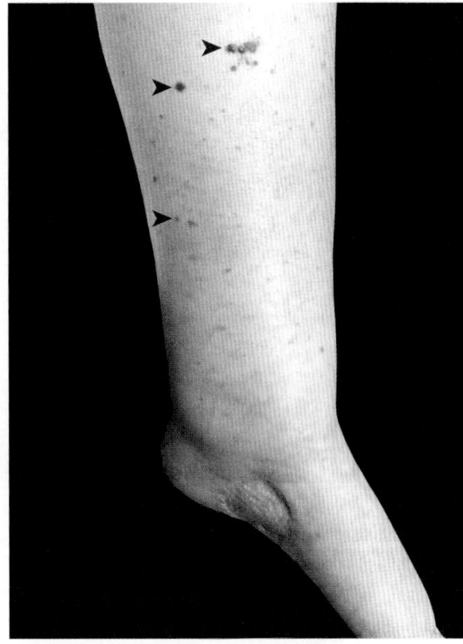

Fig. 93.15 In-transit metastases of melanoma. Multiple pink, brown and black papulonodules (see arrowheads) developed along the lymphatic drainage route following resection of a recurrent melanoma (3.2 mm Breslow depth) on the left medial foot one year prior. This patient subsequently received intralesional talimogene laherparepvec injection treatment. *Courtesy, Karynne O. Duncan, MD.*

94 Vascular Neoplasms and Reactive Proliferations

Lesions of vascular origin are broadly, and somewhat imperfectly, classified as neoplasms (tumors), malformations, reactive proliferations, or telangiectasias. The growth of a neoplasm is largely autonomous (i.e. not reactive). Malformations, in general, are not actively proliferating (see Ch. 85). Reactive proliferations represent endothelial cell proliferation that is in response to some factor (e.g. fibrin, hypoxia, trauma). Telangiectasias represent pre-existing capillaries that are persistently dilated but lack a proliferative component (see Ch. 87).

Neoplasms/Tumors

Infantile Hemangioma and Congenital Hemangioma

- See Chapter 85.

Cherry Angioma

- Bright red, 1- to 6-mm papule, commonly on the trunk or upper extremities (Fig. 94.1); appears during adulthood; early, tiny lesions can be macular.
- Dermoscopy: red to red-blue lacunas (well-demarcated round to oval, red to red-blue structures).

Glomus Tumor

- Solitary, painful papule or nodule on the extremities, or in the nail bed (beneath the nail plate) in young adults (Fig. 94.2).
- A glomus cell is a perivascular contractile cell that influences vessel diameter as a means of controlling temperature.

Tufted Angioma

- Pink to dark red patches and plaques with superimposed papules (Fig. 94.3) that slowly enlarge and occasionally regress.
- Commonly found on the neck and trunk.
- Congenital or acquired during childhood or young adulthood.
- On a spectrum with kaposiform hemangioendothelioma.
- Early-onset lesions can be associated with Kasabach–Merritt phenomenon (consumptive coagulopathy with decreased platelets) – see below.

Kaposiform Hemangioendothelioma

- Ill-defined, pink to violaceous plaques or nodules (Fig. 94.4); sometimes deeply seated; any site.
- May be congenital and generally appears by 2 years of age.
- Locally aggressive, persistent.

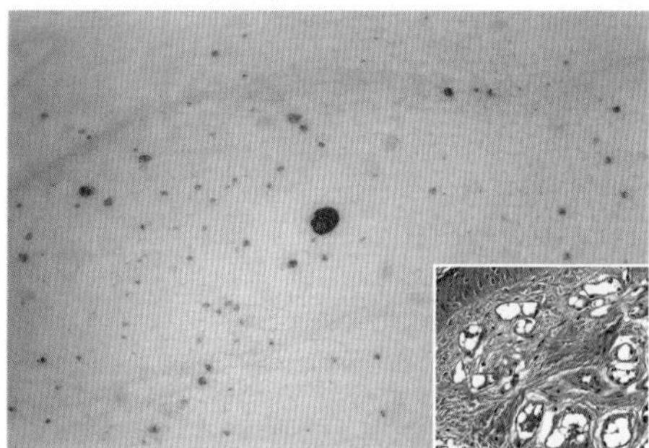

Fig. 94.1 Cherry angiomas. Multiple, slightly compressible red papules. Histologically, congested capillaries and postcapillary venules expand the papillary dermis (inset). *Courtesy, Jean L. Bolognia, MD.*

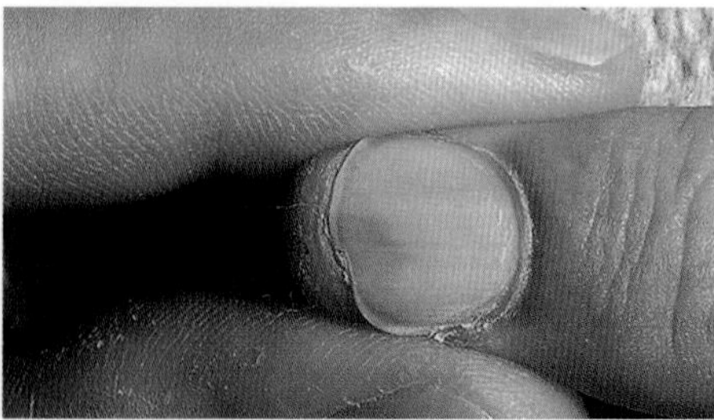

Fig. 94.2 Glomus tumor. The lesion presented with pain and ill-defined subungual erythema. *Courtesy, Ronald P. Rapini, MD.*

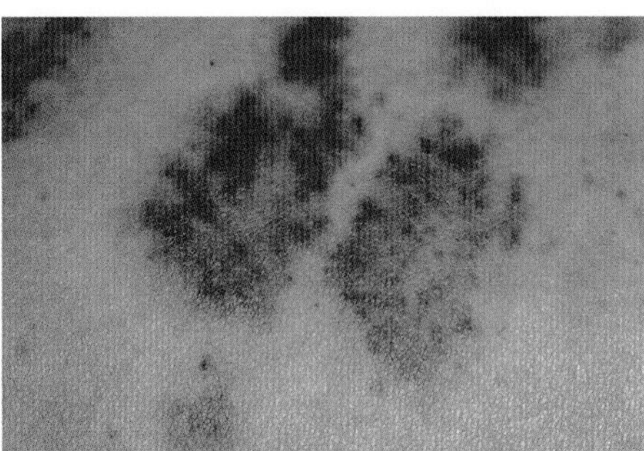

Fig. 94.3 Tufted angioma. Mottled red patches and superimposed papules are typical clinical features. *Courtesy, YDRSC.*

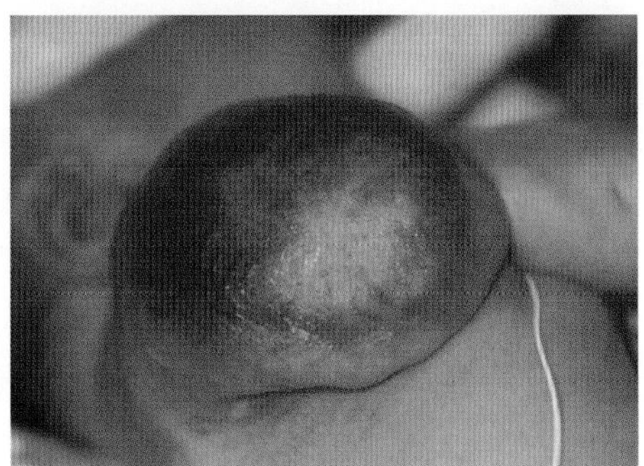

Fig. 94.4 Kaposiform hemangioendothelioma complicated by Kasabach–Merritt phenomenon. A large red-purple mass on the upper flank of an infant. *Courtesy, YDRSC.*

- Associated with Kasabach–Merritt phenomenon (KMP).
  - Life-threatening thrombocytopenic coagulopathy associated with a vascular tumor, usually a kaposiform hemangioendothelioma or tufted angioma in an infant (*not* an infantile hemangioma)
  - Presents with a rapidly enlarging, indurated, ecchymotic mass associated with marked thrombocytopenia and a consumptive coagulopathy (see Fig. 94.4)
  - **Rx:** difficult; sirolimus (rapamycin) or vincristine plus prednisone

Kaposi Sarcoma

- Multifocal systemic disease; extramucocutaneous sites include gastrointestinal tract, lymph nodes, and lungs.
- Four main variants: (1) older men from the Mediterranean basin or of Ashkenazi Jewish descent with lesions on the lower extremities (Fig. 94.5); (2) African endemic; (3) iatrogenic/immunocompromised; and (4) AIDS-related epidemic (Fig. 94.6).

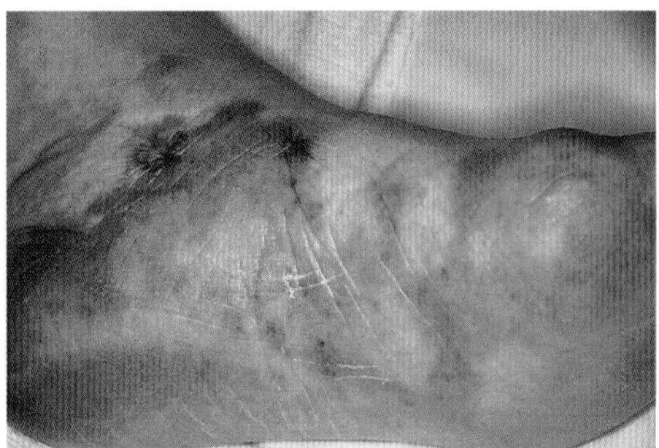

Fig. 94.5 Classic Kaposi sarcoma. Red macules and patches on the plantar surface of the foot, with violaceous plaques on the ankle. *Courtesy, Paula North, MD.*

- Pink to dark violet patches and plaques; with time, can become nodular.
- May have mucosal involvement, e.g. oral.
- Associated with human herpes virus-(HHV-) 8 infection.
- Histopathology varies from a subtle increase in slit-like vessels to nodular proliferations of spindle cells; HHV-8 can be detected in endothelial cells by immunohistochemistry.
- **Rx:** observation, surgical excision, cryotherapy, laser removal, radiotherapy, topical alitretinoin, intralesional or systemic vinblastine, taxanes, liposomal anthracyclines, pomalidomide, reduction of immunosuppression.

Angiosarcoma

- Most commonly begins as a bruise-like patch in the head and neck region of older adults with color varying from pink to dark purple (likened to the color of an eggplant); also associated with lymphedema (Fig. 94.7) or previously irradiated skin (Fig. 94.8).
- With time nodules and ulceration can develop.
- 15% survival at 5 years.
- **Rx:** wide excision ± radiotherapy; consider systemic therapy with taxanes, tyrosine kinase inhibitors (e.g. sorafenib, pazopanib), or bevacizumab for larger lesions.

Malformations (see Ch. 85)

Glomuvenous Malformation (Previously Referred to as Glomangioma)

- See Chapter 85.

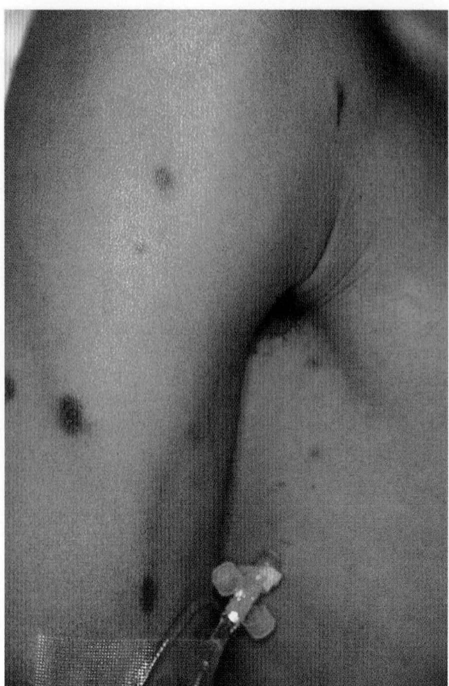

Fig. 94.6 Kaposi sarcoma in a patient with AIDS. Violet-red papules or nodules are often oval to lance-ovate and are usually more widely distributed than in classic KS. *Courtesy, Paula North, MD.*

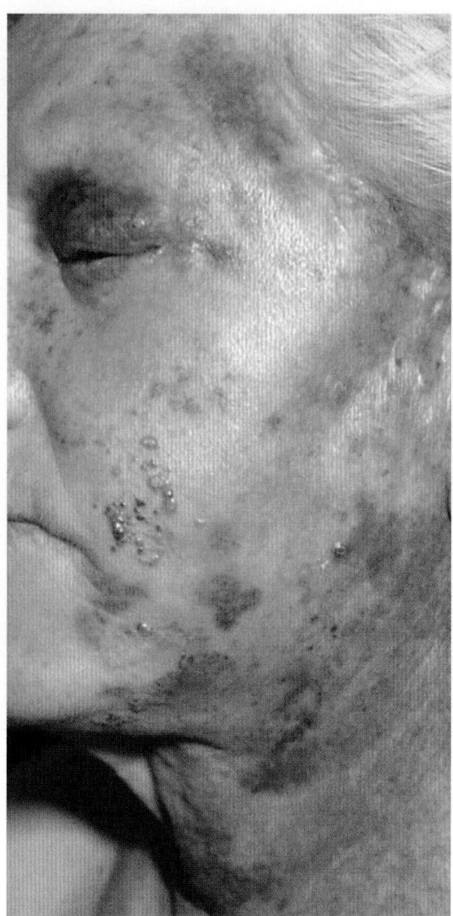

Fig. 94.7 Angiosarcoma. Erythematous and purple hemorrhagic plaques as well as grouped vesicles with clear or hemorrhagic fluid (reminiscent of microcystic lymphatic malformation) are present. There is also induration and a pink hue to the left side of the face in addition to evidence of previous excisions and radiotherapy. *Courtesy, Lorenzo Cerroni, MD.*

Targetoid Hemosiderotic Lymphatic Malformation (Previously Referred to as Hobnail "Hemangioma"/Targetoid Hemosiderotic Hemangioma)

- Uncommon red-purple papule on the trunk or extremities of children or young adults; papule may have a surrounding pale area and outer ecchymotic ring, thus creating a target lesion (Fig. 94.9).

Reactive Proliferations

- Some consider pyogenic granuloma, angiolymphoid hyperplasia with eosinophilia (epithelioid hemangioma), and glomeruloid hemangioma to be tumors.

Pyogenic Granuloma

- Rapidly growing, friable, red papulonodule that is sometimes pedunculated; often ulcerates and bleeds; common in children and young adults.
- Gingival and fingers > lips > face > tongue (Fig. 94.10).
- May arise on the gingiva of pregnant women (granuloma gravidarum).
- Multiple tumors (especially periungual) may be seen in association with medications (e.g. oral retinoids, antiretroviral protease inhibitors, EGFR inhibitors).
- **DDx:** need to distinguish from amelanotic melanoma and Spitz nevus.
- **Rx:** shave excision or saucerization followed by electrosurgery of the base under local anesthesia.

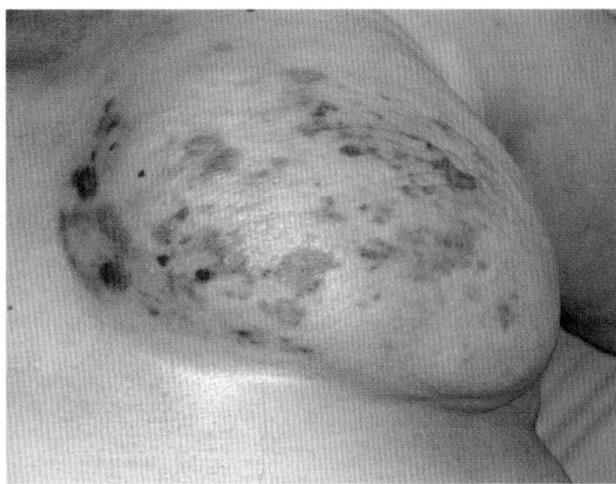

Fig. 94.8 Post-radiation angiosarcoma. Red-violet patches and plaques on the breast. The clinicopathologic differential diagnosis is primarily post-radiation atypical vascular lesions of the skin, an entity that may represent a precursor of post-radiation angiosarcoma. Development of thicker, more indurated plaques and the presence of cellular atypia, multilayering of the vessels, and positivity for c-MYC favor angiosarcoma. *Courtesy, Paula North, MD.*

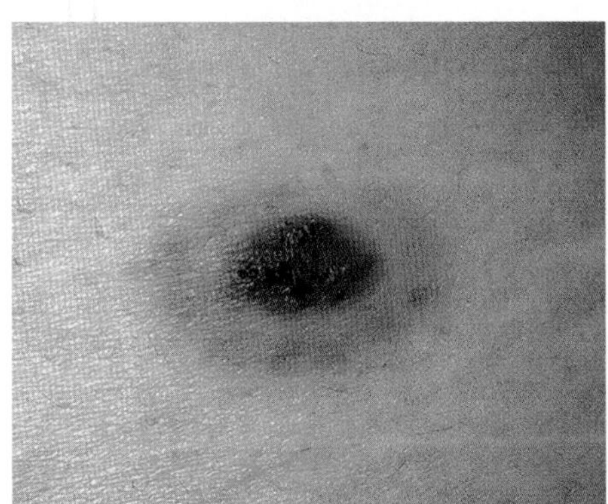

Fig. 94.9 Targetoid hemosiderotic lymphatic malformation (hobnail "hemangioma" [targetoid hemosiderotic hemangioma]). Note the target-like appearance. *Courtesy, Ronald P. Rapini, MD.*

Angiolymphoid Hyperplasia with Eosinophilia (Epithelioid Hemangioma)

- Pink to red-brown nodules or plaques, often multiple and grouped.
- Favors the head and neck region, especially around ears (Fig. 94.11).
- May be painful, pruritic, or rarely pulsatile.
- Occasionally, peripheral eosinophilia.

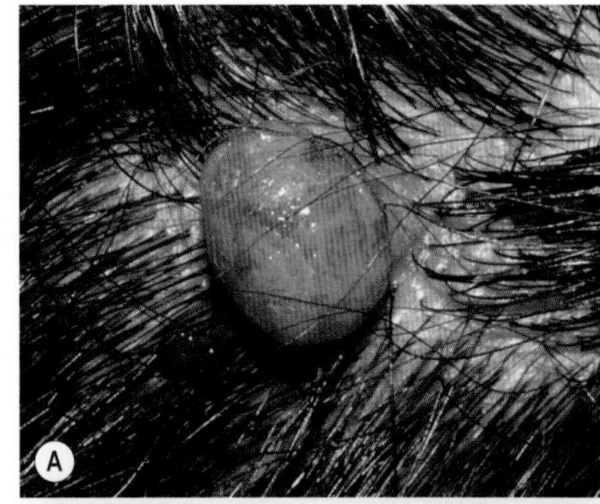

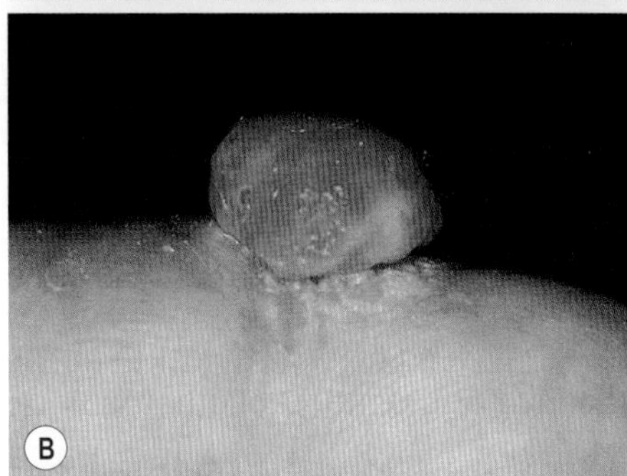

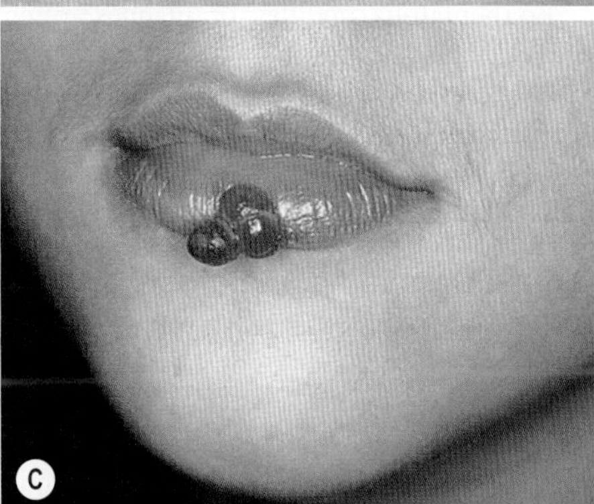

Fig. 94.10 Pyogenic granuloma. A Eroded pink-red papulonodule with a narrow base on the scalp. **B** Pedunculated papule on the finger. **C** Grouped red papules on the lip. The latter two are both common sites. By dermoscopy, red homogeneous areas are intersected by white lines. *A, Courtesy, Julie V. Schaffer, MD; B, C, Courtesy, Paula North, MD.*

Glomeruloid Hemangioma

- Firm red papules or nodules on the trunk and proximal extremities.
- Associated with POEMS (polyneuropathy, organomegaly, endocrinopathy, monoclonal gammopathy, and skin findings) syndrome.

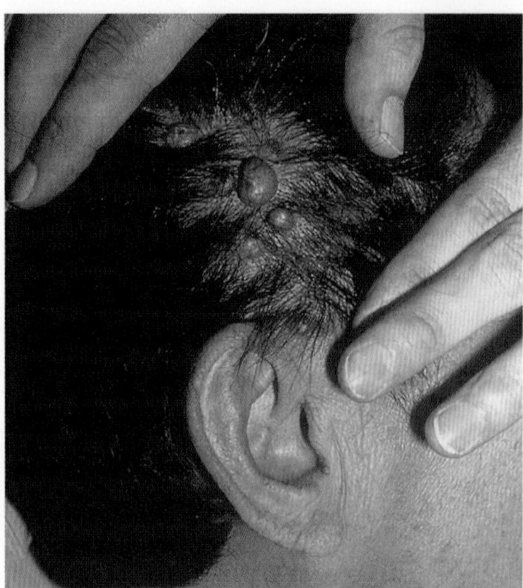

Fig. 94.11 Angiolymphoid hyperplasia with eosinophilia (epithelioid hemangioma). Multiple pink papulonodules are often seen on the scalp. *Courtesy, USCDRSC.*

Reactive Angioendotheliomatosis

- Rare, self-limited.
- Erythematous nodules or plaques, often with petechiae or purpura.
- Associated with cryoglobulinemia (type I) or systemic disorders (e.g. renal failure).
- The form due to severe atherosclerosis leads to ulceration.

Diffuse Dermal Angiomatosis

- Some consider this a variant of reactive angioendotheliomatosis.
- This term has been used to describe an ulcerated lesion in the setting of severe atherosclerosis or vascular compromise; these ulcers usually occur on the lower extremities and resolve with revascularization; less often occurs on the breast or pannus.

Telangiectasias

- See Chapter 87.

Angiokeratomas

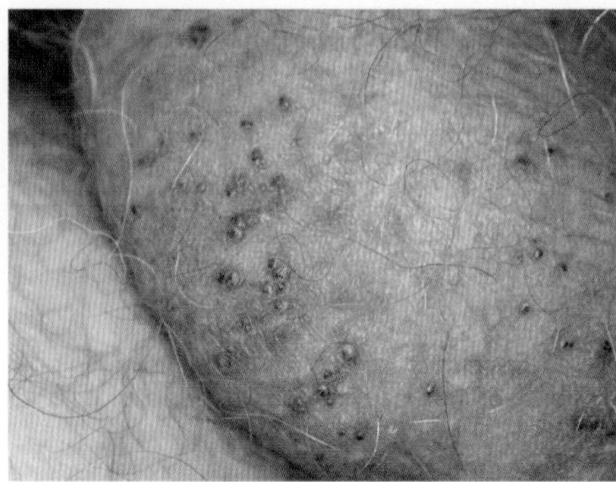

Fig. 94.12 Scrotal angiokeratomas. These lesions typically arise along superficial vessels. *Courtesy, Christopher Baker, MD, and Robert Kelly, MD.*

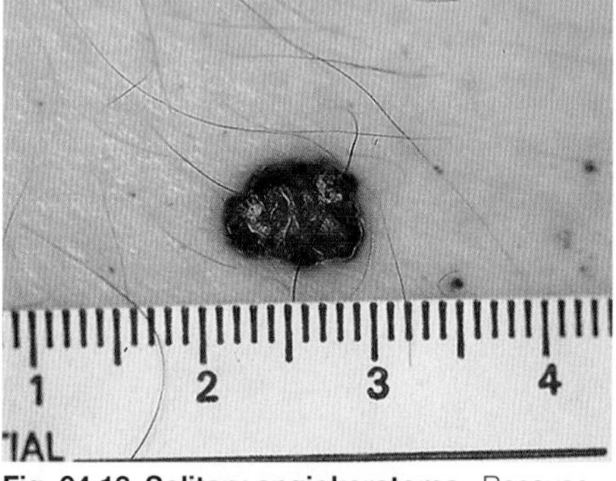

Fig. 94.13 Solitary angiokeratoma. Because of their dark color, these lesions may resemble cutaneous melanoma. Dermoscopy will readily distinguish between these two entities. *Courtesy, Jean L. Bolognia, MD.*

- Dark red to purple papules that represent vascular ectasias; the affected blood vessels are often located in the most superficial portion of the dermis.
- Most commonly occur as multiple lesions on the scrotum or vulva (Fig. 94.12) or as an isolated lesion on the lower extremity (Fig. 94.13).
- Occasionally, angiokeratomas are grouped (circumscriptum and Mibelli forms) or rarely more widely distributed (diffusum form), especially within the girdle area; the latter form is a cutaneous manifestation of several lysosomal storage disorders (e.g. Fabry disease) (see Ch. 52).

For further information see Ch. 114 from *Dermatology, Fourth Edition*.

For additional online figures visit www.expertconsult.com 

Common Soft Tissue Tumors/ Proliferations

95

Neural/Neuroendocrine

Neurofibroma

- Skin-colored to pink, soft papulonodule, often on the trunk (see Fig. 50.2).
- Compressible (the tumor often herniates inward upon palpation – this is referred to as the "button-hole" sign); it is sometimes pedunculated.
- Usually solitary in most individuals.
- When multiple, need to distinguish linear form (segmental; mosaic) from a generalized distribution pattern (neurofibromatosis type 1) (see Ch. 50).
- Histopathology: wavy, delicate spindle cells with tapered nuclei in a pink stroma.
- Plexiform type has been likened to a "bag of worms" (Fig. 95.1); it is generally on the trunk and proximal extremities, highly associated with neurofibromatosis type 1, and prone to malignant degeneration (2–13%).

Schwannoma/Neurilemmoma

- Solitary, pink-yellow, soft, smooth papulonodule; generally seen in adults.
- Often on the extremities or head (Fig. 95.2).
- Asymptomatic (rarely painful).
- Histopathology: encapsulated tumor with foci of wavy, spindled nuclei in palisades and foci of myxoid change.

Granular Cell Tumor

- Often in adults; skin-colored to brown-red, firm papulonodule; sometimes ulcerated or verrucous.
- 30% on the tongue.
- Multiple tumors in 10% of patients.
- Histopathology: polygonal cells with oval nuclei and characteristic granular cytoplasm.

Traumatic Neuroma

- Skin-colored papulonodule(s) at a site of prior trauma.
- Often painful or "sensitive" (Fig. 95.3).
- Histopathology: haphazardly distributed fascicles of spindle cells with tapered nuclei.

Merkel Cell Carcinoma

- In older adults; solitary, rapidly growing, pink to red to violaceous nodule (Fig. 95.4).
- Commonly on the head and neck.
- Pathogenesis involves clonal integration of Merkel cell polyoma virus DNA into the host genome in ~80%; UVR-signature mutations in the remainder.
- Aggressive behavior: distant metastases in 40%; 70% survival at 5 years if primary lesion is <2 cm in diameter; 18% survival at 5 years if distant metastatic disease.

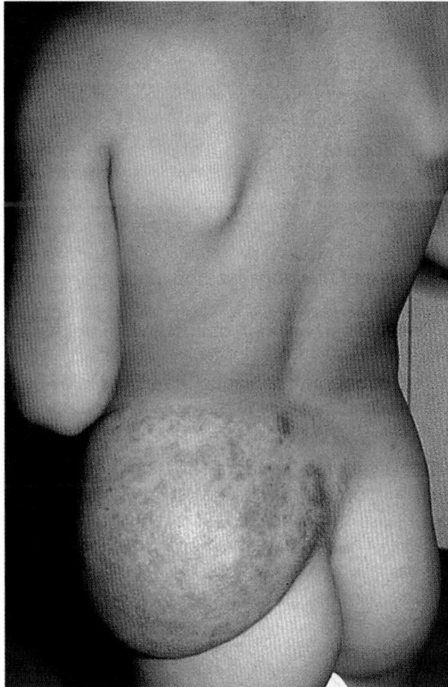

Fig. 95.1 Plexiform neurofibroma in a child with neurofibromatosis. Bag-like mass with overlying patches of hyperpigmentation. *Courtesy, Zsolt B. Argenyi, MD.*

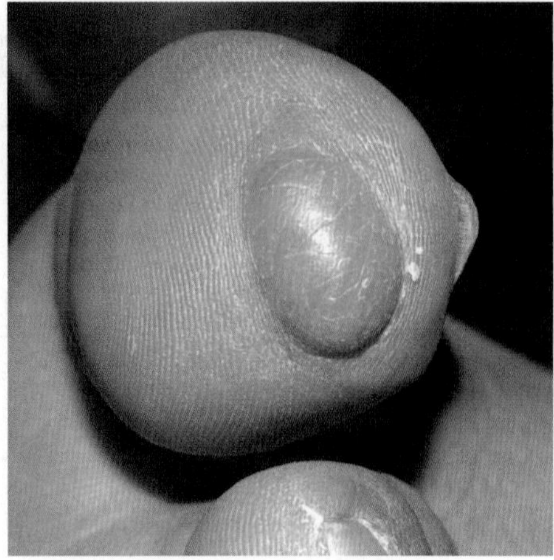

Fig. 95.2 Solitary schwannoma. Skin-colored nodule on the plantar surface of the great toe. *Courtesy, Julie V. Schaffer, MD.*

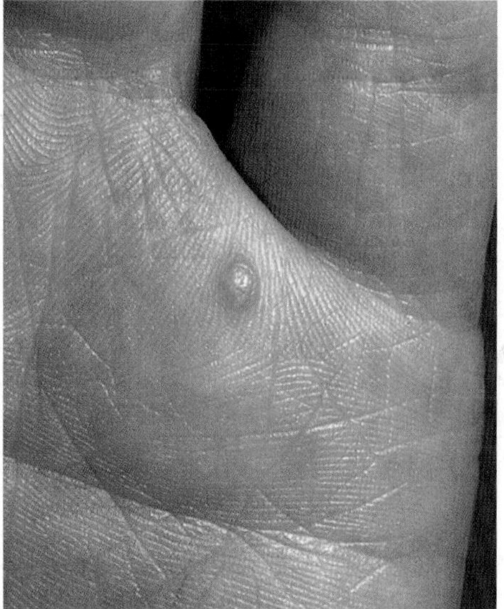

Fig. 95.3 Traumatic neuroma. A painful, firm papule that appeared after a deep puncture injury. *Courtesy, Zsolt B. Argenyi, MD.*

- Histopathology: islands or trabeculae of blue cells that on high-power magnification have chromatin that appears speckled like "salt and pepper"; characteristically cytokeratin 20 (CK20)-positive and thyroid transcription factor-1 (TTF1)-negative.
- **Rx:** consider baseline Merkel cell polyomavirus serology for prognostic significance and to track disease; optimally includes wide excision, accompanied by sentinel lymph node biopsy (SLNB); adjuvant radiation treatment recommended for most patients (exceptions: primary ≤1 cm, SLNB negative, no immunosuppression). For metastatic disease, consider a checkpoint inhibitor (e.g. pembrolizumab) or chemotherapy (e.g. etoposide and carboplatin).

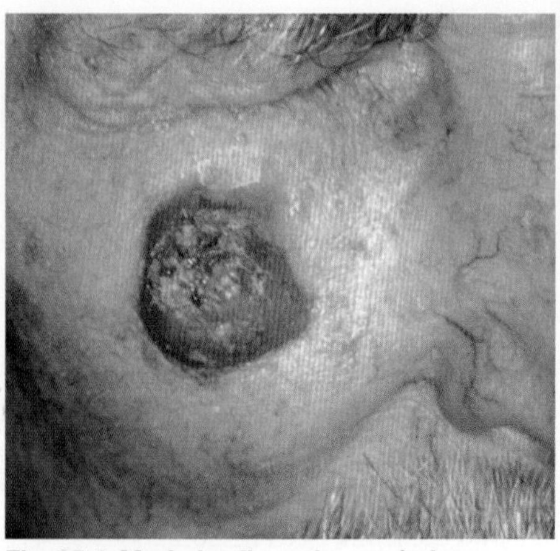

Fig. 95.4 Merkel cell carcinoma (primary cutaneous neuroendocrine carcinoma). Eroded erythematous nodule arising within sun-damaged skin of the cheek. *Courtesy, Lorenzo Cerroni, MD.*

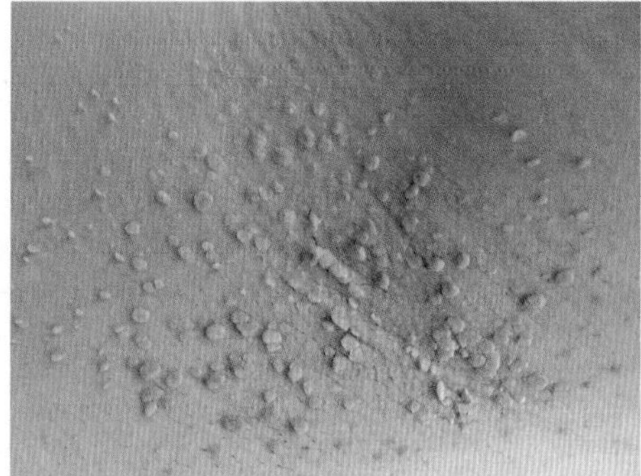

Fig. 95.5 Multiple skin tags in the axilla. The lesions are skin-colored, soft, and pedunculated. *Courtesy, YDRSC.*

Fibrous/Fibrohistiocytic

Skin Tag (Acrochordon, Fibroepithelial Polyp, Soft Fibroma)

- Common; skin-colored to pink or occasionally hyperpigmented, pedunculated papule.
- Sites of predilection: neck, axilla, groin (Fig. 95.5).
- Can become irritated or infarcted.

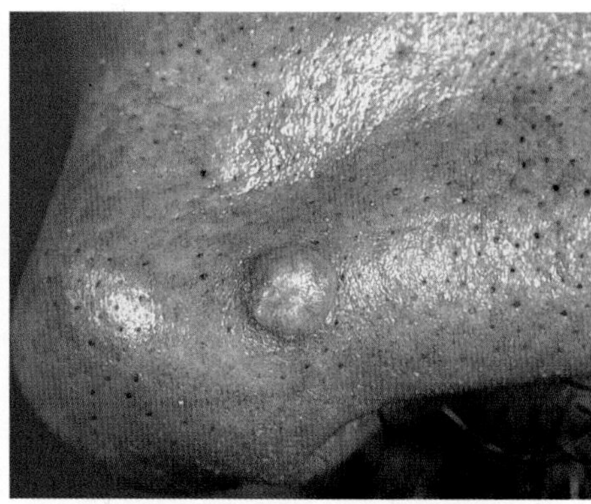

Fig. 95.6 Fibrous papule of the nose. A smooth, dome-shaped, skin-colored papule. *Courtesy, NYUDSC.*

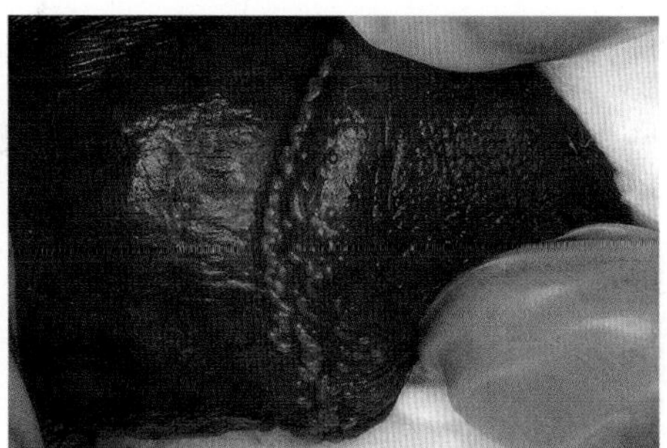

Fig. 95.7 Pearly penile papules. Multiple small white papules along the corona of the glans penis. Note the multilayered distribution. *Courtesy, Kalman Watsky, MD.*

Angiofibroma (Fibrous Papule)

- Solitary, skin-colored to pink, shiny papule; commonly on the nose (Fig. 95.6).
- When multiple, need to consider genodermatoses (e.g. tuberous sclerosis, multiple endocrine neoplasia type I).
- Histopathology: stellate spindle cells in a hyalinized stroma with dilated vessels.
- **DDx:** BCC, intradermal melanocytic nevus, adnexal tumors.

Pearly Penile Papules

- Multiple, small, white to light pink papules along the corona of the glans penis, often with a multilayered distribution (Fig. 95.7).
- **Rx:** reassurance.

Dermatofibroma

- 6- to 10-mm pink (especially in fair-skinned individuals), tan, or brown papule (Fig. 95.8; see Fig. 1.16D); firm; dimples inward with lateral pressure.
- Often on the lower extremities; women > men.
- Common; multiple lesions can be seen in normal individuals but also are associated with lupus erythematosus and immunosuppression (e.g. HIV infection).
- Histopathology: epidermal hyperplasia (sometimes with basaloid induction that resembles BCC) above a spindle cell proliferation that entraps collagen.
- Dermoscopic features are shown in Fig. 1.16D.

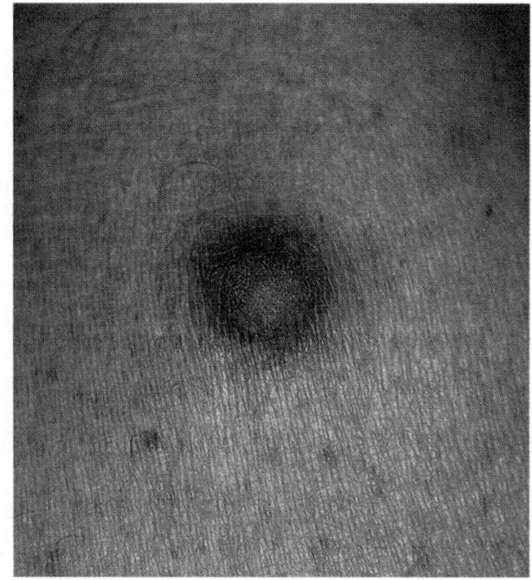

Fig. 95.8 Dermatofibroma. Hyperpigmented firm papule on the lower extremity. *Courtesy, Jean L. Bolognia, MD.*

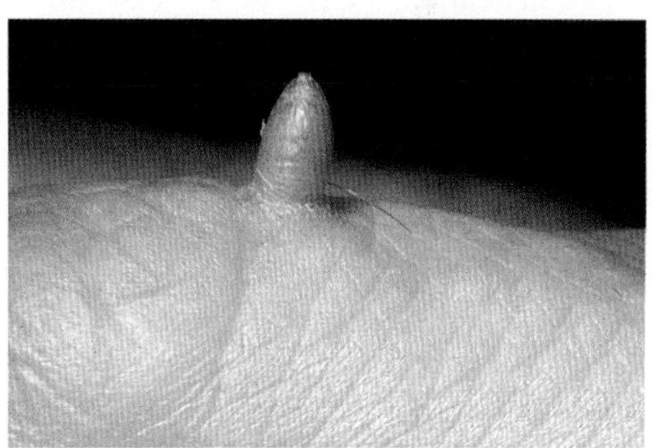

Fig. 95.9 Acral fibrokeratoma. A light pink exophytic papule arising from the dorsal surface of the finger. *Courtesy, NYUDSC.*

Acral Fibrokeratoma

- 4- to 10-mm solitary, skin-colored to pink, cone-shaped, keratotic papule with a collarette of elevated skin (Fig. 95.9).

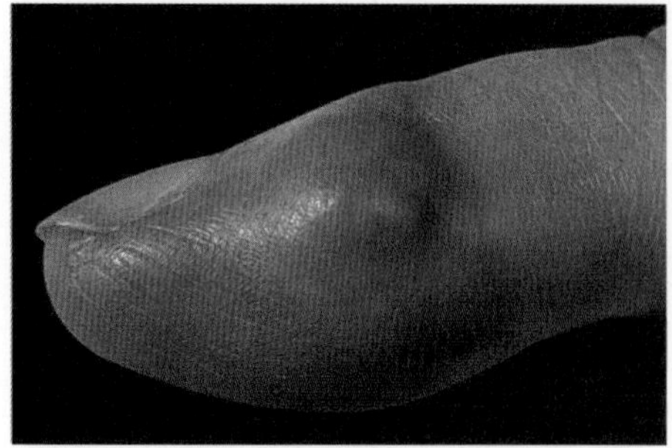

Fig. 95.10 Giant cell tumor of tendon sheath. A skin-colored nodule on the lateral aspect of the index finger. *Courtesy, NYUDSC.*

- Located on the fingers and sometimes the palms.

Sclerotic Fibroma

- 2- to 9-mm dome-shaped, pearly papule or nodule in adults.
- Slight predilection for the head and neck.
- Can be seen in patients with Cowden disease.

Giant Cell Tumor of Tendon Sheath

- Firm nodule (1–2 cm), generally on the fingers or toes (Fig. 95.10).
- 30% of tumors recur locally.

Nodular Fasciitis

- Benign, reactive process in young adults.
- Rapidly growing subcutaneous nodule (1–5 cm in diameter).
- Commonly on the distal upper extremity.
- Sometimes associated with trauma.
- Histopathology: subcutaneous nodule of elongated spindle cells in a myxoid matrix.

Connective Tissue Nevus

- Skin-colored to yellow-tan (more yellow when composed predominantly of elastic tissue), firm papulonodules or plaques; solitary or multiple (often grouped) (Fig. 95.11).
- Present at birth or arise during childhood.
- May be associated with genodermatoses (e.g. tuberous sclerosis, Buschke–Ollendorf syndrome, Proteus syndrome).
- Histopathology: increased collagen (sometimes subtle) and/or elastic tissue; diagnosis may require special stains for elastic fibers and collagen.

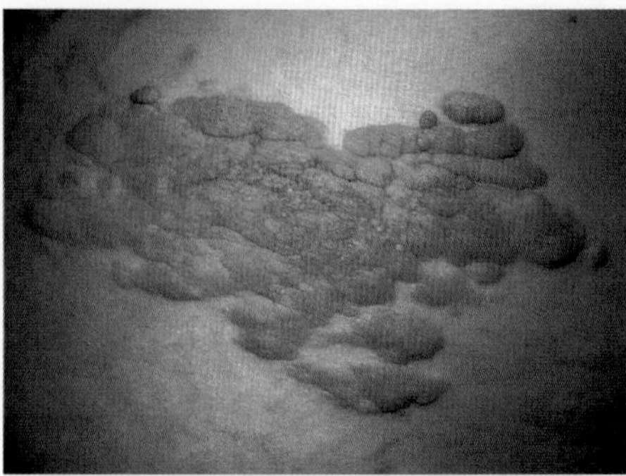

Fig. 95.11 Connective tissue nevus. Coalescence of multiple tan papules and plaques on the lower back. The lesion was firm to palpation and histologically had increased collagen. *Courtesy, YDRSC.*

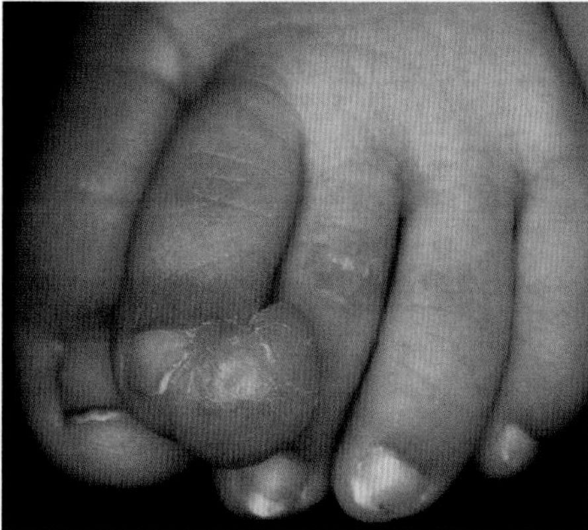

Fig. 95.12 Infantile digital fibroma. Firm skin-colored nodule on the dorsolateral aspect of the second toe in a young child. *Courtesy, YDRSC.*

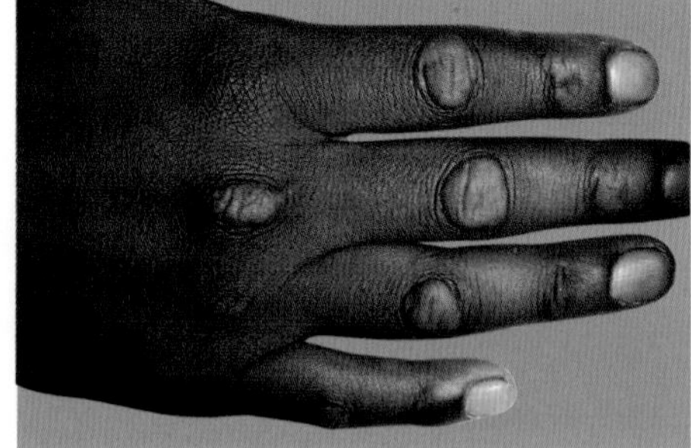

Fig. 95.13 Knuckle pads. Note the localization to the skin overlying the knuckles. *Courtesy, Ronald P. Rapini, MD.*

Infantile Digital Fibroma

- Firm, skin-colored to pink papulonodule on the fingers or toes (tends to spare the thumb and great toe) (Fig. 95.12).

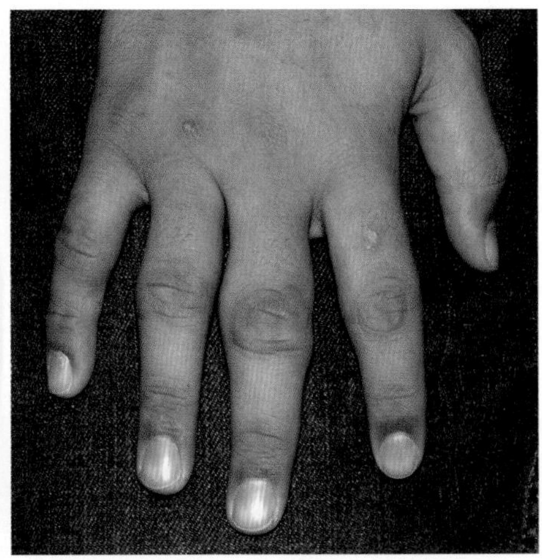

Fig. 95.14 Pachydermodactyly. A form of digital fibromatosis characterized by soft tissue swelling of the lateral aspects of the fingers, usually in the area of the proximal interphalangeal joints of the second to fourth fingers. *Courtesy, Julie V. Schaffer, MD.*

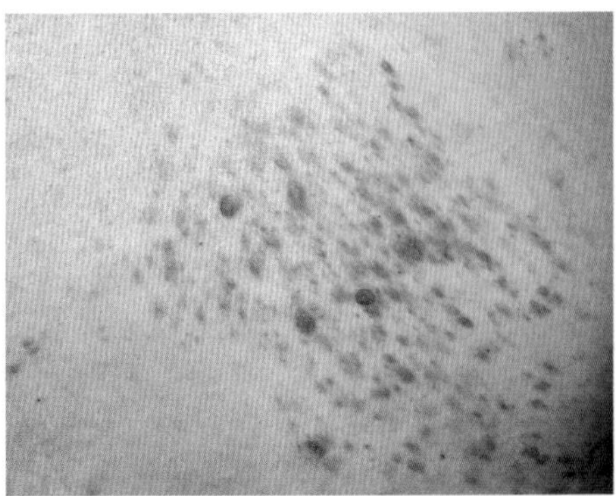

Fig. 95.15 Clustered piloleiomyomas on the back. The trunk is a common location for multiple piloleiomyomas. Patients with this clinical presentation need to be evaluated for the possibility of hereditary leiomyomatosis and renal cell cancer (Reed syndrome). *Courtesy, Julie V. Schaffer, MD.*

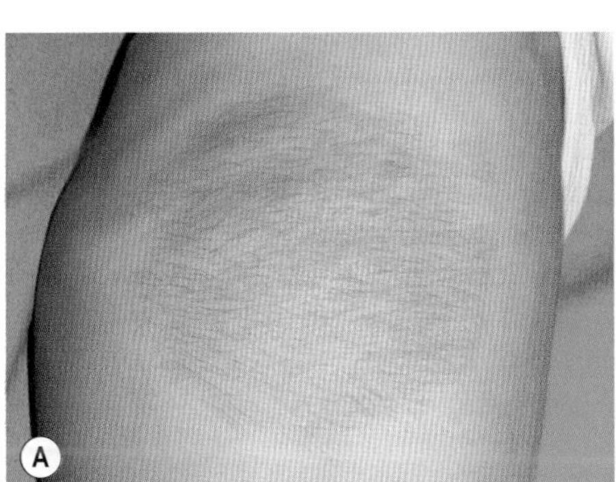

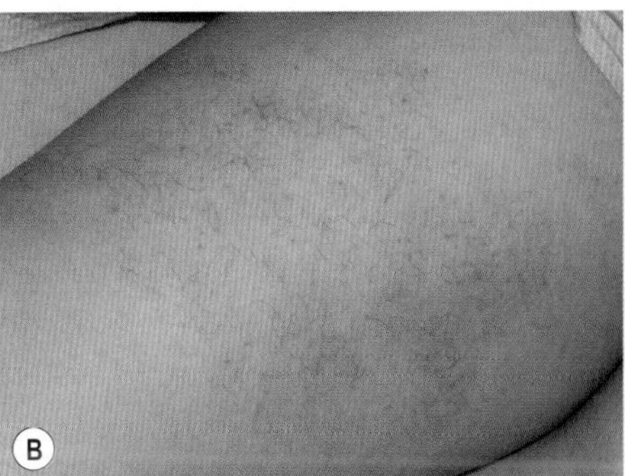

Fig. 95.16 Smooth muscle hamartoma. A A hyperpigmented plaque with hypertrichosis that can be misdiagnosed clinically as a congenital melanocytic nevus or less often a neurofibroma. **B** Sometimes the hamartoma has a broken-up appearance and there is overlap with Becker melanosis (nevus) both clinically and histologically. *A, Courtesy, Antonio Torello, MD; B, Courtesy, Julie V. Schaffer, MD.*

- Solitary or multiple; generally present before 1 year of age.
- Tend to spontaneously regress within a few years but may recur.

Infantile Myofibromatosis

- One or more skin-colored to pink to violet, firm to rubbery dermal/subcutaneous nodules.
- Most commonly on the head and neck or trunk.
- Rare; lesions present at birth or appear during the first 2 years of life.
- Can have cutaneous lesions alone or systemic involvement (bone, gastrointestinal, kidneys, lungs, heart).
- Tumors tend to self-regress.
- Histopathology: biphasic pattern of spindle cells in nodular arrangements with vessels at the periphery.

Fibromatoses

- Most subtypes are superficial: (1) palmar (Dupuytren disease); (2) plantar (Ledderhose disease); (3) penile (Peyronie disease); (4) knuckle pads (holoderma) (Fig. 95.13); and (5) pachydermodactyly (Fig. 95.14).

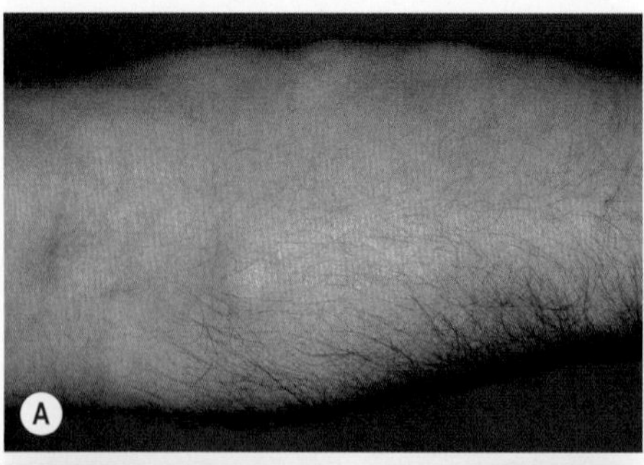

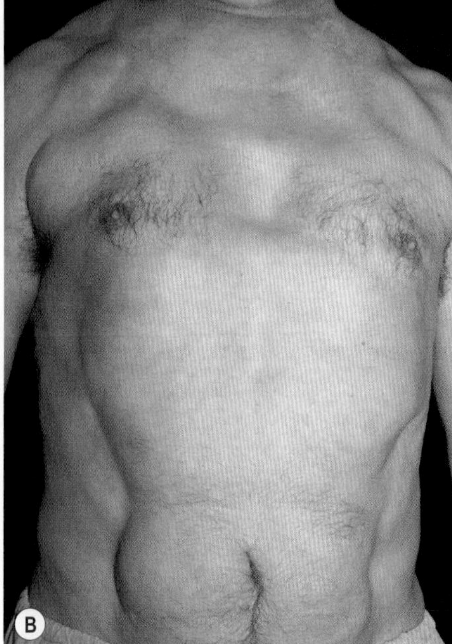

Fig. 95.17 Lipomatoses. A Familial multiple lipomatosis. Several discrete lipomas are present on the forearm. **B** Benign symmetric lipomatosis (Madelung disease). Large symmetric fatty deposits in the supraclavicular region, lateral chest, and abdomen. *A, Courtesy, YDRSC; B, Courtesy, Steven Kaddu, MD.*

- One deep form: extra-abdominal desmoid tumor.
- Slowly growing nodules or plaques or cord-like tumors.
- Palmar fibromatosis can result in flexion contractures, especially of the 4th and/or 5th finger (see Ch. 81).
- Penile fibromatosis can result in pain and erectile dysfunction.

Muscle/Adipose

Leiomyoma

- Solitary or multiple red-brown papules or nodules, often grouped (Fig. 95.15).
- Sometimes painful.
- Generally on the trunk.
- When multiple, consider association with uterine leiomyomas and papillary renal cell carcinoma (Reed syndrome: autosomal dominant familial cancer syndrome with mutation in fumarate hydratase).
- Histopathology: fascicles of spindle cells with cigar-shaped nuclei that have perinuclear vacuoles.

Smooth Muscle Hamartoma

- Congenital or acquired, skin-colored to hyperpigmented plaque on the trunk > proximal extremities (Fig. 95.16).
- Follicular prominence and hypertrichosis may be present.
- May be confused with a congenital melanocytic nevus.
- Is on a clinicopathologic spectrum with Becker nevus.

Lipoma

- Common tumor of mature fat; soft, mobile subcutaneous nodule.
- Generally on the trunk and extremities, but any site possible.
- Occasionally painful.
- Multiple lesions may be associated with a lipomatosis (e.g. familial type; Fig. 95.17) or a genodermatosis (e.g. Gardner syndrome, Proteus syndrome).
- **DDx:** see Fig. 95.18.

Angiolipoma

- Soft, mobile, subcutaneous nodule; often on the forearm in young adults.
- Often painful.

Nevus Lipomatosus

- Grouped, soft, yellow to skin-colored papulonodules on the hips and/or upper thighs (Fig. 95.19).
- Develops during infancy to the first two decades of life.

Soft Tissue Sarcomas (Table 95.1)

- Rare in comparison to benign soft tissue tumors.
- Generally presents as a nonspecific, deep-seated nodule.
- May occasionally primarily involve the dermis.

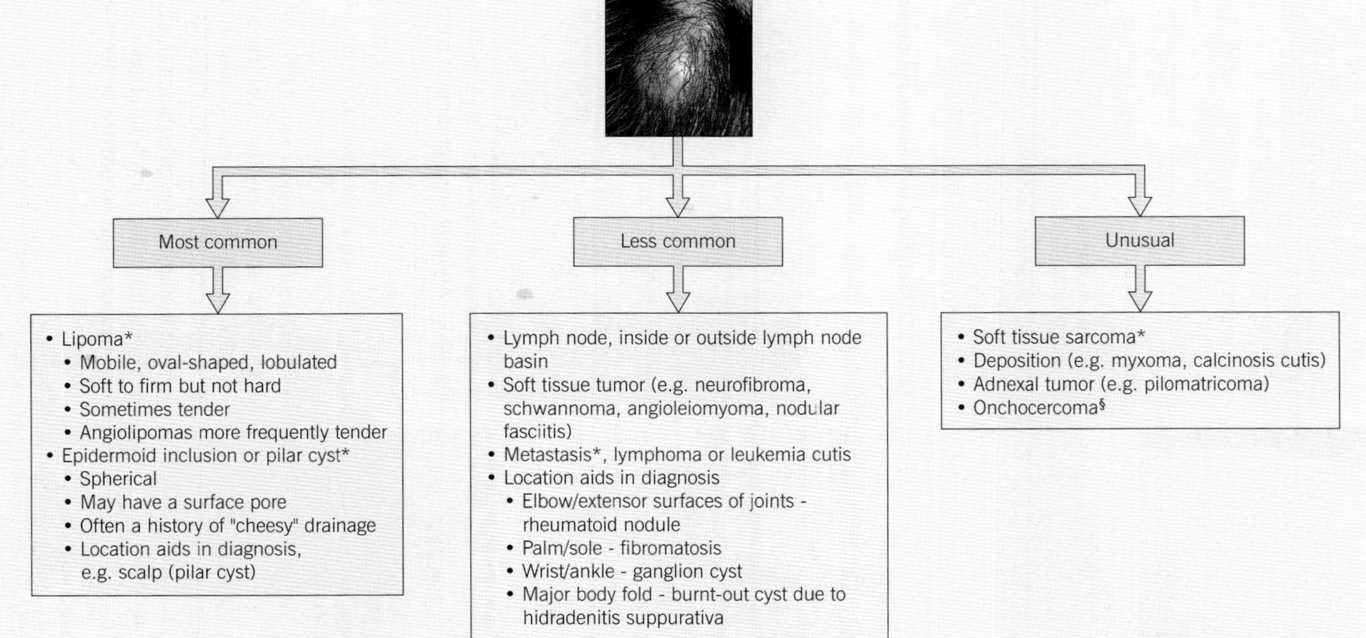

Fig. 95.18 Approach to a "lump under the skin" in adults. Incisional biopsy is preferred for the histopathologic evaluation of subcutaneous nodules while a punch biopsy suffices for dermal lesions. For bedside diagnosis of an epidermal inclusion cyst: after local anesthesia and superficial incision with a #11 blade, keratin is expressed.

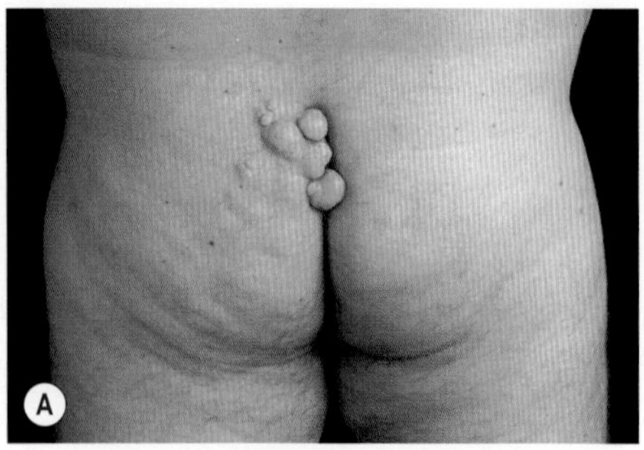

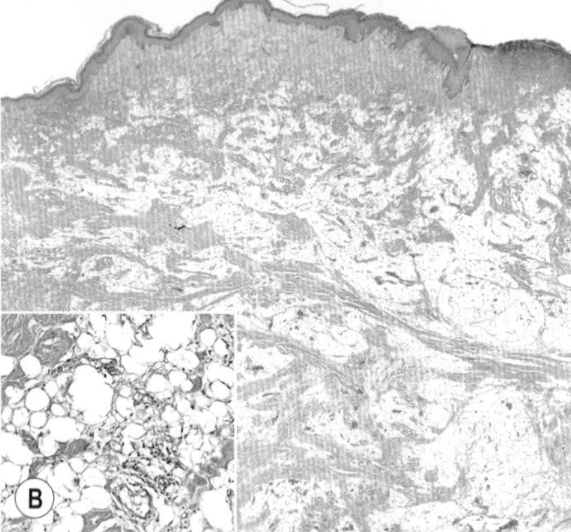

Fig. 95.19 Nevus lipomatosus superficialis. **A** This hamartoma is characterized by grouped, soft, pedunculated, skin-colored tumors. **B** Histopathologically, irregular aggregates of mature fat cells ectopically located in the dermis are the characteristic feature. *Courtesy, Steven Kaddu, MD.*

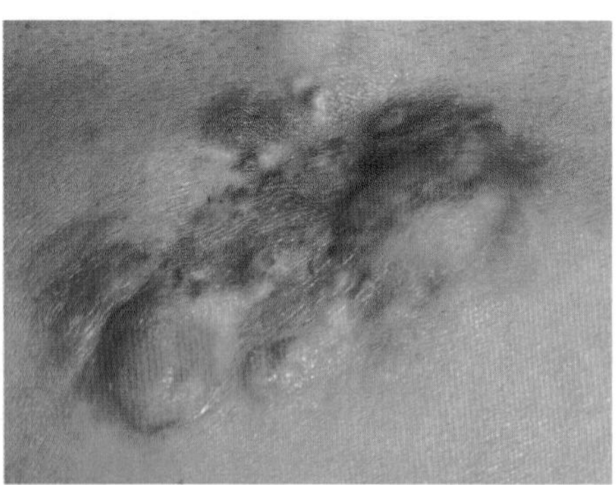

Fig. 95.20 Dermatofibrosarcoma protuberans. A broad, pink-brown, multinodular, firm plaque on the back. Histopathologically, bland spindle cells are arranged in storiform ("cartwheel") patterns. *Courtesy, NYUDSC.*

SELECTED SOFT TISSUE SARCOMAS
Angiosarcoma (can arise in setting of lymphedema and on the scalp of elderly patients) (see Ch. 94) Atypical fibroxanthoma (Fig. 95.21) Dermatofibrosarcoma protuberans (often multinodular; see Fig. 95.20)
Pleomorphic undifferentiated sarcoma (previously referred to as malignant fibrous histiocytoma*) Malignant peripheral nerve sheath tumor Epithelioid sarcoma Fibrosarcoma Leiomyosarcoma Liposarcoma

**Some pathologists consider atypical fibroxanthoma (AFX) to be a superficial variant of malignant fibrous histiocytoma (MFH); dermatologists see AFXs more commonly than MFHs.*

Table 95.1 Selected soft tissue sarcomas.

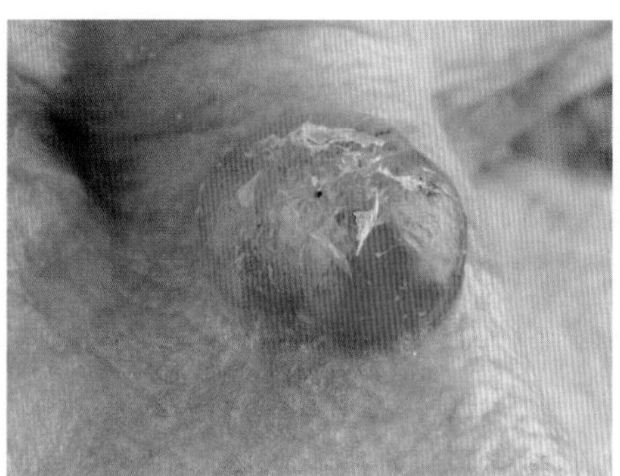

Fig. 95.21 Atypical fibroxanthoma. A red, dome-shaped nodule on the nose of an elderly man. *Courtesy, Lorenzo Cerroni, MD.*

- Dermatofibrosarcoma protuberans (DFSP) is characteristically multinodular (Fig. 95.20).
- Most DFSPs have a translocation t(17;22) that fuses the collagen I and platelet-derived growth factor genes; expression of this fusion gene results in high levels of platelet-derived growth factor that stimulates proliferation of fibroblasts.

For further information see Chs 115, 116, and 117 from *Dermatology, Fourth Edition*.

For additional online figures and tables visit www.expertconsult.com 

Mastocytosis 96

• Spectrum of disorders caused by proliferation and accumulation of mast cells in the skin and/or other tissues (Table 96.1).
• *Childhood-onset mastocytosis*, defined as presenting prior to puberty, develops before 6 months of age in ~70% of patients; it has a benign course and often remits spontaneously by adolescence (Fig. 96.1).
• *Adult-onset mastocytosis* most often develops in the third or fourth decade of life; it typically persists and may have systemic involvement (see Fig. 96.1).
• The majority of pediatric and adult mastocytosis patients have a *somatic* activating mutation (most frequently involving codon 816) in the gene encoding the KIT tyrosine kinase receptor expressed on mast cells; familial mastocytosis occasionally occurs.

Clinical Features of Cutaneous Mastocytosis

• Patients frequently experience pruritus and may have episodic urtication (redness and swelling) of mastocytosis lesions.

WHO CLASSIFICATION OF MASTOCYTOSIS
Cutaneous mastocytosis (CM)
Maculopapular CM/"urticaria pigmentosa" Diffuse CM Mastocytoma (≤3 lesions)
Systemic mastocytosis (SM)
Indolent SM* Smoldering SM* SM with associated hematologic neoplasm** Aggressive SM Mast cell leukemia
Mast cell sarcoma (e.g. larynx, colon, brain)

**Forms of SM most likely to have cutaneous involvement.*
***The associated disorder may be myeloproliferative (including the form of hypereosinophilic syndrome characterized by FIP1L1/PDGFRA fusion gene; see Ch. 25), myelodysplastic, or lymphoproliferative.*

Table 96.1 WHO classification of mastocytosis.

• Lesions in infants and preschool-aged children can blister due to release of proteases from densely packed mast cells.
• Firmly rubbing or stroking cutaneous lesions of mastocytosis often causes urtication (Darier sign) (Fig. 96.2); this is generally more pronounced in children.
• In approximately half of patients, hiving develops after stroking clinically uninvolved skin (dermatographism).
• Several clinical patterns of cutaneous mastocytosis are recognized, but overlap between these groups can occur.

Mastocytomas (≤3 Lesions)

• Typically present at birth or appear during infancy.
• One to several papules, nodules, or plaques with a yellow-tan to red-brown color and leathery (peau d'orange) texture (Fig. 96.3).
• Can occur anywhere on the skin surface, including acral sites.
• Smaller mastocytomas frequently go unrecognized and are likely underrepresented in series of pediatric mastocytosis patients.
• **DDx:** melanocytic nevus (e.g. congenital, Spitz), café-au-lait macule, juvenile xanthogranuloma, arthropod bite, pseudolymphoma, bullous impetigo.

Maculopapular Cutaneous Mastocytosis, Including "Urticaria Pigmentosa"

• Multiple (often numerous) pink-tan to red-brown macules, papules, and/or plaques (Fig. 96.4).
• Two major variants:
  – *monomorphic small* lesions ("urticaria pigmentosa") that can occur in adults or children and tend to persist

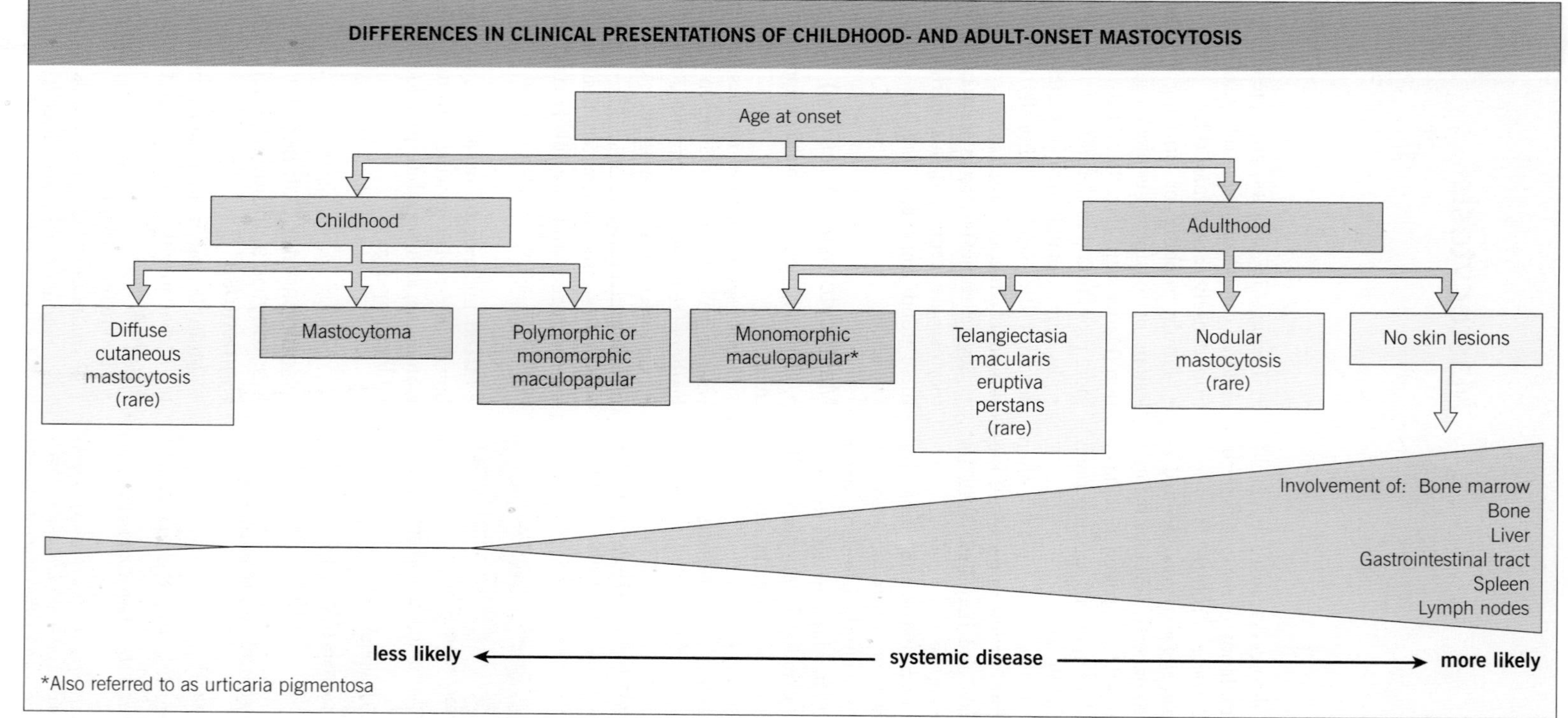

Fig. 96.1 Differences in clinical presentations of childhood- and adult-onset mastocytosis. The darker boxes represent the most common forms. *Courtesy, Michael Tharp, MD.*

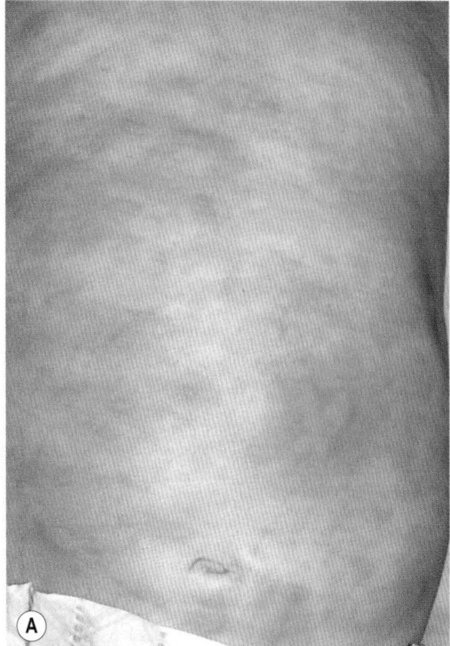

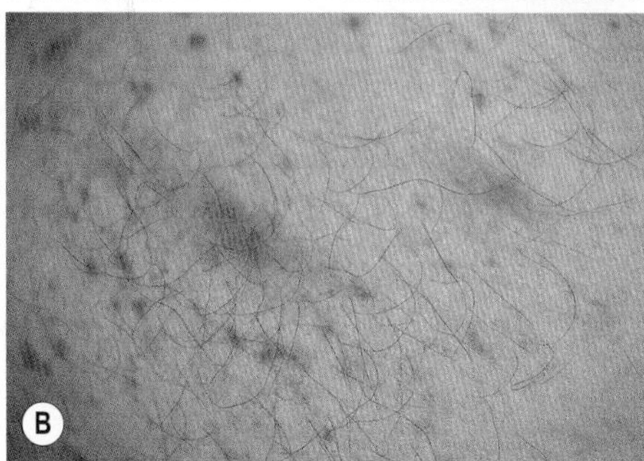

Fig. 96.2 Darier sign in mastocytosis. An infant with extensive cutaneous involvement (**A**) and an adult with macular and papular lesions (**B**). *A, Courtesy, Julie V. Schaffer, MD; B, Courtesy, Thomas Horn, MD.*

- *polymorphic larger* lesions (some >1 cm) that most often develop in infancy and typically resolve by adolescence

• Favors the trunk and proximal extremities, usually sparing the central face, palms, and soles.

• A subtle leathery texture is usually evident in larger lesions, and hyperpigmentation is less prominent in patients with lightly colored skin.

• Telangiectasias may be seen, especially in adults; ***t****elangiectasia* ***m****acularis* ***e****ruptiva* ***p****erstans* (TMEP) is a rare adult variant that presents with telangiectatic macules and patches without significant hyperpigmentation (Fig. 96.5), often with a minimal Darier sign.

• **DDx:** lentigines, melanocytic nevi; for TMEP, photodamage, poikiloderma, multiple spider telangiectasias, and other telangiectatic conditions (see Ch. 87).

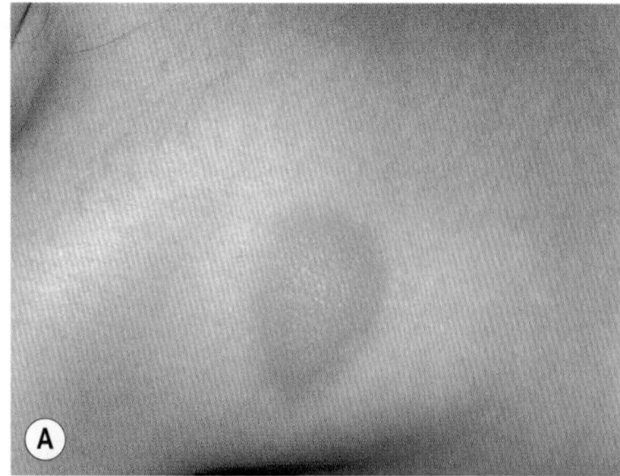

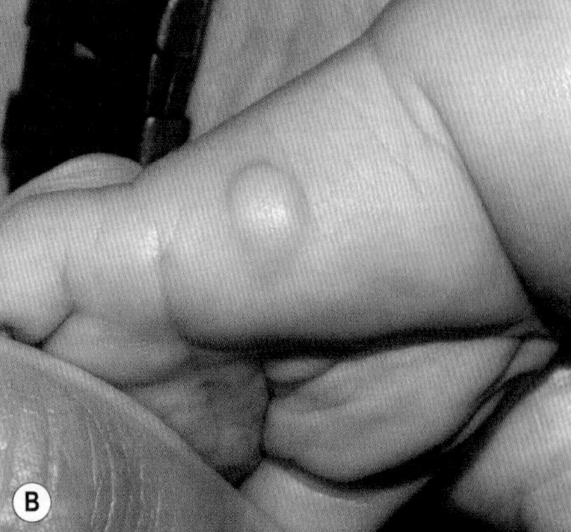

Fig. 96.3 Mastocytomas in infants. A Tan plaque with a leathery surface. **B** Swelling and a subtle rim of erythema due to urtication of a yellowish nodule on the wrist. *A, Courtesy, Antonio Torrelo, MD; B, Courtesy, Julie V. Schaffer MD.*

Diffuse Cutaneous Mastocytosis

• Occurs primarily in infants, with rare reports in adults.

• Generalized, doughy thickening of the skin with a leathery texture, sometimes with deep creases.

• Flushing, blistering, and erosions are common (Fig. 96.6), but spontaneous resolution usually occurs.

• **DDx:** epidermolysis bullosa, autoimmune bullous dermatoses.

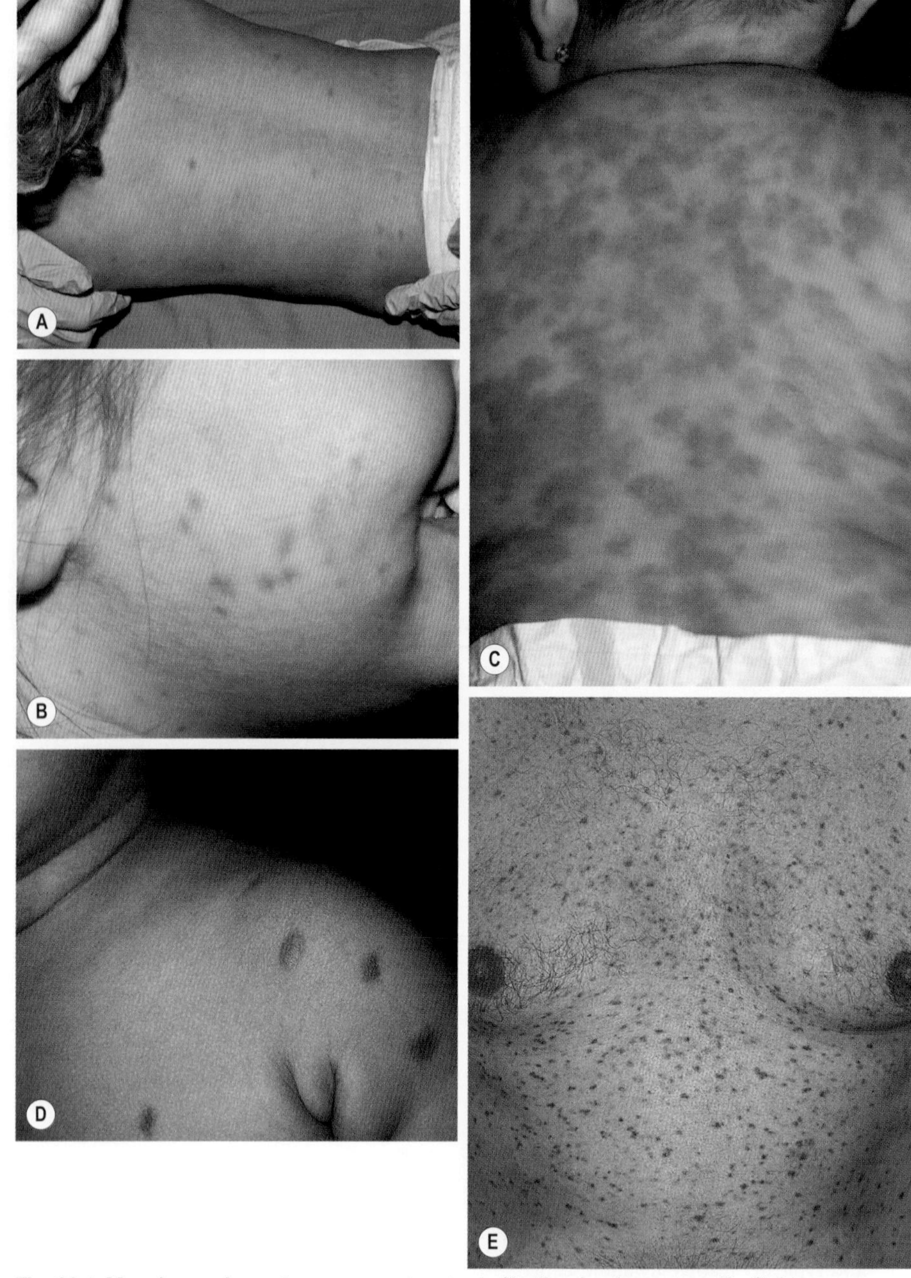

Fig. 96.4 Maculopapular cutaneous mastocytosis ("urticaria pigmentosa"). Children present with variable numbers and sizes of papules, which may be scattered (**A**) or clustered (**B**), as well as polymorphic lesions including plaques (**C**) or papulonodules (**D**). The degree of associated hyperpigmentation also varies. **E** Adults typically present with small, red-brown macules and papules. *A, Courtesy, Antonio Torrelo, MD; B, C, Courtesy Julie V. Schaffer, MD; D, E, Courtesy, Michael Tharp, MD.*

Systemic Manifestations of Mastocytosis

- In patients with a higher mast cell burden (e.g. extensive cutaneous disease, a large mastocytoma, extracutaneous involvement), release of mast cell mediators such as histamine can lead to systemic symptoms, which range from flushing to abdominal pain and diarrhea to lightheadedness and syncope (Fig. 96.7).

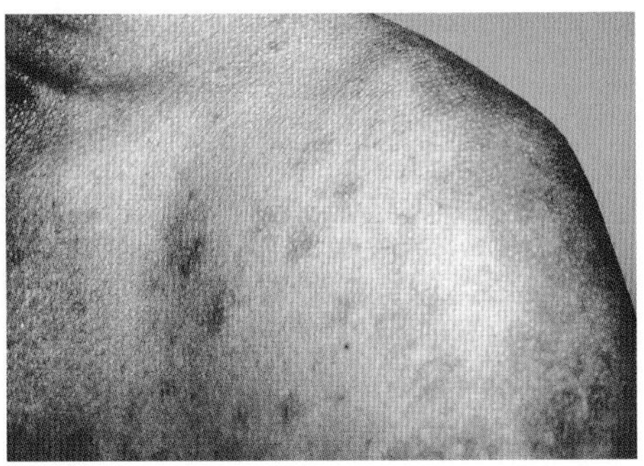

Fig. 96.5 Telangiectasia macularis eruptiva perstans. Multiple lesions composed of telangiectasias are present. *Courtesy, YDRSC.*

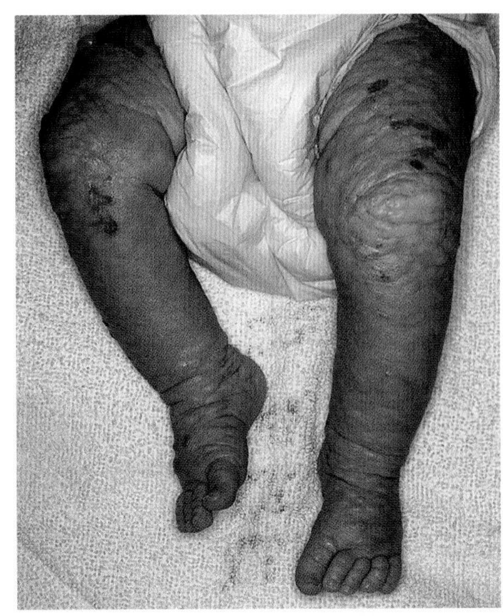

Fig. 96.6 Diffuse cutaneous mastocytosis in an infant. Diffusely infiltrated skin with multiple erosions and a leathery texture. *Courtesy, YDRSC.*

MAST CELL MEDIATORS AND ASSOCIATED SYMPTOMS OF MASTOCYTOSIS

Mast cells

Preformed mediators
Histamine
Heparin
Proteases
(e.g. tryptase)

Newly formed mediators
Prostaglandins
Leukotrienes

Cytokines and chemokines
e.g. TNF-α,
IL-4,
IL-5,
SCF

Headaches
Cognitive disorganization
Fatigue

Bullae
Flushing
Pruritus
Urticaria

Cramping
Diarrhea
Epigastric pain
Nausea
Vomiting
Weight loss

Chest pain
Dizziness
Dyspnea
Palpitations
Syncope

Bone pain
(Osteoporosis/
osteosclerosis)

Fig. 96.7 Mast cell mediators and associated symptoms of mastocytosis. SCF, stem cell factor (binds to KIT receptor).

WHO CRITERIA FOR THE DIAGNOSIS OF SYSTEMIC MASTOCYTOSIS
Requires either the major criterion plus one minor criterion or three minor criteria
Major criterion
• Multifocal dense infiltrates of mast cells (aggregates of ≥15 mast cells) in bone marrow or extracutaneous tissues
Minor criteria
• >25% of mast cells in bone marrow samples or extracutaneous tissues are spindle-shaped or otherwise atypical • Extracutaneous mast cells (CD117+) express CD2, CD25, or both (often bone marrow; determined via flow cytometry) • Presence of c-*KIT* codon 816 mutation in blood, bone marrow, or extracutaneous tissues • Serum total tryptase level is persistently >20 ng/ml (unless there is an associated clonal myeloid disorder, in which case this parameter is not valid)

Table 96.2 WHO criteria for the diagnosis of systemic mastocytosis.

- Systemic disease is extremely rare in childhood mastocytosis.
- Although the bone marrow is frequently involved in adult patients with cutaneous mastocytosis, hematologic sequelae are uncommon (see Table 96.1).
- Criteria for the diagnosis of systemic mastocytosis are presented in Table 96.2.
- Patients with systemic mastocytosis (primarily adults) occasionally develop osteoporosis, osteosclerosis, hepatosplenomegaly, lymphadenopathy, and infiltration of the GI tract.

Evaluation and Treatment

- An approach to the evaluation of a patient with cutaneous mastocytosis is presented in Fig. 96.8.
- Treatment of cutaneous and indolent systemic mastocytosis is directed at alleviating symptoms, if present.
- Triggers of mast cell degranulation (Table 96.3) should be avoided when possible.
- **Rx:** low-sedating H_1 antihistamine(s), often in higher than standard doses (e.g. up to 40 mg daily of cetirizine in adults); addition of a sedating H_1 antihistamine at night, an H_2 antagonist (especially if upper GI symptoms), or cromolyn sodium (topical or oral) may be beneficial.
- An Epipen® or Epipen Jr® for emergency use can be given to patients with a high mast cell burden.
- Topical therapy with a potent CS or calcineurin inhibitor, narrowband UVB phototherapy, or omalizumab may be helpful in patients with refractory symptoms.
- Aggressive systemic disease can be treated with agents such as midostaurin (a multikinase/KIT inhibitor), imatinib (for some KIT mutations), or cladribine.

For further information see Ch. 118 from *Dermatology, Fourth Edition*.

For additional online figures visit www.expertconsult.com 

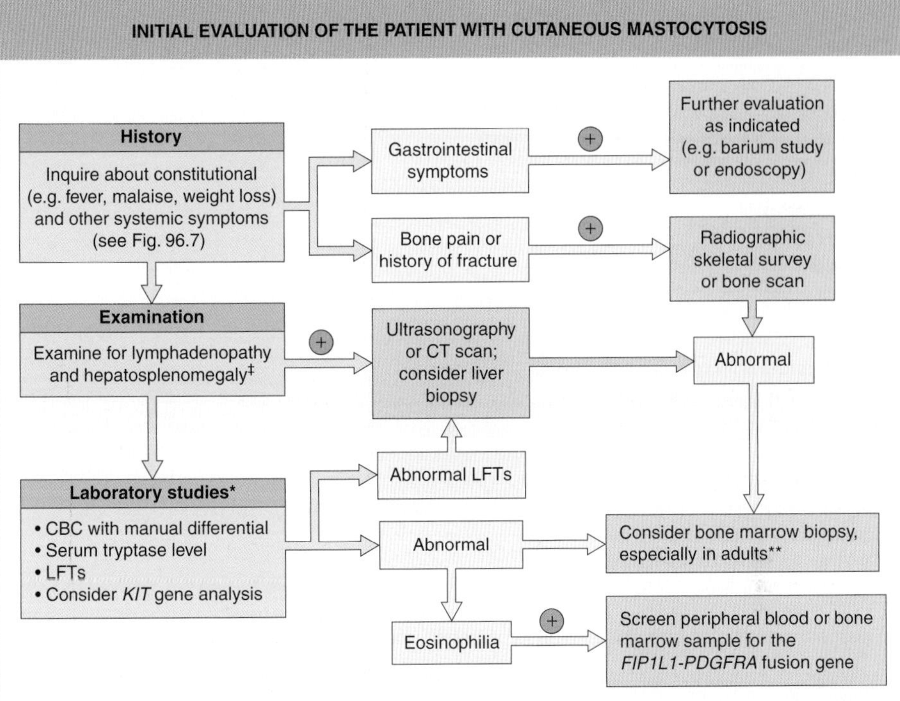

* Not typically needed for pediatric patients with a mastocytoma and optional for young children with asymptomatic or less extensive disease. *KIT* mutation detection in the peripheral blood (e.g. via allele-specific quantitative PCR for D816V) can help identify individuals at increased risk of systemic mastocytosis and follow disease progression.

** Some groups recommend in all adult mastocytosis patients, especially if extensive skin disease or persistently elevated/rising serum tryptase levels. Assessment of bone marrow should include tryptase staining, mast cell immunophenotyping (e.g. CD2, CD25), cytogenetic studies (e.g. for an associated hematologic malignancy), and *KIT* analysis.

‡ Hepatosplenomegaly represents a marker of systemic involvement in children.

Fig. 96.8 Initial evaluation of the patient with cutaneous mastocytosis. A proposed scheme for the diagnosis of mastocytosis in the skin requires the major criterion of typical skin lesions associated with the Darier sign plus one minor criterion, either an increased number of mast cells histologically or an activating *KIT* mutation in lesional skin. Patients with systemic mastocytosis should be assessed for osteoporosis with a DEXA scan.

POTENTIAL STIMULANTS OF MAST CELL DEGRANULATION
Physical
• Friction • Exercise • Heat (e.g. hot bath) or cold (e.g. swimming)
Dietary
• Hot beverages • Spicy foods • Alcohol
Medications
• Aspirin • Nonsteroidal anti-inflammatory drugs • Narcotics (e.g. morphine, codeine) • Anticholinergics (e.g. scopolamine) • Dextromethorphan (a cough suppressant) • Polymyxin B sulfate • Some systemic anesthetics (e.g. lidocaine*, etomidate, thiopental, isoflurane) • Iodine-based radiographic dyes • Dextran (in some IV solutions)
Allergic
• Allergens causing an immediate-type hypersensitivity reaction in that patient

**Local injections are safe.*

Table 96.3 Potential stimulants of mast cell degranulation.

B-Cell Lymphomas of the Skin

97

General

- Cutaneous lymphomas can involve the skin as either the exclusive site of involvement (*primary cutaneous lymphoma*) or as the result of cutaneous involvement in association with a systemic (usually nodal) lymphoma (*secondary cutaneous lymphoma*).
- Primary cutaneous lymphomas are defined as lymphomas presenting in the skin with no evidence of extracutaneous disease at the time of diagnosis.
- Primary cutaneous lymphomas differ significantly from their nodal counterparts in terms of their natural history and thus require a specialized approach to their evaluation and treatment.
- Primary cutaneous lymphomas can originate from B cells (PCBCL), T cells (CTCL), or natural killer (NK) cells.
- Unlike most extranodal lymphomas, T-cell rather than B-cell lymphomas are more prevalent in the skin.

PCBCL

- Primary cutaneous B-cell lymphomas are derived from B lymphocytes in different stages of differentiation.
- B-cell lineage is identified by the presence of CD20 and CD79a and the absence of CD3 markers.
- PCBCLs constitute approximately 20–25% of all primary cutaneous lymphomas, but there may be regional variation in incidence and specific types of CBCLs.
- Usually affects older adults of both sexes.
- Pathogenesis is unknown, but in certain areas of the world, *Borrelia* species are thought to play a role; marked immune suppression/dysregulation is also a risk factor.
- Precise classification can be achieved only after a complete synthesis of clinical, histopathologic, immunophenotypic, and molecular features.
- Once the diagnosis of a B-cell lymphoma in the skin has been made, complete staging (Table 97.1) is recommended to distinguish between primary and secondary cutaneous lymphoma.
- The World Health Organization–European Organization for Research and Treatment of Cancer (WHO–EORTC) classification provides the basis for a consistent classification of patients and divides PCBCL into three major types (Table 97.2).
- Primary cutaneous marginal zone B-cell lymphoma (PCMZL) and primary cutaneous follicle center lymphoma (PCFCL) are indolent lymphomas with 5-year survival rates of ≥95% (Table 97.3).
- Primary cutaneous diffuse large B-cell lymphoma, leg type (PCDLBCL, LT) has intermediate clinical behavior, worse 5-year survival estimates, and requires more aggressive treatment (see Table 97.3).
- An approach to the patient with a suspected diagnosis of cutaneous B-cell lymphoma is shown in Fig. 97.1.

Plasma Cell Dyscrasias, Including Multiple Myeloma

- Plasma cell dyscrasias include monoclonal gammopathy of undetermined significance (MGUS), smoldering/asymptomatic myeloma and active/symptomatic myeloma, as well as light and heavy chain deposition diseases and primary systemic amyloidosis (AL).
- While proliferations of plasma cells in the skin are unusual, cutaneous disorders associated with or thought to be related to a monoclonal gammopathy are more common (Table 97.4).

RECOMMENDED STAGING INVESTIGATIONS FOR PATIENTS WITH A CONFIRMED DIAGNOSIS OF B-CELL LYMPHOMA INVOLVING THE SKIN
History and physical examination
• Presence/absence of "B" symptoms, including fever, night sweats, weight loss, malaise • Complete lymph node examination • Palpation of abdomen for hepatosplenomegaly • Examination of oral cavity • History of organ transplantation and/or other immune suppression (e.g. HIV, iatrogenic, congenital)
Laboratory studies
• Complete blood count with differential and platelet count • Comprehensive serum chemistries including LDH • Flow cytometry of peripheral blood mononuclear cells*
Imaging studies
• Ultrasound of abdomen and superficial lymph nodes • Whole-body PET/CT scan or whole-body CT scan*
Additional studies as clinically indicated
• Bone marrow biopsy** • Excisional biopsy of enlarged lymph nodes or other suspicious lesions • PCR analysis for *Borrelia* spp. DNA in patients from endemic areas (Europe) or travelers to endemic areas

**Not required in primary cutaneous marginal zone B-cell lymphoma.*
***While recommended for follicle center lymphoma and all types of large B-cell lymphoma, in the US bone marrow biopsy has been replaced by PET scan, as the latter is a more sensitive test.*

Table 97.1 Recommended staging investigations for patients with a confirmed diagnosis of B-cell lymphoma involving the skin. PET, positron emission tomography.

CLASSIFICATION OF B-CELL LYMPHOMAS WITH PRIMARY CUTANEOUS MANIFESTATIONS
• Primary cutaneous marginal zone B-cell lymphoma (PCMZL)* • Primary cutaneous follicle center lymphoma (PCFCL)** • Primary cutaneous diffuse large B-cell lymphoma, leg type (PCDLBCL, LT)** • Intravascular large B-cell lymphoma

**Includes cases previously designated as primary cutaneous immunocytoma and primary cutaneous plasmacytoma.*
***In rare cases that cannot be classified as either PCDLBCL, LT or PCFCL, a diagnosis of primary cutaneous DLBCL-NOS (not otherwise specified) should be made.*

Table 97.2 WHO–EORTC 2018 classification of B-cell lymphomas with primary cutaneous manifestations. In addition, there is one provisional diagnosis of EBV-positive mucocutaneous ulcer (EBVMCU).

For further information see Ch. 119 from *Dermatology, Fourth Edition*.

For additional online figures visit www.expertconsult.com 

THE PRIMARY CUTANEOUS B-CELL LYMPHOMAS (PCBCLs): CLINICAL AND DIAGNOSTIC FEATURES AND RECOMMENDED TREATMENT OPTIONS						
Primary cutaneous B-cell lymphoma subtype	**Preferred location**	**Clinical features**	**Other distinguishing features**	**DDx**	**Rx**	**Outcome**
Indolent behavior						
Primary cutaneous marginal zone B-cell lymphoma (PCMZL)	• Extremities: upper > lower • Trunk • Occasionally generalized	• Multifocal, pink-violet to red-brown, asymptomatic papules, plaques and nodules (Fig. 97.2) • Rare ulceration; may resolve with anetoderma • Can occur in areas of acrodermatitis chronica atrophicans (Fig. 97.2C)	• Bcl-2 (+), Bcl-6 (–), CD10 (–) • Monoclonal rearrangement of *IGH* genes • Intracytoplasmic monotypic expression of Ig light chains (Fig. 97.3) • May be linked to infection with *Borrelia* species in endemic areas (e.g. Europe)	• Distinguish between the various PCBCLs • Benign reactive processes (e.g. lymphocytic infiltrate of Jessner, cutaneous lymphoid hyperplasia) • Leukemia cutis (e.g. cutaneous CLL) • Secondary involvement from a systemic lymphoma • Solid organ metastases	**Solitary or few lesions (trunk, occasionally more generalized)** • Watchful waiting • XRT • Surgical excision • Surgical excision plus postoperative XRT • Intralesional rituximab • Intralesional CS **Multiple lesions at different body sites or diffuse PCFCL with disseminated lesions or if located on legs** • Intralesional CS • Intralesional rituximab • Subcutaneous or intralesional interferon α-2a • Systemic rituximab • Systemic chemotherapy plus rituximab	• 5-year survival ≥95% • Skin relapse common • Occasionally spontaneous resolution • Progression to systemic involvement is rare
Primary cutaneous follicle center lymphoma (PCFCL)	• Scalp, forehead, trunk (especially back), rarely legs (~5%)	• Solitary or grouped, asymptomatic, pink to plum-colored papules, plaques, or tumors (Fig. 97.4) • May have peripheral patch of erythema (*Crosti lymphoma*) • Ulceration uncommon • Occasionally miliary, acneiform-like small papules	• Bcl-6 (+), MUM1 (–) • Usually Bcl-2 (–), t(14;18) (–) ; if either (+) suspect systemic involvement • (–) monoclonal Ig gene rearrangement • (+) monotypic surface Ig expression			

Table 97.3 The primary cutaneous B-cell lymphomas (PCBCLs): clinical and diagnostic features and recommended treatment options. *Continued*

THE PRIMARY CUTANEOUS B-CELL LYMPHOMAS (PCBCLs): CLINICAL AND DIAGNOSTIC FEATURES AND RECOMMENDED TREATMENT OPTIONS						
Primary cutaneous B-cell lymphoma subtype	**Preferred location**	**Clinical features**	**Other distinguishing features**	**DDx**	**Rx**	**Outcome**
Intermediate to aggressive behavior						
Primary cutaneous diffuse large B-cell lymphoma, leg type (PCDLBCL, LT)	• Distal leg • Unilateral > bilateral • May occur elsewhere (10–15%)	• Solitary or clustered, red to red-brown nodules • Often see small red papules adjacent to larger nodules (Fig. 97.5) • Ulceration may occur	• Bcl-2 (+), MUM1 (+), MYC (+) • Usually Bcl-6 (+) • CD10 (–) • ± monoclonal rearrangement of *IGH* genes • (+) monotypic surface and/or intracytoplasmic Ig expression	• Secondary cutaneous involvement from systemic lymphoma • Cutaneous infiltrates from AML • Solid organ metastases	• Systemic rituximab • Systemic chemotherapy plus rituximab • Consider local XRT for small solitary lesions	• 5-year survival ~50% • Extracutaneous involvement in ~50% • Multiple lesions on leg = poor prognosis
Other						
Intravascular large B-cell lymphoma	• Indurated, red to violaceous patches and plaques; favors trunk and thighs • Neoplastic CD20(+) cells are located within the lumina of blood vessels that are CD31(+) and CD34(+) • ~25% present with skin-limited disease at the time of diagnosis, predominantly in women; much better prognosis than in patients with systemic disease (e.g. CNS, lungs)					
Provisional						
EBV-positive mucocutaneous ulcer (EBVMCU)	• Solitary, sharply demarcated ulcerating lesion involving the skin, oropharyngeal mucosa or GI tract in patients with age-related or iatrogenic immunosuppression • Typically self-limited, indolent course; reduction or cessation of immunosuppressive therapy may result in complete remission					

Table 97.3 *Continued* **The primary cutaneous B-cell lymphomas (PCBCLs): clinical and diagnostic features and recommended treatment options.**
AML, acute myelogenous leukemia; CLL, chronic lymphocytic leukemia; Ig, immunoglobulin.

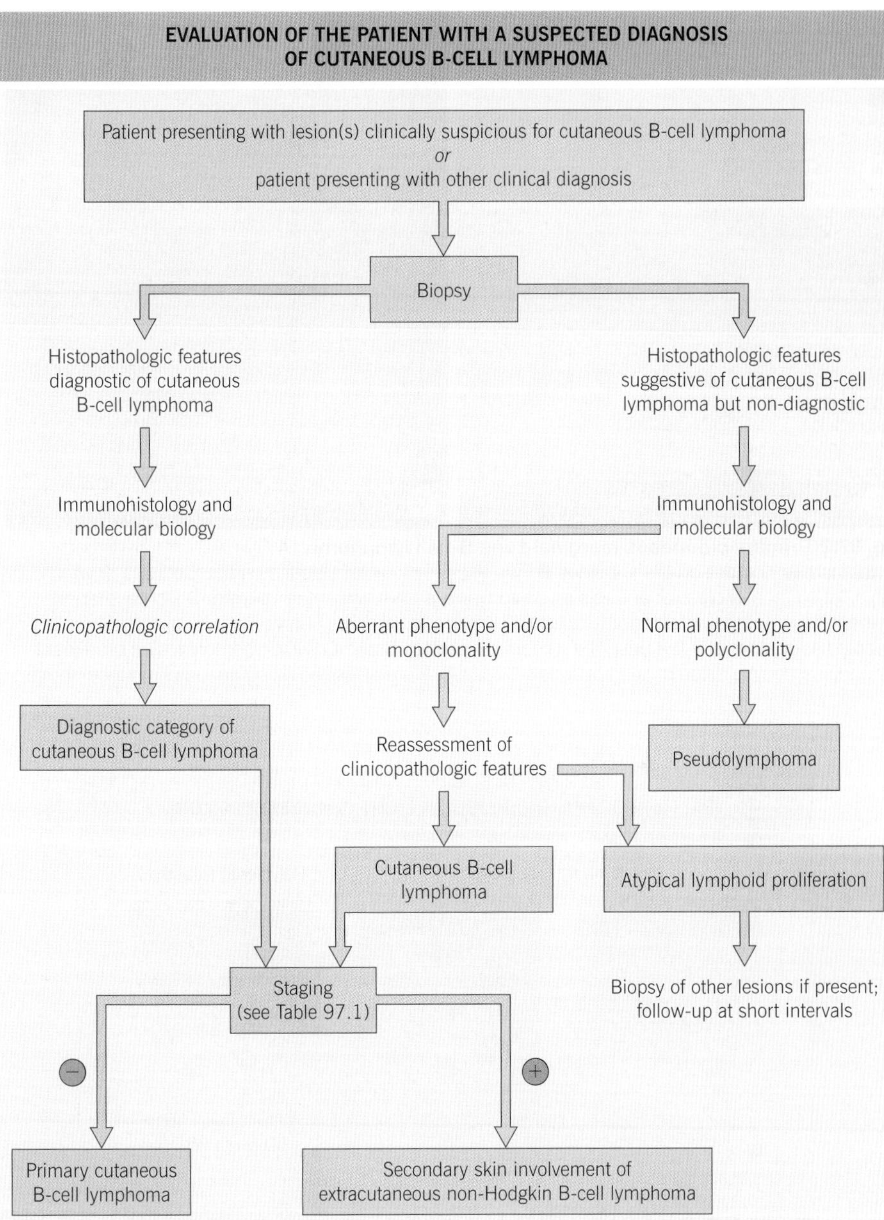

Fig. 97.1 Evaluation of the patient with a suspected diagnosis of cutaneous B-cell lymphoma. Algorithm outlining approach to the patient. *Courtesy, Lorenzo Cerroni, MD.*

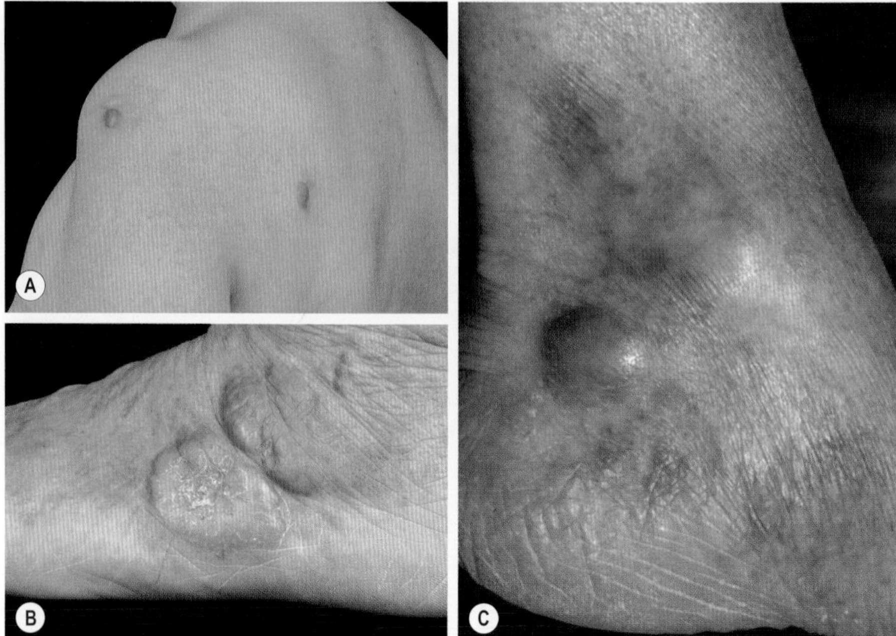

Fig. 97.2 Primary cutaneous marginal zone B-cell lymphoma. A Two well-circumscribed, erythematous nodules on the shoulder. **B** Two thick, pink-violet plaques on the foot, one of which has a flat surface. Molecular analysis revealed *Borrelia* DNA within the infiltrate. **C** Dome-shaped erythematous nodule with smooth surface. The surrounding area shows features of acrodermatitis chronica atrophicans. In the past, the tumors pictured in **B** and **C**, which demonstrated prominent lymphoplasmacytic differentiation histopathologically, were classified as cutaneous immunocytomas. *Courtesy, Lorenzo Cerroni, MD.*

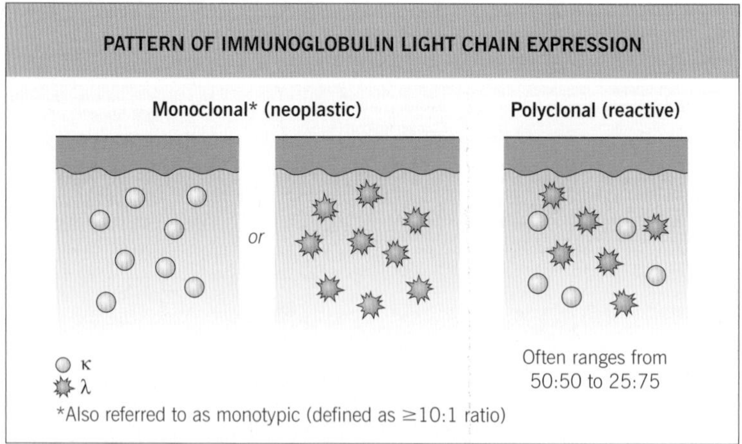

Fig. 97.3 Pattern of immunoglobulin light chain expression. Detection of monoclonal expression of immunoglobulin light chains (κ or λ) is a key diagnostic feature for primary cutaneous marginal zone B-cell lymphoma. Monoclonality is defined as a ≥10:1 ratio.

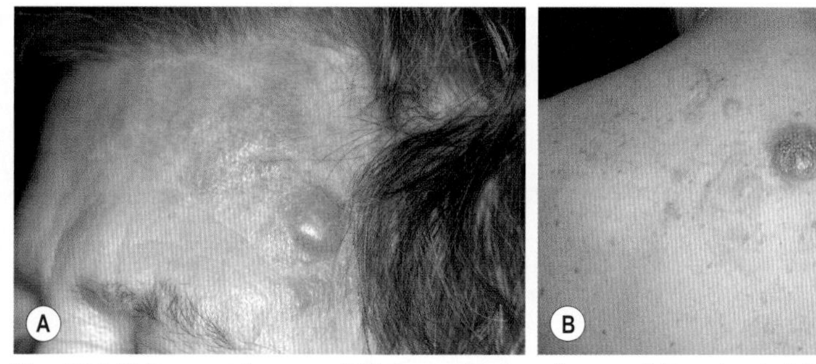

Fig. 97.4 Primary cutaneous follicle center lymphoma. A Prominent pink-violet nodule on the lateral forehead with a few telangiectasias. The nodule is surrounded by papules and large infiltrated plaques. **B** Large nodule on the upper back. Note the surrounding erythematous papules, patches, and plaques (Crosti lymphoma). *Courtesy, Lorenzo Cerroni, MD.*

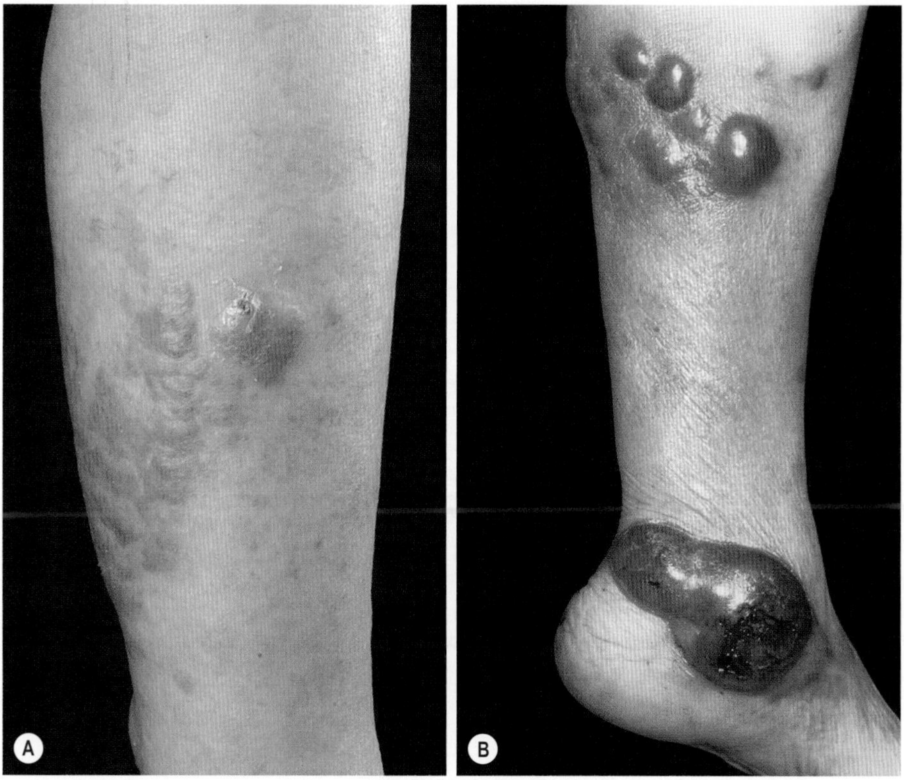

Fig. 97.5 Primary cutaneous diffuse large B-cell lymphoma, leg type. A Multiple coalescing red-brown papulonodules and plaques on the lower leg. **B** Multiple red-brown papulonodules and tumors on the lower leg. *Courtesy, Lorenzo Cerroni, MD.*

CUTANEOUS CONDITIONS ASSOCIATED WITH MONOCONAL GAMMOPATHY
Proliferation of lymphoplasmacytic cells in the skin
• Extramedullary cutaneous plasmacytoma* • Cutaneous Waldenström macroglobulinemia**
Deposition of the monoclonal protein in the skin, by definition
• Primary systemic amyloidosis (light chains) • Cryoglobulinemic occlusive vasculopathy (type I cryoglobulins†) • Hyperkeratotic spicules (follicular > nonfollicular) • Crystal-storing histiocytosis • Crystalglobulinemia • IgM storage papules (cutaneous macroglobulinosis)** • Subepidermal bullous dermatosis associated with IgM gammopathy**
Deposition of the monoclonal protein in the skin frequently observed
• Plasma cell dyscrasia-associated acquired cutis laxa, acral or generalized (amyloid and/or IgG) • Plasma cell dyscrasia-associated reactive angioendotheliomatosis (type I cryoglobulins or amyloid)
Almost always associated with monoclonal gammopathy
• Scleromyxedema • POEMS syndrome‡ • AESOP syndrome – *a*denopathy and *e*xtensive *s*kin patch *o*verlying a *p*lasmacytoma; may coexist with POEMS syndrome‡ • Schnitzler syndrome** • Necrobiotic xanthogranuloma
Frequently associated with monoclonal gammopathy
• Normolipemic plane xanthoma • Scleredema (type 2) • Angioedema secondary to acquired C1 esterase inhibitor deficiency • Clarkson syndrome (idiopathic systemic capillary leak syndrome)
Significant association with monoclonal gammopathy (at least 15% of cases)
• Erythema elevatum diutinum • Subcorneal pustular dermatosis (SPD) and SPD-type IgA pemphigus • Pyoderma gangrenosum
Occasionally associated with monoclonal gammopathy
• Sweet syndrome • Cutaneous small vessel vasculitis†, including adult IgA vasculitis with monoclonal IgA gammopathy • Xanthoma disseminatum • Epidermolysis bullosa acquisita • Paraneoplastic pemphigus

**In the current WHO–EORTC classification (see Table 97.2), primary cutaneous plasmacytoma is classified as primary cutaneous marginal zone B-cell lymphoma.*
***IgM monoclonal gammopathy is present by definition; in Schnitzler syndrome, IgG gammopathy has occasionally been observed; Waldenström macroglobulinemia is due to a lymphoplasmacytic lymphoma.*
†Cryoglobulinemic vasculitis can occur secondary to type II cryoglobulins.
‡Polyneuropathy (P), organomegaly (O), endocrinopathy (E), M-protein (M), skin changes (S) (see Ch. 45); diagnosis requires monoclonal plasmaproliferative disorder & neuropathy + one other major criterion (sclerotic bone lesions, Castleman disease, increased serum VEGF levels) and one minor criterion (extravascular volume overload, papilledema, O, E, S, thrombocytosis/polycythemia).

Table 97.4 Cutaneous conditions associated with a monoclonal gammopathy.

Cutaneous T-Cell Lymphoma 98

• *Primary* cutaneous lymphomas present in the skin without evidence of extracutaneous disease at the time of diagnosis.
• *Secondary* cutaneous lymphomas are skin manifestations of systemic (nodal) lymphomas and will not be discussed (see oncology texts).
• Primary **c**utaneous **l**ymphomas may be of **T**-**c**ell origin (75–80%) or **B**-**c**ell origin (20–25%) and are termed **CTCL** and **CBCL**, respectively.
• The term CTCL will be used herein to describe the heterogeneous group of primary cutaneous lymphomas composed of neoplastic T cells or natural killer (NK) cells (Tables 98.1–98.3).
• As different types of CTCLs, CBCLs, and even secondary cutaneous lymphomas may present with similar clinical and histopathological features, it is imperative to combine clinical and staging data with histopathologic, immunophenotypic, and genetic data before making a definitive diagnosis (classification).
• Immunophenotyping, as determined from immunohistochemical studies done on skin biopsy specimens, can help distinguish between a T-cell vs an NK-cell vs a B-cell lymphoma and can aid in subtyping.
• T-cell receptor (TCR) gene rearrangement analysis is useful in detecting the presence or absence of a clonal T-cell population in skin biopsy specimens.
• The presence of a clonal T-cell population cannot be used as an absolute criterion of malignancy, as several benign conditions may also demonstrate clonality (e.g. pityriasis lichenoides et varioliformis acuta, lichen planus, pigmented purpuric dermatosis, lichen sclerosus, and some pseudolymphomas).
• An approach to the evaluation of a patient with suspected CTCL is presented in Fig. 98.1.
• Once a diagnosis of CTCL has been made, the type of CTCL should then be determined.
• Of the various CTCLs (see Tables 98.1–98.3), approximately 65% are mycosis fungoides (MF), MF variants, or Sézary syndrome (SS); 25% are within the spectrum of CD30$^+$ lymphoproliferative disorders (Fig. 98.2); and the remainder (10%) are composed of other rare entities.
• In general, the aggressive-behaving CTCLs (see Tables 98.1 and 98.3) require more extensive staging (Table 98.4), referral to a hematologist–oncologist, and systemic chemotherapy or targeted immunotherapy (e.g. rituximab, brentuximab).

Mycosis Fungoides (MF)

• The most common subtype of CTCL, representing about 50% of all *primary* cutaneous lymphomas.
• The term MF should be restricted to the classic "Alibert–Bazin" type, characterized by the typical evolution of patches, plaques, and tumors (Fig. 98.3).
• Other clinical variants with similar behavior include hypo- and hyperpigmented MF (Fig. 98.3C) and bullous MF.
• Three rare clinical variants of MF with distinctive clinicopathologic features are considered separately, namely folliculotropic MF (Fig. 98.4), pagetoid reticulosis (Fig. 98.5), and granulomatous slack skin (Fig. 98.6).
• Classic MF is an uncommon disease; more prevalent in males (> females), older adults, and African-Americans; pathogenesis is unknown.
• Clinical presentation depends on stage at diagnosis (Tables 98.5 and 98.6), but classically patients progress from persistent patch/plaque stage to tumor stage over years to decades (see Fig. 98.3).

2018 WHO–EORTC CLASSIFICATION FOR CUTANEOUS T-CELL LYMPHOMAS		
2018 WHO–EORTC classification	**Frequency (%)***	**5-year DSS (%)***
Indolent clinical behavior		
Mycosis fungoides (MF)	39	88
Mycosis fungoides variants		
• Folliculotropic MF	5	75
• Pagetoid reticulosis	<1	100
• Granulomatous slack skin	<1w	100
Primary cutaneous CD30-positive lymphoproliferative disorders		
• Lymphomatoid papulosis (LyP)	12	99
• Primary cutaneous anaplastic large cell lymphoma (C-ALCL)	8	95
Subcutaneous panniculitis-like T-cell lymphoma (SPTCL)	1	87
Primary cutaneous CD4-positive small/medium T-cell lymphoproliferative disorder (provisional)	6	100
Primary cutaneous acral CD8-positive T-cell lymphoma (provisional)	<1	100
Aggressive clinical behavior		
Sézary syndrome (SS)	2	36
Adult T-cell leukemia/ lymphoma (ATLL)	<1	NDA
Extranodal NK/T-cell lymphoma, nasal type	<1	16
Primary cutaneous aggressive epidermotropic CD8-positive T-cell lymphoma (provisional)	<1	31
Primary cutaneous gamma/delta T-cell lymphoma (PCGD-TCL)	<1	11
Chronic active EBV infection	<1	NDA
Primary cutaneous peripheral T-cell lymphoma (PTCL), NOS	2	15

**Based on data included in Dutch and Austrian cutaneous lymphoma registries between 2002 and 2017.*

Table 98.1 2018 WHO–EORTC classification for cutaneous T-cell lymphomas. DSS, disease specific survival; NDA, no data available; NOS, not otherwise specified. *From Willemze R, Cerroni L, Berti E, et al. The 2018 update of the WHO-EORTC classification for primary cutaneous lymphomas. Blood. April 2019; 133(16):1703–14.*

- Most patients have years of nonspecific eczematous or psoriasiform skin lesions and nondiagnostic biopsies before a definitive diagnosis of MF is made.
- There can be gradual progression or relapse at a similar stage of disease; advancement to a higher stage usually transpires after years and multiple treatment failures.
- Extracutaneous disease is extremely rare in patch/plaque stage, uncommon with generalized plaques, and most likely with extensive tumors or erythroderma.
- Extracutaneous involvement almost always initially involves regional lymph nodes draining the areas of greatest skin involvement; visceral involvement can develop subsequently; bone marrow involvement is rare.
- Histopathologic examination of persistently enlarged lymph nodes can help distinguish between dermatopathic (reactive) lymphadenopathy and involvement with MF.
- Treatment is dependent on the stage at diagnosis, the host's immune status, and the general condition of the patient (Table 98.7).

CUTANEOUS T-CELL LYMPHOMAS WITH INDOLENT CLINICAL BEHAVIOR		
Clinical & diagnostic features	**DDx**	**Treatment recommendations**
Mycosis fungoides		
• Variable progression from patch to plaque to tumor stage over years–decades (see Fig. 98.3) • **Patch stage:** variably sized red, finely scaling lesions with atrophy and poikiloderma; predilection for sun-protected sites • **Plaque stage:** infiltrated red-brown scaling plaques; often annular, polycyclic or horseshoe-shaped • **Tumor stage:** often have combination of patches, plaques, and tumors; many with ulceration • $CD3^+$, $CD4^+$, $CD45RO^+$, $CD8^-$ • Occasionally $CD4^-$, $CD8^+$; rarely $CD4^-$, $CD8^-$	• **Benign dermatoses:** – Eczema – Psoriasis – Superficial fungal infections – Drug reactions • **Benign conditions with histopathologic features suggestive of MF:** – Lymphomatoid contact dermatitis – Lymphomatoid drug reactions – Actinic reticuloid • **Other types of epidermotropic CTCL**	• See Table 98.7
Mycosis fungoides variants		
Folliculotropic MF		
• Grouped follicular papules, acneiform lesions, indurated plaques (see Fig. 98.4) • Favors head and neck • Pruritus, alopecia, mucinorrhea • Pruritus often severe • $CD3^+$, $CD4^+$, $CD8^-$; occasionally $CD30^+$	• Acne vulgaris • Chloracne • Alopecia mucinosa • Seborrheic dermatitis • Atopic dermatitis	• Two subgroups: 1. Indolent clinical behavior treated similarly to early-stage MF (see Table 98.7) 2. More aggressive form requiring combination therapy (see Table 98.7)
Pagetoid reticulosis		
• Slowly progressive, solitary or localized psoriasiform or hyperkeratotic patch or plaque • Favors extremities (see Fig. 98.5) • Histologically purely intraepidermal proliferation • $CD3^+$, $CD4^+$, $CD8^-$ *-OR-* $CD3^+$, $CD4^-$, $CD8^+$; $CD30^+$ in many cases	• Isolated patch of psoriasis or eczema • Other types of CTCL	• XRT or surgical excision

Table 98.2 Cutaneous T-cell lymphomas (CTCL) with *indolent* clinical behavior: clinical and diagnostic features as well as treatment recommendations.
Continued

CUTANEOUS T-CELL LYMPHOMAS WITH INDOLENT CLINICAL BEHAVIOR		
Granulomatous slack skin		
• Circumscribed areas of pendulous, atrophic, lax skin (see Fig. 98.6) • Favors axillae and groin • $CD3^+$, $CD4^+$, $CD8^-$	• Acquired generalized cutis laxa • Pseudoxanthoma elasticum	• XRT is an option
Primary cutaneous $CD30^+$ lymphoproliferative disorders		
Lymphomatoid papulosis (LyP)		
• Red-brown papules and nodules that can develop central hemorrhage, necrosis, and crusting (Fig. 98.8) • Spontaneously disappear over 3–8 weeks • Different stages of evolution coexist • May last months to >40 years • ~20% preceded by/followed by/associated with another cutaneous lymphoma (e.g. MF, C-ALCL, Hodgkin lymphoma) • Type B may be $CD30^-$	• Pityriasis lichenoides et varioliformis acuta (PLEVA) • Pityriasis lichenoides chronica (PLC) • Folliculitis • If clustered, Majocchi granuloma • Arthropod bites	• Low-dose oral methotrexate (e.g. 5–20 mg/week) is the most effective treatment • Long-term follow-up, given risk of systemic lymphoma
Primary cutaneous anaplastic large cell lymphoma (C-ALCL)		
• Solitary or localized nodules or tumors, often with ulceration (Fig. 98.9) • Occasionally will spontaneously regress • $CD30^+$, $CD4^+$ >> $CD8^+$, ALK^-, EMA^-, $CD15^-$, $TIA\text{-}1^+$	• $CD30^+$ large cell lymphoma secondary to MF transformation • HIV-associated or post-transplant lymphoma • Skin manifestations of systemic ALCL	• Solitary lesions may resolve spontaneously • XRT or surgical excision if limited number of lesions • Brentuximab vedotin, low-dose methotrexate, retinoids, IFN-alpha; systemic chemotherapy when extensive
Subcutaneous panniculitis-like T-cell lymphoma (SPTCL)		
• Subcutaneous nodules and plaques • Extremities > trunk (Fig. 98.10) • ± Fever, fatigue, weight loss • $CD3^+$, $CD4^-$, $CD8^+$, $CD56^-$, $\beta F1^+$ (TCR α/β^+)	• Other types of panniculitis (see Ch. 83)	• XRT for solitary lesions • More conservative immunosuppressive regimens (e.g. prednisone, cyclosporine) as well as combination chemotherapy

Table 98.2 *Continued* **Cutaneous T-cell lymphomas (CTCL) with *indolent* clinical behavior: clinical and diagnostic features as well as treatment recommendations.** *Continued*

CUTANEOUS T-CELL LYMPHOMAS WITH INDOLENT CLINICAL BEHAVIOR		
Primary cutaneous CD4$^+$ small/medium T-cell lymphoproliferative disorder (provisional)		
• Most often a solitary plaque or tumor on face, neck, upper trunk • CD3$^+$, CD4$^+$, CD8$^-$, βF1$^+$ (TCR α/β^+), CD30$^-$, CD56$^-$; CD279/PD-1$^+$, BCL66$^+$, CXCL13$^+$	• Other types of CTCL	• If lesions do not resolve spontaneously after biopsy, then treat with intralesional CS, surgical excision, or rarely XRT
Primary cutaneous acral CD8$^+$ T-cell lymphoma (provisional)		
• Solitary, slowly progressive papule or nodule, typically located on the ear or less commonly other acral sites (e.g. nose, foot) • CD3$^+$, CD4$^-$, CD8$^+$, CD30$^-$,TIA-1$^+$	• Other types of CTCL	• Surgical excision or XRT

Table 98.2 *Continued* **Cutaneous T-cell lymphomas (CTCL) with *indolent* clinical behavior: clinical and diagnostic features as well as treatment recommendations.** HTLV-1, human T-lymphotrophic virus 1; IFN, interferon; NDA, no data available; TCR, T-cell receptor; TSEB, total skin electron beam irradiation.

CUTANEOUS T-CELL LYMPHOMAS WITH AGGRESSIVE CLINICAL BEHAVIOR		
Clinical and diagnostic features	**DDx**	**Treatment recommendations**
Sézary syndrome		
• Exfoliative erythroderma (see Fig. 98.7), lymphadenopathy, and circulating clonal malignant T cells • Intense pruritus with lichenification • Alopecia, palmoplantar keratoderma • $CD3^+$, $CD4^+$, $CD8^-$, $CD7^-$, $CD26^-$	• Other erythrodermic syndromes (see Ch. 8) • Actinic reticuloid	• See Table 98.7
Adult T-cell leukemia/lymphoma (ATLL)		
• Associated with HTLV-1 infection • More common in SW Japan, Caribbean islands • **Smoldering variant**: resembles MF • **Acute presentation**: leukemia, lymphadenopathy, hypercalcemia, skin lesions • $CD3^+$, $CD4^+$, $CD8^-$, $CD25^+$	**Smoldering variant** • MF **Acute variant** • Other lymphomas, leukemias	**Smoldering variant** • Skin-directed therapies as in MF (see Table 98.7) **Acute variant** • Systemic chemotherapy; occasionally zidovudine + IFN-alpha
Extranodal NK/T-cell lymphoma, nasal type		
• Almost always associated with EBV • **Nasal type**: mid-facial destructive tumor (Fig. 98.11) • **Skin only**: ulcerated plaques or tumors on trunk/extremities • $CD2^+$, CD3 epsilon$^+$, TIA-1$^+$, EBER-1$^+$, $CD56^+$, $CD4^-$, $CD8^{-/+}$	**Nasal type** • Mucormycosis • Leishmaniasis **Skin only** • Other cutaneous lymphomas	• XRT for localized disease • More advanced disease often resistant to chemotherapy
Primary cutaneous aggressive epidermotropic $CD8^+$ T-cell lymphoma (provisional)		
• Eruptive papulonodules with ulceration (Fig. 98.12) *-OR-* • Keratotic patches and plaques • $CD3^+$, $CD4^-$, $CD8^+$, TIA-1$^+$, AF1$^+$ (TCR α/β^+)	• Other $CD8^+$ CTCLs (e.g. pagetoid reticulosis, MF, LyP, C-ALCL)	• Systemic chemotherapy
Primary cutaneous gamma/delta T-cell lymphoma (PCGD-TCL)		
• Disseminated plaques and/or ulceronecrotic nodules or tumors • Hemophagocytic syndrome common • $CD4^-$, $CD8^-$, TCR γ/δ^+, TF1$^-$ (TCR α/β^-), TIA-1$^+$, $CD56^+$, $CD3^+$	• Other panniculitides (see Ch. 83)	• Aggressive, often rapidly fatal disease that is resistant to multi-agent chemotherapy

Table 98.3 Cutaneous T-cell lymphomas (CTCL) with *aggressive* clinical behavior: clinical and diagnostic features as well as treatment recommendations.
Continued

CUTANEOUS T-CELL LYMPHOMAS WITH AGGRESSIVE CLINICAL BEHAVIOR		
Chronic active EBV infection		
• Two entities with a risk of progression to systemic EBV (+) T-cell or NK-cell lymphoma; favors Asian and native Latin American children: 1. **Hydroa vacciniforme-like lymphoproliferative disorders (HV-like LPD)** – Similar presentation to HV (see Ch. 73; Fig. 73.9) but may have more extensive involvement, e.g. facial swelling and ulcerated nodules 2. **Hypersensitivity reactions to mosquito bites (HMB)** – Ulceronecrotic lesions at sites of bites • Both may have systemic symptoms such as fever, lymphadenopathy, hepatosplenomegaly	• Other photosensitizing disorders (e.g. hydroa vacciniforme (see Fig. 73.8), porphyrias, cutaneous lupus) • Other lymphomas	• Treatment of cutaneous disease similar to HV (see Ch. 73) • Referral to hematology is recommended
Primary cutaneous peripheral T-cell lymphoma (PTCL), NOS		
• Diagnosis of exclusion; refers to CTCLs that do not fit into any of the other subtypes • Generalized > solitary or localized nodules and tumors (Fig. 98.13) • $CD4^+$, $CD30^-$, $CD56^-$	• Other cutaneous lymphomas	• Systemic chemotherapy, but prognosis is poor

Table 98.3 *Continued* **Cutaneous T-cell lymphomas (CTCL) with *aggressive* clinical behavior: clinical and diagnostic features as well as treatment recommendations.** IFN, interferon; NOS, not otherwise specified.

AN APPROACH TO THE PATIENT WITH A SUSPECTED CUTANEOUS T-CELL LYMPHOMA (CTCL)

Skin lesions suspicious for CTCL
- Persistent patches and/or plaques in non-photodistributed areas
- Erythroderma
- Indurated plaques of the head and neck
- Solitary, localized, or generalized nodules or tumors, +/– ulceration and necrosis
- Subcutaneous nodules and plaques

Perform skin biopsies of multiple suspicious sites
- If patch or thin plaque: broad, deep shave biopsy
- If indurated plaque, nodule, tumor: 4–6 mm deep punch biopsy
- If isolated lesion: excisional or incisional biopsy

Send specimen(s) to experienced dermatopathologist

Benign condition

Treat accordingly

Indeterminate histopathology

Histopathology suggestive of cutaneous lymphoma*

Immunohistochemical studies of skin biopsies

Normal or non-diagnostic immunophenotype

- Clinicopathologic correlation
- Longitudinal observation and repeat biopsies

B-cell immunophenotype

Especially if papulonodules, consider CBCL (see Ch.97)

T-cell immunophenotype

T-cell receptor (TCR) gene rearrangement analysis of skin biopsy to test for clonality

+**

–

Clinicopathologic correlation

CTCL

Not CTCL

Clinicopathologic correlation

65%

25%

10%

(Continued)

Fig. 98.1 An approach to the patient with a suspected cutaneous T-cell lymphoma (CTCL). *Continued*

AN APPROACH TO THE PATIENT WITH A SUSPECTED CUTANEOUS T-CELL LYMPHOMA (CTCL)

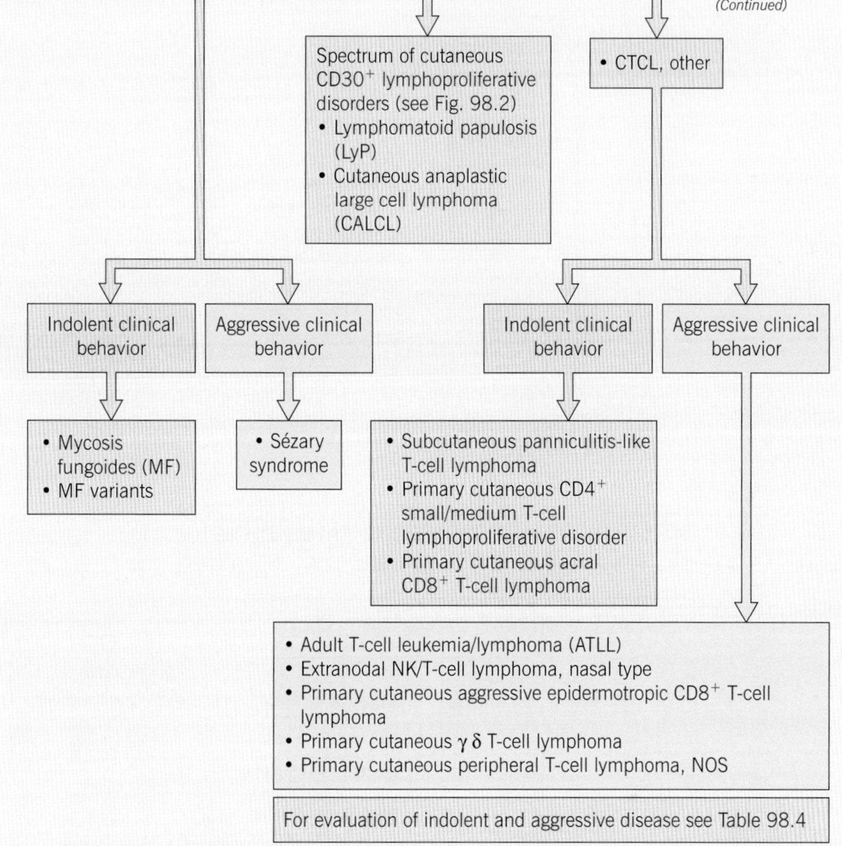

*If classic clinical and histopathological findings for MF, immunohistochemical and TCR/clonality studies may not be necessary

**The presence of a clonal T-cell population cannot be used as an absolute criterion of malignancy, as several benign conditions may also demonstrate clonality (e.g. pityriasis lichenoides et varioliformis acuta, lichen planus, pigmented purpuric dermatosis)

Fig. 98.1 *Continued* **An approach to the patient with a suspected cutaneous T-cell lymphoma (CTCL).** CBCL, cutaneous B-cell lymphoma; NOS, not otherwise specified.

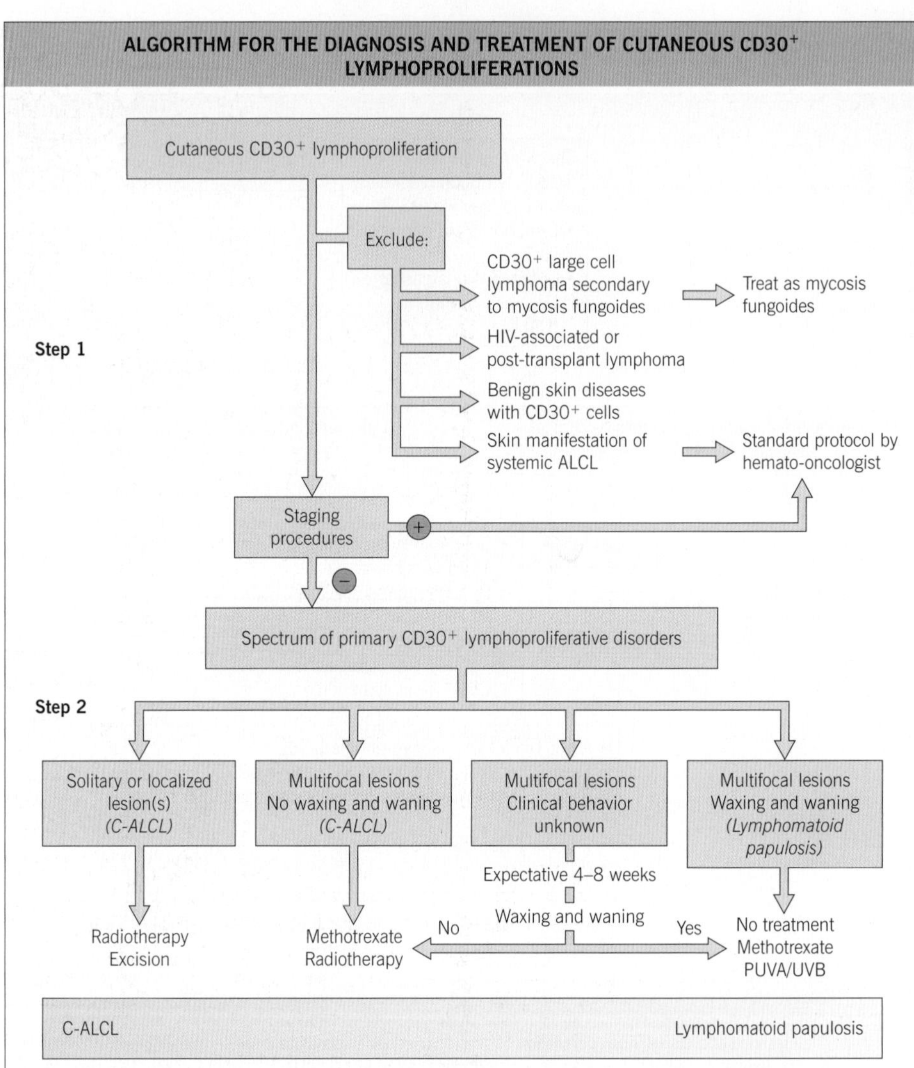

Fig. 98.2 Algorithm for the diagnosis and treatment of primary cutaneous CD30+ lymphoproliferative disorders. Cases previously designated as regressing atypical histiocytosis, as well as rare cases of primary cutaneous Hodgkin lymphoma with an indolent clinical course, also belong to this spectrum. Of note, there are reports of ALCL developing in patients with breast implants. C-ALCL, cutaneous anaplastic large cell lymphoma. *From Bekkenk M, Geelen FAMJ, van Voorst Vader PC, et al. Primary and secondary cutaneous CD30-positive lymphoproliferative disorders: long term follow-up data of 219 patients and guidelines for diagnosis and treatment. A report from the Dutch Cutaneous Lymphoma Group. Blood. 2000;95:3653–61.*

RECOMMENDED STAGING EVALUATION FOR INDOLENT- AND AGGRESSIVE-BEHAVIOR CUTANEOUS T-CELL LYMPHOMAS (CTCL)
Indolent-behavior CTCL
• Physical examination, including lymph nodes and palpation for hepatosplenomegaly • Laboratory studies: CBC with differential, platelets, chemistry panel, calcium, LDH • Biopsy of persistently enlarged lymph node(s)
Aggressive-behavior CTCL
In addition to that performed for indolent, also include:
• CT vs CT/PET scan • Referral to hematology–oncology
Special tests, if clinically indicated
• Detection of peripheral blood involvement (flow cytometry, TCR gene rearrangement, Sézary cell buffy coat preparation) • HTLV-1 serology, Southern blot analysis, or PCR in at-risk populations

Table 98.4 Recommended staging evaluation for indolent- and aggressive-behavior cutaneous T-cell lymphomas (CTCL). TCR, T-cell receptor; PET, positron emission tomography.

- Available therapies are effective in controlling disease but usually do not prolong life.
- Three main treatment categories are available: (1) skin-directed therapies (SDT); (2) systemic biologic therapies; and (3) systemic chemotherapies; combination therapy is also utilized (Table 98.7).
- Prognosis depends on stage, the type and extent of skin lesions, and the presence of extracutaneous disease (see Tables 98.5 and 98.6).
- The disease-related 10-year survival rate is approximately 95% for stage IA, 80% for stage IB, 40% for stage IIB, but only 20% for stage IV.
- An aggressive course is seen in patients with effaced lymph nodes, visceral involvement, or transformation into a large T-cell lymphoma.
- Death is usually due to systemic involvement or profound immunosuppression with resultant opportunistic infection.

Sézary Syndrome (SS)

- A leukemic, more aggressive variant of CTCL that is thought to arise from a distinct functional T-cell subset.
- Defined historically by the triad of: (1) erythroderma; (2) generalized lymphadenopathy; and (3) the presence of clonally related neoplastic T cells (Sézary cells) in the skin, lymph nodes, and peripheral blood (Fig. 98.7).
- Diagnosis is aided by the presence of one of the following: (1) absolute Sézary cell count of ≥1000 cells/mm^3; (2) CD4:CD8 ratio ≥10 and/or an abnormal immunophenotype, including the loss of CD7 (>40%) or CD26 (>30%) by flow cytometry; and (3) evidence of T-cell clonality in the blood.
- SS is distinguished from patients who begin as classic MF who then become erythrodermic (erythrodermic MF).
- Prognosis is generally poor, and most patients die from opportunistic infections due to immunosuppression.
- Systemic treatment is required, with skin-directed therapies sometimes being used as adjuvant therapy (see Table 98.7).

For further information see Ch. 120 from *Dermatology, Fourth Edition*.

For additional online figures and tables visit www.expertconsult.com

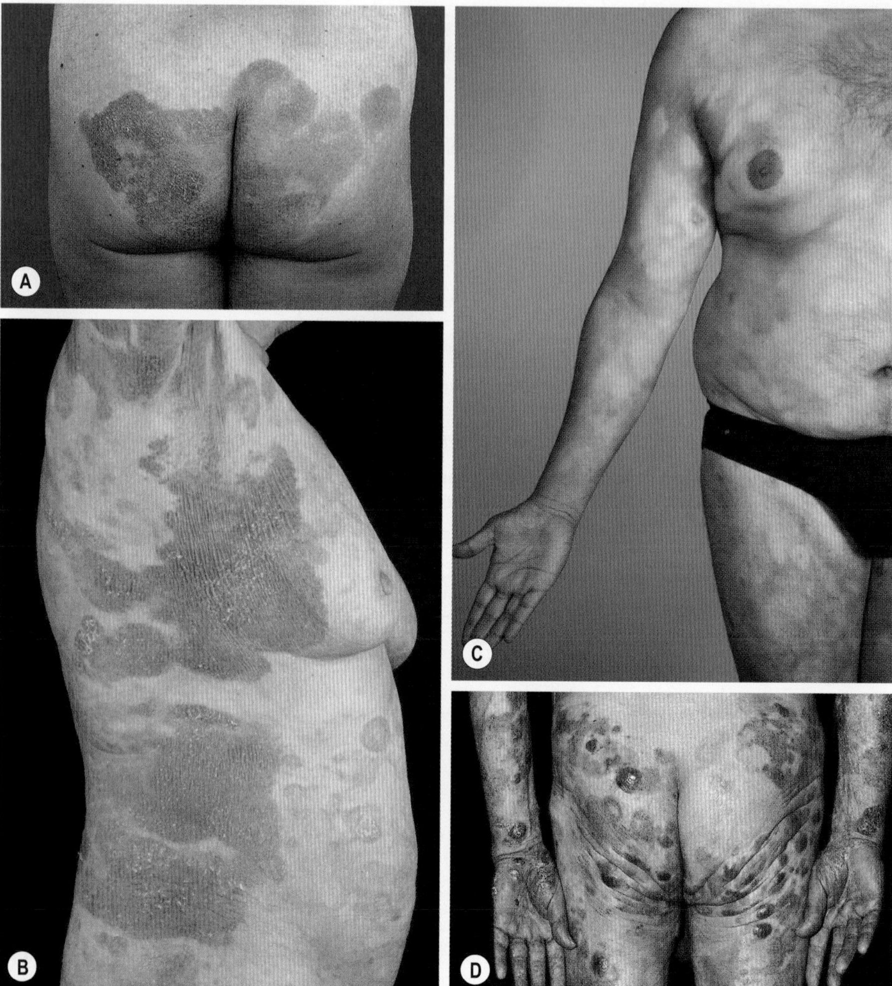

Fig. 98.3 Mycosis fungoides (MF). A Limited patch/plaque stage disease (*stage 1A*). Patches on the buttocks, involving less than 10% of the skin surface. **B** Generalized patch/plaque disease (*stage 1B*). Extensive patches and plaques with scale involving more than 10% of the skin surface. **C** Hypopigmented MF (*stage 1B*) with generalized hypopigmented lesions as well as pink to pink-brown plaques. **D** *Tumor stage.* Multiple skin tumors in combination with typical patches and plaques. *A, C, D, Courtesy, Rein Willemze, MD; B, Courtesy Lorenzo Cerroni, MD.*

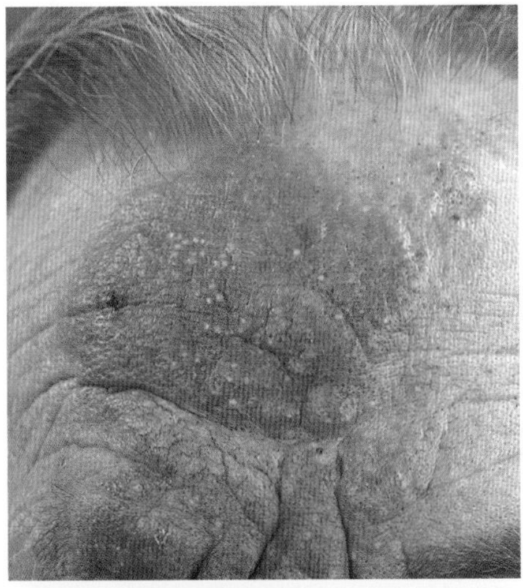

Fig. 98.4 Folliculotropic mycosis fungoides. Infiltrated erythematous plaques and acneiform lesions on the forehead and eyebrows with concurrent hair loss. The infiltration, thickening, and accentuation of the skin folds is referred to as a "leonine facies." *Courtesy, Rein Willemze, MD.*

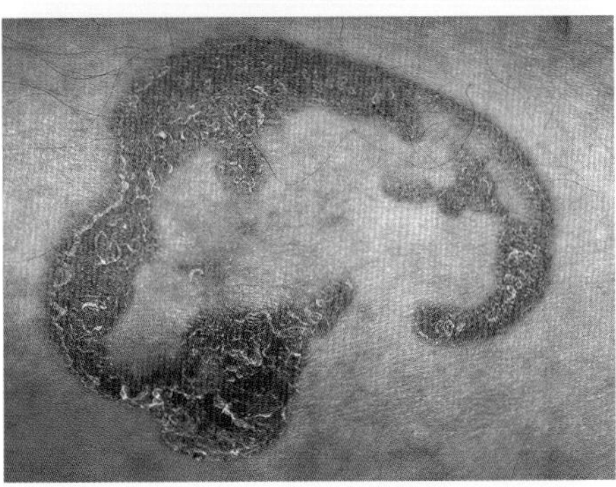

Fig. 98.5 Pagetoid reticulosis. Solitary plaque on the left upper leg. *Courtesy, Rein Willemze, MD.*

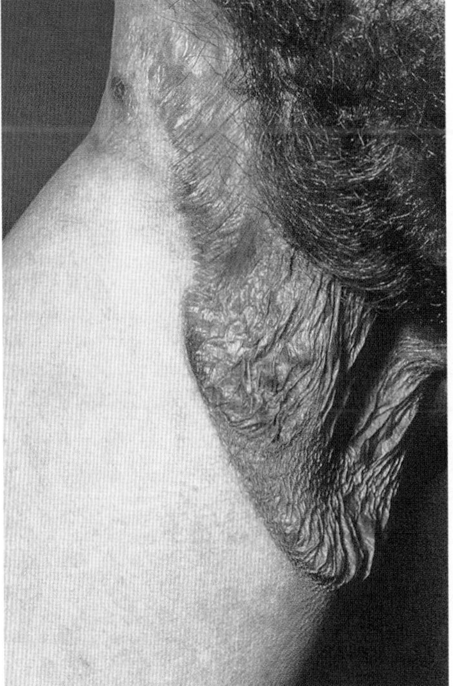

Fig. 98.6 Granulomatous slack skin. Pendulous fold of atrophic lax skin in the right inguinal area. *Courtesy, Rein Willemze, MD.*

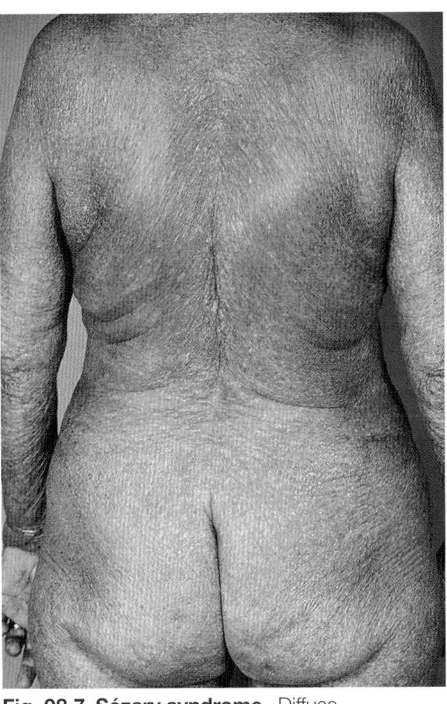

Fig. 98.7 Sézary syndrome. Diffuse erythroderma is present. *Courtesy, Rein Willemze, MD.*

TNMB CLASSIFICATION OF MYCOSIS FUNGOIDES AND SÉZARY SYNDROME	
T (skin)	
T_1	Limited patch/plaque (involving <10% of total skin surface)
T_2	Generalized patch/plaque (involving ≥10% of total skin surface)
T_3	Tumor(s)
T_4	Erythroderma
N (lymph node)	
N_0	No enlarged lymph nodes
N_1	Enlarged lymph nodes, histologically uninvolved
N_2	Enlarged lymph nodes, histologically involved (nodal architecture uneffaced)
N_3	Enlarged lymph nodes, histologically involved (nodal architecture [partially] effaced)
M (viscera)	
M_0	No visceral involvement
M_1	Visceral involvement
B (blood)	
B_0	No circulating atypical (Sézary) cells (or <5% of lymphocytes)
B_1	Low blood tumor burden (≥5% of lymphocytes are Sézary cells, but not B_2)
B_2	High blood tumor burden (≥1000/mcl Sézary cells + positive clone)

Table 98.5 TNMB classification of mycosis fungoides and Sézary syndrome.

CLINICAL STAGING SYSTEM FOR MYCOSIS FUNGOIDES AND SÉZARY SYNDROME				
Clinical stage				
IA	T_1	N_0	M_0	B_{0-1}
IB	T_2	N_0	M_0	B_{0-1}
IIA	T_{1-2}	N_{1-2}	M_0	B_{0-1}
IIB	T_3	N_{0-1}	M_0	B_{0-1}
IIIA	T_4	N_{0-2}	M_0	B_0
IIIB	T_4	N_{0-2}	M_0	B_1
IVA_1	T_{1-4}	N_{0-2}	M_0	B_2
IVA_2	T_{1-4}	N_3	M_0	B_{0-2}
IVB	T_{1-4}	N_{0-3}	M_1	B_{0-2}

Table 98.6 Clinical staging system for mycosis fungoides and Sézary syndrome. The shaded boxes highlight the required features for the three subdivisions of stage IV disease. By definition, patients with Sézary syndrome are stage IVA or IVB because of blood involvement.

TREATMENT OF MYCOSIS FUNGOIDES AND SÉZARY SYNDROME
Premycotic phase
• Topical or intralesional CS; narrowband UVB§ • If former not effective, PUVA§
Stage IA–IIA (patches/plaques)
• PUVA§; HN2 • Narrowband UVB§ (if only patches) • Topical CS or topical retinoids^ (if only limited patches/thin plaques as second-line therapy) • XRT (if single lesion) • TSEB (if generalized thick plaques)
Stage IIB (skin tumors)
• PUVA or HN2 + XRT (if only a few tumors) • TSEB (followed by skin-directed therapies) • Relapse: PUVA + IFN-α; PUVA + retinoids (acitretin; oral bexarotene*); second-line therapy: denileukin diftitox*,¶; HDACi (vorinostat, romidepsin)* • Add XRT (if persistent tumors); consider second course of TSEB (10–20 Gy)
Stage III (erythroderma)
• ECP; if not effective, add oral bexarotene, IFN-α, low-dose MTX • Low-dose chlorambucil and prednisone; low-dose methotrexate • Add skin-directed therapies (PUVA; HN2; XRT), if necessary • Second-line therapy: oral bexarotene*; denileukin diftitox*,¶; HDACi*; low-dose alemtuzumab; mogamulizumab-kpkc
Stage IV (nodal, visceral involvement)
• Multi-agent chemotherapy (e.g. CHOP) • Biological response modifiers (denileukin diftitox¶; IFN-α; oral retinoids) • Add skin-directed therapies (PUVA; HN2), if necessary • Allogeneic hematopoietic stem cell transplantation (utilizing non-myeloablative reduced-intensity conditioning regimens), in selected cases

§Address UV-shielded areas (e.g. upper inner thighs) via positioning.
^Bexarotene 1% gel, tazarotene 0.1% gel, altretinoin 0.1% gel.
**Efficacy compared to traditional treatments yet to be determined.*
¶At the time of writing, not commercially available.

Table 98.7 Treatment of mycosis fungoides (MF) and Sézary syndrome (SS). Topical bis-chloronitrosourea (BCNU; carmustine) is rarely used nowadays. Based upon one case series, topical resiquimod may be effective for Stage IA/IIA disease. SS requires systemic treatment with occasional use of skin-directed therapies as adjuvant treatment (see options listed for treatment of stage III and IV disease). Anti-PD-1 antibodies have been used to treat SS in the setting of PD-1 positivity. CHOP, cyclophosphamide, hydroxydaunomycin (doxorubicin), Oncovin® (vincristine) and prednisone; ECP, extracorporeal photopheresis; HDACi, histone deacetylase inhibitors; HN2, topical mechlorethamine (nitrogen mustard); IFN, interferon; TSEB, total skin electron beam.

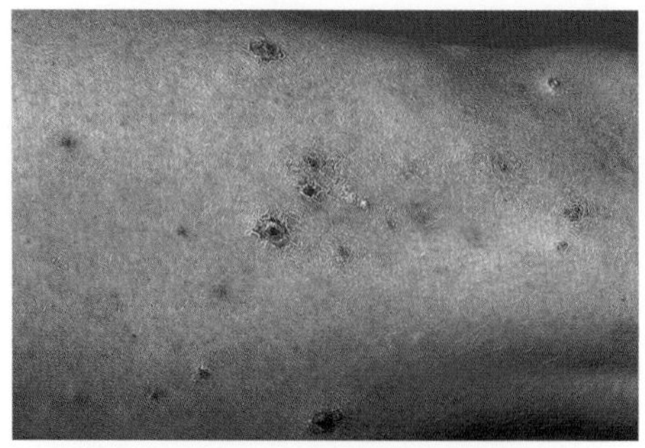

Fig. 98.8 Lymphomatoid papulosis (LyP). Clinical presentation with papulonecrotic skin lesions at different stages of evolution. *Courtesy, Rein Willemze, MD.*

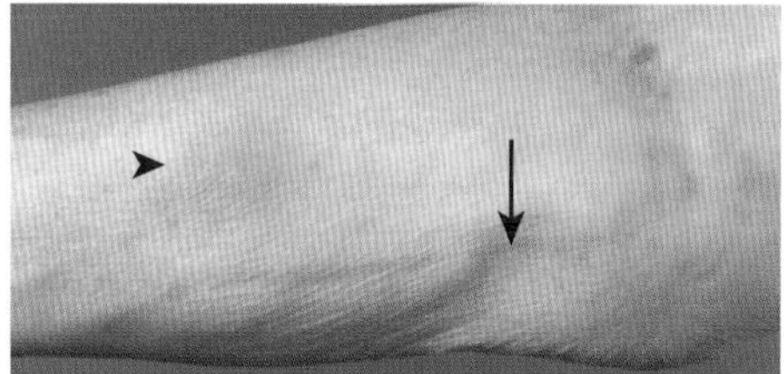

Fig. 98.10 Subcutaneous panniculitis-like T-cell lymphoma (SPTCL). Pink nodular skin lesions (arrowhead) as well as an area of lipoatrophy (arrow) at the site of a resolved nodule. *Courtesy, Rein Willemze, MD.*

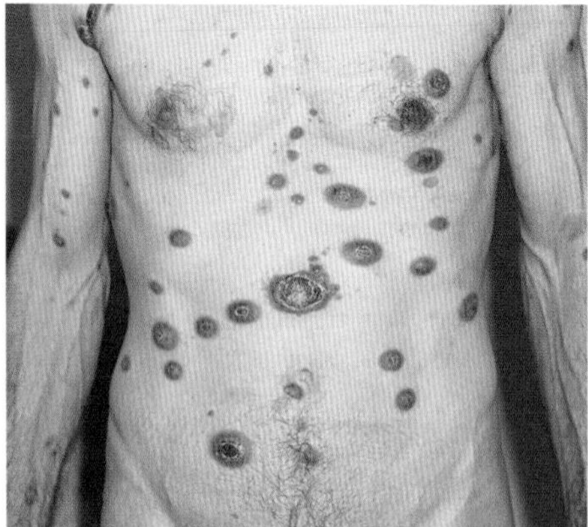

Fig. 98.12 Primary cutaneous aggressive epidermotropic CD8+ T-cell lymphoma. Generalized skin tumors with central ulceration. *Courtesy, Rein Willemze, MD.*

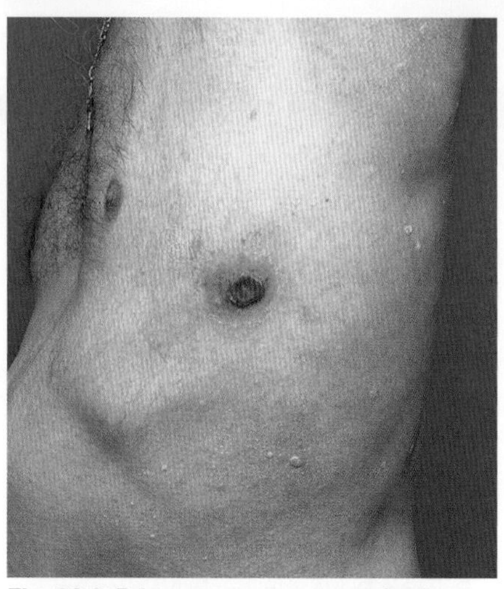

Fig. 98.9 Primary cutaneous anaplastic large cell lymphoma (C-ALCL). Characteristic clinical presentation with a solitary ulcerating tumor. *Courtesy, Rein Willemze, MD.*

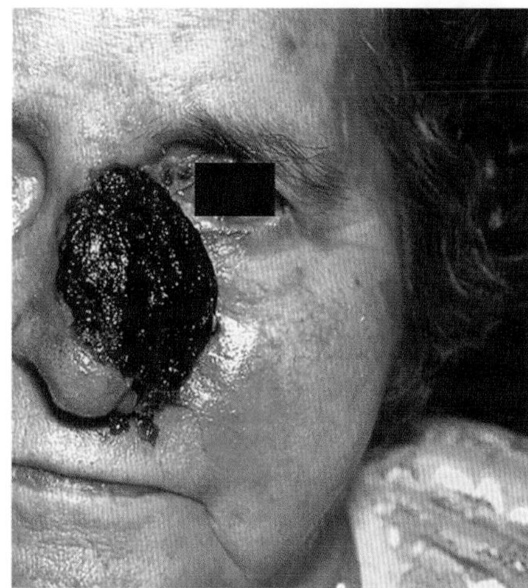

Fig. 98.11 Extranodal NK/T-cell lymphoma, nasal type. An extensive ulceronecrotic nasal mass, previously referred to as lethal midline granuloma. *Courtesy, Rein Willemze, MD.*

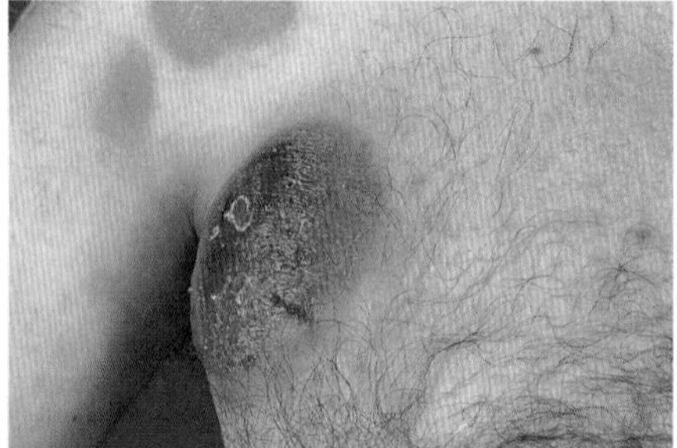

Fig. 98.13 Primary cutaneous peripheral T-cell lymphoma, not otherwise specified. Rapidly growing nodules and tumors. Note: The skin lesions in the left upper corner do not represent patches but, rather, deep plaques present for 2 weeks. *Courtesy, Rein Willemze, MD.*

Other Lymphoproliferative and Myeloproliferative Diseases

99

Benign Lymphocytic Infiltrates

Lymphocytic Infiltrate of Jessner

- A benign skin-limited disorder that overlaps with other entities, including dermal lupus erythematosus, cutaneous lymphoid hyperplasia, and polymorphic light eruption (PMLE).
- Males = females; onset typically during middle age; very rare in children.
- Most commonly appears on the head, neck, and upper back as one or several asymptomatic, erythematous papules, plaques (often annular) > nodules (Fig. 99.1); no secondary or surface changes (such as scale or crust).
- May last several weeks to months and will typically resolve spontaneously over months to years without sequelae.
- No systemic manifestations.
- **DDx:** see Fig. 99.2.
- **Rx:** watch-and-wait approach is often acceptable; if Rx desired, consider topical (class I) or intralesional CS; less often hydroxychloroquine is used.

Cutaneous Lymphoid Hyperplasia (CLH); also known as "Pseudolymphoma" or "Lymphocytoma Cutis"

- A benign, reactive lymphocytic proliferation that is thought to represent an exaggerated local immunologic reaction to a trigger that is usually unidentified.
- Inciting agents that have been reported include arthropod bites, tattoos, vaccinations, medications (e.g. antihistamines, antidepressants, angiotensin II receptor blockers), and in Europe, *Borrelia burgdorferi* infection.
- Presents most often on the head, neck, and upper extremities as one or several firm, erythematous to violaceous papules, plaques, or nodules (Fig. 99.3); usually no surface changes.
- Often spontaneously resolves without scarring.
- **DDx** (see Fig. 99.2): lymphocytic infiltrate of Jessner, lymphoma cutis, leukemia cutis, solid organ metastases, and occasionally adnexal tumors.
- **Rx:** topical (class I) or intralesional CS; excision or XRT; antibiotics if *Borrelia* infection.

Extramedullary Hematopoiesis

- Most commonly seen in neonates secondary to underlying bone marrow dysfunction; rarely in adults secondary to myelofibrosis, other myeloproliferative disorders or after splenectomy.
- Most often associated with TORCH (*t*oxoplasmosis, *o*ther [e.g. parvovirus B19], *r*ubella, *c*ytomegalovirus) infections in neonates.
- Clinically presents with erythematous to violaceous papules and nodules > plaques, ulcers, or nasal polyps (Fig. 99.4).
- When widely disseminated (typically in neonates) it leads to the classic "blueberry muffin baby" presentation (Table 99.1).
- Diagnosis is made by histopathology (dermal infiltrates of immature erythrocytes, leukocytes, and megakaryocytes).
- **DDx:** see Table 99.1 for neonates, leukemia cutis in adults.
- **Rx:** treat underlying bone marrow dysfunction; spontaneous resolution typically occurs in cases related to viral infections.

Malignant Hematopoietic Infiltrates

Leukemia Cutis

- Cutaneous lesions associated with both acute and chronic leukemias may be either (1) *nonspecific* reactive skin lesions (Table 99.2);

or (2) *specific* infiltrates, called "leukemia cutis."

- Leukemia cutis typically presents as erythematous to violaceous firm papules or nodules (Fig. 99.5); less often purpura, ulcers, and rarely bullae; lesions may be hemorrhagic due to thrombocytopenia.
- Favors head, neck, trunk, and sites of scars or trauma.
- Less common presentations of leukemia cutis: chloromas, gingival hyperplasia.
- In most patients with acute leukemia, cutaneous lesions (if present) appear at the time of diagnosis or recurrence.
- Occasionally, leukemia cutis antedates the appearance of leukemia in the peripheral smear ("aleukemic leukemia cutis"); rarely predates apparent bone marrow involvement by months.
- **DDx:** lengthy list because of the protean clinical presentations of leukemia cutis, but may include lymphoma cutis, infectious emboli, vasculitis, drug eruptions, Sweet syndrome and other neutrophilic disorders, extramedullary hematopoiesis.
- **Rx:** treat the underlying leukemia.

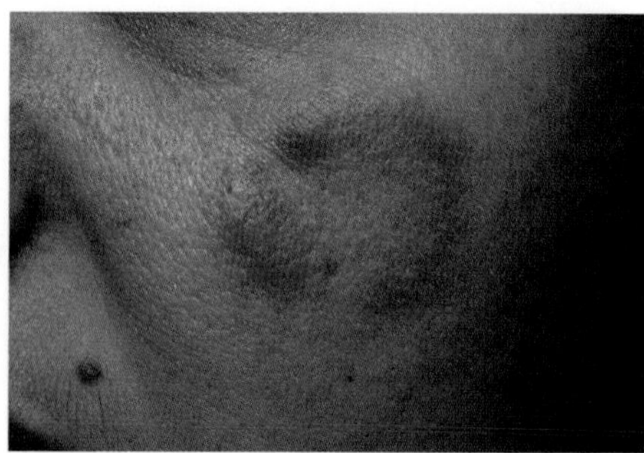

Fig. 99.1 Lymphocytic infiltrate of Jessner. Annular erythematous plaque with central clearing on the face. *Courtesy, YDRSC.*

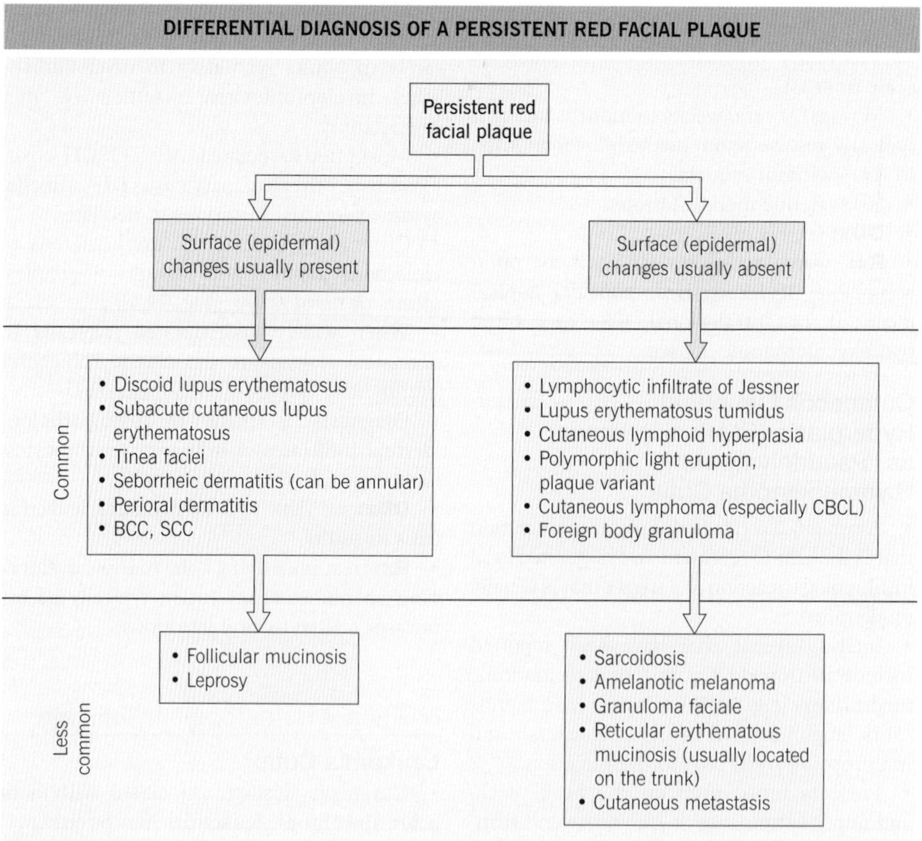

DIFFERENTIAL DIAGNOSIS OF A PERSISTENT RED FACIAL PLAQUE

Persistent red facial plaque

Surface (epidermal) changes usually present

Common
- Discoid lupus erythematosus
- Subacute cutaneous lupus erythematosus
- Tinea faciei
- Seborrheic dermatitis (can be annular)
- Perioral dermatitis
- BCC, SCC

Less common
- Follicular mucinosis
- Leprosy

Surface (epidermal) changes usually absent

Common
- Lymphocytic infiltrate of Jessner
- Lupus erythematosus tumidus
- Cutaneous lymphoid hyperplasia
- Polymorphic light eruption, plaque variant
- Cutaneous lymphoma (especially CBCL)
- Foreign body granuloma

Less common
- Sarcoidosis
- Amelanotic melanoma
- Granuloma faciale
- Reticular erythematous mucinosis (usually located on the trunk)
- Cutaneous metastasis

Fig. 99.2 Differential diagnosis of a persistent red facial plaque. CBCL, cutaneous B-cell lymphoma.

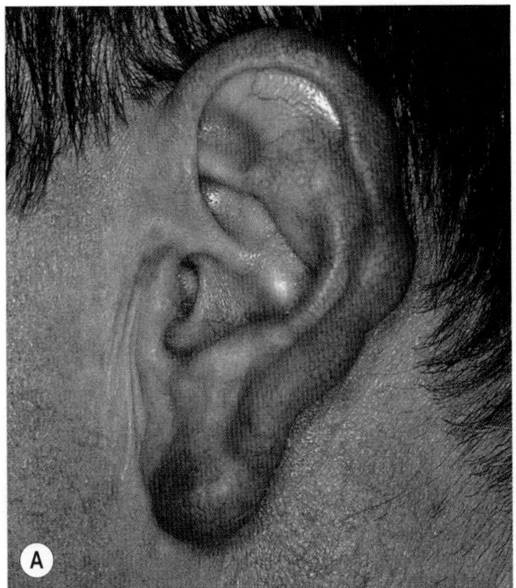

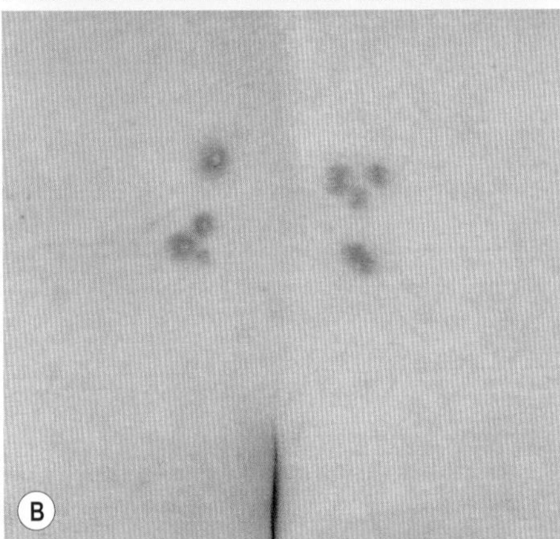

Fig. 99.3 Cutaneous lymphoid hyperplasia (pseudolymphoma of the skin; lymphocytoma cutis). A Violet papulonodules on the helix and lobe of the ear (unknown etiology). **B** Multiple red-brown to violet papules at the sites of *Hirudo medicinalis* (medicinal leech) application. *A, Courtesy, YDRSC; B, Courtesy, Cesare Massone, MD.*

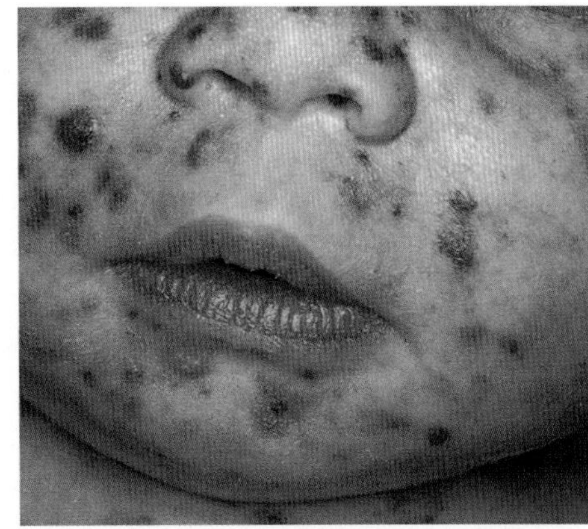

Fig. 99.4 Extramedullary hematopoiesis. "Blueberry muffin baby" secondary to congenital rubella. *Courtesy, Eugene Mirrer, MD.*

DIFFERENTIAL DIAGNOSIS OF "BLUEBERRY MUFFIN BABY"

Disseminated extramedullary hematopoiesis
• Prenatal infections
• TORCH
  - Congenital rubella
  - Cytomegalovirus
  - Toxoplasmosis
• Coxsackievirus
• Parvovirus
• Severe and chronic prenatal anemias
• Severe hemolytic anemias
  - Congenital spherocytosis
  - Rhesus hemolytic disease
  - ABO incompatibility
• Twin–twin transfusion
• Chronic fetomaternal hemorrhage
• Severe internal bleeding (e.g. intracranial)
• Myelodysplasia, congenital leukemia
Congenital leukemia cutis
Neonatal neuroblastoma
Congenital Langerhans cell histiocytosis
Congenital alveolar rhabdomyosarcoma
Hemangiomatosis, other vascular lesions (e.g. multifocal lymphangioendotheliomatosis, glomuvenous malformations)

Table 99.1 Differential diagnosis of "blueberry muffin baby." TORCH, *t*oxoplasmosis, *o*ther agents, *r*ubella, *c*ytomegalovirus and *h*erpes simplex virus.

Cutaneous Hodgkin Lymphoma (Cutaneous Hodgkin Disease; HD)

- **Primary** or isolated cutaneous HD is very unusual; typically presents as one or several ulcerated nodules and usually follows a more indolent course, with prognosis similar to those patients with early stage HD.
- **Secondary** cutaneous HD, occurring in patients with advanced systemic disease, constitutes the vast majority of cutaneous HD cases and as expected carries a worse prognosis.
- **Secondary** cutaneous HD usually presents with the rapid appearance of multiple, disseminated papulonodules and plaques, often on the trunk (Fig. 99.6), along with locations distal to affected lymph nodes.

"INFLAMMATORY" DISORDERS ASSOCIATED WITH ACUTE AND CHRONIC LEUKEMIAS	
Disorder	**Associated leukemias**
Neutrophilic dermatoses	
Sweet syndrome	AML > CML, hairy cell leukemia, CNL > ALL, CLL
Pyoderma gangrenosum*	AML, CML, hairy cell leukemia > ALL, CLL
Neutrophilic eccrine hidradenitis	AML >> ALL, CML, CLL
Reactive erythemas	
Exaggerated arthropod reactions (eosinophilic dermatosis associated with hematologic disorders)	CLL > other hematologic disorders, chronic active EBV infection (see Table 98.3)
Erythroderma	CLL†
Vasculitis	
Polyarteritis nodosa	Hairy cell leukemia >> CMML
Vasculitis (small vessel/leukocytoclastic)	Hairy cell leukemia, CLL > AMML, ALL
Erythema elevatum diutinum	Hairy cell leukemia, CLL
Panniculitis	
Erythema nodosum**	AML, CML, CMML
Other panniculitides‡	Hairy cell leukemia, AML, CMML
Other	
Paraneoplastic pemphigus	CLL

**Especially bullous.*
†Many probably represent Sézary syndrome.
***Isolated case reports; may occur concomitantly with Sweet syndrome.*
‡Including subcutaneous Sweet syndrome.

Table 99.2 "Inflammatory" disorders associated with acute and chronic leukemias. ALL, acute lymphoblastic leukemia; AML, acute myelogenous leukemia; AMML, acute myelomonocytic leukemia; CLL, chronic lymphocytic leukemia; CML, chronic myelogenous leukemia; CMML, chronic myelomonocytic leukemia; CNL, chronic neutrophilic leukemia.

Angioimmunoblastic T-Cell Lymphoma (AITCL)

• A peripheral T-cell lymphoma whose cells of origin are follicular T helper cells.

• Unique in that it characteristically presents *acutely* and at an advanced stage with fever, weight loss, sweats, lymphadenopathy, hepatosplenomegaly, and a diffuse, pruritic morbilliform eruption mimicking an acute viral infection or drug eruption.

• Other findings include polyclonal gammopathy, autoantibodies, hemolytic anemia, thrombocytopenia and eosinophilia.

• The morbilliform eruption and lymphadenopathy typically wax and wane, making suspicion and diagnosis of this malignancy even more elusive.

• The usual course is aggressive with a poor prognosis (median survival is <3 years); up to 30% may have longer-term survival.

• **DDx:** reactive lymphadenopathy due to a viral infection; drug eruptions, including DRESS; infectious mononucleosis, or other systemic inflammatory diseases.

• **Rx:** Systemic chemotherapy and allogeneic stem cell transplantation have been used but response and prognosis are poor.

Lymphomatoid Granulomatosis (LYG)

• A rare, EBV-associated, angiocentric/destructive lymphoproliferative disorder that primarily affects the lungs, skin, and nervous system (less often the kidneys and gastrointestinal tract).

• Although previously classified as a reactive process, in most patients it represents a form of large B-cell lymphoma.

• LYG can be divided into grades 1, 2, or 3 depending on the proportion of CD20(+) large lymphoid cells.

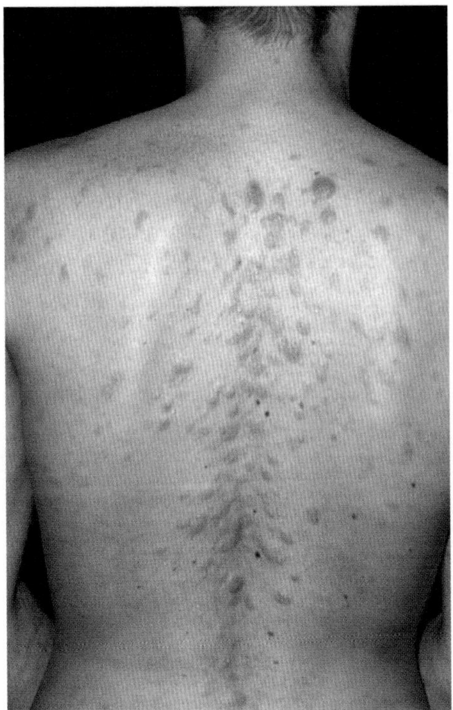

Fig. 99.5 Leukemia cutis. Numerous red-brown papules and plaques on the back of a patient with acute myelogenous leukemia. *Courtesy, Cesare Massone, MD.*

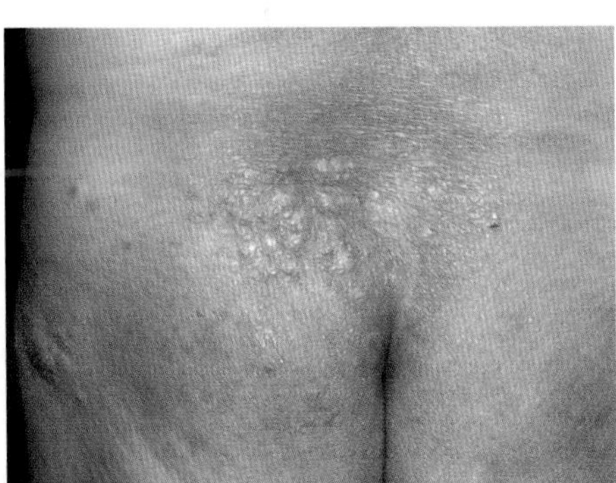

Fig. 99.6 Cutaneous Hodgkin lymphoma. Pink to red-brown papulonodules within a thin erythematous plaque; note the larger tumor on the hip. *Courtesy, Lorenzo Cerroni, MD.*

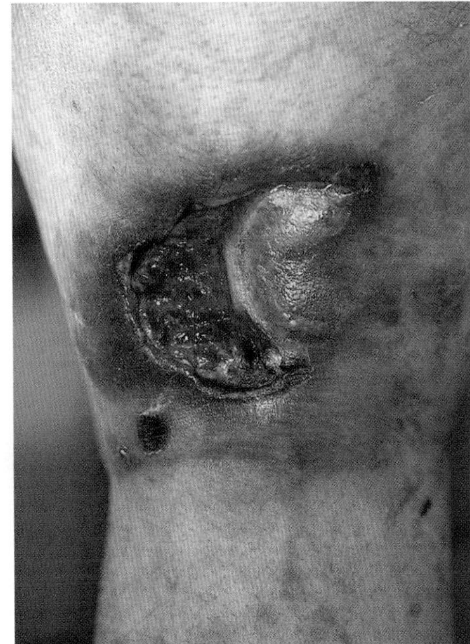

Fig. 99.7 Lymphomatoid granulomatosis. Ulcerated violaceous plaque in the popliteal fossa. *Courtesy, Jean L. Bolognia, MD.*

- Most often seen in adults; males > females; can occur in the setting of immune dysfunction (e.g. renal transplantation, HIV infection, Wiskott–Aldrich syndrome).
- Frequently presents with cough, dyspnea, chest pain, fever, weight loss, malaise, arthralgia, and myalgia; cavitary pulmonary nodules on chest radiograph.
- Nodular or ulcerative cutaneous lesions in 25–50% (Fig. 99.7); rarely an exanthematous eruption develops.
- Typically follows an aggressive, fatal course with a 5-year mortality rate of 60–90%.
- **DDx:** other cutaneous lymphomas, infections (e.g. tuberculosis), pyoderma gangrenosum, medium vessel vasculitis, granulomatosis with polyangiitis, sarcoidosis.
- **Rx:** rituximab, multidrug chemotherapy, or perhaps interferon-α in earlier stage disease.

For further information see Ch. 121 from *Dermatology, Fourth Edition*.

For additional online figures and tables visit www.expertconsult.com 

100 Cutaneous Metastases

- Relatively rare with the exception of breast cancer and melanoma metastases.
- May be the presenting sign of a malignancy.
- Often associated with a poor prognosis.
- Overall, breast carcinoma most commonly metastasizes to the skin and prostate carcinoma least commonly (Table 100.1).
- Most common skin metastases: women – breast carcinoma, melanoma; men – melanoma, squamous cell carcinoma of the head and neck and lung, and colon carcinoma (Table 100.2).
- In general, nonspecific morphology: firm, mobile, painless papulonodule(s), often skin-colored to pink or red-brown and occasionally ulcerated (Figs 100.1 and 100.2).
- Other clinical morphologies may be characteristic of a particular primary malignancy (Table 100.3).
- Melanoma metastases vary from pink to blue to black and they may develop along the lymphatic drainage between the primary site and regional lymph nodes (referred to as in-transit metastases; AJCC Stage III) or at distant sites (AJCC Stage IV) (Fig. 100.2).
- Location of cutaneous metastases is generally near the primary tumor, especially when secondary to intralymphatic spread (e.g. squamous cell carcinoma of the head and neck, breast carcinoma).

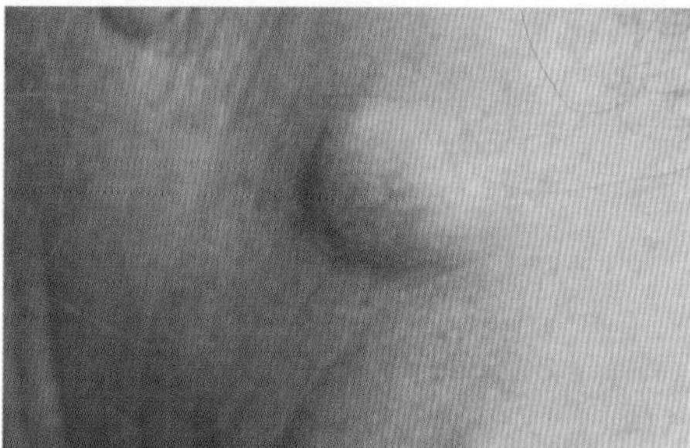

Fig. 100.1 Cutaneous metastasis of small cell lung carcinoma on the neck. This skin-colored nodule can resemble an epidermoid cyst or lipoma clinically but on palpation will be much firmer. *Courtesy, Ian Odell, MD.*

PERCENTAGES OF PATIENTS WITH METASTATIC CANCER WHO HAD CUTANEOUS METASTASES		
Primary malignancy	**Patients with metastatic disease (*n* = 4020)**	**Patients with cutaneous metastases (*n* = 420; 10%)**
Melanoma	172	77 (45%)
Breast	707	212 (30%)
Squamous cell carcinoma of the head and neck (e.g. laryngeal, oral)	221	29 (13%)
Colon/rectum	413	18 (4.5%)
Lung	802	21 (2.5%)
Prostate	207	0

Table 100.1 Percentages of patients with metastatic cancer who had cutaneous metastases. *Adapted from Lookingbill DP, Spangler N, Helm KF. Cutaneous metastases in patients with metastatic carcinoma: A retrospective study of 4020 patients.* J Am Acad Dermatol *1993;29(2 Pt 1):228–36.*

RANKING OF UNDERLYING PRIMARY MALIGNANCIES IN PATIENTS WITH CUTANEOUS METASTASES – MEN VERSUS WOMEN			
Primary malignancy	**Men with cutaneous metastases (n = 127)**	**Primary malignancy**	**Women with cutaneous metastases (n = 300)**
Melanoma	41 (32%)	Breast	212 (70%)
Squamous cell carcinoma of the head and neck	21 (16.5%)	Melanoma	36 (12%)
Lung	15 (12%)		
Colon/rectum	14 (11%)		

Table 100.2 Ranking of underlying primary malignancies in patients with cutaneous metastases – men versus women. *Adapted from Lookingbill DP, Spangler N, Helm KF. Cutaneous metastases in patients with metastatic carcinoma: A retrospective study of 4020 patients.* J Am Acad Dermatol *1993;29(2 Pt 1):228–36.*

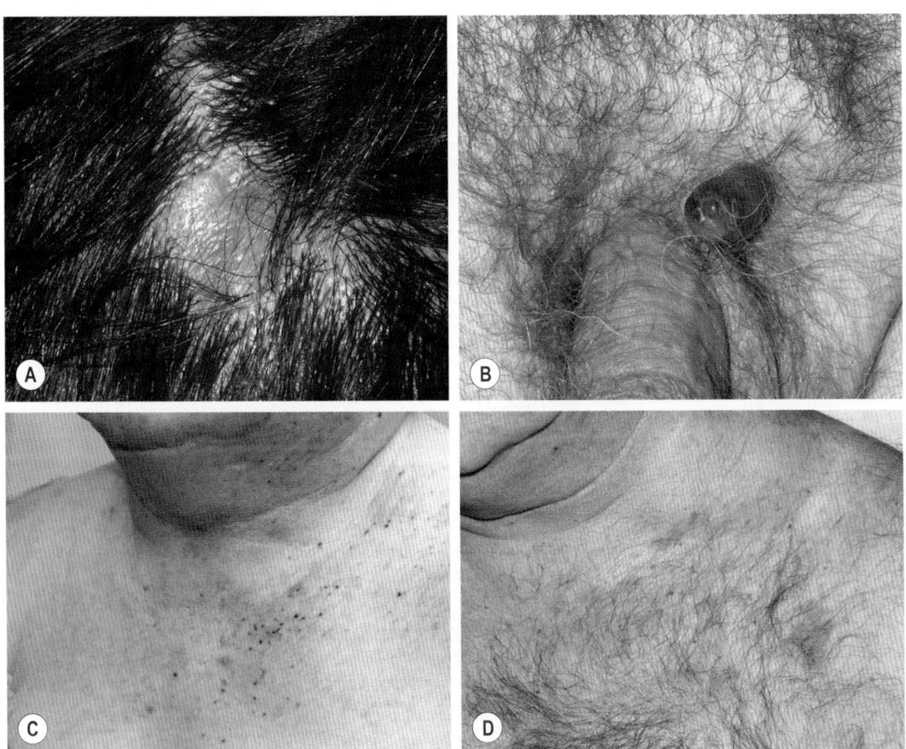

Fig. 100.2 Cutaneous metastases. A Pink nodule on the scalp with associated alopecia due to a metastasis from lung carcinoma (alopecia neoplastica). **B** Red-purple eroded nodule due to a metastasis from renal cell carcinoma; such lesions may be confused with vascular tumors. **C** Multiple small dark purple to black papules on the left neck and chest due to metastatic melanoma. **D** Pink papules and plaques on the chest due to metastases from adenocarcinoma of the colon. The patient was referred for treatment of dermatitis. *A, Courtesy, Lorenzo Cerroni, MD; B, Courtesy, Edward Cowen, MD; C, Courtesy, Christopher Bunick, MD; D, Courtesy, Kalman Watsky, MD.*

CLINICAL PRESENTATIONS OF CUTANEOUS METASTASES AND HISTOLOGIC CORRELATES			
Type	**Clinical description**	**Histology**	**Associated primary malignancy**
Dermal or subcutaneous nodules	Small miliary lesions to large tumors; single or multiple	Tumor cells infiltrating among collagen bundles or replacing dermis; grenz zone often present	Most common presentation; any type
Inflammatory carcinoma (carcinoma erysipeloides)	Erythematous patch with spreading border; resembles erysipelas	Tumor cells within dilated lymphatic vessels	Breast >> lung, ovary, prostate, GI, others
En cuirasse	Morpheaform or sclerodermoid, depending on extent; indurated with *peau d'orange* appearance	Fibrosis with infiltrating tumor cells	Breast >> lung, GI, kidney, others
Carcinoma telangiectoides	Red-violet papules	Tumor cells within superficial blood vessels and RBC sludging	Breast
Paget disease*	Patches extending from the nipple and areola that resemble dermatitis	Large, atypical epithelial cells with abundant pale cytoplasm arranged in solitary units and small nests within all layers of the epidermis	Breast
Alopecia neoplastica	Nodules or plaques on the scalp in association with alopecia	Cords of tumor cells between collagen bundles	Breast > lung, renal, others
Pyogenic granuloma-like	Rapidly growing nodule resembling a vascular tumor (particularly a pyogenic granuloma)	Neoplastic cells in cords and lobules admixed with prominent hemorrhage and "pseudovascular" spaces	Renal clear cell carcinoma, hepatocellular carcinoma > others

**Lesions of extramammary Paget disease share similar histopathologic features with those of Paget disease of the breast, but they usually represent (>75% of patients) primary cutaneous adenocarcinomas (see Table 60.6); an underlying visceral malignancy is most likely when there is perianal involvement.*

Table 100.3 Clinical presentations of cutaneous metastases and histologic correlates. An individual patient can have an admixture of the various types. Occasionally, cutaneous metastases have a zosteriform distribution pattern and clinically they can resemble dermatoses, including eczema, vasculitis, and erythema annulare centrifugum. Obviously, they can also mimic epidermoid or pilar cysts as well as cutaneous tumors, including non-melanoma skin cancers, lipomas, granular cell tumors, or angiosarcoma.

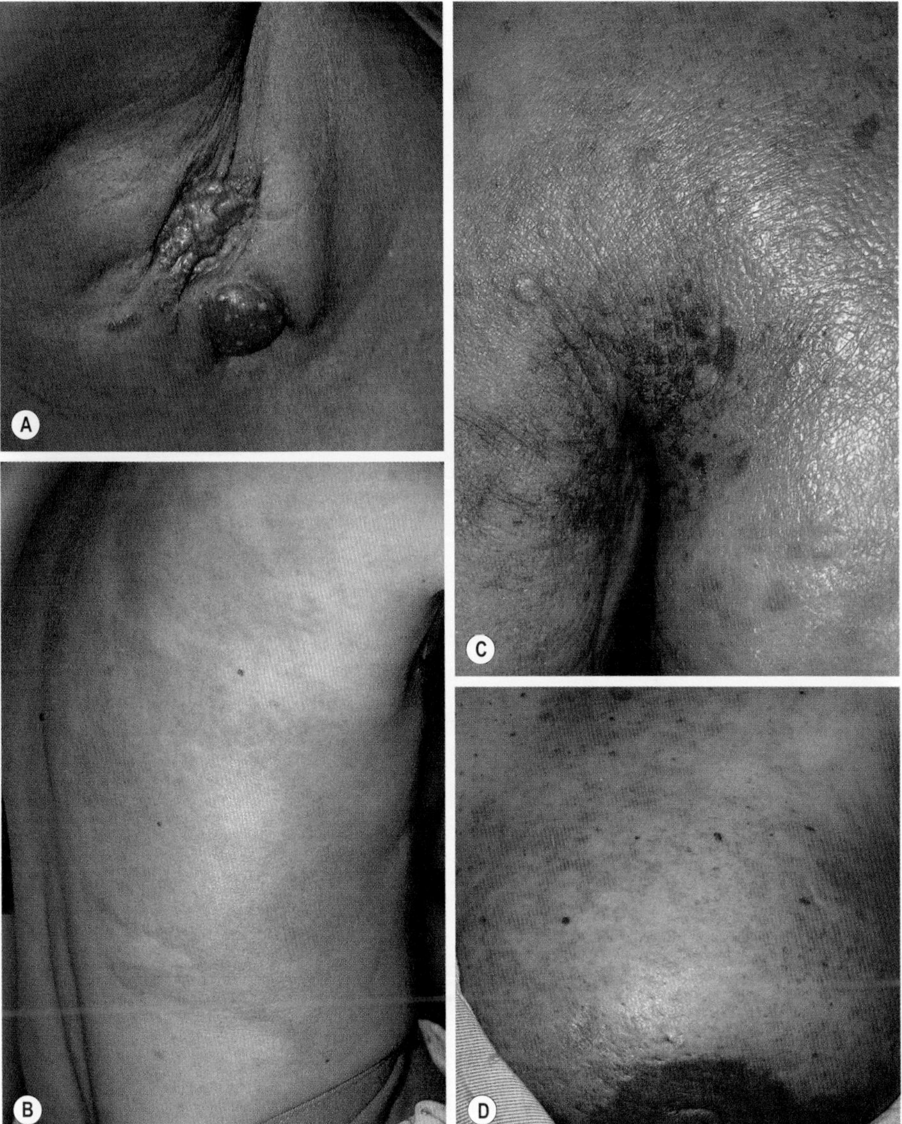

Fig. 100.3 Various presentations of cutaneous metastases of breast carcinoma. **A** Eroded erythematous nodules in the axilla. **B** Inflammatory form (carcinoma erysipeloides) with patches of erythema that may initially be misdiagnosed as infectious cellulitis. **C** Primarily *en cuirasse* form with obvious induration and *peau d'orange* appearance in addition to papulonodules. **D** Mixed pattern – reticulated erythema of carcinoma erysipeloides as well as *peau d'orange* appearance near the areola. *A, D, Courtesy, Matthew B. Zook, MD, and Stuart R. Lessin, MD; B, C, Courtesy, YDRSC.*

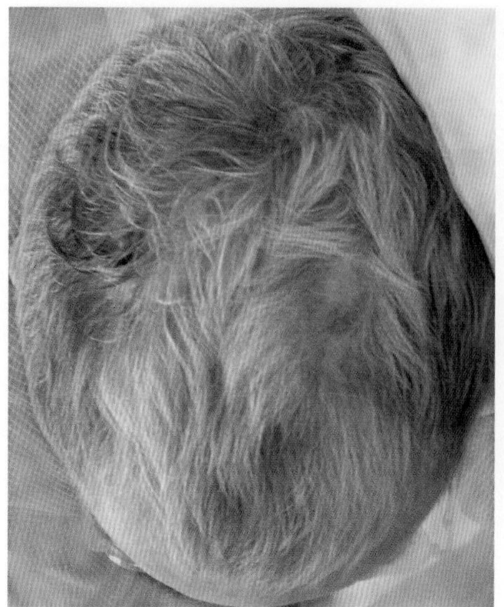

Fig. 100.4 Alopecia neoplastica secondary to metastatic breast carcinoma. Erythematous, indurated plaques of scarring alopecia on the scalp. *Courtesy, Joslyn S. Kirby, MD.*

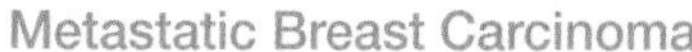

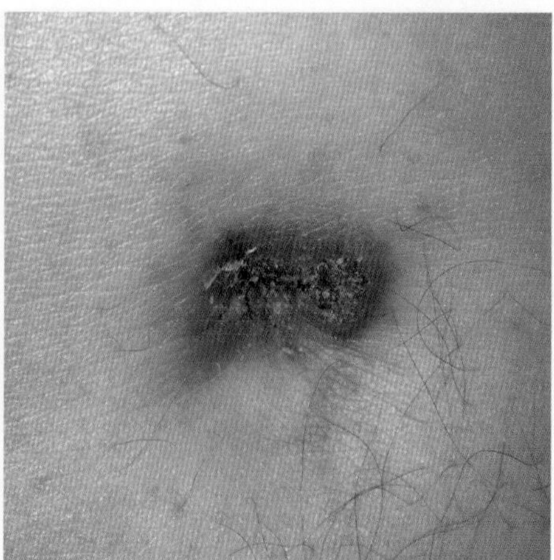

Fig. 100.5 Cutaneous metastasis of colon carcinoma. A Sister Mary Joseph nodule presenting as a pink plaque with scale-crust. *Courtesy, Matthew B. Zook, MD, and Stuart R. Lessin, MD.*

Metastatic Breast Carcinoma

• May have distinctive clinical morphologies (Fig. 100.3): (1) *carcinoma erysipeloides* – well-demarcated elevated erythema that resembles erysipelas or cellulitis; (2) *carcinoma telangiectoides* – telangiectasias and red papules; and (3) *carcinoma en cuirasse* – begins on the chest as induration with a *peau d'orange* appearance reminiscent of scleredema.

Alopecia Neoplastica

• Scarring alopecia of the scalp (Fig. 100.4).
• Associated with breast, lung, gastric, and renal carcinomas.

Sister Mary Joseph Nodule

• Pink to red-brown papule, umbilical or periumbilical (Fig. 100.5).
• Originally described in association with gastric carcinoma.
• May be associated with any abdominal malignancy.

For further information see Ch. 122 from *Dermatology, Fourth Edition*.

For additional online figures visit www.expertconsult.com 

Appendix

FITZPATRICK SCALE OF SKIN PHOTOTYPES		
Skin phototype	**Skin color**	**Response to UV irradiation**
I	White	Always burns, does not tan
II	White	Burns easily, tans with difficulty
III	Beige	Mild burns, tans gradually
IV	Brown	Rarely burns, tans easily
V	Dark brown	Very rarely burns, tans very easily
VI	Black	Never burns, gets darker

DETERMINATION OF THE SUN PROTECTION FACTOR (SPF)

- 10 human subjects
- Skin type I or II
- Irradiation: light source which mimics solar spectrum
- Procedure: determine minimal erythema dose (MED) in sunscreen-protected* and unprotected skin

$$SPF = \frac{\text{MED protected}}{\text{MED unprotected}}$$

- To test substantivity – after application and before MED testing:
  Water resistant (40): 2 × 20-min water immersions (whirlpool bath)†
  Water resistant (80): 4 × 20-min water immersions (whirlpool bath)†

*Sunscreen product applied at 2 mg/cm^2.
†Air drying in between immersions.

RELATIONSHIP OF THE SUN PROTECTION FACTOR (SPF) TO BLOCKAGE OF ERYTHEMAL RADIATION	
SPF	**Blockage of erythemal radiation (%)**
10	90
15	92.5
20	95
40	97.5

FDA PROPOSED RULE ON SUNSCREENS (2019) – ULTRAVIOLET B (UVB) AND ULTRAVIOLET A (UVA) PROTECTION AND LABELING REQUIREMENTS

Ultraviolet B (UVB) protection

- Raise the maximum proposed labeled SPF from 50+ to 60+
- Allow marketing on sunscreen products formulated up to an SPF of 80

Ultraviolet A (UVA) protection

- Require any sunscreen with SPF 15 or higher to be BROAD SPECTRUM
- Requirement for all BROAD SPECTRUM sunscreens with an SPF ≥ 15: as the SPF increases, so too does the magnitude of protection against UVA
- Require that BROAD SPECTRUM sunscreens provide adequate protection against UVA
  - UV absorbance critical wavelength of ≥ 370 nm (90% of the area under the curve [AUC])
  - UVA1/UV ratio of ≥ 0.7

Continued

FDA PROPOSED RULE ON SUNSCREENS (2019) – ULTRAVIOLET B (UVB) AND ULTRAVIOLET A (UVA) PROTECTION AND LABELING REQUIREMENTS—cont'd
Substantivity*
• WATER RESISTANT (40 minutes) or WATER RESISTANT (80 minutes) • The following designations are prohibited: "WATERPROOF", "SUNBLOCK", "ALL DAY PROTECTION", or "SWEAT PROOF"
Additional labeling
• Include an alphabetical listing of active ingredients on the front of the packaging • If the SPF of the sunscreen is <15, then it must have the following Skin Cancer/Skin Aging Alert: "Spending time in the sun increases your risk of skin cancer and early skin aging. This product has been shown only to help prevent sunburn, not skin cancer or early skin aging" • Require font and placement changes to ensure the terms SPF, BROAD SPECTRUM, and WATER RESISTANT are obvious on the label • Optional: If a sunscreen has an SPF ≥15 *and* is BROAD SPECTRUM, then can state that the product can help to reduce the risk of skin cancer and the risk of early skin aging, when used regularly and as directed in combination with other sun protection measures

**These changes were proposed and implemented in the 2011 FDA final rule for "Labeling and Effectiveness Testing: Sunscreen Drug Products for Over-the-Counter Human Use"*

Active ingredient safety and dosage forms are addressed in next table. SPF, sunscreen protection factor. *Adapted from Department of Health and Human Services/Food and Drug Administration. Sunscreen drug products for over-the-counter human use. Federal Register 2019;84:6204-75.*

FDA PROPOSED RULE (2019) FOR GRASE STATUS OF SUNSCREEN ACTIVE INGREDIENTS AND DOSAGE FORMS

	GRASE	Not GRASE	Insufficient data to support positive GRASE determination
Active sunscreen ingredients	Zinc oxide Titanium dioxide	Para-aminobenzoic acid* Trolamine salicylate*	Avobenzone, cinoxate, dioxybenzone, ensulizole, homosalate, meradimate, octinoxate, octisalate, octocrylene, oxybenzone, padimate O, sulisobenzone
Dosage forms^	Lotions, creams, ointments, oils, gels, butters, pastes, sticks, sprays^^	Sunscreen-insect repellant combinations**	Powders

**Not currently marketed in the US.*
^Wipes, towelettes, body washes, shampoos and other dosage forms are categorized as "new drugs" because the FDA has not yet received enough information about their efficacy and safety.
^^Sprays are approved as GRASE subject to testing, including particle size restrictions to avoid inhalation toxicity; flammability testing; and related safety labeling requirements.
***Data suggest that combining some sunscreen active ingredients with some insecticides may increase absorption of one or both components. CDC recommends that if applying both a sunscreen and an insect repellant, apply the sunscreen first and then the insect repellant.*

Each of the 16 approved active ingredients was assigned to one of three categories: (1) GRASE (*generally recognized as safe and effective*); (2) not GRASE; or (3) insufficient data to support positive GRASE determination. For the third group, the FDA requires additional information to determine whether or not sunscreens with these ingredients and dosage forms are GRASE. Of note, it does not mean that the FDA has concluded that these ingredients and dosage forms are unsafe. *Adapted from Department of Health and Human Services/Food and Drug Administration. Sunscreen drug products for over-the-counter human use. Federal Register 2019;84:6204-75.*

COMMONLY USED INSECT REPELLENTS	
Conventional repellents in EPA classification	
DEET (N,N-diethyl-3-methylbenzamide)*	Effective against a wide range of arthropods
	Long history of use
Picaridin (KBR 3023)	Good evidence for mosquitoes
	Fewer studies support repellent effect against ticks
Biopesticide repellents in EPA classification	
IR3535 (3-[N-butyl-N-acetyl]-aminopropionic acid, ethyl ester)	Good evidence for mosquitoes in some, but not all, studies
	Fewer studies support repellent effect against ticks
p-Menthane-3,8-diol†	Good evidence for mosquitoes
	Fewer studies support repellent effect against ticks
Botanicals (e.g. soybean oil, citronella, neem oil, fennel oil, geraniol)	Have consumer appeal as "natural" repellents
	Best published evidence is for neem oil
	Lack of evidence does not necessarily equate to lack of efficacy, but available evidence to date suggests they are inferior to the synthetic repellents listed above

**There is a plateau of efficacy at 30% with long-acting products, and higher concentrations should generally be avoided. Because sunscreens require frequent reapplication and DEET does not, combination products with these ingredients are not recommended.*
†The active ingredient of oil of lemon eucalyptus; use on children less than 3 years of age is not recommended.

Agents are listed in order of decreasing evidence of efficacy. Sunscreen, if also used, should be applied first. Treatment of clothing and other fabrics with permethrin can also be helpful, especially to repel ticks and chiggers (see Ch. 72). EPA, Environmental Protection Agency.

POTENCY RANKING OF SOME COMMONLY USED TOPICAL GLUCOCORTICOSTEROIDS
Class 1 (superpotent)
• Clobetasol propionate gel, ointment, cream, lotion, foam, spray and shampoo 0.05% • Betamethasone dipropionate gel* and ointment* 0.05% • Diflorasone diacetate ointment* 0.05% • Fluocinonide cream 0.1% • Flurandrenolide tape 4 mcg/cm^2 • Halobetasol propionate ointment and cream 0.05% and lotion 0.01%
Class 2 (high potency)
• Amcinonide ointment 0.1% • Betamethasone dipropionate cream*, lotion*, gel and ointment 0.05% • Clobetasol propionate solution ("scalp application") 0.05% • Desoximetasone ointment and cream 0.25% and gel 0.05% • Diflorasone diacetate ointment and cream* 0.05% • Fluocinonide gel, ointment, cream and solution 0.05% • Halcinonide ointment, cream and solution 0.1% • Mometasone furoate ointment 0.1% • Triamcinolone acetonide ointment 0.5%
Class 3 (high potency)
• Amcinonide cream and lotion 0.1% • Betamethasone dipropionate cream, lotion, and spray 0.05% • Betamethasone valerate ointment 0.1% • Diflorasone diacetate cream 0.05% • Fluticasone propionate ointment 0.005% • Triamcinolone acetonide ointment 0.1% and cream 0.5%

Continued

POTENCY RANKING OF SOME COMMONLY USED TOPICAL GLUCOCORTICOSTEROIDS—cont'd
Class 4 (medium potency)
• Betamethasone valerate foam 0.12% • Desoximetasone cream 0.05% • Fluocinolone acetonide ointment 0.025% • Flurandrenolide ointment 0.05% • Hydrocortisone valerate ointment 0.2% • Mometasone furoate cream and lotion 0.1% • Triamcinolone acetonide ointment (Kenalog®) and cream 0.1% or spray 0.2%
Class 5 (medium potency)
• Betamethasone dipropionate lotion 0.05% • Betamethasone valerate cream and lotion 0.1% • Clocortolone pivalate cream 0.1% • Fluocinolone acetonide cream 0.025% or oil and shampoo 0.01% • Fluticasone propionate cream and lotion 0.05% • Flurandrenolide cream and lotion 0.05% • Hydrocortisone butyrate ointment, cream and lotion 0.1% • Hydrocortisone probutate cream 0.1% • Hydrocortisone valerate cream 0.2% • Prednicarbate ointment and cream 0.1% • Triamcinolone acetonide ointment 0.025% and lotion 0.1%
Class 6 (low potency)
• Alclometasone dipropionate ointment and cream 0.05% • Triamcinolone acetonide cream 0.1% (Aristocort®) • Betamethasone valerate lotion 0.1% • Desonide gel, ointment, cream, lotion and foam 0.05% • Fluocinolone acetonide cream and solution 0.01% • Triamcinolone acetonide cream and lotion 0.025%
Class 7 (low potency)
• Topicals with hydrocortisone, dexamethasone and prednisolone

*Optimized vehicle.

INSTRUCTIONS FOR OPEN WET DRESSINGS
1. Use a single thickness of thin white cotton material such as a pillowcase, handkerchief, or bed sheet. Do not use a towel or washcloth.
2. Place the material in either (depending upon what is recommended): • Warm tap water • Domeboro® solution (one packet per 16 oz of water stored in the refrigerator, then brought to room temperature).
3. Squeeze out excess water, do not wring dry.
4. Unravel material and cover red, itchy areas with the wet dressing – **apply as only one (1) layer.** Do not apply additional materials such as a blanket.
5. Allow the wet dressing to remain on the skin for 10–15 minutes.
6. Remove the wet dressing and allow skin to air dry. When the skin is dry, apply the topical corticosteroid prescribed.
7. You may feel chilled if you have covered large areas of your body. If you are treating the entire body then place dressings to one side of the body at a time.

Open wet dressings allow cooling by continuous evaporation of water. They are used to decrease redness, itching, burning and weeping of skin lesions. They will help to make you more comfortable. Apply two to three times per day.

CORTICOSTEROID CLASSES
Group 1: non-methylated, most often non-halogenated molecules (formerly A, D2, and budesonide)
Budesonide* Cortisone acetate Fludrocortisone acetate *Hydrocortisone*^ Hydrocortisone aceponate Hydrocortisone acetate^ *Hydrocortisone-17-butyrate* Hydrocortisone-21-butyrate Methylprednisolone aceponate Methylprednisolone acetate Prednisolone Prednisone *Tixocortol pivalate* Triamcinolone
Group 2: halogenated molecules with a C_{16}/C_{17} cis ketal/diol structure (formerly B)
Amcinonide Desonide Fluocinolone acetonide Fluocinonide Halcinonide *Triamcinolone acetonide*
Group 3: halogenated and C_{16}-methylated molecules (formerly C, D1)
Aclometasone dipropionate Betamethasone Betamethasone-17-valerate Betamethasone dipropionate Betamethasone-disodium phosphate *Clobetasone butyrate* Clobetasol propionate Desoximetasone Dexamethasone Dexamethasone-disodium phosphate Fluocortolone Fluticasone propionate Mometasone furoate

**Budesonide R-isomer may cross-react with acetonides in Group 2.*
^Available without a prescription in the U.S.

Most allergic reactions are due to corticosteroids in Group 1. Suggested patch test screening agents are in *italics* for when allergic contact dermatitis to topical CS is suspected; all but hydrocortisone are in the American Contact Dermatitis Society screening series.

SPECIAL CONSIDERATIONS FOR CORTICOSTEROID AND ANTIHISTAMINE USE DURING PREGNANCY	
Corticosteroids	
Topical	• Overuse of high-potency products can lead to systemic absorption, and halogenated corticosteroids do cross the placenta; they may also add to the already considerable risk of striae • Corticosteroids that have enhanced cutaneous metabolism (e.g. mometasone furoate, prednicarbate, and methylprednisolone aceponate) can also be considered

Continued

SPECIAL CONSIDERATIONS FOR CORTICOSTEROID AND ANTIHISTAMINE USE DURING PREGNANCY—cont'd	
Corticosteroids	
Systemic	• Prednisolone is the systemic corticosteroid of choice for dermatologic indications because it is largely inactivated in the placenta (mother:fetus = 10:1) • During the first trimester, particularly between weeks 8 and 11, there is a possible (debated) slightly increased risk of cleft lip/cleft palate, especially if high doses prescribed and for >10 days; during this same period, a longer duration of therapy appears safe if dosages are <10–15 mg daily • If use is long term and extends late into gestation, fetal growth should be monitored and the risk of adrenal insufficiency in the newborn should be addressed
Antihistamines	
Systemic	• During the first trimester, the classic sedating agents (e.g. chlorpheniramine, clemastine, dimethindene) are preferred • During the second and third trimesters, if a non-sedating agent is requested, loratadine and cetirizine are considered safe

Courtesy, Christina M. Ambros-Rudolph, MD.

DOSING OF SYSTEMIC DRUGS MOST COMMONLY USED IN DERMATOLOGY	
Corticosteroids	
Duration	***Examples of three scenarios***
• Short-term	*Acute allergic contact dermatitis (e.g. poison oak), severe* Prednisone 60 mg each AM × 5–7 days, 40 mg × 5–7 days, 20 mg × 5–7 days In children, begin with ~1 mg/kg of prednisolone and taper in a similar fashion over 15–21 days
• Medium-term (requires monitoring for osteopenia)	*DRESS* Prednisone 1 mg/kg each AM then taper over ~3–4 months, following peripheral eosinophil count and any other abnormal laboratory value or systemic involvement (as well as cutaneous examination)
• Long-term (requires monitoring for osteopenia)	*Bullous pemphigoid, moderate-to-severe disease* Prednisone 0.5–1 mg/kg each AM then taper over ~7–9 months, e.g. when 1 mg/kg/day, taper by 5 mg every 10 days then when reach 30 mg daily go to alternate day and decrease by 2.5 mg every 14 days until reach 5 mg every other day
Retinoids	
Acitretin	10–50 mg/day, depending upon disorder
Isotretinoin	*Acne* 0.5–1 mg/kg/day^, often reaching a cumulative dose of 120–150 mg/kg
Antimalarials	
Chloroquine	Adult: 125–250 mg/day, up to 2.3 mg/kg actual body weight/day Children: <2.3 mg/kg actual body weight/day
Hydroxychloroquine	Adult: 200 mg daily–twice daily, up to 5 mg/kg actual body weight/day (whichever is lower) Children: ≤5 mg/kg actual body weight/day up to a maximum of 400 mg/day

Continued

DOSING OF SYSTEMIC DRUGS MOST COMMONLY USED IN DERMATOLOGY—cont'd	
Immunosuppressives	
Azathioprine	Empiric dosing after checking thiopurine methyltransferase (TPMT) level*: 0.5 mg/kg/day (TPMT level 5–13.7 U) 1.5 mg/kg/day (TPMT level 13.7–19 U) 2.5 mg/kg/day (TPMT level > 19 U)
Cyclosporine emulsion	For psoriasis, <6–12 months continual use: 2.5–5 mg/kg/day; taper at 3 months by 1 mg/kg/day every 2 weeks as tolerated
Methotrexate	5–25 mg (for children, 0.2–0.7 mg/kg) once weekly, depending upon disease and severity
Mycophenolate mofetil	1500–3000 mg (for children, 30–50 mg/kg) daily, divided into 2 doses
Rituximab	375 mg/m^2 weekly for 3–4 weeks – *or* – 1 g on days 0 and 14 repeated in 4 or more months as directed by anti-desmoglein antibody levels
Other	
Apremilast	30 mg twice daily if no renal impairment; upward titration from 10 mg/day recommended
Colchicine	0.5 or 0.6 mg two to three times daily
Dapsone	50–200 mg/day (for children, 1–2 mg/kg/day)
IVIg	Dosage, duration, and schedule vary by disease, e.g. total 2 g/kg per monthly cycle over 2–5 days in dermatomyositis
Spironolactone	For acne vulgaris or hidradenitis suppurativa: 50–200 mg/day For hirsutism or female pattern hair loss: 100–200 mg/day • Usually given in divided doses, twice daily • Often used in combination with OCPs • Clinical response may take up to 3 months
Thalidomide	25–100 mg/day, can be tapered to every other day, depending on disease

^Typically begin with ≤0.5 mg/kg the first month, with lower initial doses and slower escalation for patients with more severe inflammatory acne (especially teenage boys).
**Contraindicated if TPMT level <5 U.*

Monitoring recommendations are available online. OCP, oral contraceptive pill.

USE OF POTASSIUM IODIDE (KI)
Saturated solution of potassium iodide (SSKI)
• 1000 mg/ml • Droppers are supplied with calibrations for: 1. 0.3 ml (300 mg)* 2. 0.6 ml (600 mg) • In adults and older children, common dose = 300 mg TID PO with starting dose = 150–300 mg TID • In infants and young children, common dose = 150 mg TID PO • SSKI should be diluted in water or juice to try to minimize the bitter aftertaste • Crystallization may occur with cold temperatures, but rewarming and shaking dissolves the crystals; discard if solution turns yellow-brown
Side effects of SSKI
• Acute – nausea, bitter eructation, excessive salivation, urticaria, angioedema, cutaneous small vessel vasculitis • Chronic – enlargement of salivary and lacrimal glands, acneiform eruption, iododerma, hypothyroidism, hyperkalemia, occasionally hyperthyroidism

**0.3 ml = 10 drops from the calibrated dropper supplied with SSKI.*

BIOLOGIC AGENTS			
	Medication	Available as	Dosing
TNF inhibitors	Adalimumab	10–80 mg prefilled syringes 40 mg autoinjector	Psoriasis: 80 mg SC loading dose, then 40 mg SC at day 8, then 40 mg every other week Hidradenitis suppurativa (age ≥12 y and ≥60 kg): 160 mg SC loading dose, then 80 mg on day 15, then 40 mg weekly starting day 29
	Certolizumab	200 mg prefilled syringe	Psoriasis: 400 mg SC at weeks 0, 2, 4; then 200–400 mg every other week
	Golimumab	50 mg prefilled syringe/ autoinjector	Psoriatic arthritis: 50 mg SC monthly
	Etanercept	25–50 mg prefilled syringes 50 mg autoinjectors 25 mg multiple use vials	Adult: 25–50 mg BIW × 3 months, then 50 mg weekly Children (age ≥4 y): 0.8 mg/kg weekly (maximum 50 mg)
	Infliximab		3–10 (most commonly 5) mg/kg slow IV infusion at 0, 2, 6, 8 weeks, then every 8 weeks
IL-12/23 inhibitors	Guselkumab	100 mg prefilled syringe	100 mg SC at weeks 0, 4, 8 and every 8 weeks
	Risankizumab	75 mg prefilled syringe	150 mg SC at weeks 0 and 4 and every 3 months
	Tildrakizumab	100 mg prefilled syringe	100 mg SC at weeks 0, 4, and every 12 weeks
	Ustekinumab	45 mg and 90 mg prefilled syringes 45 mg single dose vial IV solution	Psoriasis (age ≥12 y): 90 mg (if >100 kg), 45 mg (if 60–100 kg), or 0.75 mg/kg (if <60 kg) SC at weeks 0 and 4, then every 12 weeks
IL-17 inhibitors	Brodalumab	210 mg prefilled syringe	210 mg SC every other week
	Ixekizumab	80 mg prefilled syringe/autoinjector	160 mg SC loading dose then 80 mg every other week × 12 weeks, then 80 mg monthly
	Secukinumab	150 mg prefilled syringe/autoinjector	300 mg SC weekly × 5 weeks, then every 4 weeks
Dupilumab		Adults and adolescents (age ≥12 y and ≥60 kg): 600 mg SC at week 0 then 300 mg every other week Adolescents <60 kg: 400 mg SC at week 0 then 200 mg every other week	

RECOMMENDED LABORATORY EVALUATION FOR PATIENTS RECEIVING TARGETED IMMUNOMODULATORS FOR PSORIASIS	
Prior to treatment	**During treatment**
Tuberculin skin test*/interferon-γ release assay** and/or (e.g. if immunosuppression or history of tuberculosis) chest X-ray CBC, CMP Hepatitis B and C virus serologic profiles Consider HIV testing	Annual tuberculin skin test*/interferon-γ release assay** and/or chest X-ray CBC or CMP every 3–12 months (or as clinically indicated)

*≥5 mm of induration should be considered as positive.
**e.g. QuantiFERON® TB Gold or T-SPOT®.TB.

A complete medical history and physical examination should also be performed, with particular attention to history/risk/symptoms/signs of tuberculosis, other chronic infections, malignancy, neurologic disorders and cardiac disease (especially congestive heart failure in patients receiving TNF-α inhibitors). CMP, comprehensive metabolic panel (includes liver function tests).

SLICC CLASSIFICATION CRITERIA FOR SYSTEMIC LUPUS ERYTHEMATOSUS (2012)	
Clinical criteria	**Immunologic criteria**
• Acute^ or subacute cutaneous lupus • Chronic cutaneous lupus^^ • Oral or nasal ulcers • Non-scarring alopecia • Arthritis (synovitis involving ≥2 joints) • Serositis (e.g. pleural or pericardial) • Renal (proteinuria ≥500 mg/24 hours *OR* RBC casts) • Neurologic (e.g. seizures, psychosis, mononeuritis multiplex, myelitis) • Hemolytic anemia • Leukopenia (<4000/mm^3) *OR* lymphopenia (<1000/mm^3) • Thrombocytopenia (<100,000/mm^3)	• ANA (above lab reference range) • Anti-ds-DNA (above lab reference range) • Anti-Sm positivity • Antiphospholipid antibody positivity (e.g. positive lupus anticoagulant, false-positive rapid plasma reagin, medium- or high-titer anti-cardiolipin antibody level, or positive anti-β_2-glycoprotein I antibody) • Low complement (C3, C4, CH50) • Direct Coombs test (in the absence of hemolytic anemia)
• Criteria for the classification of SLE include: ≥**4** criteria (at least 1 clinical and 1 immunologic criteria) *OR* biopsy-proven lupus nephritis with either positive ANA or anti-ds-DNA	

^Includes malar rash (but not discoid lesions), bullous lupus, toxic epidermal necrolysis variant of SLE, maculopapular lupus rash, photosensitive lupus rash (in the absence of dermatomyositis).
^^Discoid lesions (localized or generalized), hypertrophic lupus, lupus panniculitis, mucosal lupus, LE tumidus, chilblain lupus, discoid lupus/lichen planus overlap.

These revised criteria are intended to be more clinically relevant and to incorporate new immunologic information. They have not been tested for the purposes of SLE diagnosis. SLICC, Systemic Lupus International Collaborating Clinics. *Adapted from Petri M et al. Arthritis Rheum 2012;64:2677.*

For online cutaneous melanoma patient worksheet visit www.expertconsult.com 

Index

Page numbers followed by 'f' indicate figures, 't' indicate tables, and 'b' indicate boxes.

A

Index

B

C

Index

D

E

F

G

H

I

J

K

L

M

N

Index

O

P

Index

Index

Q

R

S

T

U

V

W

X

Y

Z